Linné & Ringsrud's

Clinical Laboratory Science

The Basics and Routine Techniques

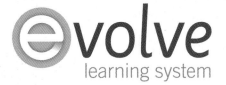 **evolve**
learning system

To access your Student Resources, visit:

http://evolve.elsevier.com/Turgeon/clinicallab/

Evolve Student Resources for Turgeon: Linné & Ringsrud's Clinical Laboratory Science: The Basics and Routine Techniques offers the following features:

- **Glossary**
  Provides definitions for essential laboratory terms.

- **Audio Glossary**
  Definitions of the key term from the text, with audio pronunciation.

- **Procedures**
  Step-by-step procedures written in CLSI format for use in the lab.

- **Weblinks**
  Links to places of interest on the web specifically for clinical laboratory science students.

 ELSEVIER
MOSBY

Linné & Ringsrud's
Clinical Laboratory Science
Sixth Edition

The Basics and Routine Techniques

Mary Louise Turgeon, EdD, MLS(ASCP)

Clinical Laboratory Education Consultant
Mary L. Turgeon & Associates
Boston, Massachusetts and St. Petersburg, Florida

Clinical Adjunct Assistant Professor
Tufts University
School of Medicine
Boston, Massachusetts

Adjunct Professor
Northeastern University
College of Professional Studies
Boston, Massachusetts

Professor
South University
Physician Assistant Program
Tampa, Florida

With 311 illustrations

ELSEVIER
MOSBY

3251 Riverport Lane
Maryland Heights, MO 63043

LINNÉ & RINGSRUD'S CLINICAL LABORATORY SCIENCE:
THE BASICS AND ROUTINE TECHNIQUES
Copyright © 2012, 2007, 1999, 1992, 1979, 1970 by Mosby, Inc., an affiliate of Elsevier Inc.

978-0-323-06782-9

Notices

Knowledge and best practice in this field are constantly changing. As new research and experience broaden our understanding, changes in research methods, professional practices, or medical treatment may become necessary.

Practitioners and researchers must always rely on their own experience and knowledge in evaluating and using any information, methods, compounds, or experiments described herein. In using such information or methods they should be mindful of their own safety and the safety of others, including parties for whom they have a professional responsibility.

With respect to any drug or pharmaceutical products identified, readers are advised to check the most current information provided (i) on procedures featured or (ii) by the manufacturer of each product to be administered, to verify the recommended dose or formula, the method and duration of administration, and contraindications. It is the responsibility of practitioners, relying on their own experience and knowledge of their patients, to make diagnoses, to determine dosages and the best treatment for each individual patient, and to take all appropriate safety precautions.

To the fullest extent of the law, neither the Publisher nor the authors, contributors, or editors, assume any liability for any injury and/or damage to persons or property as a matter of products liability, negligence or otherwise, or from any use or operation of any methods, products, instructions, or ideas contained in the material herein.

Library of Congress Cataloging-in-Publication Data
Turgeon, Mary Louise.
  Linne & Ringsrud's clinical laboratory science : the basics and routine techniques. -- 6th ed. / Mary Louise Turgeon.
     p. ; cm.
  Other title: Clinical laboratory science
  Includes bibliographical references and index.
  ISBN 978-0-323-06782-9 (pbk. : alk. paper) 1. Diagnosis, Laboratory. I. Ringsrud, Karen Munson.
II. Linné, Jean Jorgenson. Clinical laboratory science. III. Title. IV. Title: Clinical laboratory science.
  [DNLM: 1. Clinical Laboratory Techniques--methods. 2. Technology, Medical--methods.
3. Laboratory Techniques and Procedures. QY 25 T936L 2011]
  RB37.L683 2011
  616.07'56--dc22

2010022343

Publishing Director: Andrew Allen
Managing Editor: Ellen Wurm-Cutter
Publishing Services Manager: Catherine Jackson
Senior Project Manager: Rachel E. McMullen
Senior Designer: Amy Buxton

Printed in China
Last digit is the print number: 9 8 7 6 5 4 3 2 1

Contributor

CAROL L. FINN, MS, M(ASCP)
Senior Medical Technologist
Lahey Clinic
Burlington, Massachusetts
Chapter 16, Introduction to Microbiology

PATRICIA A. WRIGHT, MT(ASCP)SBB
Supervisor of Blood Bank
UMass Memorial Medical Center
Worcester, Massachusetts
Chapter 18, Immunohematology and Transfusion Medicine

About the Author

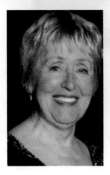

Mary Louise Turgeon, EdD, MT(ASCP) is an author, professor, and consultant in medical laboratory science. Her books are *Basic & Applied Clinical Laboratory Science*, ed 6 (2011), *Clinical Hematology*, ed 5 (2011), *Immunology and Serology in Laboratory Medicine*, ed 4, and *Fundamentals of Immunohematology*, ed 2. Foreign language editions have been published in Chinese, Spanish, and Italian.

Dr. Turgeon has fourteen years of university and fifteen years of community college teaching and program administration experience. She currently teaches on-line and on-the-ground in Massachusetts and Florida. Guest speaking and technical workshops complement teaching and writing activities. Her consulting practice (www.mlturgeon.com) focuses on new program development, curriculum revision, and increasing teaching effectiveness in the United States and internationally.

Reviewers

Keith Bellinger, PBT(ASCP), BA
Assistant Professor of Phlebotomy
Department of Clinical Laboratory Sciences
School of Health Related Professions
University of Medicine and Dentistry
  of New Jersey
Newark, New Jersey

Beth W. Blackburn, MT(ASCP), BS MT
Instructor, MLT Program
Orangeburg-Calhoun Technical College
Orangeburg, South Carolina

Debbie Heinritz, MS, MT(ASCP), CLS(NCA)
Clinical Laboratory Technician Instructor
Health Sciences Department
Northeast Wisconsin Technical College
Green Bay, Wisconsin

Amy R. Kapanka, MS, MT(ASCP)SC
MLT Program Director
Hawkeye Community College
Waterloo, Iowa

M. Lorraine Torres, EdD, MT(ASCP)
Program Director
Clinical Laboratory Science Program
College of Health Sciences
The University of Texas El Paso
El Paso, Texas

Dedication

La Dolce Vita
42° 19′ N
70° 54′ W

Preface

The intention of this sixth edition of *Clinical Laboratory Science: The Basics and Routine Techniques* is to continue to fulfill the needs of medical laboratory scientists, medical laboratory technicians, clinical laboratory assistants, medical office assistants, physician assistants, and others for a comprehensive, entry-level textbook. This type of basic and clinical information is needed by anyone engaged in ordering or performing laboratory assays, or analyzing laboratory output data in various settings.

The purpose of this edition continues to be to describe the basic concepts in laboratory medicine, to outline the underlying theory of routine laboratory procedures done in clinical laboratories of varying sizes and geographic locations, and to present applicable case studies to help students integrate theory and practice. The major topical areas are divided into two sections: Part I: Basic Laboratory Techniques, and Part II: Clinical Laboratory Specializations.

This sixth edition capitalizes on the strengths of previous editions but presents extensively revised information and new content in most chapters. The pedagogy of the book includes a topical outline and behavioral objectives at the beginning of each chapter. The outlines and objectives should be of value to students in the organization of content and delineation of learning expectations. Review questions are at the end of each chapter. Case studies are provided at the end of each chapter in Part II. Illustrations and full-color photographs are used to visually clarify concepts and arrange detailed information.

Representative procedures published in the book or on the Evolve site are written in the format suggested by the CLSI. The use of this format familiarizes students with the recommended procedural write-up encountered in a working clinical laboratory.

WHAT IS SIGNIFICANTLY NEW IN THE SIXTH EDITION?

Part I: Basic Laboratory Theory and Techniques

- The history of Clinical Laboratory Science as a profession, certification and licensure, medical ethics and ISO 15189 kick off the new content in Chapter 1.

- Up-to-date safety information is always essential. In this edition, a discussion of the Americans with Disabilities act is included. New content in Chapter 2 includes the latest information on vaccinations such as H1N1, emerging knowledge about nosocomial infections such as MRSA, and new developments in disinfection and sterilization.
- Revised order of draw of venous blood specimens and new types of blood collection tubes are presented in Chapter 3. Information related to additives and gels, and conditions related to evacuated tubes has been added to this chapter.
- English-to-Metric conversions, hazardous management information system (HMIS), and updated aspects of chemical labeling has been added to Chapter 4.
- More review questions have been added to the traditional information in Chapters 5, 6, and 7.
- In Chapter 6, *Measurement Techniques in the Clinical Laboratory*, new labeling technologies and molecular techniques have been added as essential methods in modern testing.
- Chapter 8, *Quality Assessment and Quality Control in the Clinical Laboratory*, incorporates new information on Lean Six Sigma, latent errors, and preanalytical and postanalytical errors.
- Changes in Chapter 10, *Laboratory Information Systems and Central Laboratory Automation*, are reflected in information on bar coding and radio frequency devices, autoverification of laboratory results, middleware, and molecular and genetic testing and laboratory information systems.

Part II: Clinical Laboratory Specializations

The body of knowledge of clinical laboratory theory and practice continues to expand. In this sixth edition, new information has been added to every chapter.
- Chapter 11, *Introduction to Clinical Chemistry*, features expanded descriptions of acid-base balance, and the anion gap, osmolality and gap, and diabetes.
- Chapter 12, *Principles and Practice of Clinical Hematology*, incorporates expanded coverage

of postanalytical errors, automated digital cell morphology, critical values, and histograms.

- Additional content on pre-analytical variable in coagulation testing is presented in Chapter 13, *Introduction to Hemostasis*.
- Chapter 14, *Renal Physiology and Urinalysis*, features more content on quality control, and newer types of containers, preservatives, and collection methods. In addition, content on the history of urinalysis and modern urinalysis is incorporated.
- Chapter 15, *Examination of Body Fluids*, a discussion of amniotic fluid has been added.
- Chapter 16, *Introduction to Medical Microbiology*, presents more microorganism identification characteristics.
- Chapter 17, *Immunology and Serology*, features expanded coverage of phagocytosis, prozone and postzone, antinuclear antibody photomicrographs.
- The final chapter, Chapter 18, *Immunohematology and Transfusion Medicine*, incorporates gel technology, automation, and the principles of antibody identification.

The appendices now include a list of Spanish-English Conversational Phrases for Phlebotomists as well as approved curriculum competencies for medical laboratory assistants.

No attempt has been made to replace textbooks that exclusively focus on a specific clinical laboratory specialty and written at a more detailed level for medical laboratory science (MLS) students. The sixth edition of this text is appropriate for introductory clinical laboratory science courses, laboratory techniques or basic core laboratory courses, or as a reference book. Comments from instructors, other professionals, and students are welcome at m.turgeon@neu.edu.

Mary L. Turgeon
Boston, Massachusetts
St. Petersburg, Florida

Acknowledgments

My objective in writing *Linné & Ringsrud's Clinical Laboratory Science: The Basics and Routine Techniques*, Sixth Edition, is to continue the work started by Linné and Ringsrud to share comprehensive basic concepts, theory, and applications of clinical laboratory science with beginning clinical laboratory students or others who have a need for laboratory information. This book has provided me with a challenging opportunity to expand my knowledge of the latest medical laboratory content and to share my generalist skill set and teaching experience with others.

Special thanks to my former colleagues at Northeastern University, Carol Finn, MS, M(ASCP) and Patricia A. Wright, BS, MT (ASCP), SBB, Blood Bank Supervisor, University of Massachusetts Memorial Medical Center.

Thanks to Ellen Wurm-Cutter, who was my editor for this and other books. Working with her is always a pleasure. Rachel McMullen deserves recognition for her attention to detail in the production of this book.

Mary L. Turgeon

Contents

PART I

Basic Laboratory Techniques

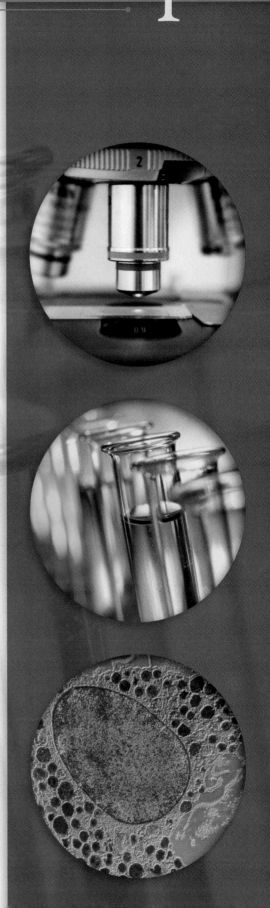

FUNDAMENTALS OF THE CLINICAL LABORATORY

Learning Objectives

At the conclusion of this chapter, the student will be able to:

- Compare the functions of the professional organizations.
- Define the term *ethics*, and discuss medical applications.
- Draw and describe the organizational structure of a health care organization.
- Name the typical departments of a clinical laboratory.
- Name and describe clinical laboratory staffing and functions.
- Define the acronyms OSHA, CLIA '88, CMS, TJC, CLSI, and CAP.
- Compare and contrast the uses of various sites for laboratory testing: central laboratory, point of care, physician office laboratory, and reference laboratory.
- Describe the importance of federal, state, and institutional regulations concerning the quality and reliability of laboratory work.
- Briefly explain the CLIA '88 regulations and the classification of laboratory testing by complexity of the test: waived, moderately

- complex, highly complex, and provider-performed microscopy.
- Describe the purpose of participation in CLIA '88–mandated proficiency testing programs and how they relate to quality assessment.
- Name and describe alternate sites of laboratory testing.
- Name and describe nonanalytical and analytical factors in quality assessment.
- Name the three most frequent inspection deficiencies over time for all CLIA-approved laboratories.
- Describe proficiency testing.
- Discuss ISO Standards in the clinical laboratory.
- Name three medical-legal issues, and discuss issues associated with each.
- Compare the four newest directions in laboratory testing.

CLINICAL LABORATORY SCIENCE

Clinical laboratory testing plays a crucial role in the detection, diagnosis, and treatment of disease. Medical laboratory scientists (MLS) and medical laboratory technicians (MLT) collect and process specimens and perform chemical, biological, hematologic, immunologic, microscopic, molecular diagnostic, and microbial testing. They may also collect and prepare blood for transfusion. Laboratory aides may also be members of the laboratory team (see Appendix A for a description of laboratory aide topics and objectives for training).

After collecting and examining a specimen, laboratory professionals analyze the results and relay them to physicians or other health care providers. In additional to routine testing, duties in the clinical laboratory include developing and modifying procedures, and monitoring programs to ensure the accuracy of test results.

The Bureau of Labor Statistics *Occupational Outlook Handbook* for Clinical Laboratory Technologists and Technicians states, "Rapid job growth and excellent job opportunities are expected. Most jobs will continue to be in hospitals, but employment will grow in other settings, as well."[1]

HISTORY OF CLINICAL LABORATORY SCIENCE AS A PROFESSION

Rudimentary examinations of human body fluids date back to the time of the ancient Greek physician Hippocrates around 300 BC, but it was not until 1896 that the first clinical laboratory was opened in a small room equipped at a cost of $50 at Johns Hopkins Hospital, Baltimore, Maryland. The diagnostic and therapeutic value of laboratory testing was not yet understood. Many physicians viewed clinical laboratories simply as an expensive luxury that consumed both valuable space and time.

Discovery of the causative agents of devastating epidemics such as tuberculosis, diphtheria, and cholera in the 1880s and the subsequent development of tests for their detection in the late 1890s highlighted the importance of laboratory testing.

Original Credentialing and Professional Organizations

World War I caused a critical shortage of qualified laboratory assistants to staff laboratories. This urgent situation prompted the creation of diversified training programs to meet the growing need for trained laboratory professionals.

The American Society of Clinical Pathologists (ASCP) created the Board of Registry (BOR) in 1928 to certify laboratory professionals and later the Board of Schools (BOS). Individuals who passed the BOR's registry exam were referred to as "medical technologists," identified by the acronym "MT (ASCP)."

In 1933, the American Society of Clinical Laboratory Technicians (ASCLT) was formed. Later, this organization was renamed the American Society of Medical Technologists (ASMT) and, finally, today's designation as the American Society for Clinical Laboratory Science (ASCLS). The catalyst for establishment of ASCLT was the desire for a greater degree of autonomy and control of the direction of the profession by nonphysician laboratory professionals. ASCLS is proud to champion the profession and ensure that other members of the health care field—as well as the public—fully recognize the contributions of clinical laboratory professionals.

In 1973, as a result of pressure from the U.S. Office of Education and the National Commission on Accrediting, ASCP agreed to disband the BOS and turn over its functions to an independently operated and governed board, the National Accrediting Agency for Clinical Laboratory Sciences (NAACLS). In 1977, the autonomous certification agency, the National Certification Agency for Medical Laboratory Personnel (NCA) was formed.[2]

Individual Professional Recognition

During the 1960s, new categories of laboratory professionals joined generalist medical technologists in performing the daily work of the clinical laboratory. These categories were created to help cope with an increased workload. The category of certified laboratory assistant (CLA) was developed as a one-year certificate program; the category of medical laboratory technician (MLT) was developed as a two-year associate degree program. Simultaneously, specialist categories in chemistry, microbiology, hematology, and blood banking were created. Specialists certified in cytotechnology, histotechnology, laboratory safety, and molecular pathology/molecular biology have evolved as well. Technicians certified as donor phlebotomists or phlebotomy technicians are part of the laboratory team. Pathologists' assistants[3] are another category of specialty certification. Certification as a Diplomat in Laboratory Management is available.[3]

Newest Professional Recognition

In September 2009, a historic step was taken when the NCA and ASCP merged into a single professional agency. Generalists are now referred to as *medical laboratory scientists* (MLSs). The technician-level designation has not changed but continues to be designated as *medical laboratory technicians* (MLTs). Continuing education is now a requirement for certified professionals.

Additional Individual Professional Certification and Licensure

Many employers prefer or are required by the Clinical Laboratory Improvement Amendments of 1988 (CLIA '88) regulations (see later discussion) to hire laboratory staff who are certified by a recognized professional association. In addition to the newly merged ASCP route, the American Medical Technologists (AMT) also offer certification.

Numerous states currently require licensure or registration of laboratory personnel, with other states considering it, thus further ensuring the integrity of the profession. The requirements vary by state and specialty. Information on licensure is available from state departments of health or boards of occupational licensing.

MEDICAL ETHICS

What is *ethics*? According to the Merriam-Webster dictionary, the definition of ethics includes the discipline dealing with what is good and bad, or a set of moral principles. Personal ethics are based on values or ideals and customs that are held in high regard by an individual or group of people. For example, many people value friendship, hard work, and loyalty.

Ethics also encompasses the principles of conduct of a group or individual, such as professional ethics. ASCLS endorses a professional Code of Ethics (Box 1-1), which states that all laboratory professionals have a responsibility for proper conduct toward the patient, colleagues and the profession, and society. In addition, ASCLS has a Pledge to the Profession (Box 1-2).

Situational ethics is a system of ethics by which acts are judged within their contexts instead of by categorical principles. Hospitals have ethics committees to evaluate situational ethics cases. Individual laboratory professionals may need to make decisions based on personal or professional values. An example of a five-step model for decision making is presented in Box 1-3.

HEALTH CARE ORGANIZATIONS

Modern health care organizations have many different configurations, depending on the geographic region and market, mix of patients (e.g., age), overall size, and affiliations. The size of health care

American Society for Clinical Laboratory Science Code of Ethics

Preamble

The Code of Ethics of the American Society for Clinical Laboratory Science sets forth the principles and standards by which clinical laboratory professionals practice their profession.

I. Duty to the Patient

Clinical laboratory professionals are accountable for the quality and integrity of the laboratory services they provide. This obligation includes maintaining individual competence in judgment and performance and striving to safeguard the patient from incompetent or illegal practice by others.

Clinical laboratory professionals maintain high standards of practice. They exercise sound judgment in establishing, performing, and evaluating laboratory testing.

Clinical laboratory professionals maintain strict confidentiality of patient information and test results. They safeguard the dignity and privacy of patients and provide accurate information to other health care professionals about the services they provide.

II. Duty to Colleagues and the Profession

Clinical laboratory professionals uphold and maintain the dignity and respect of our profession and strive to maintain a reputation of honesty, integrity, and reliability. They contribute to the advancement of the profession by improving the body of knowledge, adopting scientific advances that benefit the patient, maintaining high standards of practice and education, and seeking fair socioeconomic working conditions for members of the profession.

Clinical laboratory professionals actively strive to establish cooperative and respectful working relationships with other health care professionals, with the primary objective of ensuring a high standard of care for the patients they serve.

III. Duty to Society

As practitioners of an autonomous profession, clinical laboratory professionals have the responsibility to contribute from their sphere of professional competence to the general well-being of the community.

Clinical laboratory professionals comply with relevant laws and regulations pertaining to the practice of clinical laboratory science and actively seek, within the dictates of their consciences, to change those which do not meet the high standards of care and practice to which the profession is committed.

Reprinted with permission of the American Society for Clinical Laboratory Science, 2009. http://www.ascls.org/.

Pledge to the Profession

As a clinical laboratory professional, I strive to:
- Maintain and promote standards of excellence in performing and advancing the art and science of my profession
- Preserve the dignity and privacy of others
- Uphold and maintain the dignity and respect of our profession
- Seek to establish cooperative and respectful working relationships with other health professionals
- Contribute to the general well-being of the community

I will actively demonstrate my commitment to these responsibilities throughout my professional life.

Accessed April 2009. Reprinted with permission of the American Society for Clinical Laboratory Science. http://www.ascls.org/.

Five Steps to Decision Making

1. State the problem.
2. Establish personal and professional values regarding the problem.
3. List alternative possibilities for problem resolution.
4. Rank order your choice of possible solutions, and compare this list to a ranked-order list of applicable personal and professional values.
5. Rank order a list of the short- and long-term consequences of the problem.
6. Make a dicussion.

Courtesy Cecile Sanders, Austin Community College, Austin, TX.

(CEO) and the board of trustees, who set policy and guide the organization. The chief operating officer (COO) is responsible for implementing policies and daily activities. Other high-level positions can include the chief financial officer (CFO), chief information officer (CIO), and chief technology officer (CTO), depending on the size of a health care organization. A variable number of vice presidents (VPs) have several departments reporting to them. Organizations usually have vice

organizations range from the very large tertiary care–level teaching hospitals, to community hospitals, to freestanding specialty clinics or phlebotomy drawing stations.

A common organizational structure for a hospital (Fig. 1-1) includes the chief executive officer

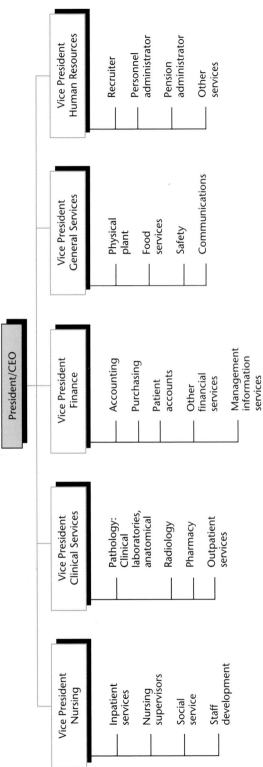

FIGURE 1-1 Hospital organizational chart. (From Kaplan LA, Pesce AJ: Clinical chemistry: theory, analysis, correlation, ed 5, St Louis, 2010, Mosby.)

presidents of Nursing, Clinical Services, General Services, and Human Resources. The Vice President of Clinical Services oversees the managers of the clinical laboratory as well as radiology and pharmacy.

LABORATORY MEDICINE (CLINICAL PATHOLOGY)

Laboratory medicine, or **clinical pathology**, is the medical discipline in which clinical laboratory science and technology are applied to the care of patients. Laboratory medicine comprises several major scientific disciplines: clinical chemistry and urinalysis, hematology including flow cytometry, clinical microbiology, immunology, molecular diagnostics, and blood banking.

Each discipline of laboratory medicine is described in more detail in later chapters of this book. Many changes are taking place in the clinical laboratory and are already affecting the types of tests being offered. Anatomic pathology, cytology, and histology are part of the overall clinical laboratory but usually function separately.

Fig. 1-2 shows a possible system for the organization of a clinical laboratory. In addition to the traditional areas already mentioned, the disciplines of cytogenetics, toxicology, flow cytometry, and other specialized divisions are present in larger

laboratories. Molecular diagnostics is done in many laboratories.

Another change has been the move from tests being done in a centralized laboratory setting to point-of-care testing (POCT). Alternative testing sites—the patient's bedside, in operating rooms or recovery areas, or even home testing—are extensions of the traditional clinical laboratory site (see Chapter 9).

The leaders and managers of the clinical laboratory must be certain all legal operating regulations have been met and all persons working in the laboratory setting are fully aware of the importance of compliance with these regulations. Those in leadership positions in a clinical laboratory must have expertise in medical, scientific, and technical areas as well as a full understanding of regulatory matters. All laboratory personnel must be aware of these regulatory considerations, but the management is responsible for ensuring that this information is communicated to everyone who needs to know.

Appropriate utilization of the clinical laboratory is critical to the practice of laboratory medicine. It is important that the laboratory serve to educate the physician and other health care providers so that the information available through the reported test results can be used appropriately. When tests are being ordered, the clinical

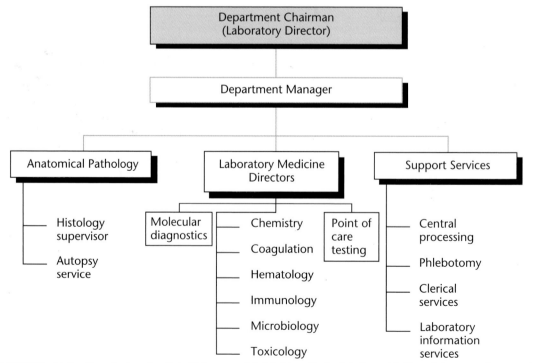

FIGURE 1-2 **Organization of a clinical laboratory.** (Modified from Kaplan LA, Pesce AJ: Clinical chemistry: theory, analysis, correlation, ed 5, St Louis, 2010, Mosby.)

laboratory should assume a role of leadership and education in assisting the physician to understand the most useful pattern of ordering, for example, to serve the best interest of the patient, the clinical decision-making process for the physician, and the costs involved.

Continuing education is always part of a laboratory's program for ensuring high-quality service and maintaining the morale of the laboratory staff. Programs are offered at professional meetings as well as online.

Hundreds of different laboratory tests are readily available in the larger laboratories, but typically only a small percentage of these tests are routinely ordered. When the results of these tests are used appropriately in the context of the patient's clinical case, physical examination findings, and the medical history, clinical decision making will be improved. It is unusual that the results from a single laboratory assay will provide a diagnosis. Certain additional laboratory tests may be needed to take decision making to the next step. Generally, a small number of appropriately chosen laboratory tests (a panel of tests) or an algorithm is sufficient to confirm or rule out one or more of the possibilities in a differential diagnosis.

LABORATORY DEPARTMENTS OR DIVISIONS

The organization of a particular clinical laboratory depends on its size, the number of tests done, and the facilities available. Larger laboratories tend to be departmentalized; there is a separate area designated for each of the various divisions. The current trend is to have a more "open" design or a core lab where personnel can work in any of several areas or divisions. Cross-training is important in a core lab model.

With either the more traditional divisions by separate areas or the open model, there are still several distinct departments or divisions in the organization of the clinical laboratory. These include hematology, hemostasis and coagulation, urinalysis, clinical chemistry, blood bank (immunohematology) and transfusion services, immunology and serology, molecular diagnostics, and microbiology. Each division is addressed in separate chapters of this book.

Hematology

Hematology is the study of blood (see Chapter 12). The formed elements of the blood, or blood cells, include erythrocytes (red blood cells [RBCs]), leukocytes (white blood cells [WBCs]), and thrombocytes (platelets). The routine hematology

screening test for abnormalities in the blood is the complete blood cell count (CBC). Most CBCs include RBC count, WBC count, platelet count, hemoglobin concentration, hematocrit, and a percentage differential of the WBCs present. The results of the CBC are useful in diagnosing anemias, in which there are too few RBCs or too little hemoglobin; in leukemias, in which there are too many WBCs or abnormal WBCs; and in infectious processes of several etiologies, in which changes in WBCs are noted. These tests are done in most hematology laboratories by use of an automated instrument. Many of these automated cell counters also provide automated WBC differential analyses, separating the types of WBCs present by size, maturity, and nuclear and cytoplasmic characteristics.

Cell counts for other body fluids, such as cerebrospinal fluid (CSF) or synovial fluid, are also performed in some hematology laboratories. The work done in the hematology laboratory also has a microscopy component. Microscopic assessment of a stained blood film is done as part of some CBCs, especially when automated instrumentation is not readily available or when a more complete morphologic examination is necessary.

Other tests done in hematology laboratories are reticulocyte counts and erythrocyte sedimentation rate (ESR) measurements. Examination of bone marrow is done in special hematology divisions where trained hematopathologists and technologists are present to examine the slides. The bone marrow from a patient is obtained by a trained physician.

Hemostasis and Coagulation

Work done in the hemostasis and coagulation laboratory assesses bleeding and clotting problems (see Chapter 13). In some laboratories, hematology and coagulation tests are part of the same laboratory department. The two tests most often performed in the coagulation laboratory are prothrombin time (PT) and activated partial thromboplastin time (APTT). These tests can be used to identify potential bleeding disorders and to monitor anticoagulant therapy. Patients who have had a heart attack or stroke, both caused by formation of blood clots, are given medications that anticoagulate their blood or slow the clotting process. These patients must be monitored because too large a dose of these drugs can lead to bleeding problems.

Urinalysis

In the urinalysis laboratory division, the routine urine screening tests are done (see Chapter 14). Historically, the routine urinalysis was one of the earliest laboratory tests performed, and it still provides valuable information for the detection of disease related to the kidney and urinary tract. By evaluating the results of the three component parts of the urinalysis—observation of the physical characteristics of the urine specimen itself (e.g., color, clarity, specific gravity), screening for chemical constituents (e.g., pH, glucose, ketone bodies, protein, blood, bilirubin, urobilinogen, nitrites, leukocyte esterase), and microscopic examination of the urinary sediment—metabolic diseases such as diabetes mellitus, kidney disease, and infectious diseases of the urinary bladder or kidney can be diagnosed and monitored.

Clinical Chemistry

The clinical chemistry laboratory performs quantitative analytical procedures on a variety of body fluids, but primarily on serum or plasma that has been processed from whole blood collected from the patient (see Chapter 11). Tests are also done on urine or, less frequently, on body fluids (e.g., CSF). Several hundred analytes can be tested in the chemistry laboratory, but a few tests are used much more often to assist in the diagnosis of disease.

One of the most commonly performed chemistry tests is blood glucose. Other frequently performed assays are cholesterol, electrolytes, and serum proteins. Blood glucose tests are used to diagnose and monitor diabetes mellitus. Cholesterol is a test that is part of a battery of tests to monitor the patient's lipid status. Electrolytes affect many of the metabolic processes in the body, including maintenance of osmotic pressure and water distribution in various body compartments, maintenance of pH, regulation of the functioning of heart and other muscles, and oxidation-reduction processes. Elevated serum protein levels can indicate disease states of several types. Serum enzyme tests are done to identify damage to or disease of specific organs, such as heart muscle damage or liver cell damage. Tests to monitor drug therapy and drug levels, or toxicology, are also performed in chemistry laboratories.

Most routine chemistry testing is done by automated methods using computerized instruments that are sophisticated and rapid and provide reliable results (see Chapter 9). Persons working in chemistry laboratories will be using automated analytical equipment; having a good working knowledge of the various types of methodologies and instrumentation used is essential.

Blood Bank (Immunohematology) and Transfusion Services

When blood is donated for transfusion purposes, it must undergo a rigorous protocol of testing to make certain it is safe for transfusion (see Chapter 18).

Proper sample identification is particularly crucial in blood-banking procedures, because a mislabeled specimen could result in a severe transfusion reaction or even death for the recipient. Most of the testing done in the blood bank laboratory is based on antigen-antibody reactions. In the specialized tests performed in the blood bank laboratory, *antigens* are specific proteins attached to red or white blood cells. The nature of specific antigens determines the blood group assigned: A, B, O, or AB. Rh typing is also done, with blood being classified as Rh positive or Rh negative. Donated blood is also screened for any unusual antibodies present and for the presence of antibodies associated with blood-borne infectious diseases such as hepatitis viruses or human immunodeficiency virus (HIV). The donor blood must be matched to the prospective recipient's to ensure that they are compatible. When a blood transfusion is ordered, it is extremely important that only properly matched blood be transfused.

Blood banks also practice transfusion medicine using components of blood or blood products. A patient does not usually need the whole unit of blood, only a particular part of it, such as the RBCs, platelets, or specific clotting factors. By using blood component therapy, one unit of donated blood can help several different patients who have different needs. The blood bank technologist separates the donated unit into components and stores them for transfusion at a later time.

Immunology and Serology

The normal immune system functions to protect the body from foreign microorganisms that may invade it. When foreign material—that is, something the body does not already have as part of itself—enters the body, the immune system works to eliminate the foreign material, which can be bacteria, viruses, fungi, or parasites. The body's defensive action is carried out by its WBCs—lymphocytes, monocytes, and other cells—through which the invading organism is eliminated or controlled. As in the blood bank laboratory, many of the immunology/serology laboratory's procedures are based on antigen-antibody reactions. When foreign material (antigen) is introduced into the body, the body reacts by means of its immune system to make antibodies to the foreign antigen. The antibodies formed can be measured in the laboratory.

In the evaluation of certain infectious diseases, the detection of antibodies in the serum of the patient is an important step in making and confirming a diagnosis and managing the illness. The usefulness of serologic testing is based on the rise and fall of specific antibody titers in response to the disease process. In many cases, serologic testing is done retrospectively because the disease must progress to a certain point before the antibody titers will rise; often it takes several days or weeks for the antibody titer to rise after the first symptoms appear. In general, serologic testing is most useful for infectious organisms that are difficult to culture, cause chronic conditions, or have prolonged incubation periods.

In addition to its value in the diagnosis of infectious disease, immunologic testing performed in a dedicated immunology laboratory or immunoassays performed in clinical chemistry departments can identify normal and abnormal levels of immune cells and serum components. Immune cellular function can also be determined (see Chapter 17).

Molecular Diagnostics

Biotechnology is a fast-growing discipline of the diagnostic laboratory. Molecular biology, or the discipline of molecular diagnostics, uses this technology. Molecular pathology applies the principles of basic molecular biology to the study of human diseases. New approaches to human disease assessment are being developed by clinical laboratories because of the new information about the molecular basis of disease processes in general. Traditional laboratory analyses give results based on a description of events currently occurring in the patient (e.g., blood cell counts, infectious processes, blood glucose concentration). But molecular biology introduces a predictive component: findings from these tests can be used to anticipate events that may occur in the future, when patients may be at risk for a particular disease or condition. More than ever, this predictive component reinforces the importance of how laboratory test results are used and emphasizes ethical considerations and the need for genetic counseling (see Chapter 6 and in the clinical chapters as appropriate).

Microbiology

In the microbiology laboratory, microorganisms that cause disease are identified; these are known as **pathogens** (see Chapter 16). Generally, the common bacteria, viruses, fungi, and parasites are identified in a typical clinical laboratory. Specimens sent to the microbiology laboratory for culture include swabs from the throat or wounds, sputum, vaginal excretions, urine, and blood. It is important that the microbiology staff be able to differentiate *normal biota* or *normal flora*—organisms that are usually present at specific sites in the body—from *pathogenic flora*. Various differential testing is done, from inoculation and incubation of the classic culture plate,

to observation of a microorganism's growth characteristics, to the use of Gram-staining techniques to separate gram-positive from gram-negative organisms. Once a pathogen is suspected, more testing is done to confirm its identity. Rapid testing methods have been developed to identify routine pathogens. For example, immunologic tests have been devised using monoclonal antibodies to identify the streptococcal organism causing pharyngitis, or "strep" throat.

Another task for the microbiology laboratory is to identify effective antibiotics for treatment of an offending pathogen. A pure culture of a potential pathogen is tested by using a panel of antibiotics of various types and dosages to determine the susceptibility of the organism to these antibiotics. With this information, the primary care provider can choose the most effective antibiotic based on *in vitro* laboratory testing.

CLINICAL LABORATORY STAFFING AND FUNCTIONS

Clinical laboratory staff members are an essential component of the medical team. In some laboratories, personnel are cross-trained to work in core laboratories; other laboratories may have specialists in certain areas of the laboratory.

Pathologist

Most clinical laboratories are operated under the direction of a **pathologist** or **PhD**. The clinical laboratory can be divided into two main sections:
- Anatomic pathology
- Clinical pathology

Most pathologists have training in both anatomic and clinical pathology, although research can be substituted for the clinical pathology portion of the pathology residency program. The *anatomic pathologist* is a licensed physician, usually trained for an additional 4 to 5 years after graduating from medical school, to examine (grossly and microscopically) all the surgically removed specimens from patients, which include frozen sections, tissue samples, and autopsy specimens. Examination of Pap smears and other cytologic and histologic examinations are also generally done by an anatomic pathologist.

A *clinical pathologist* is also a licensed physician with additional training in clinical pathology or laboratory medicine. Under the direction of the clinical pathologist, many common laboratory tests are performed on blood and urine. Consultation with physicians is also important; any information gained concerning the patient's case is actually the result of collaborative activity between the laboratory and the attending physician.

The pathologist will perform only certain services such as examination of the surgical specimens, which is done primarily by the anatomic pathologist. Other testing falls under the clinical pathologist's/medical director's responsibility and supervision.

A person holding a PhD in a scientific discipline may be recognized as a laboratory director.

Laboratory Supervisor or Manager

Typically, a laboratory has a supervisor or manager who is responsible for the technical aspects of managing the laboratory. This person is most often an MLS with additional education and experience in administration. In very large laboratories, a technical manager may supervise the technical aspects of the facility (issues involving assay of analytes), including quality control programs, off-site testing, and maintenance of the laboratory instruments. In addition, a business manager may be hired to handle administrative details.

The supervisor or administrative manager may also be the technical manager in the case of smaller laboratories. Section-supervising technologists are in place as needed, depending on the size and workload of the laboratory. A major concern of administrative technologists, regardless of the job titles used, is ensuring that all federal, state, and local regulatory mandates are being followed by the laboratory. Persons in leadership and management positions in the clinical laboratory must be certain all legal operating conditions have been met and that these conditions are balanced with the performance of work in a cost-effective manner.

It is important that the people serving in a supervisory position be able to communicate in a clear, concise manner, both to the persons working in their laboratory settings and to the physicians and other health care workers who utilize laboratory services.

Technologists, Technicians, and Specialists

Depending on the size of the laboratory and the numbers and types of laboratory tests performed, various levels of trained personnel are needed. CLIA '88 regulations set the standards for personnel, including their levels of education and training. Generally, the level of training or education of the laboratory professional will be taken into consideration in the roles assigned in the laboratory and the types of laboratory analyses performed.

The responsibilities of MLSs and MLTs vary but may include performing laboratory assays, supervising other staff, or teaching. Some are engaged in research. An important aspect of clinical laboratory science education is to understand the science behind the tests being performed, so that problems can be recognized and solved. Troubleshooting is a constant consideration in the clinical laboratory. Because of in-depth knowledge of technical aspects, principles of methodology, and instrumentation used for the various laboratory assays, the laboratory professional is able to correlate and interpret the data.

Other laboratory professionals may be assigned to specific sections of the laboratory. Although MLSs and MLTs may collect blood specimens at smaller facilities, phlebotomists collect blood specimens in larger hospitals. They may process test specimens in the specimen-processing section of the laboratory.

PRIMARY ACCREDITING ORGANIZATIONS

In current laboratory settings, many governmental regulations, along with regulations and recommendations from professional, state, and federal accreditation agencies and commissions of various types, govern the activities of the laboratory.

In the United States, there are approximately 15,206 accredited laboratories, 97% of which are inspected by three primary accrediting organizations: COLA, CAP, and TJC.[2]

Commission on Office Laboratory Accreditation

The Commission on Office Laboratory Accreditation (COLA) accredits 6179 facilities, or 40% of laboratories. COLA was founded in 1988 as a private alternative to help laboratories stay in compliance with the new CLIA regulations. In 1993, the Health Care Financing Administration (now CMS) granted COLA deeming authority under CLIA, and in 1997 the Joint Commission on Accreditation of Health care Organizations (JCAHO)—now known as The Joint Commission (TJC)—also recognized COLA's laboratory accreditation program.

COLA is the first organization to be renewed since increased government scrutiny of survey organizations and will be given permission to accredit laboratories for the next 6 years to help labs meet CLIA requirements. The increase in oversight by CMS was driven by a government investigation in 2006 into how some highly publicized laboratory errors had occurred and could have been prevented.

COLA will incorporate new standard program requirements that coincide with updated CLIA requirements and are closely aligned with quality systems methodology. The new standard program requirements are a compilation of 75 new or revised criteria to the existing 299 questions. Some of the new program features for laboratories in 2007 include:

- Revised quality control requirements
- Increased attention to laboratory information systems
- New focus on quality assessments activities that span all phases of laboratory testing
- Incorporation of quality systems processes to all categories of the laboratory's path of workflow

College of American Pathologists

The College of American Pathologists (CAP) accredits 5179, or 34% of laboratories. The CAP Laboratory Accreditation Program is an internationally recognized program and the only one of its kind that utilizes teams of practicing laboratory professionals as inspectors. Designed to go well beyond regulatory compliance, the program helps laboratories achieve the highest standards of excellence to positively impact patient care. The CAP Laboratory Accreditation Program meets the needs of a variety of laboratory settings.

The Centers for Medicare and Medicaid Services (CMS) has granted the CAP Laboratory Accreditation Program deeming authority. It is also TJC recognized and can be used to meet many state certification requirements.

The Joint Commission

TJC accredits 3467, or 23% of laboratories, and has been evaluating and accrediting hospital laboratory services since 1979 and freestanding laboratories since 1995. Laboratories eligible for accreditation include:

- Laboratories in hospitals, clinics, long-term care facilities, home care organizations, behavioral health care organizations, ambulatory sites, and physician offices
- Reference laboratories
- Freestanding laboratories, such as assisted reproductive technology labs
- Blood transfusion and donor centers
- Public health laboratories, including Indian Health Service laboratories
- Laboratories in federal facilities, such as the Department of Veteran's Affairs and the Department of Defense
- POCT sites that include blood gas labs providing services to patients in emergency rooms, surgical suites, cardiac catheterization labs, and other patient care areas

Other Agencies

Other organizations, including the American Association of Blood Banks (AABB), American Society of Histocompatibility and Immunogenetics (ASHI), and American Osteopathic Association (AOA), accredit 381 facilities, or 3% of laboratories.

EXTERNAL GOVERNMENT LABORATORY ACCREDITATION AND REGULATION

Regulations and standards are designed specifically to protect staff working in the laboratory, other health care personnel, patients treated in the health care facility, and society as a whole. **Federal regulations** exist to meet these objectives. Certain regulatory mandates have been issued externally, such as the **Clinical Laboratory Improvement Amendments of 1988 (CLIA '88)**. Others are internal, and some are both external and internal.[4-6] In addition to CLIA '88 regulations, other state and federal regulations are in place to regulate chemical waste disposal, use of hazardous chemicals, and issues of laboratory safety for personnel, including handling of biohazardous materials and application of standard precautions (see Chapter 2).

A laboratory that wants to receive payment for its services from Medicare or Medicaid must be licensed under the **Public Health Service Act**. To be licensed, the laboratory must meet the conditions for participation in those programs. The **Centers for Medicare and Medicaid Services (CMS)**, formerly the **Health Care Financing Administration (HCFA)**, has the administrative responsibility for both the Medicare and CLIA '88 programs. Facilities accredited by approved private accreditation agencies such as CAP must also follow the regulations for licensure under CLIA '88. States with equivalent CLIA '88 regulations are reviewed individually as to possible waiver for CLIA '88 licensure.

The CMS, under the U.S. **Department of Health and Human Services (HHS)**, has also established regulations to implement CLIA '88. Any facility performing quantitative, qualitative, or screening test procedures or examinations on materials derived from the human body is regulated by CLIA '88. This includes hospital laboratories of all sizes; physician office laboratories; nursing home facilities; clinics; industrial laboratories; city, state, and county laboratories; pharmacies, fitness centers, and health fairs; and independent laboratories.

As of December 29, 1993, HCFA approved the accreditation program developed by the **Commission on Office Laboratory Accreditation (COLA)** for the physician office laboratory. This means that COLA accreditation requirements are recognized by HCFA as being equivalent to those established by CLIA. The COLA accreditation established a peer review option in place of the CLIA regulatory requirements. COLA-accredited laboratories are surveyed every 2 years to ensure that they meet requirements developed by their peers in family practice, internal medicine, or pathology.

The **Clinical and Laboratory Standards Institute (CLSI)** is a nonprofit, educational organization created for the development, promotion, and use of national and international laboratory standards. CLSI employs voluntary consensus standards to maintain the performance of the clinical laboratory at the high level necessary for quality patient care. CLSI recommendations, guidelines, and standards follow the CLIA '88 mandates and therefore serve to inform and assist the laboratory in following the federal regulations.

Through labor laws and environmental regulations, assessment has been given to laboratory workers that they are in a safe atmosphere and that every precaution has been taken to maintain that safe atmosphere. The **Occupational Safety and Health Administration (OSHA)** has been involved in setting these practices into motion; through OSHA, these mandates have become part of the daily life of the laboratory workplace. Other external controls include standards mandated by public health laws and reporting requirements through the **Centers for Disease Control and Prevention (CDC)** and through certification and licensure requirements issued by the **U.S. Food and Drug Administration (FDA)**. State regulations are imposed by Medicaid agencies, state environmental laws, and state public health laws and licensure laws. Local regulations include those determined by building codes and fire prevention codes.

Two certifying agencies, the **College of American Pathologists (CAP)** and **The Joint Commission (TJC)** have been given deemed status to act (see previous discussion) on the federal government's behalf. From an external source, guidelines and standards have also been set by these organizations to govern safe work practices in the clinical laboratory. Independent agencies also have influence over practices in the clinical laboratory through accreditation policies or other responsibilities. These include groups such as CAP, TJC, and other specific proficiency testing programs.

CLINICAL LABORATORY IMPROVEMENT AMENDMENTS OF 1988

Much of how clinical laboratories perform their work is delineated by federal regulations or other external policies. CLIA '88 regulations govern most of the activities of a particular laboratory, although federal laboratories (e.g., Veterans Affairs hospitals/medical centers) are not regulated by CLIA requirements.[3,4] The goals of these amendments are to ensure that the laboratory results reported are of high quality regardless of where the testing is done: small laboratory, physician's office, large reference laboratory, or patient's home. CLIA '88 regulations include aspects of proficiency testing programs, management of patient testing, quality assessment programs, the use of quality control systems, personnel requirements, inspections and site visits, and consultations. Several federal agencies govern practices in the clinical laboratory. These regulatory agencies or organizations are primarily concerned with setting standards, conducting inspections, and imposing sanctions when necessary.

CLIA Requirements for Personnel

The personnel section of the CLIA regulations defines the responsibilities of persons working in each of the testing sites where tests of moderate or high complexity are done, along with the educational requirements and training and experience needed. Minimum education and experience needed by testing personnel to perform the specific laboratory tests on human specimens are also regulated by CLIA '88. These job requirements are listed in the CLIA '88 final regulations, along with their amendments published from 1992 to 1995.[3-5]

There are no CLIA regulations for testing personnel who work at sites performing only the waived tests or provider-performed microscopy testing. For laboratories where only tests of moderate complexity are performed, the minimum requirement for testing personnel is a high school diploma or equivalent, so long as there is documented evidence of an amount of training sufficient to ensure that the laboratory staff has the skills necessary to collect, identify, and process the specimen and perform the laboratory analysis.

For tests of the highly complex category, the personnel requirements are more stringent. Anyone who is eligible to perform highly complex tests can also perform moderate-complexity testing. OSHA requires that training in handling chemical hazards, as well as training in handling infectious materials (standard precautions), be included for all new testing personnel. The laboratory director is ultimately responsible for all personnel working in the laboratory.

Levels of Testing

External standards have been set to ensure that all laboratories provide the best, most reliable information to the physician and the patient. It was primarily to this end that CLIA '88 was enacted.

CLIA regulations divide laboratories into categories based on the "complexity" of the tests being performed by the laboratory, as follows:

- Waived tests
- Moderately complex tests
- Highly complex tests

This tiered grouping (see Chapter 9) has been devised with varying degrees of regulation for each level. The criteria for classification include:

1. Risk of harm to the patient
2. Risk of an erroneous result
3. Type of testing method used
4. Degree of independent judgment and interpretation needed
5. Availability of the particular test in question for home use

The law contains a provision to exempt certain laboratories from standards for personnel and from quality control programs, proficiency testing, or quality assessment programs. These laboratories are defined as those that perform only simple, routine tests considered to have an insignificant risk of an erroneous result. Those laboratories that receive a "certificate of waiver" can perform waived testing. Other categories include provider-performed microscopy for laboratory testing, generally performed by the physician in the office setting; this category is also exempt from some of the CLIA requirements. The two additional categories are moderate-complexity and high-complexity levels of testing. These levels are more regulated, with some minimal personnel standards required, as well as proficiency testing and quality assessment programs.

Waived Tests

As currently defined, waived laboratory tests or procedures are those cleared by the FDA for home use, which employ methodologies that are so simple the likelihood of erroneous results is negligible, and which pose no reasonable risk of harm to the patient if the test is performed incorrectly.

The list of waived tests continues to expand (http://www.fda.gov). Waived tests include dipstick or tablet reagent urinalysis (nonautomated) for bilirubin, glucose, hemoglobin, ketones, leukocytes, nitrite, pH, protein, specific gravity, and urobilinogen; fecal occult blood; ovulation tests (visual color comparison tests for human luteinizing hormone); urine pregnancy tests (visual color comparison tests); erythrocyte sedimentation rate (nonautomated); hemoglobin (copper sulfate, nonautomated, an extremely outdated testing methodology); blood glucose (by FDA-approved monitoring devices specifically for home use); spun microhematocrit; hemoglobin by single-analyte instruments (with self-contained or component features to perform specimen-reagent interaction, providing direct measurement and readout); and blood cholesterol (by FDA-approved monitoring devices for home use).[4]

Provider-Performed Microscopy

To meet the criteria for inclusion in the provider-performed microscopy (PPM) category, procedures must follow these specifications:

1. The examination must be personally performed by the practitioner (defined as a physician, a midlevel practitioner under the supervision of a physician, or a dentist).
2. The procedure must be categorized as moderately complex.
3. The primary instrument for performing the test is the microscope (limited to brightfield or phase-contrast microscopy).
4. The specimen is labile.
5. Control materials are not available.
6. Specimen handling is limited.

As currently defined, the PPM category includes all direct wet mount preparations for the presence or absence of bacteria, fungi, parasites, and human cellular elements in vaginal, cervical, or skin preparations; all potassium hydroxide (KOH) preparations; pinworm examinations; fern tests; postcoital direct qualitative examinations of vaginal or cervical mucus; urine sediment examinations; nasal smears for granulocytes (eosinophils); fecal leukocyte examinations; and qualitative semen analysis (limited to the presence or absence of sperm and detection of motility).

ALTERNATE SITES OF TESTING

The traditional setting for performance of diagnostic laboratory testing has been a centralized location in a health care facility (hospital) where specimens from patients are sent to be tested. The centralized laboratory setting remains in many institutions, but the advent of near-testing, bedside testing, or POCT has changed the organization of many laboratories. In POCT, the laboratory testing actually comes to the bedside of the patient. Any changes to implement the use of POCT should show a significant improvement in patient outcome and a total financial benefit to the patient and the institution, not only a reduction in the costs of equipment and supplies.

Point-of-Care Testing

Decentralization of testing away from the traditional laboratory setting can greatly increase the interaction of laboratory personnel with patients and with other members of the health care team. POCT is an example of an interdisciplinary activity that crosses many boundaries in the health care facility. POCT is not always performed by laboratory staff. Other health care personnel, including nurses, respiratory therapists, anesthesiologists, operating room technologists, and physician assistants, often perform near-patient testing. Even in these cases, however, the CLIA '88 regulations associated with clinical laboratory testing must be followed for POCT, even if nonlaboratory staff members are actually performing the tests.

These CLIA regulations are considered "site neutral," meaning that all laboratory testing must meet the same standards for quality of work done, personnel, proficiency testing, quality control, and so on, regardless of where the tests are performed, whether in a central laboratory or at the bedside of the patient. Regulation of the clinical laboratory (waived tests, tests of moderate complexity, tests of high complexity, and PPMs) also apply to POCT. If performed in a facility that is TJC- or CAP-accredited, these tests are regulated in essentially the same way as tests performed in a centralized laboratory.

Qualifications for POCT personnel are also set by federal, state, and local regulations.[4] The level of training varies with the analytical system being employed and the background of the individual involved, which can range from a requirement for a high school diploma with no experience to a bachelor of science degree with 2 years of experience. The director of the laboratory is responsible for setting additional requirements, so long as the federal CLIA '88 regulations are also being followed.

Because results can be reported immediately, and the patient's case management depends on these results, it is essential that POCT devices have built-in quality control and quality assessment systems to prevent erroneous data from being reported to the physician. POCT has been found to provide cost-effective improvements in medical care. In a hospital setting, POCT provides immediate assessment and management of the critically ill patient; this is its most significant use for this setting. Tests usually included in POCT are based on criteria of immediate medical need: blood gases, electrolytes (Na^+, K^+, Cl^-, $HCO3^-$), prothrombin time (PT), partial thromboplastin time (PTT) or activated clotting time (ACT), hematocrit or hemoglobin, and glucose. POCT attempts to meet the demands of intensive care units, operating rooms, and emergency departments for faster reporting of test results. Other possible benefits of POCT are improved therapeutic turnaround times, less trauma and more convenience for the patient (when blood is collected and analyzed at the bedside), decreased preanalytical errors (errors formerly caused by specimen collection, transportation, and handling by the laboratory), decreased use of laboratory personnel (use of cross-training, whereby nurses can perform the laboratory analysis, eliminating a laboratorian for this step), more collaboration of clinicians with the laboratory, and shorter intensive care unit stays. Certain tests, such as the fecal screen for blood and the routine chemical screening of urine by reagent strips, can often be done more easily on the nursing unit, if the assays are properly performed and controlled using quality assessment protocol.

POCT in outpatient settings provides the ability to obtain test results during the patient's visit to the clinic or the physician's office, enabling diagnosis and subsequent case management in a more timely manner.

When central laboratory testing is compared with POCT, consideration must be given to which site of testing will provide the most appropriate testing mechanism. Centralized laboratories can provide "stat" testing capabilities, which can report results in a timely manner. Some laboratories develop a laboratory satellite that is set up to function at the point of need, such as a laboratory located near or in the operating room or a laboratory that is portable and can be transported on a cart to the point of need.

Reference Laboratories

When a laboratory performs only routine tests, specimens for the more complex tests ordered by the physician must be sent to a **reference laboratory** for analysis. It is often more cost-effective for a laboratory to perform only certain common, repetitive tests and to send out the others for another laboratory to perform. These reference laboratories can then perform the more complex tests for many customers, giving good turnaround times; this is their service to their customers. It is important to select a reference laboratory where the mechanisms for specimen transport and results reporting are managed well. The turnaround time is important, and it often is a function of how well the specimens are handled by the reference laboratory. There must be a good means of communication between the reference laboratory and its customers. The reference laboratory should be managed by professionals who both recognize the importance of providing quality results and, when needed, can provide the patient's clinician information about utilizing the results. Messengers or couriers are engaged to transport or drive specimens within a fixed, reasonable geographic area. The various commercial delivery systems are used for transport out of the area.

Physician Office Laboratories

A **physician office laboratory (POL)** is a laboratory where the tests performed are limited to those done for the physician's own patients coming to the practice, group, or clinic. Because of the concern that some of these laboratories were lacking in quality of work done, the CLIA '88 regulations include POLs. Before CLIA '88, the POLs were largely unregulated. Most POLs perform only the waived tests or PPM, as set by CLIA (see earlier discussion). Tests most often performed in POLs are visually read reagent strip urinalysis, blood glucose, occult fecal blood, rapid streptococcus A in throats, hemoglobin, urine pregnancy, cholesterol, and hematocrit.

The convenience to the patient of having laboratory testing done in the physician's office is a driving force for physicians to include a laboratory in their office or clinic. Manufacturers of laboratory instruments have accommodated the clinic or office setting with a modern generation of instruments that require less technical skill by the user. The improved turnaround times for test results and patient convenience must be balanced, however, with cost-effectiveness and the potential for physicians to be exposed to problems that may be outside the realm of their expertise or training. Laboratory staff, including pathologists, must be available to act as consultants when the need arises.

A POL must submit an application to HHS or its designee. This application form includes details about the number of tests done, methodologies used for each measurement, and the qualifications of each of the testing personnel employed to perform the tests. Certificates are issued for up to 2 years, and any changes in tests done or methodologies used, personnel hired, and so forth, must be submitted to HHS within 30 days of the change. This application may also be made through an accreditation agency whose requirements are deemed by HHS to be equal to or more stringent than the HHS requirements. Accreditation requirements from COLA have been recognized by CMS (formerly HCFA) as being equivalent to the CLIA requirements.

When a POL performs only waived tests or PPM tests, there are no CLIA personnel requirements. The physician is responsible for the work done in the POL. When moderately or highly complex testing is done in a POL, the more stringent CLIA personnel requirements must be followed for the testing personnel; these POLs must also adhere to a program of quality assessment, including proficiency testing.

PATIENT SPECIMENS

Clinical laboratorians work with many types of specimens. Blood (see Chapter 3) and urine specimens (see Chapter 14) usually are most often tested, but tests are also ordered on body tissues and other body fluids, including synovial, cerebrospinal, peritoneal, and pericardial fluids (see Chapter 15).

The purpose of the clinical laboratory is to provide information regarding the assay results for the specimens analyzed; it is most important that the specimens be properly collected in the first place. In the testing process, analytes or constituents are measured by using only very small amounts of the specimens collected. In interpreting the results, however, it is assumed the results obtained represent the actual concentrations of the analytes in the patient. Only by using the various quality assessment systems discussed later in this book can the reliability of results be ensured. No matter how carefully a laboratory assay has been carried out, valid laboratory results can be reported only when preanalytical quality control has also been ascertained. Special patient preparation considerations for some specimen collections, along with proper transportation to and handling in the laboratory before the actual analytical assay, are very important. Appropriate quality assessment programs must be in place in the laboratory to make certain that each patient specimen is given the best analysis possible and that the results reported will benefit the patient in the best possible way.

QUALITY ASSESSMENT

External standards have been set to ensure the quality of laboratory results reported through quality assessment, as imposed by CLIA '88 and administered by CMS. A clinical laboratory must be certified by CMS, by a private certifying agency, or by a state regulatory agency that has been given approval by CMS. Once certified, the laboratory is scheduled for regular inspections to determine compliance with the federal regulations, including CLIA '88.

Quality assessment (previously called *quality assurance*) programs are now also a requirement in the federal government's implementation of CLIA '88 (see Chapter 8). The standards mandated are for all laboratories, with the intent that the medical community's ability to provide good-quality patient care will be greatly enhanced. Included in the CLIA '88 provisions are requirements for quality control and quality assessment, for the use of proficiency testing, and for certain levels of personnel to perform and supervise the work in the laboratory (see Chapter 8).

According to CLIA '88 regulations, quality assessment activities in the laboratory must be documented and must be an active part of the ongoing organization of the laboratory. Dedication of sufficient planning time to quality assessment and implementation of the program in the total laboratory operation are critical. All clinical laboratory personnel must be willing to work together to make the quality of service to the patient their top priority. It is important to develop a comprehensive program to include all levels of laboratory staff.

Local, internal programs must be in place to carry out the external mandates. Internal regulation also comes from the need to ensure quality performance and reporting of results for the many laboratory tests being done—a process of quality assessment. It is the responsibility of the clinical laboratory, to both patient and physician, to ensure that the results reported from that laboratory are reliable and to provide the physician with an estimate of what constitutes the reference range or "normal" range for an analyte being measured. Internal monitoring programs are concerned with **total quality management (TQM)**, **quality assessment (QA)**, or **continuous quality improvement (CQI)**, each of which is designed to monitor and improve the quality of services provided by the laboratory.

A quality assessment system is divided into two major components: nonanalytical factors and the analysis of quantitative data (quality control).

Nonanalytical Factors in Quality Assessment

To guarantee the highest quality of patient care through laboratory testing, a variety of preanalytical and postanalytical factors (see Chapter 8) must be considered in addition to analytical data. For laboratories to comply with CLIA '88 and be certified to perform testing, they must meet minimum standards. In some cases, deficiencies are noted and must be corrected (Table 1-1). Nonanalytical factors that support quality testing include the following:
1. Qualified personnel
2. Established laboratory policies
3. Laboratory procedure manual
4. Proper procedures for specimen collection and storage
5. Preventive maintenance of equipment
6. Appropriate methodology
7. Established quality control and quality assessment techniques
8. Accuracy in reporting results

TABLE 1-1

	Top 10 CLIA Deficiencies	
Rank	Top 10 CLIA Deficiencies	% of Labs
1	At least twice annually, the laboratory must verify the accuracy of any test or procedure it performs that is not included in subpart I or this part.	5.80%
2	Test systems must be selected by the laboratory. The testing must be performed following the manufacturer's instructions and in a manner that provides test results within the laboratory's stated performance specifications for each test system as determined under 493.1253.	5.69%
3	The laboratory must establish and follow written policies and procedures for an ongoing mechanism to monitor, assess, and when indicated, correct problems identified in the analytical systems specified in 493.1251 through 493.1283.	5.43%
4	The laboratory must define criteria for those conditions that are essential for proper storage of reagents and specimens, accurate and reliable test system operation, and test result reporting. The criteria must be consistent with the manufacturer's instructions, if provided. These conditions must be monitored and documented.	5.15%
5	The procedure manual must include the requirements for specimen acceptability, microscopic examination, step-by-step performance of the procedure, preparation of materials for testing, etc.	4.93%
6	The laboratory must establish and follow written policies and procedures for an ongoing mechanism to monitor, assess, and when indicated, correct problems identified in the general laboratory systems requirements in 493.1231 through 493.1236.	4.21%
7	The test report must indicate positive patient identification, name and address of the laboratory where the test was performed, the report date, test performed, specimen source, result, and units of measurement or interpretation.	4.06%
8	The laboratory director must ensure that the quality assessment programs are established and maintained to assure the quality of laboratory services provided.	3.80%
9	The laboratory must maintain an information or record system that includes positive identification of the specimen, date and time of specimen receipt, condition and disposition of specimens that do not meet the laboratory's criteria for acceptability, and the records and dates of all specimen testing, including the identity of the personnel who performed the test.	3.40%
10	Reagents, solutions, culture media, control materials, calibration materials, and other supplies must not be used when they have exceeded their expiration date, have deteriorated, or are of substandard quality.	3.38%

Modified from Kibak P: CMS rolls out new CLIA policy changes, Clin Lab News 34(2):1, 5-7, 2008.
CLIA, Clinical Laboratory Improvement Amendments of 1988.
Courtesy Centers for Medicare and Medicaid Services, Baltimore, MD.

Qualified Personnel

The entry-level examination competencies of all certified persons in the section(s) in which they work must be validated. Validation takes the form of both external certification and new employee orientation to the work environment. Continuing competency is equally important. Participation in continuing education activities is essential to the maintenance of competency and to maintaining professional certification (e.g., NCA).

Established Laboratory Policies

Laboratory policies should be included in a laboratory reference manual that is available to all personnel.

Laboratory Procedure Manual

Written procedures should follow CLSI protocol and should be updated regularly.

Proper Procedures for Specimen Collection and Storage

Strict adherence to correct procedures for specimen collection and storage is critical to the accuracy of any test. Preanalytical errors are the most common source of laboratory errors. For example, identification errors, either of the patient or of the specimen, are major potential sources of error. The use of computerized barcode identification of specimens is an asset to specimen identification. Correct storage of specimens is critical to obtaining accurate results. Some analyses require that specimens be refrigerated or frozen immediately or kept out of direct light.

Preventive Maintenance of Equipment

Equipment such as microscopes, centrifuges, and spectrophotometers should be cleaned and checked for accuracy on a regular schedule. A preventive maintenance schedule should be followed for all pieces of automated equipment (e.g., cell-counting instruments). Failure to monitor equipment regularly can produce inaccurate test results and lead to expensive repairs.

Appropriate Methodology

When new methods are introduced, it is important to check the procedure for accuracy and variability. Replicate analyses using control specimens are recommended to check for accuracy and to eliminate factors such as day-to-day variability, reagent variability, and differences between technologists.

Established Quality Control and Quality Assessment Techniques

Quality control oversees each procedure for an established protocol to ensure the quality of the results. Usually, normal and abnormal control samples are analyzed at the same time patient specimens are analyzed. Quality assessment is much broader in overseeing the quality of results. Quality assessment includes laboratory personnel, procedure manuals, and many other facets of the operating laboratory.

Accuracy in Reporting Results

Many laboratories have established **critical values** and the **Delta check system** to monitor individual patient results.

Appropriate communication is critical to high-quality patient care. In most situations, laboratory reports are recorded and sent to the appropriate patient area rather than conveyed by telephone; the risk of error is too great when depending on verbal reports alone. In emergency ("stat") situations, verbal reports may be necessary but must be followed by written reports as soon as possible. It is equally important in reporting results to be on the alert for clerical errors, particularly transcription errors. The introduction of computer-interfaced, online reporting is useful in communicating information correctly and efficiently (see Chapters 9 and 10).

Other Factors in Quality Assessment

It is important to understand basic statistical concepts used in quality control. Knowledge of specific elements of statistics is important for the following two reasons:

1. Application of statistical analysis of results in quality assessment protocols
2. Instrumental applications of statistics to measurements

Terms Used in Clinical Quality Assessment

The following terms are used to describe different aspects of quality assessment:

1. **Accuracy** describes how close a test result is to the true value. Reference samples and standards with known values are needed to check accuracy.
2. **Calibration** is the comparison of an instrument measurement or reading to a known physical constant.
3. **Control** (noun) represents a specimen that is similar in composition to the patient's whole blood or plasma. The value of a control specimen is known. Control specimens are

tested in exactly the same way as the patient specimen and are tested daily or in conjunction with the unknown (patient) specimen. Controls are the best measurements of precision and may represent normal or abnormal test values.

4. **Precision** describes how close the test results are to one another when repeated analyses of the same material are performed. Precision refers to the reproducibility of test results. It is important to make a distinction between precision and accuracy. The term *accuracy* implies freedom from error; the term *precision* implies freedom from variation.

5. **Standards** are highly purified substances of a known composition. A standard may differ from a control in its overall composition and in the way it is handled in the test. Standards are the best way to measure accuracy. Standards are used to establish reference points in the construction of graphs (e.g., manual hemoglobin curve) or to calculate a test result.

6. **Quality control** is a process that monitors the accuracy and reproducibility of results through the use of control specimens.

Functions of a Quantitative Quality Control Program

Assaying control specimens and standards along with patient specimens serves several major functions:

1. Provides a guide to the functioning of equipment, reagents, and individual technique
2. Confirms the accuracy of testing when compared with reference values
3. Detects an increase in the frequency of both high and low minimally acceptable values (dispersion)
4. Detects any progressive drift of values to one side of the average value for at least 3 days (trends)
5. Demonstrates an abrupt shift or change from the established average value for 3 days in a row (shift)

Proficiency Testing

According to CLIA '88, a laboratory must establish and follow written quality control procedures for monitoring and evaluating the quality of the analytical testing process of each method to ensure the accuracy and reliability of patient test results and reports. Proficiency testing (PT) is a means by which quality control between laboratories is maintained. Provisions of CLIA '88 require enrollment in an external PT program for laboratories performing moderately complex or highly complex tests. Only the waived tests under CLIA '88 are exempt from PT regulations. The PT program being used must be approved by CLIA. PT programs are available through CAP, CDC, and the health departments in some states.

Laboratories enrolled in a particular PT program test samples for specific analytes and send the results to be tabulated by the program managers. Results of the assays are graded for each participating laboratory according to designated evaluation limits, and the results are compared with those of other laboratories participating in the same PT program.

If a laboratory performs only waived tests, it is not required to participate in a PT program. However, it must apply for and be given a certificate of waiver from HHS. If a laboratory performs moderate-complexity or high-complexity tests for which no PT is available, it must have a system for verifying the accuracy and reliability of its test results at least twice a year.

ISO STANDARDS IN CLINICAL LABORATORIES

The College of American Pathologists, the second largest laboratory accrediting organization, recently adopted an optional accreditation program based on the International Organization for Standardization (ISO) 15189 standards for medical laboratories.[7] The ISO 15189 standards, designed specifically for medical laboratories, covers 15 management requirements and 8 technical requirements that are aimed at areas such as technical competency. The basic benefit to using ISO 15189 is the use of a comprehensive and highly structured approach for quality management that allows labs to use tools such as Lean or Six Sigma systems (see Chapter 8). The process used actual assessment by certified assessors who make people understand what the expectation is and what the intent is of the standard.

In the 15189 accreditation program, one of the most important steps is the gap analysis that takes place after a lab has purchased the 15189 document from ISO and conducted a preliminary internal audit of its processes. In the gap analysis, assessors look carefully at where the lab does not meet the ISO standard. This analysis reveals what facets of day-to-day lab operations warrant improvement. A preassessment from CAP may take place. Once a lab passes the final accreditation assessment, a 3-year cycle begins. During this period, two surveillance assessments are scheduled, and an onsite reaccreditation is required.

One caution about using 15189 is that it is considered to be too general, and in some cases, not as stringent or specific as CLIA regulations. Hence, ISO standards are not acceptable to the U.S. government.

MEDICAL-LEGAL ISSUES

Informed Consent

For laboratories, an important responsibility is obtaining informed consent from the patient. **Informed consent** means that the patient is aware of, understands, and agrees to the nature of the testing to be done and what will be done with the results reported. Generally, when a patient enters a hospital, there is an implied consent to the many routine procedures that will be performed while the patient is in the hospital. Venipuncture is one of the routine tests that carries this implied consent. The patient must sign specific consent forms for more complex procedures, such as bone marrow aspiration, lumbar puncture for collection of CSF, and fine-needle biopsy, as well as for nonurgent transfusion of blood or its components.

The patient should be given sufficient information about the reasons why the informed consent is needed and must be given the opportunity to ask questions. In the event the patient is incapable of signing the consent form, a guardian should be obtained—for example, when the patient is a minor, legally not competent, physically unable to write, hearing impaired, or does not speak English as the first language. Health care institutions have policies in place for handling these situations.

Confidentiality

Any results obtained for specimens from patients must be kept strictly confidential. The **Health Insurance Portability and Accountability Act (HIPAA)** enacted in 1996 requires the privacy of patient information (see Chapter 10). Any information about the patient, including the types of measurements being done, must also be kept in confidence. Only authorized persons should have access to the information about a patient, and any release of this information to non–health care persons (e.g., insurance personnel, lawyers, friends of the patient) can be done only when authorized by the patient. It is important to speak about a particular patient's situation only in the confines of the laboratory setting and not in any public place such as elevators or hospital coffee shops.

Chain of Custody

Laboratory test results that could potentially be used in a court of law, such as at a trial or judicial hearing, must be handled in a specific manner. For evidence to be admissible, each step of the analysis, beginning with the moment the specimen is collected and transported to the laboratory, to the analysis itself and the reporting of the results, must be documented; this process is known as maintaining the **chain of custody.** The links between specimen collection and presentation in court must establish certainty that the material or specimen tested had not been altered in any way that would change its usefulness as admissible evidence. Any specimen that has potential evidentiary value should be labeled, sealed, and placed in a locked refrigerator or other suitable secure storage area. Specimens that provide alcohol levels, specimens collected from rape victims, specimens for paternity testing, and specimens submitted from the medical examiner's cases are the usual types requiring chain-of-custody documentation.

Other Legal Considerations

Health care organizations and their employees are obliged to provide an acceptable *standard of care*, which is defined as the degree of care a reasonable person would take to prevent an injury to another. When a hospital, other health care provider, physician, or other medical professional does not treat a patient with the proper quality of care, and this results in serious patient injury or death, the provider has committed medical negligence. As a result, perceived negligence may result in legal action or a lawsuit or tort. A *tort* is an act that injures someone in some way and for which the injured person may sue the "wrongdoer" for damages. Legally, torts are called *civil wrongs*. Medical personnel working directly with patients (e.g., phlebotomists) are more likely than laboratory bench staff to encounter legal issues.

THE NEWEST DIRECTIONS FOR LABORATORY TESTING

Genetics was in its infancy in the 1850s with the publication of Darwin's *On the Origin of Species* and Mendel's experiments of inheritance factors in pea plants. A milestone in genetics cam in 1994 when the FDA approved FlavrSavr tomato, the first genetically engineered food to go on the market. Now, in the 21st century, molecular diagnosis is the hottest topic in the clinical laboratory.

The release of a complete mapping of the human genome in 2003 created an explosion of new testing. The Human Genome Project transformed biological science, changed the future of genetic research, and opened new doorways into the diagnosis and treatment of disease. The finished sequence covers 99% of the genome and is accurate to 99.99%.

For health care and information-solution providers, four major areas of development in the expansive field of molecular diagnostics currently exist:

1. Cytogenetics
2. Flow cytometry
3. Molecular
4. Human leukocyte antigens (HLA) (immunogenetics)

Cytogenetics

Cytogenetics, the study of all aspects of cytology including the structure of chromosomal material, involves a broad and in-depth analysis of hereditary information derived from chromosomal materials. In cancer screening and screening related to congenital abnormalities, cytogenetics has proven beneficial to both clinicians and laboratory scientists in isolating the causes of the disease and providing a starting point from which a solution is reached.

Flow Cytometry

Flow cytometry (see Chapter 12) is a technique for counting, examining, and sorting microscopic particles suspended in a stream of fluid. This unique form of genetic research utilizes concentrated light to determine the size, number, sort, and other relevant data pertaining to particulate matter suspended in fluid media. Owing to its utility and the valuable information it generates, scientists rely significantly on the information provided through this method of analysis, particularly in diagnosis of leukemias.

Molecular Genetics

The field of human **molecular genomics** is evolving literally, but the technology needed to analyze and understand the vast volume of information generated in this field is continually evolving as well. Information solutions for molecular genetics research can provide real-time information management for applications such as gene therapy, genetic screening, stem cell research, cloning, and cell culture.

Human Leukocyte Antigens/ Immunogenetics

The *human leukocyte antigen* (HLA) system is the name of the human major histocompatibility complex (MHC), a group of genes that resides on chromosome 6 and encodes cell-surface antigen-presenting proteins and many other genes. The major HLA antigens are essential elements in immune function and also have a role in disease defense, reproduction, cancer, and human disease. Histocompatibility and immunogenetics have evolved in the past 20 years to address the role of MHC genes in organ, bone marrow, and stem cell transplantation, as well as disease association to the wider realm of the central role HLA molecules play in immunologic responsiveness.[8]

The fundamentals of clinical laboratory practice have expanded in recent years to incorporate massive amounts of data related to recent revolutionary discoveries in molecular genomics. Chapter 10, Laboratory Information Systems and Automation, will address how the modern lab manages all this additional data.

REFERENCES

1. U.S. Department of Labor, Bureau of Labor Statistics: Clinical laboratory technologists and technicians. Occupational outlook handbook, 2010-11 edition (website) www.bls.gov/oco/ocos096.htm. Accessed July 1, 2010.
2. Delwiche FA: Mapping the literature of clinical laboratory science, J Med Libr Assoc 91(3):303–310, 2003 July.
3. American Society of Clinical Pathologists: www.ascp.org. Accessed August 18, 2009.
4. Health Care Financing Administration, Department of Health and Human Services: Clinical Laboratory Improvement Amendments of 1988, Fed Regist, Feb 28, 1992(CLIA '88; Final Rule. 42 CFR. Subpart K, 493.1201).
5. Health Care Financing Administration, Department of Health and Human Services: Clinical Laboratory Improvement Amendments of 1988, Fed Regist, April 24, 1995: (Final rules with comment).
6. Health Care Financing Administration, Department of Health and Human Services: Clinical Laboratory Improvement Amendments of 1988, Fed Regist Sept 15, 1995: (Proposed rules).
7. College of American Pathologists: ISO 15189. www.cap.org. Retrieved August 18, 2009.
8. Hakim G: What is on the molecular diagnostics horizon? Part 5b—a brief history of medical diagnosis and the birth of the clinical laboratory, MLO Med Lab Obs vol. 40, no. 3, March 2008.

BIBLIOGRAPHY

Berger D: "Medicare, government regulation, and competency certification: a brief history of medical diagnosis and the birth of the clinical laboratory, part 3." MLO Med Lab Obs FindArticles.com , 12 Feb, 2009.

Clinical and Laboratory Standards Institute (CLSI): Laboratory design: approved guideline, Wayne, PA, 1998, GP18-A.

Clinical and Laboratory Standards Institute (CLSI) National Committee for Clinical Laboratory Standards: Clinical laboratory technical procedure manuals: approved guideline, ed 4, Wayne, PA, 2006, GP2–A5.

Clinical and Laboratory Standards Institute (CLSI) National Committee for Clinical Laboratory Standards: CLIA specialty collection (a collection of documents), Wayne, PA, 1999-2004, SC11-L.

Clinical and Laboratory Standards Institute (CLSI) National Committee for Clinical Laboratory Standards: Continuous quality improvement: essential management approaches and their use in proficiency testing: proposed guideline, ed 2, Wayne, PA, 2004, GP22–A2.

Clinical and Laboratory Standards Institute (CLSI) National Committee for Clinical Laboratory Standards: Point-of-care testing (a collection of guidelines), Wayne, PA, 2001-2004, SC17-L.

Clinical and Laboratory Standards Institute (CLSI) National Committee for Clinical Laboratory Standards: Training and competence assessment, ed 2, Wayne, PA, 2004, GP21–A2.

Kaplan LA, Pesce AJ: Clinical chemistry: theory, analysis, and correlation, ed 5, St Louis, 2010, Mosby.

Malone B: ISO Accreditation Comes to America, Clin Lab News Vol 35, No. 1:3–4, Jan 2009:1.

Turgeon ML: Immunology and serology in laboratory medicine, ed 4, St Louis, 2009, Mosby.

RELATED WEBSITES

http://www.cola.org/newcriteria.html
http://www.jointcommission.org/accreditationprograms/laboratoryservices/lab_facts.htm

REVIEW QUESTIONS

1. Which of the following acts, agencies, or organizations was created to make certain the quality of work done in the laboratory is reliable?
   a. Centers for Medicare and Medicaid Services (CMS)
   b. Occupational Safety and Health Administration (OSHA)
   c. Clinical Laboratory Improvement Amendments of 1988 (CLIA '88)
   d. Centers for Disease Control and Prevention (CDC)

Questions 2-6: Match each of the following agencies or organizations with the best description of its purpose pertaining to the clinical laboratory (a to e).

2. ___ Centers for Medicare and Medicaid Services (CMS)

3. ___ The Joint Commission (TJC)

4. ___ College of American Pathologists (CAP)

5. ___ Commission on Office Laboratory Accreditation (COLA)

6. ___ CLSI
   a. Sets accreditation requirements for physician office laboratories (POLs)
   b. Administers both the CLIA '88 and Medicare programs
   c. CMS has given it deemed status to act on the government's behalf to certify clinical laboratories.
   d. Nonprofit educational group that establishes consensus standards for maintaining a high-quality laboratory organization
   e. Accredits health care facilities and sets standards for quality assessment programs in those facilities

7. Laboratories performing which of the following types of tests need to be enrolled in a CLIA-approved proficiency testing program?
   a. Waived
   b. Moderately complex
   c. Highly complex
   d. Both b and c

Questions 8-11: Match the following terms with the best descriptive statement (a to d).

8. ___ Proficiency testing (PT)

9. ___ Quality assessment (QA)

10. ___ Provider-performed microscopy (PPM)

11. ___ Point-of-care testing (POCT)
    a. Continuing process of evaluating and monitoring all aspects of the laboratory to ensure accuracy of test results
    b. Specific microscopic tests (wet mounts) performed by a physician for his or her own patients
    c. Means by which quality control between laboratories is maintained
    d. Process of performing laboratory testing at the bedside of the patient; a means of decentralizing some of the laboratory testing

12. Which of the following is an analytical factor in a quality assessment system?
    a. Qualified personnel and established laboratory policies
    b. Monitoring the standard deviation and reporting results of normal and abnormal controls
    c. Maintaining a procedure manual and use of appropriate methodology
    d. Preventive maintenance of equipment and correct specimen collection

13. In which of the following laboratory situations is a verbal report permissible?
    a. When the patient is going directly to the physician's office and wants to have the report available
    b. When the report cannot be found at the nurse's station
    c. When preoperative test results are needed by the anesthesiologist
    d. None of the above

Questions 14-16: Match the following terms with the best description (a to d).

14. ___ Accuracy

15. ___ Calibration

16. ___ Control
    a. Value is known
    b. Closeness to the true value
    c. Process of monitoring accuracy
    d. Comparison to a known physical constant

Questions 17-19: Match the following terms with the best description (a to d).

17. ___ Precision

18. ___ Standards

19. ___ Quality control
    a. How close test results are when repeated
    b. Purified substance of a known composition
    c. Process of monitoring accuracy and reproducibility of known control results
    d. Value is unknown

CHAPTER 2

SAFETY IN THE CLINICAL LABORATORY

Learning Objectives

At the conclusion of this chapter, the student will be able to:

- Define the acronyms of various governmental and professional agencies.

- Describe the purpose of the National Health care Safety Network.

- Explain the purpose of the Americans with Disabilities Act and Amendments of 2008.

- Explain the general safety regulations governing the clinical laboratory, including components of the OSHA-mandated plans for chemical hygiene and for occupational exposure to bloodborne pathogens, the importance of the safety manual, and general emergency procedures.

- Describe the basic aspects of infection control policies, including how and when to use personal protective equipment or devices (e.g., gowns, gloves, goggles) and the reasons for using Standard Precautions.

- Compare and contrast how to take the necessary precautions to avoid exposure to the many potentially hazardous situations in the clinical laboratory: biohazards; chemical, fire, and electrical hazards; and certain supplies and equipment (e.g., broken glassware).

- Explain successful implementation of chemical hazards "right-to-know" rules.

Continued

The importance of safety and correct first-aid procedures cannot be overemphasized. Many accidents do not just happen; they are caused by carelessness, lack of attention to detail, or lack of proper communication. For this reason, the practice of safety should be uppermost in the mind of all persons working in a clinical laboratory. Most laboratory accidents are preventable by exercising good technique, staying alert, and using common sense.

SAFETY STANDARDS AND GOVERNING AGENCIES

Safety standards for patients and/or clinical laboratories are initiated, governed, and reviewed by several agencies or committees:

1. U.S. Department of Labor's Occupational Safety and Health Administration (OSHA)
2. Clinical and Laboratory Standards Institute (CLSI)
3. Centers for Disease Control and Prevention (CDC), part of the U.S. Department of Health and Human Services (DHHS), Public Health Service
4. College of American Pathologists (CAP)
5. The Joint Commission (formerly The Joint Commission on Accreditation of Health care Organizations).[1-5] The Commission has established National Patient Safety Goals. One of the goals of particular interest to laboratorians addresses the issue of critical laboratory assay values. Urgent clinician notification of critical results is the responsibility of the laboratory (Box 2-1).

Americans With Disabilities Amendments Act of 2008

In 1990, Congress enacted the Americans with Disabilities Act (ADA) to provide a clear and comprehensive national mandate for eliminating discrimination against individuals with disabilities.

BOX 2-1
National Patient Safety Goals

Goal 02.03.01

1. Organizations are required to measure, assess, and if needed, take action to improve the timeliness of reporting and receipt of critical tests and critical results* or values by the responsible licensed caregiver, e.g., laboratory.
2. Once critical tests and critical results or values are identified, the organization determines how the tests, results, or values will be processed.
3. The organization determines the acceptable length of time from ordering to reporting of critical tests, results, or values and the acceptable length of time between availability of critical tests, results, or values and receipt by the responsible caregiver.
4. When the responsible caregiver is not available, a back-up reporting system is required to provide the results in a timely manner to another qualified caregiver to prevent avoidable delays in treatment or decision-making response.
5. The organization collects, aggregates, and analyzes data on the critical test, result, or value process. If needed, action to improve timeliness of report and/or the timeliness of receipt of critical results must be taken.

Retrieved from www.jointcommission.org. Accessed September 11, 2009.
*Critical results or critical limits define the high and low boundaries of the life-threatening values of laboratory test results.
Copyright The Joint Commission, 2010. Reprinted with permission.

The ADA prohibits discrimination on the basis of disability in several different areas, including employment.

The term *disability* means, with respect to an individual:

- A physical or mental impairment that substantially limits one or more major life activities of such individual
- A record of such an impairment
- Being regarded as having such an impairment[6]

The ADA Amendments Act of 2008 (ADAAA) does not change the working definition of a disability but effectively expands the scope of the original law. The new ADAAA has its greatest impact in the employment context, requiring employers with 15 or more employees covered by the ADA to adjust their policies and procedures to comply with the ADAAA.

National Health care Safety Network

In 2006, the CDC introduced the new National Health care Safety Network (NHSN). This new voluntary system integrates a number of surveillance systems and provides data on devices, patients, and staff. The NHSN expands legacy patient and health care personnel safety surveillance systems managed by the Division of Health care Quality Promotion (DHQP) at CDC. NHSN also includes a new component for hospitals to monitor adverse reactions and incidents associated with receipt of blood and blood products. Enrollment is open to all types of health care facilities in the United States.

The National Nosocomial Infections Surveillance (NNIS) System of the CDC performed a survey from October 1986 to April 1998. The highest rates of infection occurred in the burn intensive care unit (ICU), the neonatal ICU, and the pediatric ICU. Within hours of admission, colonies of hospital strains of bacteria develop in the patient's skin, respiratory tract, and genitourinary tract. Risk factors for the invasion of colonizing pathogens can be categorized into three areas: iatrogenic, organizational, and patient related.

- Iatrogenic risk factors include pathogens on the hands of medical personnel, invasive procedures (e.g., intubation and extended ventilation, indwelling vascular lines, urine catheterization), and antibiotic use and prophylaxis.
- Organizational risk factors include contaminated air-conditioning systems, contaminated water systems, and staffing and physical layout of the facility (e.g., nurse-to-patient ratio, open beds close together).
- Patient risk factors include the severity of illness, underlying immunocompromised state, and length of stay.

Nosocomial infections are estimated to occur in 5% of all acute-care hospitalizations. In the United States, the incidence of hospital acquired infection (HAI) is more than 2 million cases per year. Nosocomial infections are caused by viral, bacterial, and fungal pathogens. In pediatric patient units surveyed between 1992 and 1997, the incidence of nosocomial invasive bacterial and fungal infections was highest in bloodstream infections, with coagulase-negative staphylococci found in the majority of cases. Infections caused by methicillin-resistant *Staphylococcus aureus* (MRSA) are not worse than those caused by susceptible *S. aureus*. MRSA requires treatment with different families of antibiotics. Although the pathogenicity does not generally differ from that of susceptible strains of *S. aureus*, MRSA strains that carry the loci for Panton-Valentine leukocidin can be hypervirulent and can cause lymphopenia, rapid tissue necrosis, and severe sepsis.

Many hospitals have reorganized the physical layout of handwashing stations (see Handwashing) and have adopted patient cohorting to prevent the spread of pathogens. They have also restricted or rotated the administration of many antibiotics that are used to combat nosocomial infections. A special concern in regard to bacterial agents is that multiple-resistant organisms, such as vancomycin-resistant enterococci, glycopeptide-resistant *S. aureus*, and inducible or extended-spectrum beta-lactamase gram-negative organisms, are a constant threat.[7]

Occupational Safety and Health Administration Acts and Standards

To ensure that workers have safe and healthful working conditions, the U.S. Federal government created a system of safeguards and regulations under the **Occupational Safety and Health Act of 1970**, and in 1988 expanded the **Hazard Communication Standard** to apply to hospital staff.[8] Occupational Safety and Health Act regulations apply to all businesses with one or more employees and are administered by the U.S. Department of Labor through OSHA. The programs deal with many aspects of safety and health protection, including compliance arrangements, inspection procedures, penalties for noncompliance, complaint procedures, duties and responsibilities for administration and operation of the system, and how the many standards are set. Responsibility for compliance is placed on both the administration of the institution and the employee.

The **OSHA standards**, where appropriate, include provisions for warning labels or other appropriate forms of warning to alert all workers to potential hazards, suitable protective equipment, exposure control procedures, and implementation of training and education programs. The primary purpose of OSHA standards is to ensure safe and healthful working conditions for every American worker.

OSHA and the CDC have published numerous safety standards and regulations that are applicable to clinical laboratories (e.g., 1988 OSHA Hazard

TABLE 2-1

Recommended Safety Training Schedule		
Topic	Who Needs to Be Trained	Frequency
All laboratory safety policies and procedures	All laboratory staff	Upon employment
Fire extinguisher practice	All laboratory staff	Upon employment
Spill cleanup	All technical staff	Upon employment
Fire prevention and preparedness	All laboratory staff	Annually
Fire drill evacuation	All laboratory staff	Annually
Chemical safety	All staff who handle or transport chemicals	Annually
Biological hazard	All laboratory staff	Annually
Infection control	All laboratory staff	Annually
Radiation safety	Only employees who use or transport radioactive materials	Annually
Specimen packaging and shipping procedures	Staff who package specimens for shipping by ground or air	Every 24 months

From Gile TJ: Complete guide to laboratory safety, Marblehead, MA, 2004, HCPro.

Communication Standard). Ensuring safety in the clinical laboratory includes the following measures:

- A formal safety program
- Specifically mandated plans (e.g., chemical hygiene, bloodborne pathogens)
- Identification of various hazards (e.g., fire, electrical, chemical, biological)

Safety Officer

A designated safety officer is a critical part of a laboratory safety program. This individual is responsible for initial orientation of staff and the periodic updating of staff (Table 2-1). In addition, the safety officer is responsible for compliance with existing regulations affecting the laboratory and staff, such as labeling of chemicals and providing supplies for the proper handling and disposal of biohazardous materials.

OSHA-Mandated Plans

In 1991, OSHA mandated that all clinical laboratories must implement a chemical hygiene plan and an exposure control plan. As part of the chemical hygiene plan, a copy of the material safety data sheet must be on file and readily accessible and available to all employees at all times.

Chemical Hygiene Plan

A chemical hygiene plan (CHP) is the core of the OSHA safety standard. Existing safety and health plans may meet the CHP requirements. A written

CHP is to be developed by each employer and must specify the following:

- The training and information requirements of the OSHA standard
- Designation of a chemical hygiene officer and committee
- Appropriate work practices
- A list of chemicals in inventory
- Availability of material safety data sheets
- Labeling requirements
- Record-keeping requirements
- Standard operating procedures and housekeeping requirements
- Methods of required engineering controls (e.g., eyewashes, safety showers)
- Measures for appropriate maintenance and list of protective equipment
- Requirements for employee medical examinations
- Special precautions for working with particularly hazardous substances
- Information on waste removal and disposal
- Other information deemed necessary for safety assurance

MATERIAL SAFETY DATA SHEETS

The 1991 CHP is designed to ensure that laboratory workers are fully aware of the hazards associated with chemicals in their workplaces. This information is provided in the **material safety data sheet (MSDS)** (see Fig. 4-9), which describes hazards, safe handling, storage, and disposal of hazardous chemicals. The information is provided by chemical manufacturers and suppliers about each chemical and accompanies the shipment of each chemical.

Each MSDS contains basic information about the specific chemical or product, including trade name, chemical name and synonyms, chemical family, manufacturer's name and address, emergency telephone number for further information about the chemical, hazardous ingredients, physical data, fire and explosion data, and health hazard and protection information. The MSDS describes the effects of overexposure or exceeding the threshold limit value of allowable exposure for an individual employee in an 8-hour day. The MSDS also describes protective personal clothing and equipment requirements, first-aid practices, spill information, and disposal procedures.

"RIGHT-TO-KNOW" LAWS

Legislation on chemical hazard precautions, such as state **"right-to-know" laws**, and OSHA document 29 CFR 1910 set the standards for chemical hazard communication (HAZCOM) and determine the types of documents that must be on file in a laboratory. For example, a yearly physical inventory of all hazardous chemicals must be performed, and MSDSs should be made available in each department for use. Each institution should also have at least one centralized area where all MSDSs are stored.

LABELING

Labeling may be the simplest and most important step in the proper handling of any hazardous substance. A label for a container should include a date and the contents of the container. When the contents of one container are transferred to another container, this information should also be transferred to the new container. OSHA recommends that all chemically hazardous material be properly labeled with the hazardous contents and severity of the material, as well as bear a hazard symbol. A substance can be classified as hazardous by the Department of Transportation (DOT), the Environmental Protection Agency (EPA), or the National Fire Protection Association (NFPA). The labels of chemicals in the original containers must not be removed or altered.

For chemicals not in the original container, the labeling information for all substances with a rating of 2 or greater according to the hazards identification system developed by NFPA (the scale is 0 to 4, with 4 being the most severe risk) must include the following:

- Identity of the hazardous chemical
- Route of body entry (eyes, nose, mouth, skin)
- Health hazard
- Physical hazard
- Target organ affected

The hazards identification system consists of four small, diamond-shaped symbols grouped into

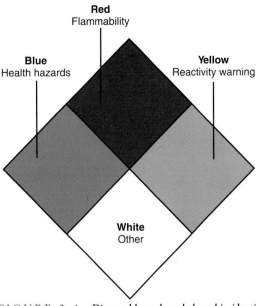

FIGURE 2-1 Diamond hazard symbol used in identification system of National Fire Protection Association.

a larger diamond shape (Fig. 2-1 and Box 2-2; also see Chemical Hazards).

THRESHOLD LIMITS

Many toxic chemicals now have limits that must be met within the laboratory, specifically threshold limit values (TLVs) and permissible exposure limits (PELs). TLVs are the maximum safe exposure limits as set down by the federal government. OSHA sets PELs to protect workers against the health effects of exposure to hazardous substances. PELs are regulatory limits on the amount or concentration of a substance in the air. PELs may also contain a skin designation. OSHA PELs are based on an 8-hour time-weighted average (TWA) exposure.[9]

Exposure Control Plan

The OSHA-mandated program, **Occupational Exposure to Bloodborne Pathogens**, became law in March 1992.[1] This regulation requires that laboratories:

- Develop, implement, and comply with a plan that ensures the protective safety of laboratory staff to potential infectious bloodborne pathogens.
- Manage and handle medical waste in a safe and effective manner.

Government regulations require that all employees who handle hazardous material and waste must be trained to use and handle these materials. Chemical hazard education sessions must be presented to new employees and conducted annually for all employees. Each laboratory is required to evaluate

BOX 2-2
Hazards Identification System: Diamond-Shaped Symbols

Position	Color	Indication
Left	Blue	Health hazard
Top	Red	Flammability
Right	Yellow	Reactivity-stability hazard*
Bottom	White	Special hazard information

Within each section, a number ranks the degree of hazard:
- 4: extreme hazard
- 3: serious hazard
- 2: moderate hazard
- 1: slight hazard
- 0: no or minimal hazard

The white section alerts the user to special hazards the material may possess, such as:
- Water reactivity
- Strong oxidizer
- Corrosivity
- Radioactivity

*Used for substances that are capable of explosion or violent chemical change.

BOX 2-3
Categories and Characteristics of Bioterrorism Agents

Category A

Pathogens that are rarely seen in the United States. These agents have the highest priority; organisms in this category pose a risk to national security because they:
- Can be easily disseminated or transmitted from person to person
- Result in high mortality rates and have the potential for major public health impact
- Might cause public panic and social disruption
- Require special action for public health preparedness

Category B

These agents have the second-highest priority and include pathogens that:
- Are moderately easy to disseminate
- Result in moderate morbidity rates and low mortality rates
- Require specific enhancements of the CDC's diagnostic capacity and enhanced disease surveillance

Category C

These agents have the third-highest priority and include emerging pathogens that could be engineered for mass dissemination in the future because of:
- Availability
- Ease of production and dissemination
- Potential for high morbidity and mortality rates and major health impact

Modified from Centers for Disease Control and Prevention: Bioterrorism agents/diseases (website). http://www.bt.cdc.gov/agent/agentlist-category.asp. Accessed February 2005.

the effectiveness of its plan at least annually and to update it as necessary. The written plan must be available to employees. A laboratory's written plan must include the purpose and scope of the plan, references, definitions of terms and responsibilities, and detailed procedural steps to follow.

The CDC also recommends safety precautions concerning the handling of all patient specimens, known as **Standard Precautions** (formerly "universal precautions" or "universal blood and body fluid precautions"). CLSI has also issued guidelines for the laboratory worker in regard to protection from bloodborne diseases spread through contact with patient specimens.[3] In addition, the CDC provides recommendations for treatment after occupational exposure to potentially infectious material. These agencies are working to reduce the risk of exposure of health care workers to bloodborne pathogens.

BIOHAZARDS

Because many hazards in the clinical laboratory are unique, a special term, **biohazard**, was devised. This word is posted throughout the laboratory to denote infectious materials or agents that present a risk or even a potential risk to the health of humans or animals in the laboratory. The potential risk can be either through direct infection or through the environment. Infection can occur during the process of specimen collection or from handling, transporting, or testing the specimen. Safe collection and transportation of specimens to the

laboratory must take priority in any discussion of safety in the laboratory (see Chapter 3).

Bioterrorism agents are a concern to laboratories. These agents are divided into categories A, B, and C (Box 2-3 and Table 2-2). The OSHA categories of risk classifications are now obsolete, but the Public Health Service (PHS) Biosafety Levels 1, 2, and 3 are used to describe the relative risk that may be encountered in a work area. Biosafety Level 1 is the least threatening.

Infections are frequently caused by accidental aspiration of infectious material, accidental inoculation with contaminated needles or syringes, animal bites, sprays from syringes, aerosols from the uncapping of specimen tubes, and centrifuge accidents. Other sources of laboratory infections are cuts or scratches from contaminated glassware, cuts from instruments used during animal surgery or autopsy, and spilling or spattering of pathogenic

TABLE 2-2

Examples of Bioterrorism Agents and Diseases	
Agent	Disease
Category A	
Anthrax	*Bacillus anthracis*
Botulism	*Clostridium botulinum* toxin
Plague	*Yersinia pestis*
Smallpox	*Variola major*
Tularemia	*Francisella tularensis*
Viral Hemorrhagic Fevers	
Filoviruses	Ebola, Marburg
Arenaviruses	Lassa, Machupo
Category B	
Brucellosis	*Brucella* species
Epsilon toxin	*Clostridium perfringens*
Food contaminants	*Salmonella* species, *Escherichia coli* O157:H7, *Shigella*
Glanders	*Pseudomonas (Burkholderia) mallei*
Melioidosis	*Pseudomonas (Burkholderia) pseudomallei*
Psittacosis	*Chlamydia psittaci*
Q fever	*Coxiella burnetii*
Ricin toxin	*Ricinus communis* (castor beans)
Staphylococcal Enterotoxin B	
Typhus fever	*Rickettsia prowazekii*
Viral encephalitis	Alphaviruses, e.g., Venezuelan equine encephalitis Eastern equine encephalitis, Western equine encephalitis
Water safety threats	*Vibrio cholerae, Cryptosporidium parvum*

Modified from Centers for Disease Control and Prevention: Bioterrorism agents/diseases (website). http://www.bt.cdc.gov/agent/agentlist-category.asp. Retrieved February 2005.

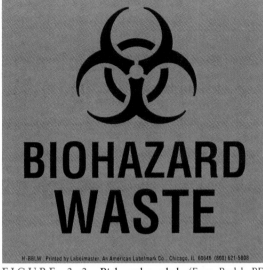

FIGURE 2-2 **Biohazard symbol.** (From Rodak BF, Fritsma GA, Keohane EM: Hematology: clinical principles and applications, ed 4, St Louis, 2012, Saunders.)

of patients identified with **human immunodeficiency virus (HIV)** was partially responsible for a change in the initial recommendations issued by the CDC. More specific regulations in regard to the handling of blood and body fluids from patients suspected or known to be infected with a bloodborne pathogen were originally issued in 1983.

Current safety guidelines for the control of infectious disease are based on the original CDC 1987 recommendations[10] and 1988 clarifications.[4] Safety practices were further clarified by OSHA[1] in 1991 and DHHS[9] in 1992.

The purpose of the standards for bloodborne pathogens and occupational exposure is to provide a safe work environment. OSHA mandates that an employer:

1. Educate and train all health care workers in Standard Precautions and preventing bloodborne infections.
2. Provide proper equipment and supplies (e.g., gloves).
3. Monitor compliance with the protective biosafety policies.

HIV has been isolated from blood, semen, vaginal secretions, saliva, tears, breast milk, cerebrospinal fluid (CSF), amniotic fluid, and urine, but only blood, semen, vaginal secretions, and breast milk have been implicated in transmission of HIV to date. Evidence for the role of saliva in transmission of the virus is unclear; however, Standard Precautions do not apply to saliva uncontaminated with blood.

The latest statistics on acquired immunodeficiency syndrome (AIDS) and HIV in the United States were published in February 2009 by the

samples on the work desks or floors. Persons working in laboratories on animal research or other research involving biologically hazardous materials are also susceptible to the problems of biohazards. Fig. 2-2 shows the symbol used to denote the presence of biohazards.

AVOIDING TRANSMISSION OF INFECTIOUS DISEASES

Transmission of various bloodborne pathogens (e.g., hepatitis) has always been a concern for laboratory staff, but the rapid increase in the number

CDC.[11] Since the beginning of the HIV/AIDS epidemic, health care workers across the world have become infected with HIV as a result of their work. The main cause of infection in occupational settings is exposure to HIV-infected blood via a percutaneous injury (i.e., from needles, instruments, bites which break the skin, etc.). The average risk for HIV transmission after such exposure to infected blood is low—about 3 per 1000 injuries. Nevertheless, this understandably remains an area of considerable concern for many health care workers.

Certain specific factors may mean a percutaneous injury carries a higher risk, for example:

- A deep injury
- Late-stage HIV disease in the source patient
- Visible blood on the device that caused the injury
- Injury with a needle that had been placed in a source patient's artery or vein

There are a small number of instances when HIV has been acquired through contact with nonintact skin or mucous membranes (i.e., splashes of infected blood in the eye). Research suggests that the risk of HIV infection after mucous membrane exposure is less than 1 in 1000 infections. Scientists estimate that the risk of infection from a needle-stick is less than 1%, a figure based on the findings of several studies of health care workers who received punctures from HIV-contaminated needles or were otherwise exposed to HIV-contaminated blood. The CDC emphasizes that over 90% of health care workers infected with HIV also have nonoccupational risk factors for acquiring their infection.[11]

Blood is the single most-important source of HIV, **hepatitis B virus (HBV)**, and other bloodborne pathogens in the occupational setting. HBV may be stable in dried blood and blood products at 25°C for up to 7 days. HIV retains infectivity for more than 3 days in dried specimens at room temperature and for more than 1 week in an aqueous environment at room temperature.

HBV and HIV may be indirectly transmitted. Viral transmission can result from contact with inanimate objects such as work surfaces or equipment contaminated with infected blood or certain body fluids. If the virus is transferred to the skin or mucous membranes by hand contact between a contaminated surface and nonintact skin or mucous membranes, it can produce viral exposure.

Medical personnel should be aware that HBV and HIV are totally different diseases caused by completely unrelated viruses. The most feared hazard of all, the transmission of HIV through occupational exposure, is among the least likely to occur. The modes of transmission for HBV and HIV are similar, but the potential for transmission in the occupational setting is greater for HBV than HIV.

Since the late 1980s, the incidence of acute hepatitis B has declined steadily. During 1990 to 2002, the incidence of acute hepatitis B declined 67%. Although the number of cases has sharply declined since hepatitis B vaccine became available, unvaccinated health care workers can become infected with HBV following occupational exposure.

The likelihood of infection after exposure to blood infected with HBV or HIV depends on a variety of factors, including:

1. The concentration of HBV or HIV virus; viral concentration is higher for HBV than for HIV
2. The duration of the contact
3. The presence of skin lesions or abrasions on the hands or exposed skin of the health care worker
4. The immune status of the health care worker for HBV

HBV and HIV may be directly transmitted by various portals of entry. In the occupational setting, however, the following situations may lead to infection:

1. Percutaneous (parenteral) inoculation of blood, plasma, serum, or certain other body fluids from accidental needlesticks
2. Contamination of the skin with blood or certain body fluids without overt puncture, caused by scratches, abrasions, burns, weeping, or exudative skin lesions
3. Exposure of mucous membranes (oral, nasal, conjunctival) to blood or certain body fluids as the direct result of pipetting by mouth, splashes, or spattering
4. Centrifuge accidents or improper removal of rubber stoppers from test tubes, producing droplets. If these aerosol products are infectious and come in direct contact with mucous membranes or nonintact skin, direct transmission of virus can result.

The CDC estimates that more than 380,000 needlestick injuries occur in U.S. hospitals each year; approximately 61% of these injuries are caused by hollow-bore devices. An *occupational exposure* is defined as a percutaneous injury (e.g., needlestick or cut with a sharp object) or contact by mucous membranes or nonintact skin (especially when the skin is chapped, abraded, or affected with dermatitis or the contact is prolonged or involves an extensive area) with blood, tissues, blood-stained body fluids, body fluids to which Standard Precautions apply, or concentrated virus. Blood is the most frequently implicated infected body fluid in HIV and HBV exposure in the workplace.

Most exposures do not result in infection. The risk varies not only with the type of exposure but also may be influenced by other factors such as the amount of infected blood in the exposure, the length of contact with infectious material, and the amount of virus in the patient's blood, body fluid, or tissue at the time of exposure. Studies suggest that the average risk of HIV transmission is approximately 0.3% after a percutaneous exposure to HIV-infected blood and approximately 0.09% after mucous membrane exposure.[10]

SAFE WORK PRACTICES FOR INFECTION CONTROL

Standard Precautions represent an approach to infection control used to prevent occupational exposures to bloodborne pathogens. This approach eliminates the need for separate isolation procedures for patients known or suspected to be infectious. The application of Standard Precautions also eliminates the need for warning labels on specimens. According to the CDC concept of Standard Precautions, all human blood and other body fluids are treated as potentially infectious for HIV, HBV, and other bloodborne microorganisms that can cause disease in humans. The risk of nosocomial transmission of HBV, HIV, and other bloodborne pathogens can be minimized if laboratory personnel are aware of and adhere to essential safety guidelines.

Personal Protective Equipment

OSHA requires laboratories to have a **personal protective equipment (PPE)** program. The components of this regulation include:
- A workplace hazard assessment with a written hazard certification
- Proper equipment selection
- Employee information and training, with written competency certification
- Regular reassessment of work hazards

Laboratory personnel should not rely solely on devices for PPE to protect themselves against hazards. They also should apply PPE standards when using various forms of safety protection. A clear policy on institutionally required Standard Precautions is needed. For usual laboratory activities, PPE consists of gloves and a laboratory coat or gown. Other equipment, such as masks, would normally not be needed.

Standard Precautions are intended to supplement rather than replace handwashing recommendations for routine infection control. The risk of nosocomial transmission of HBV, HIV, and other bloodborne pathogens can be minimized if laboratory personnel are aware of and adhere to essential safety guidelines.

Selection and Use of Gloves

Gloves for phlebotomy and laboratory work are made of vinyl or latex. There are no reported differences in barrier effectiveness between intact latex and intact vinyl gloves. Either type is usually satisfactory for phlebotomy and as a protective barrier when performing technical procedures. Latex-free gloves should be available for personnel with sensitivity to the typical glove material.

Care must be taken to avoid indirect contamination of work surfaces or objects in the work area. Gloves should be properly removed (Fig. 2-3) or covered with an uncontaminated glove or paper towel before answering the telephone, handling laboratory equipment, or touching doorknobs.

Guidelines for the use of gloves during phlebotomy procedures are:
1. Gloves must be worn when performing fingersticks or heelsticks on infants and children.
2. Gloves must be worn when receiving phlebotomy training.
3. Gloves should be changed between each patient contact.

Facial Barrier Protection and Occlusive Bandages

Facial barrier protection should be used if there is a potential for splashing or spraying of blood or certain body fluids. Masks and facial protection should be worn if mucous membrane contact with blood or certain body fluid is anticipated. All disruptions of exposed skin should be covered with a water-impermeable occlusive bandage. This includes defects on the arms, face, and neck.

Laboratory Coats or Gowns as Barrier Protection

A color-coded, two–laboratory coat or equivalent system should be used whenever laboratory personnel are working with potentially infectious specimens. The coat worn in the laboratory must be changed or covered with an uncontaminated coat when leaving the immediate work area. If a lab coat becomes grossly contaminated with blood or body fluids, it should be changed immediately to prevent seepage through street clothes to the skin. Contaminated coats or gowns should be placed in an appropriately designated biohazard bag for laundering. Disposable plastic aprons are recommended if blood or certain body fluids might be splashed. Aprons should be discarded into a biohazard container.

> When the hand hygiene indication occurs before a contact requiring glove use, perform hand hygiene by rubbing with an alcohol-based handrub or by washing with soap and water.

I. How to don gloves:

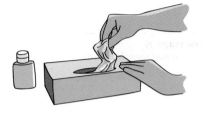

1. Take out a glove from its original box

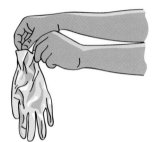

2. Touch only a restricted surface of the glove corresponding to the wrist (at the top edge of the cuff)

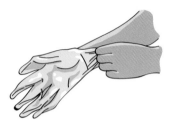

3. Don the first glove

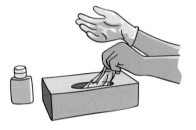

4. Take the second glove with the bare hand and touch only a restricted surface of glove corresponding to the wrist

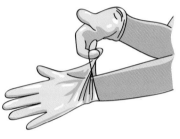

5. To avoid touching the skin of the forearm with the gloved hand, turn the external surface of the glove to be donned on the folded fingers of the gloved hand, thus permitting to glove the second hand

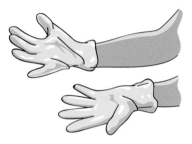

6. Once gloved, hands should not touch anything else that is not defined by indications and conditions for glove use

II. How to remove gloves:

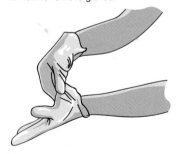

1. Pinch one glove at the wrist level to remove it, without touching the skin of the forearm, and peel away from the hand, thus allowing the glove to turn inside out

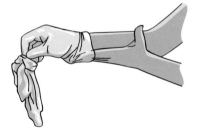

2. Hold the removed glove in the gloved hand and slide the fingers of the ungloved hand inside between the glove and the wrist. Remove the second glove by rolling it down the hand and fold into the first glove

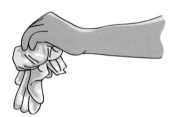

3. Discard the removed gloves

> 4. Then, perform hand hygiene by rubbing with an alcohol-based handrub or by washing with soap and water.

FIGURE 2-3 **Technique for donning and removing nonsterile examination gloves.** (From World Health Organization: Glove use information leaflet, Geneva, Switzerland, August 2009, WHO.)

Handwashing

Frequent handwashing[12] is an important safety precaution. It should be performed after contact with patients and laboratory specimens. Gloves should be used as an adjunct to, not a substitute for, handwashing. The Association for Professionals in Infection Control and Epidemiology reports extreme variability in the quality of gloves, with leakage in 4% to 63% of vinyl gloves and 3% to 52% of latex gloves.

The efficacy of handwashing in reducing transmission of microbial organisms has been demonstrated. At the very minimum, hands should be washed with soap and water (if visibly soiled) or with soap and water or by hand antisepsis with an alcohol-based handrub (if hands are not visibly soiled) in the following situations:

- After completing laboratory work and before leaving the laboratory
- After removing gloves
- Before eating, drinking, applying makeup, and changing contact lenses, and before and after using the bathroom
- Before all activities that involve hand contact with mucous membranes or breaks in the skin
- Immediately after accidental skin contact with blood, body fluids, or tissues

Two important points in the practice of hand hygiene technique are:

1. When decontaminating hands with a waterless antiseptic agent (e.g., alcohol-based hand rub), apply product to the palm of one hand and rub hands together, covering all surfaces of hands and fingers, until hands are dry.
2. When washing with a nonantimicrobial or antimicrobial soap, wet hands first with warm water, apply 3 to 5 mL of detergent to hands, and rub hands together vigorously for at least 15 seconds, covering all surfaces of the hands and fingers. Rinse hands with warm water, and dry thoroughly with a disposable towel. Use the towel to turn off the faucet.

Box 2-4 provides guidelines for handwashing and hand antisepsis in health care settings.

Decontamination of Work Surfaces, Equipment, and Spills

Disinfection[13] describes a process that eliminates many or all pathogenic microorganisms, except bacterial spores, on inanimate objects. In health care settings, objects usually are disinfected by liquid chemicals or wet pasteurization. Factors that affect the efficacy of both disinfection and sterilization include:

1. Prior cleaning of the object
2. Organic and inorganic load present

BOX 2-4

Guidelines for Handwashing and Hand Antisepsis in Health Care Settings

1. Wash hands with a nonantimicrobial soap and water or an antimicrobial soap and water when hands are visibly dirty or contaminated with proteinaceous material.
2. Use an alcohol-based waterless antiseptic agent for routine decontamination of hands if not visibly soiled.
3. Waterless antiseptic agents are highly preferable, but hand antisepsis using antimicrobial soap may be considered in certain circumstances.
4. Decontaminate hands after contact with patient's skin.
5. Decontaminate hands after contact with blood and body fluids.
6. Decontaminate hands if moving from a contaminated area to clean body site during patient care.
7. Decontaminate hands after contact with inanimate objects in the immediate vicinity of a patient.
8. Decontaminate hands after removing gloves.

Modified from Centers for Disease Control and Prevention: Guideline for Hand Hygiene in Health care Settings, MMWR Morb Mortal Wkly Rep 51(RR-16):1, 2002.

---

3. Type and level of microbial contamination
4. Concentration of and exposure time to the germicide
5. Physical nature of the object (e.g., crevices, hinges, and lumens)
6. Presence of biofilms
7. Temperature and pH of the disinfection process
8. In some cases, relative humidity of the sterilization process (e.g., ethylene oxide)

The effective use of disinfectants is part of a multibarrier strategy to prevent health care–associated infections. Surfaces are considered noncritical items because they contact intact skin. Use of noncritical items or contact with noncritical surfaces carries little risk of causing an infection in patients or staff.

Disinfecting Solutions

Hypochlorites, the most widely used of the chlorine disinfectants, are available in liquid (e.g., sodium hypochlorite) or solid (e.g., calcium hypochlorite) forms. The most prevalent chlorine products in the United States are aqueous solutions of 5.25% to 6.15% sodium hypochlorite, usually called *household bleach*. They have a broad spectrum of antimicrobial activity, do not leave toxic residues, are unaffected by water hardness, are inexpensive and fast acting, remove dried or fixed organisms and biofilms from surfaces, and have a low incidence of serious toxicity. Sodium hypochlorite at the concentration used in household bleach can produce ocular irritation or oropharyngeal, esophageal, and gastric burns. The EPA has determined the currently registered uses of hypochlorites will not result in unreasonable adverse effects to the environment.

Hypochlorites are widely used in health care facilities in a variety of settings. Inorganic chlorine solution is used for spot disinfection of countertops and floors. A 1:10 to 1:100 dilution of 5.25% to 6.15% sodium hypochlorite (i.e., household bleach) or an EPA-registered tuberculocidal disinfectant has been recommended for decontaminating blood spills. For small spills of blood (i.e., drops) on noncritical surfaces, the area can be disinfected with a 1:100 dilution of 5.25% to 6.15% sodium hypochlorite or an EPA-registered tuberculocidal disinfectant. Because hypochlorites and other germicides are substantially inactivated in the presence of blood, large spills of blood require that the surface be cleaned before an EPA-registered disinfectant or a 1:10 (final concentration) solution of household bleach is applied. If a sharps injury is possible, the surface initially should be decontaminated then cleaned and disinfected (1:10 final concentration).

An important issue concerning use of disinfectants for noncritical surfaces in health care settings is that the contact time specified on the label of the product is often too long to be practically followed. The labels of most products registered by EPA for use against HBV, HIV, or *Mycobacterium tuberculosis* specify a contact time of 10 minutes. Such a long contact time is impractical for disinfection of environmental surfaces in a health care setting, because most health care facilities apply a disinfectant and allow it to dry (~1 minute). Multiple scientific papers have demonstrated significant microbial reduction with contact times of 30 to 60 seconds.

Hypochlorite solutions in tap water at a pH above 8 stored at room temperature (23°C) in closed, opaque plastic containers can lose up to 40% to 50% of their free available chlorine level over 1 month. Sodium hypochlorite solution does not decompose after 30 days when stored in a closed brown bottle.[12]

Disinfecting Procedure

While wearing gloves, employees should clean and sanitize all work surfaces at the beginning and end of their shift with a 1:10 dilution of household bleach. Instruments such as scissors or centrifuge carriages should be sanitized daily with a diluted solution of bleach. It is equally important to clean and disinfect work areas frequently during the workday as well as before and after the workday. Studies have demonstrated that HIV is inactivated rapidly after being exposed to common chemical germicides at concentrations that are much lower than those used in practice. Disposable materials contaminated with blood must be placed in containers marked "Biohazard" and properly discarded.

Neither HBV (or HCV) nor HIV has ever been documented as being transmitted from a housekeeping surface (e.g., countertops). However, an area contaminated by either blood or body fluids must be treated as potentially hazardous, with prompt removal and surface disinfection. Strategies differ for decontaminating spills of blood and other body fluids; the cleanup procedure depends on the setting (e.g., porosity of the surface) and volume of the spill. The following protocol is recommended for managing spills in a clinical laboratory:

1. Wear gloves and a laboratory coat.
2. Absorb the blood with disposable towels. Remove as much liquid blood or serum as possible before decontamination.
3. Using a diluted bleach (1:10) solution, clean the spill site of all visible blood.
4. Wipe down the spill site with paper towels soaked with diluted bleach.
5. Place all disposable materials used for decontamination into a biohazard container.

Decontaminate nondisposable equipment by soaking overnight in a dilute (1:10) bleach solution and rinsing with methyl alcohol and water before reuse. Disposable glassware or supplies that have come in contact with blood should be autoclaved or incinerated.

General Infection-Control Safety Practices

All laboratories need programs to minimize risks to the health and safety of employees,[14] volunteers, and patients. Suitable physical arrangements, an acceptable work environment, and appropriate equipment should be available to maintain safe operations.

Laboratories should adhere to the following safety practices to reduce the risk of inadvertent contamination with blood or certain body fluids:

1. All devices in contact with blood and capable of transmitting infection to the donor or recipient must be sterile and nonreusable.
2. Food and drinks should not be consumed in work areas or stored in the same area as specimens. Containers, refrigerators, or freezers used for specimens should be marked as containing a biohazard.
3. Specimens needing centrifugation should be capped and placed into a centrifuge with a sealed dome.

4. Rubber-stoppered test tubes must be opened slowly and carefully with a gauze square over the stopper to minimize aerosol production (the introduction of substances into the air).
5. Autodilutors or safety bulbs should be used for pipetting. Pipetting of any clinical material by mouth is strictly forbidden (see following discussion).
6. No tobacco products can be used in the laboratory.
7. No manipulation of contact lenses or teeth-whitening strips should be done with gloved or potentially infectious hands.
8. No lipstick or makeup should be applied in the laboratory.
9. All personnel should be familiar with the location and use of eyewash stations and safety showers.

Pipetting Safeguards: Automatic Devices

Pipetting must be done by mechanical means, either mechanical suction or aspirator bulbs. Another device, a bottle top dispenser, can be used to deliver repetitive aliquots of reagents. It is designed as a bottle-mounted system that can dispense selected volumes in an easy, precise manner. It is usually trouble free and requires minimal maintenance.

Safety Manual

Each laboratory must have an up-to-date safety manual. This manual should contain a comprehensive listing of approved policies, acceptable practices, and precautions, including Standard Precautions. Specific regulations that conform to current state and federal requirements (e.g., OSHA regulations) must be included in the manual. Other sources of mandatory and voluntary standards include TJC, CAP, and CDC.

Sharps Safety and Needlestick Prevention

OSHA estimates that approximately 600,000 to 1 million needlestick injuries, the majority of which are unreported, occur in the United States each year. The most widespread control measure required by OSHA and CLSI is the use of puncture-resistant sharps containers[1,3] (Fig. 2-4). The primary purpose of using these containers is to eliminate the need for anyone to transport needles and other sharps while looking for a place to discard them. Sharps containers are to be located in patient areas as well as conveniently placed in the laboratory. Phlebotomists should carry these red, puncture-resistant containers in their collection

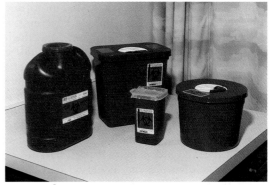

FIGURE 2-4 Sharps containers. (From Kinn ME, Woods M: The medical assistant: administrative and clinical, ed 8, Philadelphia, 1999, Saunders.)

trays. Needles should not be overfilled and should not project from the top of the container. Overfilling can result in a needle bouncing back at the employee and potential needlestick injury. To discard them, sharps containers are closed and placed in the biohazard waste.

Use of the special sharps container permits quick disposal of a needle without recapping and safe disposal of other sharp devices that may be contaminated with blood. This supports the recommendation against recapping, bending, breaking, or otherwise manipulating any sharp needle or lancet device by hand. Most needlestick accidents have occurred during recapping of a needle after a phlebotomy. Injuries also can occur to housekeeping personnel when contaminated sharps are left on a bed, concealed in linen, or disposed of improperly in a waste receptacle. Most accidental disposal-related exposures can be eliminated by the use of sharps containers. An accidental needlestick must be reported to the supervisor or other designated individual.

To help laboratories make informed decisions about sharps safety, needlestick prevention, and device selection, ECRI (www.ecri.org), formerly the Emergency Care Research Institute, a nonprofit health services research agency, conducts comparative ratings of available protective devices. This service assists laboratories in determining whether and to what degree a product can protect staff from injury without compromising the patient's safety or comfort.

Specimen-Processing Protection

Specimens should be transported to the laboratory in plastic leakproof bags. Protective gloves should always be worn for handling any type of biological specimen.

Substances can become airborne when the stopper (cap) is popped off a blood-collecting container, a serum sample is poured from one tube to another, or a serum tube is centrifuged. When the cap is being removed from a specimen tube or a blood collection tube, the top should be covered with a disposable gauze pad or a special protective pad. Gauze pads with an impermeable plastic coating on one side can reduce contamination of gloves. The tube should be held away from the body and the cap gently twisted to remove it. Snapping off the cap or top can cause some of the contents to aerosolize. When not in place on the tube, the cap should be kept in the gauze, not placed directly on the work surface or countertop.

Specially constructed plastic splash shields are used in many laboratories for the processing of blood specimens. Tube caps are removed behind or under the shield, which acts as a barrier between the person and the specimen tube. This is designed to prevent aerosols from entering the nose, eyes, or mouth. Laboratory safety boxes are commercially available and can be used to remove stoppers from tubes or perform other procedures that might cause spattering. Splash shields and safety boxes should be periodically decontaminated.

When specimens are being centrifuged, the tube caps should always be kept on the tubes. Centrifuge covers must be used and left on until the centrifuge stops. The centrifuge should be allowed to stop by itself and should not be manually stopped by the worker.

Another step that should be taken to control the hazard from aerosols is to exercise caution in handling pipettes and other equipment used to transfer human specimens, especially pathogenic materials. These materials should be discarded properly and carefully.

Specimen Handling and Shipping Requirements

Proper handling of blood and body fluids is critical to the accuracy of laboratory test results, and the safety of all individuals who come in contact with specimens must be guaranteed.

If a blood specimen is to be transported, the shipping container must meet OSHA requirements for shipping clinical specimens (Federal Register 29, CAR 1910.1030). Shipping containers must meet the packaging requirements of major couriers and Department of Transportation hazardous materials regulations. Approved reclosable plastic bags for handling biohazardous specimens (Fig. 2-5) and amber bags for specimens for analysis of light-sensitive drugs are available. These bags must meet the NCCLS M29-A3 specimen-handling guidelines. Approved bags (e.g., LabGuard Reclosable Bags) have bright orange and black graphics that

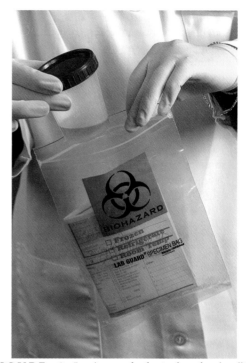

FIGURE 2-5 **Approved plastic bag for handling biohazardous materials.** (From Warekois RS, Robinson R: Phlebotomy: worktext and procedures manual, ed 3, St Louis, 2012, Saunders.)

clearly identify bags as holding hazardous materials. Some products have an additional marking area that allows phlebotomists to identify contents that must be kept frozen, refrigerated, or at room temperature.

Maintaining specimens at the correct preanalytical temperature is extremely important. Products such as the Insul-Tote (Palco Labs, Scotts Valley, CA) are convenient for specimen transport from the field to the clinical laboratory. This particular product has a reusable cold gel pack that keeps temperatures below 70°F for 8 hours even if the exterior temperature is above 100°F. Many laboratory courier services use common household coolers. Blood specimen collection and processing should conform to the current checklist requirements adopted by the College of American Pathologists (http://www.cap.org). Errors in specimen collection and handling (preanalytical errors) are a significant cause of incorrect patient results.

Once the specimen has been collected and properly labeled, it must be transported to the laboratory for processing and analysis. In many institutions, a specimen container is placed in a leakproof plastic bag as a further protective measure to prevent pathogen transmission—the implementation of the Standard Precautions policy and the use of barriers. The request form must be placed on the outside of this bag; many transport bags have a special pouch for this purpose.

PREVENTION OF DISEASE TRANSMISSION

Immunization/Vaccination

A well-planned and properly implemented immunization program is an important component of a health care organization's infection prevention and control program. When planning these programs, valuable information is available from the Advisory Committee on Immunization Practices (ACIP), the Hospital Infection Control Practices Advisory Committee (HICPAC) and the Centers of Disease Control and Prevention (CDC). Major considerations include the characteristics of the health care workers employed, the individuals served, and the requirements of regulatory agencies and local, state, and federal regulations.

Preemployment health profiles with baseline screening of students and laboratory staff should include an immune status evaluation for hepatitis B, rubella, and measles at a minimum. In their recommendations for immunization of health care workers, ACIP and HICPAC identify those employees whose maintenance of immune status is important; this includes laboratory staff. Individuals are recognized for being at risk for exposure to, and possible transmission of, diseases that can be prevented by immunizations.

The ACIP/HICPAC recommendations are divided into the following three categories:
1. Immunizing agents strongly recommended for health care workers.
2. Other immunologics that are or may be indicated for health care workers.
3. Other vaccine-preventable diseases.

All health care organizations should include those immunizations that are strongly recommended. To determine whether or not to include those immunologics that may or may not be included, the incidence of the vaccine-preventable diseases within the community served needs to be reviewed. Also, comparing the demographics of the workforce pool with the disease pattern within the community will determine which of these immunologics are indicated for the specific organization's program. Some vaccines may not be routinely administered but may be considered after an injury or exposure incident or for immunocompromised or older health care workers.

The ACIP/HICPAC recommendations determine which vaccines are included in this category based on documented nosocomial transmission and significant risk for acquiring or transmitting these

---

BOX 2-5

Vaccines Recommended for Teens and College Students

- Tetanus-diphtheria-pertussis vaccine
- Meningococcal vaccine
- HPV vaccine series
- Hepatitis B vaccine series
- Polio vaccine series
- Measles-mumps-rubella (MMR) vaccine series
- Varicella (chickenpox) vaccine series
- Influenza vaccine
- Pneumococcal polysaccharide (PPV) vaccine
- Hepatitis A vaccine series
- Annual flu + H1N1 flu shot

From Centers for Disease Control and Prevention (website): www.cdc.gov. Accessed May 12, 2009. And from Centers for Disease Control and Prevention: H1N1 flu advisory (website). www.cdc.gov. Accessed Sept. 11, 2009.
  Note: For complete statements by the Advisory Committee on Immunization Practices (ACIP), visit www.cdc.gov/vaccines/pubs/ACIP-list.htm.

---

diseases.[1] Box 2-5 lists vaccines recommended for teens and college students.

Hepatitis B

Before the advent of the hepatitis B vaccine, the leading occupationally acquired infection in health care workers was hepatitis B. OSHA issued a federal standard in 1991 mandating employers to provide the hepatitis B vaccine to all employees who have or may have occupational exposure to blood or other potentially infective materials. The vaccine is to be offered at no expense to the employee, and if the employee refuses the vaccine, a declination form must be signed.

Influenza

Influenza has been shown to be transmitted in health care facilities during community outbreaks of this disease. Annual influenza vaccination programs are carried out in the fall. Programs that immunize both the health care worker and the individuals served have been extremely effective in reducing morbidity and mortality and staff absenteeism. It has been demonstrated that when the vaccine is available free to the health care worker and at a convenient location and time, the number of recipients increases significantly.

In addition to the annual flu vaccine, a newly developed H1N1 flu vaccine became available in Fall 2009. The general populations, including health care workers and students, are advised to receive this vaccination.

Measles

Although ongoing measles transmission was declared eliminated in the United States in 2000 and in the World Health Organization (WHO) Region of the Americas in 2002, approximately 20 million cases of measles occur each year worldwide. As a result of a successful U.S. vaccination program, measles elimination (i.e., interruption of endemic measles transmission) was declared in the United States in 2000.

However, during January 1 to April 25, 2008, a total of 64 confirmed measles cases were preliminarily reported to CDC, the most reported by this date for any year since 2001. Of the 64 cases, 54 were associated with importation of measles from other countries into the United States, and 63 of the 64 patients were unvaccinated or had unknown or undocumented vaccination status. The findings underscore the ongoing risk for measles among unvaccinated persons and the importance of maintaining high levels of vaccination.[15]

The 2008 upsurge in measles cases serves as a reminder that measles is still imported into the United States and can result in outbreaks unless population immunity remains high through vaccination. Among the 64 confirmed measles cases, prior vaccination could be documented for only one person.

Mumps

Mumps transmission has been reported in medical settings. Programs that ensure that the worker is immune to mumps are easily linked to measles and rubella control.

Rubella

Vaccination programs have significantly decreased the overall risk for rubella transmission in all age groups. All workers who are likely to have contact with pregnant women should be immune to rubella. Because it is not harmful for people who are already immune to measles, mumps, or rubella to receive the vaccine, the trivalent MMR (measles, mumps, rubella) should be given rather than the monovalent vaccine.

Varicella

Postexposure procedures to address varicella-zoster virus are usually costly and disruptive to a health care organization. A program that (1) identifies susceptible workers, patients, and visitors; (2) applies restrictions when necessary; and (3) provides the immunization can help prevent the need to manage such exposure incidents.

Optional Immunizations

Hepatitis A

Standard Precautions are recommended and often a part of the isolation practices of U.S. health care facilities. When these are followed, nosocomial transmission of the hepatitis A virus (HAV) is rare.[3] Also, most patients hospitalized with hepatitis A are admitted when they are beyond the point of peak infectivity, which is after the onset of jaundice. Health care workers have not demonstrated an elevated prevalence of HAV compared with other occupational groups who were serologically tested. In communities that have high rates of hepatitis A or that are experiencing an outbreak, immunizing the health care worker population may need to be considered in certain settings. This vaccine has also been recommended for preexposure prophylaxis for the following groups who may be included in a health care worker population[3]:

- Those who travel to an endemic country
- Household and sexual contacts of HAV-infected people
- Those who have contact with active cases
- Laboratory workers who handle live HAV; workers and attendees at day care centers where attendees wear diapers; food handlers, staff, and residents of institutions for mentally handicapped patients; chronic carriers of hepatitis B; and people with chronic liver diseases

Meningococcal Disease

Routine vaccination of health care workers against meningococcal disease is not recommended. If an outbreak of serogroup C meningococcal disease is identified, use of the meningococcal vaccine may be warranted.

Pertussis

No vaccine against pertussis is licensed for use in an adult population. If one becomes available in the future, booster doses of adult formulations may be recommended because pertussis is highly contagious.

Typhoid

Typhoid vaccine should be administered to workers in microbiology laboratories who frequently work with *Salmonella typhi*.

Vaccinia

Vaccinia vaccine should be administered to the few people who work with orthopoxviruses, such as the laboratory workers who directly handle cultures or animals contaminated or infected with vaccinia.

Other Immunizations

Other vaccine-preventable diseases include diphtheria, pneumococcal disease, and tetanus. Because health care workers are not at increased risk for acquiring these diseases over the general population, they should seek these immunizations from their primary care provider.

Screening Tests

Tuberculosis: Purified Protein Derivative (PPD, Mantoux) Skin Test

If health care workers have recently spent time with and been exposed to someone with active tuberculosis (TB), their TB skin test reaction may not yet be positive. They may need a second skin test 10 to 12 weeks after the last time they had contact with the infected person. It can take several weeks after infection for the immune system to react to the TB skin test. If the reaction to the second test is negative, the worker probably does not have latent TB infection. Workers who have strongly positive reactions, a skin test diameter greater than 15 mm, and symptoms suggestive of TB should be evaluated clinically and microbiologically. Two sputum specimens collected on successive days should be investigated for TB by microscopy and culture.

QuantiFERON TB Gold (QFT) is a blood test used to determine if a person is infected with TB bacteria. The QFT measures the response to TB proteins when they are mixed with a small amount of blood. Currently, few health departments offer the QFT. If the worker's health department does offer the QFT, only one visit is required, at which time the person's blood is drawn for the test.

Rubella

All phlebotomists and laboratory staff need to demonstrate immunity to rubella. If antibody is not demonstrable, vaccination is necessary.

Hepatitis B Surface Antigen

All phlebotomists and laboratory staff need to demonstrate immunity to hepatitis B. If antibodies are not demonstrable, vaccination is necessary.

Prophylaxis, Medical Follow-Up, and Records of Accidental Exposure

If accidental occupational exposure occurs, laboratory staff members should be informed of options for treatment. Because a needlestick can trigger an emotional response, it is wise to think about a course of action before the occurrence of an actual incident. If a "source patient" can be identified, part of the workup could involve testing the patient for various infectious diseases. Laws addressing patient's rights in regard to testing of a source patient can vary from state to state.

Although the most important strategy for reducing the risk of occupational HIV transmission is to prevent exposure, plans for postexposure management of health care personnel should be in place. Occupational exposures should be considered urgent medical concerns by the employee health department.

CDC has issued guidelines for the management of health care personnel exposure to HIV and recommendations for **postexposure prophylaxis (PEP)**.[16,17] Considerations include whether personnel should receive PEP and which type of PEP regimen to use.

Hepatitis B Virus Exposure

After skin or mucosal exposure to blood, the ACIP recommends immunoprophylaxis, depending on several factors. If an individual has not been vaccinated, HBIG is usually given, within 24 hours if practical, and concurrently with hepatitis B vaccine postexposure injuries. HBIG contains antibodies to HBV and offers prompt but short-lived protection.

Recommendations for HBV postexposure management include initiation of the hepatitis B vaccine series to any susceptible, unvaccinated person who sustains an occupational blood or body fluid exposure. PEP with HBIG and hepatitis B vaccine series should be considered for occupational exposures after evaluation of the hepatitis B surface antigen status of the source and the vaccination and vaccine response status of the exposed person. The specific protocol for these measures is determined by the institution's infection control division. Postvaccination testing for the development of antibody to surface HB antigen (anti-HBsAg) for persons at occupational risk who may have had needlestick exposures necessitating postexposure prophylaxis should be done to ensure that the vaccination has been successful.

Hepatitis C Virus Exposure

Immune globulin and antiviral agents (e.g., interferon with or without ribavirin) are not recommended for PEP of hepatitis C. For **hepatitis C virus (HCV)** postexposure management, the HCV status of the source and the exposed person should be determined. For health care personnel exposed to an HCV-positive source, follow-up HCV testing should be performed to determine if infection develops. After exposure to blood of a patient with (or with suspected) HCV infection, immune globulin should be given as soon as possible. No vaccine is currently available.

In special circumstances (e.g., delayed exposure report, unknown source person, pregnancy in exposed person, resistance of source virus to antiretroviral agents, toxicity of PEP regimen), consultation with local experts and the National Clinicians' Post-Exposure Prophylaxis Hotline (PEPline, 1-888-448-4911) is recommended.

Human Immunodeficiency Virus

Transmission of HIV is believed to result from intimate contact with blood and body fluids from an infected person. Casual contact with infected persons has not been documented as a mode of transmission. If there has been occupational exposure to a potentially HIV-infected specimen or patient, the antibody status of the patient or specimen source should be determined if allowed by law and not already known. If the source is a patient, voluntary consent should be obtained, if possible, for testing for HIV antibodies as soon as possible. High-risk exposure prophylaxis includes the use of a combination of antiretroviral agents to prevent seroconversion. For most HIV exposures that warrant PEP, a basic 4-week, two-drug regimen is recommended. For HIV exposures that pose an increased risk of transmission, a three-drug regimen may be recommended. Special circumstances (e.g., delayed exposure report, unknown source person, pregnancy in exposed person, resistance of source virus to antiviral agents, toxicity of PEP regimens) are discussed in the CDC guidelines.

PEP guidelines from the CDC are based on the determined risks of transmission (stratified as "highest," "increased," and "no risk"). Highest risk has been determined to exist when there has been occupational exposure both to a large volume of blood (as with a deep percutaneous injury or cut with a large-diameter hollow needle previously used in the source patient's vein or artery) and to blood containing a high titer of HIV (known as a *high viral load*), to fluids containing visible blood, or to specific other potentially infectious fluids or tissue, including semen, vaginal secretions, and cerebrospinal, peritoneal, pleural, pericardial, and amniotic fluids.[13]

If a known or suspected parenteral exposure takes place, a technician or technologist may request follow-up monitoring for HIV (or HBV) antibodies. This monitoring and follow-up counseling must be provided free of charge. If voluntary informed consent is obtained, the source of the potentially infectious material and the technician/technologist should be tested immediately. The laboratory technologist should also be tested at intervals after exposure. An injury report must be filed after parenteral exposure.

An enzyme immunoassay (EIA) screening test is used to detect antibodies to HIV. Before any HIV result is considered positive, the result is confirmed by Western blot (WB) analysis. A negative antibody test for HIV does not confirm the absence of virus. There is a period after infection with HIV during which detectable antibody is not present. In these cases, detection of antigen is important; a polymerase chain reaction (PCR) assay for HIV deoxyribonucleic acid (DNA) can be used for this purpose, and a p24 antigen test is used for screening blood donors for HIV antigen.

If the source patient is seronegative, the exposed worker should be screened for antibody again at 3 and 6 months. If the source patient is at high risk for HIV infection, more extensive follow-up of both the worker and the source patient may be needed.

If the source patient or specimen is HIV positive (HIV antibodies, WB assay, HIV antigen, or HIV DNA by PCR), the blood of the exposed worker should be tested for HIV antibodies within 48 hours if possible. Exposed workers who are initially seronegative for the HIV antibody should be tested again 6 weeks after exposure. If this test is negative, the worker should be tested again at 12 weeks and 6 months after exposure. Most reported seroconversions have occurred between 6 and 12 weeks after exposure. PEP should be started immediately and according to policies set by the institution's infection control program. A policy of "hit hard, hit early" should generally be in place.

During the early follow-up period after exposure, especially the first 6 to 12 weeks, the worker should follow the recommendations of the CDC regarding the transmission of AIDS, including the following[1]:

1. Refrain from donating blood or plasma.
2. Inform potential sex partners of the exposure.
3. Avoid pregnancy.
4. Inform health care providers of their potential exposure so they can take necessary precautions.
5. Do not share razors, toothbrushes, or other items that could become contaminated with blood.
6. Clean and disinfect surfaces on which blood or body fluids have spilled.

The exposed worker should be advised of the risks of infection and evaluated medically for any history, signs, or symptoms consistent with HIV infection. Serologic testing for HIV antibodies should be made available to all health care workers who are concerned they may have been infected with HIV.

Occupational exposures should be considered urgent medical concerns to ensure timely postexposure management and administration of HBIG, hepatitis B vaccine, and HIV PEP.

Respirators or Masks for Tuberculosis Control[18]

A person must be exposed to M. *tuberculosis* to be infected with TB. This occurs through close contact over a period of time, when contaminated droplet nuclei from an infected person's respiratory tract enter another person's respiratory tract.

A commonsense way to control transmission of these contaminated droplets is to cover the mouth during coughing and to use tissues. In addition, specialized types of masks or respirators are now OSHA-mandated measures for use by persons who are occupationally exposed to patients with suspected or confirmed cases of pulmonary TB. A "Special Respiratory Precautions" sign should identify rooms where there are patients fitting this criterion. Health care personnel caring for these patients must be fitted with and trained to use the proper respirator.[13]

Protection from Aerosols

Biohazards are generally treated with great respect in the clinical laboratory. The adverse effects of pathogenic substances on the body are well documented. The presence of pathogenic organisms is not limited to the culture plates in the microbiology laboratory. Airborne infectious particles, or aerosols, can be found in all areas of the laboratory where human specimens are used.

Biosafety Cabinets

Biosafety cabinets are protective workplace devices used to control the presence of infectious agents in the air. Microbiology laboratories selectively use biological safety cabinets for performing procedures that generate infectious aerosols. Several common procedures in the processing of specimens for culture—grinding, mincing, vortexing, centrifuging, and preparation of direct smears—are known to produce aerosol droplets. Air containing the infectious agent is sterilized by heat or ultraviolet light or, most often, by passage through a high-efficiency particulate air (HEPA) filter. Biosafety cabinets not only remove air contaminants through a local exhaust system but also provide an added measure of safety by confining the aerosol contaminant within an enclosed area, thereby isolating it from the worker.

Negative-Pressure Isolation Rooms

Another infectious disease control measure [19] is the use of negative-pressure isolation rooms. This type of room is used to control the direction of airflow between the room and adjacent areas, preventing contaminated air from escaping from the room into other areas of the facility. The minimum pressure difference necessary to achieve and maintain negative pressure that will result in airflow into the room is very small (0.001 inch of water), but higher pressures (>0.001 inch of water) are satisfactory. Negative pressure in a room can be altered by changing the ventilation system operation or by opening and closing the room's doors, corridor doors, or windows. When an operating configuration has been established, it is essential that all doors and windows remain properly closed in the isolation room and other areas (e.g., doors in corridors that affect air pressure), except when persons need to enter or leave the room or area.

ADDITIONAL LABORATORY HAZARDS

It cannot be overemphasized that clinical laboratories present many potential hazards simply because of the nature of the work done there. In addition to biological hazards, other hazards present in the clinical laboratory include open flames, electrical equipment, glassware, chemicals of varying reactivity, flammable solvents, and toxic fumes.

In addition to the safety practices common to all laboratory situations, such as the proper storage of flammable materials, certain procedures are mandatory in a medical laboratory. Proper procedures for the handling and disposal of toxic, radioactive, and potentially carcinogenic materials must be included in the safety manual. Information regarding the hazards of particular substances must be addressed both as a safety practice and to comply with the legal right of workers to know about the hazards associated with these substances. Some chemicals (e.g., benzidine) previously used in the laboratory are now known to be carcinogenic and have been replaced with safer chemicals.

Chemical Hazards

Hazard assessment is an important OSHA requirement. The MSDS (see Fig. 4-9 and Chapter 4) accompanies all hazardous chemicals and contains information relevant to possible hazards, safe handling, storage, and proper disposal.

Proper storage and use of chemicals are essential to avoid a potential fire hazard and other health hazards resulting from inhalation of toxic vapors or skin contact. Fire and explosion are a concern when flammable solvents (e.g., ether, acetone) are used. These materials should always be stored in special OSHA-approved metal storage cabinets that are properly ventilated. Storage of organic solvents is regulated by OSHA rules.

Organic solvents should be used in a fume hood. Proper precautions must be taken to avoid vaporization. Disposal of flammable solvents in sewers is prohibited. Chemical waste must be deposited in appropriately labeled receptacles for eventual disposal.

Specific Hazardous Chemicals

Specific chemicals that must be handled with care because of potential hazards in their use are:

- Sulfuric acid: at a concentration above 65% may cause blindness; may produce burns on the skin; if taken orally, may cause severe burns, depending on the concentration.
- Nitric acid: gives off yellow fumes that are extremely toxic and damaging to tissues; overexposure to vapor can cause death, loss of eyesight, extreme irritation, itching, and yellow discoloration of the skin; if taken orally, can cause extreme burns, may perforate the stomach wall, or cause death.
- Acetic acid: severely caustic; continuous exposure to vapor can lead to chronic bronchitis.
- Hydrochloric acid: inhalation of vapors should be avoided; any acid on the skin should be washed away immediately to prevent a burn.
- Sodium hydroxide: extremely hazardous in contact with the skin, eyes, or mucous membranes (mouth), causing caustic burns; dangerous even at very low concentrations; any contact necessitates immediate care.
- Phenol (a disinfectant): can cause caustic burns or contact dermatitis even in dilute solutions; wash off skin with water or alcohol.
- Carbon tetrachloride: damaging to the liver even at an exposure level with no discernible odor.
- Trichloroacetic acid: severely caustic; respiratory tract irritant.
- Ethers: cause depression of central nervous system.

Select Carcinogens

OSHA regulates select substances as carcinogens. Carcinogens are any substances that cause the development of cancerous growths in living tissue. They are considered hazardous to personnel working with these substances in laboratories. When

possible, substances that are potentially carcinogenic have been replaced by ones that are less hazardous. If necessary, with the proper safeguards in place, potentially carcinogenic substances can be used in the laboratory. Lists of potential carcinogens used in a particular laboratory must be available to all personnel who work there; these lists can be long.

Hazard Warning System

As noted earlier, the hazards identification system developed by the National Fire Protection Association (NFPA) provides at a glance—in words, symbols, and pictures—information on the potential health, flammability, and chemical-reactivity hazards of materials used in the laboratory. This information is provided on the labels of all containers of hazardous chemicals.

The hazards identification system consists of four small, diamond-shaped symbols grouped into a larger diamond shape (see Fig. 2-1). The top diamond is red and indicates a flammability hazard. The diamond on the right is yellow and indicates a reactivity-stability hazard; these materials are capable of explosion or violent chemical reactions. The diamond on the left is blue and indicates a possible health hazard. The diamond on the bottom is white and provides special hazard information (e.g., radioactivity, special biohazards, other dangerous elements). The system also indicates the severity of the hazard by using numerical designations from 4 to 0, with 4 being extremely hazardous and 0 being no hazard (Fig. 2-6).

The Hazard Communication Standard (HCS) and the process of assigning Hazardous Materials Identification System (HMIS) ratings help to meet OSHA requirements. HMIS ratings may appear on the surface to be similar to several recognized rating systems such as NFPA, but each of these systems serves a slightly different purpose. The rating criteria of other systems (e.g., health rating) differ, and the resulting ratings are not interchangeable with those generated by the HMIS ratings criteria. For detailed information on HMIS III, refer to www.paint.org.

Protective Measures

When any potentially hazardous solution or chemical is being used, protective equipment for the eyes, face, head, and extremities, as well as protective clothing or barriers, should be used. Volatile or fuming solutions should be used under a fume hood. In case of accidental contact with a hazardous solution or a contaminated substance, quick action is essential. The laboratory should have a safety shower where quick, "all-over" decontamination can take

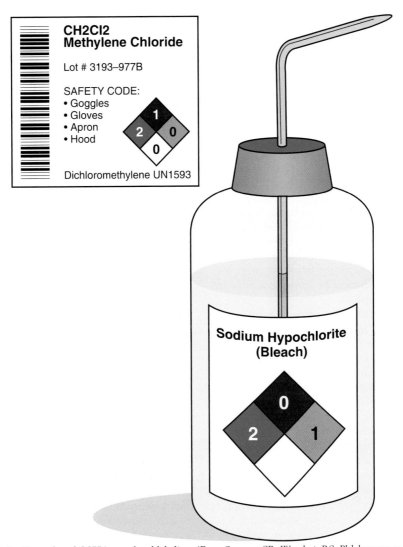

CH2Cl2
Methylene Chloride

Lot # 3193–977B

SAFETY CODE:
• Goggles
• Gloves
• Apron
• Hood

Dichloromethylene UN1593

Sodium Hypochlorite
(Bleach)

FIGURE 2-6   **Examples of OSHA-mandated labeling.** (From Sommer SR, Warekois RS: Phlebotomy: worktext and procedures manual, Philadelphia, 2002, Saunders.)

place immediately. Another essential safety device in all laboratories is a face or eye washer that streams aerated water directly onto the face and eyes to prevent burns and loss of eyesight. Any such action must be undertaken immediately, so these safety devices must be present in the laboratory area.

Measures to limit exposure to hazardous chemicals must be implemented. All personnel must use appropriate work practices, emergency procedures, and PPE. Many of the measures taken are also those needed for protection from biological hazards, as discussed previously (see Personal Protective Equipment). These measures include the use of gloves, keeping the work area clean and uncluttered, proper and complete labeling of all chemicals, and use of proper eye protection, fume hood, respiratory equipment, and any other emergency or protective equipment as necessary.

General equipment (e.g., safety showers, eyewashes) must be present in each laboratory. Routine verification of equipment operation and maintenance must be established.

Electrical Hazards

Shock or fire hazards from electrical apparatus in the clinical laboratory can be a source of injury. OSHA regulations stipulate that the requirements for grounding electrical equipment published in the NFPA's National Electrical Code must be met. Some local codes are more stringent.

All electrical equipment must be Underwriters Laboratories (UL) approved. Regular inspection of electrical equipment decreases the likelihood of electrical accidents. Grounding of all electrical equipment is essential. Personnel should not handle electrical equipment and connections with wet hands, and electrical equipment should not be used after liquid has been spilled on it. Any equipment used in an area of where organic solvents are present must be equipped with explosion-free fittings (e.g., outlets, plugs).

Fire Hazards

NFPA and OSHA publish standards related to fire safety. In addition, NFPA also publishes the National Fire Codes, which may be adopted instead of OSHA regulations.

Personnel need to be trained in the use of safety equipment and procedures. Annual retraining is mandatory. Each laboratory must have equipment to extinguish or confine a fire in laboratory as well as on an individual's clothing. Safety showers are essential. Fire blankets must be easily accessible in wall-mounted cabinets.

Fires are classified into five different basic types:
Class A Ordinary combustibles
Class B Flammable liquids and gases
Class C Electrical equipment
Class D Powdered metal (combustible) material
Class E Cannot be extinguished

Fires can be classified as a combination of A, B, and C classes (Fig. 2-7). The type of recommended extinguisher is determined by the class of fire. There are four different types or classes of fire extinguishers, each of which extinguishes specific types of fire. Newer fire extinguishers use a picture/labeling system to designate which types of fires they are to be used on. Older fire extinguishers are labeled with colored geometrical shapes and letter designations. Additionally, class A and class B fire extinguishers have a numerical rating based on UL-conducted tests and designed to determine the extinguishing potential for each size and type of extinguisher.

Many extinguishers available today can be used on different types of fires and will be labeled with more than one designator, such as A-B, B-C, or A-B-C. Class D and E fires should be handled only by trained personnel. Many clinical laboratories are installing computerized systems to minimize fire damage in temperature- and humidity-controlled rooms.

The various types of fire extinguishers are water, carbon dioxide, Halon 1211 or 1301 foam, loaded steam, dry chemical, and triplex dry chemical. Dry chemical extinguishers are the most common all-purpose extinguishers.

The local fire marshal determines where the equipment will be stored, the locations of fire alarms, and maps of evacuation routes. A fire extinguisher should be located near each laboratory door and also at the end of the room opposite

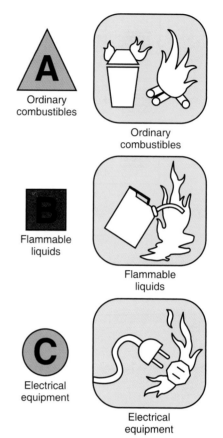

FIGURE 2-7　Classes of fire extinguisher with corresponding types of fire.

the door in large laboratories. Fire extinguishers must be tested by qualified personnel at intervals specified by the manufacturer. Even though extinguishers come in various shapes and sizes, they all operate in a similar manner. An easy acronym for use of fire extinguishers is PASS: pull, aim, squeeze, and sweep.

Glassware Hazards

Many forms of glassware are basic implements in the clinical laboratory. Caution must be used to prevent unnecessary or accidental breakage. Most glassware currently used is discarded when broken. Any broken or cracked glassware should be discarded in a special container for broken glass, not thrown in the regular waste container. Common sense should be used in storing glassware, with heavy pieces placed on lower shelves and tall pieces placed behind smaller pieces. Shelves should be installed at reasonable heights; glassware should not be stored out of reach. Broken or cracked glassware is the cause of many lacerations, and care should be taken to avoid this laboratory hazard.

Infectious Waste

The purpose of waste disposal control is to confine or isolate any possible hazardous material from all workers, laboratory personnel as well as custodial and housekeeping personnel. CLSI has also published guidelines on management of clinical laboratory waste.[20]

OSHA Standards

OSHA standards provide for the implementation of a **waste disposal program.**[21] On the Federal level, the storage and management of medical waste is primarily regulated by OSHA. Laws and statutes are defined by The Occupational Health and Safety Act and The Clean Air Act. For more information, refer to www.fedcenter.gov.

States often expand the definition of medical waste or blood to include animals. State-by-state guidance concerning regulated medical waste and mercury issues can be found at www.encap.org. The OSHA regulations only apply to human blood, human infectious wastes, and human pathological wastes. Under OSHA:

- Contaminated reusable sharps must be placed in containers that are: closeable, puncture resistant, labeled or color coded, and leakproof on the sides and bottom (see Fig. 2-2). Reusable sharps that are contaminated with blood or other potentially infectious materials must not be stored or processed in a manner that requires employees to reach by hand into the containers.
- Specimens of blood or other potentially infectious material are required to be placed in a container that is labeled and color coded and closed prior to being stored, transported, or shipped. Contaminated sharps must be placed in containers that are: closeable, puncture resistant, leakproof on sides and bottoms, and labeled or color coded (see Fig. 2-2).
- Regulated wastes (liquid or semi-liquid blood or other potentially infectious materials
- Contaminated items that would release blood or other potentially infectious materials in a liquid or semi-liquid state if compressed
- Items that are caked with dried blood or other potentially infectious materials and are capable of releasing these materials during handling
- Contaminated sharps
- Pathological and microbiological wastes containing blood or other potentially infectious materials) must be placed in containers that are: closeable, constructed to contain all contents and prevent leakage of fluids, labeled or color coded, and closed prior to removal (see a full discussion below of biohazard containers and biohazard bag).
- All bins, pails, cans, and similar receptacles intended for reuse that have the likelihood of becoming contaminated with blood or other potentially infectious materials are required to be inspected and decontaminated on a regularly scheduled basis. Waste containers must be easily accessible to personnel and must be located in laboratory areas where they are typically used. Containers for waste should be constructed so that their contents will not be spilled if the container is tipped over accidentally.
- Labels affixed to containers of regulated wastes, refrigerators and freezers containing blood or other potentially infectious materials, and other containers used to store, transport, or ship blood or other potentially infectious materials must: include the biohazard symbol; be fluorescent orange or orange-red or predominantly so, with lettering and symbols in contrasting color; and be affixed as closely as possible to the container by adhesive or wire to prevent loss or removal.[8]

Biohazard Containers

Body fluid specimens, including blood, must be placed in well-constructed biohazard containers with secure lids to prevent leakage during transport and for future disposal. Contaminated specimens and other materials used in laboratory tests should be decontaminated before reprocessing for disposal, or they should be placed in special impervious bags for disposal in accordance with established waste removal policies. If outside contamination of the bag is likely, a second bag should be used.

Hazardous specimens and potentially hazardous substances should be tagged and identified as such. The tag should read "Biohazard," or the biological hazard symbol should be used. All persons working in the laboratory area must be informed about the meaning of the tags and the precautions that should be taken for each tag.

Contaminated equipment must be placed in a designated area for storage, washing, decontamination, or disposal. With the increased use of disposable protective clothing, gloves, and other PPE, the volume of waste for discard will also increase.

Biohazard Bags

Plastic bags are appropriate for disposal of most infectious waste materials, but rigid, impermeable containers should be used for disposal of sharps and broken glassware (see Fig. 2-4). Plastic bags with the biohazard symbols and lettering prominently visible can be used in secondary metal or plastic containers. These containers can be decontaminated or disposed of on a regular basis or immediately when visibly contaminated. These biohazard containers should be used for all blood, body fluids, tissues, and other disposable materials contaminated with infectious agents and should be handled with gloves.

FINAL DECONTAMINATION OF WASTE MATERIALS

The control of infectious, chemical, and radioactive waste is regulated by a variety of government agencies, including OSHA and the U.S. Food and Drug Administration (FDA). Legislation and regulations that affect laboratories include the Resource Recovery and Conservation Act (RCRA), the Toxic Substances Control Act (TOSCA), clean air and water laws, "right-to-know" laws, and HAZCOM (chemical hazard communication). Laboratories should implement applicable federal, state, and local laws that pertain to hazardous material and waste management by establishing safety policies. Laboratories with multiple agencies should follow the guidelines of the most stringent agency. Safety policies should be reviewed and signed annually or whenever a change is instituted. Employers are responsible for ensuring that personnel follow the safety policies.

Infectious Waste

Infectious waste, such as contaminated gauze squares and test tubes, must be discarded in proper biohazard containers. These containers should have the following characteristics:

1. Conspicuously marked "Biohazard" and bear the universal biohazard symbol
2. Display the universal color: orange, orange and black, or red
3. Rigid, leakproof, and puncture resistant; cardboard boxes lined with leakproof plastic bags are available
4. Used for blood and certain body fluids, as well as for disposable materials contaminated with blood and fluids

If the primary infectious waste containers are red plastic bags, they should be kept in secondary metal or plastic cans. Extreme care should be taken not to contaminate the exterior of these bags. If they do become contaminated on the outside, the entire bag must be placed into another red plastic bag. Secondary plastic or metal cans should be decontaminated regularly and immediately after any grossly visible contamination, with an agent such as a 1:10 solution of household bleach.

Terminal disposal of infectious waste should be by incineration, but an alternate method of terminal sterilization is autoclaving. Material that is to be autoclaved should be loosely packed so the steam can circulate freely around it. Autoclaving depends on humidity, temperature, and time. Under pressure, steam becomes hotter than boiling water and kills bacteria much more quickly; therefore, autoclaves must be used with caution. Autoclaves should be monitored regularly for their performance in adequately sterilizing the materials to be decontaminated. This monitoring procedure should be part of the ongoing quality assurance program for the laboratory.

If incineration is not done in the health care facility or by an outside contractor, all contaminated disposable items should be autoclaved before leaving the facility for disposal with routine waste. Disposal of medical waste should be done by licensed organizations that will ensure that no environmental contamination or esthetically displeasing incident occurs. The U.S. Congress has passed various acts and regulations regarding the proper handling of medical waste to assist the EPA to carry out this process in the most prudent manner.

Radioactive Waste

The Nuclear Regulatory Commission (NRC) regulates the methods of disposal of radioactive waste. Radioactive waste associated with the radioimmunoassay (RIA) laboratory must be disposed of with special caution. In general, low-level RIA radioactive waste can be discharged in small amounts into the sewer with copious amounts of water. This practice will probably be illegal in the future; therefore the best method of disposal is to store the used material in a locked, marked room until the background count is down to 10 half-lives for radioiodine (^{125}I). It can then be disposed with other refuse. Meticulous records are required to document the amounts and methods of disposal.

BASIC FIRST-AID PROCEDURES

Because of the many potential hazards in a clinical laboratory, knowledge of basic first aid should be an integral part of any educational program in the clinical laboratory. The first priority should be removal of the accident victim from further injury, followed by definitive action or first aid to the victim. By definition, *first aid* is the immediate care of a person who has been injured or acutely ill. Any person who attempts to perform first aid before professional treatment can be arranged should remember that such assistance is only temporary. Stop bleeding, prevent shock, and then treat the wound—in that order.

A rule to remember in dealing with emergencies in the laboratory is to keep calm. This is not always easy but is important to the victim's well-being. Keep crowds of people away, and give the victim plenty of fresh air. Because many injuries may be extreme, and because immediate care is critical with such injuries, all laboratory personnel must thoroughly understand the application of the proper first-aid procedures. Every student or person working in the medical laboratory should learn the following more common emergencies and appropriate first-aid procedures:

1. **Alkali or acid burns on the skin or in the mouth**. Rinse thoroughly with large amounts of running tap water. If the burns are serious, consult a physician.
2. **Alkali or acid burns in the eye**. Wash out eye thoroughly with running water for a minimum of 15 minutes. Help the victim by holding the eyelid open so water can make contact with the eye. An eye fountain is recommended for this purpose, but any running water will suffice. Use of an eyecup is discouraged. A physician should be notified immediately, while the eye is being washed.
3. **Heat burns**. Apply cold running water (or ice in water) to relieve the pain and stop further tissue damage. Use a wet dressing of 2 tablespoons of sodium bicarbonate in 1 quart of warm water. Apply the bandage securely but not tightly. In the case of a third-degree burn (the skin is burned off), do not use ointments or grease, and consult a physician immediately.
4. **Minor cuts**. Wash the wound carefully and thoroughly with soap and water. Remove all foreign material, such as glass, that projects from the wound, but do not gouge for embedded material. Removal is best accomplished by careful washing. Apply a clean bandage if necessary.
5. **Serious cuts**. Apply direct pressure to the wound area to control the bleeding, using the hand over a clean compress covering the wound. Call for a physician immediately.

For victims of serious laboratory accidents such as burns, medical assistance should be summoned while first aid is being administered. With general accidents, competent medical help should be sought as soon as possible after the first-aid treatment has been completed. In cases of chemical burns, especially when the eyes are involved, speed in treatment is most essential.

Remember that first aid is useful not only in your working environment, but also at home and in your community. It deserves your earnest attention and study.

CASE STUDY

CASE STUDY 1-1

Charlie is a laboratory technologist on the midnight shift at a 125-bed rural community hospital. He has worked at this institution for 25 years, always on the midnight shift. He is known for taking shortcuts to get his work out faster, but he is reliable, and management is reluctant to counsel him. It is difficult to find qualified employees in the rural areas. The work gets done quickly, and Charlie has ample time to work in a stress-free environment. A typical night for Charlie is as follows:

Charlie arrives at 10:55 PM to clock in for his shift, which begins at 11 PM. He is wearing his usual clothes: jeans, a red plaid flannel shirt with the long sleeves rolled up to just below the elbow, heavy white socks, and sandals that he has worn for years. He has an unkempt 2-inch beard and dirty fingernails. His hair is thinning and often smells because he only washes it when he has his hair cut. He puts on his lab coat but removes it as soon as the evening shift is gone. He is responsible for collecting blood from patients in the emergency department (ED) as well as STATs on the nursing divisions. He has been assigned additional PM tasks to perform during the downtimes at night.

Tonight Charlie is updating the chemical inventory. His supervisor has asked him to collect any chemicals that are out of date or no longer used and to box them up for disposal. As he scans the shelves, Charlie notices that there is a liter of glacial acetic acid on the top shelf that has been in the lab for years. He is not sure when it was opened because the date is missing, but he knows the chemical is no longer used, and he puts it in the box for disposal. He also finds a small bottle of sodium azide and puts it in the disposal box as well. He continues to check the inventory, and all chemicals on the list are accounted for in the upper cabinets in the lab. There are two new chemicals that come with the chemistry kits, but he doesn't bother to add them to the list. He will leave that for the day shift.

Evaluation time is next month, and Charlie wants to make a good impression on his supervisor. She has made a few comments on his appearance, which he has chosen to ignore, but he wants to be on her good side. Charlie decides to save the lab money and dispose of the acetic acid and sodium azide himself by pouring them down the drain. Charlie knows that lab packs are expensive, and the "stuff" just goes into the septic tank used by the hospital.

Charlie receives a call from the ED. A 17-year-old girl with severe abrasions about the head and

Continued

face has been brought in by her mother. The physician orders a CBC and BMP. When Charlie goes to collect the blood, he does not wear any personal protective equipment (PPE). He never wears gloves to draw blood; he says it interferes with his ability to find the vein. The night nurse insists that he wear gloves, and he reluctantly puts them on. After she leaves the room, he pulls off the index finger of the glove on his left hand so he can feel the vein. After he gets the sample, he discards the needle in the sharps container by unscrewing the needle, then sticks the single-use needle holder in his jeans pocket. He draws the blood, placing the unlabeled tubes in his shirt pocket, grabs the paperwork, and hurries off to the lab to begin the tests.

When Charlie returns to the lab, he opens the EDTA tube for the CBC and checks the tube for clots before placing it on the instrument. He puts the sticks used to rim the tube on the counter. He runs the CBC on the instrument without running a set of controls. He knows that the evening shift just left an hour ago and that the controls they ran were "OK." He puts the sticks in the trash can, then cleans up a spill with a dry paper towel. He doesn't notice that the sleeve at the elbow of his shirt absorbed some of the blood before he could clean it up.

Charlie's supervisor left him a note to change the gas tank on the incubator. Charlie removes the valves and replaces the tank. He leaves the empty tank sitting beside the newly installed tank. His supervisor also asked him to check the eyewash; Charlie was supposed to do this 2 weeks ago but forgot. He removes the eyewash caps, turns the water on and off quickly, and replaces the caps.

Now that the ED work is over, Charlie decides to have his supper. Just as he is about to eat, the phone rings regarding a STAT in the ICU. Charlie puts his lunch on the counter and goes to collect the samples. When he returns, he puts the samples in the centrifuge. While the samples spin, he uses the restroom and finishes his food. He puts the specimens on the chemistry analyzer and continues to drink his soda while waiting for the results.

At 6:45 AM, Charlie puts on his lab coat again as the day shift arrives. At 7:30 AM, he hangs the coat up with the lab coats that have just been delivered from the laundry and hurries out the door, happy to be heading home.

The Challenge
Sorry, Charlie, but you need an extreme makeover of your safety habits. As a laboratory administrator, identify the issues and how you would handle the situation.

Terry Jo Gile is an internationally recognized consultant, speaker, and author. She helps organizations create "safety savvy" laboratories. She may be reached through her website www.safetylady.com.

REFERENCES

1. Occupational Safety and Health Administration, US Department of Labor: Occupational exposure to bloodborne pathogens: final rule, Federal Register 56(235), 1991:(29 CFR 1910.1030, 64003-64182; Part 1910 to title 29 of Code of Federal Regulations).
2. Occupational Safety and Health Administration, Department of Labor: Occupational exposure to hazardous chemicals in laboratories: final rule, Federal Register 55(21), 1990:(29 CFR 1910.1450, 3327–3335).
3. Clinical and Laboratory Standards Institute (CLSI) Protection of laboratory workers from infectious disease transmitted by blood, body fluids, and tissue: tentative guideline, ed 3, Wayne, PA, 2005, CLSI, M29–A3.
4. Centers for Disease Control and Prevention, US Department of Health and Human Services: Update: universal precautions for prevention of transmission of human immunodeficiency virus, hepatitis B virus, and other bloodborne pathogens in health-care settings, MMWR Morb Mortal Wkly Rep 37(24):377, 1988.
5. Centers for Disease Control and Prevention US Department of Health and Human Services: Guidelines for environmental infection control in health-care facilities, Washington, D.C, 2003, HHS.
6. Americans with Disabilities Act and Amendments, www.ada.gov, retrieved August 13, 2009.
7. National Health care Safety Network, www.cdc, retrieved August 15, 2009
8. Occupational Safety and Health Administration, US Department of Labor: Occupational safety and health standards, Fed Regist 43:52952–53014, 1978.
9. Occupational Safety and Health Administration, US Department of Labor: Permissible exposure limits (PELs), www.osha.gov/SLTC/pel/(retrieved August 2005).
10. Centers for Disease Control and Prevention, US Department of Health and Human Services: Recommendations for prevention of HIV transmission in health-care settings, MMWR Morb Mortal Wkly Rep 36(suppl):3s, 1987.
11. HIV and AIDS in America, www.avert.org/aids-america.htm (retrieved August 15, 2009).
12. Centers for Disease Control and Prevention, US Department of Health and Human Services: Guideline for hand hygiene in health care settings, MMWR Morb Mortal Wkly Rep 51(RR-16):1–44, 2002.
13. Rutala WA, DJ: Weber and the Health care Infection Control Practices Advisory Committee (HICPAC), Guideline for Disinfection and Sterilization in Health care Facilities, 2008:retrieved August 16, 2009 www.cdc.gov.
14. Clinical Laboratory and Standards Institute (CLSI) Protection of laboratory workers from infectious disease transmitted by blood, body fluids and tissue: approved guideline, ed 3, Wayne, PA, 2005, CLSI, M29–A3.
15. Centers for Disease Control and Prevention, US Department of Health and Human Services MMWR 57(18): 494–498, 2008.
16. Centers for Disease Control and Prevention, US Department of Health and Human Services: MMWR Updated US Public Health Service guidelines for the management of occupational exposure to HIV and recommendations for postexposure prophylaxis, www.cdc.gov (retrieved April 2006).
17. Centers for Disease Control and Prevention, US Department of Health and Human Services: Updated US Public Health Service guidelines for the management of occupational exposures to HBV, HCV, and HIV and recommendations for postexposure prophylaxis, MMWR Morb Mortal Wkly Rep 50(RR-11), 2001.
18. Roark J: HICPAC revises isolation and TB guidelines, www.infectioncontroltoday.com (retrieved May 2005).

19. Centers for Disease Control and Prevention, US Department of Health and Human Services: Hospital Infection Control Practices Advisory Committee (HICPAC): Guidelines for isolation precautions in hospitals, Philadelphia, 1996, HHS.
20. Clinical and Laboratory Standards Institute (CLSI): Clinical laboratory waste management; approved guideline, ed. 2, Wayne, PA, 2002, CLSI, GP5–A2.
21. Occupational Safety and Health Administration, Department of Labor: Standards for the tracking and management of medical waste: interim final rule and request for comments, Fed Regist 54(107):24310–24311, 1989.

BIBLIOGRAPHY

All you ever wanted to know about fire extinguishers, www.handord.gov/fire/safety/extingrs.htm (retrieved May 2005).

Burtis CA, Ashwood ER, Bruns DE: Tietz fundamentals of clinical chemistry, ed 6, St Louis, 2008, Saunders.

Centers for Disease Control and Prevention, US Department of Health and Human Services: Protection against viral hepatitis: recommendations of the Immunization Practices Advisory Committee, MMWR Morb Mortal Wkly Rep 39:1, 1990.

Centers for Disease Control and Prevention, US Department of Health and Human Services: Provisional public health service recommendations for chemoprophylaxis after occupational exposure to HIV, MMWR Morb Mortal Wkly Rep 45:468, 1996.

Centers for Disease Control and Prevention, US Department of Health and Human Services: Surveillance of health care personnel with HIV/AIDS, as of December 2002, http://www.cdc.gov/ncidod/dhqp/bp_hiv_hp_with.html (retrieved Nov 2009).

Clinical Laboratory and Standards Institute (CLSI): Clinical laboratory safety: approved guideline, ed 2, Wayne, PA, 2004, CLSI, GP17–A2.

Downer K: The debate on HIV screening, Clin Lab News 31(8):1, 2005.

Gile TJ: Laboratory training: safety at any age, MLO Med Lab Obs 37(8):28, 2005.

Harty-Golder B: Prepare for occupational bloodborne pathogen exposure, MLO Med Lab Obs vol. 41, no. 4:40, April 2009.

Kaplan LA, Pesce AJ: Clinical chemistry: theory, analysis, and correlation, ed 5, St Louis, 2010, Mosby.

Sebazcp S: Considerations for immunization programs, www.infectioncontroltoday.com/articles/0a1feat4.html (retrieved May 2005).

Williams D: Address deficiencies in bloodborne pathogens exposure management, MLO Med Lab Obs vol. 41, no. 7:24, July, 2009:26.

REVIEW QUESTIONS

Questions 1-4: Match each of the following acronyms with the agency it represents (a to e).

1. ___ **CAP**

2. ___ **CLSI**

3. ___ **CDC**

4. ___ **OSHA**
   a. College of American Pathologists
   b. Occupational Safety and Health Administration
   c. Clinical and Laboratory Standards Institute
   d. Centers for Disease Control and Prevention
   e. Communicable Disease Center

5. **Which of the following acts, agencies, or organizations is primarily responsible for safeguards and regulations to ensure a safe and healthful workplace?**
   a. Health care Finance Administration
   b. Occupational Safety and Health Administration
   c. Clinical Laboratory Improvement Act, 1988
   d. Centers for Disease Control and Prevention

6. **The OSHA hazard communication standard, the "right-to-know" rule, is designed for what purpose?**
   a. To avoid lawsuits
   b. To protect laboratory staff
   c. To protect patients
   d. To establish safety standards

7. **Where appropriate, the OSHA standards provide:**
   a. provisions for warning labels.
   b. exposure control procedures.
   c. implementation of training and education programs.
   d. all of the above.

8. **To comply with various federal safety regulations, each laboratory must have which of the following?**
   a. A chemical hygiene plan
   b. A safety manual
   c. Biohazard labels in place
   d. All of the above

9. **The simplest and single most important step in proper handling of any hazardous substance is:**
   a. wearing disposable gloves.
   b. wearing safety glasses.
   c. properly labeling containers.
   d. using a biosafety hood.

Questions 10-13: Match the color triangles of the hazards identification system with the following hazards (a to d).

10. ___ **Blue**

11. ___ **Red**

12. ___ **Yellow**

13. ___ **White**
    a. Flammability
    b. Reactivity-stability hazard
    c. Special hazard information
    d. Health hazard

14. **The term *Standard Precautions* refers to:**
    a. treating all specimens as if they are infectious.
    b. assuming that every direct contact with a body fluid is infectious.

c. treating only blood or blood-tinged specimens as infectious.
d. both a and b.

15. **The term *biohazard* denotes:**
    a. infectious materials that present a risk to the health of humans in the laboratory.
    b. infectious materials that present a potential risk to the health of humans in the laboratory.
    c. agents that present a chemical risk or potential risk to the health of humans in the laboratory.
    d. both a and b

16. **The CDC Bloodborne Pathogen Standard and the OSHA Occupational Exposure Standard mandate:**
    a. education and training of all health care workers in Standard Precautions.
    b. proper handling of chemicals.
    c. calibration of equipment.
    d. fire extinguisher maintenance.

17. **The most common source of human immunodeficiency virus (HIV) in the occupational setting is:**
    a. saliva.
    b. urine.
    c. blood.
    d. cerebrospinal fluid.

Questions 18 and 19: Transmission to medical personnel of (18) ___ is more probable than (19) ___ in unvaccinated individuals.

18. a. Human immunodeficiency virus (HIV)
    b. Hepatitis B virus (HBV)
    c. Hepatitis C virus (HCV)
    d. Malaria

19. a. Human immunodeficiency virus (HIV)
    b. Hepatitis B virus (HBV)
    c. Hepatitis C virus (HCV)
    d. Malaria

Questions 20-22: A = True or B = False.

20. ___ Sterile gloves should be worn for all laboratory procedures.

21. ___ Gloves must be worn when receiving phlebotomy training.

22. ___ Gloves should be changed between each patient contact.

Questions 23-25: A = True or B = False.
Hands should be washed:

23. ___ after removing gloves.

24. ___ after leaving the laboratory.

25. ___ before and after using the bathroom.

26. **Decontaminate hands after:**
    a. contact with patient's skin.
    b. contact with blood or body fluids.
    c. removing gloves.
    d. all of the above.

27. **All work surfaces should be sanitized at the end of the shift with a solution of:**
    a. 5% bleach
    b. 5% phenol
    c. 10% bleach
    d. concentrated bleach

28. **Clinical laboratory personnel need to have demonstrable immunity to:**
    a. rubella.
    b. polio.
    c. hepatitis B.
    d. both a and c.

Questions 29-31: Match the type of fire extinguisher with the class of fire (a to c).

29. ___ Class A

30. ___ Class B

31. ___ Class C
    a. Paper
    b. Electrical
    c. Gasoline

32. **Terminal waste of infectious material can be processed by autoclaving or by:**
    a. incineration.
    b. soaking in bleach.
    c. ethylene dioxide gas.
    d. normal garbage disposal.

33. **Immediate first aid for acid burns on the skin is:**
    a. ice.
    b. running water.
    c. Vaseline.
    d. butter.

CHAPTER 3

PHLEBOTOMY: COLLECTING AND PROCESSING BLOOD

Learning Objectives

At the conclusion of this chapter, the student will be able to:

- Identify seven factors that should be monitored by quality assessment methods.
- Demonstrate and describe the skills needed to interact with patients when collecting specimens.
- Explain the Patient Care Partnership and its importance.
- Describe the principles and applications of Standard Precautions.

Continued

- Describe the equipment used for venous blood collection.

- Explain and demonstrate the proper collection technique for venous blood.

- Identify the color codes of evacuated tubes with the additives contained in the tubes.

- Compare common anticoagulants and additives used to preserve blood specimens and the general use of each type of anticoagulant.

- Describe the mode of action of EDTA and heparin.

- Identify the major potential type of error in specimen collection.

- List and explain five specific situations that could complicate venipuncture site selection.

- Identify eight typical phlebotomy problems, and describe the solution for each problem.

- Explain some techniques for obtaining blood from small or difficult veins.

- Describe special blood-collection considerations for pediatric and geriatric patients.

- List the six categories of phlebotomy complications, and describe the symptoms and treatment for each type of complication.

- Demonstrate and describe the proper technique for collecting a capillary blood specimen.

- Describe relevant medical-legal issues related to specimen collection.

QUALITY ASSESSMENT

The term **quality assessment** or the older term, **quality assurance**, is used to describe management of the treatment of the whole patient (see Chapter 8). As it applies to the clinical laboratory, quality assessment requires establishing policies that maintain and control processes involving the patient and laboratory analysis of specimens. Quality assessment includes monitoring the following specimen collection measures:

- Preparation of a patient for any specimens to be collected
- Collection of valid samples
- Proper specimen transport
- Performance of the requested laboratory analyses
- Validation of test results
- Recording and reporting the assay results
- Transmitting test results to the patient's medical record
- Documentation, maintenance, and availability of records describing quality assessment practices and quality control measures

The accuracy of laboratory testing begins with the quality of the specimen received by the laboratory. This quality depends on how a specimen was collected, transported, and processed. A laboratory assay will be no better than the specimen on which it is performed. If a preanalytical error occurs , the most perfect analysis is invalid and cannot be used by the physician in diagnosis or treatment.

Venous or arterial blood collection, phlebotomy, and capillary blood collect remain an error prone phase of the testing cycle. In the United States, it is estimated that more than 1 billion venipunctures

are performed annually, and errors occurring within this process may cause serious harm to patients, either directly or indirectly. The top 5 causes of preanalytical errors have been reported as:[1]

1. Specimen collection tube not filled properly.
2. Patient identification error.
3. Inappropriate specimen collection tube or container.
4. Test request error.
5. An empty collection tube.

Patient Care Partnership

The delivery of health care involves a partnership between patients and physicians and other health care professionals. When collecting blood specimens, it is important that the phlebotomist consider the rights of the patient at all times. The American Hospital Association[2] has developed the **Patient Care Partnership** document, which replaces the former Patient's Bill of Rights. This document stresses:

- High-quality hospital care
- A clean and safe environment
- Involvement by patients in their care
- Protection of patients' privacy
- Help for patients when leaving the hospital
- Help for patients with billing claims

Patients themselves or another person chosen by the patient can exercise these patient rights. A proxy decision maker can act on the patient's behalf if the patient lacks decision-making ability, is legally incompetent, or is a minor.

The partnership nature of health care requires that patients—or their families or surrogates—take part in their care. As such, patients are responsible for providing an accurate medical history and any written advance directives, following hospital rules and regulations, and complying with activities that contribute to a healthy lifestyle.

Pediatric Patients

When working with children, it is important to be gentle and compassionate. Attempt to interact with the pediatric patient, realizing that both the patient and the parent (if present) may have anxiety about the procedure and may be unfamiliar with the clinical setting. Acknowledge both the parent and the child.

Don't hurry; allow enough time for the procedure. It is important to take extra time to gain a child's confidence before proceeding with specimen collection. When working with pediatric patients, it is important to bolster their morale as much as possible. Ask for help in restraining a very small or uncooperative child. Older children may be more responsive when permitted to "help" (e.g., by holding the gauze).

In the nursery, each hospital will have its own rules, but a few general precautions apply. After working with an infant in a crib, the crib sides must be returned to the precollection position. If an infant is in an incubator, the portholes should be closed as much as possible. When oxygen is in use, do not forget to close the openings when the collection process is completed. Dispose of all waste materials properly.

Adolescent Patients

When obtaining a blood specimen from an adolescent, it is important to be relaxed and alert to possible anxiety. Adolescents may mask their anxiety. General interaction techniques include allowing enough time for the procedure, establishing eye contact, and allowing the patient to maintain a sense of control.

Adult Patients

Adult patients must be told briefly what is expected of them and what the test involves. Complete honesty is important. The patient should be greeted in a friendly and tactful manner. Without becoming overly familiar, a pleasant conversation can be started. The patient should be told about the purpose of the blood collection. Any personal information revealed by the patient is told in confidence. The patient's religious beliefs should be respected, laboratory reports kept confidential, and any personal information also kept in confidence. Information about other patients or physicians is always kept

confidential. If the same patient is seen frequently, the phlebotomist may become familiar with the patient's interests, hobbies, or family and use these as topics of conversation. Many patients in the hospital are lonely; kindness is greatly appreciated. Occasionally, especially if extremely ill, the patient will not want to talk at all, and this should be respected. It is important to be honest but also attempt to boost the patient's morale as much as possible.

Even if the patient is disagreeable, the phlebotomist should remain pleasant. A smile can often work miracles. It is important to be firm when the patient is unpleasant, to remain cheerful, and to express confidence in the work to be done.

In a hospital setting, before leaving the patient's room, the area should be checked to see that everything is in place in the laboratory tray and that the room has been left as it was found. The tray holding the blood collection supplies and equipment should always be kept out of reach of the patient. All sharps and supplies should be disposed of properly.

Geriatric Patients

It is extremely important to treat geriatric patients with dignity and respect and not demean them. It is best to address the patient with a more formal title, such as Mrs., Ms., or Mr., rather than by his or her first name. As with patients in general, older patients may enjoy a short conversation. Keep a flexible agenda so enough time is allowed. If a patient appears to be having difficulty hearing, speak slightly slower and louder.

Problem Patients

Occasionally, a patient will be combative. This may be the result of alcohol ingestion, drug use, or a psychiatric condition. In some of these cases, such as with mentally challenged patients, the phlebotomist would need the written permission of a parent, guardian, or conservator. This is the same requirement as drawing blood from a minor—a patient younger than 18 years of age. Because injury to the patient or the phlebotomist could result from performing a phlebotomy, a supervisor should be consulted. The supervisor could consult with the patient's physician regarding how to proceed with this patient.

INFECTION CONTROL
Isolation as Safety System

Isolation was once understood as the separation of a seriously ill patient to stop the spread of infection to others or to protect the patient from irritating factors. The term *isolation* has changed from meaning a special set of precautions performed by a few health care providers for a select few patients to a safety system that is practiced by everyone in the course of routine patient care. Isolation precautions are now a routine part of the everyday work process.

Modern isolation techniques incorporate a broad-based theory that addresses the needs of both patients and employees to ensure that the safest possible environment is maintained throughout the health care facility. Current guidelines use a two-tiered strategy to create this safety system.

Standard and Additional Precautions

The concept of Standard Precautions forces health care professionals to change the way they view infection control. A two-tiered system has been developed, the goal of which is to minimize the risk of infection and maximize the safety level within the health care facility's environment.

The first tier of infection control is the practice of Standard Precautions. Standard Precautions theory recognizes the need to reduce the risk of microbial transmission, including HIV, from both identified and unidentified sources of infection. These precautions require that protective protocols be followed whenever contact is made with blood and body fluids.

A second tier of an infection control system was developed to provide additional precautions to control the transmission of infectious agents under special circumstances when Standard Precautions alone may not be enough. Transmission-based precautions are divided into three basic categories: contact, airborne, and droplet.

Contact Precautions

Contact precautions are designed to stop the spread of microorganisms via direct contact, such as skin-to-skin contact and indirect contact, which is usually the result of a person making contact with a contaminated inanimate object. Contact precautions include wearing gloves when making contact with the patient's skin or with inanimate objects that have been in direct contact with the patient. The use of gowns may be mandated when the health care worker's clothing is likely to come in contact with the patient or items in the patient's room.

Airborne Precautions

Airborne precautions are designed to provide protection from extremely tiny airborne bacteria or dust particles, which may be suspended in the air for an extended period. Guidelines include the use of respiratory protection and the use of special air-handling systems to control airborne bacteria.

Droplet Precautions

Droplet precautions protect health care workers, visitors, and other patients from droplets, which may be expelled during coughing, sneezing, or talking. Guidelines include using a mask when working close to the patient. Guidelines for patient placement, from the use of a private room to using a room with special air-handling capabilities, should be implemented as well. Specific guidelines for transport and placement of patients and the environmental management of equipment should be implemented according to each category's requirements.

SPECIMEN COLLECTION

Blood is the type of specimen most frequently analyzed in the clinical laboratory. Urine specimens and body fluids are also frequently analyzed (see Chapters 14 and 15). Fecal specimens (see Chapter 9, POCT) and other specimens such as throat cultures and swabs from wound abscesses are sent to the microbiology laboratory for study (see Chapter 16).

Knowledge of proper collection, preservation, and processing of specimens is essential. A properly collected blood specimen is crucial to quality performance in the laboratory. In addition to specimen procurement, related areas of specimen transportation, handling, and processing must also be fully understood by anyone who collects or handles blood specimens.

Strict adherence to the rules of specimen collection is critical to the accuracy of any test. Errors such as identification errors, either of the patient or the specimen, are major potential sources of error.

The Phlebotomist

Blood specimens may be collected by health care personnel with several different educational backgrounds, depending on the facility. In some institutions, blood specimen collection is done by the clinical laboratory scientist/medical technologist or the clinical laboratory technician/medical laboratory technician. In other institutions, specially trained individuals, phlebotomists, perform blood collections.

The role of the phlebotomist has never been more important to the patient and the laboratory. Phlebotomists in the hospital, clinic, or drawing station have a major impact on the impression patients develop of the entire laboratory. Phlebotomists are laboratory ambassadors These members of the team must demonstrate professionalism by their conduct, appearance, composure, and communication skills. Critical thinking skills are essential for phlebotomists. They must make effective decisions and solve problems, frequently under conditions of stress.[3]

More than two-thirds of laboratory errors are caused by mistakes before testing, or preanalytical errors (see Chapter 8). Phlebotomists can reduce these mistakes by being well trained and constantly alert to sources of error.

The phlebotomist is expected to deliver unexcelled customer satisfaction. It is important to understand and know the patient's expectations, manage unrealistic expectations through patient education, and be diplomatic with patient complaints. If a patient is unhappy, the phlebotomist should listen with interest, express genuine concern, and make an attempt to resolve the issue of concern. If the phlebotomist is directly at fault, an apology would be appropriate.

Blood Collection Variables

Most clinical laboratory determinations are done on whole blood, plasma, or serum. Blood specimens may be drawn from fasting or nonfasting patients. The **fasting state** is defined as having no food or liquid other than water for 8 to 12 hours before blood collection. Fasting specimens are not necessary for most laboratory determinations. Blood from fasting patients is usually drawn in the morning before breakfast.

Blood collected directly after a meal is described as a **postprandial specimen**. In the case of blood glucose, a sample may be collected 2 hours postprandially. After 2 hours, blood glucose levels should return to almost fasting levels in patients who are not diabetic. Blood should not be collected while intravenous solutions are being administered, if possible.

Food intake, medication, activity, and time of day can all influence the laboratory results for blood specimens. It is critically important to control preanalytical variables such as timed drawing of a specimen, peak and trough drug levels, and postmedication conditions. Other controllable biological variations in blood include:

- Posture (whether the patient is lying in bed or standing up)
- Immobilization (e.g., resulting from prolonged bed rest)
- Exercise
- Circadian/diurnal variations (cyclical variations throughout the day)
- Recent food ingestion (e.g., caffeine effect)
- Smoking (nicotine effect)
- Alcohol ingestion

Blood Collection Procedures

There are two general sources of blood for clinical laboratory tests: venous blood and peripheral (or capillary) blood. The CLSI has set standards for the collection of **venous blood (venipuncture, or phlebotomy)** and **capillary blood (skin puncture)**.[4-5] Arterial blood may be needed to perform specific procedures such as blood gas analysis.

Layers of Normal Anticoagulated Blood

In vivo (in the body) the blood is in a liquid form, but in vitro (outside the body) it will clot in a few minutes. Blood that is freshly drawn into a glass tube appears as a translucent, dark red fluid. In minutes it will start to clot, or coagulate, forming a semisolid jelly-like mass. If left undisturbed in the tube, this mass will begin to shrink, or retract, in about 1 hour. Complete retraction normally takes place within 24 hours.

When coagulation occurs, a pale yellow fluid called *serum* separates from the clot and appears in the upper portion of the tube. During the process of coagulation, certain factors present in the original blood sample are depleted, or used up. Fibrinogen is one important substance found in circulating blood (in the plasma portion) that is necessary for coagulation to occur. Fibrinogen is converted to fibrin when clotting occurs, and the fibrin lends structure to the clot in the form of fine threads in which the red blood cells (RBCs, erythrocytes) and the white blood cells (WBCs, leukocytes) are embedded. To assist in obtaining serum, collection tubes with a separator gel additive are used. Serum is used extensively for chemical, serologic, and other laboratory testing and can be obtained from the tube of clotted blood by centrifuging.

When fresh whole blood is mixed with substances that prevent blood clotting, called **anticoagulants**, the blood can be separated into plasma, a straw-colored fluid, and the cellular components: erythrocytes, leukocytes, and platelets (thrombocytes). Whole blood that is allowed to clot normally produces the straw-colored serum.

When an anticoagulated blood specimen is allowed to stand for a time, the components will settle into three distinct layers (Fig. 3-1):

1. Plasma, the top layer, a liquid that normally represents about 55% of the total blood volume
2. Buffy coat, a grayish white cellular middle layer composed of WBCs and platelets, normally about 1% of the total blood volume
3. Erythrocytes, the bottom layer, consisting of packed RBCs and normally about 45% of the total blood volume

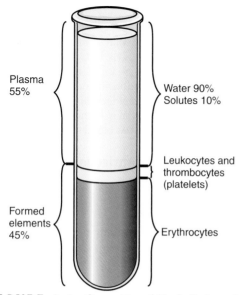

FIGURE 3-1 **Composition of blood.** (Redrawn from Applegate E: The anatomy and physiology learning system, ed 4, St Louis, 2011, Saunders.)

Environmental Factors Associated With Evacuated Blood Collection Tubes

A variety of environment factors can affect the quality of evacuated tubes used to collect blood. These factors can then influence the published expiration dates of the evacuated tubes.[6] Environmental factors affecting evacuated tubes include:

- Ambient temperature
- Altitude
- Humidity
- Sunlight

Ambient Temperature

If evacuated tubes are stored at low temperature, the pressure of the gas inside the tube will decrease. This would lead to an increase in draw volume for the evacuated tube. Conversely, higher temperatures could cause reductions in draw volume.

Increased temperatures in evacuated tubes can also have a negative impact on the stability of certain tube additives such as biochemicals or gel. Gel is a compound that could potentially degrade when exposed to high temperatures.

Altitude

In situations where blood is drawn at high altitudes (>5000 feet), the draw volume may be affected. Because the ambient pressure at high altitude is lower than at sea level, the pressure of the residual gas inside the tube will reach this reduced ambient pressure during filling earlier than if the tube were drawn at sea level. The resulting draw volume will be lower.

Humidity

The impact of storage under different humidity conditions can affect only plastic evacuated tubes, owing to the greater permeability of these materials to water vapor relative to glass. Conditions of very high humidity could lead to the migration of water vapor inside a tube that contains a moisture-sensitive material, such as a lyophilized additive. Conditions of very low humidity could hasten the escape of water vapor from a tube containing a wet additive. It is possible that such storage conditions could compromise the accuracy of clinical results.

Light

A special additive mixture for coagulation testing that is sensitive to light and found only in glass evacuated tubes is called CTAD (citric acid, theophylline, adenosine, and dipyridamole). The CTAD mixture minimizes platelet activation after blood collection. Normally, this additive has a slightly yellow appearance that becomes clear when no longer viable. These tubes are generally packaged in small quantities to minimize exposure to light.

Expiration Dates of Evacuated Tubes

Expiration dates are determined through shelf-life testing performed under known environmental conditions. Shelf life of an evacuated tube is defined by (1) the stability of the additive and (2) vacuum retention. Most evacuated tubes on the market have at least a 12-month shelf life. It is important that tubes be stored under recommended conditions.

The expiration dates of glass tubes are generally limited by the shelf life of the additives, because vacuum and water vapor losses are minimal over time. Exposure to irradiation during sterilization of tubes and to moisture or light during the shelf life of the product can limit the stability of biochemical additives. The expiration dates of evacuated plastic tubes are also limited by the same factors that affect glass tubes. Evacuated plastic tubes do sustain a measurable loss of vacuum over time, and some evacuated plastic blood collection tubes may have their expiration dates determined by their ability to assure a known draw volume.

It is important to understand that evacuated blood collection tubes are not completely evacuated. There is a small amount of gas (air) still residing in the tube, at low pressure. The higher the pressure of the gas inside the tube on the date of manufacture, the lower the intended draw volume will be for a tube of a given size. The draw volume specified for a given tube is achieved by manufacturing the tube at a designated evacuation pressure.

The dynamics of blood collection inside the tube are based on the ideal gas law:

$$PV = nRT$$

In the equation, P is the pressure inside the tube, V is the volume that the gas occupies, n is the number of moles of gas inside the tube, R is the universal gas constant, and T is the temperature inside the tube.

According to the equation, if the moles of gas and the temperature do not change, the product of pressure and volume is a constant. When blood starts filling the tube, the residual gas inside is confined into a decreasing volume, causing the pressure of the gas to increase. When the pressure of this gas reaches ambient pressure, the collection process is completed for that tube. The specially designed, single-use needle holder is used to secure the needle. It is no longer acceptable to wash and reuse this plastic needle holder device.[6]

Anticoagulants and Additives in Evacuated Blood Tubes

Evacuated blood collection tubes (see inside front cover) without additives are used to yield serum (or used as a discard tube), other evacuated tubes contain some type of anticoagulant or additive (Table 3-1). The additives range from those that promote faster clotting of the blood to those that preserve or stabilize certain analytes or cells. The inclusion of additives at the proper concentration in evacuated tubes greatly enhances the accuracy and consistency of test results and facilitates faster turnaround times in the laboratory.

The CLSI and International Organization for Standardization (ISO) standards define the concentrations of these additives dispensed into tubes per milliliter of blood.

Anticoagulants

There are several different types of inorganic additives, biochemical additives, or gel in blood collection tubes. Some frequently used anticoagulants are dipotassium ethylenediaminetetraacetic acid (K_2EDTA), sodium citrate, and heparin. Each of the anticoagulant types prevents the coagulation of whole blood. The proper proportion of anticoagulant to whole blood is important to avoid the introduction of errors into test results. The specific type

TABLE 3-1

Examples of Stopper Colors for Venous Blood Collection*	
Color	Additive
Lavender	K 2 EDTA (spray-coated plastic tube) K 3 EDTA (liquid in glass tube)
Pink	K 2 EDTA (spray-coated plastic tube)
Green	Sodium heparin, lithium heparin
Light blue or clear (hemogard closure)	Buffered sodium citrate, citrate, theophylline, adenosine, dipyridamole (CTAD)
White†	K2 EDTA with gel
Red/light gray‡ or clear (hemogard closure)	None (plastic)
Red	Silicone coated (glass) Clot activator, silicone coated (plastic)
Red/gray	
Gold (hemogard closure)	Clot activators and gel

From BD Vacutainer Venous Blood Collection Tube Guide, Courtesy and © Becton, Dickinson and Company.
*See inside book cover for the comprehensive BD Vacutainer Venous Blood Collection Tube Guide including additives, inversions of blood collection and laboratory use.
†New tube for use in molecular diagnostic test methods.
‡New red/light gray for use as a discard tube or secondary specimen tube.

of anticoagulant needed for a procedure should be stated in the laboratory procedure manual.

DIPOTASSIUM EDTA

The salts of the chelating (calcium-binding) agent K_2EDTA are recommended by the International Council for Standardization in Haematology (ICSH) and CLSI as the anticoagulant of choice for blood cell counting and sizing, because they produce less shrinkage of RBCs and less of an increase in cell volume on standing. For hematology applications, EDTA is available in three forms, including dry additives (K_2EDTA) and a liquid additive (K_3EDTA). EDTA prevents clotting by chelating calcium, an important cofactor in coagulation reactions. The amount of EDTA per milliliter of blood is essentially the same for all three forms of EDTA.

EDTA is spray-dried on the interior surface of evacuated plastic tubes. The proper ratio of EDTA to whole blood is important because some test results will be altered if the ratio is incorrect. Excessive EDTA produces shrinkage of erythrocytes, thus affecting tests such as the manually performed packed cell volume or microhematocrit.

SODIUM CITRATE

Sodium citrate in the concentration of a 3.2% solution has been adopted as the appropriate concentration by the ICSH and the International Society for Thrombosis and Hemostasis for coagulation studies. The College of American Pathologists (CAP) also recommends the use of 3.2% sodium citrate.

Sodium citrate is also used as an anticoagulant for activated partial thromboplastin time (APTT) and prothrombin time (PT) testing and for the Westergren erythrocyte sedimentation rate (ESR). The correct ratio of one part anticoagulant to nine parts of whole blood in blood collection tubes is critical. An excess of anticoagulant can alter the expected dilution of blood and produce errors in the results. Because of the dilution of anticoagulant to blood, sodium citrate is generally unacceptable for most other hematology tests.

Citrate, theophylline, adenosine, dipyridamole (CTAD) is used for selected platelet functions and routine coagulation determination.

HEPARIN

Heparin is used as an in vitro and in vivo anticoagulant. It acts as a substance that inactivates the blood-clotting factor, thrombin. It prevents blood coagulation by inhibiting thrombin and factor Xa. Heparin is a common anticoagulant used in chemistry and special chemistry testing. It is the only anticoagulant that should be used in a blood collection device for the determination of pH, blood gases, electrolytes, and ionized calcium. Heparin should not be used for coagulation or hematology testing. It is the recommended anticoagulant for many determinations using whole blood or plasma specimens because of its minimal chelating properties, minimal effects on water shifts, and relatively low cation concentration.

Heparin is available as sodium, lithium, and ammonium salts. Lithium heparin is the recommended form of heparin for use because it is least likely to interfere when performing tests for other ions. Lithium heparin is essentially free of extraneous ions. It should not be used for collection of blood for lithium levels. Only a small amount of heparin is needed, so simply coating the insides of tubes or syringes is often enough to give a good anticoagulant effect. Tubes containing heparin should be inverted 8 times after collection to ensure thorough mixing of the additive with the blood and thus complete anticoagulation of the sample.

Additives

THROMBIN

One type of additive is thrombin, an enzyme that converts fibrinogen to fibrin. Thrombin tubes are often used for STAT serum testing owing to the short clotting time.

SODIUM FLUORIDE

A dry additive and weak anticoagulant, sodium fluoride is used primarily for preservation of blood glucose specimens to prevent glycolysis or destruction of glucose (see Chapter 11).

GEL

The function of additive gel is to provide a physical and chemical barrier between the serum or plasma and the cells. Their use offers significant benefits in collecting, processing, and storage of the specimen in the primary tube.

Separator gels are capable of providing barrier properties because of the way they respond to applied forces. After blood is drawn into the evacuated gel tube, and once centrifugation begins, the g-force applied to the gel causes its viscosity to decrease, enabling it to move or flow. Materials with these flow characteristics are often called *thixotropic*. Once centrifugation ceases, the gel becomes an immobile barrier between the supernatant and the cells. The composite nature of gels gives these gel tubes an infinite shelf life.[6]

ADVERSE EFFECTS OF ADDITIVES

The additives chosen for specific determinations must not alter the blood components or affect the laboratory tests to be done. The following are some adverse effects of using an improper additive or using the wrong amount of additive:

- Interference with the assay. The additive may contain a substance that is the same, or reacts in the same way, as the substance being measured. An example would be the use of sodium oxalate as the anticoagulant for a sodium determination.
- Removal of constituents. The additive may remove the constituent to be measured. An example would be the use of an oxalate anticoagulant for a calcium determination; oxalate removes calcium from the blood by forming an insoluble salt, calcium oxalate.
- Effect on enzyme action. The additive may affect enzyme reactions. An example would be the use of sodium fluoride as an anticoagulant in an enzyme determination; sodium fluoride destroys many enzymes.
- Alteration of cellular constituents. An additive may alter cellular constituents. An example would be the use of an older anticoagulant additive, oxalate, in hematology. Oxalate distorts the cell morphology; RBCs become crenated (shrunken), vacuoles appear in the granulocytes, and bizarre forms of lymphocytes and monocytes appear rapidly when oxalate is used as the anticoagulant. Another example is the use of heparin as an anticoagulant for blood to be used in the preparation of blood films that

will be stained with Wright's stain. Unless the films are stained within 2 hours, heparin gives a blue background with Wright's stain.

- Incorrect amount of anticoagulant. If too little additive is used, partial clotting of whole blood will occur. This interferes with cell counts. By comparison, if too much liquid anticoagulant is used, it dilutes the blood sample and thus interferes with certain quantitative measurements.

Venipuncture Procedure

Safe Blood Collection: Equipment and Supplies

An increased emphasis on safety has led to new product development by various companies. The Becton Dickinson (BD) blood collection products (www.bd.com) include the following:

1. BD Vacutainer Eclipse Blood Collection Needle
2. BD Blood Transfer Device
3. BD Vacutainer Safety-Lok Blood Collection Set
4. BD Vacutainer Plastic Tubes
5. BD Genie Safety Lancets
6. BD Quikheel Safety Lancet

The standard needle for blood collection with a syringe or evacuated blood collection tubes is a 21-gauge needle. Butterfly needles are being used more frequently as the acuity of patients increases. The collecting needle is double pointed; the longer end is for insertion into the patient's vein, and the shorter end pierces the rubber stopper of the collection tube. Sterile needles that fit a standard holder are used. Various needle sizes are available. In addition to length, needles are classified by gauge size; the higher the gauge number, the smaller the inner diameter, or bore.

The specially designed, single-use needle holder is used to secure the needle. It is no longer acceptable to wash and reuse this plastic needle holder device. The BD Vacutainer One Use Holder is a clear plastic needle holder prominently marked with the words "Do Not Reuse" and "Single Use Only." Once a venipuncture is completed, the entire needle and holder assembly is disposed in a sharps container. The needle should not be removed from the holder. No change in venipuncture technique is required with a single-use holder.

On November 6, 2000, the Needlestick Safety and Prevention Act became law. It:

- Requires health care employers to provide safety-engineered sharps devices and needleless systems to employees to reduce the risk of occupational exposure to HIV, hepatitis C, and other bloodborne disease

- Expands the definition of engineering controls to include devices with engineered sharps injury protection
- Requires that exposure-control plans document consideration and implementation of safer medical devices designed to eliminate or minimize occupational exposure; plans must be reviewed and updated at least annually
- Requires each health care facility to maintain a sharps injury log, with detailed information regarding percutaneous injuries
- Requires employers to solicit input from health care workers when identifying and selecting sharps and document process

Later, on October 15, 2003, the U.S. Occupational Safety and Health Administration (OSHA) posted a Safety and Health Information Bulletin (SHIB) to clarify the OSHA position on reusing tube holders during blood collection procedures, a clarification of the OSHA Bloodborne Pathogens Standard [29 CFR 1910.1030 (d) (2) (vii) (A)]. The standard prohibits the removal of a contaminated needle from a medical device. Prohibition of needle removal from any device is addressed in the 1991 and 2001 standards, the OSHA compliance directive (CPL 2-2.69), and in a 2002 letter of interpretation. Blood collected into the syringe would then need to be transferred into a tube before disposing of the contaminated syringe. In these situations, a syringe with an engineered sharps injury prevention feature and safe work practices should be used whenever possible. Transfer of the blood from the syringe to the test tube must be done using a needleless blood transfer device.

As with any OSHA rule or regulation, noncompliance may result in the issuance of citations by an OSHA compliance officer after the completion of a site inspection. It is the responsibility of each facility to evaluate their work practices, implement appropriate engineering controls, and institute all other applicable elements of exposure control to achieve compliance with current OSHA rules and regulations. The OSHA SHIB provides a step-by-step Evaluation Toolbox for a facility to follow (Box 3-1).

Evacuated Blood Collection Tubes

Evacuated tubes are the most extensively used system for collecting venous blood samples. An evacuated blood collection system consists of a collection needle, a nonreusable needle holder, and a tube containing enough vacuum to draw a specific amount of blood (Fig. 3-2). Evacuated tubes and microtainer tubes have various color-coded stoppers. The stopper color denotes the type of anticoagulant, additive or the presence of a gel

OSHA Safety and Health Information Bulletin: Evaluation Toolbox

1. Employers must first evaluate, select, and use appropriate engineering controls (e.g., sharps with engineered sharps injury protection), which includes single-use blood tube holders with sharps with engineered sharps injury protection (SESIP) attached.
2. The use of engineering and work practice controls provide the highest degree of control in order to eliminate potential injuries after performing blood draws. Disposing of blood tube holders with contaminated needles attached after the activation of the safety feature affords the greatest hazard control.
3. In very rare situations, needle removal is acceptable.
   * If the employer can demonstrate that no feasible alternative to needle removal is available (e.g., inability to purchase single-use blood tube holders because of a supply shortage of these devices).
   * If the removal is necessary for a specific medical or dental procedure.
   * In these rare cases, the employer must ensure that the contaminated needle is protected by a SESIP before disposal. In addition, the employer must ensure that a proper sharps disposal container is located in the immediate area of sharps use and is easily accessible to employees. This information must be clearly detailed and documented in the employer's Exposure Control Plan.
4. If it is necessary to draw blood with a syringe, a syringe with engineered sharps injury protection must be used, in which the protected needle is removed using safe work practices, and transfer of blood from the syringe to the tube must be done using a needleless blood transfer device.

Disposal of Contaminated Needles and Blood Tube Holders Used for Phlebotomy.
   Safety and Health Information Bulletins, SHIB 10-15-03.
   From Occupational Safety and Health Administration http://www.osha.gov/dts/shib/shib101503.html.

separator. Increasingly, glass collection tubes are being replaced with safer plastic tubes.

BD recommends that storage temperature for all BD Vacutainer blood collection tubes not exceed 25°C or 77°F. If plastic tubes reach higher temperatures, the tubes may lose their vacuum or implode. Evacuated tubes are intended for one-time use.

When collecting multiple tubes of blood, a specified "order of draw" protocol should be followed to diminish the possibility of cross-contamination between tubes caused by the presence of different additives (Table 3-2). Errors in the order of draw can affect laboratory test results.

Syringe Technique

Disposable plastic syringes are used for special cases of venous blood collection. If a patient has particularly difficult veins, or if other special circumstances exist, the syringe technique may be used. Some facilities recommend an order of draw with a syringe that varies from the evacuated-tube protocol. It is more common today to use wing-tip (butterfly) blood collection sets for difficult patients or some pediatric patients.

General Protocol

1. Phlebotomists should pleasantly introduce themselves to the patient and clearly explain the procedure to be performed. It is always a courtesy to speak a few words in a patient's native language if English is not their first language. Ethnic populations vary geographically, but many patients are now Spanish speaking. Appendix B lists some English-Spanish medical phrases for the phlebotomist.
2. Patient identification is the critical first step in blood collection. In the 2007 Laboratory Services National Patient Safety Goals from The Joint Commission, goal #1 is accuracy in patient identification. Patient misidentification errors are potentially associated with the worst clinical outcomes because of the possibility of misdiagnosis and mishandled therapy.[1]
   It is necessary to have the patient state and speak his or her name. If a patient cannot provide this information, he or she must provide some form of identification or be identified by a family member or caregiver. Check the identification band that is physically attached to the patient. Wristbands with unique barcoded patient identifiers have great potential for reducing patient misidentification. Unfortunately, wristband errors do occur. A CAP-conducted study identified six major types of wristband errors:
   * Absent wristband
   * Wrong wristband
   * More than one wristband with different information
   * Partially missing information on the wristband
   * Erroneous information on the wristband
   * Illegible information on the wristband
   When the patient is unable to give his or her name, or when identification is attached to the bed or is missing, nursing personnel should be asked to identify the patient physically. Any variations in protocol should be noted on the test requisition. A CAP recommendation is that phlebotomists should refuse to collect blood from a patient when a wristband error is detected.[1]
3. Test requisitions should be checked and the appropriate evacuate tubes assembled. All

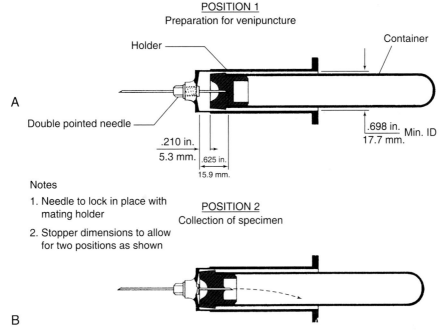

POSITION 1
Preparation for venipuncture

Holder

Container

A

Double pointed needle

.210 in.
5.3 mm.

.625 in.
15.9 mm.

.698 in. Min. ID
17.7 mm.

Notes

1. Needle to lock in place with mating holder

2. Stopper dimensions to allow for two positions as shown

POSITION 2
Collection of specimen

B

FIGURE 3-2 **Standard double-ended blood-collecting needle with holder using vacuum tube system. A, Preparation for venipuncture. B, Collection of specimen.** (NCCLS H1-A4: Evacuated tubes and additives for blood specimen collection—fourth edition; approved standard, 1996.)

TABLE 3-2

Order of Draw of Multiple Evacuated Tubes Collections*			
Order	Closure Color	Type of Tube	Mix by Inverting
1	Yellow	Blood cultures-SPS—aerobic and anaerobic	8-10×
2	Light blue	Citrate tube†	3-4×
3	Gold or red/gray	BD vacutainer SST gel separator tube	5×
	Red	Serum tube (plastic)	5×
	Red	Serum tube (glass)	none
	Orange	BD vacutainer rapid serum tube (RST)	5-6×
4	Light green or green/gray	BC vacutainer PST gel separator tube with heparin	8-10×
	Green	Heparin	8-10×
5	Lavender	EDTA	8-10×
6	White	BD vacutainer PPT separator tube	
		K_2 EDTA with gel	8-10×
7	Gray	Fluoride (glucose) tube	8-10×

From Becton, Dickinson and Company, 2010, with permission. Courtesy and © Becton, Dickinson and Company.
*The order of draw has been revised to reflect the increased use of plastic evacuated collection tubes. Plastic serum tubes containing a clot activator may cause interference in coagulation testing. Some facilities may continue using glass serum tubes without a clot activator as a waste tube before collecting special coagulation assays. Reflects change in CLSI recommended Order of Draw (H3-A5, Vol 23, No 32, 8.10.2).
†If a winged blood collection set for venipuncture and a coagulation (citrate) tube is the first specimen tube to be drawn, a discard tube should be drawn first. To ensure a proper blood to citrate ratio, use the discard tube to fill the air space with blood. The discard tube does not need to be completely filled.

specimens should be properly labeled immediately after the specimen is drawn. Prelabeling is unacceptable.

4. The patient's name, unique identification number, room number or clinic, and date and time of collection are usually found on the label. In some cases, labels must include the time of collection of the specimen and the type of specimen. A properly completed request form should accompany all specimens sent to the

laboratory. NOTE: Capillary blood collection is performed with a sterile, disposable lancet. These lancets should be properly discarded in a puncture-proof container after a single use.

Labels

Quality assessment policies are implemented in the clinical laboratory to protect the patient from any adverse consequences of errors resulting from an improperly handled specimen, beginning with the collection of that specimen. Laboratory quality assessment and accreditation require that specimens be properly labeled at the time of collection. All specimen containers must be labeled by the person doing the collection to ensure the specimen is actually collected from the patient whose identification is on the label.

An unlabeled container or one labeled improperly should not be accepted by the laboratory. Specimens are considered improperly labeled when there is incomplete or no patient identification on the tube or container holding the specimen. Many specimen containers are transported in leakproof plastic bags. It is unacceptable practice for only the plastic bags to be labeled; the container actually holding the specimen must be labeled as well. If the identification is illegible, the specimen is unacceptable. A specimen is also unacceptable if the specimen container identification does not match exactly the identification on the request form for that specimen.

In many laboratories, labels are computer generated, which helps ensure that the proper identification information is included for each patient. Bar-coded labels facilitate this process. One automated computer system, BD.id Patient Identification System (http://www.bd.com) eliminates mislabeling because the system reads the patient's bar-coded wristband. The software indicates the tests, appropriate tubes, and quantity of tubes required for the patient, then generates bar-coded laboratory labels for tube identification at the patient's bedside. Each laboratory has a specific protocol for the handling of mislabeled or "unacceptable" specimens.

VENOUS BLOOD COLLECTION (PHLEBOTOMY)

Supplies and Equipment

The following is a list of supplies and equipment that will be needed in venipuncture (Procedure 3-1):

- Test requisition
- Tourniquet and disposable gloves
- Sterile disposable needles and needle holder
- Various evacuated blood tubes
- Alcohol (70%) and gauze square or alcohol wipes
- Any special equipment
- Adhesive plastic strips

Special Site-Selection Situations

Five specific situations may result in a difficult venipuncture or may be sources of preanalytical error: intravenous lines, edema, scarring or burn patients, dialysis patients, and mastectomy patients.

Intravenous Lines

A limb with an IV line running should not be used for venipuncture because of contamination to the specimen. The patient's other arm or an alternate site should be selected.

Edema

Edema is the abnormal accumulation of fluid in the intracellular spaces of the tissue.

Scarring or Burn Patients

Veins are very difficult to palpate in areas with extensive scarring or burns. Alternate sites or capillary blood collection should be used.

Dialysis Patients

Blood should never be drawn from a vein in an arm with a cannula (temporary dialysis access device) or fistula (a permanent surgical fusion of a vein and an artery). A trained staff member can draw blood from a cannula. The preferred venipuncture site is a hand vein or a vein away from the fistula on the underside of the arm.

Mastectomy Patients

If a mastectomy patient has had lymph nodes adjacent to the breast removed, venipuncture should not be performed on the same side as the mastectomy.

Phlebotomy Problems

Occasionally a venipuncture is unsuccessful. Do not attempt to perform the venipuncture more than two times. If two attempts are unsuccessful, notify the phlebotomy supervisor. Problems encountered in phlebotomy can include:

1. Refusal by the patient to have blood drawn
2. Difficulty obtaining a specimen because the bore of the needle is against the wall of the vein or going through the vein

Venipuncture

INITIATION OF THE VENIPUNCTURE PROCEDURE

1. Properly identify the patient (see General Protocol, #2).
2. Assemble all necessary equipment and evacuated tubes at the patient's bedside.
3. Put on disposable gloves (see Fig. 2-3 for proper method of donning gloves).
4. The plastic shield on a needle is to remain on the needle until immediately before the venipuncture. The evacuated tube is placed into the holder and gently pushed until the top of the stopper reaches the guideline on the holder. Do not push the tube all the way into the holder, or a loss of vacuum will result.

SELECTION OF AN APPROPRIATE SITE

Obtaining a blood specimen from an intravenous (IV) line should be avoided because it increases the risk of mixing the fluid with the blood sample and producing incorrect test results.

1. Visually inspect both arms. Choose a site that has not been repeatedly used for phlebotomy. In the arm, three veins are typically used for venipuncture: the cephalic, basilic, and median cubital (Fig. 3-3).
2. Apply the tourniquet (Fig. 3-4). Do not leave the tourniquet on for more than 2 minutes. Prolonged tourniquet application can elevate certain blood chemistry analytes, including albumin, aspartate aminotransferase (AST), calcium, cholesterol, iron, lipids, total bilirubin, and total protein.
3. To make the veins more prominent, ask the patient to make a fist. With the index finger, palpate (feel) for an appropriate vein (see Fig. 3-4). The ideal site is generally near or slightly below the bend in the arm. Palpation is important for identifying the vein, which has a resilient feeling compared with the surrounding tissues. Large veins are not always a good choice because they tend to roll as you attempt the venipuncture. Superficial and small veins should also be avoided. If no appropriate veins are found in one arm, examine the other arm by applying the tourniquet and palpating the arm. Veins in other areas, such as the wrist, hands, and feet, can only be used by experienced phlebotomists.

PREPARATION OF THE VENIPUNCTURE SITE

1. After an appropriate site has been chosen, release the tourniquet.
2. Using an alcohol pad saturated with 70% alcohol, cleanse the skin in the area of the venipuncture site. Using a circular motion, clean the area from the center and move outward. Do not go back over any area of the skin once it has been cleansed.
3. Allow the site to air dry.

PERFORMING THE VENIPUNCTURE

Avoid touching the cleansed venipuncture site.

1. Use one hand to hold the evacuated tube assembly. Position the patient's arm in a slightly downward position. Use one or more fingers of the other hand to secure the skin area of the forearm below the intended venipuncture site. This will tighten the skin and secure the vein.
2. Hold the needle with attached holder about 1 to 2 inches below and in a straight line with the intended venipuncture site. Position the blood-drawing unit at an angle of about 20 degrees. The bevel of the needle should be upward (Fig. 3-5).
3. Insert the needle through the skin and into the vein. This insertion motion should be smooth. One hand should steady the needle holder unit while the other hand pushes the tube to the end of the plastic holder. It is important to hold the needle steady during the phlebotomy to avoid interrupting the flow of blood. Multiple samples can be drawn by inserting each additional tube as soon as the tube attached to the needle holder has filled. (See Table 3-2 for the order of drawing multiple evacuated tubes.) If required, gently invert tubes with anticoagulant or additive to mix.

TERMINATION OF THE PROCEDURE

1. The tourniquet can be released as soon as the blood begins to flow into the evacuated tube or syringe or immediately before the final amount of blood is drawn.
2. Ask the patient to open the hand.

Continued

PROCEDURE **3-1** (Continued)

3. Withdraw the blood-collecting unit with one hand, and immediately press down on the gauze pad with the other hand after the desired amount of blood has been drawn.

4. If possible, have the patient elevate the entire arm and press on the gauze pad with the opposite hand. If the patient is unable to do this, apply pressure until bleeding ceases.

5. Place a nonallergenic adhesive spot or strip over the venipuncture site. Failure to apply sufficient pressure to the venipuncture site could result in a hematoma (a collection of blood under the skin that produces a bruise).

6. Mix tubes with anticoagulant by inverting the tubes several times. Do not shake the tubes. Discard the used equipment into an appropriate puncture-proof container.

7. Label all test tubes as required by the laboratory.

8. Clean up supplies from the work area, remove gloves (see Fig. 2-3 for correct method of glove removal), and wash hands. If the patient is an outpatient, wait a few minutes after the venipuncture is complete, and check to be sure the patient does not feel dizzy or nauseated before discharge.

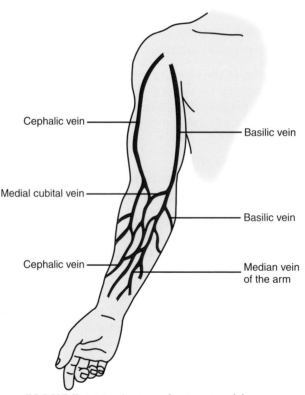

FIGURE 3-3   Anatomy of major veins of the arm.

3. Movement of the vein
4. Sudden movement by the patient or phlebotomist that causes the needle to come out of the arm prematurely
5. Improper anticoagulant
6. Inadequate amount of blood in an evacuated tube
7. Fainting or illness subsequent to venipuncture

Phlebotomy Complications

Patients can experience complications resulting from a phlebotomy procedure. These complications can be divided into six major categories:

1. **Vascular complications.** Bleeding from the site of the venipuncture and hematoma formation are the most common vascular complications.

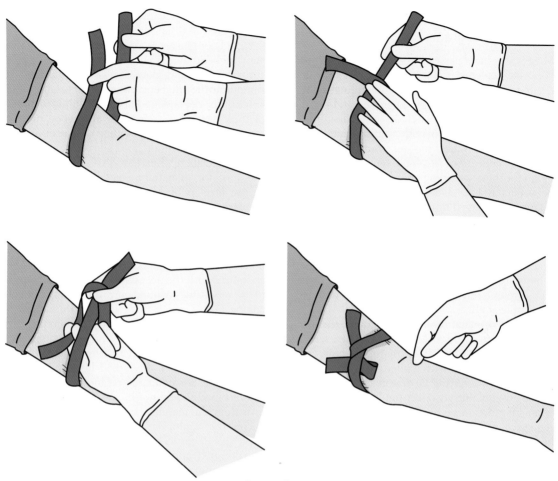

FIGURE 3-4   Selection of appropriate venipuncture site.

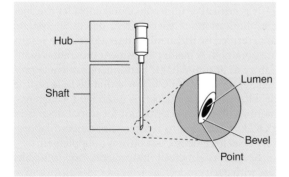

FIGURE 3-5   **Parts of a needle.** (From Warekois RS, Robinson R: Phlebotomy: worktext and procedures manual, ed 3, St Louis, 2012, Saunders.)

2. **Infections**. The second most common complication of venipuncture is infection.
3. **Anemia**. Iatrogenic anemia is also known as *nosocomial anemia, physician-induced anemia,* or *anemia resulting from blood loss for testing.* This can be a particular problem with pediatric patients.

4. **Neurologic complications**. Postphlebotomy patients can exhibit some neurologic complications, including seizure or pain.
5. **Cardiovascular complications**. Cardiovascular complications include orthostatic hypotension, syncope, shock, and cardiac arrest.
6. **Dermatologic complications**. The most common dermatologic consequence of phlebotomy is an allergic reaction to iodine in the case of blood donors.

CAPILLARY OR PERIPHERAL BLOOD COLLECTION BY SKIN PUNCTURE

Capillary blood can be used for a variety of laboratory assays. Capillary blood is often used for point-of-care tests (POCTs). A common POCT is bedside testing for glucose using one of several available reading devices and the accompanying reagent strips, as done at home by diabetic patients (see POCT discussion).

Blood Spot Collection for Neonatal Screening Programs

Most states have passed laws requiring that newborns be screened for certain diseases that can result in serious abnormalities, including mental retardation, if they are not diagnosed and treated early. These diseases include phenylketonuria (PKU), galactosemia, hypothyroidism, and hemoglobinopathies. CLSI has set standards for filter paper collection, or **blood spot collection**, of blood for these screening programs.[7] Blood should be collected 1 to 3 days after birth, before the infant is discharged from the hospital, and at least 24 hours after birth and after ingestion of food for a valid PKU test. There is an increased chance of missing a positive test result when an infant is tested for PKU before 24 hours of age. When infants are discharged early, however, many physicians prefer to take a sample early rather than risk no sample at all.

In most **neonatal screening programs**, the specimen is collected on filter paper and then sent to the approved testing laboratory for analysis. Special collection cards with a filter paper portion are supplied by the testing laboratory; these are kept in the hospital nursery or central laboratory. There is an information section on these cards, and all requested information must be provided and should be treated as any other request form. The filter paper section of the card contains circles designed to identify the portion of the paper onto which the specimen should be placed, where the filter paper will properly absorb the amount of blood necessary for the test.

Collection is usually done by heel puncture (see Procedure 3-2), following the accepted procedure for the institution. When a drop of blood is present, the circle on the filter paper is touched against the drop until the circle is completely filled. A sufficiently large drop should be formed so that the process of filling the circle can be done in only one step. The filter paper is allowed to air dry and then is transported to the testing laboratory in a plastic transport bag or other acceptable container. The procedure established by the testing laboratory should be followed for the collection step.

Capillary Blood for Testing at the Bedside (Point-of-Care Testing)

Capillary blood samples for glucose testing and for other assays are used frequently in many health care facilities for **bedside testing**, or **point-of-care testing (POCT).** Quantitative determinations for glucose are made available within 1 or 2 minutes, depending on the system employed. CLSI has set guidelines for these tests because they are performed in acute care and long-term care facilities.[8] (POCT is discussed in Chapter 9.)

POCT for glucose is also performed at home by many diabetic outpatients, using their own blood and one of several glucose-measuring devices. It is important for diabetic patients, especially those with insulin-dependent diabetes mellitus, to monitor their own blood glucose levels several times a day and to be able to adjust their dosage of insulin accordingly to maintain good glucose control.

For the diabetic inpatient, POCT is also a valuable tool for diabetes management. The blood glucose level is often unstable in these patients, a situation that may necessitate frequent adjustments of insulin dosage. POCT provides results that are immediate, so dosages can be adjusted more quickly. Ordering and collecting venous blood specimens for glucose tests done by a central laboratory, with the necessary frequency and rapidity of reporting required, are often impractical, making POCT much more useful. Good quality-control programs must be used to ascertain the reliability of the POCT results. Whole blood samples should be collected by puncture from the heel (for infants only), finger, or flushed heparinized line, using policies for standard precautions. Arterial or venous blood should not be used unless the directions from the manufacturer of the POCT device specify the appropriateness of these alternative blood specimens. The POCT instrument should be calibrated and the test performed according to the manufacturer's directions. Results should be recorded permanently in the patient's medical record in a manner that distinguishes between bedside test results and central laboratory test results.

It is critical to understand and consider the specific limitations of each POCT detection system, as described by the manufacturer, so reliable results are obtained. A quality assessment program is mandatory to ensure reliable performance of these procedures. The use of POCT, whether bedside testing or self-testing for glucose, is intended for management of diabetic patients, not for initial diagnosis. POCT is not used to replace the standard laboratory tests for glucose, but only as a supplement.

Several commercial instruments are available, and with each product, a meter provides quantitative determination of glucose present when used with an accompanying reagent strip. A drop of capillary blood is touched to the reagent strip pad and, according to the specific procedure, read in the meter. The instrument provides an accurate and standardized reading when used according to the manufacturer's directions. The reagent strips must be handled with care and used within their proper shelf life. The strips are specific only for glucose. The meters are packaged in convenient carrying cases and are small enough to be placed in a pocket or briefcase.

Capillary Blood Collection

SELECTION OF AN APPROPRIATE SITE

1. Usually the fingertip of the third or fourth finger, heel, and big toe are appropriate sites for the collection of small quantities of capillary blood. The earlobe may be used as a site of last resort in adults. Do not puncture the skin through previous sites, which may be infected. The plantar surface (sole) of the heel or big toe is an appropriate site in infants or in special cases such as burn victims. The ideal site in infants is the medial or lateral plantar surface of the heel, with a puncture no deeper than 2 mm beneath the plantar heel skin surface and no more than half this distance at the posterior curve of the heel (Fig. 3-6). CLSI recommendations are not to use fingers of infants. The back of the heel should never be used because of the danger of injuring the heel bone, cartilage, and nerves in this area.

2. The site of blood collection must be warm to ensure the free flow of blood.

PREPARATION OF THE SITE

1. Hold the area to be punctured with the thumb and index finger of a gloved hand.

2. Wipe the area with a 70% alcohol pad and allow to air-dry.

3. Wipe the area with a dry gauze square. If the area is not dry, the blood will not form a rounded drop and will be difficult to collect.

PUNCTURING THE SKIN

1. Use a disposable sterile lancet once, and discard it properly in a puncture-proof container.

2. Securely hold the area, and puncture once (perpendicular) with a firm motion (Fig. 3-7). NOTE: the incision must be perpendicular to the fingerprint or heelprint.

3. Wipe away the first drop of blood, because the first drop of blood is mixed with lymphatic fluid and possibly alcohol.

4. Apply gentle pressure to the area to obtain a suitable specimen.

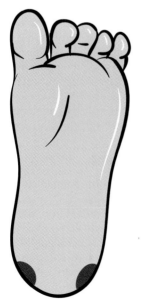

FIGURE 3-6 **Sites for heel puncture in infants.** (From Warekois RS, Robinson R: Phlebotomy: worktext and procedures manual, ed 3, St Louis, 2012, Saunders.)

CAPILLARY BLOOD COLLECTION

Supplies and Equipment

The following is a list of supplies and equipment that will be needed in capillary blood collection (see Procedure 3-2):

- Alcohol (70%) and gauze squares or alcohol wipes
- Disposable gloves and sterile small gauze squares
- Sterile disposable blood lancets
- Equipment specific to the test ordered (e.g., glass slides for blood smears, micropipette and diluent for CBCs, microhematocrit tubes)

Special Capillary Blood Collection

Unopette

The Unopette system (Becton Dickinson Company, Franklin Lakes, NJ) is only a microsample collection system for use in reticulocyte counts. This product is no longer manufactured for RBC

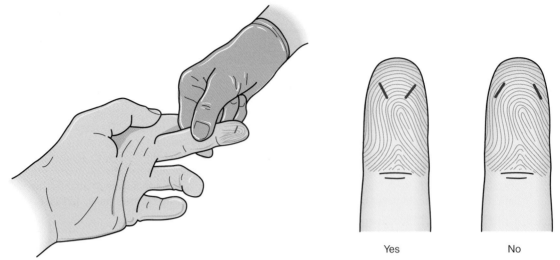

FIGURE 3-7 **Sites for finger puncture.** (From Warekois RS, Robinson R: Phlebotomy: worktext and procedures manual, ed 3, St Louis, 2012, Saunders.)

or WBC/platelet counts. An alternative equivalent product is manufactured by Bioanalytic GmbH. These FDA-approved products have been on the Europeon market since 1978 (www.bioanalytic.de).

A product insert describes the collection and processing procedure used in special capillary blood collection.

Capillary Blood for Slides

To collect capillary blood for slides, a finger or heel puncture is made, and after the first drop is wiped away, the glass slide is touched to the second drop formed. The slide is placed on a flat surface and a spreader slide used to prepare the smear (see Chapter 12). The slide is allowed to air dry, is properly labeled, and then transported to the laboratory for examination.

Collecting Microspecimens

At times, only small amounts of capillary blood can be collected (Box 3-2), and many laboratory determinations have been devised for testing small amounts of sample. In general, the same procedure is followed as for any other drawing of capillary blood. For chemistry procedures, blood can be collected in a capillary tube or microcontainers (Figs. 3-8 and 3-9) by touching the tip of the tube to a large drop of blood while the tube is held in a slightly downward position. The blood enters the collection unit by capillary action. Several tubes can be filled from a single skin puncture if needed. Tubes are capped and brought to the laboratory for testing. Careful centrifugation technique must be used if serum is needed. Microcontainers are available with various additives, including serum separator gels (Table 3-3).

Laser Equipment

Laser technology is the first radical change in phlebotomy in more than 100 years. Revolutionary devices received approval from the U.S. Food and Drug Administration (FDA) in 1997. The Lasette (Cell Robotics, Albuquerque, NM) and the Laser Lancet (Transmedica International, Little Rock, AR) can draw blood without the use of sharp objects (Fig 3-10).

A laser device emits a pulse of light energy that lasts a fraction of a second. The laser concentrates on a very small portion of skin, literally vaporizing

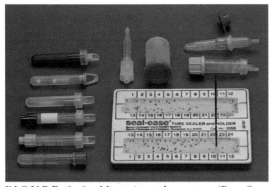

FIGURE 3-8 Microtainer tube system. (From Sommer SR, Warekois RS: Phlebotomy: worktext and procedures manual, ed 2, St Louis, 2007, Saunders.)

TABLE 3-3

Order of Draw for BD Microtainer Tubes with BD Microgard Closure

Closure Color	Additive	Mix by Inverting
1. Lavender	K₃EDTA	10×
2. Green	Lithium heparin	10×
3. Mint green	Lithium heparin and gel for plasma separation	10×
4. Grey	NaFl	
	Na₂EDTA	10×
5. Gold	Clot activator and gel for serum separation	5×
6. Red	No additive	0×

From LabNotes: BD Diagnostics, 20(1):7, 2009, with permission. Courtesy and © Becton, Dickinson and Company.
Note: Hold tube upright, gently invert 180 degrees and back, and repeat movement as recommended. If not mixed properly, tubes with anticoagulants will clot and specimen will often need to be recollected.

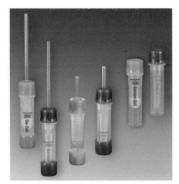

FIGURE 3-9 Microvette ® capillary blood collection system. (Courtesy Sarstedt Inc, Newton, NC.)

the tissue about 1 to 2 mm to the capillary bed. The device can draw a 100-μL blood sample, a sufficient amount for certain tests. The laser process is less painful and heals faster than when blood is drawn with traditional lancets. The patient feels a sensation similar to heat rather than the prick of a sharp object.

SPECIMENS: GENERAL PREPARATION

Accurate chemical analysis of biological fluids depends on proper collection, preservation, and preparation of the sample, in addition to the technique and method of analysis used. The most quantitatively perfect determination is of no use if the specimen is not properly handled in the initial steps of the procedure.

Processing Blood Specimens

Blood specimens must be properly handled after collection. CLSI has published standards for handling blood specimens after collection by venipuncture.[7] If no anticoagulant is used, the blood will clot, and serum is obtained. After being placed in a plain

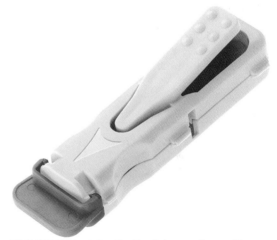

FIGURE 3-10 OneTouch lancing device. (Courtesy LifeScan Inc, Milpitas, CA.)

tube with no additives, the blood is allowed to clot. The serum is then removed from the clot by centrifugation. To prevent excessive handling of biological fluids, many laboratory instrumentation systems can now use the serum directly from the centrifuged tube, without another separation step and without removing the stopper.

It is important to remove the plasma or serum from the remaining blood cells, or clot, as soon as possible. Because biological specimens are being handled, the need for certain safety precautions is stressed. The Standard Precautions policy should be used because all blood specimens should be considered infectious and must be handled with gloves. The outside of the tubes may be bloody, and initial laboratory handling of all specimens necessitates direct contact with the tubes. When stoppers must be removed from the tubes, they must be removed carefully and not popped off, because this could cause infection by inhalation or by contact of the infectious aerosol with mucous membranes. Stoppers should be twisted gently while being covered with protective gauze to minimize the risk from aerosolization. This processing step can be done using a protective plastic shield to prevent direct splashes. To separate the serum and plasma from the remaining blood cells, the tube must be centrifuged.

It is generally best to test specimens as quickly as possible. Specimens should be processed to the point where they can be properly stored so that the constituents to be measured will not be altered. Specimens collected at collection stations away from the testing laboratory need to guarantee that delivery will be made in less than 2 hours from collection and that specimens have been stored properly, including refrigeration or freezing if necessary.

If the centrifuged serum or plasma must be removed into a separate tube or vial, pipette the serum or plasma by using mechanical suction and a disposable pipette; use a protective plastic shield to prevent direct splashes. All serum and plasma tubes, as well as the original blood tubes, should be discarded properly in biohazard containers when they are no longer needed for the determination.

Centrifuging the Specimens

After clotting has taken place, the tube is centrifuged with its cap on (Fig. 3-11). It is important to use Standard Precautions, which require all persons handling specimens to wear gloves. When necessary, stoppers must be carefully removed from blood collection tubes to prevent aerosolization of the specimen. Centrifuges (see Chapter 4) must be covered and placed in a shielded area. When serum or plasma samples must be removed from the blood cells or clot, mechanical suction is used for pipetting, and all specimen tubes and supplies must be discarded properly in biohazard containers.

The use of automated analyzers often allows the use of the primary collection tube for the analysis itself. In these cases, the primary blood tube is centrifuged with its cap on, and the serum is aspirated directly into the analyzer.

Unacceptable Specimens

Various conditions render a blood specimen unsuitable for testing. Clotted specimens are not suitable for cell counts because the cells are trapped in the clot and are therefore not counted. A cell count on a clotted sample will be falsely low.

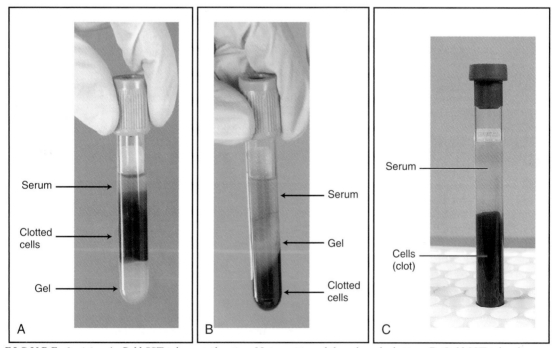

FIGURE 3-11   **A**, Gold SST tube centrifugation. Note position of the gel on the bottom. **B**, Gold SST tube after centrifugation. **Note that the gel now separates the serum from the clotted cells. C**, Centrifuged red-topped "clot" tube with no gel **or clotting additive.** (Modified from Bonewit-West K: Clinical procedures for medical assistants, ed 6, Philadelphia, 2004, Saunders.)

Hemolyzed Specimens

Hemolysis in specimens is the most common cause of an abnormal appearance. Hemolyzed serum or plasma is unfit as a specimen for several chemistry determinations.

A specimen that is hemolyzed appears red (usually clear red) because the RBCs have been lysed, and the hemoglobin has been released into the liquid portion of the blood. Often the cause of hemolysis in specimens is the technique used for venipuncture. A poor venipuncture with excessive trauma to the blood vessel can result in a hemolyzed specimen. Inappropriate needle bore size and contact with alcohol on the skin are other causes. Hemolysis of blood can also result from freezing, prolonged exposure to warmth, or allowing the serum or plasma to remain too long on the cells before testing or removal to another tube. A determination of whether the hemolysis is in vitro or in vivo is also useful. Although relatively rare, in vivo hemolysis is a clinically significant finding.

Hemolyzed serum or plasma is unsuitable for several chemistry determinations because substances usually present within cells (e.g., K^+) can be released into the serum or plasma if serum is left on the cells for a prolonged period. In addition, several other constituents, including the enzymes acid phosphatase, lactate dehydrogenase (LDH), and aspartate aminotransferase (AST, GOT), are present in large amounts in RBCs, so hemolysis of red cells will significantly elevate the value obtained for these substances in serum. Hemoglobin is released during hemolysis and may directly interfere with a reaction, or its color may interfere with photometric analysis of the specimen. The procedure to be done should always be checked to determine whether abnormal-looking specimens can be used.

Icteric Specimens

Icteric (yellow) serum or plasma is another specimen with an abnormal appearance. When serum or plasma takes on an abnormal brownish yellow color, there has most likely been an increase in bile pigments, namely bilirubin. Excessive intravascular destruction of RBCs, obstruction of the bile duct, or impairment of the liver leads to an accumulation of bile pigments in the blood, and the skin becomes yellow. Those performing clinical laboratory determinations should note any abnormal appearance of serum or plasma and record it on the report form. The abnormal color of the serum can interfere with photometric measurements.

Lipemic Specimens

Lipemic plasma or serum takes on a milky white color. The presence of lipid, or fats, in serum or plasma can cause this abnormal appearance. Often, the lipemia results from collecting the blood from the patient too soon after a meal. Use of a lipemic serum specimen does not interfere with some chemical determinations but may interfere with others (e.g., triglyceride assay).

Drug Effect on Specimens

Blood drawn from patients taking certain types of medication can give invalid chemistry results for some constituents. Drugs can alter several chemical reactions and can affect laboratory results in two general ways: some action of the drug or its metabolite can cause an alteration (in vivo) in the concentration of the substance being measured, or some physical or chemical property of the drug can alter the analysis directly (in vitro). The number of drugs that affect laboratory measurements is increasing.

Logging and Reporting Processes

As part of the processing and handling of laboratory specimens, a careful, accurate logging and recording process must be in place in the laboratory, regardless of the size of the facility. A log sheet and a printed report form are vital to the operation of any laboratory. The log sheet documents on a daily basis the various patient specimens received in the laboratory. Log sheets and result reports are generated by laboratory information systems when used (see Chapter 10).

Items to be listed on the log sheet are the patient's name, identification number, type of specimen collected (description of the specimen and its source), date and time of specimen collection, and laboratory tests to be done. The log sheet should also indicate the time when the specimen arrived in the laboratory and may include a column for test results and the date when the tests are completed. Results can be documented by hand, by use of laboratory instrument–printed reports, or by computer printouts. The log sheet data are part of the permanent record of the laboratory and must be stored and available for future reference.

A printed report is often sent to the physician, with the vital data pertaining to the test results. Result reports are also available electronically in many facilities. The following information should be included in the report: patient's name, identification number, date and time of specimen collection, description and source of specimen, the initials of the person who collected the specimen, tests requested, the name of the physician requesting the tests, the test results, and the initials or signature of the person who performed the test. Much of this documentation of data is being done with the use of laboratory computerized information systems. Copies of this laboratory report may be sent to the medical records department and to the accounting office for patient billing purposes.

Preserving and Storing Specimens

Some chemical constituents change rapidly after the blood is removed from the vein. The best policy is to perform tests on fresh specimens. When the specimen must be preserved until the test can be done, there are ways to impede alteration. For example, sodium fluoride can be used to preserve blood glucose specimens because it prevents glycolysis.

With few exceptions, the lower the temperature, the greater the stability of the chemical constituents. Furthermore, the growth of bacteria is considerably inhibited by refrigeration and completely inhibited by freezing. Room temperature is generally considered to be 18°C to 30°C, the refrigerator temperature about 4°C, and freezing about 5°C or less. Refrigeration is a simple and reliable means of impeding alterations, including bacteriologic action and glycolysis, although some changes still take place. Refrigerated specimens must be brought to room temperature before chemical analysis. Removing cells from plasma and serum is another means of preventing some changes. Some specimens needed for certain assays, such as bilirubin, must be shielded from the light or tested immediately. Bilirubin is a light-sensitive substance.

Serum or plasma may be preserved by freezing. Whole blood cannot be frozen satisfactorily because freezing ruptures the RBCs (hemolysis). Freezing preserves enzyme activities in serum and plasma. Serum and plasma freeze in layers with different concentrations, and therefore these specimens must be well mixed before they are used in a chemical determination.

If the results are to be meaningful, every precaution must be taken to preserve the chemical constituents in the specimen from the time of collection to the time of testing in the laboratory. In general, tubes for collecting blood for chemical determinations do not have to be sterile, but they should be chemically clean. Serum is usually preferred to whole blood or plasma when the constituents to be measured are relatively evenly distributed between the intracellular and extracellular portions of the blood.

Storage of Processed Specimens

The processing of individual serum or plasma tubes will depend on the analysis to be done and the time that will elapse before analysis. Serum or plasma may be kept at room temperature, refrigerated, frozen, or protected from light, depending on the circumstances and the determination to be done. Some specimens must be analyzed immediately after they reach the laboratory, such as specimens for blood gas and pH analyses. Blood specimens for hematology studies can be stored in the refrigerator for 2 hours before being used in testing. After storage, anticoagulated blood, serum, or plasma must be thoroughly mixed after it has reached room temperature.

As already noted, plasma and serum often can be frozen and preserved satisfactorily until a determination can be done, but whole blood cannot because RBCs rupture on freezing. Freezing preserves most chemical constituents in serum and plasma and provides a method of sample preservation for the laboratory. In general, refrigerating specimens impedes alterations of many constituents. With all biological specimens, however, preservation should be the exception rather than the rule. A laboratory determination is best done on a fresh specimen.

CHAIN-OF-CUSTODY SPECIMEN INFORMATION

When specimens are involved in possible medicolegal situations, certain specimen-handling policies are required. Medicolegal or forensic implications require that any data pertaining to the specimen in question be determined in such a way that the information will be recognized by a court of law. Processing steps for such specimens—initial collection, transportation, storage, and analytical testing—must be documented by careful record keeping. Documentation ensures that there has been no tampering with the specimen by any interested parties, that the specimen has been collected from the appropriate person, and that the results reported are accurate. Each step of the collection, handling, processing, testing, and reporting processes must be documented; this is called the *chain of custody*.

Chain-of-custody documentation must be signed by every person who has handled the specimens involved in the case in question. The actual process may vary in different health care facilities, but the general purpose of this process is to make certain any data obtained by the clinical laboratory will be admissible in a court of law, and all the proper steps have been taken to ensure the integrity of the information produced.

REFERENCES

1. Carraro P, Plebani M: Errors in a state laboratory: types and frequences 10 years later, Clin Chem 53:1338–1342, 2007.
2. American Hospital Association: Patient care partnership, www.aha.org (retrieved August 2005).

3. Ogden-Grable, H: Phlebotomy A to Z: Using critical thinking and making ethical decisions, Chicago, 2008, American Society for Clinical Pathology.
4. Clinical and Laboratory Standards Institute: Procedures and devices for the collection of diagnostic capillary blood specimens: approved standard, ed 5, Wayne, Pa, 2004, H4-A5.
5. Clinical and Laboratory Standards Institute: Tubes and additives for venous blood specimen collection: approved standard, ed 5, Wayne, Pa, 2003, H1-A5.
6. Bush V, Cohen R: The evolution of evacuated blood collection tubes, lab med 34:304–310, 2003.
7. Clinical and Laboratory Standards Institute: Blood collection on filter paper for newborn screening programs: approved standard, ed 4, Wayne, Pa, 2003, LA4-A3.
8. Clinical and Laboratory Standards Institute: Procedures for the collection of diagnostic blood specimens by venipuncture: approved standard, ed 5, Wayne, Pa, 2003, H3-A5.

BIBLIOGRAPHY

Burtis CA, Ashwood ER, editors: Tietz fundamentals of clinical chemistry, ed 6, St. Louis, 2008, Saunders.
Bush V: Why doesn't my heparinized plasma specimen remain anticoagulated? Lab Notes 13(2):9–10, 2003: Spring www.bd.com.
Bush V, Mangan L: The hemolyzed specimen: causes, effects and reduction, Lab Notes 13(1):1–5, 2003:Winter www.bd.com.
Dale JC: Phlebotomy complications, Boston, August 1996, Paper presented at Mayo Laboratory's Phlebotomy Conference.
Ernst D, Calam R: NCCLS simplifies the order of draw: a brief history, MLO Med Lab Obs 36:26, 2004.
Faber V: Phlebotomy and the aging patient, Adv Med Lab Prof 29:24, 1998.
Forbes BA, Sahm DF, Weissfeld A: Bailey & Scott's diagnostic microbiology, ed 12, St Louis, 2007, Mosby.
Foubister V: Quick on the draw: coagulation tube response, Cap Today 16:38, 2002.
Gerberding JL: Occupational exposure to HIV in health care settings, N Engl J Med 348:826, 2003.
Haraden L: Pediatric phlebotomy: great expectations, Adv Med Lab Prof 28:12, 1997.
Hurley TR: Considerations for the pediatric and geriatric patient, Boston, August 1996, Paper presented at Mayo Laboratory's Phlebotomy Conference.
Latshaw J: Laser takes sting out of phlebotomy, Adv Med Lab Prof 28:40, 1997.
Lee F, Lind N: Isolation guidelines, Infection Control Today (www.infectioncontroltoday.com/articles/051col5.html. retrieved May 2005).
Magee LS: Preanalytical variables in the chemistry laboratory, Lab Notes 15(1):1–4, 2005.
Norberg A, et al: Contamination rates of blood cultures obtained by dedicated phlebotomy vs intravenous catheter, JAMA 289:726, 2003.
Occupational Safety and Health Administration, US Department of Labor: Disposal of contaminated needles and blood tube holders used in phlebotomy, Safety and Health Information Bulletin (www.osha.gov/dts/shib/shib101503.html, retrieved May 2005).
Occupational Safety and Health Administration, US Department of Labor: Best practice: OSHA's position on the reuse of blood collection tube holders, Safety and Health Information Bulletin (www.osha.gov/dts/shib/shib101503.html, retrieved May 2005).
Ogden-Grable H, Gill GW: Preventing phlebotomy errors-potential for harming your patients, Lab Med 36:430, 2005.
Turgeon M: Clinical hematology: theory and procedures, ed 4, Philadelphia, 2005, Lippincott Williams & Wilkins, p 18.
Understanding additives: heparin, Lab Notes 14(1):7, 2004www.bd.com/vacutainer/labnotes/2004winterspring/additives_heparin.asp:retrieved May 2005.

REVIEW QUESTIONS

1. _____ One of the top 5 causes of preanalytical errors is:
   a. improperly filled blood collection tube
   b. patient incorrectly identified
   c. test request error
   d. all the above

Questions 2-4: Match transmission-based infection control precautions with the appropriate application (a to c).

2. ___ Contact precautions

3. ___ Airborne precautions

4. ___ Droplet precautions
   a. Stop spread of bacteria via direct contact
   b. Used to protect from agents dispersed by talking, coughing, or sneezing
   c. Provide protection from dust particles

5. When the coagulation of fresh whole blood is prevented through the use of an anticoagulant, the straw-colored fluid that can be separated from the cellular elements is:
   a. serum.
   b. plasma.
   c. whole blood.
   d. platelets.

6. Which characteristic is inaccurate with respect to the anticoagulant dipotassium ethylenediaminetetraacetic acid (K2 EDTA)?
   a. Removes ionized calcium (Ca^{2+}) from fresh whole blood by the process of chelation
   b. Is used for most routine coagulation studies
   c. Is the most often used anticoagulant in hematology
   d. Is conventionally placed in lavender-stoppered evacuated tubes

7. Heparin inhibits the clotting of fresh whole blood by neutralizing the effect of:
   a. platelets.
   b. ionized calcium (Ca^{2+}).
   c. fibrinogen.
   d. thrombin.

Questions 8-11: *Match the conventional color-coded stopper with the appropriate anticoagulant.*

8. ___ EDTA

9. ___ Heparin

10. ___ Sodium citrate

11. ___ No anticoagulant
    a. Red
    b. Lavender
    c. Blue
    d. Green

Questions 12-16: *The following five procedural steps (a to e) are significant activities in the performance of a venipuncture. Place these steps in the correct sequence (12-16).*

12. ___

13. ___

14. ___

15. ___

16. ___
    a. Select an appropriate site, and prepare the site.
    b. Identify the patient, check test requisitions, assemble equipment, wash hands, and put on latex gloves.
    c. Remove tourniquet, remove needle, apply pressure to site, and label all tubes.
    d. Reapply the tourniquet, and perform the venipuncture.
    e. Introduce yourself, and briefly explain the procedure to the patient.

17. **The appropriate veins for performing a routine venipuncture are the:**
    a. cephalic, basilic, and median cubital.
    b. subclavian, iliac, and femoral.
    c. brachiocephalic, jugular, and popliteal.
    d. saphenous, suprarenal, and tibial.

18. **A blood sample is needed from a patient with intravenous (IV) fluid lines running in one arm. Which of the following is an acceptable procedure?**
    a. Any obtainable vein is satisfactory.
    b. Disconnect the IV line.
    c. Obtain sample from the other arm.
    d. Do not draw a blood specimen from this patient.

19. **The bevel of the needle should be held _____ during a venipuncture.**
    a. Sideways
    b. Upward
    c. Downward
    d. In any direction

20. **A hematoma can form if:**
    a. improper pressure is applied to a site after the venipuncture.
    b. the patient suddenly moves, and the needle comes out of the vein.
    c. the needle punctures both walls of the vein.
    d. all of the above.

21. **Phlebotomy problems can include:**
    a. the use of improper anticoagulants.
    b. misidentification of patients.
    c. inadequate filling of an evacuated tube containing anticoagulant.
    d. all of the above.

22. **Which of the following area(s) is (are) acceptable for the collection of capillary blood from an infant?**
    a. Previous puncture site
    b. Posterior curve of the heel
    c. The arch
    d. Medial or lateral plantar surface

23. **The proper collection of capillary blood includes:**
    a. wiping away the first drop of blood.
    b. occasionally wiping the site with a plain gauze pad to avoid the buildup of platelets.
    c. avoiding the introduction of air bubbles into the column of blood in a capillary collection tube.
    d. all of the above.

24. **Blood specimens are unacceptable for laboratory testing when:**
    a. there is no patient name or identification number on the label.
    b. the label on the request form and the label on the collection container do not match.
    c. the wrong collection tube has been used (i.e., anticoagulant additive instead of tube for serum).
    d. all of the above.

25. **If serum is allowed to remain on the clot for a prolonged period, which of the following effects will be noted?**
    a. Elevated level of serum potassium
    b. Decreased level of serum potassium
    c. Elevated level of glucose
    d. None of the above.

Questions 26-28: *Match each of the abnormal serum appearances with the likely cause for the color change (a to c).*

26. ___ Red-pink

27. ___ Yellow

28. ___ Milky white
    a. Elevated bilirubin (jaundice; icteric serum)
    b. Lysis of red blood cells (hemolyzed serum)
    c. Presence of lipids or fat (lipemic serum)

Questions 29-32: *A = True or B = False.*
This factor can influence a laboratory test result.

29. ___ Posture

30. ___ Exercise

31. ___ Recent food ingestion

32. ___ Ingestion of drugs

CHAPTER 4

SYSTEMS OF MEASUREMENT, LABORATORY EQUIPMENT, AND REAGENTS

Learning Objectives

At the conclusion of this chapter, the student will be able to:

- Convert metric units of measurement for weight, length, volume, and temperature to English units and English units to metric units.

- Convert temperatures from degrees Celsius to degrees Fahrenheit and vice versa.

- Describe the various types of and uses for laboratory volumetric glassware, the techniques for their use, and the various types of glass used to manufacture them.

- Explain how laboratory volumetric glassware is calibrated, how the calibration markings are indicated on the glassware, and proper cleaning protocol.

- Discuss the operation and uses of common laboratory balances.

Learning Objectives—cont'd

- Compare various types and uses of laboratory centrifuges.
- Contrast various forms and grades of water used in the laboratory and how each is prepared.
- List and describe the various grades of chemicals used in the laboratory, including their levels of quality and purpose.

- Define the terms *solute* and *solvent,* and calculate problems related to these constituents.
- Identify the components of a properly labeled container used to store a laboratory reagent or solution.

If the results of laboratory analyses are to be useful to the physician in diagnosing and treating patients, the tests must be performed accurately. Many factors contribute to the final laboratory result for a single determination.

To unify physical measurements worldwide, the International System of Units (SI units) has been adopted. Many of these units also relate to the metric system. A coherent system of measurement units is vital to precise clinical laboratory analyses. This chapter discusses SI units of measure and the use of metric measurements in the laboratory; Chapter 7 discusses other laboratory calculations.

The use of high-quality analytical methods and instrumentation is essential to laboratory work. The importance of knowing the correct use of the various pieces of glassware must be thoroughly appreciated. The three basic pieces of volumetric glassware—volumetric flasks, graduated measuring cylinders, and pipettes—are specialized designs, with each having its own particular use in the laboratory. Many different pieces of laboratory equipment are used in performing clinical determinations, and knowledge of the proper use and handling of this equipment is an important part of any laboratory work. Use of balances and measurement of volume using pipettes are important basic analytical procedures in the clinical laboratory. Centrifuges also have a variety of uses in the laboratory.

The accuracy of laboratory analyses depends to a great extent on the accuracy of the reagents used. Traditional preparation of reagents makes use of balances and volumetric measuring devices such as pipettes and volumetric flasks—examples of fundamental laboratory apparatus. When reagents and standard solutions are being prepared, it is imperative that only the purest water supply be used in the procedure. Chapter 7 discusses the calculation of required constituents of solutions.

SYSTEMS OF MEASUREMENT

The ability to measure accurately is the keystone of the scientific method, and anyone engaged in performing clinical laboratory analyses must have a working knowledge of measurement systems and units of measurement. It is also necessary to understand how to convert units of one system to units of another system. Systems of measurement included here are the English, metric, and SI systems.

English and Metric Systems

The metric system has not been widely used in the United States, except in the scientific community. Because the English system is common in everyday use, English/metric system equivalents are presented in Table 4-1.

Traditionally, measurements in the clinical laboratory have been made in metric units. The **metric system** is based on a decimal system, a system of divisions and multiples of tens. The meter (m) is the standard metric unit for measurement of length, the gram (g) is the unit of mass, and the liter (L) is the unit of volume. Multiples or divisions of these reference units constitute the various other metric units.

International System (SI System)

Another system of measurement, the **International System of Units** (from Système International d'Unités, or **SI**) has been adopted by the worldwide scientific community as a coherent, standardized system based on seven base units. In addition, derived units and supplemental units are used as well. The SI base units describe seven fundamental but independent physical quantities. The derived units are calculated mathematically from two or more base units.

The SI system was established in 1960 by international agreement and is now the standard international language of measurement. The **International Bureau of Weights and Measures** is responsible for maintaining the standards on which the SI system of measurement is based.

The term *metric system* generally refers to the SI system, and for informational purposes, metric terms that remain in common usage are described here as needed.

TABLE 4-1

Common Conversions Between English and Metric Systems	
English to Metric Conversions	
English	Metric
1 inch	2.54 centimeters
1 foot	0.3 meters
1 yard	0.9 meters
1 quart	0.9 liters
1 gallon	0.004 liters
1 pound	0.5 kilograms
Metric to English Conversions	
Metric	English
1 centimeter	0.39 = inches
1 meter	3.3 feet
1 meter	1.1 yard
1 liter	1.1 quarts
1 kilogram	2.2 pounds

TABLE 4-2

Basic Units of the SI System		
Measurement	Unit Name	Abbreviation
Length	metre*	m
Mass	kilogram	kg
Time	second	s
Amount of substance	mole	mol
Electric current	ampere	A
Temperature	kelvin†	K
Luminous intensity	candela	cd

*The spelling *meter* is more common in the United States and is used in this book.
†Although the basic unit of temperature is the kelvin, the degree Celsius is regarded as an acceptable unit, because kelvins may be impractical in many cases. Celsius is used more often in the clinical laboratory.

TABLE 4-3

Prefixes of the SI System			
Prefix	Symbol	Factor	Decimal
Tera	T	10^{12}	1 000 000 000 000
Giga	G	10^{9}	1 000 000 000
Mega	M	10^{6}	1 000 000
Kilo	k	10^{3}	1 000
Hecto	d	10^{2}	100
Deka	da	10^{1}	10
Deci	d	10^{-1}	0.1
Centi	c	10^{-2}	0.01
Milli	m	10^{-3}	0.001
Micro	μ	10^{-6}	0.000 001
Nano	n	10^{-9}	0.000 000 001
Pico	p	10^{-12}	0.000 000 000 001
Femto	f	10^{-15}	0.000 000 000 000 001
Atto	a	10^{-18}	0.000 000 000 000 000 001

The CLSI recommends an extensive educational effort to implement the SI system in clinical laboratories in the United States.[1,2] Any changes in units used to report laboratory findings should be done with great care to avoid misunderstanding and confusion in interpreting laboratory results.

Base Units of SI System

In the SI system, the base units of measurement are the metre (meter), kilogram, second, mole, ampere, kelvin, and candela (Table 4-2). All SI units can be qualified by standard prefixes that serve to convert values to more convenient forms, depending on the size of the object being measured (Table 4-3).

Various rules should be kept in mind when combining these prefixes with their basic units and using the SI system. An *s* should not be added to form the plural of the abbreviation for a unit or for a prefix with a unit. For example, 25 millimeters should be abbreviated as 25 mm, not 25 mms. Do not use periods after abbreviations (use mm, not mm.). Do not use compound prefixes; instead, use the closest accepted prefix. For example, 24×10^{-9} gram (g) should be expressed as 24 nanograms (24 ng) rather than 24 millimicrograms. In the SI system, commas are not used as spacers in recording large numbers, because they are used in place of decimal points in some countries. Instead, groups of three digits are separated by spaces. When recording temperature on the Kelvin scale, omit the degree sign. Therefore, 295 kelvins should be recorded as 295 K, not 295°K. However, the symbol for degrees Celsius is °C, and 22 degrees Celsius should be recorded as 22°C. Multiples and submultiples should be used in steps of 10^{3} or 10^{-3}. Only one solidus, or slash (/), is used when indicating per or a denominator: thus, meters per second squared (m/s^2), not meters per second per second (m/s/s), and millimoles per liter-hour (mmol/L hour), not millimoles per liter per hour (mmol/L/ hour). Finally, although the preferred SI spellings are "metre" and "litre," the spellings *meter* and *liter* remain in common usage in the United States and are used in this book.

The base units of measurement that are used most often in the clinical laboratory are those for length, mass, and volume.

Length

The standard unit for the measurement of length or distance is the **meter (m)**. The meter is standardized as 1,650,763.73 wavelengths of a certain orange light in the spectrum of krypton-86. One meter equals 39.37 inches (in), slightly more than a yard in the English system. There are 2.54 centimeters in 1 inch.

Using the system of prefixes previously discussed, further common divisions and multiples of the meter follow. One-tenth of a meter is a *decimeter* (dm), one hundredth of a meter is a *centimeter* (cm), and one-thousandth of a meter is a *millimeter* (mm). One thousand meters equals 1 *kilometer* (km). The following examples show equivalent measurements of length:

    25 mm = 0.025 m
    10 cm = 100 mm
    1 m = 100 cm
    1 m = 100 mm

Other units of length that were in common usage in the metric system but are no longer recommended in the SI system are the angstrom and the micron. The micron (m), which is equal to 10^{-6} m, has been replaced by the micrometer (mm).

Mass (and Weight)

Mass denotes the quantity of matter, whereas weight takes into account the force of gravity and should not be used in the same sense as mass. These terms are often used interchangeably.

The standard unit for the measurement of mass in the SI system is the **kilogram (kg)**. This is the basis for all other mass measurements in the system. One kilogram weighs approximately 2.2 pounds (lb) in the English system.

The kilogram is divided into thousandths, called *grams* (g). One thousand grams equals 1 kg. The gram is used much more often than the kilogram in the clinical laboratory. The gram is divided into thousandths, called *milligrams* (mg). Grams and milligrams are units commonly used in weighing substances in the clinical laboratory. The following are examples of weight measurement equivalents:

    10 mg = 0.01 g
    0.055 g = 55 mg
    25 g = 25,000 mg
    1.5 kg = 1500 g

Volume

In the clinical laboratory the standard unit of volume is the **liter (L)**. It was not included in the list of base units of the SI system, because the liter is a derived unit. The standard unit of volume in the SI system is the *cubic meter* (m^3). However, this unit is quite large, and the cubic decimeter (dm^3) is a more convenient size for use in the clinical laboratory. In 1964, the Conférence Générale des Poids et Mésures (CGPM) accepted the litre (liter) as a special name for the cubic decimeter. Previously, the standard liter was the volume occupied by 1 kg of pure water at 4°C (the temperature at which a volume of water weighs the most) and at normal atmospheric pressure. On this basis, 1 L equals 1000.027 cubic centimeters (cm^3), and the units, milliliters and cubic centimeters, were used interchangeably, although there is a slight difference between them. One liter is slightly more than 1 quart (qt) in the English system (1 L = 1.06 qt).

The liter is divided into thousandths, called *milliliters* (mL); millionths, called *microliters* (mL); and billionths, called *nanoliters* (nL). The following examples show volume equivalents:

    500 mL = 0.5 L
    0.25 L = 250 mL
    2 L = 2000 mL
    500 mL = 0.5 mL

Because the liter is derived from the meter (1 L = 1 dm^3), it follows that 1 cm^3 is equal to 1 mL and that 1 millimeter cubed (mm^3) is equal to 1 mL. The former abbreviation for cubic centimeter (cc) has been replaced by cm^3. Although this is a common means of expressing volume in the clinical laboratory, milliliter (mL) is preferred.

Amount of Substance

The standard unit of measurement for the amount of a (chemical) substance in the SI system is the mole (mol). The *mole* is defined as the quantity of a chemical equal to that present in 0.0120 kg of pure carbon-12. A mole of a chemical substance is the relative atomic or molecular mass unit of that substance. Formerly, the terms *atomic weight* and *molecular weight* were used to describe the mole (see later discussion).

Temperature

Three scales are used to measure temperature: the Kelvin, Celsius, and Fahrenheit scales. The **Celsius scale** is sometimes referred to as the *centigrade scale*, which is an outdated term.

The basic unit of temperature in the SI system is the **kelvin (K)**. The kelvin may be impractical in many cases. The Celsius scale is used most often in the clinical laboratory. The Kelvin and Celsius scales are closely related, and conversion between them is simple because the units (degrees) are equal in magnitude. The difference between the

Kelvin and Celsius scales is the **zero point**. The zero point on the Kelvin scale is the theoretical temperature of no further heat loss, which is absolute zero. The zero point on the Celsius scale is the freezing point of pure water. Remember, however, that the magnitude of the degree is equal in the two scales. Therefore, because water freezes at 273 kelvins (273 K), it follows that 0 degrees Celsius (0°C) equals 273 kelvins (273 K) and that 0 Kelvin (0 K) equals minus 273 degrees Celsius (−273°C). Thus, to convert from kelvins to degrees Celsius, add 273; to convert from degrees Celsius to kelvins, subtract 273, as follows:

$$K = °C + 273$$
$$°C = K − 273$$

Because the Celsius scale was devised so that 100°C is the boiling point of pure water, the boiling point on the Kelvin scale is 373 K.

Converting from Celsius to Fahrenheit is not as simple, because the degrees are not equal in magnitude on these two scales. The Fahrenheit scale was originally devised with the zero point at the lowest temperature attainable from a mixture of table salt and ice, and the body temperature of a small animal was used to set 100°F. Thus, on the Fahrenheit scale, the freezing point of pure water is 32°F, and the temperature at which pure water boils is 212°F. It is rare that readings on one of these scales must be converted to the other, because almost always, readings taken and used in the clinical laboratory are on the Celsius scale.

Table 4-4 provides examples of comparative readings of the three temperature scales, with common reference points.

It is possible to convert from one scale to the other. The most common conversions are between Celsius and Fahrenheit and vice versa (Box 4-1). The basic conversion formulas are:

To convert Fahrenheit to Celsius:

$$°C = \frac{5}{9} °F − 32$$

To convert Celsius to Fahrenheit:

$$°F = \frac{9}{5} (°C) + 32$$

TABLE 4-4

Common Reference Points on the Three Temperature Scales			
Reference Point	Degrees Fahrenheit	Kelvin	Degrees Celsius
Boiling point of water	212	373	100
Body temperature	98.6	310	37
Room temperature	68	293	20
Freezing point of water	32	273	0
Absolute zero*	−459	0	−273

*Coldest possible temperature.

Box 4-2 provides sample calculations between Celsius and Fahrenheit.

Non-SI Units

Several non-SI units are relevant to clinical laboratory analyses, such as minutes (min), hours (hr), and days (d). These units of time have such historic use in everyday life that it is unlikely new SI units derived from the second (the base unit for time in the SI system) will be implemented. Another non-SI unit is the liter (L), as already discussed with the base SI units of volume. Pressure is expressed in **millimeters of mercury (mm Hg)** and enzyme activity in **international units (IU)**. *One unit* (U) is defined as the amount of enzyme that will catalyze the transformation of 1 μmol of substrate/minute, or 1 unit (U) is the amount of enzyme that catalyses the reaction of 1 nmol of substrate/minute.

Reporting Results in SI Units

To give a meaningful laboratory result, it is important to report both the numbers and the units by which the result is measured. The unit expresses or defines the dimension of the measured substance—concentration, mass, or volume—and it is an important part of any laboratory result. Table 4-5 shows conversions between metric and SI units.

LABORATORY PLASTICWARE AND GLASSWARE

The general laboratory supplies described in this chapter are used for storage, measurement, and containment. Regardless of composition, most laboratory supplies must meet certain tolerances of accuracy. Those that satisfy specifications of the National Institute of Standards and Technology (NIST) are categorized as Class A. Vessels holding or transferring liquid are designed either "to contain" (TC) or "to deliver" (TD) a specified volume. Most laboratory glassware and other laboratory ware can be divided into two main categories according to use:

- Containers and receivers (e.g., beakers, test tubes, Erlenmeyer flasks, reagent bottles)
- Volumetric ware (e.g., pipettes, automatic and manual; volumetric flasks; graduated cylinders; burets)

Plasticware

The clinical laboratory has benefited greatly from the introduction of plasticware. It is cheaper and more durable, but glassware is frequently preferred because of its chemical stability and clarity. Plastic

BOX 4-1
Temperature Conversions

From Fahrenheit to Centigrade

To convert from degrees Fahrenheit to degrees Centigrade, subtract 32 degrees from the temperature and multiply by $\frac{5}{9}$:

Fahrenheit	0	10	20	30	40	50	60	70	80	90	100
Centigrade	−18	−12	−7	−1	4	10	16	21	27	32	38

From Centigrade to Fahrenheit

To convert from degrees Centigrade to degrees Fahrenheit, multiply the temperature by 1.8 and add 32 degrees:

Centigrade	−10	−5	0	5	10	15	20	25	30	35	40
Fahrenheit	14	23	32	41	50	59	68	77	86	95	104

BOX 4-2
Sample Temperature Conversion Problems

What is 50°F in degrees Celsius?
$°C = \frac{5}{9} °F - 32$
$x = \frac{5}{9} 50°F - 32$
$x = \frac{5}{9} 18°F$
$x = 10°C$

What is 18°C in degrees Fahrenheit?
$°F = \frac{9}{5} (°C) + 32$
$x = \frac{9}{5} (18°C) + 32$
$x = 32.4 + 32$
$x = 64°F$

TABLE 4-5

Examples of Conversions Between Metric and SI Units

	Metric Unit ×	Factor =	SI units
Gram	g/mL	$\frac{10^{15}}{MW}$	pmol/L
	g/100 mL	10	g/L
	g/100 mL	$\frac{10^4}{MW}$	mmol/L
Microgram	μg/100 mL	$\frac{10}{MW}$	μmol/L
Milligram	mg/100 mL	10^{-2}	g/L
Milliliter	mL/100 g	10	mL/kg

MW, Molecular weight; *mmol*, millimole.

is unbreakable, which is its greatest advantage. It is preferred for certain analyses in which glass can be damaged by chemicals used in the testing. Alkaline solutions must be stored in plastic.

The disadvantages of plastic are that there is some leaching of surface-bound constituents into solutions, some permeability to water vapor, some evaporation through breathing of the plastic, and some absorption of dyes, stains, or proteins. Because evaporation is a significant factor in using plastic-ware, small volumes of reagent should never be stored in oversized plastic bottles for long periods.

Glassware

Although disposable plasticware has largely replaced glassware because of high resistance to corrosion and breakage, clinical and research laboratories still use glassware for analytical work. Glassware is used in all departments of the laboratory, and special types of glass apparatus have been devised for special uses. Certain types of glass can be attacked by reagents to such an extent that the determinations done in them are not valid. It is therefore important to use the correct type of glass for the determinations being done.

Types of Glass

Clinical laboratory glassware can be divided into several types: glass with high thermal resistance, high-silica glass, glass with a high resistance to alkali, low-actinic glass, and standard flint glass.

THERMAL-RESISTANT (BOROSILICATE) GLASS

High-thermal-resistant glass is usually a boro-silicate glass with a low alkali content. This type of glassware is resistant to heat, corrosion, and thermal shock and should be used whenever heating or sterilization by heat is employed. Borosilicate glass, known by the commercial name of *Pyrex* (Corning Glass Works, Corning, NY) or *Kimax*, (Kimble Glass Co., Vineland, NJ) is used widely in the laboratory because of its high qualities of resistance. Laboratory apparatus such as beakers, flasks, and pipettes are usually made from borosilicate glass. Other brands of glassware are made from lower-grade borosilicate glass and may be used when a high-quality borosilicate glass is not necessary.

One or more of these brand names will be found on many different types of glassware in the laboratory. It is essential to choose glassware that has a reliable composition and will be resistant to laboratory chemicals and conditions. In borosilicate glassware, mechanical strength and thermal and chemical resistance are well balanced.

ALUMINA-SILICATE GLASS

Alumina-silicate glass has a high silica content, which makes it comparable to fused quartz in its heat resistance, chemical stability, and electrical characteristics. It is strengthened chemically rather than thermally. Corex brand (Corning) is made from alumina-silica. This type of glassware is used for high-precision analytical work; it is radiation resistant and can also be used for optical reflectors and mirrors. It is not used for the general type of glassware found in the laboratory.

ACID-RESISTANT AND ALKALI-RESISTANT GLASS

Glass with high resistance to acids or alkali was developed particularly for use with strong acid or alkaline solutions. It is boron free. It is often referred to as *soft glass* because its thermal resistance is much less than that of borosilicate glass, and it must be heated and cooled very carefully. Its use should be limited to times when solutions of, or digestions with, strong acids or alkalis are made.

LOW-ACTINIC (AMBER-COLORED) GLASS

Low-actinic glassware contains materials that usually impart an amber or red color to the glass and reduce the amount of light transmitted through to the substance in the glassware. It is used for substances that are particularly sensitive to light, such as bilirubin and vitamin A.

FLINT GLASS

Standard flint glass, or soda-lime glass, is composed of a mixture of the oxides of silicon, calcium, and sodium. It is the most inexpensive glass and is readily made into a variety of types of glassware. This type of glass is much less resistant to high temperatures and sudden changes in temperature, and its resistance to chemical attack is only fair. Glassware made from soda-lime glass can release alkali into solutions and can therefore cause considerable errors in certain laboratory determinations. For example, manual pipettes made from soda-lime glass may release alkali into the pipetted liquid.

DISPOSABLE GLASSWARE

The widespread use of relatively inexpensive disposable glassware has greatly reduced the need to clean glassware. Disposable glassware is made to be used and discarded, and no cleaning is necessary either before or after use in most cases. Disposable glass and plastic are used to manufacture many laboratory supplies, including test tubes of all sizes, pipettes, slides, Petri dishes for microbiology, and specimen containers.

Containers and Receivers

This category of glassware includes many of the most frequently used and most common pieces of glassware in the laboratory. Containers and receivers must be made of good-quality glass. They are not calibrated to hold a particular or exact volume, but rather are available for various volumes, depending on the use desired. Beakers, Erlenmeyer flasks, test tubes, and reagent bottles are made in many different sizes (Fig. 4-1). This glassware, as with the volumetric glassware, has certain information indicated directly on the vessel. The volume and the brand name, or trademark, are two pieces of information found on items such as beakers and test tubes. Containers and receivers are not as expensive as volumetric glassware because the process of exact volume calibration is not necessary.

BEAKERS

Beakers are wide, straight-sided cylindrical vessels and are available in many sizes and in several forms. The most common form used in the clinical laboratory is known as the *Griffin low form*. Beakers should be made of glass that is resistant to the many chemicals used in them and also resistant to heat. Beakers are used along with flasks for general mixing and reagent preparation.

ERLENMEYER FLASKS

Erlenmeyer flasks are often used in the laboratory for preparing reagents and for titration procedures. As with beakers, these flasks come in various sizes and must be made from a resistant form of glass.

TEST TUBES

Test tubes come in many sizes, depending on the use for which they are intended. Test tubes without lips are the most satisfactory because there is less chance of chipping and eventual breakage. Disposable test tubes are used for most laboratory purposes. Because chemical reactions occur in test tubes used in the chemistry laboratory, test tubes intended for such use should be made of borosilicate glass, which is resistant to thermal shock.

REAGENT BOTTLES

All reagents should be stored in reagent bottles of some type. These can be made of glass or some other material; some of the more common bottles are now made of plastic. Reagent bottles come in

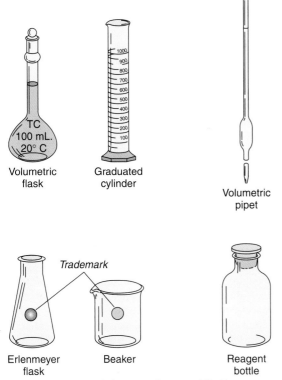

FIGURE 4-1 Laboratory glassware. *TC, To contain.*

various sizes. The size used should meet the needs of the particular situation.

Volumetric Glassware

Volumetric glassware must go through a rigorous process of volume calibration to ensure the accuracy of the measurements required for laboratory determinations. In very precise work, it is never safe to assume the volume contained or delivered by any piece of equipment is exactly that indicated on the equipment. The calibration process is lengthy and time consuming, so the cost of volumetric glassware is relatively high compared to the cost of uncalibrated glassware.

CALIBRATION OF VOLUMETRIC GLASSWARE

Calibration is the means by which glassware or other apparatus used in quantitative measurements is checked to determine its exact volume. To *calibrate* is to divide the glassware or mark it with graduations (or other indices of quantity) for the purpose of measurement. Calibration marks will be seen on every piece of volumetric glassware used in the laboratory. Specifications for the calibration of glassware are established by the **National Bureau of Standards (NBS)**.[3,4] High-quality volumetric glassware is calibrated by the manufacturer; this

calibration can be checked by the laboratory using the glassware.

Each piece of volumetric glassware must be checked and must comply with these specifications before it can be accurately used in the clinical laboratory. Pipettes, volumetric flasks, and other types of volumetric glassware are supposed to hold, deliver, or contain a specific amount of liquid. This specified amount, or volume, is known as the *units of capacity* and is indicated by the manufacturer directly on each piece of glassware.

Volumetric glassware is usually calibrated by weight, using distilled water. Water is typically used as the liquid for calibration because it is readily available and similar in viscosity and speed of drainage to the solutions and reagents used in the clinical laboratory. The units of capacity determined will therefore be the volume of water contained in, or delivered by, the glassware at a particular temperature. The manufacturer knows what the weights of various amounts of distilled water are at specific temperatures. This information is used in the manual calibration of volumetric glassware. If a manufacturer wants a volumetric flask to contain 100 mL, a sensitive balance such as an analytical balance is used. Weights corresponding to what 100 mL of distilled water weighs at a specific temperature are placed on one side of the balance. The flask to be calibrated is placed on the other side of the balance, and distilled water is gradually added to it until equilibrium is achieved. The manufacturer then makes a permanent calibration mark on the neck of the flask at the bottom of the water meniscus level. This flask is then calibrated to contain 100 mL. Other sizes and types of volumetric glassware are similarly calibrated.

The volume of a particular piece of glassware varies with the temperature. For this reason, it is necessary to specify the temperature at which the glassware was calibrated. Glass will swell or shrink with changes in temperature, and the volume of the glassware will therefore vary. Most volumetric glassware for routine clinical use is calibrated at 20°C. This means that the calibration process and checking took place at a controlled temperature of 20°C. On all volumetric glassware, the inscription "20°C" will be seen. Although 20°C has been almost universally adopted as the standard temperature for calibration of volumetric glassware, each piece of glassware will have the temperature of calibration inscribed on it. The volume of a volumetric flask is smaller at a low temperature than at a high temperature. A 50-mL volumetric flask that was calibrated at 20°C would contain less than 50 mL at 10°C.

Because the laboratory depends so greatly on the quality of its glassware to produce reliable results, it is necessary to be certain that the glassware is of the best quality. The glass used for volumetric glassware must meet certain standards of quality. It must be transparent and free from striations and other surface irregularities. It should have no defects that would distort the appearance of the liquid surface or the portion of the calibration line seen through the glass.

The design and workmanship for volumetric glassware are also specified by NBS. The shape of the glassware must permit complete emptying and thorough cleaning, and it must stand solidly on a level surface.

Volumetric Flasks

Volumetric flasks are flasks with a round bulb at the bottom. This tapers to a long neck on which the calibration mark is found. The NBS specifications apply to all volumetric glassware and therefore to volumetric flasks[3] (see Fig. 4-1). Volumetric flasks are calibrated *to contain* a specific amount or volume of liquid, and therefore the letters *TC* are inscribed somewhere on the neck of the flask. Many different sizes of volumetric flasks are available for the different volumes of liquid used. Sizes in which volumetric flasks can be purchased include 10, 25, 50, 100, and 500 mL and 1 and 2 L.

Volumetric flasks have been calibrated individually "to contain" the specified volume at a specified temperature; they are not calibrated "to deliver" this volume. For each size of volumetric flask, there are certain allowable limits within which its volume must lie. These limits are called the **tolerance** of the flask. All volumetric glassware has a specific tolerance, the capacity tolerance, which is dependent on the size of the glassware. For example, if a 100-mL volumetric flask has a tolerance of 0.08 mL, conditions are controlled during the calibration of a 100-mL volumetric flask to guarantee these limits. A tolerance of 0.08 mL indicates that the allowable limits for the volume of a 100-mL volumetric flask are from 99.92 to 100.08 mL. A tolerance of 0.05 mL for a 50-mL volumetric flask indicates allowable limits of 49.95 to 50.05 mL for the volume of the flask. Volumetric flasks are used in the preparation of specific volumes of reagents or laboratory solutions. They should be used with reagents or solutions at room temperature. Solutions diluted in volumetric flasks should be repeatedly mixed during the dilution so the contents are homogeneous before they are made up to volume. In this way, errors caused by the expansion or contraction of liquids during mixing become negligible. An important factor in the use of any volumetric apparatus is an accurate reading of the meniscus level (see later discussion on pipetting technique).

Graduated Measuring Cylinders

A graduated measuring cylinder is a long, straight-sided, cylindrical piece of glassware with calibrated markings. Graduated cylinders are used to measure volumes of liquids when a high degree of accuracy is not essential. They can be made from plastic or polyethylene as well as from glass (see Fig. 4-1). Graduated cylinders come in various sizes according to the volumes they measure: 10, 25, 50, 100, 500, and 1000 mL. A 100-mL graduated cylinder can measure 100 mL or a fraction of this amount, depending on the calibration, or graduation, marks on it. Most graduated cylinders are calibrated *to deliver*, as indicated directly on the glassware by the inscription "TD." The letters *TD* can be found on many types of volumetric glassware, especially on the numerous pipettes used in the laboratory.

Graduated cylinders can be used to measure a specified volume of a liquid, such as water, in the preparation of laboratory reagents. The calibration marks on the cylinder indicate its capacity at different points. If 450 mL of water is to be measured, the most satisfactory cylinder to use would be one with a capacity of 500 mL. Graduated cylinders are not calibrated as accurately as volumetric flasks. Therefore, the capacity tolerance for graduated cylinders allows a greater variation in volume. The capacity tolerance is greater for the larger graduated cylinders. A 100-mL graduated cylinder (TD) has a tolerance of 0.40 mL, meaning that the allowable limits are 99.60 to 100.40 mL.

Pipettes

Pipettes are another type of volumetric glassware used extensively in the laboratory. Although many types of pipettes are available, it is important to use only pipettes manufactured by reputable companies. Care and discretion should be used in selecting pipettes for clinical laboratory use, because their accuracy is one of the determining factors in the accuracy of the procedures done. A pipette is a cylindrical glass tube used in measuring fluids. Pipettes are calibrated to deliver, or transfer, a specified volume from one vessel to another (see Fig. 4-1). Manual and automatic pipettes are available.

Each manual pipette has at least one calibration or graduation mark on it, as does all volumetric glassware. A pipette is filled by using mechanical suction or an aspirator bulb. Mouth suction is never used. Strong acids, bases, solvents, or human specimens are much too potent or contaminated to risk pipetting them by mouth. Caustic liquids and some solvents are very dangerous; some destroy tissue immediately on contact. Some solvents have harmful vapors.

For most general laboratory use, there are two main types of manual pipettes: the **volumetric (or transfer) pipette** and the **graduated (or measuring) pipette**. They are classified according to whether they contain or deliver a specified amount; they may be called **to-contain pipettes** or **to-deliver pipettes**. A to-contain pipette is identified by the inscribed letters TC and a to-deliver pipette by the letters *TD*. The TD pipette is filled properly and allowed to drain completely into a receiving vessel. Portions of nonviscous samples are accurately measured by allowing the volumetric pipette to drain while it is held in the vertical position, using only the force of gravity. For most volumetric glassware, the temperature of calibration is usually 20°C, and this is inscribed on the pipette.

The opening (orifice) at the delivery tip of the pipette is of a certain size to allow a specified time for drainage when the pipette is held vertically. A pipette must be held vertically to ensure proper drainage. It will not drain as fast when held at a 45-degree angle.

VOLUMETRIC PIPETTES

A volumetric, or transfer, pipette has been calibrated to deliver a fixed volume of liquid by drainage. These pipettes consist of a cylindrical bulb joined at both ends to narrow glass tubing. A **calibration mark** is etched around the upper suction tube, and the lower delivery tube is drawn out to a fine tip. Some important considerations concerning volumetric pipettes are that the calibration mark should not be too close to the top of the suction tube, the bulb should merge gradually into the lower delivery tube, and the delivery tip should have a gradual taper. To reduce drainage errors, the orifice should be of such a size that the outflow of the pipette is not too rapid. These pipettes should be made from a good-quality Kimax or Pyrex glass (Fig. 4-2).

Volumetric pipettes are suitable for all accurate measurements of volumes of 1 mL or more. They are calibrated to deliver the amount inscribed on them. This volume is measured from the calibration mark to the tip. A 5-mL volumetric pipette will deliver a single measured volume of 5 mL, and a 2-mL volumetric pipette will deliver 2 mL. The tolerance of volumetric pipettes increases with the capacity of the pipette. A 10-mL volumetric pipette will have a greater tolerance than a 2-mL one. The tolerance of a 5-mL volumetric pipette is 0.01 mL. When volumes of liquids are to be delivered with great accuracy, a volumetric pipette is used. Volumetric pipettes are used to measure standard solutions, unknown blood and plasma filtrates, serum, plasma, urine, cerebrospinal fluid, and some reagents.

Measurements with volumetric pipettes are done individually, and the volumes can be only whole milliliters, as determined by the pipette selected (e.g., 1, 2, 5, and 10 mL). To transfer 1 mL of a standard solution into a test tube volumetrically, a 1-mL volumetric pipette is used. To transfer 5 mL of the same solution, a 5-mL volumetric pipette is used. After a volumetric pipette drains, a drop remains inside the delivery tip. The specific volume the pipette is calibrated to deliver is dependent on the drop left in the pipette tip. Information inscribed on the pipette includes the temperature of calibration (usually 20°C), capacity, manufacturer, and use (TD). The technique involved in using volumetric pipettes correctly is very important, and a certain amount of skill is required (see Pipetting Technique Using Manual Pipettes).

GRADUATED PIPETTES

Another way to deliver a particular amount of liquid is to deliver the amount of liquid contained between two calibration marks on a cylindrical tube or pipette. Such a pipette is called a *graduated pipette*, or measuring pipette. It has several graduation, or calibration, marks (see Fig. 4-2). Many measurements in the laboratory do not require the precision of the volumetric pipette, so graduated pipettes are used when great accuracy is less critical. This does not mean that these pipettes may be used with less care than the volumetric pipettes. Graduated pipettes are used primarily in measuring reagents, but they are not calibrated with sufficient tolerance to use in measuring standard or control solutions, unknown specimens, or filtrates.

A graduated pipette is a straight piece of glass tubing with a tapered end and graduation marks on the stem, separating it into parts. Depending on the size used, graduated pipettes can be used to measure parts of a milliliter or many milliliters. These pipettes come in various sizes or capacities, including 0.1, 0.2, 1.0, 2.0, 5.0, 10, and 25 mL. If 4 mL of deionized water is to be measured

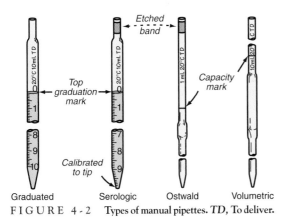

FIGURE 4-2 **Types of manual pipettes.** *TD*, To deliver.

into a test tube, a 5-mL graduated pipette would be the best choice. Graduated pipettes require draining between two marks; they introduce one more source of error compared with the volumetric pipettes, which have only one calibration mark. This makes measurements with the graduated pipette less precise. Because of this relatively poor precision, the graduated pipette is used when speed is more important than precision. It is used for measurements of reagents and is generally not considered accurate enough for measuring samples and standard solutions.

Two types of graduated pipettes are calibrated for delivery (see Fig. 4-2). A Mohr pipette is calibrated between two marks on the stem, and a serologic pipette has graduation marks down to the delivery tip. The serologic pipette has a larger orifice and therefore drains faster than the Mohr pipette.

The volume of the space between the last calibration mark and the delivery tip is not known in the Mohr pipette. In Mohr graduated pipettes, this space cannot be used for measuring fluids. Graduated pipettes are calibrated in much the same manner as volumetric pipettes, but they are not constructed to as strict specifications, and they have larger tolerances. The allowable tolerance for a 5-mL graduated pipette is 0.02 mL.

SEROLOGIC PIPETTES

The **serologic pipette** is similar to the graduated pipette in appearance (see Fig. 4-2). The orifice, or tip opening, is larger in the serologic pipette than in other pipettes. The rate of the fall of liquid is much too fast for great accuracy or precision. Using the serologic pipette in chemistry would require impeding the flow of liquid from the delivery tip. The serologic pipette is graduated to the end of the delivery tip and has an etched band on the suction piece. It is therefore designed to be blown out mechanically. The serologic pipette is less precise than any of the pipettes discussed earlier. It is designed for use in serology, in which relative values are sought.

Specialized Pipettes

MICROPIPETTES (TO-CONTAIN PIPETTES)

The micropipette, or to-contain pipette, when used properly, is one of the more precise pipettes used in the clinical laboratory. This type of pipette is calibrated to contain a specified amount of liquid. If a pipette contains only 10 mL (0.1 mL), and 10 mL of blood is needed for a laboratory determination, then none of the blood can be left inside the pipette. The entire contents of the pipette must be emptied. If this pipette is rinsed well with a diluting solution, all the blood or similar specimen will be removed from it. The correct way to use a TC

pipette is to rinse it with a suitable diluent. Thus, a TC pipette cannot be used properly unless the receiving vessel contains a diluent; that is, a TC pipette should not be used to deliver a specimen into an empty receiving vessel. Because all the liquid in a TC pipette is rinsed out and used, there is only one graduation mark.

Micropipettes are used when small amounts of blood or specimen are needed. Many procedures require only a small amount of blood, and a micropipette is used for this measurement. Because even a minute volume remaining in the pipette can cause a significant error in microwork, most micropipettes are calibrated to contain the stated volume rather than to deliver it. They are generally available in small sizes from 1 to 500 mL.

UNOPETTE

A special disposable micropipette used in the hematology laboratory is a self-filling pipette accompanied by a polyethylene reagent reservoir (see Chapter 12). This unit is called a *Unopette* (Becton Dickinson [BD], Franklin Lakes, NJ). Although this device is no longer manufactured for red, white, and platelet counts, a product for reticulocyte counts continues to be manufactured. A capillary pipette is fitted in a plastic holder and fills automatically with blood by means of capillary action. The plastic reagent bottle (called the *reservoir*) is squeezed slightly while the pipette is inserted. On release of pressure, the sample is drawn into the diluent in the reservoir. Intermittent squeezing fills and empties the pipette to rinse out the contents.

CAPILLARY PIPETTES

This inexpensive, disposable micropipette is made of capillary tubing with a calibration line marking a specified volume. The capillary micropipette is filled to the line by capillary action, and the measured liquid is delivered by positive pressure, as with a medicine dropper. These pipettes are usually calibrated TC and require rinsing to obtain the stated accuracy.

Pipetting

Care and discretion should be used in selecting pipettes for clinical laboratory use; their accuracy is one of the determining factors in the accuracy of the procedures done. As previously mentioned, several types of pipettes are used in the laboratory. Qualified personnel must understand their uses and gain experience in how to handle pipettes in clinical determinations. Practice is the key to success in the use of laboratory pipettes. To reiterate, the two categories of manual pipettes are to-contain (TC) and to-deliver (TD).

To-Contain Pipettes

TC pipettes are calibrated to contain a specified amount of liquid but are not necessarily calibrated to deliver that exact amount. A small amount of fluid will cling to the inside wall of the TC pipette, and when these pipettes are used, they should be rinsed out with a diluting fluid to ensure that the entire contents have been emptied.

To-Deliver Pipettes

TD pipettes are calibrated to deliver the amount of fluid designated on the pipette; this volume will flow out of the pipette by gravity when the pipette is held in a vertical position with its tip against the inside wall of the receiving vessel. A small amount of fluid will remain in the tip of the pipette; this amount is left in the tip because the calibrated portion has been delivered into the receiving vessel.

Another category of pipette is called *blowout*. The calibration of these pipettes is similar to that of TD pipettes, except that the drop remaining in the tip of the pipette must be "blown out" into the receiving vessel. If a pipette is to be blown out, an etched ring will be seen near the suction opening. A mechanical device or safety bulb must be used to blow out the entire contents of the pipette.

Pipetting Technique Using Manual Pipettes

It is important to develop a good technique for handling pipettes (Fig. 4-3); only through practice can this be accomplished (Procedure 4-1). With few exceptions, the same general steps apply to pipetting for all manual pipettes.

Laboratory accidents frequently result from improper pipetting techniques. The greatest potential hazard is when mouth pipetting is done instead of mechanical suction. Mouth pipetting is *never* acceptable in the clinical laboratory. Caustic reagents, contaminated specimens, and poisonous solutions are all pipetted at some point in the laboratory, and every precaution must be taken to ensure the safety of the person doing the work (see Chapter 2).

After the pipette has been filled above the top graduation mark, removed from the vessel, and held in a vertical position, the meniscus must be adjusted (Fig. 4-4). The **meniscus** is the curvature in the top surface of a liquid. The pipette should be held in such a way that the calibration mark is at eye level. The delivery tip is touched to the inside wall of the original vessel, not the liquid, and the meniscus of the liquid in the pipette is eased, or adjusted, down to the calibration mark.

When clear solutions are used, the bottom of the meniscus is read. For colored or viscous solutions, the top of the meniscus is read. All readings must be made with the eye at the level of the meniscus (see Fig. 4-4). Note that the pipette should be held steady with a finger of the opposite hand while the liquid is allowed to drain into a container.

Before the measured liquid in the pipette is allowed to drain into the receiving vessel, any liquid adhering to the outside of the pipette must be wiped off with a clean piece of gauze or tissue. If this is not done, any drops present on the outside of the pipette might drain into the receiving vessel along with the measured volume. This would make the volume greater than that specified, and an error would result.

Pipetting Technique Using Automatic Pipettes

AUTOMATIC MICROPIPETTORS

These **automatic pipetting devices** allow rapid, repetitive measurements and delivery of predetermined volumes of reagents or specimens. The most common type of micropipette used in many laboratories is one that is automatic or semiautomatic, called a *micropipettor*. These piston-operated devices allow repeated, accurate, reproducible delivery of specimens, reagents, and other liquids requiring measurement in small amounts. Many pipettors are continuously adjustable so that variable volumes of liquids can be dispensed with the same device. Delivery volume is selected by adjusting the settings on the device. Different types or models are available and allow volume delivery ranging from 0.5 to 500 mL, for example. The calibration of these micropipettes should be checked periodically.

The piston (usually in the form of a thumb plunger) is depressed to a "stop" position on the pipetting device, the tip is placed in the liquid to be measured, and then slowly the plunger is allowed to rise back to the original position (Fig. 4-5). This will fill the tip with the desired volume of liquid. The tips are usually drawn along the inside wall of the vessel from which the measured volume is drawn so that any adhering liquid is removed from the end of the tip. These pipette tips are not usually wiped, as is done with the manual pipettes, because the plastic surface is considered nonwettable. The tip of the pipette device is then placed against the inside wall of the receiving vessel, and the plunger is depressed. When the manufacturer's directions for the device are followed, sample delivery volume is judged to be extremely accurate.

The pipette tips are usually made of disposable plastic, so no cleaning is necessary. Various types of tips are available. Some pipetting devices automatically eject the tip after use. These will also allow the user to insert a new tip as well as remove the

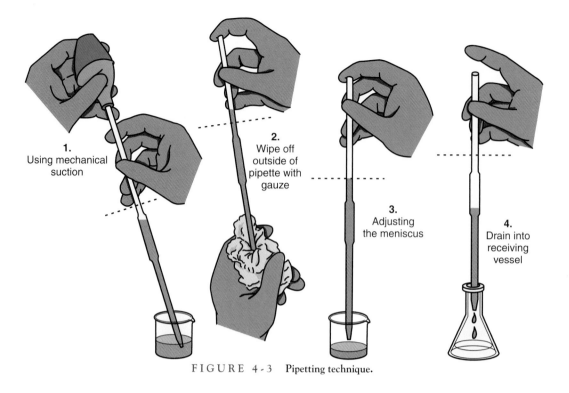

FIGURE 4-3 Pipetting technique.

PROCEDURE **4-1**

Pipetting With Manual Pipettes

1. Check the pipette to ascertain its correct size, being careful also to check for broken delivery or suction tips.
2. Wearing protective gloves, hold the pipette lightly between the thumb and last three fingers, leaving the index finger free.
3. Place the tip of the pipette well below the surface of the liquid to be pipetted.
4. Using mechanical suction or an aspirator bulb, carefully draw the liquid up into the pipette until the level of liquid is well above the calibration mark.
5. Quickly cover the suction opening at the top of the pipette with the index finger.
6. Wipe the outside of the pipette dry with a piece of gauze or tissue to remove excess fluid.
7. Hold the pipette in a vertical position, with the delivery tip against the inside of the original vessel. Carefully allow the liquid in the pipette to drain by gravity until the bottom of the meniscus is exactly at the calibration mark. (The meniscus is the concave or convex surface of a column of liquid as seen in a laboratory pipette, buret, or other measuring device.) To do this, do not entirely remove the index finger from the suction-hole end of the pipette; rather, by rolling the finger slightly over the opening, allow slow drainage to take place.
8. While still holding the pipette in a vertical position, touch the tip of the pipette to the inside wall of the receiving vessel. Remove the index finger from the top of the pipette to permit free drainage. Remember to keep the pipette in a vertical position for correct drainage. In TD pipettes, a small amount of fluid will remain in the delivery tip.
9. To be certain the drainage is as complete as possible, touch the delivery tip of the pipette to another area on the inside wall of the receiving vessel.
10. Remove the pipette from the receiving vessel, and place it in the appropriate place for washing (see Cleaning Laboratory Glassware and Plasticware).

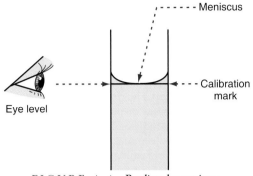

Meniscus

Calibration mark

Eye level

F I G U R E   4 - 4   **Reading the meniscus.**

used tip without touching it, minimizing infectious biohazard exposures.

Automatic and semiautomatic micropipettors are useful in many areas of laboratory work. Each of the different types must be carefully calibrated before use. The problems encountered with automatic pipetting depend largely on the nature of the solution to be pipetted. Some reagents cause more bubbles than others, and some are more viscous. Bubbles and viscous solutions can cause problems with measurement and delivery of samples and solutions.

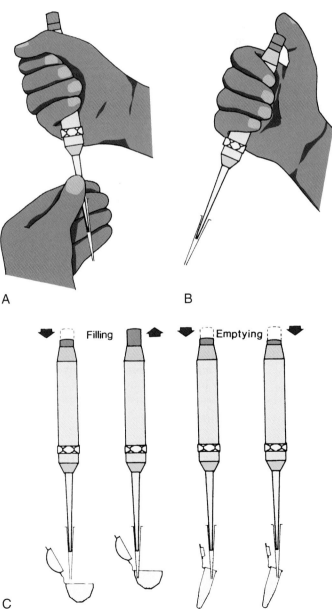

A   B

Filling   Emptying

C

F I G U R E   4 - 5   **Steps in using piston-type automatic micropipette. A,** Attaching proper tip size for range of pipette volume and twisting tip as it is pushed onto pipette to give an airtight, continuous seal. **B,** Holding pipette before use. **C,** Detailed instructions for filling and emptying pipette tip. (From Kaplan LA, Pesce AJ: Clinical chemistry: theory, analysis, correlation, ed 5, St Louis, 2010, Mosby.)

Micropipettors contain or deliver from 1 to 500 mL. It is important to follow the manufacturer's instructions for the device being used because each may be slightly different. In general, the following steps apply for use of a micropipettor (see Fig. 4-5):

1. Attach the proper tip to the pipettor, and set the delivery volume.
2. Depress the piston to a stop position on the pipettor.
3. Place the tip into the solution, and allow the piston to rise slowly back to its original position. (This fills the pipettor tip with the desired volume of solution.)
4. Some tips are wiped with a dry gauze at this step, and some are not wiped. Follow the manufacturer's directions.
5. Place the tip on the wall of the receiving vessel and depress the piston, first to a stop position where the liquid is allowed to drain, then to a second stop position where the full dispensing of the liquid takes place.
6. Dispose of the tip in the waste disposal receptacle. Some pipettors automatically eject the used tips, thus minimizing biohazard exposure.

AUTOMATIC DISPENSERS OR SYRINGES

Many types of automatic dispensers or syringes are used in the laboratory for repetitive adding of multiple doses of the same reagent or diluent. These devices are used for measuring serial amounts of relatively small volumes of the same liquid. The volume to be dispensed is determined by the pipettor setting. Dispensers are available with a variety of volume settings. Some are available as syringes and others as bottle-top devices. Most of these dispensers can be cleaned by autoclaving.

DILUTER-DISPENSERS

In automated instruments, diluter-dispensers are used to prepare a number of different samples for analysis. These devices pipette a selected aliquot of sample and diluent into the instrument or receiving vessel. These devices are mostly of the dual-piston type, one being used for the sample and the other for the diluent or reagent.

Cleaning Laboratory Glassware and Plasticware

Among the many factors that ensure accurate results in laboratory determinations is the use of clean, unbroken glassware. There is no point in exercising care in obtaining specimens, handling the specimens, and making the laboratory determination if the laboratory ware used is not extremely clean. Plasticware must also be clean.

Since the widespread adoption of disposable glassware and plasticware, few pieces are cleaned for reuse. Only larger pieces of glassware (e.g., volumetric flasks, pipettes, graduated cylinders) are usually cleaned. Various methods are used; general cleaning methods involve the use of a soap, detergent, or cleaning powder. In most laboratories, detergents are used. Laboratory ware that cannot be cleaned immediately after use should be rinsed with tap water and left to soak in a basin or pail of water to which a small amount of detergent has been added. If the dirty glassware has been soaking in a solution of the detergent water, the cleaning job will be much easier.

Glassware that is contaminated, as by use with patient specimens, must be decontaminated before it is washed. This can be done by presoaking in 5% bleach or by boiling, autoclaving, or some similar procedure.

Most plasticware can be cleaned in the same manner as glassware and using ordinary glassware washing machines, but the use of any abrasive cleaning materials should be avoided.

Cleaning Pipettes

Nondisposable pipettes used in the laboratory are cleaned in a special way. Immediately after use, the pipettes should be placed in a special pipette container or cylinder containing water; the water should be high enough to cover the pipettes completely. Pipettes should be placed in the container carefully with the tip up to avoid breakage. When the pipettes are to be cleaned, they are removed from the cylinder and placed in another cylinder containing a cleaning solution. This cleaning solution can be a detergent or a commercial analytical cleaning product. The pipettes are allowed to soak in the cleaning solution for 30 minutes.

The next step involves thorough rinsing of the pipettes. This can be accomplished by hand, but more often an automatic pipette washer is used. The pipettes are rinsed with tap water, using the automatic washer, for 1 to 2 hours. They are then rinsed in deionized or distilled water two or three times and dried in a hot oven.

Glass Breakage

It is important in the clinical laboratory to check all glassware periodically to determine its condition. No broken or chipped glassware should be used; many laboratory accidents are caused this way. Serious cuts may result, and infections may develop.

Each time a laboratory procedure is carried out, the glassware used should be checked. Equipment such as beakers, pipettes, test tubes, and flasks should not have broken edges or cracks. To prevent breakage, glassware should be handled carefully, and personnel should avoid carrying too much glassware at one time in the laboratory.

LABORATORY BALANCES

General Use of Balances

Some of the most important measurement devices are the various balances used in the **measurement of mass or weight** in preparing the reagents and standard solutions used in the laboratory. This is one method of **quantitative analysis** in the clinical laboratory. Almost every procedure performed in the laboratory depends to some extent on the use of a balance. Laboratory balances function by either mechanical or electronic means.

In the traditional clinical laboratory, **gravimetric analysis** (analysis by measurement of mass or weight) was used in the preparation of some reagents and standard solutions. In many laboratories now, reagents, standard solutions, and control solutions are purchased ready to use, and the actual laboratory preparation of reagents and solutions is limited. Because measurement of mass remains fundamental to all analyses, the technique of weighing should continue to be fundamental to the base of knowledge for all persons working in a clinical laboratory. Some laboratories routinely prepare their own standard solutions. Another use for weighing is the calibration of volumetric equipment. The measurement of mass continues to be the quantitative means by which this equipment is calibrated.

Some solutions require more accurately weighed chemicals than others. The accuracy needed depends on the planned use of the solution. The worker must decide what type of balance (or scale) is most appropriate for the precision or reproducibility required in weighing the chemicals to be used for a particular solution. The different balances available are suited to particular needs.

Most clinical laboratories have replaced mechanical balances with electronic types that are either top loading or analytical in design. The balance considered the "backbone" of the clinical laboratory is the analytical balance.

Analytical Balance

Many types of analytical balances are made by different companies and have various degrees of automatic operation. In this discussion, analytical balances are divided into two types: manually operated (mechanical) and automatic or electronic (Fig. 4-6). Each company that manufactures analytical balances has its own trade name for each of the balances produced. Some of the fine analytical balances used in the clinical laboratory are the Ainsworth, Voland, Christian-Becker, Mettler, Ohaus, and Sartorius balances. Others are also available. It is important to investigate carefully several different analytical balances before deciding on one for use in a particular laboratory.

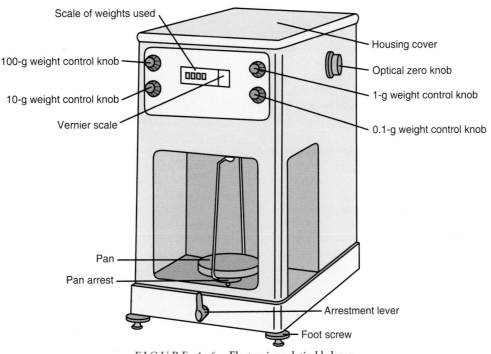

FIGURE 4-6 Electronic analytical balance.

General Principles

The basic principle in the quantitative measurement of mass is to balance an unknown mass (the substance being weighed) with a known mass. The **electronic analytical balance** is a single-pan balance that uses an electromagnetic force to counterbalance the load placed on the pan (see Fig. 4-6). This pan is mechanically connected to a coil that is suspended in the field of a permanent cylindrical electromagnet. When a load is placed on the pan, a force is produced that displaces the coil within the magnetic field. A photoelectric cell scanning device changes position and generates a current just sufficient to return the coil to its original position; this is called *electromagnetic force compensation*. This current is proportional to the weight of the load on the pan and is displayed for the person using the balance to see visually, or it can be interfaced with a data output device. The greater the mass placed on the pan, the greater the deflecting force and the stronger the compensating current required to return the coil to its original position. A direct linear relationship exists between the compensation current and the force produced by the load placed on the pan. Electronic balances permit fast, accurate weighings with a high degree of resolution. They are easy to use and have replaced the traditional mechanically operated analytical balance in most clinical laboratories.

Uses

Almost every procedure performed in the traditional clinical laboratory depends on the use of balances, and the most important one is the analytical balance. Before any procedure is started, reagents and standard solutions are prepared. Standard solutions are always very accurately prepared, and the analytical balance is used to weigh the chemicals for these solutions. The analytical balance might be called the "starting point" of each method used in the laboratory.

The analytical balance should be cleaned and adjusted at least once a year to ensure its continued accuracy and sensitivity. Its accuracy is what makes this instrument so essential in the clinical laboratory. The accuracy to which most analytical balances used in the clinical laboratory should weigh chemicals is usually 0.1 mg, or 0.0001 g. With the electronic balance, the weights are added by manipulating a series of dials.

General Rules for Positioning and Weighing

Weighing errors will occur if the analytical balance is not properly positioned. Therefore, the balance must be located and mounted in an optimal position. The balance must be level; this is usually accomplished by adjusting the movable screws on the legs of the balance. The firmness of support is also important. The bench or table on which the balance rests must be rigid and free from vibrations. Preferably, the room in which the balance is set up should have constant temperature and humidity. Ideally, the analytical balance should be in an air-conditioned room. The temperature factor is most important. The balance should not be placed near hot objects such as radiators, flames, stills, or electric ovens. Neither should it be placed near cold objects and especially not near an open window. Sunlight or illumination from high-power lamps should be avoided in choosing a good location for the analytical balance.

The analytical balance is a delicate precision instrument that will not function properly if abused. When learning to use an analytical balance, personnel should be responsible for knowing and adhering to the rules for the use of that particular balance. The following general rules apply:

1. Set up the balance where it will be free from vibration.
2. Close the balance case before observing the reading; any air currents present will affect the weighing process.
3. Never weigh any chemical directly on the pan; a container of some type must be used for the chemical.
4. Never place a hot object on the balance pan. If an object is warm, the weight determined will be too little because of convection currents set up by the rising heated air.
5. Whenever the shape of the object to be weighed permits, handle it with tongs or forceps. Round objects such as weighing bottles may be handled with the fingers, but take care to prevent weight changes caused by moisture from the hand. Do not hold any object longer than necessary.
6. On completion of weighing, remove all objects and clean up any chemical spilled on the pan or within the balance area. Close the balance case.
7. Weighed materials should be transferred to labeled containers or made into solutions immediately.

Achieving speed in the weighing process is obtained only through practice (Procedure 4-2).

Basic Parts of Analytical Balance

The parts of the analytical balance must be thoroughly understood so that the weighing process can be carried out to the degree of accuracy necessary. Once the correct use of an analytical balance has been mastered, the worker should be able to

Weighing With an Electronic Analytical Balance

1. Before doing any weighing, make certain the balance is properly leveled. Observe the spirit level (leveling bubble), and adjust the leveling screws on the legs of the balance if necessary.

2. To check the zero-point adjustment, fully release the balance, and turn the adjustment knob clockwise as far as it will go. The optical scale zero should indicate three divisions below zero on the vernier scale. Using the same adjustment knob, adjust the optical scale zero so it aligns exactly with the zero line on the vernier scale. Arrest the balance.

3. With the balance arrested, place the weighing vessel on the pan, using tongs if possible so no humidity or heat is brought into the weighing chamber by the hands. Close the balance window.

4. Weigh the vessel in the following manner. Partially release the balance, and turn the 100-g weight control knob clockwise. When the scale moves up, turn the knob back one step. Repeat this operation with the 10-g, 1.0-g, and 0.1-g knobs, in that order. Arrest the balance. After a short pause, release the balance, and allow the scale to come to rest. Read the result and arrest the balance. With the balance arrested, unload the pan and bring all knobs back to zero.

5. Add the weight of the sample desired to the weight of the vessel just weighed to obtain the total to be weighed. Set the knobs (100, 10, 1.0, and 0.1 g) to the correct total weight needed. When the 0.1-g knob has been set at its proper reading, the balance should be placed in partial release. Slowly add the chemical to the vessel until the optical scale begins to move downward. When the optical scale starts downward, fully release the beam and continue to add the chemical until the optical scale registers the exact position desired. To obtain the reading to the nearest 0.1 mg (the sensitivity of most analytical balances), the vernier scale must be used in conjunction with the chain scale.

6. With the balance arrested, unload the pan, and bring all the knobs back to zero. Clean up any spilled chemical in the balance area.

use any of the available types, because they all have the same basic parts. Each manufacturer supplies a complete manual of operating directions, as well as information on the general use and care of the balance, with each balance purchased. These directions should be followed. The following parts are common to most analytical balances, electronic or mechanical (manually operated):

1. *Glass enclosure.* The analytical balance is enclosed in glass to prevent currents of air and collection of dust from disturbing the process of weighing.

2. *Balancing screws.* Before any weighing is done on the balance, it must be properly leveled. This is done by observing the leveling bubbles, or spirit level, located near the bottom of the balance. If necessary, adjust the balancing screws on the bottom of the balance case (usually found on each leg of the balance).

3. *Beam.* This is the structure from which the pans are suspended.

4. *Knife edges.* These support the beam at the fulcrum during weighing and provide sensitivity for the balance. Knife edges are vital parts and are constructed of hard metals to cause minimal friction.

5. *Pans for weighing.* The manually operated analytical balance has two pans: the weights are placed on the right-hand pan, and the object to be weighed is placed on the left-hand pan. The electronic analytical balance has only one pan; the object to be weighed is placed on this pan. The pans are suspended from the ends of the beam.

6. *Weights.* With the manual analytical balance, the weights are found in a separate weight box. These weights are never handled with the fingers but are removed from the box and placed on the balance pan by using special forceps. Mishandling of weights, either by using the fingers or by dropping, can result in an alteration of the actual and true mass of the weight. Weights come in units ranging from 100 mg to 50 g. The values of the weights are stamped directly on top of them.

   With the electronic analytical balance, the weights are inside the instrument and are not seen by the operator unless there is a need to remove the casing for repair or adjustment. The weights are added by manipulating specific dials calibrated for the weighing process. The built-in weights are on the same end of the beam as the sample pan and are counterbalanced by a fixed weight at the opposite end. There is always a constant load on the beam, and the projected scale has the same weight regardless of the load. The total weight of an object is registered automatically by a digital counter or in conjunction with an optical scale.

7. *Pan arrest.* This is a means of arresting the pan so that sudden movement or addition of weights or chemical will not injure the delicate knife edges. The pan arrests (usually found under the pans) can absorb any shock resulting from weight inequalities so that the knife edges are not subjected to this shock. The pan must be released to swing freely during actual weighing. In the electronic analytical balance, the arresting mechanism for both the pan and the beam is operated by a single lever. Partial release or full release can be obtained, depending on how the lever is moved.

8. *Damping device.* This is necessary to arrest the swing of the beam in the shortest practical time, thus reducing the time required in the weighing process.

9. *Vernier scale.* This is the small scale used to obtain precise readings to the nearest 0.1 mg. The vernier scale is used in conjunction with the large reading scale to obtain the necessary readings (Fig. 4-7).

10. *Reading scale.* In the manual analytical balance, this scale is actually the reading scale for the chain that is used for weighing 100 mg or less. It is used in conjunction

with the vernier scale to obtain readings to the nearest 0.1 mg. In the electronic analytical balance, this is usually a lighted optical scale, giving a high magnification and sharp definition for easier reading. The total weight of the object in question is registered automatically on this viewing scale.

Top-Loading Balance

A single-pan top-loading balance is one of the most common balances used in the laboratory. It is usually electronic and self-balancing. It is much faster and easier to use than some of the analytical balances previously described. A substance can be weighed in just a few seconds. These balances are usually modified torsion or substitution balances. Top-loading balances are used when the substance being weighed does not require as much analytical precision, as when reagents of a large volume are being prepared.

LABORATORY CENTRIFUGES

Centrifugation is used in the separation of a solid material from a liquid through the application of increased gravitational force by rapid rotation or spinning. It is also used in recovering solid materials from suspensions, as in the microscopic examination of urine. The solid material or sediment packed at the bottom of the centrifuge tube is sometimes called the *precipitate,* and the liquid or top portion is called the *supernatant.* Another important use for the centrifuge is in the separation of serum or plasma from cells in blood specimens. The suspended particles, solid material, or blood cells usually collect at the bottom of the centrifuge tube because the particles are heavier than the liquid. Occasionally the particles are lighter than the liquid and will collect on the surface of the liquid when it is centrifuged. Centrifugation is employed in many areas of the clinical laboratory, including chemistry, urinalysis, hematology, and blood banking. Proper use of the centrifuge is important for anyone engaged in laboratory work.

Types of Centrifuges

Centrifuges facilitate the separation of particles in suspension by the application of centrifugal force. Several types of centrifuges are usually found in the same laboratory; each is designed for special uses. The various types include table-model and floor-model centrifuges (some small and others very large), refrigerated centrifuges, ultracentrifuges, cytocentrifuges, and other centrifuges adapted for special procedures.

Two traditional types of centrifuges are used in routine laboratory determinations: a conventional

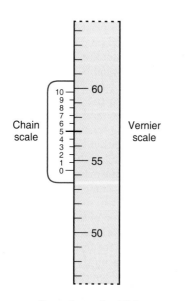

Chain scale   Vernier scale

Example reading 54.5 mg

FIGURE 4-7   **Readings obtained with a vernier scale.**

horizontal-head centrifuge with swinging buckets and a fixed angle–head centrifuge.

With the **horizontal-head centrifuge**, the cups holding the tubes of material to be centrifuged occupy a vertical position when the centrifuge is at rest but assume a horizontal position when the centrifuge revolves (Fig. 4-8). The horizontal-head, or swinging-bucket, centrifuge rotors hold the tubes being centrifuged in a vertical position when the centrifuge is at rest. When the rotor is in motion,

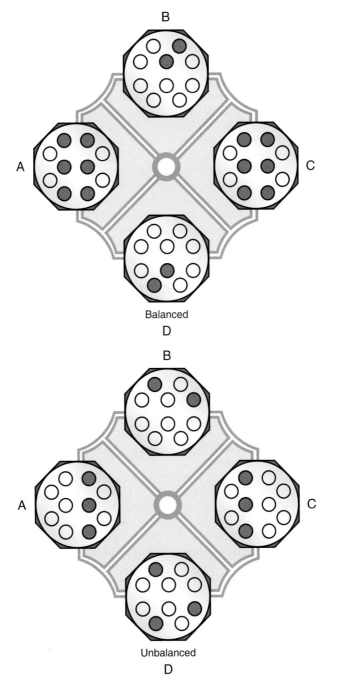

FIGURE 4-8 Examples of balanced and unbalanced loads in a horizontal-head centrifuge. A, Assuming all tubes have been filled with an equal amount of liquid, this rotor load is balanced. Opposing bucket sets A-C and B-D are loaded with equal numbers of tubes and balanced across the center of rotation. Each bucket is also balanced with respect to its pivotal axis. B, Even if all the tubes are filled equally, this rotor is improperly loaded. None of the bucket loads is balanced with respect to its pivotal axis. At operating speed, buckets A and C will not reach the horizontal position. Buckets B and D will pivot past the horizontal. Also note that the tube arrangement in the opposing buckets, B and D, is not symmetrical across the center of rotation. (From A centrifuge primer, Palo Alto, CA, 1980, Spinco Division of Beckman Instruments.)

the tubes move and remain in a horizontal position. During the process of centrifugation, when the tube is in the horizontal position, the particles being centrifuged constantly move along the tube, and any sediment is distributed evenly against the bottom of the tube. When centrifugation is complete and the rotor is no longer turning, the surface of the sediment is flat, with the column of liquid resting above it.

For the **fixed angle–head centrifuge**, the cups are held in a rigid position at a fixed angle. This position makes the process of centrifuging more rapid than with the horizontal-head centrifuge. There is also less chance that the sediment will be disturbed when the centrifuge stops. During centrifugation, particles travel along the side of the tube to form a sediment that packs against the bottom and side of the tube. Fixed angle–head centrifuges are used when rapid centrifugation of solutions containing small particles is needed; an example is the microhematocrit centrifuge. The microhematocrit centrifuge used in many hematology laboratories for packing red blood cells attains a speed of about 10,000 to 15,000 rpm.

A **cytocentrifuge** uses a very high-torque and low-inertia motor to spread monolayers of cells rapidly across a special slide for critical morphologic studies. This type of preparation can be used for blood, urine, body fluid, or any other liquid specimen that can be spread on a slide. An advantage of this technology is that only a small amount of sample is used, producing evenly distributed cells that can then be stained for microscopic study. The slide produced can be saved and examined at a later time, in contrast to "wet" preparations, which must be examined immediately.

Refrigerated centrifuges are available with internal refrigeration temperatures ranging from −15°C to −25°C during centrifugation. This permits centrifugation at higher speeds because the specimens are protected from the heat generated by the rotors of the centrifuge. The temperature of any refrigerated centrifuge should be checked regularly, and the thermometers should be checked periodically for accuracy.

Centrifuge Speed

Directions for use of a centrifuge are most frequently given in terms of speed, or revolutions per minute (rpm). The number of revolutions per minute and the centrifugal force generated are expressed as **relative centrifugal force (RCF)**. The number of revolutions per minute is related to the relative centrifugal force by the following formula:

$$RCF = 1.12 \times 10^{-5} \times r \times (rpm)^2$$

where r is the radius of the centrifuge expressed in centimeters. This is equal to the distance from the center of the centrifuge head to the bottom of the tube holder in the centrifuge bucket.

General laboratory centrifuges operate at speeds of up to 6000 rpm, generating RCF up to 7300 times the force of gravity (g). The top speed of most conventional centrifuges is about 3000 rpm. Conventional laboratory centrifuges of the horizontal type attain speeds of up to 3000 rpm, about 1700 g, without excessive heat production caused by friction between the head of the centrifuge and the air. Angle-head centrifuges produce less heat and may attain speeds of 7000 rpm (about 9000 g).

Ultracentrifuges are high-speed centrifuges generally used for research projects, but for certain clinical uses, a small air-driven ultracentrifuge is available that operates at 90,000 to 100,000 rpm and generates a maximum RCF of 178,000 g. Ultracentrifuges are often refrigerated.

A rheostat is used to set the desired speed; the setting on the rheostat dial does not necessarily correspond directly to revolutions per minute. The setting speeds on the rheostat can also change with variations in weight load and general aging of the centrifuge.

The College of American Pathologists (CAP) recommends that the number of revolutions per minute for a centrifuge used in chemistry laboratories be checked every 3 months. This periodic check can be done most easily by using a photoelectric tachometer or strobe tachometer. Timers and speed controls must also be checked periodically, with any corrections posted near the controls for the centrifuge.

Uses for Centrifuges

A primary use for centrifuges in clinical laboratories is to process blood specimens. Separation of cells or clotted blood from plasma or serum is done on an ongoing basis in the handling and processing of the many specimens needed for the various divisions of the clinical laboratory. The relative centrifugal force is not critical for the separation of serum from clot for most laboratory determinations. A force of at least 1000 g for 10 minutes will usually give a good separation. When serum separator collection tubes are used that contain a silicone gel needing displacement up the side of the tube, a greater centrifugal force is needed to displace this gel: 1000 to 1300 g for 10 minutes. An RCF less than 1000 g may result in an incomplete displacement of the gel. It is always important to follow the manufacturer's directions when special collection tubes or serum separator devices are being used. These may require different conditions for centrifugation (see Processing Blood Specimens, Chapter 3).

In the hematology laboratory, a tabletop version of the centrifuge has been specially adapted for determination of microhematocrit values. This centrifuge accelerates rapidly and can be stopped in seconds. Centrifugation is needed to prepare urinary sediment for microscopic examination. The urine specimen is centrifuged, the supernatant decanted, and the remaining sediment examined. Refrigerated centrifuges are used in the blood bank and for other temperature-sensitive laboratory procedures. Ultracentrifuges, which can generate G forces in the hundreds of thousands, are used in laboratories where tissue receptor assays and other assays requiring high-speed centrifugation are needed.

Technical Factors in Using Centrifuges

The most important rule to remember in using any centrifuge is: *Always balance the tubes placed in the centrifuge.* To balance the centrifuge, in the centrifuge cup opposite the material to be centrifuged, a container of equivalent size and shape with an equal volume of liquid of the same specific gravity as the load must be placed. (See Fig. 4-8 for examples of a properly balanced and an unbalanced centrifuge.) For most laboratory determinations, water may be placed in the balance load.

Tubes being centrifuged must be capped. Open tubes of blood should never be centrifuged because of the risk of aerosol spread of infection (see Chapter 2). Aerosols produced from the heat and vibration generated during the centrifugation process can increase the risk of infection to the laboratory personnel. Some evaporation of the sample can occur during centrifugation in uncapped specimen tubes.

Special centrifuge tubes can be used. These tubes are constructed to withstand the force exerted by the centrifuge. They have thicker glass walls or are made of a stronger, more resistant glass or plastic. Some of these tubes are conical, and some have round bottoms.

Before placing the centrifuge tubes in the cups or holders, check the cups to make certain the rubber cushions are in place. If some cushions are missing, the centrifuge will not be properly balanced. In addition, without the cushions, the tubes are more likely to break.

When a tube breaks in the centrifuge cup, both the cup and the rubber cushion in the cup must be cleaned well to prevent further breakage by glass particles left behind.

Covers specially made for the centrifuge should be used, except in certain specified instances. Using the cover prevents possible danger from aerosol spread and from flying glass, should tubes break in the centrifuge. Keep the centrifuge cover closed at all times, even when not using the machine. In addition to the danger from broken glass, using the centrifuge without the cover in place may cause the revolving parts of the centrifuge to vibrate, which causes excessive wear of the machine.

Do not try to stop the centrifuge with your hands. It is generally best to let the machine stop by itself. A brake may be applied if the centrifuge is equipped with one. The brake should be used with caution, because braking may cause some resuspension of the sediment. Many laboratories discourage use of the brake except when it is evident that a tube or tubes have broken in the centrifuge.

Centrifuges should be checked, cleaned, and lubricated regularly to ensure proper operation. Centrifuges that are used routinely must be checked periodically with a photoelectric or strobe tachometer to comply with quality assurance guidelines set by CAP.

LABORATORY REAGENT WATER

Water is one of the most important and frequently used reagents in the clinical laboratory. The quality of water used in the laboratory is crucial. Its use in reagent and solution preparation, reconstitution of lyophilized materials, and dilution of samples demands specific requirements for its level of purity. All water used in the clinical laboratory should be free from substances that could interfere with the tests being performed. Significant error can be introduced into a laboratory assay if inorganic or organic impurities in the water supply have not been removed before analysis.

Levels of Water Purity

CLSI[5] and CAP[6] recommend three levels of laboratory water: type I, type II, and type III (Table 4-6).

Type I Reagent Water

Type I reagent water is the most pure and should be used for procedures that require maximum water purity. For preparation of standard solutions, buffers, and controls and in quantitative analytical procedures (especially when nanograms or subnanogram measurements are required), electrophoresis, toxicology screening tests, and high-performance liquid chromatography, type I reagent water must be used. Type I water should be used immediately after it is produced; it cannot be stored.

Type II Reagent Water

For qualitative chemistry procedures and for most procedures done in hematology, immunology, microbiology, and other clinical test areas, type II reagent

TABLE 4-6

Characteristics of the Three Grades of Reagent Water			
Characteristic	Type I	Type II	Type III
Maximum colony count (CFU/mL)	<10	1000	Not specified
pH	Not specified	Not specified	5.0 to 8.0
Silicate (mg/L SiO₂)	0.05	0.1	1.0

Modified from National Committee for Clinical Laboratory Standards: Preparation and testing of reagent water in the clinical laboratory, ed 2, Villanova, PA, 1997, NCCLS Document C3-A3.
CFU, Colony-forming units.

water is suitable. Type II water is used for general laboratory tests that do not require type I water.

Type III Reagent Water

Type III water can be used for some qualitative laboratory tests, such as those done in general urinalysis. Type III reagent water can be used as a water source for preparation of type I or type II water and for washing and rinsing laboratory glassware. Any glassware should be given a final rinse with either type I or type II water, depending on the intended use for the glassware.

Quality Control and Impurity Testing

Water must be monitored at regular intervals to evaluate the performance of the water purification system. Testing at periodic intervals should include:

- Microbial monitoring
- Resistivity
- pH
- Pyrogens
- Silica
- Organic contaminants

There are several ways to test for water purity. With regard to the presence of inorganic ionized materials, as the purity of the water increases, the amount of dissolved ionized substances decreases, and the ability of the water to conduct an electrical current decreases. This principle is used in commercially available resistance test analyzers for water purity. As the ability of the water to conduct an electrical current decreases, the resistance increases. The presence of ionizable contaminants in distilled water or deionized water is most easily determined by measuring the conductance, or electrical resistance, of the water. This is the basis for having purity meters or conductivity warning lights on distillation and deionization apparatus.

Water of the highest purity will vary with the method of preparation and may be referred to as *nitrogen-free water, double-distilled water,* or *conductivity water,* depending on the actual method used. However, a measure of conductance does not consider the presence of nonionized substances

(organic contaminants) such as dissolved gases. Especially important in the clinical laboratory is dissolved carbon dioxide. Water free of such dissolved gases may be obtained by boiling it immediately before use and is often referred to as *gas-free* or *carbon dioxide–free water.* Such water may be necessary for the preparation of strongly alkaline solutions. Another contaminant of water may be substances dissolved from the storage container.

Accreditation or certification requirements for clinical laboratories, set up by state and federal agencies, have resulted in specific, well-defined criteria for water purity. The classification of and specifications for water purity are designed, for example, to enable laboratory personnel to specify the quality of the water needed for particular laboratory analyses and reagent preparation. Each test performed in the laboratory must be evaluated as to the type of water needed, to avoid potential interference with specificity, accuracy, and precision. It is well known, for example, that water contaminated with metal, when used in analyses of enzymes, can have a dramatic effect on the values obtained.

Storage of Reagent Water

It is important to store reagent water appropriately. Type I water must be used immediately after its production to prevent carbon dioxide from being absorbed into it. Types II and III water can be stored in borosilicate glass or polyethylene bottles but should be used as soon as possible to prevent contamination with airborne microbes. Containers should be tightly stoppered to prevent absorption of gases. It is also important to keep the delivery system for the water protected from chemical or microbiological contamination.

Purification of Water Process

The original source of water varies greatly with the health care facility. Water originating from rivers, lakes, springs, or wells contains a variety of inorganic, organic, and microbiological contaminants. No single purification system can remove all the contaminants. For this reason, a variety of methods in differing combinations are used to obtain the particular types of water used in a laboratory facility. Two general methods are employed to prepare water for laboratory use: deionization and distillation. Sometimes it is necessary to treat distilled water further with a deionization process to obtain water with the degree of purity needed.

Distilled Water

In the process of distillation, water is boiled and the resulting steam is cooled; condensed steam is distilled water. Many minerals are found in natural water, most often iron, magnesium, and calcium. Water from which these and other minerals have been removed by distillation is known as *distilled water*. The process of distillation also removes microbiological organisms, but volatile impurities such as carbon dioxide, chlorine, and ammonia are not removed. Water that has been distilled meets the specifications for type II and type III water.

DOUBLE-DISTILLED WATER

Distilled or deionized water is not necessarily pure water. There may be contamination by dissolved gases, by nonvolatile substances carried over by steam in the distillation process, or by dissolved substances from storage containers. For example, in tests for nitrogen compounds (e.g., urea nitrogen, a common clinical chemistry determination) it is important to use ammonia-free (nitrogen-free) water. This may be specially purchased by the laboratory for such determinations or prepared in the laboratory by a specific method, double distillation, to remove the contaminating ammonia.

Deionized Water

In the process of deionization, water is passed through a resin column containing positively (+) and negatively (−) charged particles. These particles combine with ions present in the water to remove them; this water is known as *deionized water*. Only substances that can ionize will be removed in the process of deionization. Organic substances and other substances that do not ionize are not removed. Further treatment with membrane filtration and activated charcoal is necessary to remove organic impurities, particulate matter, and microorganisms to produce type I water from deionized water.

Combinations of Deionization and Distillation

Water of higher purity is also produced by special distillation units in which the water is first deionized and then distilled, eliminating the need for double distillation. Other systems may first distill the water then deionize it.

Reverse Osmosis

The process of reverse osmosis passes water under pressure through a semipermeable membrane made of cellulose acetate or other materials. This treatment removes approximately 90% of dissolved solids, 98% of organic impurities, insoluble matter, and microbiological organisms. It does not remove dissolved gases and only about 10% of ionized particles.

Other Processes of Purification

Other processes for water purification include ultrafiltration, ultraviolet oxidation and sterilization (used after other purification processes), and ozone (used primarily in industrial settings). Filtration of water through semipermeable membranes will remove insoluble matter, pyrogens, and microorganisms if the pore size of the membrane is small enough. Adsorption by activated charcoal, clays, silicates, or metal oxides can remove organic matter. Type I water can be processed through a combination of deionization, filtration, and adsorption.

REAGENTS USED IN LABORATORY ASSAYS

Reagent Preparation

Instructions for preparing a reagent resemble a cooking recipe in that they specify what quantities of ingredients to mix together. The instructions identify the names of the chemicals needed, the number of grams or milligrams needed, and the total volume to which the particular reagent should be diluted. The solvent most often used for dilution is deionized or distilled water.

A *reagent* is defined as any substance employed to produce a chemical reaction. In highly automated clinical laboratories, very few reagents are prepared by laboratory staff. In many cases, only water or buffer needs to be added to a prepackaged reagent. In some cases, clinical laboratories and research laboratories may need to prepare a reagent or solution for method validation or specialized analyses. In-house reagent preparation may be done because of reagent deterioration considerations, supply and demand, or as a verified aspect of cost containment.

Grades of Chemicals

A chemical is a substance that occurs naturally or is obtained through a chemical process; it is used to produce a chemical effect or reaction. Chemicals are produced in various purities or grades. Analytical chemicals exist in varying grades of purity, as follows:

- Analytical reagent (AR) grade
- Chemically pure (CP) grade
- U.S. Pharmacopeia (USP) and National Formulary (NF) grade
- Technical or commercial grade

The label on the bottle and the supplier's catalog may give important information, such as the maximum limits of impurities or an actual analysis of the chemical. Directions for reagent preparation usually specify the grade and often state the particular brand of chemical.

Analytical Reagent Grade

AR-grade chemicals are of a high degree of purity and are used often in the preparation of reagents in the clinical laboratory. The American Chemical Society (ACS) has developed specifications for many reagent-grade or AR-grade chemicals, and those that meet its standards are designated by the letters ACS.

Chemically Pure Grade

CP-grade chemicals are sufficiently pure to be used in many analyses in the clinical laboratory. However, the CP designation does not reveal the limits of impurities that are tolerated. Therefore, CP chemicals may not be acceptable for research and various clinical laboratory techniques unless they have been specifically analyzed for the desired procedure. It may be necessary to use CP grade when higher-purity biochemicals are not available.

USP and NF Grade

USP-grade and NF-grade reagents meet the specifications stated in the U.S. Pharmacopeia or the National Formulary. They are generally less pure than CP-grade chemicals, because the tolerances specified are such that USP and NF chemicals are not injurious to health, rather than chemically pure.

Technical or Commercial Grade

These chemicals are used only for industrial purposes and are generally not used in the preparation of reagents for the clinical laboratory.

Hazardous Chemicals Communication Policies

Information and training regarding hazardous chemicals must be provided to all persons working with them in the clinical laboratory. Occupational Safety and Health Administration (OSHA) regulations ensure that all sites where hazardous chemicals are used comply with the necessary safety precautions. Any information about signs and symptoms associated with exposures to hazardous chemicals used in the laboratory must be communicated to all persons. Reference materials about the individual chemicals are provided by all chemical manufacturers and suppliers by means of the **material safety data sheet (MSDS)** (Fig. 4-9). This information accompanies the shipment of all hazardous chemicals and should be available in the laboratory for anyone to review. The MSDS contains information about possible hazards, safe handling, storage, and disposal of the particular chemical it accompanies (see Chapter 2).

Storage of Chemicals

It is important that chemicals kept in the laboratory be stored properly. Chemicals that require refrigeration should be refrigerated immediately. Solids should be kept in a cool, dry place. Acids and bases should be stored separately in well-ventilated storage units. Flammable solvents (e.g., alcohol, chloroform) should be stored in specially constructed, well-ventilated storage units with appropriate labeling in accordance with OSHA regulations. Flammable solvents such as acetone and ether should always be stored in special safety cans or other appropriate storage devices and in approved storage units. Fuming and volatile chemicals such as solvents, strong acids, and strong bases should be opened, and reagent preparation resulting in fumes should be done only under a fume hood so vapors will not escape into the room. Chemicals that absorb water should be weighed only after desiccation or drying in a hot oven; otherwise the weights will not be accurate.

It is very important that the label on a chemical be read for instructions about storage details. Most chemicals are stable at room temperature without desiccation. Some must be stored at refrigeration temperature, some must be frozen, and some that are light sensitive must be stored in brown bottles.

Reference Materials

NBS, CAP, and CLSI supply certified clinical laboratory standards. The highest-grade or purest chemicals are available from NBS. Very few such compounds are available to the clinical laboratory, and they are known as *standards, clinical type*.

Chemicals used to prepare **standard solutions** are the most highly purified types of chemicals available. This group includes primary, reference, and certified standards. Primary standards meet

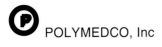 POLYMEDCO, Inc   **MATERIAL SAFETY DATA SHEET**

Commercial product name:	SED-CHEK®2ESR CONTROLS

1. INFORMATION OF THE SUBSTANCE/PREPARATION AND OF THE COMPANY

1.1 Commercial product name	**SED-CHEK®2 ESR CONTROLS**
Cat. No.:	**ESR-2CT, ESR-2CTN, ESR-2CTA, ESR-5CT, ESR-5CTN, ESR-5CTA, ESR-SSA, ESR-SSN**
1.2 Company:	**POLYMEDCO, Inc.** 510 Furnace Dock Road Cortland Manor, NY 10567 (914) 739-5400
1.3 Emergency Telephane No-:	(914) 739-5400 Attention: Safety Officer

2. CHEMICAL CHARACTERIZATION/INFORMATION ON INGREDIENTS:

Kit Contents:	Chemical characterization: CAS No. Description Human source material Identification number(s) EINECS No: 268-338-3 Chemical characterization Description: mixture of the substances listed below with nonhazardous additions Additional information contains human sourced and/or potentially infectious components.

3. HAZARDS IDENTIFICATION:

Warnings:	Routes of exposure: Ingestion, inhalation, and skin Information pertaining to particular dangers for man and environment The product does not have to be labeled due to the calculation procedures of the "General Classification system." The classification was made according to the latest editions of the EU-lists, and expanded upon from company and literature data.

FIGURE 4-9 **Sample material safety data sheet (MSDS).** (Courtesy Polymedco, Inc, Cortland Manor, NY.)

Continued

Commercial product name:	SED-CHEK®2ESR CONTROLS

4. FIRST AID MEASURES:

General information: no special measures required
After inhalation, supply fresh air; consult doctor in case of complaints after skin contact
Immediately wash with water and soap and rince thoroughly.
Generally the product does not irritate the skin.
After eye contact, rinse opened eye for several minutes under running water. Then consult a doctor.
After swallowing, rinse mouth with water. Seek medical attention and appropriate follow-up information for doctor.
The following symptoms may occur: Skin and eye irritation.
Medical conditions aggravated by exposure: None expected.

5. FIRE-FIGHTING MEASURES:

Extinguishing media:	CO_2 extinguishing powder or water spray. Fight larger fires with water spray or alcohol-resistant foam.

6. ACCIDENTAL RELEASE MEASURES:

After spillage:	Measures for cleaning/collecting: Absorb liquid components with liquid-binding material. Pick up mechanically. Clean the affected area carefully. Suitable cleaners are disinfectant. Dispose contaminated material as waste. Additional information: No dangerous substances are released.

7. HANDLING AND STORAGE:

7.1 Handling:	Information for safe handling: No special precautions are necessary if used correctly. Information about protection against explosions and fires: No special measures required
7.2 Storage	Further information about storage conditions: None Requirements to be met by storerooms and receptacles: No special requirements
Do not store together:	No restrictions

FIGURE 4-9, cont'd   Sample material safety data sheet (MSDS). (Courtesy Polymedco, Inc, Cortland Manor, NY.)

Commercial product name:	SED-CHEK®2ESR CONTROLS

8. EXPOSURE CONTROLS/PERSONAL PROTECTION:

TLV:	Threshold Limit Value established by ACGIH: Substance not listed
Respiratory protection:	Not required
Eye protection:	Safety glasses
Hand protection:	Protective gloves

9. PHYSICAL AND CHEMICAL PROPERTIES:

Physical state:	LIQUID REAGENTS
Color:	Red
Odor:	Light
pH value at 20°C	7.0-9.0
Boiling point:	N/A
Melting point:	N/A
Flash point:	N/A
Substance does not have any oxidizing properties:	N/A
Ignition temperature:	N/A
Explosion limits:	N/A
Vapor pressure:	N/A
Density:	N/A
Solubility in water:	Fully
Viscosity:	N/A

10. STABILITY AND REACTIVITY:

Hazardous Reactions:	None when used appropriately.
Hazardous decomposition products:	N/A

FIGURE 4-9, cont'd   Sample material safety data sheet (MSDS). (Courtesy Polymedco, Inc, Cortland Manor, NY.)

Continued

Commercial product name:	SED-CHEK®2ESR CONTROLS

11. TOXICOLOGICAL INFORMATION:

Acute toxicity:	Primary irritant effect: On the skin: No irritant effect
On the eye:	No irritant effect sensitization: No sensitizing effect known
Additional toxicological information:	The product is not subject to classification according to the calculation method of the General EU Classification Guidelines for Preparations as issued in the latest version. When used and handled according to specifications, the product does not have any harmful effects according to our experience and the information provided to us.
Target organs:	Not applicable

12. ECOLOGICAL INFORMATION:

Water hazard class:	(German regulations) (self-assessment): Slightly hazardous for water. Do not allow undiluted product or large quantities of it to reach ground water, water source, or sewer system.

13. DISPOSAL CONSIDERATIONS:

	Recommendation: Dispose of waste in accordance with applicable regional or local regulations. **Uncleaned Packagings:** Recommendation: Disposal must be made according to official regulations. Recommended cleansing agent: Water, if necessary with cleansing agents.

14. TRANSPORT INFORMATION:

DOT Regulations	Hazard Class		
Land transport ADR/RID (cross border)	ADR/RID class		
Maritime transport IMDG:	IMDG class		
Marine pollutant:	No		

FIGURE 4-9, cont'd   Sample material safety data sheet (MSDS). (Courtesy Polymedco, Inc, Cortland Manor, NY.)

Commercial product name:	SED-CHEK®2ESR CONTROLS

15. REGULATORY INFORMATION:	
Hazard symbol:	T, I
Warnings:	See section 3: Hazards Identification
Precautions:	Wear protective clothing upon contact, wash thoroughly with soap and water. Re-wash w/a detergent that contains anti-microbial agents.

16. OTHER INFORMATION:	
	The information herein is believed to be correct as of the date hereof but is provided without warranty of any kind. The recipient of our products is responsible for observing any laws and guidelines applicable.

FIGURE 4-9, cont'd   **Sample material safety data sheet (MSDS).** (Courtesy Polymedco, Inc, Cortland Manor, NY.)

specifications set by the ACS Committee on Analytical Reagents. Each lot of these chemicals is assayed, and the chemicals must be stable substances of definite composition. Reference standards are chemicals whose purity has been ensured by the NBS list of standard reference materials (SRM). Certified standards are also available[3]; for example, CAP certifies bilirubin and cyanmethemoglobin standards, and CLSI certifies a standardized protein solution.

Concentration of Solutions

Using solutions of the correct concentrations is of the greatest importance in attaining good results in the laboratory (see Chapter 7). Quantitative transfer, along with accurate initial measurement of a chemical, helps ensure that a solution will be of the correct concentration. The **concentration of a solution** may be expressed in different ways.

In the clinical chemistry laboratory, where the vast majority of the total laboratory analyses are performed, most measurements are concerned with the concentrations of substances in solutions. The solution is usually blood, serum, urine, cerebrospinal fluid, or other body fluid, and the substance to be measured is dissolved in the solution. Therefore, the substances being measured in the analyses (whether organic or inorganic or of high or low molecular weight) are **solutes.** In comparison, the substance in which a solute is dissolved is called the **solvent.**

When a reagent is being prepared and the solution is being diluted with water, its volume increases and concentration decreases, but the amount of solute remains unchanged.

Buffers and pH

Buffers are weak acids or bases and their related salts that, as a result of their dissociation characteristics, minimize changes in the hydrogen ion concentration. Hydrogen ion concentration is often expressed as *pH.* The pH scale ranges from 0 to 14 and is a convenient way of expressing hydrogen ion concentrations. Measurement of the pH of blood and various body fluids (e.g., urine) is important in laboratory analyses.

A buffer's capacity to minimize changes in pH is related to the dissociation characteristics of the weak acid or base in the presence of its respective salt.

Transfer and Dilution of Chemicals for Reagents

In preparing any solution in the clinical laboratory, it is necessary to use the practice known as **quantitative transfer** (Procedure 4-3). It is essential that the entire amount of the weighed or measured substance be used in preparing the solution. In quantitative transfer, the entire amount of the measured substance is transferred from one vessel to another for dilution. The usual practice in preparing most laboratory reagents is to weigh the chemical in a beaker (or other suitable vessel, such as a disposable weighing boat) and quantitatively transfer the chemical to a volumetric flask for dilution with deionized or distilled water. The volumetric flask chosen must be the correct size; that is, it must hold the amount of solution desired for the total volume of the reagent being prepared.

The most common amount of solution prepared at one time is 1 L. If 1 L of reagent is needed, the

Quantitative Transfer

1. Place a clean, dry funnel in the mouth of the volumetric flask.
2. Carefully transfer the chemical in the measuring vessel into the funnel.
3. Wash the chemical into the flask with small amounts of deionized water or the required solvent for the reagent.
4. Rinse the measuring vessel (beaker) three to five times with small portions of deionized water or the required solvent until all the chemical has been transferred from the vessel into the volumetric flask (add each rinsing to the flask).
5. Rinse the funnel with deionized water or the required solvent, and remove the funnel from the volumetric flask.
6. Dissolve the chemical in the flask by swirling or shaking it. Some chemicals are more difficult to dissolve than others; dissolving the chemical occasionally becomes a problem and requires additional attention.
7. Add deionized water or the required solvent to about 0.5 inches below the calibration line on the flask, allow a few seconds for drainage of fluid above the calibration line, and then carefully add deionized water or the required solvent to the calibration line (the bottom of the meniscus must be exactly on the calibration mark).
8. Stopper the flask with a ground-glass stopper, and mix well by inverting at least 20 times.
9. Rinse a properly labeled reagent bottle with a small amount of the mixed reagent in the volumetric flask. Transfer the prepared reagent to the labeled reagent bottle for storage.

measured chemical must be transferred quantitatively to a 1-L volumetric flask and diluted to the calibration mark with deionized water or the required solvent. The method of quantitative transfer requires great care and accuracy.

Dissolving the Chemical into Solution

Several methods can be used to hasten the dissolution of solid materials. Heating usually increases the solubility of a chemical, and heat also causes the fluid to move (currents help in dissolving materials). Even mild heat, however, will decompose some chemicals, so heat must be used with caution. Agitation by a stirring rod or swirling by means of a mechanical shaker increases solubility by removing the saturated solution from contact with the chemical. Rapid addition of the solvent is another means of hastening the dissolution of solid materials. Some chemicals tend to cake and form aggregates as soon as the solvent is added. By adding the solvent quickly and keeping the solids in motion, aggregation may be prevented. Because the flask is calibrated at 20°C, the solution must be returned to room temperature before final adjustment is made.

Labeling the Reagent Container

Containers for storage of reagents (usually reagent bottles) should be labeled before the material is added. A reagent should never be placed in an unlabeled bottle or container. If an unlabeled container is found, the reagent in it must be discarded. Proper labeling of reagent bottles is of the greatest importance. All labels should include the following information (Fig. 4-10):

1. Name and concentration of the reagent
2. Date the reagent was prepared
3. Initials of the person who made the reagent

In addition to standard label information, the Hazardous Materials Identification System (HMIS)[7] that was originally developed by the National Paint & Coatings Association (NPCA), (www.paint.org) is a system for compliance with OSHA's Hazard Communication Standard (HCS). The program uses a numerical hazard rating system, icons, and labels with colored bars to inform workers of chemical hazards in the workplace. HMIS III labels contain fields for Health, Flammability, and Physical Hazard, along with Personal Protective Equipment (PPE) requirements. HMIS III labels are also distinguished by a unique yellow border surrounding the entire label. This distinctive border not only identifies the label as an HMIS III label, but visually separates the information on the label from the background.

OSHA recommends that labels prepared in accordance with the NPCA Hazardous Materials Identification System are in compliance with this standard. OSHA previously confirmed the acceptability of HMIS as a hazard communication tool.

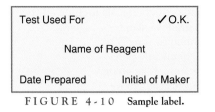

FIGURE 4-10   **Sample label.**

In the preamble to the 1994 revised HCS, OSHA indicated that this type of system continues to be an acceptable means of complying with the standard.

Checking a Reagent Before Use

After the prepared reagent is in the reagent bottle, it must be checked before it is put into actual use in any procedure. This can be done in one of several ways, depending on the reagent itself. New lots or batches of reagents are generally run in parallel testing with existing reagents. Controls, standards, and calibrators are means of testing the new lot or batch with the existing reagent.

In addition, a reagent log should be kept to indicate date in use and expiration date of the reagent. This log should also note the lot numbers of controls. After the reagent has been checked, this is indicated on the label, and the solution can be used for laboratory testing.

Ready-Made Reagents

Many laboratories use ready-made reagents, especially those using large automated instruments. The manufacturers of these instruments usually provide the necessary specific reagents for use with their instruments. These reagents must be handled with extreme care and always must be used according to the manufacturer's directions.

Immunoreagents

Special commercial reagent kits are often used for clinical immunology tests. A typical test kit will contain all necessary reagents, including standards, labeled antigen, and antibody, plus any other associated reagents needed. The laboratory must maintain strict evaluation policies for these kits to ensure their reliability. The disadvantage of such kits is that the laboratory is dependent on the supplier to produce and maintain components, which must meet the necessary standards. Each new kit must be evaluated by the laboratory according to a strict protocol, then a periodic monitoring program must be maintained to ensure the reliability of the results produced.

REFERENCES

1. National Committee for Clinical Laboratory Standards: Quantities and units (SI): committee report, Villanova, Pa, 1983, NCCLS document C11-CR.
2. National Bureau of Standards: International System of Units, Washington, DC, 1972, US Department of Commerce, No 330.
3. National Bureau of Standards: Standard reference materials: summary of the Clinical Laboratory Standards, Washington, DC, 1981, US Department of Commerce, NBS special publication.
4. National Bureau of Standards: Testing of glass volumetric apparatus, Washington, DC, 1959, US Department of Commerce, NBS circ 602.
5. Clinical Laboratory Standards Institute: Preparation and testing of reagent water in the clinical laboratory: proposed guideline, ed 4, Wayne, Pa, 2005, CLSI, C3-P4.
6. Commission on Laboratory Inspection and Accreditation: Reagent water specifications, Chicago, 1985, College of American Pathologists.
7. Hazardous Information System. www.paint.org. retrieved July 9, 2009.

BIBLIOGRAPHY

Bishop ML, Fody EP, Schoeff L: Clinical chemistry: techniques, principles, correlations, ed 6, Philadelphia, 2010, Lippincott Williams & Wilkins.
Burtis CA, Ashwood ER, Bruns DE: Tietz fundamentals of clinical chemistry, ed 6, St Louis, 2008, Saunders.
Campbell JM, Campbell JB: Laboratory mathematics: medical and biological applications, ed 5, St Louis, 1997, Mosby.
Kaplan LA, Pesce AJ: Clinical chemistry: theory, analysis, correlation, ed 5, St Louis, 2010, Mosby.

REVIEW QUESTIONS

Questions 1-3: *Match the units of measurements (a to c) and provide accepted abbreviations.*

1. ___ **Volume**

2. ___ **Length**

3. ___ **Mass**
   a. Meter (abbreviation)
   b. Gram (abbreviation)
   c. Liter (abbreviation)

4. 20°C = ___ °F
   a. 25
   b. 53
   c. 68
   d. 86

5. 75°F = ___ °C
   a. 15
   b. 21
   c. 25
   d. 32

Questions 6-8: *Match each type of volumetric glassware with its primary use (a to c).*

6. ___ **1-mL volumetric pipette**

7. ___ 10-mL graduated pipette

8. ___ 100-mL volumetric flask
   a. To prepare a reagent of specific total volume
   b. To measure an unknown serum sample
   c. To add a reagent to a reaction tube

9. **An etched ring on a to-deliver (TD) pipette indicates:**
   a. a small amount of fluid will remain in the tip of the pipette.
   b. the drop remaining in the tip must be blown out.
   c. either a or b.
   d. no significance.

Questions 10-12: *A = True or B = False.*

10. ___ **An electronic analytical balance has two pans.**

11. ___ **An analytical balance has a glass enclosure.**

12. ___ **Top-loading balances can be used to weigh reagents.**

13. **A cytocentrifuge is used to spread:**
    a. liquid specimen evenly over a slide.
    b. monolayers of cells.
    c. a large volume of specimen.
    d. both a and b.

14. **The purest type of reagent water is:**
    a. type I.
    b. type II.
    c. type III.
    d. all are equal.

15. **Water from which minerals have been removed is called:**
    a. distilled water.
    b. deionized water.
    c. reagent-grade water.
    d. charcoal-activated water.

16. **Grades of chemicals include all the following grades except:**
    a. analytical reagent.
    b. chemically pure.
    c. commercial grade.
    d. industrial grade.

17. **Reference standards are chemicals whose purity has been ensured by the:**
    a. National Bureau of Standards.
    b. Centers for Disease Control and Prevention.
    c. Occupational and Safety Health Agency.
    d. state licensing agencies.

Questions 18 and 19: *Match the term with its definition (a and b).*

18. ___ **Solute**

19. ___ **Solvent**
    a. The substance dissolved in the solution
    b. The substance that does the dissolving

Questions 20-23: *A = True or B = False.*
All labels should include:

20. ___ **the name and concentration of the reagent.**

21. ___ **the date on which the reagent was prepared.**

22. ___ **the initials of the person who made the reagent.**

23. ___ **the date that reagent expires.**

Questions 24 and 25: *Match*

24. ___ **Prefix *milli-***

25. ___ **Prefix *micro-***
    a. 10^{-2}
    b. 10^{-3}
    c. 10^{-6}
    d. 10^{-9}

CHAPTER 5

THE MICROSCOPE

DESCRIPTION
PARTS OF THE MICROSCOPE
Framework
Illumination System
Magnification System
Focusing System
CARE AND CLEANING OF THE MICROSCOPE
Cleaning the Microscope Exterior
Cleaning Optical Lenses: General Comments
Cleaning the Objectives
Cleaning the Ocular
Cleaning the Condenser
Cleaning the Stage and Adjustment Knobs
USE OF THE MICROSCOPE
Alignment
Light Adjustment
Focusing

OTHER TYPES OF MICROSCOPES (ILLUMINATION SYSTEMS)
Phase-Contrast Microscope
Interference-Contrast Microscope
Polarizing Microscope
Darkfield Microscope
Fluorescence Microscope
Electron Microscope
DIGITAL IMAGING
Artificial Neural Networks
Digital Cell Morphology

Learning Objectives

At the conclusion of this chapter, the student will be able to:

- Identify the parts of the microscope.
- Compare magnification and resolution.
- Define *parfocal*, and describe how it is used in microscopy.
- Define *alignment*, and describe the process of aligning a microscope.
- Explain the procedure for correct light adjustment to obtain maximum resolution with sufficient contrast.

- Name the components of a phase-contrast microscope, and explain how they differ from the components of a brightfield microscope.
- Identify the components of the compensated polarizing microscope, and describe their locations and functions.
- Compare and contrast darkfield, fluorescent, and electron microscopy.
- Describe the function and applications of artificial neural networks.

The microscope is probably the piece of equipment that receives the most use (and misuse) in the clinical laboratory. Microscopy is a basic part of the work in many areas of the laboratory, including hematology, urinalysis, and microbiology. Because the microscope is such a precision instrument and an important piece of equipment, it must be kept in excellent condition, optically and mechanically. It must be kept clean, and it must be kept aligned.

DESCRIPTION

In simple terms, a microscope is a magnifying glass. The compound light microscope, or the **brightfield microscope**—the type used in most clinical laboratories—consists of two magnifying lenses, the objective, and the eyepiece (ocular). It is used to magnify an object to a point where it can be seen with the human eye.

The total magnification observed is the product of the magnifications of these two lenses. In other words, the magnification of the objective times the magnification of the ocular equals the total magnification. For example, the total magnification of an object seen with a 10× ocular and a 10× objective is 100 times (100×). Magnification units are in terms of *diameters*, so 10× means the diameter of an object is magnified to 10 times its original size. The object itself or its area is not magnified 10 times; only the diameter of the object is magnified.

Because of the manner in which light travels through the compound microscope, the image seen is upside down and reversed. The right side appears as the left, the top as the bottom, and vice versa. This should be kept in mind when one is moving the slide (or object) being observed.

As with magnification, *resolution* is a basic term in microscopy. **Resolution** indicates how small and how close individual objects (dots) can be and still be recognizable. Practically, the resolving power is the limit of usable magnification. Further magnification of two dots that are no longer resolvable would be "empty magnification" and would result in a dumbbell appearance, as shown in Fig. 5-1.

The relative resolving powers of the human eye, the light microscope, and the electron microscope are:

Human eye
0.25 mm 0.25×10^3 m   0.00025 m
Light microscope
0.25 mm 0.25×10^6 m   0.00000025 m
Electron microscope
0.5 nm 0.5×10^9 m   0.0000000005 m

Another term encountered in microscopy is **numerical aperture (NA)**. The light-gathering ability of a microscope objective is quantitatively expressed in terms of the NA, which is a measure of the number of highly diffracted image-forming light rays captured by the objective. Higher values of numerical aperture allow increasingly oblique rays to enter the objective front lens, producing a more highly resolved image.

As the NA increases, objects can be positioned closer and still be distinguished from each other; that is, the greater the NA, the greater the resolving power of a lens. Any particular lens has a constant-rated NA, and this value depends on the radius of the lens and its focal length (the distance from the

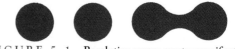

FIGURE 5-1   Resolution versus empty magnification.

BOX 5-1		
Typical Numerical Aperture (NA) Values		
Magnification	Term	NA Value
4×	Scanning	0.1
10×	Low power	0.25
40×	High power	0.65
100×	Oil immersion	1.25

object being viewed to the lens or the objective), but decreasing the amount of light passing through a lens will decrease the actual NA. The importance of this becomes apparent in the later discussion of proper light adjustments with the microscope. The magnification and NA are inscribed on each lens as a number (Box 5-1).

PARTS OF THE MICROSCOPE

The structures basic to all types of compound microscopes fall into four main categories:
1. Framework
2. Illumination system
3. Magnification system
4. Focusing system (Fig. 5-2)

Framework

The framework of the microscope consists of several units. The *base* is a firm, horseshoe-shaped foot on which the microscope rests. The *arm* is the structure that supports the magnifying and adjusting systems. It is also the handle by which the microscope can be carried without damaging the delicate parts. The *stage* is the horizontal platform, or shelf, on which the object being observed is placed. Most microscopes have a mechanical stage, which makes it much easier to manipulate the object being observed.

Illumination System

Good microscope work cannot be accomplished without proper illumination. The illumination system is an important part of the compound light microscope. Different illumination techniques or systems that are useful in the clinical laboratory include:
1. Brightfield
2. Phase contrast

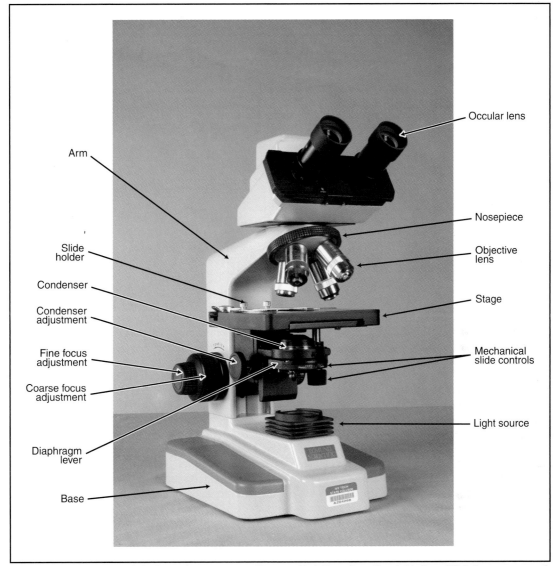

F I G U R E 5 - 2 **Parts of the binocular microscope.** (Courtesy Zack Bent, from Garrels M, Oatis CS: Laboratory testing for ambulatory settings: a guide for health care professionals, Philadelphia, 2006, Saunders.)

3. Interference contrast
4. Polarized and compensated polarized
5. Fluorescence
6. Darkfield

The brightfield microscope is the type of illumination system most often employed in the clinical laboratory. The electron microscope is also useful but requires a more specialized laboratory than the routine clinical laboratory.

The illumination system begins with a source of light. The clinical microscope most often has a built-in light source (or bulb). The bulb is turned on with an on/off switch (or in some cases by a rheostat, which turns on the bulb and adjusts the intensity of light). The light intensity is controlled by a rheostat, dimmer switch, or slide, ensuring both adequate illumination and comfort for the microscopist. When there is a separate on/ off switch, to lengthen the life of the bulb, the light intensity should be lowered before the bulb is turned off. The light source is located at the base of the microscope, and the light is directed up through the condenser system. It is important that the bulb be positioned correctly for proper alignment of the microscope. Proper alignment means that the parts of the microscope are adjusted so the light path from the source of light through the microscope and the ocular is physically correct. Microscopes are designed so the light bulb filament will be centered if the bulb is installed properly. Many styles or types of bulbs are available (generally tungsten or tungsten-halogen), and it is important that the bulb designed for a particular microscope be used.

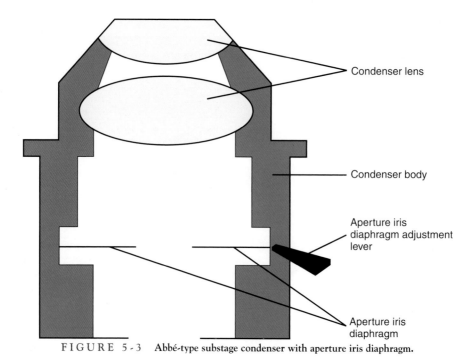

FIGURE 5-3   Abbé-type substage condenser with aperture iris diaphragm.

Condenser

Another part of the illumination system is the **condenser**. Microscopes generally use a substage Abbé-type condenser. The condenser directs and focuses the beam of light from the bulb onto the material under examination. The Abbé condenser is a conical lens system (actually consisting of two lenses) with the point planed off (Fig. 5-3). The condenser position is adjustable; it can be raised and lowered beneath the stage by means of an adjustment knob. It must be appropriately positioned to focus the light correctly on the material being viewed. When it is correctly positioned, the image field is evenly lighted.

When the microscope is properly used, the apparent NA of the condenser should be equal to or slightly less than the rated NA of the objective being used. The apparent or actual NA of the condenser can be varied by changing its position; as it is lowered, the apparent NA is reduced. The condenser position must be adjusted with each objective used to maximize the light focus and the resolving power of the microscope. When the apparent NA of the condenser is decreased below that of the rated NA of the objective, contrast and depth of field are gained and resolution is lost. This manipulation is often necessary in the clinical laboratory when wet, unstained preparations are being observed, such as urine sediment. In this case, to gain contrast when a specimen is being scanned, the condenser is lowered (or the aperture iris diaphragm partially closed), thus reducing the apparent NA of the condenser. Preferably, the

condenser should be left in a generally uppermost position, at most only 1 or 2 mm below the specimen, and the light adjusted primarily by opening or closing the aperture iris diaphragm located in the condenser. The practice of "racking down" the condenser when one is looking at wet preparations is not acceptable.

Some microscopes are equipped with a condenser element, which is used in place for low-power work and swings out for high power. Other models employ an element that swings out for low-power work and is used in place for higher magnification. This changes the apparent NA of the condenser, matching it with that of the objective. Other illumination systems employ different types of condensers, such as phase-contrast, differential interference-contrast, and darkfield condensers.

Aperture Iris Diaphragm

The **aperture iris diaphragm** also controls the amount of light passing through the material under observation. It is located at the bottom of the condenser, under the lenses but within the condenser body, as seen in Fig. 5-3. This aperture diaphragm consists of a series of horizontally arranged interlocking plates with a central aperture (Fig. 5-4). It can be opened or closed as necessary to adjust the intensity of the light by means of a lever or dial. The size of the aperture, and consequently the amount of light permitted to pass, is regulated by the microscopist. Such regulation of the light

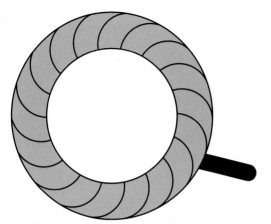

FIGURE 5-4 Aperture iris diaphragm. By opening or closing the aperture iris diaphragm, you let more or less light into the field of view.

affects the apparent NA of the condenser, decreasing the size of the field under observation, with the iris diaphragm decreasing the apparent NA of the condenser. Thus, proper illumination techniques involve a combination of proper light intensity regulation, condenser position, and field-size regulation.

Field Diaphragm

Better microscopes have a field iris diaphragm, located in the light port in the base of the microscope, through which light passes up to the condenser. The **field diaphragm** controls the area of the circle of light in the field of view when the specimen and condenser have been properly focused. It is also used in the alignment of the microscope.

Magnification System

The magnification system contains several important parts. It plays an extremely important role in the use of the microscope.

Ocular (Eyepiece)

The **ocular**, or **eyepiece**, is a lens that magnifies the image formed by the objective. The usual magnification of the ocular is 10 (10×); however, 5× and 20× oculars are also generally available. Most microscopes have two oculars and are called *binocular microscopes*. Some microscopes have only one ocular and are called *monocular microscopes*. The magnification produced by the ocular, when multiplied by the magnification produced by the objective, gives the total magnification of the object being viewed. The distance between the two oculars **(interpupillary distance)** is adjustable, as is the focus on one of the oculars **(diopter adjustment)**.

Objectives

Microscope **objectives** are probably the most important components of an optical microscope. Objectives are responsible for primary image formation and play a central role in determining the quality of images the microscope is capable of producing. Objectives are also instrumental in determining the magnification of a particular specimen and the resolution under which fine specimen detail can be observed in the microscope.

Objective lenses are inscribed with certain information, including type of lens, magnification, rated NA, body tube length, and coverglass thickness or requirement for immersion oil. Most microscopes have three, sometimes four, objectives. With three objectives, the magnifying powers are 10×, 40×, and 100×. The objectives are mounted on the **nosepiece**, which is a pivot that enables a quick change of objectives.

Objectives are described or rated according to **focal length**, which is inscribed on the outside of the objective. Microscopes used in the clinical laboratory most often have 16-mm, 4-mm, and 1.8-mm objectives. The focal length is a physical property of the objective lens and is slightly less than the distance from the object being examined to the center of the objective lens. Practically speaking, the focal length of a lens is very close in value to the **working distance**, the distance from the bottom of the objective to the material being studied. The greater the magnifying power of a lens, the smaller the focal length and thus the working distance. This becomes very important when the microscope is being used, because the working distance is very short for the 40× (4-mm) and 100× (1.8-mm) objectives. For this reason, correct focusing habits are necessary to prevent damaging the objectives against the slide on the stage.

ACHROMAT AND PLANACHROMAT OBJECTIVES

Generally, two types of objectives are available in clinical microscopes: **achromats** and **planachromats**. The least expensive and most common objectives used on most laboratory microscopes are the achromatic objectives, which correct for color (chromatic) aberrations. Although achromats are adequate for most laboratory work, the center of the field of view will be in sharp focus, but the edges appear out of focus, and the field does not appear to be flat. Achromatic objectives yield their best results with light passed through a green filter (often an interference filter). The lack of correction for flatness of field further hampers achromat objectives.

In the past few years, most manufacturers have been providing flat-field corrections for achromat objectives and have given these corrected objectives the name *plan achromats*. Plan achromatic objectives, although more expensive, are more appropriate for high-magnification work using a 40× or 100× objective, because the field of view is in focus and flat throughout. **Apochromatic** objectives are also available. This type of objective corrects for chromatic and spherical aberrations. These are the finest lenses available and may be necessary for photomicroscopy, but because they are significantly more expensive, they are unnecessary for routine laboratory microscopy (Table 5-1).

LOW-POWER OBJECTIVE

The **low-power objective** is usually a 10× lens with a 16-mm working distance. This objective is used for the initial scanning and observation in most microscope work. For example, blood films and urine sediment are routinely examined using the low-power objective first. This is also the lens employed for the initial focusing and light adjustment of the microscope. Some routine microscopes also have a very low-power 4× magnification lens. This is used in the initial scanning in the morphologic examination of histologic sections.

A term often used in discussing microscopes is *parfocal*, which means that if one objective is in focus and a change is made to another objective, the focus will not be lost. Thus, the microscope can be focused under low power and then changed to the high-power or oil-immersion objective (by rotating the nosepiece), and it will still be in focus except for fine adjustment.

The rated NA of the low-power objective is significantly less than that of the condenser on most microscopes (for the 10× objective, the NA is approximately 0.25; for the condenser, it is approximately 0.9). To achieve focus, the NAs must be more closely matched by reducing the light to the specimen. This is done by focusing or lowering the condenser slightly (1 or 2 mm below the specimen) and then reducing the size of the field of light to about 70% to 80% with the aperture iris diaphragm.

HIGH-POWER OBJECTIVE

The **high-power objective**, or high-dry objective, is usually a 40× lens with a 4-mm working distance. This objective is used for more detailed study; the total magnification with a 10× eyepiece is 400× rather than the 100× of the low-power system. The high-power objective is used to study histologic sections and wet preparations (e.g., urine sediment) in more detail. The working distance of the 4-mm lens is quite short, so care must be taken in focusing. The NA of the high-power lens is fairly close to (although slightly less than) that of most frequently used condensers (for most high-power objectives, NA = 0.85; for the condenser,

TABLE 5-1

Examples of Objective Correction for Optical Aberration			
Objective Type	Spherical Aberration	Chromatic Aberration	Field Curvature
Achromat	1 Color	2 Colors	No
Plan achromat	1 Color	2 Colors	Yes
Plan apochromat	3-4 Colors	4-5 Colors	Yes

Modified from Nikon Microscopy U, www.microscopyu.com. Accessed July 8, 2009.

NA = 0.9). Therefore, the condenser should generally be all the way up (or very slightly lowered) and the light field slightly closed, with the aperture iris diaphragm for maximum focus.

OIL-IMMERSION OBJECTIVE

The **oil-immersion objective** is generally a 100× lens with a 1.8-mm working distance. This is a very short focal length and working distance. In fact, the objective lens almost rests on the microscope slide when the microscope is in use. An oil-immersion lens requires that a special grade of oil called *immersion oil* be placed between the objective and the slide or coverglass. Oil is used sparingly to increase the NA and thus the resolving power of the objective. Because the focal length of this lens is so small, there is a problem in getting enough light from the microscope field to the objective. Light travels through air at a greater speed than through glass, and it travels through immersion oil at the same speed as through glass. Thus, to increase the effective NA of the objective, oil is used to slow down the speed at which light travels, increasing the gathering power of the lens.*

Because the NA of the oil-immersion objective is greater than that of the condenser in most systems (for the 100× objective, NA = 1.2; for the condenser, NA = 0.9), the condenser should be used in the uppermost position, and the aperture iris diaphragm should generally be open. Practically speaking, however, partially closing the iris diaphragm may be necessary. The oil-immersion lens, with a total magnification of 1000× when used with a 10× eyepiece, is generally the limit of magnification with the light microscope.

The oil-immersion lens is routinely used for morphologic examination of blood films and

---

*The speed at which light travels through a substance is measured in terms of the refractive index. The refractive index is calculated as the speed at which light travels through air divided by the speed at which it travels through the substance. The refractive index of air is therefore 1.00. The refractive index of glass is 1.515; immersion oil, 1.515; and water, 1.33.

microbes. The short working distance requires dry films. Wet preparations (e.g., urine sediment) cannot be examined under an oil-immersion lens.

The high-power lens is also referred to as a *high-dry lens* because it does not require the use of immersion oil. Other objectives that might be present on a microscope in the clinical laboratory are a lower-power 4× scanning lens and a 50× or 63× oil-immersion lens.

Focusing System

Oculars are a component of the focusing system. There is an interocular adjustment as well as an adjustment for the left ocular to focus for the left eye.

The **body tube** is the part of the microscope through which the light passes to the ocular. The tube length from the eyepiece to the objective lens is generally 160 mm. This is the tube that actually conducts the image. The required body tube length is also inscribed on each objective.

The adjustment system enables the body tube to move up or down for focusing the objectives. This usually consists of two adjustments: coarse and fine. The coarse adjustment gives rapid movement over a wide range and is used to obtain an approximate focus. The fine adjustment gives very slow movement over a limited range and is used to obtain exact focus after coarse adjustment.

CARE AND CLEANING OF THE MICROSCOPE

The microscope is a precision instrument and must be handled with great care. When it is necessary to transport the microscope, it should always be carried with both hands; it should be carried by the arm and supported under the base with the other hand. When not in use, the microscope should be covered and put away in a microscope case or in a desk or cupboard. It should be left with the low-power (10×) objective in place and the body tube barrel adjusted to the lowest possible position.

Cleaning the Microscope Exterior

The surface of most microscopes is finished with black or gray enamel and metal plating that is resistant to most laboratory chemicals. It may be kept clean by washing with a neutral soap and water. To clean the metal and enamel, a gauze or soft cloth should be moistened with the cleaning agent and rubbed over the surface with a circular motion. The surface should be dried immediately with a clean, dry piece of gauze or cloth. Gauze should never be used to clean the optical parts of the microscope.

Cleaning Optical Lenses: General Comments

The glass surfaces of the ocular, the objectives, and the condenser are hand-ground optical lenses. These lenses must be kept meticulously clean (Procedure 5-1). Optical glass is softer than ordinary glass and should never be cleaned with paper tissue or gauze; these materials will scratch the lens. To clean the lenses of the microscope, use lens paper. Before polishing with lens paper, take care that nothing is present that will scratch the optical glass in the polishing process. Such potentially abrasive dirt, dust, or lint can easily be blown away before polishing. Cans of compressed air are commercially available, or an air syringe can be made simply by fitting a plastic eyedropper or a 1-mL plastic tuberculin syringe with the tip cut off into a rubber bulb of the type used for pipetting. This air syringe is used to blow away dust or lint that might otherwise scratch the optical glass in the polishing process.

Cleaning the Objectives

Oil must be removed from the oil-immersion (100×) objective immediately after use by wiping with clean lens paper. If not removed, oil may seep inside the lens or dry on the outside surface of the objective. The high-dry (40×) objective should never be used with oil, but if this or any other objective or microscope part comes into contact with oil, it should be cleaned immediately. If a lens is especially dirty, it may be cleaned with a small amount of commercial lens cleaner, methanol, or manufacturer-recommended solution applied to lens paper then wiped across the surface. Xylene should not be used; it can damage the lens mounting if allowed beyond the front seal, and its fumes are toxic.

To clean the oil-immersion lens properly, first lower the stage, then rotate the objective to the front and wipe gently with clean lens paper. Clean off the immersion oil with lens paper dampened with special lens cleaner or methanol. Alternatively, the cleaning agent may be applied to a wooden applicator stick wrapped with cotton or lens paper and moistened with the cleaning agent. Do not use a plastic applicator stick; it will be dissolved by the solvent, ruining the objective. Apply the cleaning agent by blotting and using a circular motion, beginning at the center and moving outward. Repeat with new dampened lens paper as necessary. Finally, blot dry with clean lens paper. Do not rub; this may scratch the surface of the lens.

Lenses should never be touched with the fingers. Objectives must not be taken apart because even a slight alteration of the lens setting may ruin

Summary of Basic Steps for Cleaning the Microscope Lens

Regular cleaning is important not only in maintaining the life of the microscope and lenses but also in obtaining good-quality images.

Lens cleaning in particular requires great care. All glass surfaces should be cleaned in the following sequence:

1. Blowing. Use air source to blow dust off lenses. This removes all larger particles of dust that could scratch the lens in the later cleaning stages.
2. Brushing. Use clean, soft camel's hair or sable brush to remove particles of dust that blowing does not displace.
3. Wiping. Use only clean lens paper to wipe lenses. Lens paper is specially made with soft fibers that will not scratch the glass. Moisten the lens paper with water or lens cleaner and wipe carefully; moistening further softens the paper fibers. Never use alcohol as a cleaning agent, because some lens adhesives are soluble in alcohol. Always first clean the objectives that were not used with oil (10×, 40× [high dry]), then follow with cleaning the oil-immersion objectives (50× or 100×). Care should be taken to use a separate lens paper for dry and oil objectives so there is no transfer of oil, which may ruin the objectives.

the objective. Merely clean the outer surface of the lens as described. An especially dirty objective may be removed (unscrewed) from the nosepiece then held upside down and checked for cleanliness by using the ocular (removed from the body tube) as a magnifying glass. Dust or lint can also be removed from the rear lens of the objective by blowing it away with an air syringe. Such removal of the objective from the nosepiece is not a routine cleaning procedure. The final step after using the microscope should always be to wipe off all objectives with clean lens paper.

Cleaning the Ocular

The ocular, or eyepiece, is especially vulnerable to dirt because of its location on the microscope and contact with the observer's eye. Mascara presents a constant cleaning problem. Dust can be removed from the lens of the ocular with an air syringe or camel's hair brush; air is probably easier to use and more efficient. The lens should then be polished with lens paper. The ocular can be checked for additional dirt by holding it up to a light and looking through it. When looking into the microscope, dirt on any part of the ocular will rotate with the ocular when it is turned. The ocular should not be removed for more than a few minutes; dust can collect in the body tube and settle on the rear lens of an objective.

Cleaning the Condenser

The light source and condenser should also be free of dust, lint, and dirt. First, blow away the dust with an air syringe or camel's hair brush, then polish the light source and condenser with lens paper. It may be necessary to clean these parts further with lens paper moistened with a commercial lens cleaner or methanol before polishing them with lens paper.

Cleaning the Stage and Adjustment Knobs

The stage of the microscope should be cleaned after each use by wiping with gauze or a tissue. After it has been cleaned thoroughly, the stage should be wiped dry.

The coarse and fine adjustments occasionally need attention, as does the mechanical stage adjustment mechanism. When there is unusual resistance to any manipulation of these knobs, force must not be used to overcome the resistance. Such force might damage the screw or rack-and-pinion mechanism. Instead, the cause of the problem must be found. A small drop of oil may be needed.

It is best to call in a specialist to repair the microscope when a serious problem occurs. In addition, the microscope should be cleaned at least once a year by a professional microscope service company.

USE OF THE MICROSCOPE

When a microscope is being used, two conditions must be met: the microscope must be clean, and it must be aligned. The cleaning procedure is described in the previous section; alignment is discussed next (Procedure 5-2).

General Alignment Procedure for Microscope use

For optimal results, set the alignment each time you sit down at the microscope and "touch up" the focus from one area of the sample to another. The protocol varies from person to person, but the general steps are as follows:

1. Eyepieces (preliminary step): The eyepieces have focus rings on them (turn the very top). Set the "0" to the white dot.

2. Objective: Bring the objective into focus for the sample by "focusing away." Start by looking outside the microscope at the distance between the front of the objective and the sample. Rotate the coarse focus knob away from you to raise the stage as close as possible to the objective. Then, while looking in the microscope, rotate the knob gently toward you until the image comes into sharp focus. Touch up with the fine focus.

3. Condenser: Look under the stage for the small focusing knob for the condenser carrier. Raise the condenser until it is almost touching the back of the slide. Note which direction you turned the knob to raise the condenser.

    a. Close the field iris diaphragm. While watching in the microscope, gently rotate the condenser focus in the other direction until the dark edges of the field iris image come into focus.
    b. Open the field iris just outside the field of view. (Note: If you have a highly scattering sample, try moving the feature of interest to the center of the field and leaving the field iris mostly closed.)
    c. Adjust the condenser aperture iris until you have clean, crisp edges and as clear a background as possible.

4. Final setting for eyepieces:

    a. Leave the microscope controls set for the dominant eye, and adjust the eyepiece focus to bring the image into focus for the other eye.

SUMMARY

1. Set the eyepieces to "0."

2. Focus away with the coarse focus to obtain a sharp image of the specimen.

3. a. Bring the condenser full up to the top using its own focus.
    b. Close the field iris, and while looking in the microscope, focus away to obtain a sharp image of the field iris superimposed on the image of the specimen.
    c. Set the field iris (usually just outside the field of view).
    d. Set the aperture iris (sharp, crisp, clean image).

4. For final setting of eyepiece, focus for nondominant eye.

This process should take you about 30 seconds. Touch up the two irises as you move from one section of the sample to another or one magnification to another. Because many confocal sections are highly scattering, you only may be able to approximate these settings, but doing the best you can will greatly help the quality of your images and results.

Alignment

When properly aligned, the microscope is adjusted in such a way that the light path through the microscope, from the light source to the eye of the observer, is correct. This is referred to as *Köhler illumination*. If a microscope is misaligned, the field of view will seem to swing—a very uncomfortable situation, often described as making the observer feel seasick. This can be corrected by properly aligning or adjusting the light path through the microscope. Many microscopes produced for student use are aligned by the manufacturer, and realignment requires special knowledge and experience because the field diaphragm, condenser-centering adjustment screws, and removable eyepieces are not present. In such microscopes, realignment should be done by a professional microscope service company.

If the microscope has a field diaphragm, it is used in the alignment procedure. A field diaphragm is an iris diaphragm that is part of the built-in illuminator. With the low-power objective in place, close down the field diaphragm to a minimum, then focus the condenser by adjusting the condenser height with the condenser focus knob until the image of the field diaphragm is sharply visible in the field of view (Fig. 5-5, A). Next, bring the

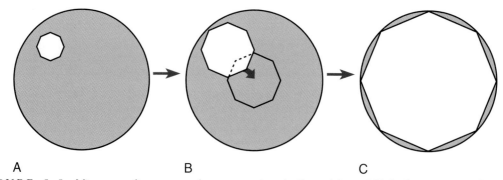

FIGURE 5-5 Microscope alignment; condenser centration. A, Stopped-down field diaphragm image, off center or misaligned. B, Field diaphragm image widened and moved toward center by means of condenser adjustment knobs. C, Field diaphragm image diameter widened and centered.

image of the field diaphragm into the center of the field by means of the centering screws located on the condenser (see Fig. 5-5, B). Open the field diaphragm until it is just contained within the field of view (see Fig. 5-5, C). At this point, it may be necessary to repeat the centering procedure. Finally, open the diaphragm until the leaves are just out of view.

Light Adjustment

With the low-power objective in position, the object to be examined, usually on a glass microscope slide, is placed on the stage and secured. Care must be taken to avoid damaging the objective when the specimen is placed on the stage. The slide is positioned so the portion of the slide containing the specimen to be examined is in the light path, directly over the condenser lens.

The greatest concern in learning how to use a microscope is the lighting and fine-adjustment maneuvers. The user must be certain that the light source, condenser, and aperture iris diaphragm are in correct adjustment. Light adjustment is made before any focusing is done. The power supply is turned on and the light intensity adjusted to a bright but comfortable level. Light adjustment is further accomplished by raising and lowering the condenser and opening and closing the aperture iris diaphragm. At the start of this initial light adjustment, the low-power (10×) objective should be in place. The condenser should be near its highest position, no more than 1 to 2 mm below the slide, with the aperture and field diaphragms open all the way and the body tube down so the lens is approximately 16 mm from the slide (the working distance for the low-power lens). If the microscope is equipped with a field diaphragm, the condenser height should be adjusted so as to bring the field diaphragm into sharp focus, as described in the alignment procedure.

To adjust the aperture iris diaphragm, while looking through the ocular, close the diaphragm until the light just begins to be reduced. Alternately, if possible, remove the eyepiece and darken out approximately 20% to 30% of the light by closing the iris diaphragm while looking down the body tube (Fig. 5-6). Further closing of the iris diaphragm (or lowering of the condenser), although it may increase contrast and depth of focus, will reduce resolution.

Focusing

Focusing is the next technique to be mastered. If using a binocular microscope, adjust the interpupillary distance between the oculars so the left and right fields merge into one. With the object to be examined on the stage, and while watching from the side, bring the low-power (10×) objective down as far as it will go so it almost meets the top of the specimen. Use the coarse adjustment for this procedure. The objective must not be in direct contact with the specimen. Watch from the side to avoid damaging the objective. Once the objective is just at the top of the specimen, slowly focus upward, using the coarse-adjustment knob and looking through the ocular. When the object is almost in focus, bring it into clear focus with the fine-adjustment knob. Do this procedure with the right eye, then set the ocular diopter to the left eye by rotating until the left eye is in clear focus; the object should now be in focus for both eyes.

Further light adjustment can now be made to ensure maximum focus and resolution. Adjust the light intensity with the brightness control so the background light is sufficiently bright (white) but comfortable. Next, adjust the iris diaphragm by opening it completely and then slowly closing it until the light intensity just begins to be reduced. Alternatively, remove the eyepiece and close the aperture iris diaphragm until about 80% of the body tube is filled with light.

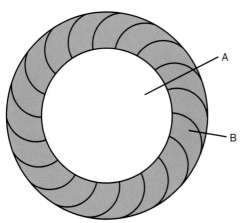

FIGURE 5-6 Adjusting the aperture iris diaphragm. A, 70% to 80% of light presented to objective. B, 20% to 30% of light restricted by stopping down the aperture iris diaphragm.

When changing to another objective, changing the barrel distance is unnecessary. As noted, most microscopes are parfocal. The only adjustment necessary should be made with the fine-adjustment knob. It is essential to remember that fine adjustment is used continuously during microscopic examination, especially when wet preparations such as urine sediment are being examined.

When greater magnification is needed, more light is necessary. It is obtained by repositioning the condenser and aperture iris diaphragm in the manner previously described. In general, the condenser will be raised and the aperture iris diaphragm opened as the objective magnification increases. When the oil-immersion lens is used, the condenser should be raised to its maximum position.

Additional light is provided by the use of immersion oil, which is placed on the viewing slide when the oil-immersion (100×) objective is used. The oil directs the light rays to a finer point, reducing spherical aberration. When the oil-immersion lens is to be used, first find the desired area on the slide by using the low-power (10×) objective. Once this area is located, pivot the objective out of position, place a drop of immersion oil on the slide, and pivot the oil-immersion lens into the oil while observing it from the side. Next, move the objective from side to side to ensure contact with the oil and avoid the presence of air bubbles. To prevent damage to the objective, the nosepiece rather than the objective itself should be grasped when lenses are being changed. The ocular should not be looked through during this adjustment procedure. After the initial adjustment has been made, adjust the fine focus while looking through the ocular. After the study has been completed, clean off the oil remaining on the objective with lens paper, as described earlier.

OTHER TYPES OF MICROSCOPES (ILLUMINATION SYSTEMS)

With few exceptions, brightfield illumination has been the primary type of microscope illumination system used in the routine clinical laboratory. Other illumination systems are also available: phase-contrast, interference-contrast, polarizing, darkfield, fluorescence, and electron microscopy. The basic principles of microscopy and rules for usage apply to all these variations. The primary difference from brightfield microscopy is the character of light delivered to the specimen and illuminating the microscope.

Phase-Contrast Microscope

Another extremely useful illumination system is the phase-contrast microscope. A disadvantage of brightfield illumination is that it is necessary to stain (or dye) many objects to give sufficient contrast and detail. **Phase contrast** facilitates the study of unstained structures, which can be alive, because wet preparations of cells or organisms are observed without prior dehydration and staining. As the name implies, the structures observed with this system show added contrast compared with the brightfield microscope.

The phase-contrast microscope is basically a brightfield microscope with changes in the objective and the condenser. An annular diaphragm, or ring, is put into (or below) the condenser. This condenser annulus is designed to let a hollow cone or "doughnut" of light pass through the condenser to the specimen. A corresponding absorption ring is fitted into the objective. Each phase objective must have a corresponding condenser annulus (Fig. 5-7). In microscopes with multiple phase objectives, the annular diaphragms are usually placed in a rotating condenser arrangement (Fig. 5-8). Use of each phase objective requires an adjustment of the condenser to "match" the annular diaphragm and the phase absorption ring.

The phase-contrast microscope may also be used as a brightfield microscope by setting the condenser to a standard brightfield (or open) position, which contains no annulus. Because the phase objective blocks out a ring of light, the resolution or detail that can be achieved when using phase objectives is compromised for brightfield examination. For more exact work, an additional brightfield objective should be employed in the microscope.

The annulus and absorption ring must be perfectly aligned or adjusted so they are concentric and superimposed; a problem with the phase-contrast microscope is the need for perfect alignment. The microscope must first be aligned for brightfield

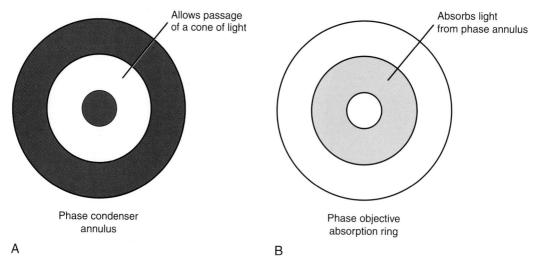

FIGURE 5-7   Phase annulus and absorption ring. A, Phase condenser annulus. B, Phase objective absorption ring.

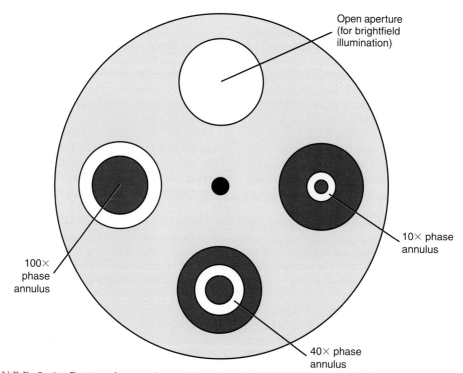

FIGURE 5-8   Rotating phase condenser with settings for brightfield, low power, high power, and oil immersion.

work. To align the phase annulus, match the phase objective to the corresponding phase annulus in the condenser by rotating the phase turret. Insert the aperture viewing unit, either by insertion into the body tube or by inserting a phase telescope into an ocular tube. Focus the viewing apparatus until the phase annulus (seen as a white ring of light) is in focus. There will be a bright (white) ring and a dark ring, which should be superimposed (Fig. 5-9). If not perfectly superimposed,

the phase annulus can be repositioned by means of the annulus-centering knobs located on the condenser. Each microscope will have a slightly different means of adjustment, and the operation directions for that microscope should be followed.

However, all phase-contrast microscopes require alignment the same as for brightfield, plus alignment of the phase annulus to the matching phase objective.

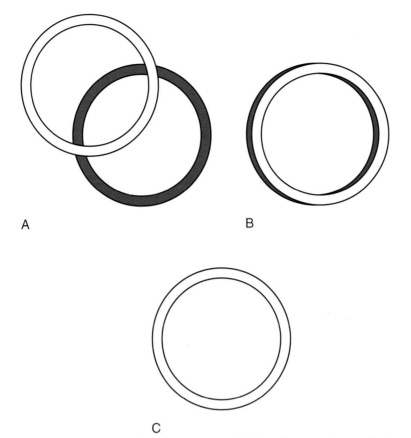

FIGURE 5-9 Alignment of phase annulus to phase absorption ring. A, Before alignment, phase annulus is out of phase adjustment. B, Phase annulus moved so it is nearly aligned. C, Alignment: phase annulus is superimposed on phase absorption ring.

The net effect of phase contrast is to slow down the speed of light by one-fourth of a wavelength. This diminution of the speed of light makes the system very sensitive to differences in refractive index. Objects with differences in refractive index, shape, and absorption characteristics show added differences in the intensity and shade of light passing through them. The end result is that the viewer can observe unstained wet preparations with good resolution and detail, as shown in Fig. 5-10. In the clinical laboratory, phase contrast is especially useful for counting platelets and observing cellular structures and casts in wet preparations of urine sediment and vaginal smears. Because of its superior visualization and ease of operation, the phase-contrast microscope has become a common tool in routine urinalysis. However, the microscopist must be proficient in changing from brightfield to phase contrast, because in a given specimen, some structures are better visualized with phase contrast and others with brightfield.

Interference-Contrast Microscope

Another illumination technique gaining clinical use is interference-contrast illumination. This technique gives the viewer a three-dimensional (3D) image of the object under study. As with phase contrast, interference contrast is especially useful for wet preparations such as urine sediment, showing finer details without the need for special staining techniques.

For the interference-contrast microscope, the brightfield microscope is modified by the addition of a special beam-splitting (Wollaston) prism to the condenser. The two split beams are then polarized; one passes through the specimen, which alters the amplitude (or height) of the light wave, and the other (which serves as a reference) does not pass through the specimen. The two dissimilar light beams then pass separately through the objective and are recombined by a second Wollaston (beam-combining) prism. This recombination of light waves gives the 3D image to the additive or subtractive effects of the light waves as they are combined.

Polarizing Microscope

Another useful adaptation of the brightfield microscope is the polarizing microscope. A *polarizer* (or polarizing filter) may be defined as a sieve that takes ordinary light waves, which vibrate in all orientations (or directions), and allows only light waves

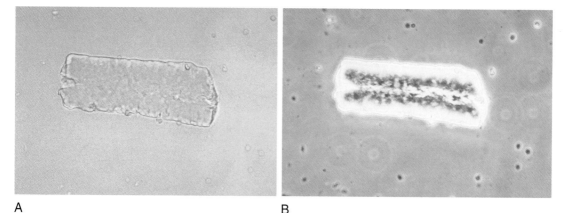

A   B

FIGURE 5-10   Brightfield versus phase-contrast illumination. A, Waxy cast with brightfield illumination, 100×. B, Same field with phase-contrast illumination, 100×. Note the central fissure and increased detail. (From Brunzel NA: Fundamentals of urine and body fluid analysis, ed 2, Philadelphia, 2004, Saunders.)

of one orientation (north-south or east-west) to pass through the filter (Fig. 5-11, A). In a polarizing microscope, a polarizing filter is placed between the light source (bulb) and the specimen. A second polarizing filter (called an *analyzer*) is placed above the specimen, between the objective and the eyepiece (either at some point in the microscope tube or in the eyepiece). One of the polarizers is then rotated until the two are at right angles to each other (see Fig. 5-11, B). When the viewer is looking through the eyepieces, this will be seen as the extinction of light (viewer sees a dark or black field), since all light is blocked out of the light path when the polarizing filters are at right angles to each other. However, certain objects have a property termed **birefringence**, which means they rotate (or polarize) light. An object that polarizes bends light so it can be visualized when viewed through crossed polarizers. Objects that do not bend light will not be observed in the microscope. An object that polarizes light (or is birefringent) will appear light against a dark background.

A further modification of the polarizing microscope involves the use of **compensated polarized light**. A compensator, also referred to as a *first-order red plate* (filter) or *full-wave retardation plate*, is placed between the two crossed polarizing filters and positioned 45 degrees to the crossed polarizer and analyzer (see Fig. 5-11, C and D). With this addition, the field background appears red or magenta, whereas objects that are birefringent (polarize light) appear yellow or blue in relation to their orientation to the compensator and their optical properties.

The compensated polarized microscope is especially useful clinically for differentiating between monosodium urate (MSU) and calcium pyrophosphate dihydrate (CPPD) crystals in synovial fluid. It is also becoming useful in the routine study of urine sediment and in some histologic work.

Polarizing microscopy is often used in geology for particle analysis and in forensic medicine clinically. With the polarizing microscope, the optical properties of an object can be determined.

Darkfield Microscope

With darkfield microscopy, a special substage condenser is used that causes light waves to cross on the specimen rather than pass in parallel waves through the specimen. When the user looks through the microscope, the field in view will be black, or dark, because no light passes from the condenser to the objective. When an object is present on the stage, however, light will be deflected as it hits the object and will pass through the objective and be seen by the viewer. As a result, the object under study appears light against a dark background. Any brightfield microscope may be converted to a darkfield microscope by use of a special darkfield condenser in place of the usual condenser.

The darkfield microscope has long been used in the routine clinical laboratory to observe spirochetes in exudates from leptospiral or syphilitic infections. A more recent use, facilitated by newer microscope design technology, is as a low-power scanner for urine sediment. A darkfield effect may be achieved by using a mismatched phase annulus and phase objective, such as a low-power phase objective with a high-power phase annulus.

Fluorescence Microscope

The transmitted-light fluorescence microscope is a further refinement of the darkfield microscope. It is basically a darkfield microscope with wavelength selection. Certain objects have the ability to fluoresce, which means they absorb light of certain very short (ultraviolet) wavelengths and emit light of longer (visible) wavelengths. In

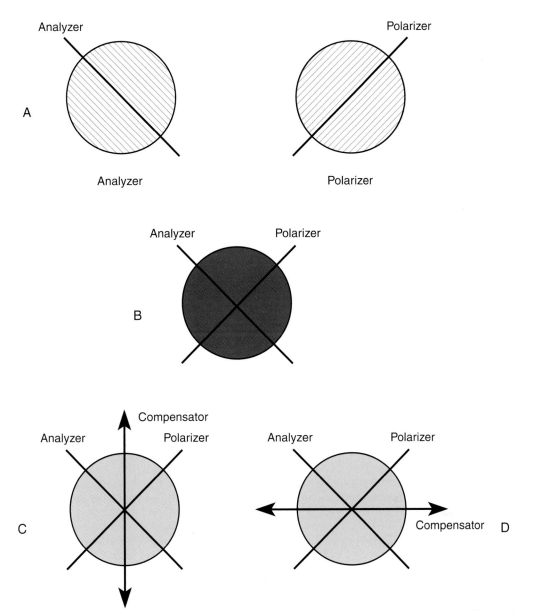

FIGURE 5-11   Principle of polarized light and compensated polarized light. A, Polarizing lenses or filters. Polarizer is placed between light source and specimen; analyzer is placed between specimen and eye of the observer. B, Polarized light, obtained by placing analyzer and polarizer at right angles to each other. Position of analyzer is fixed, and polarizer is rotated until light is extinguished (seen as a black or dark background). C, Compensated polarized light. Compensator is placed at 45 degrees to the crossed polarizers, resulting in a red or magenta background color. Here, direction of slow wave of compensation is in north-south (N-S) orientation. D, Compensated polarized light. Here, direction of slow wave of compensation is in east-west (E-W) orientation.

fluorescence microscopy with transmitted light and a compound microscope, the darkfield condenser is preceded by a special exciter filter that allows only shorter-wavelength blue light to pass and cross on the specimen plane. If the specimen contains an object that fluoresces (either naturally or because of staining or labeling with certain fluorescent dyes), it will absorb the blue light and emit light of a longer yellow or green wavelength. A special barrier filter is placed in the microscope tube or eyepiece. This barrier filter will pass only the desired wavelength of emitted light for the particular fluorescent system, so the fluorescence technique shows only the presence or absence of the fluorescing object. The barrier filter used must be carefully chosen so that only light of the desired wavelength will be passed through the microscope to the observer. Objects in the specimen that do not fluoresce will not emit light of that wavelength and will not be seen.

Fluorescence techniques, in particular fluorescent antibody (FA) techniques, are especially useful in the clinical laboratory. They are used particularly in the clinical microbiology laboratory and for various immunologic studies. Different FA techniques may be used in primary identification of microorganisms or in the final identification of bacteria such as group A streptococci, replacing older serologic methods. Such techniques have the advantage of saving time, allowing earlier diagnosis for the patient, and they are often more sensitive than other techniques. Fluorescent techniques may also be useful in identifying organisms that cannot be cultured (e.g., *Treponema pallidum*).

Electron Microscope

The limit of magnification with any of the variations of the light microscope is about 1500× to 2000×. Above this, there is decreased resolving power. For magnification of up to about 50,000×, the electron microscope may be used with good resolution.

In general, the principle of the electron microscope is the same as for the light microscope. Rather than a beam of light, however, the specimen is illuminated with a beam of electrons produced by an electron "gun." The electrons are accelerated by a high-voltage potential and pass through a condenser lens system, usually composed of two magnetic lenses. The electron beam is concentrated onto the specimen, and the objective lens provides the primary magnification. The final image is not visible and cannot be viewed directly; rather, it is projected onto a fluorescent screen or a photographic plate. This is the principle of the **transmission electron microscope (TEM)**.

Another variation is the **scanning electron microscope (SEM)**. SEM focuses on the surface of the specimen and produces a 3D image by striking the sample with a focused beam of electrons. Electrons emitted from the surface of the sample, in addition to deflected electrons from the focused beam of electrons, are focused onto a cathode ray tube or photographic plate and visualized as a 3D image.

In both TEM and SEM, specimens need special preparation not done in routine clinical laboratories. Specimens must be extremely thin. With TEM, the electron beam must pass through the specimen, and electrons have very poor penetrating power. With SEM, the specimen can be slightly thicker because the beam of electrons does not pass through the specimen. In either case, it is impossible to study living cells with electron microscopy because of the high vacuum to which the specimen is subjected, and because the electron beam itself is highly damaging to living tissue. Despite this limitation, electron microscopy has provided much information about cell structure and function.

DIGITAL IMAGING

Recent advances in artificial neural networks, image analysis, and slide handling have combined to produce instruments that automate manual differentials in new ways. This new technology, referred to as *automated digital cell morphology*, provides an unprecedented level of efficiency and consistency. In its simplest form, automated digital cell morphology is a process where blood cells are automatically located and preclassified into categories of blood cells. Images of these cells are retained for confirmation by a technologist and can be shared electronically and stored as digital images. This adaptability allows for future review and comparisons by laboratory professionals and physicians.

Artificial Neural Networks

An artificial neural network (ANN) is an information-processing model that simulates the way the human brain processes information. ANN emulates the neural structure of the brain, which is composed of a large number of highly interconnected processing elements (neurons) working together to solve specific problems.

ANNs are the result of research in artificial intelligence (AI) and its attempt to mimic the capacity to learn, as seen in biological neural systems. AI systems resulted in the development of so-called expert systems. Although very useful in some applications, AI failed to capture key aspects of the human brain's ability to critically compare and contrast complex objects.

ANNs have been around since the 1940s, but it was not until the mid-1980s that algorithms became sophisticated enough and computers powerful enough for general applications to develop. Applications of ANNs in which their pattern-recognition capabilities are used include speech recognition and analysis, handwriting, fingerprints, faces, and cellular morphology.

Digital Cell Morphology

The use of image analysis in hematology has been more difficult to achieve for several reasons: the need for higher magnifications and image resolution, high throughput due to volume, turnaround time (TAT) demands, and existing established procedures for slide review. New hardware and the development of databases have aided in developing image-analysis systems that can finally meet the demands of the hematology laboratory.

The most dramatic change in microscopy over the last 3 decades is the ability to digitize images of specimens and transmit these images electronically for remote analysis. Recent progress in microscope design is opening new doors to multidimensional microscopy. Digitalization increases our ability to enhance features, extract information, or modify images. Digitized images can be shared with remote observers for workflow automation, image acquisition, storage, and retransmission. This capability is now called *virtual microscopy*.

In 2000, CellaVision (Lund, Sweden) launched the DiffMaster Octavia. The system consists of an automated microscope with a 100× objective; a stepper motor and light control unit; and a progressive three-chip CCD color camera connected to a computer with software for localization, segmentation, and classification of white and red blood cells. The system processes eight slides per batch, utilizing a slide holder. It allows for remote review of a smear and storage of up to 20,000 slides with images in a database.

In comparison with earlier attempts by other manufacturers, the DiffMaster Octavia handles wedged smears stained according to the Wright, Wright-Giemsa, or May Grünwald–Giemsa staining protocols and uses ANNs trained on a large database of cells. It was the first image analysis system to locate and preclassify cells into 15 different categories and automatically precharacterized six red blood cell (RBC) morphologic characteristics. The platelet estimates and erythrocyte precharacterization are performed in an overview image corresponding to eight high-power fields (100×). Review and release of results can be done remotely.

BIBLIOGRAPHY

Benford JR: The theory of the microscope, Rochester, NY, 1965, Bausch & Lomb.

CellaVision: http://www.cellavision.com (retrieved July, 2009).

Gill GW: Microscope cleaning tips, techniques and timing, Lab Med 36(8):460, 2005.

Hagner R, Wilson P: Chapter 5 Automated Digital Cell Morphology: Taking the "Manual" out of the Manual Differential in Clinical Diagnostic Technology, Corey-Ward, (Ed.), Vol. 3, 2006, AACC Press.

Schwartz S: Trends in digital bioscience imaging, Bio-It World 4(7):48, 2005.

RELATED WEBSITES

http://www.microscopy-analysis.com/

REVIEW QUESTIONS

1. **Identify the parts of the microscope.**
   a. _____
   b. _____
   c. _____
   d. _____
   e. _____
   f. _____

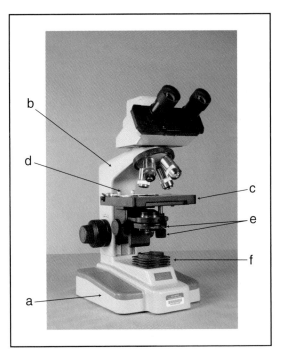

Questions 2-4: Match the common working distances with their objectives (a to c).

2. ___ 4 mm

3. ___ 1.8 mm

4. ___ 16 mm
   a. Oil-immersion objective
   b. High-power objective
   c. Low-power objective

Questions 5-7: Match the objectives with their common numerical apertures (a to c).

5. ___ **Oil-immersion objective**

6. ___ **High-power objective**

7. ___ **Low-power objective**
   a. 0.25 NA
   b. 0.85 NA
   c. 1.2 NA

Questions 8-10: *Match the objectives with how the condenser should be positioned (a to c), assuming the NA of the condenser is 0.85.*

8. ___ Oil-immersion objective

9. ___ High-power objective

10. ___ Low-power objective
    a. Highest position possible or very slightly decreased
    b. Highest position possible
    c. Decreased to 1 or 2 mm below the slide

11. **What objective must you always use when you first start looking at a slide?**
    a. High power
    b. 100×
    c. 40×
    d. 10×

12. **Which focusing adjustment do you first use when you begin looking at a slide?**
    a. Small focusing knob
    b. Coarse focus
    c. Fine focus
    d. 4× objective

13. **Which objective allows you to see the largest area of the object you are viewing?**
    a. 4×
    b. 10×
    c. 100×
    d. 40×

14. **Describe how to *decrease* light intensity.**
    a. Adjust the coarse focusing knob.
    b. Close the iris diaphragm.
    c. Adjust the dimmer switch.
    d. Open the iris diaphragm.

15. **What do you adjust if you can see through one ocular and not the other?**
    a. The fine focus
    b. The coarse focus
    c. Change to a different objective
    d. The other ocular

16. **What do you adjust if you can see two overlapping circles, with part of the object in each circle?**
    a. The focus
    b. The iris diaphragm
    c. The width of the oculars
    d. Change to a different objective

17. **How do you increase depth of field?**
    a. Increase the amount of light.
    b. Open the aperture of the iris diaphragm.
    c. Close one eye.
    d. Use fine focusing.

18. **Which focusing knob do you use with the 10× and 40× objectives?**
    a. Fine-focusing knob
    b. Respectively coarse and fine focusing knobs
    c. Both fine focusing knob and the iris diaphragm
    d. Coarse focusing knob

19. **How much are you magnifying something when you are using 10× oculars and the 40× objectives?**
    a. 40×
    b. 400×
    c. 4000×
    d. Cannot calculate without additional information.

Questions 20-25: *A = True, B = False.*

20. ___ An adaptation of the brightfield microscope is the polarizing microscope.

21. ___ In darkfield microscopy, light waves pass in parallel waves through the specimen.

22. ___ A transmitted-light fluorescence microscope is a refinement of the darkfield microscope.

23. ___ SEM focuses on the surface of the specimen and produces a three-dimensional image.

24. ___ An artificial neural network (ANN) simulates the way the human brain processes information.

25. ___ Digital microscopy allows for preclassifying leukocytes, producing platelet estimates, and precharacterizing erythrocytes.

CHAPTER 6

BASIC AND NEW TECHNIQUES IN THE CLINICAL LABORATORY

Learning Objectives

At the conclusion of this chapter, the student will be able to:

- Compare and contrast the four basic categories of measurement techniques, with examples of methods for each category.
- Describe the principle of absorbance spectrophotometry.

- Compare the observed colors of the visible spectrum and the corresponding wavelengths.
- Define Beer's law.

Continued

Learning Objectives—cont'd

- Name criteria for the preparation and use of a standard curve.
- Name the components of a spectrophotometer.
- Identify and describe the three quality control tests for spectrophotometers.
- Describe the principle of reflectance spectrophotometry.
- Describe the principle, advantages, and disadvantages of nephelometry.
- Explain the principle of flow (cell) cytometry and its clinical application.
- Describe the characteristics of enzyme immunoassay.
- Identify and compare the three basic immunofluorescent labeling techniques.
- List at least three potential benefits of automated immunoassay.
- Describe the polymerase chain reaction (PCR) amplification technique.

- Compare various PCR modifications.
- Discuss the general concept of nucleic acid blotting.
- Compare the characteristics and clinical applications of Southern blotting, Northern blotting, and Western blotting techniques.
- Compare a pH electrode with an ion-selective electrode.
- Explain the techniques of coulometry and chromatography.
- Describe the electrophoresis technique.
- Compare immunoelectrophoresis and immunofixation electrophoresis.
- Compare capillary electrophoresis and microchip capillary electrophoresis.
- Name the analytical techniques used in point-of-care testing.

In the clinical laboratory, there is a continual need for quantitative techniques of measurement. Instrumentation has become miniaturized, enabling the development of point-of-care devices. The methodologies used in technologically sophisticated automated analyzers are based on traditional approaches and technologies. General methods for most automated and manual assays in the chemistry laboratory include the use of spectrophotometry, ion-selective electrodes, electrophoresis, nephelometry, and immunoassays.

Analytical techniques and instrumentation provide the foundation for all measurements made in a modern clinical laboratory. Most measurement techniques fall into one of four basic categories:

1. Spectrometry, including spectrophotometry, atomic absorption, and mass spectrophotometry
2. Luminescence, including fluorescence, chemiluminescence, and nephelometry
3. Electroanalytical methods, including electrophoresis, potentiometry, and amperometry
4. Chromatography, including gas, liquid, and thin-layer techniques

PHOTOMETRY

Instruments that measure electromagnetic radiation have several concepts and components in common. One of the techniques used most frequently in the clinical laboratory is photometry, or specifically, absorbance or reflectance spectrophotometry. **Photometry** employs color and color variation to determine the concentrations of various substances. A photometric component is employed in many of the automated analyzers currently in use in the clinical laboratory, and any person doing clinical laboratory techniques should understand the principles of photometry.

Photometry is the measurement of the luminous intensity of light, or the amount of luminous light falling on a surface from a light source. Photometric instruments measure this intensity of light without consideration of wavelength. In contrast, spectrophotometry is the measurement of the intensity of light at selected wavelengths.

ABSORBANCE SPECTROPHOTOMETRY

In **absorbance spectrophotometry,** the concentration of an unknown sample is determined by measuring its absorption of light at a particular wavelength and comparing it with the absorption of light by known standard solutions measured at the same time and with the same wavelength. The intensity of the color is directly proportional to the concentration of the substance present.

The use of **spectrophotometry,** or **colorimetry,** as a means of quantitative measurement depends primarily on two factors: the color itself and the intensity of the color. Any substance to be measured by spectrophotometry must be naturally colored or capable of being colored. An example of a substance that is colored to begin with is hemoglobin (determined by spectrophotometry in the hematology laboratory). Sugar, specifically glucose, is an example of a substance that is not colored to begin with but is capable of being colored by certain reagents and reactions. Sugar content can therefore be measured by spectrophotometry.

When spectrophotometry is used as a method for quantitative measurement, the unknown colored substance is compared with a similar substance of known strength (a standard solution). In absorbance spectrophotometry, the absorbance units or values for several different concentrations of a standard solution are determined by spectrophotometry and plotted on graph paper. The resulting graph is known as a **standard calibration curve** or a Beer's law plot. Unknown specimens can then be read in the spectrophotometer, and using their absorbance values, their concentrations can be determined from the calibration curve.

The Nature of Light

To understand the use of absorbance spectrophotometry (and photometry in general), one must first understand the fundamentals of color. To understand color, one must also understand the nature of light and its effect on color as we see it. Light is a type of radiant energy, and it travels in the form of waves. The distance between waves is the **wavelength of light.** The term *light* is used to describe radiant energy with wavelengths visible to the human eye or wavelengths bordering on those visible to the human eye.

Electromagnetic radiation includes a spectrum of energy from short-wavelength, highly energetic gamma rays and x-rays on the left side of the spectrum to wavelengths of radio frequencies on the right side (Fig. 6-1). Visible light passes between these frequencies, with the color violet at the 400-nm wavelength and red at the 700-nm wavelength. As discussed next, these are the approximate limits of the visible spectrum.

The human eye responds to radiant energy, or light, with wavelengths between about 380 and 750 nm. A nanometer is 1×10^9 m. With modern photometric apparatus, shorter (ultraviolet) or longer (infrared) wavelengths can be measured. Modern instruments isolate a narrow wavelength range of the spectrum for measurements. Most instruments use filters (photometers) or prisms or gratings (spectrometers) to select or isolate a narrow range of the incident wavelength. The wavelength of light determines the color of the light seen by the human eye. Every color seen is light of a particular wavelength. A combination or mixture of light energy of different wavelengths is known as *daylight* or *white light.* When light is passed through a filter, a prism, or a diffraction grating, it can be broken into a spectrum of visible colors ranging from violet to red. The **visible spectrum** consists of the following range of colors: violet, blue, green, yellow, orange, and red. If white light is diffracted or partially absorbed by a filter or prism, it becomes visible as certain colors. The different portions of the spectrum may be identified by wavelengths ranging from 380 to 750 nm for the visible colors. Wavelengths below approximately 380 nm are ultraviolet, and those above 750 nm are infrared; these light waves are not visible to the human eye. Table 6-1 compares and contrasts the colors of the visible spectrum in terms of their respective wavelengths.

The color of light seen in the visible spectrum depends on the wavelength that is not absorbed.

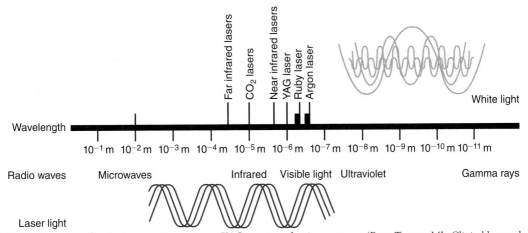

FIGURE 6-1 **The electromagnetic spectrum. YAG, yttrium-aluminum-garnet.** (From Turgeon ML: Clinical hematology: theory and procedures, ed 3, Philadelphia, 1999, Lippincott Williams & Wilkins.)

TABLE 6-1

Observed Colors of Visible Spectrum and Corresponding Wavelengths	
Approximate Wavelength (nm)	Color Observed
<380	Not visible (ultraviolet light)
380-440	Violet
440-500	Blue
500-580	Green
580-600	Yellow
600-620	Orange
620-750	Red
>750	Not visible (infrared light)

When light is not absorbed, it is transmitted. A colored solution has color because of its physical properties, which result in its absorbing certain wavelengths and transmitting others. When white light is passed through a solution, part of the light is absorbed, and the remaining light is transmitted. A rainbow is seen when there are droplets of moisture in the air that refract or filter certain rays of the sun and allow others to pass through. The colors of the rainbow range from red to violet—the visible spectrum.

Absorbance and Transmittance of Light: Beer's Law

Many solutions contain particles that absorb certain wavelengths and transmit others. Solutions appear to the human eye to have characteristic colors. The wavelength of light transmitted by the solution is recognized as color by the eye. A blue solution appears blue because particles in the solution absorb all the wavelengths except blue; the blue is the color transmitted and seen. A red solution appears red because all other wavelengths except red have been absorbed by the solution; the red wavelength passes through the solution.

Measurement by spectrophotometry is based on the reaction between the substance to be measured and a reagent, or chemical, used to produce color. The amount of color produced in a reaction between the substance to be measured and the reagent depends on the concentration of the substance. Therefore, the intensity of the color is proportional to the concentration of the substance.

Beer's law states that the concentration of a substance is directly proportional to the amount of light absorbed or inversely proportional to the logarithm of the transmitted light. (*Percent transmittance* and *absorbance* are related photometric terms; see following discussion.) Beer's law is the

basis for the use of photometry in quantitative measurement. If one saw a solution with a very intense red color, one would be correct in assuming the solution had a high concentration of the substance that made it red. Another way of stating Beer's law is that any increase in the concentration of a color-producing substance will increase the amount of color seen.

As the law states, the depth at which the color is determined must be constant. The depth of the solution is regulated by the cuvette or container used to hold it. Increasing the depth of the solution through which the light must pass (by using a cuvette with a larger diameter) is the same as placing more particles between the light and the eye, thereby creating an apparent increase in the concentration, or intensity, of color.

Expressions of Light Transmitted or Absorbed

There are two common methods of expressing the amount of **light transmitted** or **light absorbed** by a solution. (Another term for absorbed light is *optical density* [OD], which is not generally used.) The units used to express the readings obtained by the electronic measuring device are either **absorbance (A) units** or **percent transmittance (%T) units.** Most spectrophotometers give readings in both units. Absorbance units are sometimes more difficult to read directly from the reading scale because it is divided logarithmically rather than in equal divisions (Fig. 6-2).

Absorbance is an expression of the amount of light absorbed by a solution. Absorbance values are directly proportional to the concentration of the solution and can be plotted on **linear graph paper** to give a straight line (Fig. 6-3, A). Most spectrophotometers also give the percent transmittance readings on the viewing scale. **Percent transmittance** is the amount of light that passes through a colored solution compared with the amount of light that passes through a blank or standard solution. The blank solution contains all the reagents used in the procedure, but it does not contain the unknown substance being measured.

Percent transmittance varies from 0 to 100 (usually abbreviated %T), with equal divisions on the viewing scale (see Fig. 6-2). As the concentration of the colored solution increases, the amount of light absorbed increases, and the percentage of light transmitted decreases. Transmitted light does not decrease in direct proportion to the concentration or color intensity of the solution being measured. Percent transmittance readings plotted against concentration will not give a straight line on linear graph paper (see Fig. 6-3, B). A logarithmic relationship exists between percent transmittance

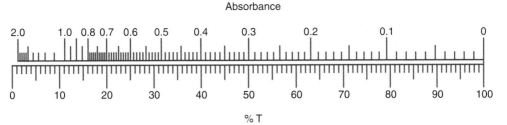

FIGURE 6-2 Viewing scales showing divisions for reading percent transmittance versus absorbance. Absorbance is the measure of light stopped or absorbed. Percent transmittance is the measure of light transmitted through the solution. (From Campbell JB, Campbell JM: Laboratory mathematics: medical and biological applications, ed 5, St Louis, 1997, Mosby.)

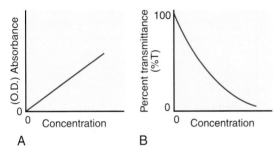

FIGURE 6-3 Relationships of absorbance (A) and percent transmittance (B) to concentration when plotted using linear graph paper. (From Kaplan LA, Pesce AJ: Clinical chemistry: theory, analysis, correlation, ed 5, St Louis, 2010, Mosby.)

and concentration, so when percent transmittance is plotted against concentration, **semilogarithmic graph paper** is used to obtain a straight line (see Fig. 6-3). Absorbance and percent transmittance are related in the following way:

Absorbance = 2 minus the logarithm of the percent transmittance

or

$$A = 2 - \log \% T$$

Therefore, 2 is the logarithm of 100%T. One can obtain a convenient conversion table for transmittance and absorbance from a standard chemistry reference textbook.

Preparation and Use of a Standard Curve

The preparation of a standard curve in today's clinical laboratory is usually not constructed manually. The steps formerly done with graph paper to calculate the relationship between spectrophotometric readings for the standards and the unknowns have been automated. In research laboratories or in the preparation of a new or special procedure, it may be necessary to prepare a standard curve manually. To understand the concept of a standard curve and

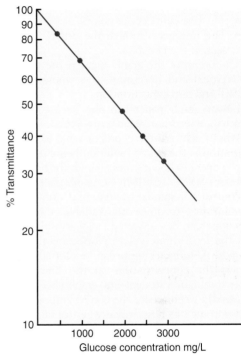

FIGURE 6-4 Use of semilogarithmic graph paper showing percent transmittance plotted against concentration. (From Kaplan LA, Pesce AJ: Clinical chemistry: theory, analysis, correlation, ed 5, St Louis, 2010, Mosby.)

its use, the principles of how a standard curve is constructed and used should be known.

Types of Graph Paper

Semilogarithmic graph paper is used to plot percent transmittance readings from the photometer, because a logarithmic relationship exists between percent and concentration, as previously described. The horizontal axis of semilogarithmic graph paper is a linear scale, and the vertical axis is a logarithmic scale (Fig. 6-4). Concentrations of the standard solutions are plotted on the horizontal axis. The transmittance or absorbance readings from the photometer are plotted along the vertical axis. When used, percent transmittance readings can be plotted directly on the logarithmic scale of the semilogarithmic graph paper (the horizontal axis) because the concentration is proportional to the logarithm of the galvanometer reading. In this way, percent transmittance readings are converted to the appropriate numbers on the logarithmic scale. When percentages are plotted against concentrations on semilogarithmic graph paper, the proportional relationship is direct, and the necessary straight-line graph is obtained when the individual standard points are connected.

The criteria for a good standard curve are:
- The line is straight.
- The line connects all points.
- The line goes through the origin, or intersect, of the two axes.

The origin of the graph paper is the point on the vertical and horizontal axes where there is 100%T and zero concentration.

Linear graph paper can also be used to plot absorbance readings because absorbance of wavelengths of light is directly proportional to the concentration of the colored solution being read. This graph paper has linear scales on both the horizontal and the vertical axis. If linear graph paper is used to construct a standard curve, and only percent transmittance readings are available, these readings must first be converted to logarithmic values and the logarithmic values plotted on the vertical axis. Absorbance units can be plotted directly against the concentration on the linear graph paper to obtain a straight-line graph (Beer's law is followed). To eliminate the conversion of percent transmittance to absorbance when obtaining the necessary straight-line graph, the use of semilogarithmic graph paper is recommended.

Plotting a Standard Curve

When points are plotted on graph paper, whether they represent concentrations or galvanometer readings, care must be taken to note the intervals on the graph paper. Many errors result from carelessness in the initial plotting of points on the graph paper. Also, when a standard curve is prepared, the axes must be properly labeled, along with other information pertaining to the graph.

Using a Standard Curve

Once the standard curve has been plotted, it is used to calculate the concentrations of any unknowns that were included in the same batch as the standards used to make the graph. Determining the concentration of a solution requires some way of comparing it with a solution of known concentration.

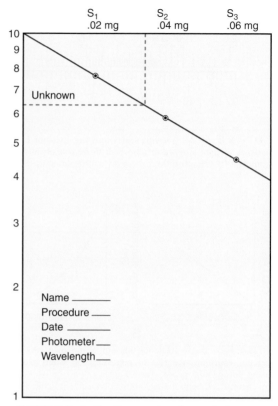

FIGURE 6-5   Construction of a standard curve.

Fig. 6-5 shows a simplified example of the construction and use of a standard curve. In this example, three standard solutions are prepared with the following concentrations: standard 1 (S_1), 0.02 mg; standard 2 (S_2), 0.04 mg; and standard 3 (S_3), 0.06 mg. These concentrations are plotted on the linear (horizontal) scale of the semilogarithmic graph paper.

The three standard tubes are read in a photometer, giving the following readings in percent transmittance: $S_1 = 76\%$T, $S_2 = 58\%$T, and $S_3 = 45\%$T. The percent transmittance readings are plotted under their respective concentrations on the logarithmic (vertical) scale of the paper. The points are connected using a ruler. An undetermined substance gives a reading of 63%T. Using the graph in Fig. 6-5, the 63%T point on the vertical scale is found, followed horizontally to the graph line just drawn, and then followed vertically to the concentration scale. The degree of accuracy with which an unknown concentration can be read depends on the concentrations of the standards used. The accuracy of the unknown can be no greater than the accuracy of the standard solutions used. Standard solutions are usually weighed to the fourth decimal place. In this example, if the graph lines were present, the unknown concentration would be read as 0.0343 mg (the figure in the fourth decimal place is approximate).

Rather than relying on a permanently established calibration curve, using standard solutions to standardize the analyses of each batch allows the clinical laboratory to produce more reliable results. It compensates for variables such as time, temperature, age of reagents, and condition of instruments. It is always best to use several different concentrations of the standard solution, not just one. To obtain reliable photometric information about the concentration of a substance, standard solutions must be used as the basis for comparison.

Instruments Used in Spectrophotometry

The instrument used to show the quantitative relationship between the colors of the undetermined solution and the standard solution is called a **spectrophotometer** or **colorimeter.** A spectrophotometer is used to measure the light transmitted by a solution to determine the concentration of the light-absorbing substance in the solution.

Most of the instruments used in photometry have some means of isolating a narrow wavelength, or range, of the color spectrum for measurements. Instruments using filters for this purpose are referred to as *filter photometers,* and those using prisms or diffraction gratings are called *spectrophotometers* or *photoelectric colorimeters.* Both types are used frequently in the clinical laboratory. Older colorimetric procedures used visual comparison of the color of an unknown with that of a standard. In general, visual colorimetry has been replaced by the more specific and accurate photoelectric methods.

One current application of visual colorimetry employs various dry reagent strip tests prevalent in many clinical chemistry tests (e.g., urinalysis). These strips can be read visually, although instruments are also available to read the developed color electronically.

Many types of spectrophotometers are in common use in the clinical laboratory (Fig. 6-6). The principle of most of these instruments is the same: the amount of light transmitted by the standard solution is compared with the amount of light transmitted by the solution of unknown concentration.

Photometers utilize an electronic device to compare the actual color intensities of the solutions measured. As the name implies, a spectrophotometer is really two instruments in a single case: a spectrometer, a device for producing light of a specific wavelength, the monochromator; and a photometer, a device for measuring light intensity. In the automated analyzing instruments used in many laboratories, a photometer is still a necessary component so that absorbance values for unknown

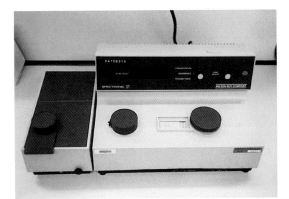

FIGURE 6-6 **Spectrophotometer.** (From Rodak BF, Fritsma GA, Doig K: Hematology: clinical principles and applications, ed 3, St Louis, 2007, Saunders.)

and standard solutions can be determined. Some instruments contain a filter wheel that allows measurement of absorbance at any wavelength for which there is a filter on the wheel. Microprocessors control the location of the correct filter for the particular analyte being measured. From the absorbance information, the computer microprocessor calculates the unknown concentration.

Parts Essential to All Spectrophotometers

The parts necessary to all spectrophotometers are light source, means to isolate light of a desired wavelength, fiber optics, cuvettes, photodetector, readout device, recorder, and microprocessor (Fig. 6-7).

Light Source

Each spectrophotometer must have a light source. This can be a light bulb constructed to give the optimum amount of light. The light source must be steady and constant; therefore, use of a voltage regulator or an electronic power supply is recommended. The light source may be movable or stationary. The most common source of light for work in the visible or near-infrared region is the incandescent tungsten or tungsten-iodide lamp. Most emitted radiant energy is near-infrared. Often, a heat-absorbing filter is inserted between the lamp and sample to absorb the infrared radiation. The most common lamps for ultraviolet work are deuterium-discharge and mercury arc lamps.

Wavelength Isolator

Before the light from the light source reaches the sample of solution to be measured, the interfering wavelengths must be removed. A system of isolating a desired wavelength and excluding others is

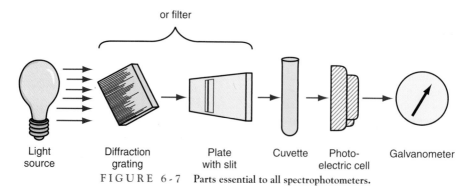

FIGURE 6-7 Parts essential to all spectrophotometers.

called a *monochromator;* the light is actually being reduced to a particular wavelength. Filters can be used to accomplish this. Some are very simple, composed of one or two pieces of colored glass. The more complicated filters are found in the better spectrophotometers. The filter must transmit a color the solution can absorb. A red filter transmits red, and a green filter transmits green. Filters are available to cover almost any point in the visible spectrum, and each filter has inscribed on it a number that indicates the wavelength of light that it transmits. For example, a filter inscribed with "540 nm" absorbs all light except that of wavelengths around 540 nm. Because the filter must transmit a color the solution can absorb, for a red solution, the filter chosen should *not* be red (all colors except red are absorbed). The wavelength of light transmitted is therefore the important factor to consider in choosing the correct filter for a procedure.

Light of a desired wavelength can also be provided by other means. One common instrument employs a diffraction grating with a special plate and slit to reduce the spectrum to the desired wavelength. The grating consists of a highly polished surface with numerous lines that break up white light into the spectrum. By moving the spectrum behind a slit (the light source must be movable), only one particular portion of the spectrum is allowed to pass through the narrow slit. The particular band of light, or wavelength, transmitted through the slit is indicated on a viewing scale on the machine. Certain wavelengths are more desirable than others for a particular color and procedure. The wavelength chosen is determined by running an absorption curve and selecting the correct wavelength after inspecting the curve obtained. Only when new methods are being developed is it necessary to run an absorption curve.

Cuvettes (Absorption Cells or Photometer Tubes)

Any light (of the wavelength selected) coming from the filter or diffraction grating will pass on to the solution in the cuvette. Glass cuvettes are

relatively inexpensive and satisfactory, provided they are matched or calibrated. **Calibrated cuvettes** are tubes that have been optically matched so that the same solution in each will give the same reading on the photometer. In using calibrated cuvettes, the depth factor of Beer's law is kept constant. Depending on the concentration and thus the color of the solution, a certain amount of light will be absorbed by the solution. The light not absorbed by the solution is transmitted and passed on to an electronic measuring device of some type. Alternatively, to eliminate the cuvette entirely, a flow-through apparatus can be used.

Electronic Measuring Device

In the more common spectrophotometers, the electronic measuring device consists of a photoelectric cell and a galvanometer. The amount of light transmitted by the solution in the cuvette is measured by a **photoelectric cell,** a sensitive instrument producing electrons in proportion to the amount of light hitting it. The electrons are passed on to a **galvanometer,** where they are measured. The galvanometer records the amount of current (in the form of electrons) it receives from the photoelectric cell on a special viewing scale on the spectrophotometer. Results are reported in terms of percent transmittance (or in some cases, absorbance). The percent transmittance depends on the concentration of the solution and its depth. If the solution is very concentrated (the color appearing intense), less light will be transmitted than if it is dilute (pale). Therefore, the reading on the galvanometer viewing scale will be lower for a more concentrated solution than for a dilute solution. This is the basis for the comparison of color intensity with the spectrophotometer.

Calibration of Cuvettes

If cuvettes are used, it is essential for their diameters to be uniform; that is, the depth of the cuvettes or tubes used in the spectrophotometer must be constant for Beer's law to apply. Precalibrated cuvettes must be checked before actual use in the laboratory. Calibrated cuvettes are optically matched so the same solution in each will give the same percent transmittance reading on the galvanometer viewing scale.

For use in spectrophotometry, the cuvette is carefully checked to ensure that the solution in it gives the same reading as in other calibrated cuvettes. To check cuvettes for uniformity, the same solution is read in many cuvettes. Readings are taken, and cuvettes that match within an established tolerance are used.

If new, plain glass tubes are being calibrated for use as cuvettes, the tubes are rotated in the cuvette well to observe any changes in reading with the position in the well, because all tubes may not be perfectly round. The cuvette is etched at the point where the reading corresponds with the established tolerance for the absorption reading. Cuvettes that do not agree or do not correspond are not used for spectrophotometry. Different sizes of cuvettes can be used, depending on the spectrophotometer.

Care and Handling of Spectrophotometers

When using a spectrophotometer, error caused by color in the reagents must be eliminated. Because color is so important, and because the color produced by the undetermined substance is the desired color, any color resulting from the reagents themselves or from interactions between the reagents could cause confusion and error. By using a blank solution, a correction can be made for any color resulting from the reagents used. The blank solution contains the same reagents as the unknown and standard tubes, with the exception of the substance being measured.

As with any expensive, delicate instrument, a spectrophotometer must be handled with care. The manufacturer supplies a manual of complete instructions on the care and use of a particular machine. Care should be taken to not spill reagents on the spectrophotometer. Spillage could damage the instrument, especially the photoelectric cell. Any reagents spilled must be wiped up immediately. Spectrophotometers with filters should not be operated without the filter in place; the unfiltered light from the light source may damage the photoelectric cell and the galvanometer. A spectrophotometer should be placed on a table with good support where it will not be bumped or jarred.

Quality Control Tests for Spectrophotometers

Quality control testing for spectrophotometry consists of checking:
- Wavelength accuracy
- Stray light
- Linearity

Wavelength accuracy is ensured when the wavelength indicated on the control dial is the actual wavelength of light passed by the monochromator. This is checked with standard absorbing solution or filters with maximum absorbance of known wavelength. Wavelength calibration can be tested by using a rare-earth glass filter (e.g., didymium) or a stable chromogen solution. Calibration at two wavelengths is necessary for instruments with diffraction gratings and at three wavelengths for instruments with prisms. Photoelectric accuracy can be checked by reading standard solutions of potassium dichromate or potassium nitrate. As an alternative, the National Bureau of Standards (NBS) has sets of three neutral-density glass filters that have known absorbance at four wavelengths for each filter. These filters are not completely stable, however, and require periodic recalibration.

Stray light refers to any wavelengths outside the band transmitted by the monochromator. The most common causes of stray light are (1) reflections of light from scratches on optical surfaces or from dust particles anywhere in the light path and (2) higher-order spectra produced by diffraction gratings. Stray light is detected by using cutoff filters.

Linearity is demonstrated when a change in concentration results in a straight-line calibration curve, as discussed under Beer's law. Neutral-density filters to check linearity over a range of wavelengths are commercially available, as are sealed sets of different colors and concentrations.

REFLECTANCE SPECTROPHOTOMETRY

Reflectance spectrophotometry is another quantitative spectrophotometric technique; the light reflected from the surface of a colorimetric reaction is used to measure the amount of unknown colored product generated in the reaction. A beam of light is directed at a flat surface, and the amount of light reflected is measured in a reflectance spectrophotometer. A photodetector measures the amount of reflected light directed to it. This technology has been employed in automated instrumentation, including many of the handheld instruments for bedside testing and smaller instruments used in physicians' offices and clinics.

Principle and Quality Control

Different surfaces have different optical properties. The optical properties of plastic strips or test paper are different from those of dry film. To use a reflectance spectrophotometer, the system must employ a standard with the same specific surface optical properties as the specific surface used in the test system. The use of reflectance spectrophotometry provides the quantitative measurement of reactions on such surfaces as strips, cartridges, and dry film.

The amount of light reflected and then measured depends on the specific instrumentation employed. Variables include the angles at which the reflected light is measured and the area of the surface being used for the measurement. Because this technology depends on products manufactured for use in the specific instrumentation, manufacturing processes (quality control considerations) as well as shipping and handling or storage problems can affect the resulting measurements.

Quality control for single-test instruments (using instrument-based systems) has been integrated into the instruments by the manufacturer. As long as the reagent packs or tabs have been properly stored and are used within the stated outdate, the manufacturer assures the user that calibration of the instrument will function automatically, that crucial quality control information has been encoded via the bar code on the unit packs, and that real-time processing is monitored. Use of the laboratory's usual quality control measures can be problematic for this technology because when the single-test, instrument-based systems are used, a new test system is created each time a new cartridge, pack, or strip is inserted into the instrument.

Parts of a Reflectance Spectrophotometer

The instrumentation necessary for a reflectance spectrophotometer is similar to that of a filter photometer, in which the filter serves to direct the selected wavelength for the methodology. A lamp generates light, which passes through the filter and a series of slits and is focused on the test surface (Fig. 6-8). As with a filter photometer, some light is absorbed by the filter; in the reflectance spectrophotometer, the remaining light is reflected. The light reflected is analogous to the light transmitted by the filter spectrophotometer. The reflected light then passes through a series of slits and lenses and on to the photodetector device where the amount of light is measured and recorded as a signal. The signal is then converted to an appropriate readout.

Applications of Reflectance Spectrophotometry

This technology is used in bedside or point-of-care testing (POCT) with smaller handheld instruments; it is also used for home testing. Common POCT and self-testing instruments include those for quantitation of blood glucose (employing single-test methodology) in maintaining good diabetic control. Chemistry and therapeutic drug-monitoring analyzer systems also employ this technology (e.g., Vitros). In urinalysis testing, various instruments use dry reagent reflectance spectrophotometry.

Fluorescence Spectrophotometry

On receiving ultraviolet (UV) radiation, the electrons of some substances absorb the radiation and become excited. After about 7 to 10 seconds, when the electron has returned to its ground state, this energy is given up as a photon of light. Fluorescent light is the result of the absorbance of a photon of radiant energy by a molecule. Once the photon is absorbed by the molecule, the molecule has an increased level of energy. It will seek to eject this excess energy because the energy of the molecule is greater than the energy of its environment. When this excess energy is ejected as a photon, the result is fluorescence emission. Generally, this emitted light is in the visible part of the spectrum.

The intensity of the fluorescence is determined by using a *fluorometer*, sometimes called a *spectrofluorometer* or *fluorescence spectrophotometer*. This measurement is governed by the same factors that affect the absorption of light (i.e., light path through the solution, concentration of the solution, wavelength of light being used) and also by the intensity of the UV exciting light. Only a few compounds can fluoresce, and of those that do, not all photons absorbed will be converted to fluorescent light. The list of fluorochromes is constantly

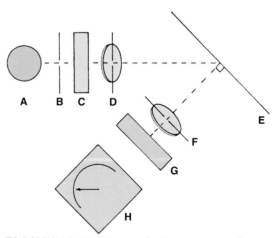

FIGURE 6-8 Diagram of reflectance spectrophotometer. A, Light source; B, slit; C, filter or wavelength selector; D, lens or slit; E, test surface; F, lens or slit; G, detector/photodetector device; H, readout device. (From Kaplan LA, Pesce AJ: Clinical chemistry: theory, analysis, correlation, ed 5, St Louis, 2010, Mosby.)

changing, but common fluorochromes are fluorescein isothiocyanate (FITC, green) and phycoerythrin (PE, red).

NEPHELOMETRY

Light can be absorbed, reflected, scattered, or transmitted when it strikes a particle in a liquid. **Nephelometry** is the measurement of light that has been scattered. **Turbidimetry** is the measurement of loss of intensity of light transmitted through a solution as a result of the light being scattered (the solution becomes turbid). Turbidimetry will measure light that is scattered, not absorbed or reflected by the particles in the suspension. Nephelometers are used to detect the amount of light scattered.

Nephelometry has become increasingly popular in diagnostic laboratories and depends on the light-scattering properties of antigen-antibody complexes (Fig. 6-9). The quantity of cloudiness or turbidity in a solution can be measured photometrically. When specific antigen-coated latex particles acting as reaction intensifiers are agglutinated by their corresponding antibody, the increased light scatter of a solution can be measured by nephelometry as the macromolecular complexes form. The use of polyethylene glycol (PEG) enhances and stabilizes the precipitates, thus increasing the speed and sensitivity of the technique by controlling the particle size for optimal light angle deflection. The kinetics of this change can be determined when the photometric results are analyzed by computer.

Principles of Use

Formation of a macromolecular complex is a fundamental prerequisite for nephelometric protein quantitation. The procedure is based on the reaction between the protein being assayed and a specific antiserum. Protein in a patient specimen reacts with specific nephelometric antisera to human proteins and forms insoluble complexes. When light is passed through such a suspension, the resulting complexes of insoluble precipitants scatter incident light in solutions. The scattered light can be detected with a photodiode. The amount of scattered light is proportional to the number of insoluble complexes and can be quantitated by comparing the unknown patient values with standards of known protein concentration.

The relationship between the quantity of antigen and the measuring signal at a constant

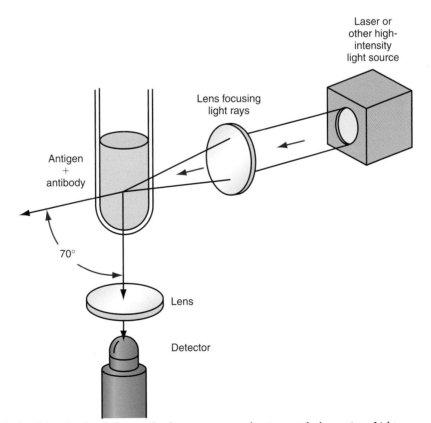

FIGURE 6-9 Principle of nephelometry for the measurement of antigen-antibody reactions. Light rays are collected in a focusing lens and can ultimately be related to the antigen or antibody concentration in a sample. (From Turgeon ML: Immunology and serology in laboratory medicine, ed 4, St Louis, 2009, Mosby.)

antibody concentration is given by the Heidelberger curve. If antibodies are present in excess, a proportional relationship exists between the antigen and the resulting signal. If the antigen overwhelms the quantity of antibody, the measured signal decreases.

By optimizing the reaction conditions, the typical antigen-antibody reactions as characterized by the Heidelberger curve are effectively shifted in the direction of high concentration. This ensures that these high concentrations will be measured on the ascending portion of the curve. At concentrations higher than the reference curve, the instrument will transmit an out-of-range warning.

Optical System and Measurement

In the nephelometric method, an infrared high-performance light-emitting diode (LED) is used as the light source. Because an entire solid angle is measured after convergence of this light through a lens system, an intense measuring signal is available when the primary beam is blocked off. In connection with the lens system, this produces a light beam of high colinearity. The wavelength is 840 nm. Light scattered in the forward direction in a solid angle to the primary beam ranges between 13 and 24 feet and is measured by a silicon photodiode with an integrated amplifier. The electrical signals generated are digitized, compared with reference curves, and converted into protein concentrations.

A fixed-time method of measurement is used routinely for precipitation reactions. Ten seconds after all reaction components have been mixed, an initial blank measurement with a cuvette is taken. Six minutes later a second measurement is taken, and after subtraction of the original 1-second blanking value, a final answer is calculated against the multiple-point or single-point calibration in the computerized program memory for the assay.

Advantages and Disadvantages

Nephelometry represents an automated system that is rapid, reproducible, relatively simple to operate, and very common in higher-volume laboratories. It has many applications in the immunology laboratory. Currently, instruments using a rate method and fixed-time approach are commercially available, with tests including C-reactive protein and rheumatoid factor.

Disadvantages include high initial equipment cost. Interfering substances such as microbial contamination may cause protein denaturation and erroneous test results. Intrinsic specimen turbidity or lipemia may exceed the preset limits. In these cases, a clearing agent may be needed before an accurate assay can be performed.

FLOW (CELL) CYTOMETRY
Fundamentals of Laser Technology

In 1917, Einstein speculated that under certain conditions, atoms or molecules could absorb light or other radiation and then be stimulated to shed this gained energy. Since then, lasers have been developed with numerous medical and industrial applications.

The electromagnetic spectrum ranges from long radio waves to short, powerful gamma rays. Within this spectrum is a narrow band of visible or white light, composed of red, orange, yellow, green, blue, and violet light. **Laser** (*light amplification by stimulated emission of radiation*) light ranges from the ultraviolet and infrared spectrum through all the colors of the rainbow. In contrast to other diffuse forms of radiation, laser light is concentrated. It is almost exclusively of one wavelength or color, and its parallel waves travel in one direction. Through the use of fluorescent dyes (e.g., FITC, green), laser light can occur in numerous wavelengths. Types of lasers include glass-filled tubes of helium and neon (most common); YAG (yttrium-aluminum-garnet, an imitation diamond), argon, and krypton.

Lasers sort the energy in atoms and molecules, concentrate it, and release it in powerful waves. In most lasers, a medium of gas, liquid, or crystal is energized by high-intensity light, an electrical discharge, or even nuclear radiation. When an atom extends beyond the orbits of its electrons, or when a molecule vibrates or changes its shape, it instantly snaps back, shedding energy in the form of a photon. The photon is the basic unit of all radiation. When a photon reaches an atom of the medium, the energy exchange stimulates the emission of another photon in the same wavelength and direction. This process continues until a cascade of growing energy sweeps through the medium.

Photons travel the length of the laser and bounce off mirrors. First a few and eventually countless photons synchronize themselves until an avalanche of light streaks between the mirrors. In some gas lasers, transparent disks (Brewster windows) are slanted at a precise angle that polarizes the laser's light. The photons, which are reflected back and forth, finally gain so much energy they exit as a powerful beam. The power of lasers to pass on energy and information is rated in watts.

Principles of Flow Cytometry

Flow cytometry is based on staining cells in suspension with an appropriate fluorochrome, which may be an immunologic reagent, a dye that stains a specific component, or some other marker with specified reactivity. Fluorescent dyes used in flow cytometry must bind or react specifically with the cellular component of interest, such as reticulocytes, peroxidase enzyme, or DNA content. Fluorescent dyes include acridine orange and PE.

Laser light is the most common light source used in flow cytometers because of its properties of intensity, stability, and monochromaticity. Argon is preferred for FITC labeling. Krypton is often used as a second laser in dual-analysis systems and serves as a better light source for compounds labeled by tetramethylrhodamine isothiocyanate (TRITC) and tetramethylcyclopropylrhodamine isothiocyanate (XRITC).

The stained cells then pass through the laser beam in single file. The laser activates the dye, and the cell fluoresces. Although the fluorescence is emitted throughout a 360-degree circle, it is usually collected by optical sensors located 90 degrees relative to the laser beam. The fluorescence information is then transmitted to a computer. Flow cytometry performs fluorescence analysis on single cells at the general rate of 500 to 5000 cells per second.

Fig. 6-10 illustrates the parts of the laser flow cytometer. The computer is the heart of the instrument; it controls all decisions regarding data collection, analysis, and cell sorting. The major applications of this technology are that cells can be sorted from the main cellular population into subpopulations for further analysis, such as T lymphocytes and B lymphocytes.

IMMUNOFLUORESCENT LABELING TECHNIQUES

The original technique of using antigen-coated cells or particles in agglutination techniques may be considered the earliest method for labeling components in immunoassays. The applications of labels in enzyme immunoassays, chemiluminescence, and fluorescent substances (Table 6-2) are presented in this chapter. Ideal characteristics of a label include the quality of being measurable by several methods, including visual inspection. The properties of a label used in an immunoassay determine the ways in which detection is possible. For example, coated latex particles can be detected by various methods: visual inspection, light scattering (nephelometry), and particle counting. The conversion of a colorless substrate into a colored product in enzyme immunoassay allows for two methods of detection, colorimetry and visual inspection.

The radioimmunoassay (RIA) method—use of a radioactive label that could identify an immunocomponent at very low concentrations—was developed by Yalow and Berson in 1959. In the 1960s, researchers began to search for a substitute for the successful RIA method because of the inherent drawbacks of using radioactive isotopes as labels (e.g., radioactive waste and short shelf life). Today, chemiluminescent reactions have replaced most RIAs in the clinical laboratory. This relatively simple, cost-effective technology has sensitivity at least as good as that of RIA without the problems (e.g., disposal of radioactive waste).

Immunoassays

Immunoassays utilize antigen-antibody reactions. When foreign material (called *antigens* or *immunogens*) is introduced into the body, protein molecules (called *antibodies*) are formed in response. For example, certain bacteria, when introduced into the body, elicit the production of specific

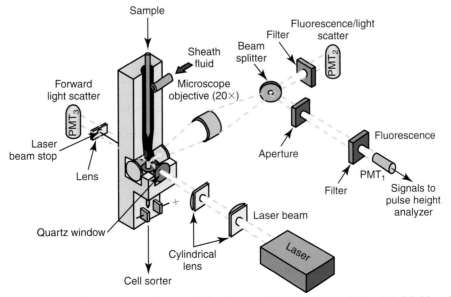

FIGURE 6-10 **Laser-flow cytometry.** (Courtesy Ortho Diagnostic Systems, Westwood, Mass.) Modified from Burtis CA, Ashwood ER, Bruns DE: Tietz fundamentals of clinical chemistry, ed 6, St Louis, 2008, Saunders.

Examples of Immunoassay Types		
Type of Immunoassay	Antibody	Comments
Enzyme Immunoassay	Enzyme-labeled antibody e.g. horseradish peroxidase	Competitive EIA Non-competitive, such as direct EIA, indirect ELISA
Chemiluminescence	Chemiluminescent molecule-labeled antibody, such as isoluminol- or acridinium ester– labeled antibodies	
Electrochemiluminescence immunoassay	Electrochemiluminescent molecule-labeled antibody, such as ruthenium-labeled antibodies	
Fluoroimmunoassay	Fluorescent molecule-labeled antibody, such as europium-labeled antibodies or fluorescein-labeled antigens	Heterogeneous, such as time-resolved immunofluoroassay, or homogeneous, such as fluorescence polarization immunoassay

antibodies. These antibodies combine specifically with the substance that stimulated the body to produce them initially, producing an *antigen-antibody complex*. In the laboratory, an antigen may be used as a reagent to detect the presence of antibodies in the serum of a patient. If the antibody is present, it shows that the person's body has responded previously to that specific antigen. This response can be elicited by exposure to a specific microorganism or by the presence of a drug or medication in the patient's serum. Antigens and antibodies are used as very specific reagents. In the clinical chemistry laboratory, antibodies are used to detect and measure an antigen (e.g., drug, medication) present in the patient's serum.

Immunoassays can be divided into heterogeneous and homogeneous immunoassays.

- Heterogeneous immunoassays involve a solid phase (microwell, bead) and require washing steps to remove unbound antigens or antibodies. Heterogeneous immunoassays can have a competitive or noncompetitive format.
- Homogeneous immunoassays consist of only a liquid phase and do not require washing steps. Homogeneous immunoassays are faster and easier to automate than heterogeneous immunoassays and have competitive formats.

Enzyme Immunoassay

There are two general approaches to diagnosing diseases or conditions by immunoassay: testing for specific antigens or testing for antigen-specific antibodies. Some enzyme immunoassay (EIA) procedures provide diagnostic information and measure antibodies to detect immune status (e.g., detect either total antibody IgM or IgG). Enzyme-linked immunosorbent assay (ELISA), a type of

EIA, is an assay designed to detect antigens or antibodies by producing an enzyme-triggered color change.

The EIA method uses a nonisotopic label, which has the advantage of safety. EIA is usually an objective measurement that provides numerical results (Fig. 6-11). It uses the catalytic properties of enzymes to detect and quantitate immunologic reactions. An enzyme-labeled antibody or enzyme-labeled antigen conjugate is used in immunologic assays (Box 6-1). The enzyme with its substrate detects the presence and quantity of antigen or antibody in a patient specimen. In some tissues, an enzyme-labeled antibody can identify antigenic locations.

Various enzymes are used in enzyme immunoassay (see Table 6-2). Commonly used enzyme labels are horseradish peroxidase, alkaline phosphatase, glucose-6-phosphate dehydrogenase, and beta-galactosidase. To be used in EIA, an enzyme must fulfill a number of criteria, including:

- A high amount of stability
- Extreme specificity
- Absence from the antigen or antibody
- No alteration by inhibitor with the system

EIAS FOR ANTIGEN DETECTION

EIAs for antigen detection (e.g., hepatitis B surface antigen) have four steps.

(1) Antigen-specific antibody is attached to a solid-phase surface such as plastic beads,

(2) patient serum that may potentially contain the antigen is added.

(3) An enzyme-labeled antibody specific to the antigen (conjugate) is added next, and

(4) followed by chromogenic substrate, which in the presence of the enzyme changes color. The amount of color that develops is proportional to the amount of antigen in the patient specimen.

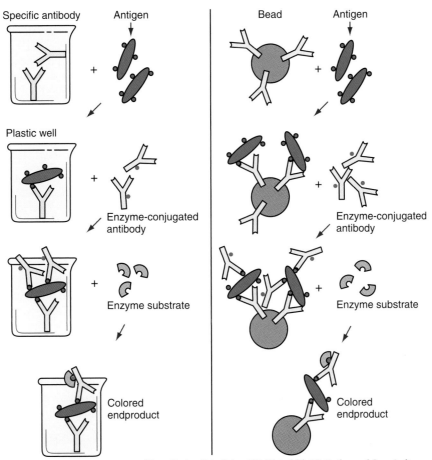

FIGURE 6-11   **Enzyme immunoassay.** (From Forbes BA, Sahm DF, Weissfeld AS: Bailey and Scott's diagnostic microbiology, ed 12, St Louis, 2007, Mosby.)

EIAs FOR ANTIBODY DETECTION

Two major types of reaction formats are used in immunochemical assays:

- Competitive (limited reagent assays)
- Noncompetitive (excess reagent, two-site, and sandwich assays)

In a *competitive* assay, all reactants are added and mixed together either simultaneously or sequentially. In a simultaneous situation, the labeled antigen and unlabeled antigen compete to bind with antibody. In a *sequential* competitive reaction, unlabeled antigen is mixed with excess antibody and binding is allowed to reach equilibrium. Labeled antigen is then added sequentially and allowed to equilibrate. After separation, the bound label is measured and used to calculated the unlabeled antigen concentration.

In *noncompetitive* assays, polyclonal or monoclonal antibides are used. These assays are performed in either simultaneous or sequentiala modes. If a simultaneous mode is used, a high concentration of analyte saturates both the capture and labeled antibodies. To avoid problems associated with high concentrations of antibody, e.g., chorionic

gonadotropin (CG), a sequential procedure is used. In a typical *noncompetitive* assay, the *capture* antibody is initially passively adsorbed or covalently bound to the surface of a solid phase. Then, the antigen from the specimen is allowed to react and is captured by the solid-phase antibody. Other proteins then are washed away, and a labeled antibody (conjugate) is added that reacts with the bound antigen through a second and distinct antigen site, epitope. After additional washings to remove the excess unbound labeled antibody, the bound label is measured, and its concentration or activity is directly proportional to the concentration of antigen.

Immunofluorescent Techniques

Fluorescent labeling is another method of demonstrating the complexing of antigens and antibodies. Fluorescent techniques are extremely specific and sensitive. Antibodies may be conjugated to other markers in addition to fluorescent dyes; the use of these markers is called *colorimetric immunologic probe detection*. The use of enzyme-substrate marker systems has been expanded, and horseradish peroxidase can be used as a visual tag for the presence of antibody. These reagents have the advantage of requiring only a standard light microscope for analysis.

Fluorescent conjugates are used in the following basic methods:

1. Direct immunofluorescent assay
2. Inhibition immunofluorescent assay
3. Indirect immunofluorescent assay

Direct Immunofluorescent Assay

In the direct technique, a conjugated antibody is used to detect antigen-antibody reactions at a microscopic level (Fig. 6-12, A). This technique can be applied to tissue sections or smears for microorganisms. Direct immunofluorescent assay can be used to detect nucleic acids in organisms such as cytomegalovirus (CMV), hepatitis B virus (HBV), Epstein-Barr virus (EBV), and *Chlamydia*.

When absorbing light of one wavelength, a fluorescent substance emits light of another (longer) wavelength. In fluorescent antibody microscopy (see Chapter 5), the incident or exciting light is often blue-green to ultraviolet. The light is provided by a high-pressure mercury arc lamp with a primary (e.g., blue-violet) filter between the lamp and the object that passes only fluorescein-exciting wavelengths. The color of the emitted light depends on the nature of the substance. Fluorescein gives off yellow-green light, and the rhodamines fluoresce in the red portion of the spectrum. The color observed in the fluorescent microscope depends on the secondary or barrier filter used in the eyepiece. A yellow filter absorbs the green fluorescence of fluorescein and transmits only yellow. Fluorescein fluoresces an intense apple-green color when excited.

Inhibition Immunofluorescent Assay

The inhibition immunofluorescent assay is a blocking test in which an antigen is first exposed to unlabeled antibody, then to labeled antibody, and is finally washed and examined. If the unlabeled and labeled antibodies are both homologous to the antigen, there should be no fluorescence. This result confirms the specificity of the fluorescent antibody technique. Antibody in an unknown serum can also be detected and identified by the inhibition test.

Indirect Immunofluorescent Assay

The indirect method is based on the fact that antibodies (immunoglobulins) not only react with homologous antigens but also can act as antigens and react with antiimmunoglobulins (see Fig. 6-12, B). The serologic method most widely used for the detection of diverse antibodies is the indirect fluorescent antibody assay (IFA). Immunofluorescence is used extensively in the detection of autoantibodies and antibodies to tissue and cellular antigens. For example, antinuclear antibodies (ANAs) are frequently assayed by indirect fluorescence. By using tissue sections that contain a large number of antigens, it is possible to identify antibodies to several different antigens in a single test. The antigens are differentiated according to their different staining patterns.

Immunofluorescence can also be used to identify specific antigens on live cells in suspension (i.e., flow cytometry). When a live stained-cell suspension is put through a fluorescent active-cell sorter (FACS), which measures its fluorescent intensity, the cells are separated according to their particular fluorescent brightness. This technique permits isolation of different cell populations with different surface antigens (e.g., CD4+ and CD8+ lymphocytes).

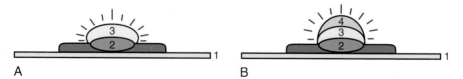

FIGURE 6-12 Principles of direct and indirect fluorescent techniques. **A,** Direct fluorescence. **B,** Indirect fluorescence. **1,** microscopic slide; **2,** cell (cytoplasm and nucleus); **3,** antiserum, conjugate in A and unconjugated in B; **4,** conjugated antiglobulin serum. (From Turgeon ML: Immunology and serology in laboratory medicine, ed 4, St Louis, 2009, Mosby.)

In the indirect immunofluorescent assay, the antigen source (e.g., whole *Toxoplasma* microorganism or virus in infected tissue culture cells) to the specific antibody being tested is affixed to the surface of a microscope slide. The patient's serum is diluted and placed on the slide to cover the antigen source. If antibody is present in the serum, it will bind to its specific antigen. Unbound antibody is then removed by washing the slide. In the second phase of the procedure, antihuman globulin (directed specifically against IgM or IgG) conjugated to a fluorescent substance that will fluoresce when exposed to UV light is placed on the slide. This conjugated marker for human antibody will bind to the antibody already bound to the antigen on the slide and serve as a marker for the antibody when viewed under a fluorescent microscope.

Time-Resolved Fluoroimmunoassay

Time-resolved assay means that the measurement of fluorescence should occur after a certain time frame in order to exclude background interference fluorescence. This form of immunoassay is heterogeneous with a direct format (sandwich assay) similar to direct ELISA.

Fluorescence Polarization Immunoassay

This immunoassay method is a homogeneous competitive fluoroimmunoassay. The polarization of the fluorescence from a fluorescein-antigen conjugate is determined by its rate of rotation during the lifetime of the excited state in solution.

Fluorescence In Situ Hybridization

Fluorescence in situ hybridization (FISH) uses fluorescent molecules to brightly paint genes or chromosomes. FISH is a molecular cytogenetic technique that uses recombinant DNA technology. Probes, short sequences of single-stranded DNA that are complementary to the DNA sequences being examined, hybridize (bind) to the complementary DNA; because of the labeled fluorescent tags, the location of those sequences can be seen. Probes can be locus specific, centromeric repeat probes, or whole chromosome probes. This protocol has potentially broad applications for clinical immunoassays and DNA hybridization analysis.

New Labeling Technologies

QUANTUM DOTS (Q DOTS)

One example of an advanced labeling technique is quantum dots (Q dots). Q dots are semiconductor nanocrystals used as fluorescent labeling reagents for biological imaging. A valuable property of Q dots is that different sizes of crystals produce different signals with a single laser excitation. Q dots are just the next step in the evolution of luminescence-based assays.

SQUID TECHNOLOGY

A novel method of target labeling is to tag antibodies with superparamagnetic particles, allow the tagged antibodies to bind with the target antigen, and use a superconducting quantum interference device (SQUID) to detect the tagged antigen-antibody complex. A current application of this technology is its use in the detection of *Listeria monocytogenes*.

LUMINESCENT OXYGEN CHANNELING IMMUNOASSAY

This novel detection technology is based on two different 200-nm latex particles: a sensitizer particle that absorbs energy at 680 nm with generation of singlet oxygen (the donor bead), and a chemiluminescer molecule that shifts the emission wavelength to 570 nm (the receptor bead). When these particles are in close proximity during excitation, singlet oxygen moves from the donor bead to the receptor bead, where it triggers the generation of a luminescent signal. Luminescent oxygen channeling immunoassay (LOCI) technology is broadly applicable to any molecule that can be determined in a binding assay.

SIGNAL AMPLIFICATION TECHNOLOGY

Tyramide signal amplification (TSA) may be used in a wide variety of both fluorescent and colorimetric detection applications. The technique's protocols are simple and require very few changes to standard operating procedures.

MAGNETIC LABELING TECHNOLOGY

Magnetic labeling technology is an application of the high-resolution magnetic recording technology already developed for the computer disk drive industry. Increased density of microscopic magnetically labeled biological samples (e.g., nucleic acid on a biochip) translates directly into reduced sample processing times. Magnetic labeling can be applied to automated DNA sequences, DNA probe technology, and gel scanners/electrophoresis.

Chemiluminescence

Chemiluminescence is the emission of light by molecules in on excited state with a limited amount of emitted heat (luminescence) as the result of a chemical reaction. Chemilumirescent assays are ultrasensitive and are widely used in automated immunoassays and DNA probe assay systems. Most immunodiagnostic manufacturers are pursuing chemiluminescence as the technology of choice. Chemiluminescence has excellent sensitivity and dynamic range. It does not require sample radiation, and nonselective excitation and source instability are eliminated. Most chemiluminescent reagents and conjugates are stable and relatively nontoxic.

In immunoassays, chemiluminescent labels can be attached to an antigen or an antibody. Chemiluminescent labels are being used to detect proteins, viruses, oligonucleotides, and genomic nucleic acid sequences in immunoassays, DNA probe assays, DNA sequencing, and electrophoresis. Two immunoassay formats are used: competitive and sandwich.

Current Trends in Immunoassay Automation

Technical advances in methodologies, robotics, and computerization have led to expanded immunoassay automation. Newer systems are using chemiluminescent labels and substrates rather than older fluorescent labels and detection systems. Immunoassay systems have the potential to improve turnaround time with enhanced cost-effectiveness (Box 6-2).

MOLECULAR TECHNIQUES

Molecular testing is one of the fastest-growing diagnostic disciplines in the clinical laboratory. Since the complete human genome (sequence) became available in 2003, molecular testing has been expanded extensively.

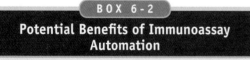

BOX 6-2

Potential Benefits of Immunoassay Automation

Ability to provide better service with less staff
Savings on controls, duplicates, dilutions, and repeats
Elimination of radioactive labels and associated regulations
Better shelf life of reagents, with less disposal caused by outdating
Better sample identification with bar code labels and primary tube sampling
Automation of sample delivery possible

Modified from Blick KE: Current trends in automation of immunoassays, J Clin Ligand Assay 22:6–12, 1999.

Amplification Techniques in Molecular Biology

Polymerase Chain Reaction

PCR is an in vitro method that amplifies low levels of specific DNA sequences in a sample to higher quantities suitable for further analysis (Fig. 6-13). To use this technology, the target sequence to be amplified must be known. Typically, a target sequence ranges from 100 to 1000 base pairs in length. Two short DNA "primers" that are typically 16 to 20 base pairs in length are used. Namely, the oligonucleotides (small portions of a single DNA strand) act as a template for the new DNA. These primer sequences are complementary to the 3′ ends of the sequence to be amplified.

This enzymatic process is carried out in cycles. Each repeated cycle consists of:
- DNA denaturation—separation of the double DNA strands into two single strands through the use of heat.
- Primer annealing—recombination of the oligonucleotide primers with the single-stranded original DNA.
- Extension of the primed DNA sequence—the enzyme DNA polymerase synthesizes new complementary strands by the extension of primers.

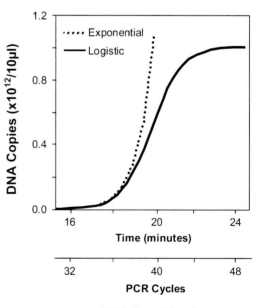

DNA Amplification

FIGURE 6-13 **Exponential and logistic curves for DNA amplified by PCR.** (Modified with permission of the publisher from Wittwer CT, Kusukawa N: Real-time PCR. In Persing DH, Tenover FC, Versalovic J, et al (eds), Molecular microbiology: diagnostic principles and practice, Washington, DC, 2004, ASM Press, pp 71–84, © 2004 ASM Press.)

Each cycle theoretically doubles the amount of specific DNA sequence present and results in an exponential accumulation of the DNA fragment being amplified (amplicons). In general, this process is repeated approximately 30 times. At the end of 30 cycles, the reaction mixture should contain about 2^{30} molecules of the desired product. After cycling is completed, the amplification products can be examined in various ways. Typically the contents of the reaction vessel are subjected to gel electrophoresis. This allows visualization of the amplified genwe segments (e.g., PCR products, bands) and a determination of their specificity. Additional product analysis by probe hybridization or direct DNA sequencing is often performed to further verify the authenticity of the amplicon.

The three important applications of PCR are:
1. Amplification of DNA
2. Identification of a target sequence
3. Synthesis of a labeled antisense probe

Adaptations of the PCR technique have been developed. One adaptation uses nested primers and a two-step amplification process. Polymerase chain reaction modifications include reverse transcriptase PCR, multiplex, and real-time PCR. Other amplification techniques are:

- Strand displacement amplification (SDA), a fully automated method that amplifies target nucleic acid without the use of a thermocycler. A double-strand DNA fragment is created and becomes the target for exponential amplification.
- Transcription-mediated amplification (TMA), another isothermal assay that targets either DNA or RNA but generates RNA as its amplified product. This method is currently being used to detect microorganisms (e.g., *Mycobacterium tuberculosis*).
- Nucleic acid sequence–based amplification (NASBA), which is similar to TMA, but only RNA is targeted for amplification. Applications of this technique are detection and quantitation of HIV and detection of CMV.
- Ligase chain reaction (LCR) nucleic acid amplification. Oligonucleotide pairs hybridize to target sequences within the gene or the cryptic plasmid. The bound oligonucleotides are separated by a small gap at the target site. The enzyme DNA polymerase uses nucleotides in the LCR nucleic acid amplification reaction mixture to fill in this gap, creating a ligatable junction. Once the gap is filled, DNA ligase joins the oligonucleotide pairs to form a short, single-stranded product that is complementary to the original target sequence. This product can itself serve as a target for hybridization and ligation of

a second pair of oligonucleotides present in the LCR reaction mixture. Subsequent rounds of denaturation and ligation lead to the geometric accumulation of amplification product. The amplified products are detected by microparticle enzyme immunoassay.

Analysis of Amplification Products

Many of the revolutionary changes that have occurred in research in the biological sciences, particularly the Human Genome Project, can be directly attributed to the ability to manipulate DNA in defined ways. Molecular genetic testing focuses on examination of nucleic acids (DNA or RNA) by special techniques to determine if a specific nucleotide base sequence is present. Nucleic acid testing has expanded, despite higher costs associated with testing, in various areas of the clinical laboratory. Clinical applications include genetic testing, hematopathology diagnosis and monitoring, and identification of infectious agents. The distinct advantages of molecular testing include:

- Faster turnaround time
- Smaller required sample volumes
- Increased specificity and sensitivity

Conventional Analysis

Detection of DNA products that result from PCR can be conventionally analyzed using **agarose gel electrophoresis** after ethidium bromide staining. This simple-to-perform technique is simply an extra step after a PCR assay has been run.

Other Techniques

Other techniques are used to enhance both the sensitivity and specificity of amplification techniques. Probe-based DNA detection systems have the advantage of providing sequence specificity and decreased detection limits. Other techniques include hybridization protection assay, DNA enzyme immunoassay, automated DNA sequencing technology, single-strand conformational polymorphisms, and restriction fragment length polymorphism (RFLP) analysis. The selection of one technique over another is often based on a variety of factors (e.g., sensitivity and specificity profiles, cost, turnaround time, and local experience).

DNA SEQUENCING

DNA sequencing is considered to be the gold-standard method by which other molecular methods are compared. DNA sequencing displays the exact nucleotide or base sequence of a targeted fragment of DNA. The Sanger method, which uses a series of enzymatic reactions to produce segments of DNA complementary to the DNA being sequenced, is the most frequently used method for DNA sequencing. Automated sequencing techniques use primers with four different fluorescent labels.

1. The first step to sequencing a target is to amplify it in some way, either by cloning or in vitro amplification—usually PCR. Once the amplified DNA is purified from the clinical specimen (the target DNA), it is heat denatured to separate the double-stranded DNA (dsDNA) into single-strand DNA (ssDNA).

2. The second step involves adding primers, short synthetic segments of ssDNA that contain a nucleotide sequence complementary to a short sequence of the target DNA, to the ssDNA. The patient's DNA serves as a template to copy. DNA polymerase catalyzes the addition of the appropriate nucleotides to the preexisting primer. DNA synthesis is terminated when the deoxynucleotide is embodied into a growing DNA chain.

HYBRIDIZATION TECHNIQUES

Probe-hybridization assays involving the complementary pairing of a probe with a DNA or RNA strand derived from the patient specimen exist in many forms. The common feature of probe hybridization assays is the use of a labeled nucleic acid probe to examine a specimen for a specific homologous DNA or RNA sequence. The clinical probes are most often labeled with nonradioisotopic molecules such as digoxigenin, alkaline phosphatase, biotin, or a fluorescent compound. The detection systems are conjugate dependent and include chemiluminescent, fluorescent, and calorimetric methodologies.

Blotting Protocols

The Southern blot and Northern blot are used to detect DNA and RNA, respectively. These procedures share some common procedural steps: electrophoretic separation of patient's nucleic acid, transfer of nucleic acid fragments to a solid support (e.g., nitrocellulose, hybridization with a labeled probe of known nucleic acid sequence), and autoradiographic or colorimetric detection of the bands created by the probe–nucleic acid hybrid.

Southern Blot

In the Southern blot procedure, specimen DNA is denatured and treated with restriction enzymes to result in DNA fragments; the ssDNA fragments are then separated by electrophoresis (Fig. 6-14). The electrophoretically separated fragments are then blotted to a nitrocellulose membrane, retaining their electrophoretic position and hybridized with radiolabeled ssDNA fragments with sequences complementary to those being sought. The resulting dsDNA bearing the radiolabel is then, if present, detected by radiography.

The Southern blot procedure has clinical diagnostic applications for diseases/disorders associated

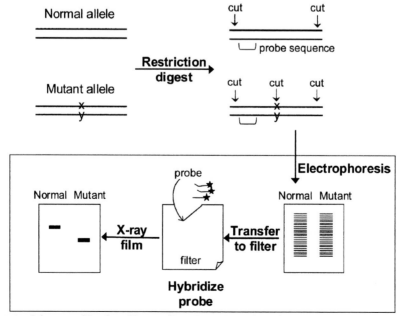

FIGURE 6-14 Schematic of Southern blotting. (From Burtis CA, Ashwood ER, Bruns DE: Tietz textbook of clinical chemistry and molecular diagnostics, ed 4, Philadelphia, 2006, Saunders.)

with significant changes in DNA, a deletion or insertion of at least 50 to 100 base pairs (e.g., fragile X syndrome or determination of clonality in lymphomas of T- or B-cell origin). If a single-base mutation changes an enzyme restriction site on the DNA, resulting in an altered band or fragment size, the Southern blot procedure can be used to detect these changes in DNA sequences (referred to as *restriction fragment length polymorphisms*). Single-base mutations that can be determined by Southern blot include sickle cell anemia and hemophilia A.

Northern Blot

Messenger RNA (mRNA) from the specimen is separated by electrophoresis and blotted to a specially modified paper support to result in covalent fixing of the mRNA in the electrophoretic positions. Radiolabeled ssDNA fragments complementary to the specific mRNA being sought are then hybridized to the bound mRNA. If the specific mRNA is present, the radioactivity is detected by autoradiography. The derivation of this technique from the Southern blot used for DNA detection has led to the common usage of the term *Northern blot* for the detection of specific mRNA. The Northern blot is not routinely used in clinical molecular diagnostics.

Western Blot

In comparison to the Southern blot, which separates and identifies RNA fragments and proteins, and the Northern blot, which concentrates on isolating m-RNA, Western blot is a technique in which proteins are separated electrophoretically, transferred to membranes, and identified through the use of labeled antibodies specific for the protein of interest. The Western blot technique is used to detect antibodies to specific epitopes of electrophoretically separated subspecies of antigens. It is a technique in which electrophoresis of antigenic material yields separation of the antigenic components by molecular weight. Blotting the separated antigen to nitrocellulose, retaining the electrophoretic position, and causing it to react with patient specimen will result in the binding of specific antibodies, if present, to each antigenic "band." Electrophoresis of known molecular weight standards allows for determining the molecular weight of each antigenic band to which antibodies may be produced. These antibodies are then detected using EIA reactions that characterize antibody specificity. This technique is often used to confirm the specificity of antibodies detected by ELISA screening procedures.

Microarrays

Microarray (DNA chip) technology has catapulted into the limelight, promising to accelerate genetic analysis in much the same way that microprocessors have sped up computation. Microarrays are basically the product of bonding or direct synthesis of numerous specific DNA probes on a stationary, often silicon-based support. The chip may be tailored to particular disease processes. It is easily performed and readily automated. Microarrays are miniature gene fragments attached to glass chips. These chips are used to examine gene activity of thousands or tens of thousands of gene fragments and to identify genetic mutations, using a hybridization reaction between the sequences on the microarray and a fluorescent sample. After hybridization, the chips are scanned with high-speed fluorescent detectors, and the intensity of each spot is quantitated. The identity and amount of each sequence are revealed by the location and intensity of fluorescence displayed by each spot. Computers are used to analyze the data.

The applications of microarrays in clinical medicine include analysis of gene expression in malignancies (e.g., mutations in *BRCA1*, mutations of the tumor-suppressor gene p53, genetic disease testing, and viral resistance mutation detection).

ELECTROCHEMICAL METHODS

When chemical energy is converted to an electrical current (a flow of electrons) in a galvanic cell, the term **electrochemistry** is used. Electrochemical reactions are characterized by a loss of electrons (oxidation) at the positive pole (*anode*) and a simultaneous gain of electrons (reduction) at the negative pole (*cathode*). The galvanic cell is made up of two parts called *half-cells*, each containing a metal in a solution of one of its salts. These methods involve the measurement of electrical signals associated with chemical systems that are within an electrochemical cell.

Electroanalytical chemistry uses electrochemistry for analysis purposes. In the clinical laboratory, electroanalytical methods are used to measure ions, drugs, hormones, metals, and gases. Methods are available for the rapid analysis of analytes present in relatively high concentrations in blood and urine, such as blood electrolytes (Na^+, K^+, Cl, HCO_3^-), and other analytes present in very low concentrations, such as heavy metals and drug metabolites. There are three general electrochemical techniques used in the clinical laboratory: potentiometric, voltammetric, and coulometric. This section discusses the electrochemical methods of potentiometry, coulometry, and electrophoresis.

Potentiometry

Potentiometry measures the potential of an electrode compared with the potential of another electrode. The method is based on the measurement of a voltage potential difference between two electrodes immersed in a solution under zero-current conditions. This difference in voltage between the two electrodes is usually measured on a pH or voltage meter. One electrode is called the *indicator electrode*; the other is the *reference electrode*. The reference electrode is an electrochemical half-cell that is used as a fixed reference for the cell potential measurements. One of the most common reference electrodes used for potentiometry is the silver or silver chloride electrode. The indicator electrode is the main component of potentiometric techniques. It is important that the indicator electrode be able to respond selectively to analyte species. The most common indicator electrode used in clinical chemistry is the *ion-selective electrode* (ISE).

The use of ion-selective electrodes (ISEs) is based on the measurement of a potential that develops across a selective membrane. The electrochemical cell response is based on an interaction between the membrane and the analyte being measured that alters the potential across the membrane. The specificity of the membrane interaction for the analyte determines the selectivity of the potential response to an analyte.

Electrodes and Ionic Concentration

Potentiometric methods of analysis involve the direct measurement of electrical potential caused by the activity of free ions. ISEs are designed to be sensitive toward individual ions. An ISE universally used in the clinical laboratory is the pH electrode. Specialized probes such as ISEs can measure concentrations of ionic species other than hydrogen ions [H^+], including fluoride, chloride, ammonia, sodium, potassium, calcium, sulfide, and nitrate ions.

An *electrode* is an electronic conductor in contact with an ionic conductor, the *electrolyte*. Passive (inert) electrodes act as electron donors or electron acceptors; *active* (participating) electrodes act as ion donors or ion acceptors. The electrode reaction is an electrochemical process in which charge transfer takes place at the interface between the electrode and the electrolyte.

By means of its potential, an indicator electrode shows the activity of an ion in a solution. The relationship between the potential and the activity is given by the Nernst equation (see later). The potential between an electrode and a solution cannot be directly measured; a reference electrode is needed. The reference electrode should have a known, or at least a constant, potential value under the prevailing experimental conditions.

The most essential component of a pH electrode is a special sensitive glass membrane that permits the passage of hydrogen ions but no other ionic species. When the electrode is immersed in a test solution containing hydrogen ions, the external ions diffuse through the membrane until an equilibrium is reached between the external and internal concentrations. Thus there is a buildup of charge on the inside of the membrane that is proportional to the number of hydrogen ions in the external solution.

Because of the need for equilibrium conditions, there is very little current flow. Therefore, this potential difference between electrode and solution can only be measured relative to a separate and stable reference system that is also in contact with the test solution but is unaffected by it. A sensitive, high-impedance millivolt meter or digital measuring system must be used to measure this potential difference accurately.

In fact, the potential difference developed across the membrane is directly proportional to the logarithm of the ionic concentration in the external solution. To determine the pH of an unknown solution, it is only necessary to measure the potential difference in two standard solutions of known pH, construct a straight-line calibration graph by plotting millivolts versus pH = (log [H^+]), then read off the unknown pH from the measured voltage.

To measure the electrode potential developed at the ion-selective membrane, the ISE/pH electrode must be immersed in the test solution together with a separate reference system, and the two must be connected by a millivolt measuring system. At equilibrium, the electrons added or removed from the solution by the ISE membrane (depending on whether it is cation or anion sensitive) are balanced by an equal and opposite charge at the reference interface. This causes a positive or negative deviation from the original stable reference voltage that is registered on the external measuring system.

The relationship between the ionic concentration (activity) and the electrode potential is given by the Nernst equation, as follows:

$$E = E^0 + (2.303RT/nF) \times Log(A)$$

where:

E = Total potential (in mV) developed between the sensing and reference electrodes

E^0 = Constant that is characteristic of the particular ISE/reference pair (sum of all the liquid junction potentials in the electrochemical cell; see later)

2.303 = Conversion factor from natural to base-10 logarithm

R = Gas constant (8.314 joules/degree/mole)

T = Absolute temperature

n = Charge on the ion (with sign)

F = Faraday constant (96,500 coulombs)

Log(A) = Logarithm of the activity of the measured ion

Note that *2.303RT/nF* is the **slope** of the line (from the straight-line plot of E versus log[A], which is the basis of ISE calibration graphs). This is an important diagnostic characteristic of the electrode; generally the slope gets lower as the electrode gets old or contaminated, and the lower the slope, the higher the errors on the sample measurements.

For practical use in measuring pH, it is not normally necessary for the operator to construct a calibration graph and interpolate the results for unknown samples. Most pH electrodes are connected directly to a special pH meter, which performs the calibration automatically. This determines the slope mathematically and calculates the unknown pH value for immediate display on the meter.

These basic principles are exactly the same for all ISEs, so it would appear that all can be used as easily and rapidly as the pH electrode—simply by calibrating the equipment by measuring two known solutions, then immersing the electrodes in any test solution and reading the answer directly from a meter. Some other ions can be measured in this simple way, but this is not the case for most ions.

pH Electrodes and Meters

The pH measurement was originally used by the Danish biochemist Soren Sorensen to represent the hydrogen ion concentration, expressed in equivalents per liter, of an aqueous solution: pH = log[H$^+$]. In expressions of this type, enclosure of a chemical symbol within square brackets denotes that the concentration of the symbolized species is the quantity being considered.

The first commercially successful electronic pH meter was invented by Dr. Arnold Beckman in 1934. This instrument was the forerunner of modern electrochemical instrumentation and became an indispensable tool in analytical chemistry. Beginning in the 1950s, electrodes were also developed for other ions, such as F, Na$^+$, K$^+$, and Ag$^+$. The pH meter and ISE have now become indispensable scientific tools. Today, Beckman Coulter pH meters provide precise pH and concentration (ISE) measurements in handheld, bench-top, and high-performance meters for research, pharmaceutical, chemical, and environmental applications.

The term **pH** refers to the concentration of hydrogen ions ([H$^+$], also called protons) in a solution. For aqueous solutions, the scale ranges from 0 to 14, with pure water in the middle at 7. The more acid a solution is, the lower the pH reading (0-6.9), and alkaline solutions come in at the high end of the scale (7.1-14).

Paper test strips (e.g., urine dipsticks) are good for measuring approximate pH values, but chemical laboratories require more exact measurements. A pH meter is a boxy-looking instrument attached to a glass or plastic tube called a *probe*. Handheld pH meters have a probe directly attached to the instrument body. The probe has a glass bulb on one end and an electrical wire on the other. The wire sends data to the instrument when the glass bulb is dipped into a sample solution.

The pH meter measures H$^+$ concentration by sensing differences in the electric charges inside and outside the probe. The glass bulb is made from silica (SiO$_2$) that contains added metal ions. Most of the oxygen atoms in the glass are surrounded by silicon and metal atoms. However, the oxygen atoms on the inside and outside surfaces of the bulb are not completely surrounded, and they can "grab" positively charged ions from the solution. When the bulb is dipped into an acid solution, H$^+$ ions bond with the outside surface of the glass bulb, forming electrically neutral Si–OH groups. The Si–O– groups on the inside surface are in contact with a reference solution. The difference in electrical charge between the two surfaces creates an electrical potential, or voltage, and this causes an electric current to flow through the wire at the other end of the probe.

Alkaline solutions have low concentrations of H$^+$ ions and higher concentrations of negative ions such as OH. The excess negative charges are balanced with positively charged metal ions such as Na$^+$, and these positive ions hover close to the surface of the bulb rather than binding to the Si–O– groups. This sets up a different sort of charge separation, and the resulting electrical signal registers a high pH.

Types of Meters

ANALOG METERS

The earliest type of pH meters were simple analog devices with a resolution of only 1 or 2 mV. The original meters were calibrated in millivolts, and the corresponding pH value was read from a calibration graph. Because pH electrodes are reasonably uniform and reproducible instruments, it was discovered that it is not necessary to have a unique calibration graph for each electrode. In this case, the meters can be calibrated directly in pH units by the manufacturer and can simply be recalibrated each time they are used (to compensate for temperature changes or slight differences in electrode response) by immersing the electrode in just one pH buffer solution and adjusting the meter output to give the correct reading. This type of meter is simple and quick to use and is perfectly adequate for many pH measurements because it requires a change of more than 5 mV to change the pH value by more than 0.1 pH units.

Simple precalibrated analog meters are not appropriate for ISE measurements.

DIGITAL METERS

A major advance was made when digital meters were introduced with a resolution of 0.1 or even 0.01 mV. This enabled the analyst to measure and read the voltage with much greater accuracy and meant that the stability and reproducibility of the electrode response became the main limiting factors in determining the accuracy and precision.

SELF-CALIBRATING, DIRECT-READING ION METERS

The next major advance occurred when microprocessors were introduced. These contained simple programs to calculate the slope and intercept from the calibration data, which were then used to calculate the sample concentration from the millivolt reading in the sample. The analyst can simply enter the concentrations of the standards and measure the millivolts, then immerse the electrodes in the sample and read the sample concentration directly from the meter. These meters are often confusing to operate, with small keypads and multifunction switches, and they are not suitable for working in the nonlinear range of the electrodes, using different slopes for different parts of the calibration range, or measuring more than one ion at a time. It is often difficult for the analyst to assess the quality of the calibration or detect errors in data entry, and it is still necessary for the results to be transferred manually to a permanent record.

Coulometry

Coulometry measures the amount of current passing between two electrodes in an electrochemical cell. The principle of coulometry involves the application of a constant current to generate a titrating agent; the time required to titrate a sample at constant current is measured and is related to the amount of analyte in the sample. The amount of current is directly proportional to the amount of substance produced or consumed by the electrode. Clinical applications of coulometry include the FreeStyle Connect blood glucose monitoring system (Abbott Labs) in the point-of-care setting (hospitals and medical clinics) and an older application for the measurement of chloride ions in serum, plasma, urine, and other body fluids.

Electrophoresis

Electrophoresis is the migration of charged solutes or particles in an electrical field. When charged particles are made to move, differences in molecular structure can be seen because different molecules have different velocities in an electrical field. The assay using electrophoresis involves the movement of charged particles when an external electric current is produced in a liquid environment.

The electrical field is applied to the solution through oppositely charged electrodes placed in the solution. Specific ions then travel through the solution toward the electrode of the opposite charge. Cations (positively charged particles) move toward the negatively charged electrode (cathode), and anions (negatively charged particles) move toward the positively charged electrode (anode) (Fig. 6-15).

Electrophoresis is a technique for separation and purification of ions, proteins, and other molecules of biochemical interest. It is used frequently in the clinical chemistry laboratory to

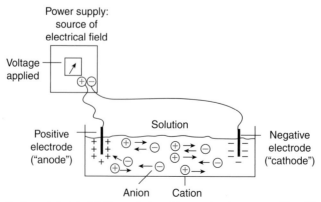

FIGURE 6-15 **Application of electrical field to solution of ions makes ions move.** (From Kaplan LA, Pesce AJ: Clinical chemistry: theory, analysis, correlation, ed 5, St Louis, 2010, Mosby.)

separate serum proteins. The equipment needed for electrophoresis generally consists of a sample applicator; a solid medium (e.g., agar gel); a buffer system; an electrophoresis chamber, which houses the solid medium and the sample; electrodes and wicks; a timer; and a power supply. Additional supplies might be stains for proteins or other substances being assayed and reagents used to remove the stains and to transform the solid media into a stable carrier for further densitometry studies or for preservation needs, depending on the requirements of the laboratory.

Serum proteins including immunoglobulins are commonly separated by electrophoresis. Serum electrophoresis results in the separation of proteins into five fractions using cellulose acetate as a support medium (Fig. 6-16). The immunologic applications of electrophoresis include identification of monoclonal proteins in either serum or urine, immunoelectrophoresis, and various blotting techniques.

Immunoelectrophoresis

Immunoelectrophoresis (IEP) involves the electrophoresis of serum or urine followed by immunodiffusion. The size and position of precipitin

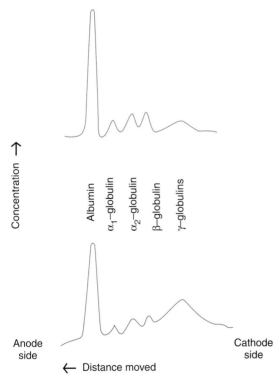

FIGURE 6-16 Example of effect of disease (hepatic cirrhosis) on serum protein electrophoretic pattern. Upper profile, distribution characteristic of healthy people. (From Kaplan LA, Pesce AJ: Clinical chemistry: theory, analysis, correlation, ed 5, St Louis, 2010, Mosby.)

bands provide the same type of information regarding equivalence or antibody excess as the double immunodiffusion method. Proteins are differentiated not only by their electrophoretic mobility but by their diffusion coefficient and antibody specificity.

IEP is a combination of the techniques of electrophoresis and double immunodiffusion (Fig. 6-17) and consists of two phases: electrophoresis and diffusion. In the first phase, serum is placed in an appropriate medium (e.g., cellulose acetate or agarose), then electrophoresed to separate its constituents according to electrophoretic mobilities: albumin, $alpha_1$-, $alpha_2$-, beta-, and gammaglobulin fractions. In the second phase after electrophoresis, the fractions are allowed to act as antigens and interact with their corresponding antibodies. When a favorable antigen-to-antibody ratio exists (equivalence point), the antigen-antibody complex becomes visible as precipitin lines or bands. Diffusion is halted by rinsing the plate in 0.85% saline. Unbound protein is washed from the agarose with saline, and the antigen-antibody precipitin arcs are stained with a protein-sensitive stain.

Each line represents one specific protein. Proteins are thus differentiated not only by their electrophoretic mobility but by their diffusion coefficient and antibody specificity. Antibody diffuses as a uniform band parallel to the antibody trough. If the proteins are homogeneous, the antigen diffuses in a circle, and the antigen-antibody precipitation line resembles a segment or arc of a circle. If the antigen is heterogeneous, the antigen-antibody line assumes an elliptical shape. One arc of precipitation forms for each constituent in the antigen mixture. This technique can be used to resolve the protein of normal serum into 25 to 40 distinct precipitation bands. The exact number depends on the strength and specificity of the antiserum used.

NORMAL APPEARANCE OF PRECIPITIN BANDS

Immunoprecipitation bands should be of normal curvature, symmetry, length, position, intensity, and distance from the antigen well and antibody trough. In normal serum, IgG, IgA, and IgM are present in sufficient concentrations of 10 mg/mL, 2 mg/mL, and 1 mg/mL, respectively, to produce precipitin lines. The normal concentrations of IgD and IgE are too low to be detected by IEP.

CLINICAL APPLICATIONS OF IEP

IEP is most commonly used to determine qualitatively the elevation or deficiency of specific classes of immunoglobulins. It is a reliable and

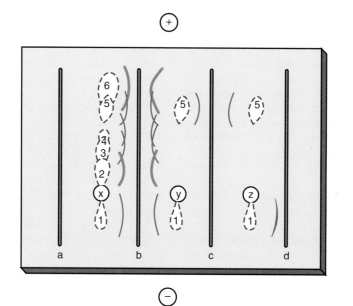

FIGURE 6-17 Configuration for immunoelectrophoresis. Sample wells are punched in agar/agarose, sample is applied, and electrophoresis is carried out to separate proteins in sample. Antiserum is loaded into troughs, and gel is incubated in a moist chamber at 4°C for 24 to 72 hours. Track *x* represents shape of protein zones after electrophoresis. Tracks *y* and *z* show reaction of proteins 5 and 1 with their specific antisera in troughs *c* and *d*. Antiserum against proteins 1 through 6 is present in trough *b*. (From Burtis CA, Ashwood ER, Bruns DE: Tietz fundamentals of clinical chemistry, ed 6, St Louis, 2008, Saunders.)

accurate method for detecting both structural abnormalities and concentration changes in proteins. The most common application of IEP is in the diagnosis of a monoclonal gammopathy, a condition in which a single clone of plasma cells produces elevated levels of a single class and type of Ig. The most important application of IEP of urine is the demonstration of Bence Jones (BJ) protein, a diagnostic sign of multiple myeloma.

Immunofixation Electrophoresis

Immunofixation electrophoresis (IFE), or simply immunofixation, has replaced IEP in the evaluation of monoclonal gammopathies because of its rapidity and ease of interpretation. It is a two-stage procedure using agarose gel protein electrophoresis in the first stage and immunoprecipitation in the second. The test specimen may be serum, urine, cerebrospinal fluid, or other body fluids. The primary use of IFE in clinical laboratories is for the characterization of monoclonal Igs.

Capillary Electrophoresis

In capillary electrophoresis, the classic separation techniques of zone electrophoresis, isotachophoresis, isoelectric focusing, and gel electrophoresis are performed in small-bore (10 to 100 μm) fused-silica capillary tubes from 20 to 200 cm in length. This method is efficient, sensitive, and rapid.

CHROMATOGRAPHY

The word *chromatography* comes from the Greek words *chromatos*, "color," and *graphein*, "to write." In **chromatography**, mixtures of solutes dissolved in a common solvent are separated from one another by a differential distribution of the solutes between two phases. The solvent, the first phase, is mobile and carries the mixture of solutes through the second phase. The second phase is a fixed or stationary phase. There are a number of variations in chromatographic techniques, in which the mobile phase ranges from liquids to gases and the stationary phase from sheets of cellulose paper to internally coated, fine capillary glass tubes. The varieties of chromatographic techniques as well as their applications to clinical assays have grown rapidly.

Chromatographic methods are usually classified according to the physical state of the solute carrier phase. The two main categories of chromatography are *gas chromatography*, in which the solute phase is in a gaseous state, and *liquid chromatography*, in which the solute phase is a solution or liquid. The methods are further classified according to how the stationary-phase matrix is contained. For example, liquid chromatography is subdivided into flat and column methods. In flat chromatography, the stationary phase is supported on a flat sheet, such as cellulose paper (paper chromatography), or in a thin layer on a mechanical backing, such as glass or plastic (thin-layer chromatography). Column methods are classically liquid chromatography. Gas chromatography is done by a column method.

The chromatographic method is used to separate the components of a given sample within a reasonable amount of time. The purpose of this separation technique is to detect or quantitate the particular component or group of components to be assayed in a pure form. By convention, the concentrations of solutes in a chromatographic system are plotted versus time or distance. The bands or zones of the various analytes separated in the technique are usually termed *peaks*.

ANALYTICAL TECHNIQUES FOR POINT-OF-CARE TESTING

Point-of-care testing (POCT) is defined as laboratory assays performed near the patient. Development of new POCT assays is increasing at a phenomenal rate. It can include home test kits and handheld monitors. The major advantage is the speed of obtaining results. The major drawback is cost, particularly if a large volume of testing is done. The same steps needed to perform an analysis from the central laboratory are needed for POCT (see Chapter 9):

- Instrument validation
- Periodic assay calibration
- Quality control testing
- Operator training
- Proficiency testing

Techniques include reflectance photometry and paper chromatography. A biosensor couples a specific biodetector (e.g., enzyme, antibody, nucleic acid probe) to a transducer for the direct measurement of a target analyte, without the need to separate it from the matrix. Commercial POCT devices use electrochemical (e.g., micro-ISEs) and optical biosensors for the measurement of glucose, electrolytes, and arterial blood gases. Biosensor probes are also available for immobilization of antibodies and specific protein sequences.

BIBLIOGRAPHY

Abbott Laboratories: Worldwide introduction of the new point-of-care glycemic control technology, Orlando, Fla, July 2005, Paper presented at AACC Symposium.

Astion ML, Wener MH, Hutchinson K: Autoantibody testing: the use of immunofluorescence assays and other assays, Clin Lab News 30, July 2000.

Bakke AC: The principles of flow cytometry, Lab Med 32(4):207, 2001.

Bakker E: Is the DNA sequence the gold standard in genetic testing? Quality of molecular genetic tests assessed, Clin Chem 52:557–558, 2006.

Behring nephelometer system folder, Branchburg, NJ, 1987, Behring Diagnostics.

Bishop ML, Fody EP, Schoeff L: Clinical chemistry: techniques, principles, correlations, ed 6, Philadelphia, 2010, Lippincott Williams & Wilkins.

Blick KE: Current trends in automation of immunoassays, J Clin Ligand Assay 22(1):6, 1999.

Bruns DE, Ashwood ER, Burtis CA: Fundamentals of molecular diagnostics, St Louis, 2007, Saunders.

Burtis CA, Ashwood ER, Bruns DE: Tietz fundamentals of clinical chemistry, ed 6, St. Louis, 2008, Saunders.

Forbes BA, Sahm DF, Weissfeld AS: Bailey and Scott's diagnostic microbiology, ed 12, St Louis, 2007, Mosby.

Helena Laboratories: Educational slide series. Protein electrophoresis and IFE and immunofixation for identification of monoclonal gammopathies. www.helena.com retrieved November 12, 2007.

Hyde A: Enzyme-Linked Immunosorbent Assay (ELISA): An overview, Advance for Med Lab Professionals :13–16, Oct. 9, 2006.

Jandreski MA: Chemiluminescence technology in immunoassays, Lab Med 29(9):555, 1998.

Kaplan LA, Pesce AJ: Clinical chemistry: theory, analysis, correlation, ed 5, St Louis, 2010, Mosby.

Killingsworth LM, Warren BM: Immunofixation for the identification of monoclonal gammopathies, Beaumont, Tex, 1986, Helena Laboratories.

Li SFY, Kricka LJ: Clinical analysis by microchip capillary electrophoresis, Clin Chem 52:42, 2006.

Mark HFL: Fluorescent in situ hybridization as an adjunct to conventional cytogenetics, Ann Clin Lab Sci 24(2): 153–163, 1994.

Ritzmann EE: Immunoglobulin abnormalities. In Ritzman S, editor: Serum protein abnormalities, diagnostic and clinical aspects, Boston, 1976, Little, Brown.

Sun T: Immunofixation electrophoresis procedures, Protein abnormalities, Physiology of immunoglobulins diagnostic and clinical aspects, vol. 1New York, 1982, Alan R Liss.

Turgeon ML: Immunology and serology in laboratory medicine, ed 4, St Louis, 2009, Mosby.

Turgeon ML: Clinical hematology, ed 4, Philadelphia, 2005, Lippincott Williams & Wilkins.

Wang Z, et al: In Situ Amplified Chemiluminescent Detection of DNA and Immunoassay of IgG Using Special-Shaped Gold Nanoparticles as Label, Clin Chem 52:1958–1962, 2006.

REVIEW QUESTIONS

Questions 1 and 2: Match the photometry instrument with its most general use (a to c).

1. ___ Absorbance spectrophotometer

2. ___ Reflectance spectrophotometer
   a. To measure the concentration of sodium or potassium in a body fluid or serum
   b. To measure the concentration of glucose in blood by using dry film technology
   c. To measure the concentration of hemoglobin in a solution

3. In the visible light spectrum, the color red is in what nanometer range?
   a. 380-440 nm
   b. 500-580 nm
   c. 600-620 nm
   d. 620-750 nm

Questions 4 and 5: Beer's law states that the concentration of a substance is (4) ___ proportional to the amount of light absorbed or (5) ___ proportional to the logarithm of the transmitted light.

4. a. directly
b. inversely

5. a. directly
b. inversely

Questions 6-8: Match the term with the appropriate definition (a to c).

6. ___ Absorbance

7. ___ Percent transmittance

8. ___ Standard solution
a. ___ Decreases as the concentration of a colored solution decreases
b. ___ Increases as the concentration of a colored solution increases
c. ___ Contains a known strength

Questions 9-11: Match the quality control tests for spectrophotomentus with the appropriate description.

9. ___ Wavelength accuracy

10. ___ Stray light

11. ___ Linearity
a. ___ Checked with standard absorbing solution or filters
b. ___ Any wavelength outside of the band transmitted
c. ___ Demonstrated when a change in concentration results in a straight-line calibration curve

12. Nephelometry measures the light scatter of:
a. ions.
b. macromolecules complexes.
c. antibodies.
d. soluble antigens.

13. *LASER* is an acronym for:
a. light amplification by stimulated emission of radiation.
b. light augmentation by stimulated emission of radiation.
c. light amplification of stimulated energy radiation.
d. large-angle stimulated emission of radiation.

14. All the following are descriptive characteristics of laser light except:
a. intensity.
b. stability.
c. polychromaticity.
d. monochromaticity.

15. A photon is a:
a. basic unit of light.
b. basic unit of all radiation.
c. component of an atom.
d. component of laser light.

Questions 16 and 17: Match the assay with its definition (a and b).

16. ___ Competitive immunoassay

17. ___ Sandwich immunoassay
a. A fixed amount of labeled antigen competes with unlabeled antigen from a patient specimen for a limited number of antibody-binding sites.
b. The sample antigen binds to an antibody; a second antibody, labeled with a chemiluminescent label, binds to the antigen-antibody complex.

18. Which enzyme label is often used in immunoassay procedures?
a. Acid phosphatase
b. Horseradish peroxidase
c. β-Galactose
d. All of the above

Questions 19 and 20: Match the assay with the label it uses (a to c).

19. ___ Enzyme immunoassay (EIA)

20. ___ Immunofluorescent technique
a. Uses a nonisotopic label
b. Uses antibody labeled with fluorescein isothiocyanate (FITC)
c. Uses a colloidal particle consisting of a metal or an insoluble metal compound

Questions 21-23: Match the assay with the appropriate statement (a to c).

21. ___ Direct immunofluorescent assay

22. ___ Inhibition immunofluorescent assay

23. ___ Indirect immunofluorescent assay
a. Based on the fact that antibodies can act as antigens and react with antiimmunoglobulins
b. Uses conjugated antibody to detect antigen-antibody reactions at a microscopic level
c. Antigen first exposed to unlabeled antibody, then labeled antibody

24. For an enzyme to be used in an enzyme immunoassay, it must meet all the following criteria except:
a. high amount of stability.
b. extreme specificity.
c. presence in antigen or antibody.
d. no alteration by inhibitor with the system.

Questions 25 and 26: A fluorescent substance is one that while (25) ___ light of one wavelength, (26) ___ light of another (longer) wavelength.

25. a. emitting
    b. absorbing
    c. generating bright
    d. generating dull

26. a. emits
    b. absorbs
    c. reduces
    d. increases

Match questions 27-29.

27. ___ Quantum dots (Q dots)

28. ___ SQUID technology

29. ___ Luminescent oxygen channeling immunoassay (LOCI)

30. ___ Fluorescent in situ hybridization (FISH)
    a. Semiconductor nanocrystals
    b. A method of tagging antibodies with superparamagnetic particles
    c. Technology based on two different 200-nm latex particles
    d. A molecular cytogenetic technique

31. **Chemiluminescence:**
    a. has excellent sensitivity and dynamic range.
    b. does not require sample radiation.
    c. uses unstable chemiluminescent reagents and conjugates.
    d. both a and b.

32. **In comparison to serologic assays, nucleic acid testing offers all of the following benefits except:**
    a. reduced cost.
    b. enhanced specificity.
    c. increased sensitivity.
    d. all of the above.

33. **PCR testing is useful in:**
    a. forensic testing.
    b. genetic testing.
    c. identification of the disease.
    d. all of the above.

34. **The traditional PCR technique:**
    a. extends the length of the genomic DNA.
    b. alters the original DNA nucleotide sequence.
    c. amplifies the target region of DNA.
    d. amplifies the target region of RNA.

35. **For the PCR reaction to take place, one must provide which of the following?**
    a. Oligonucleotide primers
    b. Individual deoxynucleotides

c. Thermostable DNA polymerase
d. All of the above

36. **The enzyme reverse transcriptase converts:**
    a. mRNA to cDNA.
    b. tRNA to DNTP.
    c. dsDNA to ssDNA.
    d. mitochondrial to nuclear DNA.

37. **DNA polymerase catalyzes:**
    a. primer annealing.
    b. primer extension.
    c. hybridization of DNA.
    d. hybridization of RNA.

Questions 38-40: *Match the method with the appropriate description.*

38. ___ Southern blot immunoassay

39. ___ Northern blot immunoassay

40. ___ Western blot immunoassay
    a. Messenger RNA is studied.
    b. Called *immunoblot*, it is used to detect antibodies to subspecies of antigens.
    c. Single-stranded DNA is studied.

41. **Which ion-selective electrode is universally used in the clinical laboratory?**
    a. pH electrode
    b. Fluoride electrode
    c. Chloride electrode
    d. Sodium electrode

Questions 42 and 43: *Match the term with its definition (a and b).*

42. ___ Indicator electrode

43. ___ Reference electrode
    a. The main component of potentiometric techniques
    b. An electrochemical half-cell that is used as a fixed reference for the cell potential measurements

Questions 44-46: *Match each term with its definition.*

44. ___ Coulometry

45. ___ Electrophoresis

46. ___ Chromatography
    a. Mixtures of solutes dissolved in a common solvent are separated from one another by a differential distribution of the solutes between two phases.
    b. Different molecules have different velocities in an electrical field.
    c. Measures the amount of current passing between two electrodes in an electrochemical cell.

47. Protein can be separated into ___ fractions by use of serum electrophoresis.
    a. three
    b. four
    c. five
    d. six

48. Which of the following is the most common application of immunoelectrophoresis (IEP)?
    a. Identification of the absence of a normal serum protein
    b. Structural abnormalities of proteins
    c. Screening for circulating immune complexes
    d. Diagnosis of monoclonal gammopathies

49. Immunofixation electrophoresis is best used in:
    a. the workup of a polyclonal gammopathy.
    b. the workup of a monoclonal gammopathy.
    c. screening for circulating immune complexes.
    d. identification of hypercomplementemia.

50. Immunoelectrophoresis involves:
    a. separation of proteins based on the rate of migration of individual components in an electrical field.
    b. electrophoresis of serum or urine.
    c. double immunodiffusion following electrophoresis.
    d. all of the above.

51. In immunoelectrophoresis (IEP), proteins are differentiated by:
    a. electrophoresis.
    b. diffusion coefficient.
    c. antibody specificity.
    d. all of the above.

52. The most important application of IEP of urine is:
    a. diagnosis of monoclonal gammopathy.
    b. diagnosis of polyclonal gammopathy.
    c. diagnosis of autoimmune hemolysis.
    d. demonstration of Bence Jones (BJ) protein.

53. Immunofixation electrophoresis (IFE) can test:
    a. serum and urine.
    b. cerebrospinal fluid.
    c. whole blood.
    d. a and b.

54. The primary use of IFE is:
    a. characterization of monoclonal immuno-globulins.
    b. characterization of polyclonal immuno-globulins.
    c. identification of monoclonal immuno-globulins.
    d. identification of polyclonal immuno-globulins.

CHAPTER 7

LABORATORY MATHEMATICS AND SOLUTION PREPARATION

Learning Objectives

At the conclusion of this chapter, the student will be able to:

- Explain and apply the rules for rounding off numbers and using significant figures.
- Describe the use of exponents.
- Calculate proportions and ratios.
- Define the terms *density* and *specific gravity*.
- Calculate the requirements for solutions of a given volume and molarity.
- Describe the procedures for making a single dilution and a serial dilution.

- Calculate the amount of one solution needed to make a solution of a lesser concentration from it.
- Compare the expressions of solution concentration, *weight per unit weight* and *weight per unit volume*.
- Prepare a percent solution.

Today's clinical laboratory requires a minimal amount of solution preparation and mathematical calculations. Most reagents are prepackaged for immediate use, and microprocessors perform various mathematical calculations. Calculations specific to hematology or clinical chemistry are discussed in discipline-specific chapters in Part II. In special circumstances, or more often in research laboratories, laboratory staff are required to calculate and prepare solutions for analytical assays or calculate results.

SIGNIFICANT FIGURES

Using more digits than necessary to calculate and report the results of a laboratory determination has several disadvantages. It is important that the number used contain only the digits necessary for precision of the determination. Using more is misleading in that it ascribes more accuracy to the determination than is actually the case. There is also the danger of overlooking a decimal point and making an error in judging the magnitude of the answer. Digits in a number that are needed to express the precision of the measurement from which the number is derived are known as **significant figures.** A significant figure is known to be reasonably reliable. Judgment must be exercised in determining how many figures should be used. Some rules to assist in making such decisions are:

1. Use the known accuracy of the method to determine the number of digits that are significant in the answer, and as a general rule, retain one more figure than this. For example, a urea nitrogen result was reported as 11.2 mg/dL. This would indicate that the result is accurate to the nearest tenth and that the exact value lies between 11.15 and 11.25. In reality, the accuracy of most urea nitrogen methods is ±10%, so the result reported as 11.2 mg/dL could actually vary from 10 to 12 mg/dL and should be reported as 11 mg/dL. In addition, if the decimal point were omitted or overlooked, the result could be taken as 112 mg/dL.

2. Take the accuracy of the least accurate measurement, or the measurement with the least number of significant figures, as the accuracy of the final result. In doing so, certain adjustments must be made in the addition and subtraction or multiplication and division of numerals. With addition or subtraction, for example, to add the following numerals:

$$206.1$$
$$7.56$$
$$0.8764$$

rewrite them as:

$$206.1$$
$$7.6$$
$$0.9$$

In this example, the least accurate figure is accurate to one decimal place; this is therefore the determining factor. To determine the least accurate figure, use this rule: In a column of addition or subtraction in which the decimal points are placed one above the other, the number of significant figures in the final answer is determined by the first digit encountered going from left to right that terminates any one numeral.

In multiplication or division, using this example:

$$32.973 \div 4.3 =$$

the result should be reported as 7.7, following this rule: The number of significant figures in the final product or quotient should not exceed the smallest number of significant figures in any one factor.

Rounding Off Numbers

Test results sometimes produce insignificant digits. It is then necessary to **round off the numbers** to a chosen number of significant value so as not to imply an accuracy of precision greater than the test is capable of delivering.

Some general rules may be used in rounding off decimal values to the proper place. When the digit next to the last one to be retained is less than 5, the last digit should be left unchanged. When the digit next to the last one to be retained is greater than 5, the last digit is increased by 1. If the additional digit is 5, the last digit reported is changed to the nearest even number. Examples are as follows:

2.31463 g is rounded off to 2.3146 g.
5.34659 g is rounded off to 5.3466 g.
23.5 mg is rounded off to 24 mg.
24.5 mg is rounded off to 24 mg.

EXPONENTS

Exponents are used to indicate that a number must be multiplied by itself as many times as indicated by the exponent. The number to be multiplied by itself is called the *base.* Usually the exponent is written as a small superscript figure to the immediate right of the base figure and is sometimes referred to as the *power* of the base. The exponent figure can have either a plus or a minus sign before it. The plus sign is usually implied and does not actually appear.

A **positive exponent** indicates the number of times the base is to be multiplied by itself. Examples of exponents with no sign or a plus sign (positive exponents) are:

$$10^2 = 10 \times 10 = 100$$
$$10^5 = 10 \times 10 \times 10 \times 10 \times 10 = 100,000$$
$$5^3 = 5 \times 5 \times 5 = 125$$

Clinical laboratory values in hematology cell counts are expressed exponentially. For example, the average of the reference range of the total erythrocyte count in an adult female is 4.8×10^{12}/L. The low end of the reference range of the total leukocyte count in an adult is 4.5×10^9/L.

A **negative exponent** indicates the number of times the *reciprocal* of the base is to be multiplied by itself. In other words, a negative exponent indicates a fraction. Examples of exponents with a minus sign (negative exponents) are:

$$10^{-1} = \frac{1}{10} = 0.1$$

$$10^{-4} = \frac{1}{10} \times \frac{1}{10} \times \frac{1}{10} \times \frac{1}{10}$$

$$= \frac{1}{10,000}$$

$$= 0.0001$$

DENSITY AND SPECIFIC GRAVITY

Density is defined as the amount of matter per unit volume of a substance. All substances have this property, not only solutions. An example of the expression of density is the specific gravity of a substance.

Specific gravity can be used to determine the mass (weight) of solutions. It relates the weight of 1 mL of a solution and the weight of 1 mL of pure water at 4°C (1 g). Specific gravity is used in the clinical or research laboratory when preparing dilutions made from concentrated acids.

Specific gravity × Percent assay =
Grams of compound / mL

Example: Concentrated HCl has a specific gravity of 1.25 g/mL and an assay value of 38%. What is the amount of HCl/mL?

$$1.25 \text{ g} / \text{mL} \times 0.38 = 0.475 \text{ g of HCl} / \text{mL}$$

Once the grams (g) of HCl in the concentrated acid is known, further calculations can be performed to determine how many milliliters (mL) of the acid are needed to prepare various concentrations of HCl solutions.

EXPRESSIONS OF SOLUTION CONCENTRATION

Solutions are made up of a mixture of substances. Making up a solution usually involves two main parts: the substance that is being dissolved (the **solute**) and the substance into which the solute is being dissolved (the **solvent**). In working with solutions, it is necessary to know or be able to measure the relative amounts of the substance in solution, known as the **concentration of the solution.** Concentration is the amount of one substance relative to the amounts of the other substances in the solution.

Solution concentration is expressed in several different ways. The most common methods used in clinical laboratories involve either weight per unit weight (w/w), also known as mass per unit mass (m/m); weight per unit volume (w/v), also known as mass per unit volume (m/v); or volume per unit volume (v/v). *Weight* is the term commonly used, although *mass* is really what is being measured. Mass is the amount of matter

in something, and weight is the force of gravity on something. The most accurate measurement is weight per unit weight, because weight (or mass) does not vary with temperature as does volume. Probably the most common measurement is weight per unit volume. The least accurate measurement is volume per unit volume because of the changes in volume resulting from temperature changes. Volume per unit volume is used in preparing a liquid solution from another liquid substance.

Weight (Mass) Per Unit Volume

The most common way of expressing concentration is by **weight (mass) per unit volume (w/v).** When weight (mass) per unit volume is used, the amount of solute (the substance that goes into solution) per volume of solution is expressed. Weight per unit volume is used most often when a solid chemical is diluted in a liquid. The usual way to express weight per unit volume is as *grams per liter* (g/L) or *milligrams per milliliter* (mg/mL). If a concentration of a certain solution is given as 10 g/L, it means there are 10 g of solute for every liter of solution. If a solution with a concentration of 10 mg/mL is desired, and 100 mL of this solution is to be prepared, a proportion formula can be applied. Example:

$$\frac{10 \text{ mg}}{1 \text{ mL}} = \frac{x \text{ mg}}{100 \text{ mL}} = 1000 \text{ mg, or } 1 \text{ g}$$

One gram of the desired solute is weighed and diluted to 100 mL.

In working with standard solutions, you will see that their concentrations, almost without exception, are expressed as milligrams per milliliter (mg/mL).

Volume Per Unit Volume

Another way of expressing concentration is by volume per unit volume (v/v). Volume per unit volume is used to express concentration when a liquid chemical is diluted with another liquid. The concentration is expressed as the number of milliliters of liquid chemical per unit volume of solution. The usual way to express volume per unit volume is as *milliliters per milliliter* (mL/mL) or *milliliters per liter* (mL/L). The number of milliliters of liquid chemical in 1 mL or 1 L of solution uses the volume per unit volume expression of concentration. If 10 mL of alcohol is diluted to 100 mL with water, the concentration is expressed as 10 mL/100 mL, or 10 mL/dL, or 0.1 mL/mL, or 100 mL/L. If a solution with a concentration of 0.5 mL/mL is desired, and 1 L is to be prepared, a proportion can again be used to solve the problem. Example:

$$\frac{0.5\ mL}{1\ mL} = \frac{x\ mL}{1000\ mL}$$

$$x = 500\ mL$$

Therefore, 500 mL of the liquid chemical is measured accurately and diluted to 1000 mL (1 L). To express concentration in milliliters per liter, one needs to know how many milliliters of liquid chemical there are in 1 L of the solution.

Any chemical (liquid or solid) can be made into a solution by diluting it with a solvent. The usual solvent is deionized or distilled water (see Laboratory Reagent Water, Chapter 4). If the desired chemical is a liquid, the amount needed is measured in milliliters or liters. On occasion, liquids are weighed, but the usual method is to measure their volume. If the desired chemical is a solid, the amount needed is weighed in grams or milligrams.

Percent

Another expression of concentration is the percent solution (%), although in the International System of Units (SI system) the preferred units are kilograms (or fractions thereof) per liter (w/v) or milliliters per liter (v/v). A description of the percent solution follows, because this expression of concentration is still used in some instances. **Percent** is defined as parts per hundred parts (the part can be any particular unit). Unless otherwise stated, a percent solution usually means grams or milliliters of solute per 100 mL of solution (g/100 mL or mL/100 mL). Recall that 100 mL is equal to 1 deciliter (dL). Percent solutions can be prepared using either liquid or solid chemicals. Percent solutions can be expressed either as weight per unit volume percent (w/v%) or as volume per unit volume percent (v/v%), depending on the state of the solute (chemical) used, that is, whether it is a solid or a liquid. When a solid chemical is dissolved in a liquid, *percent* means grams of solid in 100 mL of solution. If 10 g of NaCl is diluted to 100 mL with deionized water, the concentration is expressed as 10% (10 g/dL). If 2.5 g is diluted to 100 mL, the concentration is 2.5% (2.5 g/dL).

The following is an example of concentration expressed in percent: 10 grams of NaOH is diluted to 200 mL with water. What is the concentration in percent? A proportion can be set up to solve this problem:

$$\frac{10\ g}{200\ mL} = \frac{x\ g}{100\ mL}$$

$$x = 5\%\ \text{solution (preferably expressed as 5 g/dL)}$$

Remember that the percent expression is based on how much solute is present in 100 mL (or 1 dL) of the solution.

Some concentrations of solutions are expressed as milligrams of solute in 100 mL of solution (mg%). When this method of expression is used, mg% is always specifically stated. If 25 mg of a chemical is diluted to 100 mL, the concentration in milligrams percent would be 25 mg% (preferably expressed as 25 mg/dL).

If a liquid chemical is used to prepare a percent solution, the concentration is expressed as volume per unit volume percent, or milliliters of solute per 100 mL of solution. If 10 mL of hydrochloric acid (HCl) is diluted to 100 mL with water, the concentration is 10% (preferably expressed as 10 ml/dL). If 10 mL of the same acid is diluted to 1 L (1000 mL), the concentration is 1% (preferably expressed as 1 mL/dL).

Molarity

The **molarity of a solution** is defined as the gram-molecular mass (or weight) of a compound per liter of solution. This is a weight-per-unit-volume method of expressing concentration. A basic formula is:

$$\text{Molecular weight} \times \text{Molarity} = \text{Grams/liter}$$

Another way to define *molarity* is number of moles per liter (mol/L) of solution. A *mole* is the molecular weight of a compound in grams (1 mole = 1 gram-molecular weight). The number of moles of a compound equals the number of grams divided by the **gram-molecular weight** of that compound. One gram-molecular weight equals the sum of all atomic weights in a molecule of the compound, expressed in grams.

To determine the gram-molecular weight of a compound, the correct chemical formula must be known, then the sum of all the atomic weights in the compound can be found by consulting a periodic table of the elements or a chart with atomic masses of the elements.

Examples of Molarity Calculations

1. Sodium chloride has one sodium ion and one chloride ion; the correct formula is written as NaCl. The gram-molecular weight is derived by finding the sum of the atomic weights:

$$Na = 23$$
$$Cl = 35.5$$
$$\text{Gram-molecular weight} = 58.5$$

If the gram-molecular weight of NaCl is 58.5 g, a 1 molar (1 M) solution of NaCl would contain 58.5 g of NaCl per liter of solution, because molarity equals moles per liter, and 1 mol of NaCl equals 58.5 g.

2. For barium sulfate ($BaSO_4$), the gram-molecular weight equals 233 (the formula indicates that there are one barium, one sulfur, and four oxygen ions):

$$
\begin{aligned}
1\ Ba &= 137 \times 1 = 137\\
1\ S &= 32 \times 1 = 32\\
4\ O &= 16 \times 4 = 64\\
137 &+ 32 + 64 = 233
\end{aligned}
$$

Since the gram-molecular weight is 233, a 1 M solution of $BaSO_4$ would contain 233 g of $BaSO_4$ per liter of solution.

The quantities of solutions needed will not always be in units of whole liters, and often fractions or multiples of a 1 M concentration will be desired. Parts of a molar solution are expressed as decimals. If a 1 M solution of NaCl contains 58.5 g of NaCl per liter of solution, a 0.5 M solution would contain one half of 58.5 g, or 29 g/L, and a 3 M solution would contain 3 times 58.5 g, or 175.5 g/L.

What is the molarity of a solution containing 30 g of NaCl per liter? Molarity equals the number of moles per liter, and the number of moles equals the grams divided by the gram-molecular weight.

Step 1: Find the gram-molecular weight of NaCl. It is 58.5 g (Na = 23 and Cl = 35.5).

Step 2: Find the moles per liter.

$$
\frac{30\ g/L}{x} = \frac{58.5\ g/L}{1\ mol}
$$

$$
x = \frac{30\ g/L \times 1\ mol}{58.5\ g/L} = 0.513\ mol\ NaCl
$$

Step 3: The number of moles per liter of solution equals the molarity; the solution in the example is therefore 0.513 M, rounded off to 0.5 M.

Equations might prove useful to some in working with molarity solutions, but all these equations can be derived by applying the commonsense proportion approach to molarity problems described later under Proportions and Ratios. Some equations are:

$$
Molarity = \frac{Moles\ of\ solute}{Liters\ of\ solution}
$$

$$
Molarity = \frac{Grams\ of\ solute}{Gram-molecular\ weight} \times \frac{1}{Liters\ of\ solution}
$$

$$
Moles\ of\ solute = Molarity \times Liters\ of\ solution
$$

$$
Grams\ of\ solute = Molarity \times Gram-molecular\ weight \times Liters\ of\ solution
$$

NOTE: These equations are all on the basis of 1 L of solution; if something other than 1 L is used, refer back to the 1-L basis (e.g., 500 mL = 0.5 L, 2000 mL = 2 L).

Molarity does not provide a basis for direct comparison of strength for all solutions. For example, 1 L of 1 M NaOH will exactly neutralize 1 L of 1 M HCl, but it will neutralize only 0.5 L of 1 M sulfuric acid (H_2SO_4). It is therefore more convenient to choose a unit of concentration that will provide a basis for direct comparison of strengths of solutions. Such a unit is referred to as an *equivalent* (or equivalent weight or mass), and this term is used in describing normality.

Millimolarity

A **milligram-molecular weight** (the molecular weight expressed in milligrams) is a **millimole (mmole).** This is in contrast to the molarity described previously, which is the number of moles per liter. The following formulas compare the two:

$$
Molarity\ (moles/liter) = \frac{g/L}{Molecular\ weight}
$$

$$
Millimoles/liter = \frac{mg/L}{Molecular\ weight}
$$

Osmolarity

Osmolarity is defined as the number of osmoles of solute per liter of solution. An osmole (osm) is the amount of a substance that will produce 1 mole (mol) of particles having osmotic activity. An osmole of any substance is equal to 1 gram-molecular weight (1 mol) of the substance divided by the number of particles formed by the dissociation of the molecules of the substance. For materials that do not ionize, 1 osm is equal to 1 mol. This gives an estimate of the osmotic activity of the solution—the relative number of particles dissolved in the solution. Osmolarity is an expression of weight per unit volume concentration.

For a solution of glucose, a substance that does not ionize or dissociate in aqueous solution, 1 osm of glucose is equal to 1 mol of glucose. For a solution of sodium chloride, which does ionize, 1 osm of sodium chloride is equal to 1 gram-molecular weight divided by the number of particles formed on ionization. Sodium chloride completely ionizes in water to form one sodium ion and one chloride ion, or a total of two particles. The molecular weight of NaCl is 58.5. To calculate the osmolarity of NaCl, the following formula is used:

$$
1\ osm\ NaCl = \frac{58.2}{2} = 29.25\ g
$$

The *osmolal gap* is discussed in detail in Chapter 11, Introduction to Clinical Chemistry. The major contributors to the gap are glucose, sodium (Na^+), and blood urea nitrogen (BUN).

PROPORTIONS AND RATIOS

The use of proportions involves a commonsense approach to problem solving. **Proportions** are used to determine a quantity from a given ratio. A **ratio** is an amount of something compared to an amount of something else.

Ratios always describe a relative amount, and at least two values are always involved. For example, 5 g of something dissolved in 100 mL of something else can be expressed by the ratios 5/100 or 5:100, or by the decimal 0.05. Proportion is a means of saying that two ratios are equal. Thus, the ratio 5:100 is equal, or proportional to, the ratio 1/20. This proportion can be expressed as 5:100 = 1:20. In the laboratory, proportions and ratios are useful when it is necessary to make more (or less) of the same thing. However, ratios and proportions can be used only when the concentration (or any other type of relationship) does not change.

The following is an example of a proportion or ratio problem: A formula calls for 5 g of sodium chloride (NaCl) in 1000 mL of solution. If only 500 mL of solution is needed, how much NaCl is required?

$$\frac{5\,g}{1000\,mL} = \frac{x\,g}{500\,mL}$$

$$x = \frac{5\,g \times 500\,mL}{1000\,mL}$$

$$x = 2.5\,g\,NaCl$$

In setting up ratio and proportion problems, the two ratios being compared must be written in the same order, and they must be in the same units. When specimens are diluted in various laboratory analyses, the ratio principle is applied (see later).

CONCENTRATIONS OF SOLUTIONS

To relate different concentrations of solutions that contain the same amount of substance (or solute), a basic relationship, or ratio, is used. The volume of one solution (V_1) times the concentration of that solution (C_1) equals the volume of the second solution (V_2) times the concentration of the second solution (C_2), as follows:

$$V_1 \times C_1 = V_2 \times C_2$$

If any three of the values are known, the fourth may be determined. This relationship shows that when a solution is diluted, the volume is increased as the concentration is decreased. The total amount of substance (or solute) remains unchanged. Several applications of this relationship are used in the clinical laboratory, such as dilution of specimens or preparation of weaker solutions from stronger solutions.

An example of making a less concentrated solution from a more concentrated solution follows. A sodium hydroxide (NaOH) solution is available that has a concentration of 10 g of NaOH per deciliter (dL) of solution (1 dL = 100 mL). To calculate the volume of the 10 g/dL NaOH solution required to prepare 1000 mL of 2 g/dL NaOH:

$$V_1 \times C_1 = V_2 \times C_2$$

$$x\,mL \times 10\,g/dL = 1000\,mL \times 2\,g/dL$$

$$x = \frac{2\,g/dL \times 1000\,mL}{10\,g/dL} = 200\,mL$$

$$10\,g/dL = 200\,mL$$

Note that this relationship is not a direct proportion but an inverse proportion. Because this is a proportion problem, it is important to remember that the concentrations and volumes on both sides of the equation must be expressed in the same units.

DILUTIONS

It is often necessary to make **dilutions** of specimens being analyzed or to make weaker solutions from stronger solutions in various laboratory procedures. A laboratory professional must be capable of working with various dilution problems and **dilution factors**. In these problems, one must often be able to determine the concentration of material in each solution, the actual amount of material in each solution, and the total volume of each solution. All dilutions are a type of ratio. Dilution is an indication of relative concentration.

Diluting Specimens

In performing a laboratory assay, it may be necessary to dilute a specimen because of a high concentration of a constituent. The needed dilution will vary according to the procedure (see Use of Dilution Factors section).

Dilution Factor

A dilution factor is used to correct for having used a diluted sample in a determination rather than the undiluted sample. The result (answer) using the dilution must be multiplied by the reciprocal of the dilution made.

For example, a dilution factor by which all determination answers are multiplied to give the concentration per 100 mL of sample (blood) may be calculated as follows:

First, determine the volume of blood that is actually analyzed in the procedure. By use of a simple proportion, it is evident that 0.5 mL of blood diluted to 10 mL is equivalent to 1 mL of blood diluted to 20 mL.

$$\frac{0.5 \text{ mL blood}}{10 \text{ mL solution}} = \frac{1 \text{ mL blood}}{x \text{ mL solution}}$$

$$x = \frac{1 \text{ mL blood} \times 10 \text{ mL}}{0.5 \text{ mL}} = 20 \text{ mL}$$

Using another simple proportion, the concentration of specimen (blood) in each milliliter of solution may be determined to be 0.05 mL of blood per milliliter of solution:

$$\frac{1 \text{ mL blood}}{20 \text{ mL solution}} = \frac{x \text{ mL blood}}{1 \text{ mL solution}}$$

$$x = \frac{1 \text{ mL} \times 1 \text{ mL}}{20 \text{ mL}} = 0.05 \text{ mL}$$

Because 1 mL of the 1:20 dilution of blood is analyzed in the remaining steps of the procedure, 0.05 mL of blood is actually analyzed (1 mL of the dilution used × 0.05 mL/mL = 0.05 mL of blood analyzed).

To relate the concentration of the substance measured in the procedure to the concentration in 100 mL of blood (the units in which the result is to be expressed), another proportion may be used:

$$\frac{100 \text{ mL(volume of blood desired)}}{0.05 \text{ mL (volume of blood used)}} =$$

$$\frac{\text{Concentration desired}}{\text{Concentration used or determined}}$$

Concentration desired =
$$\frac{100 \text{ mL} \times \text{Concentration determined}}{0.05 \text{ mL}}$$
Concentration desired =
$$2000 \times \text{Value determined}$$

The concentration of the substance being measured in the volume of blood actually tested (0.05 mL) must be multiplied by 2000 to report the concentration per 100 mL of blood.

The preceding material may be summarized by the following statement and equations. In reporting results obtained from laboratory determinations, one must first determine the amount of specimen actually analyzed in the procedure, and then calculate the factor that will express the concentration in the desired terms of measurement. For the previous example:

$$\frac{0.5 \text{ mL (volume of blood used)}}{10 \text{ mL (volume of total dilution)}} =$$

$$\frac{x \text{ mL (volume of blood analyzed)}}{1 \text{ mL (volume of dilution used)}}$$

$$x = 0.05 \text{ mL (volume of blood actually analyzed)}$$

$$\frac{100 \text{ mL (volume of blood required for expression of result)}}{0.05 \text{ mL (volume of blood actually analyzed)}} =$$
$$2000 \text{ (dilution factor)}$$

Single Dilutions

When the concentration of a particular substance in a specimen is too great to be accurately determined, or when there is less specimen available for analysis than the procedure requires, it may be necessary to dilute the original specimen or further dilute the initial dilution (or filtrate). Such **single dilutions** are usually expressed as a ratio, such as 1:2, 1:5, or 1:10, or as a fraction, ½, ⅕, or ¹⁄₁₀. These ratios or fractions refer to 1 unit of the original specimen diluted to a final volume of 2, 5, or 10 units, respectively. A **dilution** therefore refers to the volume or number of parts of the substance to be diluted in the total volume, or parts, of the final solution. A dilution is an expression of concentration, not an expression of volume; it indicates the relative amount of substance in solution. Dilutions can be made singly or in series.

To calculate the concentration of a single dilution, multiply the original concentration by the dilution expressed as a fraction.

Calculation of the Concentration of a Single Dilution

A simple dilution uses the formula:

$$\frac{\text{Sample volume}}{\text{Sample volume} + \text{Diluent volume}}$$

or:

$$\frac{\text{Sample volume}}{\text{Total volume}}$$

A specimen contains 500 mg of substance per deciliter of blood. A 1:5 dilution of this specimen is prepared by volumetrically measuring 1 mL of the specimen and adding 4 mL of diluent. The concentration of substance in the dilution is:

$$500 \text{ mg/dL} \times \tfrac{1}{5} = 100 \text{ mg/dL}$$

Note that the concentration of the final solution (or dilution) is expressed in the same units as the original solution.

To obtain a dilution factor that can be applied to the determination answer to express it as a concentration per standard volume, proceed as follows. Rather than multiply by the dilution expressed as a fraction, multiply the determination value by the reciprocal of the dilution fraction. In the case of a 1:5 dilution, the dilution factor that would be applied to values obtained in the procedure would be 5, since the original specimen was five times more concentrated than the diluted specimen tested in the procedure.

Use of Dilution Factors

A 1:5 dilution of a specimen is prepared, and an aliquot (one of a number of equal parts) of the dilution is analyzed for a particular substance. The concentration of the substance in the **aliquot** is multiplied by 5 to determine its concentration in the original specimen. If the concentration of the dilution is 100 mg/dL, the concentration of the original specimen is:

$$100 \text{ mg/dL} \times 5 \text{ (dilution factor)} = $$
$$500 \text{ mg/dL in blood}$$

Serial Dilutions

As mentioned previously, dilutions can be made singly or in series, in which case the original solution is further diluted. A general rule for calculating the concentrations of solutions obtained by dilution in series is to multiply the original concentration by the first dilution (expressed as a fraction), this by the second dilution, and so on until the desired concentration is known.

Several laboratory procedures, especially serologic tests, make use of a dilution series in which all dilutions, including or following the first one, are the same. Such dilutions are referred to as **serial dilutions.** A complete dilution series usually contains five or ten tubes, although any single dilution may be made directly from an undiluted specimen or substance. In calculating the dilution or concentration of substance or serum in each tube of the dilution series, the rules previously discussed apply.

A five-tube twofold dilution may be prepared as follows (Fig. 7-1). A serum specimen is diluted 1:2 with buffer. A series of five tubes are prepared, in which each succeeding tube is rediluted 1:2. This is accomplished by placing 1 mL of diluent into each of four tubes (tubes 2 to 5). Tube 1 contains 1 mL of undiluted serum. Tube 2 contains 1 mL of undiluted serum plus 1 mL of diluent, resulting in a 1:2 dilution of serum. A 1-mL portion of the 1:2 dilution of serum is placed in tube 3, resulting in a 1:4 dilution of serum ($\frac{1}{2} \times \frac{1}{2} = \frac{1}{4}$). A 1-mL portion of the 1:4 dilution from tube 3 is placed in tube 4, resulting in a 1:8 dilution ($\frac{1}{4} \times \frac{1}{2} = \frac{1}{8}$). Finally, 1 mL of the 1:8 dilution from tube 4 is added to tube 5, resulting in a 1:16 dilution ($\frac{1}{8} \times \frac{1}{2} = \frac{1}{16}$). One milliliter of the final dilution is discarded so that the volumes in all the tubes are equal. Note that each tube is diluted twice as much as the previous tube, and the final volume in each tube is the same. The undiluted serum may also be given a dilution value: 1:1.

The concentration of serum in terms of milliliters in each tube is calculated by multiplying the previous concentration (mL) by the succeeding dilution. In the Fig. 7-1 example, tube 1 contains

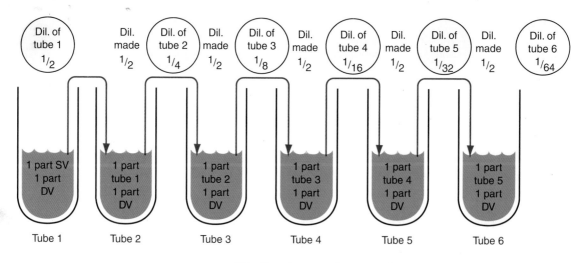

SV = Sample volume (e.g., serum)
DV = Diluent volume (e.g., saline)

FIGURE 7-1 **Schematic of a twofold serial dilution.** (From Doucette LJ: Mathematics for the clinical laboratory, ed 2, St Louis, 2011, Saunders.)

1 mL of serum, tube 2 contains 1 mL × ½ = 0.5 mL of serum, and tubes 3 to 5 contain 0.25, 0.125, and 0.06 mL of serum, respectively.

Other serial dilutions might be fivefold or tenfold; that is, each succeeding tube is diluted five or ten times. A fivefold series would begin with 1 mL of serum in 4 mL of diluent and a total volume of 5 mL in each tube. A tenfold series would begin with 1 mL of serum in 9 mL of diluent and a total volume of 10 mL in each tube. Other systems might begin with a 1:2 dilution and then dilute five succeeding tubes 1:10. The dilutions in such a series would be 1:2, 1:20 (½ × ⅟₁₀ = ⅟₂₀), 1:200 (⅟₂₀ × ⅟₁₀ = ⅟₂₀₀), 1:2000, 1:20,000, and 1:200,000.

Calculation of the Concentration After a Series of Dilutions

A working solution is prepared from a stock solution (see next section). In so doing, a stock solution with a concentration of 100 mg/dL is diluted 1:10 by volumetrically adding 1 mL of the solution to 9 mL of diluent. The diluted solution (intermediate solution) is further diluted 1:100 by volumetrically measuring 1 mL of intermediate solution and diluting to the mark in a 100-mL volumetric flask. The concentration of the final or working solution is:

$$100 \text{ mg/dL} \times {}^{1}\!/_{10} \times {}^{1}\!/_{100} = 0.1 \text{ mg/dL}$$

Standard Solutions

To determine the concentration of a substance in a specimen, there must be a basis of comparison. For analyses that result in a colored solution, a spectrophotometer is used to make this comparison (see Chapter 6). A **standard solution** is one that contains a known, exact amount of the substance being measured. It is prepared from high-quality reference material with measured, known amounts of a fixed and known chemical composition that can be obtained in a pure form. The **standard solution** is measured accurately and then treated in the testing procedure as if it were a specimen whose concentration is to be determined.

Standard solutions are purchased "ready made," already prepared from high-quality chemicals, or they can be prepared in the laboratory from high-quality chemicals that have been dried and stored in a desiccator. The standard chemical is weighed on the analytical balance and diluted volumetrically. This standard solution is usually most stable in a concentrated form, in which case it is usually referred to as a **stock standard.**

Working Standards

Working standards are prepared from the stock, and sometimes an intermediate form is prepared. The working standard (a more dilute form of the stock standard) is the one employed in the actual determination. Stock and working standards are usually stored in the refrigerator. The accuracy of a procedure is absolutely dependent on the standard solution used, so extreme care must be taken whenever these solutions are prepared or used in a clinical laboratory.

Standards Used in Spectrophotometry

To use the standard solution as a basis of comparison in quantitative analysis with the spectrophotometer, a series of calibrated cuvettes (or tubes) are prepared. Each cuvette contains a known, different amount of the standard solution. In this way, a series of cuvettes is available containing various known amounts of the standard. Standard cuvettes are carried through the same developmental steps as cuvettes containing specimens to be measured. This set of standard cuvettes is read in the spectrophotometer, and the galvanometer readings are recorded. These readings can be recorded in percent transmittance or in absorbance units (see Chapter 6). Standard solutions are also included in automated analytical methods.

Blank Solutions

For every procedure using the spectrophotometer, a blank solution must be included in the batch. The **blank solution** contains reagents used in the procedure, but it does not contain the substance to be measured. It is treated with the same reagents and processed along with the unknown specimens and the standards. The blank solution is set to read 100%T on the galvanometer viewing scale. In other words, the blank tube is set to transmit 100% of the light. The other cuvettes in the same batch (e.g., unknown specimens and standards) transmit only a fraction of this light because they contain particles that absorb light (particles of the unknown substance), so only part of the 100% is transmitted (see Chapter 6). Using a blank solution corrects for any color that may be present because of the reagents used or an interaction between those reagents.

PRACTICE PROBLEMS

1. **A 200-mg/dL solution was diluted 1:10. This diluted solution was then additionally diluted 1:5. What is the concentration of the final solution?**

Answer:

$$200 \text{ mg/dL} \times {}^1\!/_{10} \times {}^1\!/_{5} = 200/50 = 4 \text{ mg/dL}$$

2. **What is the molarity of an unknown HCl solution with a specific gravity of 1.10 and an assay percentage of 18.5%? (Atomic weights: H = 1.00794, Cl = 35.4527.)**

Answer:

$$\text{Specific gravity} \times \text{Assay percentage} = \text{g/mL}$$
$$1.10 \times 0.185 = 0.2035 \text{ g/mL}$$
$$0.2035 \text{ g/mL} \times 1000 = 203.5 \text{ g/L}$$

$$\text{Molarity} = \frac{\text{g/L}}{\text{Molecular weight (MW)}}$$

$$= \frac{203.5}{36.5} = 5.6 \text{ M}$$

3. **A 4.0-mg/dL standard solution is needed. To prepare 100 mL of the working standard, how much stock standard of a 1-mg/mL solution is needed?**

Answer:

$$\text{Volume } (V_1) \times \text{Concentration } (C_1) =$$
$$\text{Volume } (V_2) \times \text{Concentration } (C_2)$$
$$1 \text{ mg/1 mL} = 100 \text{ mg/100 mL (dL)}$$

$$100 \text{ mL} \times 4 \text{ mg/dL} = x \text{ mL} \times 100 \text{ mg/dL}$$

$$x = \frac{100 \times 4}{100} = 4 \text{ mL}$$

4. **How many milliliters (mL) of 0.25 M NaOH are needed to make 100 mL of a 0.05 M solution of NaOH?**

Answer:

$$\text{Volume } (V_1) \times \text{Concentration } (C_1) =$$
$$\text{Volume } (V_2) \times \text{Concentration } (C_2)$$
$$x \text{ mL} \times 0.25 \text{ M} = 100 \text{ mL} \times 0.05 \text{ M}$$

$$x = \frac{100 \times 0.05}{0.25} = 20 \text{ mL}$$

5. **How many grams of H_2SO_4 (MW = 98) are in 750 mL of 3M H_2SO_4?**
Answer:

$$3\text{M} \times 98 = 3 \times 98 = 294 \text{ g/L}$$

$$\frac{294}{1000 \text{ mL}} = \frac{x \text{ g}}{750 \text{ mL}}$$

$$x \text{ g} = \frac{750 \times 294}{1000} = 220 \text{ g}$$

6. **How many grams of sulfosalicylic acid (MW = 254) are required to prepare 1L of a 3% (w/v) solution?**

Answer:

$$3\% \text{ w/v} = 3\text{g/100 mL} = x \text{ g/1000 mL}$$

$$x = \frac{1000 \times 3}{100} = \frac{3000}{100} = 30 \text{ g}$$

7. **How many milliliters of a 3% solution can be made if 6 grams of solute are available?**

Answer:

$$3\% = \frac{3 \text{ g}}{100 \text{ mL}} = \frac{6 \text{ g}}{x \text{ mL}}$$

$$\frac{6 \times 100}{3} = \frac{600}{3} = 200 \text{ mL}$$

8. **Calculate the molarity of a solution that contains 18.7 g of KCl (MW: 74.5) in 500 mL of water.**

Answer:

$$\text{Molarity (M)} = \frac{\text{Gram/liter}}{\text{Molecular weight}}$$

$$M = \frac{18.7 \text{ g}}{500 \text{ mL}} = \frac{37.4 \text{ g}}{1000 \text{ mL}}$$

$$M = \frac{37.42 \text{ g/L}}{74.5} = 0.5$$

BIBLIOGRAPHY

Adams DS: Lab math: a handbook of measurements, calculations and other quantitative skills for use at the bench, Cold Spring Harbor, NY, 2003, Cold Spring Harbor Press.

Campbell JB, Campbell JM: Laboratory mathematics: medical and biological applications, ed 5, St Louis, 1997, Mosby.

Doucette LJ: Basic mathematics for the health-related professions, Philadelphia, 2000, Saunders.

Doucette LJ: Mathematics for the clinical laboratory, ed 2, St. Louis, 2011, Saunders.

Johnson CW, Timmons DL, Hall PE: Essential lab math, concepts and applications for the chemical and clinical lab technician, Clifton Park, NY, 2003, Thomson Delmar Learning.

Kaplan LA, Pesce AJ: Clinical chemistry: theory, analysis, correlation, ed 5, St Louis, 2010, Mosby.

REVIEW QUESTIONS

Questions 1 through 4: Match the terms with their respective definitions (a to d).

1. ___ Ratio

2. ___ Concentration

3. ___ Molarity

4. ___ Dilution
   a. The amount of one substance relative to the amounts of other substances in the solution
   b. Relative concentrations of the components of a mixture
   c. The gram-molecular mass (or weight) of a compound per liter of solution
   d. Expression of one amount relative to another amount

5. How would each of the following numbers be rounded off to one less decimal place?
   a. 6.32
   b. 15.57
   c. 10.02
   d. 25.96
   e. 23.7

6. To dilute a serum specimen 1:10, _____ parts of serum would be added to _____ parts distilled water.
   a. 1, 10
   b. 1, 9
   c. 0.5, 4.5
   d. Both b and c

7. 3 grams of solute in 100 mL of solvent equals _____% (w/v).
   a. 0.3
   b. 3
   c. 30
   d. 300

8. 20 grams of solute dissolved in 1 L of solvent equals _____% (w/v).
   a. 0.2
   b. 2
   c. 20
   d. 200

9. If 6 mL of liquid is placed in a volumetric flask and the volume is brought to 100 mL total, the solution is _____% of liquid.
   a. 0.6
   b. 6
   c. 60
   d. None of the above.

10. How many grams of NaCl would be used to prepare 1000 mL of a 5% (w/v) solution of NaCl?
    a. 0.5 g
    b. 5 g
    c. 50 g
    d. 500 g

11. If there is 25 g of NaCl per liter of solution, what is the molarity?
    a. 025 M
    b. 0.43 M
    c. 0.5 M
    d. 1.0 M

12. How many grams of NaCl are needed to prepare 1000 mL of a 0.5 M solution of NaCl?
    a. 5 g
    b. 15 g
    c. 29 g
    d. 58.4 g

13. How much $CaCl_2$ is needed to prepare 500 mL of a 0.5 M solution of $CaCl_2$?
    a. 27.7 g
    b. 40.0 g
    c. 57.8 g
    d. 115.6 g

14. If 0.1 mL of serum, 5 mL of reagent, and 4.9 mL of distilled water are mixed together, what is the dilution of the serum in the final solution?
    a. 1:5
    b. 1:10
    c. 1:50
    d. 1:100

15. What is the correct formula for calculating a percent (w/v) solution?
    a. Grams of solute/Volume of solution × 100
    b. Grams of solute × Volume of solvent × 100
    c. Volume of solvent/Grams of solute × 100
    d. Grams of solute × Volume of solvent/100

16. If a solution contains 20 g of solute dissolved in 0.5 L of water, what is the percentage of this solution?
    a. 2%
    b. 4%
    c. 6%
    d. 8%

17. If a glucose standard solution contains 10 mg/dL of glucose, a 1:10 dilution of this standard contains how much glucose?
    a. 0.01 mg/dL
    b. 0.1 mg/dL
    c. 1 mg/dL
    d. None of the above.

18. How is a 25% w/w solution prepared?
    a. 0.25 g solute and 75 g solvent
    b. 2.5 g solute and 97.5 g solvent
    c. 25 g solute and 75 g solvent
    d. 75 g solute and 25 g solvent

19. How many milliliters (mL) of bleach in an original bottle are needed to prepare a 10% solution?
    a. 0.1 mL bleach and 100 mL water
    b. 1.0 mL bleach and 90 mL water
    c. 10 mL bleach and 90 mL water
    d. Bleach is already a 10% solution in the original bottle.

20. What is the dilution factor if 4 mL of serum is added to 12 mL of diluent?
    a. 3
    b. 4
    c. 12
    d. 15

21. What is the dilution factor if 0.5 mL of serum is added to 2 mL of diluent?
    a. 0.5
    b. 1.5
    c. 2.5
    d. 5

22. Serum is diluted with an equal amount of diluent (e.g., tube #1, 1:2 and tube #2, 1:2). What is the concentration in tube #2 if the original concentration was 100 mg/dL?
    a. 12.5 mg/dL
    b. 25.0 mg/dL
    c. 50.0 mg/dL
    d. 75.0 mg/dL

23. If a total of 125 mL of a 10% solution is diluted to 500 mL in a 500 mL volumetric flask, what is the concentration of the resulting new solution?
    a. 0.25%
    b. 2.5%
    c. 25%
    d. None of the above.

24. If only 25 mL of a 9% saline solution is available in the laboratory, how many mL of 5% saline solution can be prepared using all available saline solution?
    a. 4.5 mL
    b. 25.0 mL
    c. 45.0 mL
    d. 100 mL

25. What volume of 25% alcohol is needed to prepare 500 mL of 15% alcohol?
    a. 30 mL
    b. 300 mL
    c. 350 mL
    d. 375 mL

CHAPTER 8

QUALITY ASSESSMENT AND QUALITY CONTROL IN THE CLINICAL LABORATORY

Learning Objectives

At the conclusion of this chapter, the student will be able to:

- Discuss how federal and professional regulations require the implementation of quality assessment programs in the clinical laboratory.

- Define terms used in quality assessment.

- Identify the components necessary to a laboratory's quality assessment program, including its quality control program and the use of control specimens.

- Assess the diagnostic usefulness of results reported, which requires an understanding of accuracy and precision as well as specificity and sensitivity, for laboratory tests and methodologies.

- Explain the sources of variance or error in a laboratory procedure.

- Explain the importance of a quality control program, including using control samples, determining control range, and using quality control charts.

- Describe the use of reference values, including using the mean and standard deviation in determining reference range.

Quality can be defined as the worth of services. Six Sigma[1] and Lean define the components critical to quality as the key measurable characteristics of a product or process whose performance standards or specification limits must be met to satisfy the customer. This process may include the upper and lower specification limits or any other factors related to the product or service. The assessment of quality results for the various analyses is critical and an important component of the operation of a high-quality laboratory.

Quality and safety are of the utmost importance in a clinical laboratory. Diagnostic laboratory test results play a decisive role not only in patient safety but in public health, clinical medical decisions, and research. It is estimated that approximately 6.8 billion laboratory tests are performed annually in the United States, with revenue of $52 billion in 2007. Although this is an impressive amount of money, it represents only 2.3% of U.S. health care expenditures and 2% of Medicare expenditures. Over 4000 laboratory tests are available for clinical use and around 500 of them are performed on a regular basis.[2]

CLINICAL LABORATORY IMPROVEMENT AMENDMENTS

In 1988, the U.S. Congress enacted the **Clinical Laboratory Improvement Amendments of 1988 (CLIA '88)** in response to concerns about laboratory testing errors.[3] The final CLIA rule, Laboratory Requirements Relating to Quality Systems and Certain Personnel Qualifications, was published in the Federal Register on January 24, 2003.[4] Enactment of CLIA established a minimum threshold for all aspects of clinical laboratory testing.

The introduction of routine **quality control (QC)** in the clinical laboratory was a major advance in improving the accuracy and reliability of clinical laboratory testing. Errors occurring during the analytical phase of testing within clinical laboratories are now relatively rare. Effective April 24, 2003, all laboratories are required to meet and follow the final QC requirements. These regulations established minimum requirements with general QC systems for all nonwaived testing. In addition, a controversial regulation published in January 2004 allows the Centers for Medicare and Medicaid Services (CMS) to consider acceptable alternative approaches to QC practices, called **equivalent quality control (EQC),** for laboratory testing.

VOLUNTARY ACCREDITING ORGANIZATIONS

The public's focus on health care delivery is relevant to most areas of work done in clinical laboratories. Standards have been set by **The Joint Commission (TJC),** formerly the Joint Commission on Accreditation of Healthcare Organizations, reflecting the commission's focus on quality assessment programs. TJC requires hospital laboratories to be accredited by TJC itself, the Commission on Office Laboratory Accreditation (COLA), or the College of American Pathologists (CAP).

TJC has announced that a **periodic performance review (PPR)** will be required for the laboratory accreditation program.[5] The PPR is a formal standards evaluation tool intended to support continuous compliance and is being added to the accreditation process at the request of accredited laboratories. Effective January 1, 2006, a laboratory must participate in either the full PPR or one of the three approved PPR options. Laboratories in complex organizations (e.g., hospital and laboratory) are required to participate in the PPR using the same methodology or selection of submission choice as the primary program. For example, if the primary program completes the full PPR, the laboratory will also complete the full PPR. Laboratories in TJC-accredited organizations that are accredited by a cooperative partner (e.g., CAP or COLA) are not required to complete the laboratory PPR. These laboratories need to participate in an equivalent intracycle assessment process. For TJC-accredited organizations that only provide waived-testing laboratory services, the standard requirements are addressed in the organizational PPR.

ISO 15189

The International Organization for Standardization (ISO) is the world's largest developer and publisher of international standards. ISO is a network of the national standards institutes of 159 countries, with one member per country and a Central Secretariat in Geneva, Switzerland, that coordinates the system. ISO is a nongovernmental organization that forms a bridge between the public and private sectors. It enables problem solving by consensus building on solutions that meet both the requirements of business and the needs of society.

ISO standards and certification are widely used by industry, but now ISO 15189 has been formulated for clinical laboratories. The standard, ISO 15189, is based on ISO/IEC 17025, the main standard used by testing and calibration laboratories and ISO 9001. Introduced in 2003 and developed with the input of the CAP, ISO 15189 has gained some standing abroad as a mandatory accreditation, such as in Australia, the Canadian province of Ontario, and many European countries. In the United States, ISO 15189 accreditation remains optional.

Requirements for quality and competence in ISO 15189 are unique because it takes into consideration the specific requirements of the medical environment and the importance of the medical laboratory to patient care (Box 8-1). ISO 15189:2007 is for use by medical laboratories in developing their quality management systems and assessing their own competence, and for use by accreditation bodies in confirming or recognizing the competence of medical laboratories. ISO 15189 contains the general requirements for testing and calibration laboratories. This working group included provision of advice to users of the laboratory service, the collection of patient samples, the interpretation of test results, acceptable turnaround times, how testing is to be provided in a medical emergency, and the lab's role in the education and training of health care staff. [6]

CAP 15189 is a voluntary, nonregulated accreditation to the ISO 15189:2007 Standard as published by the International Organization of Standardization. CAP 15189 requires a steadfast commitment to the laboratory management system and all interacting departments. CAP 15189 does not replace CAP's CLIA-based Laboratory Accreditation Program, but rather complements CAP accreditation and other quality systems by optimizing processes to improve patient care, strengthen the deployment of quality standard, reduce errors and risk, and control costs. CAP 15189 promotes sustainable quality by looking beyond individual procedures and discovering ways to continuously improve the structure and function of laboratory operations. As a management philosophy, CAP 15189 raises the bar on quality as it drives decisions throughout an entire institution.[7]

LEAN AND SIX SIGMA

Pioneering clinical laboratories in the United States that use management systems such as Lean (Box 8-2), which focuses on reducing waste, and Six Sigma, a metric and methodology that focuses on reducing variability, can have an immediate and recognizable impact when properly applied. When either of these systems was used to redesign workflow in high-volume core hematology and chemistry labs, a 50% reduction in average test turnaround time, a 40% to 50% improvement in labor productivity, and a comparable improvement in the quality of results were observed.[8]

Lean principles of reduction of unnecessary and non–value-added activities to reduce total production time and effort can be appropriately applied in all sections of the laboratory (e.g., urinalysis). Lean tools focus on identifying steps in a procedure that are error prone. If these steps cannot be eliminated, they must be controlled. Lean principles support the concept of doing activities right the first time, with minimal wasted time and effort. One highly effective tool in applying Lean principles is a process map or external and internal activities related to a specific laboratory assay. This mapping (see Chapter 14) allows for a step-by-step analysis. Knowledge of a detailed process allows for improvement in outcomes.[8]

BOX 8-1
ISO 15189 Overview

Management Requirements	Technical Requirements
Organization and management	Personnel
Quality management system	Accommodation and environmental conditions
Document control	Laboratory equipment
Review of contracts	Preexamination Procedures
Examination by referral laboratories	Examination Procedures
External services and supplies	Assuring quality of examination procedures
Advisory services	Postexamination procedures
Resolution of complaints	Reporting of results
Identification and control of nonconformities	
Corrective action	
Preventive action	
Continual improvement	
Quality and technical records	
Internal audits	
Management review	

From Malone B: ISO accreditation comes to America, Clin Lab News 35:1–4, 2009.

BOX 8-2
Key Lean Lessons

- It is not possible to overcommunicate.
- Continuously focus on improvement.
- Engage all facets of an organization, not just a core team.
- Actions speak louder than words.
- Ideas flow from the bottom up.
- Be respectful to every individual. Listen to and seriously consider their ideas.
- A feedback loop is critical to overcome challenges.
- Staff must be accountable to achieve success.

From Coons J, Courtois H: LEAN lab puts patient safety first, MLO Med Lab Obs 41:35, 2009.

QUALITY ASSESSMENT—ERROR ANALYSIS

Two types of errors occur in error analysis[9]: active error and latent error. An active error is obvious. It occurs at the interface between a health care worker and the patient (Box 8-3). In comparison, a latent error is less obvious. Latent failures are related to the organization or design of a laboratory (Box 8-4).

Ways to improve overall errors include at least three strategies:

1. Formal patient safety training, including discussion of disconnect between laboratory personnel and the patient
2. Enhanced communication between patients and laboratory staff and providers directly caring for patients
3. Quality improvement projects that involve patient outcomes data and feedback of this data to laboratory staff, with an analysis of the consequences of high- and low-quality work

QUALITY ASSESSMENT—PHASES OF TESTING

The total testing process (TTP) serves as the primary point of reference for focusing on quality in the clinical laboratory.[10] TTP is defined by activities in three distinct phases related to workflow outside and inside the laboratory:

1. Preanalytical, (Preexamination)
2. Analytical, (Examination)
3. Postanalytical, (Postexamination)

Currently, the majority of laboratory errors are related to the preexamination or postexamination phases of testing rather than the examination phase. Specimen-related errors continue to be a major problem[2] (Fig. 8-1), leading to unnecessary costs to hospitals estimated at $200 to $400 million annually.[11]

BOX 8-3
Examples of Active Errors

- Failing to identify a patient before phlebotomy
- Missing blood vessel during phlebotomy
- Errors with collection tubes
- Errors with transportation system (e.g., pneumatic tube)
- Errors with data entry
- Errors with instrument or computer (e.g., ignoring instrument flag)

Modified from Astion M: Latent errors in lab services, Clin Lab News 35:15, 2009.

BOX 8-4
Examples of Latent Errors

- Staffing problems (e.g., chronic shortages)
- Information technology (e.g., no interface with technology)
- Equipment malfunctions (e.g., old error-prone analyzers)
- Work environment (e.g., multitasking, poor lab layout, disconnect between lab and patients)
- Policy and procedures (e.g., relabeling of mislabeled or unlabeled tubes, lab requisition variation)
- Teamwork factors (e.g., poor communication between shifts, departmental "silos")
- Management/organization (e.g., when profit is a goal, ignoring patient safety, deemphasis on incident reports and interventions based on analysis)

Modified from Astion M: Latent errors in lab services, Clin Lab News 35:15, 2009.

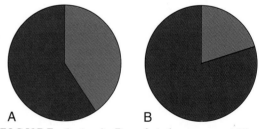

FIGURE 8-1 **A,** Preanalytical errors are **46%** to **68.2%** of total errors. **B,** Postanalytical errors are **18.5%** to **47%** of total errors. (From Plebani M: Errors in clinical laboratories or errors in laboratory medicine? Clin Chem Lab Med 44:750–759, 2006.)

To reduce and potentially eliminate laboratory errors, a quality assessment program is mandated. A **quality assessment program** can be divided into two major components: nonanalytical factors and the analysis of quantitative data (quality control). CAP[7] includes a variety of considerations in quality assessment management (Box 8-5). The Institute for Quality Laboratory Medicine (IQLM)[11] has developed 12 measures to evaluate quality in

BOX 8-5

College of American Pathologists Quality Assessment Considerations

- Supervision
- Procedure manual
- Specimen collection and handling
- Results reporting
- Reagents, calibration, and standards
- Controls
- Instruments and equipment
- Personnel
- Physical facilities
- Laboratory safety

From College of American Pathologists: Chemistry-coagulation, chemistry and toxicology, and point-of-care checklists, revised 10/06/2005, www.cap.org. Accessed October 2005.

BOX 8-6

Institute for Quality Laboratory Medicine Proposed Quality Assessment Measures

Preanalytical (Preexamination) Phase

- Test order accuracy
- Patient identification
- Blood culture contamination

Test System/Preanalytical (Preexamination)

- Adequacy of specimen information

Analytical Phase (Examination)

- Accuracy of point-of-care testing
- Cervical cytology/biopsy correlation

Test System/Analytical (Examination)

- Diabetes monitoring
- Hyperlipidemia screening

Postanalytical (Postexamination) Phase

- Critical value reporting
- Turnaround time

Test System/Postanalytical (Postexamination)

- Clinician satisfaction
- Clinician follow-up

From Institute for Quality Laboratory Medicine (IQLM), www.phppo.cdc.gov. Accessed October 2005.

the laboratory, based on the phase of testing (Boxes 8-6 and 8-7).

Nonanalytical Factors in Quality Assessment

To guarantee the highest-quality laboratory results and to comply with CLIA regulations, a variety of preanalytical and postanalytical factors need to be considered.

Qualified Personnel

The competence of personnel is an important determinant of the quality of the laboratory result.[12] Only properly certified personnel can perform nonwaived assays. CLIA '88 requirements for laboratory personnel in regard to levels of education and experience or training must be followed for laboratories doing moderately complex or highly complex testing.

In addition to the actual performance of analytical procedures, competent laboratory personnel must be able to perform QC activities, maintain instruments, and keep accurate and systematic records of reagents and control specimens, equipment maintenance, and patient and analytical data. For new laboratory personnel, a thorough orientation to the laboratory procedures and policies is vital.

Periodic opportunities for personal upgrading of technical skills and obtaining new relevant information should be made available to all persons working in the laboratory. This can be accomplished through in-service training classes, opportunities to attend continuing education courses, and by encouraging independent study habits by means of scientific journals and audiovisual materials.

Personnel performance should be monitored with periodic evaluations and reports. Quality

BOX 8-7

Examples of Potential Preanalytical/ Analytical/Postanalytical Errors

Preanalytical (Preexamination)

- Specimen obtained from wrong patient
- Specimen procured at the wrong time
- Specimen collected in the wrong tube or container
- Blood specimens collected in the wrong order
- Incorrect labeling of specimen
- Improper processing of specimen

Analytical (Examination)

- Oversight of instrument flags
- Out-of-control quality control results
- Wrong assay performed

Postanalytical (Postexamination)

- Verbal reporting of results
- Instrument: Laboratory Information System (LIS) incompatibility error
- Confusion about reference ranges

assessment demands that a supervisor monitor the results of daily work and that all analytical reports produced during a particular shift be evaluated for errors and omissions.

Established Laboratory Policies

Laboratory policies should be included in a laboratory reference manual available to all hospital personnel. Each laboratory must have an up-to-date safety manual. This manual contains a comprehensive listing of approved policies, acceptable practices, and precautions, including standard blood and body fluid precautions. Specific regulations that conform to current state and general requirement, such as Occupational Safety and Health Administration (OSHA) regulations, must be included in the manual. Other sources of mandatory and voluntary standards include TJC, CAP, and the Centers for Disease Control and Prevention (CDC).

Laboratory Procedure Manual

A complete laboratory procedure manual for all analytical procedures performed within the laboratory must be provided. The manual must be reviewed regularly, in some cases annually, by the supervisory staff and updated as needed.

The Clinical and Laboratory Standards Institute (CLSI)[13] recommends that these procedure manuals follow a specific pattern in how the procedures in the manual are organized. Each assay done in the laboratory must be included in the manual. The minimal components are as follows:

- Title of the assay
- Principle of the procedure and statement of clinical applications
- Protocol for specimen collection and storage
- QC information
- Reagents, supplies, and equipment
- Procedural protocol
- "Normal" reference ranges
- Technical sources of error
- Limitations of the procedure
- Proper procedures for specimen collection and storage

Test Requisitioning

A laboratory test can be requested by a primary care provider or, in some states, the patient. The request, either hard copy or electronic, must include the patient identification data, time and date of specimen collection, source of the specimen, and analyses to be performed. The information on the accompanying specimen container must match exactly the patient identification on the test request. The information needed by the physician to assist in ordering tests must be included in a database or handbook.

Patient Identification, Specimen Procurement, and Labeling

Maintaining an electronic database or handbook of specimen requirement information is one of the first steps in establishing a quality assessment program for the clinical laboratory. Current information about obtaining appropriate specimens, special collection requirements for various types of tests, ordering tests correctly, and transporting and processing specimens appropriately should be included in the database.

Patients must be carefully identified. For outpatients, identification may be validated with two forms of identification. Using established specimen requirement information, the clinical specimens must be properly labeled or identified once they have been obtained from the patient. Computer-generated labels assist in making certain that proper patient identification is noted on each specimen container sent to the laboratory. An important rule to remember is that the analytical result can only be as good as the specimen received (see Specimen Collection, Chapter 3).

Specimen Transportation and Processing

Specimens must be efficiently transported to the laboratory. Some assays require special handling conditions, such as placing the specimen on ice immediately after collection. Specimens should be tested within 2 hours of collection to produce accurate results. Documentation of specimen arrival times in the laboratory as well as other specific test request data are important aspects of the quality assessment process. It is important that the specimen status can be determined at any time—that is, where in the laboratory processing system a given specimen can be found.

Preventive Maintenance of Equipment

Monitoring the temperatures of heat blocks and refrigerators is important to the quality of test performance. Microscopes, centrifuges, and other pieces of equipment must be regularly cleaned and checked for accuracy. A preventive maintenance schedule should be followed for all automated equipment. Failure to monitor equipment regularly can produce inaccurate test results and lead to expensive repairs.

Manufacturers will recommend a calibration frequency determined by measurement system stability and will communicate in product inserts the specific criteria for mandatory recalibration of instrument systems. These may include:

- Reagent lot change
- Major component replacement
- Instrument maintenance
- New software installation

Clinical laboratories must follow CLIA or the manufacturer's requirements for instrument calibration frequency, whichever is most stringent. CLIA requires that laboratories recalibrate an analytical method at least every 6 months.

Quality Assessment Procedures

Documentation of an ongoing quality assessment program in clinical laboratories is mandated by CLIA regulations.[3] Quality assessment programs monitor test request procedures; patient identification, specimen procurement, and labeling; specimen transportation and processing procedures; laboratory personnel performance; laboratory instrumentation, reagents, and analytical test procedures; turnaround times; and the accuracy of the final result. Complete documentation of all procedures involved in obtaining the analytical result for the patient sample must be maintained and monitored in a systematic manner.

Proficiency Testing

Proficiency testing (PT) is incorporated into the CLIA requirements.[3] In addition to the use of internal QC programs, each laboratory should participate in an external PT program as a means of verification of laboratory accuracy.

Periodically a laboratory tests a specimen that has been provided by a government agency, professional society, or commercial company; identical samples are sent to a group of laboratories participating in the PT program. Each laboratory analyzes the specimen, reports the results to the agency, and is evaluated and graded on those results in comparison to results from other laboratories. In this way, quality control between laboratories is monitored.

TJC has an accreditation participation requirement (ORYX requirement) for proficiency testing in the laboratory. Laboratory proficiency testing is required by federal CLIA regulations.

Accuracy in Reporting Results and Documentation

Many laboratories have established critical values or the Delta check system to monitor individual patient results. The difference between a patient's present laboratory result and consecutive previous results which exceed a predefined limit is referred to as a *Delta check*. An abrupt change, high or low, can trigger this computer-based warning system and should be investigated before reporting a patient result. Delta checks are investigated by the laboratory internally to rule out mislabeling, clerical error, or possible analytical error.

Highly abnormal individual test values and significant differences from previous results in the Delta check system alert the technologist to a potential problem. At times, a phone call to the physician or charge nurse may be made by the laboratory technologist to investigate possible preanalytical errors such as obtaining specimens from IV lines, mislabeling a specimen, or actual changes in a patient's condition. Other quantitative control systems (discussed later) are also used to ensure the quality of test results.

The ongoing process of making certain the correct laboratory result is reported for the right patient in a timely manner and at the correct cost is known as *continuous quality improvement* (CQI). This process assures the clinician ordering the test that the testing process has been done in the best possible way to provide the most useful information in diagnosing or managing the particular patient in question. Quality assessment indicators are evaluated as part of the CQI process to monitor the laboratory's performance. Each laboratory will set its own indicators, depending on the specific goals of the laboratory. Any quality assessment indicators should be appreciated as a tool to ensure that reported results are of the highest quality.

An important aspect of quality assessment is documentation. CLIA regulations mandate that any problem or situation that might affect the outcome of a test result be recorded and reported. All such incidents must be documented in writing, including the changes proposed and their implementation, and follow-up monitored. Reportable incidents can involve specimens that are improperly collected, labeled, or transported to the laboratory or problems concerning prolonged turnaround times for test results. There must be a reasonable attempt to correct the problems or situation, and all steps in this process must be documented.

Another valuable quality assessment technique is to look at the data generated for each patient and inspect the relationships between them. These many relationships include the mathematical association between anions and cations in the electrolyte report, the correlation between protein and casts in urine, and the relationship between hemoglobin and hematocrit and the appearance of the blood smear in hematologic studies.

Laboratory computer systems and electronic information processing expedites record keeping. Quality assessment programs require documentation, and computer record-keeping capability assists in this effort. When control results are within the acceptable limits established by the laboratory, these data provide the necessary link between the control and patient data, thus giving reassurance that the patient results are reliable, valid, and reportable. This information is necessary to document that uniform protocols have been established and are being followed. The data can also support the proper functioning capabilities of the test systems being used at the time patient results are produced.

Quality Control

As mentioned earlier, QC consists of procedures used to detect errors that result from test system failure, adverse environmental conditions, and variance in operator performance, as well as procedures to monitor the accuracy and precision of test performance over time.[10] Accrediting agencies require monitoring and documentation of quality assessment records. CLIA states, "The laboratory must establish and follow written quality control procedures for monitoring and evaluating the quality of the analytical testing process of each method to assure the accuracy and reliability of patient test results and reports."[3] For tests of moderate complexity, CLIA states that laboratories comply with the more stringent of the following requirements:

- Perform and document control procedures using at least two levels of control material each day of testing.
- Follow the manufacturer's instructions for QC.

QC activities include monitoring the performance of laboratory instruments, reagents, other testing products, and equipment. A written record of QC activities for each procedure or function should include details of deviation from the usual results, problems, or failures in functioning or in the analytical procedure and any corrective action taken in response to these problems.

Documentation of QC includes preventive maintenance records, temperature charts, and QC charts for specific assays. All products and reagents used in the analytical procedures must be carefully checked before actual use in testing patient samples. Use of QC specimens, proficiency testing, and standards depends on the specific requirements of the accrediting agency.

In addition to in-house QC, laboratories may be asked to assist other departments in the health care facility in their QC measures. This can include checking the effectiveness of autoclaves in surgery or in the laundry or providing aseptic checks for the pharmacy, blood bank, or dialysis service.

Control Specimens

A QC program for the laboratory makes use of a **control specimen,** which is a material or solution with a known concentration of the analyte being measured in the testing procedure. Most clinical laboratories use multiconstituent controls because these require less storage space, offer ease of inventory, and increase manufacturer services through peer laboratory comparisons. Lyophilized and liquid control materials offer good stability and reasonable expiration dating. Liquid controls may offer greater reproducibility between bottles because, unlike lyophilized controls, no pipetting error is added on reconstitution. Suppliers often offer to sequester a specific quantity (estimated usage) of control material to be sent to the laboratory at the customer's request. This ensures that the customer can continue to receive the same lot for a long time.

A control specimen must be carried through the entire test procedure and treated in exactly the same way as any unknown specimen; it must be affected by all the variables that affect the unknown specimen. The use of control specimens is based on the fact that repeated determinations on the same or different portions (or aliquots) of the same sample will not, as a rule, give identical values for any particular constituent. Many factors can produce variations in laboratory analyses. With a properly designed control system, it is possible to monitor testing variables.

According to CLIA regulations, a minimum of two control specimens (negative or normal and positive or increased) must be run in every 24-hour period when patient specimens are being run. Alternately, when automated analyzers are in use, the bilevel controls are run once every 8 hours of operation (or once per shift).[3]

The use of QC specimens is an indication of the overall reliability (both accuracy and precision) of the results reported by the laboratory, a part of the quality assessment process. If the value of the QC specimen for a particular method is not within the predetermined acceptable range, it must be assumed that the values obtained for the unknown specimens are also incorrect, and the results are not reported. After the procedure has been reviewed for any indication of error, and the error has been found and corrected, testing must be repeated until the control value falls within the acceptable range. In controlling the reliability of laboratory determinations, the objective is to reject results when there is evidence that more than the permitted amount of error has occurred. The clinical laboratory has several ways of controlling the reliability of its reported results.

QUALITY ASSESSMENT DESCRIPTORS

The ability of the reported laboratory results to substantiate a diagnosis, lead to a change in diagnosis, or provide follow-up on patient management is what makes laboratory assays useful to the clinician. The diagnostic usefulness of a test and its procedure is assessed by using statistical evaluations, such as descriptions of the accuracy and reliability of the test and its methodology. To describe the **reliability** of a particular procedure, two terms are often used: accuracy and precision. The reliability of a procedure depends on a combination of these two factors, although they are different and are not dependent on each other. *Variance* is another general term that describes the factors or fluctuations that affect the measurement of the substance in question. Statistical methods available also can assess the usefulness of a test result in terms of its sensitivity, specificity, and predictive value.

Aspects of Clinical Quality Assessment

- *Accuracy* describes how close a test result is to the true value.
- *Calibration* is the comparison of an instrument measure or reading to a known physical constant.
- *Control* (noun) represents a specimen with a known value that is similar in composition, for example, to the patient's blood.
- *Precision* describes how close the test results are to one another when repeated analyses of the same material are performed.
- *Quality control* is a process that monitors the accuracy and reproducibility of results through the use of control specimens.
- *Standards* are highly purified substances of a known composition.

Accuracy versus Precision

The **accuracy** of a procedure refers to the closeness of the result obtained to the true or actual value (Fig. 8-2), whereas **precision** refers to repeatability, or reproducibility, of obtaining the same value in subsequent tests on the same sample (Fig. 8-3). It is possible to have great precision, with all laboratory personnel who perform the same procedure arriving at the same answer, but without accuracy if the answer does not represent the actual value being tested. The precision of a test, or its reproducibility, may be expressed as *standard deviation* (SD) or the derived *coefficient of variation* (CV). A procedure may be extremely accurate but so difficult to perform that laboratory personnel are

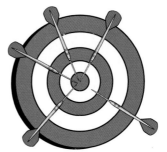

Accurate, less precise

FIGURE 8-2 **Accuracy.** (From Doucette LJ: Basic mathematics for the health related professions, Philadelphia, 2000, Saunders.)

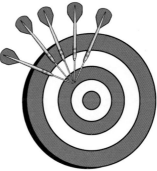

Precise, less accurate

FIGURE 8-3 **Precision.** (From Doucette LJ: Basic mathematics for the health related professions, Philadelphia, 2000, Saunders.)

unable to arrive at values close enough to be clinically meaningful.

In general terms, accuracy can be aided by the use of properly standardized procedures, statistically valid comparisons of new methods with established reference methods, the use of samples of known values (controls), and participation in PT programs.

Precision can be ensured by the proper inclusion of standards, reference samples, or control solutions; statistically valid replicate determinations of a single sample; and duplicate determinations of sufficient numbers of unknown samples. Day-to-day and between-run precision is measured by inclusion of control specimens.

Sensitivity and Specificity of a Test

Laboratory results that give medically useful information, including the specificity and sensitivity of the tests being ordered and reported, are important. Both specificity and sensitivity are desirable characteristics for a test, but in different clinical situations, one is generally preferred over the other.

For assessing the sensitivity and specificity of a test, four entities are needed: tests positive, tests negative, disease present (positive), and disease

Common Avoidable Causes of False-Positive and False-Negative Results

- Use of a test at an inappropriate time
- Use of an obsolete test
- Use of a test with inherently poor sensitivity or specificity
- Use of a test on a patient population with low or high prevalence of the disease under consideration
- Use of a test that lacks extensive clinical validation
- Use of a test on a patient population that differs from the intended or studied population

From Jackson B: The dangers of false-positive and false-negative test results: false-positive results as a function of pretest probability, Clin Lab Med 28:306, 2008.

Potential Consequences of False-Positive and False-Negative Results

- No impact in some cases
- Cascade of increasingly expensive or invasive follow-up testing
- Lengthened hospital stay
- Additional office visits
- Inappropriate therapy
- Psychological trauma caused by false belief of having a disease

From Jackson B: The dangers of false-positive and false-negative test results: false-positive results as a function of pretest probability, Clin Lab Med 28:306, 2008.

absent (negative). **True positives** are those subjects who have a positive test result and who also have the disease in question. **True negatives** represent those subjects who have a negative test result and who do not have the disease. **False positives** are those subjects who have a positive test result but do not have the disease. **False negatives** are those subjects who have a negative test result but do have the disease.

Every assay in the clinical laboratory is subject to false-positive and false-negative results. Common avoidable causes of false-positive and false-negative are presented in Boxes 8-8 and 8-9.

Sensitivity

The **sensitivity** of a test is defined as the proportion of cases with a specific disease or condition that give a positive test result (i.e., the assay correctly predicts with a positive result), as follows:

$$\text{Sensitivity \%} = \frac{\text{True positives}}{\text{True positives} + \text{False negatives}} \times 100$$

Practically, sensitivity represents how much of a given substance is measured; the more sensitive the test, the smaller the amount of assayed substance that is measured.

Specificity

The **specificity** of a test is defined as the proportion of cases with absence of the specific disease or condition that gives a negative test result (i.e., the assay correctly excludes with a negative result), as follows:

$$\text{Specificity \%} = \frac{\text{True negatives}}{\text{False positive} + \text{True negatives}} \times 100$$

Practically, specificity represents what is being measured. A highly specific test measures only the assay substance in question; it does not measure interfering or similar substances.

Predictive Values

To assess the **predictive value (PV)** for a test, the sensitivity, specificity, and prevalence of the disease in the population being studied must be known. The **prevalence** of a disease is the proportion of a population who has the disease. This is in contrast to the incidence of a disease, which is the number of subjects found to have the disease within a defined period, such as a year, in a population of 100,000.

A **positive predictive value (PPV)** for a test indicates the number of patients with an abnormal test result who have the disease, compared with all patients with an abnormal result, as follows:

$$\text{Positive predictive value} = \frac{\begin{array}{c}\text{Number of patients with disease}\\\text{and with abnormal test results}\end{array}}{\begin{array}{c}\text{Total number of patients with}\\\text{abnormal test results}\end{array}}$$

$$\text{Positive predictive value} = \frac{\text{True positives}}{\text{True positives} + \text{False positives}}$$

A **negative predictive value (NPV)** for a test indicates the number of patients with a normal test result who do not have the disease, compared with all patients with a normal (negative) result, as follows:

$$\text{Negative predictive value} = \frac{\text{True negatives}}{\text{True negatives} + \text{False negatives}}$$

QUALITY CONTROL STATISTICS

Statistically, the reference range for a particular measurement in most cases is related to a normal bell-shaped curve[14-16] (Fig. 8-4). This **gaussian curve** or **gaussian distribution** has been shown to be correct for virtually all types of biological, chemical, and physical measurements. A statistically valid series of individuals who are thought to represent a normal healthy group are measured, and the average value is calculated. This mathematical average is defined as the mean (x, called the *x-bar*). The distribution of all values around the average for the particular group measured is described statistically by the standard deviation.

Mean, Median, and Mode

Often used in laboratory measurements, the **mean** is the mathematical average calculated by taking the sum of the values and dividing by the number of values in the list. CLSI describes several methods for estimating the mean and precision for a control level.[15] CLSI recommends that at a minimum, 20 data points from 20 or more separate testing runs be obtained to determine an estimate of mean and precision. If 20 runs cannot be completed, a minimum of seven runs (three replicates per run) may be used to set provisional ranges. A mean and standard deviation can be calculated and used to set provisional ranges. The mean and limits derived from the abbreviated data collection should be replaced by a new mean and limits calculated when data from 20 separate runs becomes available.

The **median** is the middle value of a body of data. If all the variables are arranged in order of increasing magnitude in a body of data, the median is the variable that falls halfway between the highest and the lowest variables. The median equals the middle value. To find the median, the list of numbers must first be ranked according to magnitude, such as 2, 2, 3, 4, 5, 6, 7. The median number is the middle value in the list; in this example, of the seven numbers in the list, the median is 4.

The **mode** is the value most frequently occurring in a list of numbers. In the example of 2, 2, 3, 4, 5, 6, 7, the mode is 2.

Standard Deviation

Standard deviation (SD) is a measure of the spread, or variability, in a data set. Most scientific calculators contain a feature for calculating standard deviation.

The SD is the square root of the variance of the values in any one observation or in a series of test results. In any normal population, 68% of the values will be clustered above and below the average

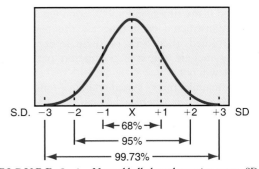

FIGURE 8-4 Normal bell-shaped gaussian curve. *SD,* Standard deviation.

and defined statistically as falling within the first standard deviation (±1 SD). The second standard deviation represents 95% of the values falling equally above and below the average (±2 SD), and 99.7% will be included within the third standard deviation (±3 SD). (Again, variations occur equally above and below the average value [or mean] for any measurement.) Thus, in determining reference values for a particular measurement, a statistically valid series of people are chosen and assumed to represent a healthy population. These people are then tested, and the results are averaged. The term *reference range* therefore means the range of values that includes 95% of the test results for a healthy reference population. This term replaces "normal values" or "normal range." The limits (or range) of normal are defined in terms of the standard deviation from the average value.

In evaluating an individual's state of health, values outside the third SD value are considered clearly abnormal. When the distribution is gaussian, the reference range closely approximates the mean ±2 SD. Values within the first (68%) and second (95%) SD limits are considered normal, whereas those between the second (95%) and third (99.7%) SD limits are questionable. The reference values are stated as a range of values. This stated range is in terms of SD units.

Confidence Intervals

When the reference range is expressed using 2 SD on either side of the mean, with 95% of the values falling above and below the mean, the term **confidence interval** or **confidence limits** is used. This interval should be kept in mind when there are day-to-day shifts in values for a particular analytical procedure. The **95% confidence** interval is used, in part, to account for certain unavoidable error caused by sampling variability and imprecision of the methods themselves.

As an example, for a population study, the 95% confidence interval can be interpreted in the following way. If the procedure or experiment is repeated many times, and a 95% confidence interval is constructed each time for the parameter being studied, then 95% of these intervals will actually include the true population parameter, and 5% will not.

The manufacturer's stated reference ranges give an indication of where a laboratory's mean and ranges may be established. Individual laboratories must establish an appropriate mean and QC limits based on the patient population. New lots of control material should be analyzed for each analyte in parallel with the control material in current use.

Coefficient of Variation

The **coefficient of variation (CV)** in percent (%CV) is equal to the standard deviation divided by the mean. The CV normalizes the variability of a data set by calculating the SD as a percent of the mean (Box 8-10). The CV can be used to compare the standard deviations of two samples. SDs cannot be compared directly without considering the mean. The %CV is helpful in comparing precision differences that exist among assays and assay methods.

After estimating the mean and total precision (SD) of the analytical measuring system, the next step is to set control limits as some multiple of the total precision around the mean. In many laboratories, the standard procedure is to set these control limits at ±2 SD; however, setting limits at ±2 SD can lean to certain problems. It is evident that ±2 SD ranges result in unnecessarily high false rejection rates. CLIA '88 does not explicitly recommend a method for determining when a system is "out of control," but this federal law does explain that laboratories must establish written procedures for monitoring and evaluating analytical testing processes (see Monitoring Quality Control).

With strict ±2 or ±3 SD limits, an out-of-control condition is marked by one QC value falling outside the limit of 2 or 3 SD. A ±2 SD limit offers a method that is sensitive to detecting a change but also presents a problem for a laboratory: a high rate of false rejection.

Determination of Control Range

Once a control solution has been purchased unassayed, it is necessary for the laboratory to determine the **acceptable control range** for a particular analysis, and there are various ways of establishing it. One method to establish a control range is to assay an aliquot of the control serum with the regular batch of assays for 15 to 25 days. In testing the control sample, it is important to treat it exactly like an unknown specimen; it must not be treated any more or less carefully than the unknown specimen.

Repeated determinations on different aliquots of the same sample will often not give identical values for any particular constituent. It has been shown that if a sufficient number of repeated determinations are made, the values obtained will fall into a normal bell-shaped curve. When a statistically sufficient number of determinations have been run (the number is different for averaged duplicate determinations and single tests), the mathematical mean (x) or average value can be calculated. The acceptable limits or variation from the mean for the control solution are then calculated on the basis of the standard deviation from the mean, using statistical formulas. Most laboratories use 2 SD above and below the mean as the allowable range of the control specimen, whereas others use this range as a warning limit. According to the normal bell-shaped curve, setting 2 SD as the allowable range for the control sample means that 95% of all determinations on that sample will fall within the allowable range, and 5% will be out of control. It may not be desirable to disallow this many batches, however, and the third SD may be chosen as the limit of control, or the action limit. Once the range of acceptable results has been established, one of the control specimens is included in each batch of determinations. If the control value is not within the limits established, the procedure must be repeated, and no patient results may be reported until the control value is acceptable.

Sources of Variance or Error

In general, it is impossible to obtain exactly the same result each time a determination is performed on a particular specimen. This may be described as the **variance,** or **error,** of a procedure. These factors include limitations of the procedure itself and limitations related to the sampling mechanism used.

Sampling Factors

One of the major difficulties in guaranteeing reliable results involves the sampling procedure. Sources of variance that involve the sample include the time of day when the sample is obtained, the

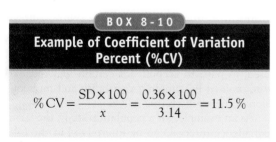

BOX 8-10

Example of Coefficient of Variation Percent (%CV)

$$\% \, CV = \frac{SD \times 100}{x} = \frac{0.36 \times 100}{3.14} = 11.5\%$$

SD, Standard deviation.

patient's position (lying down or seated), the patient's state of physical activity (in bed, ambulatory, or physically active), the interval since last eating (fasting or not), and the time interval and storage conditions between the collection of the specimen and its processing by the laboratory. The aging of the sample is another source of error.

Procedural Factors

Other sources of variance involve aging of chemicals or reagents, personal bias or limited experience of the person performing the determination, and laboratory bias because of variations in standards, reagents, environment, methods, or apparatus. There may also be experimental error resulting from changes in the method used for a particular determination, changes in instruments, or changes in personnel.

MONITORING QUALITY CONTROL

Levey-Jennings Charts

Most laboratories plot the daily control specimen values on a **quality control chart.** Levey-Jennings (Shewhart) QC plots[17] have traditionally been used to identify unacceptable runs and then evaluate the source and magnitude of the deviation to decide if results are to be released to patient charts (Fig. 8-5). The main purpose for control charting in the clinical laboratory is to aid in maintaining stability of the analytical measuring system (Fig. 8-6). The control chart attempts to detect changes in the analytical system (i.e., detect special causes of variation). After detecting such changes, an attempt is made to restore the measurement system to its previous level of performance.

Software designed for laboratory information systems (LIS) and personal computers is available to automate the plotting of control values. The software's complexity and capabilities (for multiple QC options) will vary among supplier, but typically all suppliers provide a graphical presentation of data using the traditional Levey-Jennings chart.

The mean value for the determination in question is then indicated on the chart, in addition to the limits of acceptable error. Control limits are generally set at ±2 SD or ±3 SD on either side of the mean. The 2- and 3-SD values might be indicated, with the 2-SD value as a warning limit and the 3-SD value as an action limit. Each day the control value is plotted on the chart, and any value falling "out of control" can easily be seen. The control chart serves as visual documentation of the information derived from using control specimens. A different control chart is plotted for each substance being determined. It is possible to observe trends and drift (see later discussion) leading toward trouble by plotting the control values daily. When procedural changes are made (e.g., addition of new reagents, standards, or instruments), these are also noted on the control chart.

Appropriate Testing Methods

Another part of the QC program concerns the way new procedures are validated before they are included among the methods routinely used by the laboratory. Each laboratory must determine the reproducibility (or confidence limits) for each procedure used and establish acceptable limits of variation for control specimens. The QC program includes calculation of the mean (or average value) and standard deviation and the

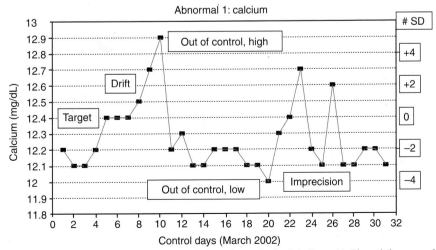

FIGURE 8-5 **Levey-Jennings quality control (QC) chart.** (From Kaplan LA, Pesce AJ: Clinical chemistry: theory, analysis, correlation, ed 5, St Louis, 2010, Mosby.)

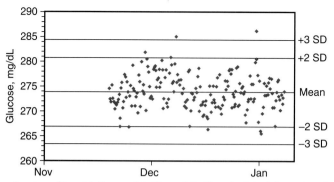

FIGURE 8-6 Levey-Jennings. (From McPherson RA, Pincus MR: Henry's clinical diagnosis and management by laboratory methods, ed 21, Philadelphia, 2006, Saunders.)

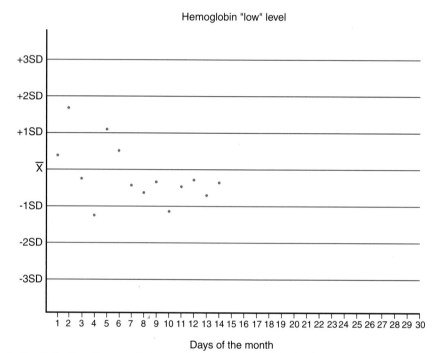

FIGURE 8-7 Shift. (From Doucette LJ: Basic mathematics for the health related professions, Philadelphia, 2000, Saunders.)

generation of control charts for each procedure. To detect problems, each laboratory must have an assessment routine for all procedures performed on a daily, weekly, or monthly basis. When such problems are indicated, they must be corrected as soon as possible and before patient results are reported.

Shifts, Trends, and Dispersion

Regular visual inspection of the control chart is useful for observing a shift, trend, or increased dispersion of results in the assay results of the control specimen. A **shift** (Fig. 8-7) is defined as a sudden and sustained change in one direction in control sample values. A **trend or drift** (Fig. 8-8) is a gradual change in the control sample results. A systematic drift or trend is displayed when the control value direction moves progressively in one direction from the mean for at least 3 days. By comparison, **dispersion** is observed when random error or lack of precision increases. Each type of change is indicative of particular problems. A shift or abrupt change may be observed with the sudden malfunction of an instrument. A trend error suggests a progressive problem with the testing system or control sample, such as deterioration of reagents or control specimen. Dispersion may indicate instability problems. The frequency of various error conditions is presented in Fig. 8-9.

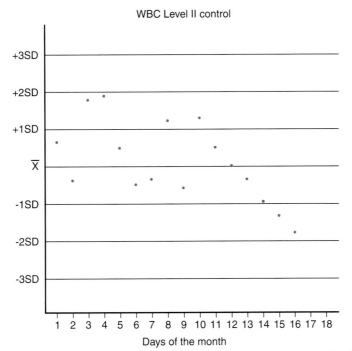

WBC Level II control

Days of the month

FIGURE 8-8   Trend. (From Doucette LJ: Basic mathematics for the health related professions, Philadelphia, 2000, Saunders.)

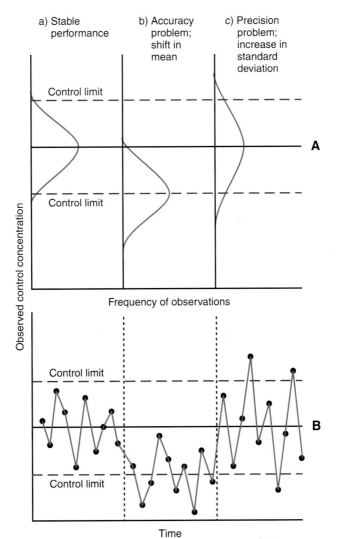

FIGURE 8-9   Conceptual basis of control charts. (From Burtis CA, Ashwood ER, Bruns DE: Tietz fundamentals of clinical chemistry, ed 6, St Louis, 2008, Saunders.)

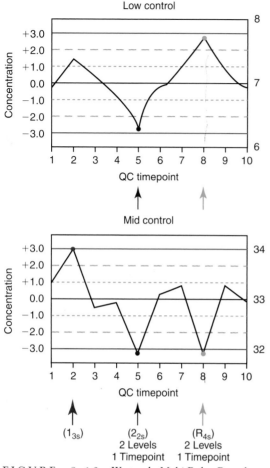

FIGURE 8-10 **Westgard Multi-Rule Procedure.** Example for 1_{3s}, 2_{2s}, and R_{4s}. QC, Quality control.

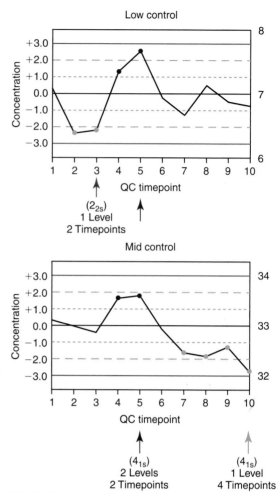

FIGURE 8-11 **Westgard Multi-Rule Procedure.** Example for 2_{2s}, 4_{1s} (across two levels), and 4_{1s} (across one level). QC, Quality control.

Westgard Rules

Westgard rules are often formulated to analyze data in control charts based on statistical methods[18] (Figs. 8-10, 8-11, and 8-12). These rules define specific performance limits for a particular assay and can be used to detect both random and systematic errors. The Westgard Multi-Rule Procedure is designed to improve the power of QC methods using ±3 SD limits to detect trends or shifts. While maintaining a low false rejection rate, Westgard's procedure examines individual values and determines the status of the measuring system. Proper use of the Westgard Multi-Rule Procedure can substantially reduce the incidence of false rejection by as much as 88% compared with strict ±2 SD limits.

Six Westgard rules are typically used; three are warning rules, and three are mandatory rules (Box 8-11). The violation of a warning rule should trigger a review of test procedures, reagent performance, and equipment calibration.

If a violation of a Westgard rule occurs, actions to take are:

1. Accept the results of the testing run if only a warning is violated.
2. Reject the results of the testing run when a mandatory rule is violated.
3. Increase the retesting range for a particular assay if either a warning or a mandatory rule is violated.

It is important to remember that CLIA requires laboratories to establish written procedures for monitoring and evaluating analytical testing processes, including procedures for resolving an out-of-control situation. Some possible control procedures include:

- Review the procedures used.
- Search for recent events that could cause change, such as a new reagent kit or lot, component replacement, or environmental condition (e.g., temperature, humidity).
- Prepare new control materials.

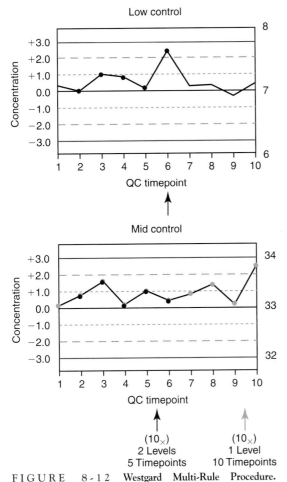

FIGURE 8-12 **Westgard Multi-Rule Procedure.** Examples for 10_x across two levels and 10_x for one level. QC, Quality control.

BOX 8-11

Six Westgard Rules for Analysis of Quality Control Charts

- 1 point is outside 2 SD (1_{2s})

If 1 point is outside 2 SD, then reject when:

- 1 point is outside 3 SD (1_{3s})
- 2 consecutive points are outside 2 (2_{2s})
  SD on same side of the center line
- Range of 2 points is greater than 4 (R_{4s})
  SD
- 4 consecutive points exceed 1 SD (4_{1s})
  on same side of the center line
- 10 consecutive points are above or $(10\ \bar{x})$
  below the mean

SD, Standard deviation.
From Westgard JO, Barry PL, Hunt MR, et al: A multi-rule Shewhart chart for quality control in clinical chemistry, Clin Chem 27:493, 1981.

- Follow the manufacturer's troubleshooting guide.
- Contact manufacturers of instruments, reagent materials, and controls.

The set of rules just outlined can be used together to form the Westgard Multi-Rule Procedure. However, a number of different configurations are possible for this same set of rules. When selecting a set of rules, the key is understanding how the set of rules performs statistically. Many software packages also apply multirule sets such as those described by Westgard. Automated monitoring of QC makes the Westgard Multi-Rule Procedure much easier to apply correctly.

TESTING OUTCOMES

It is important to realize that reference values will vary with innumerable factors, but especially between laboratories and between geographic locations. Each laboratory must provide the physician with information on the range of reference values for that particular laboratory. The values will be related to an overall reference range, but the values may be more refined or narrow and may be skewed in the particular situation in question.

Before physicians can determine whether a patient has a disease, they must know what is acceptable for a representative population of similar patients (e.g., same age, same gender, same ethnicity) as well as the analytical method used for an assay. To complicate matters, an individual may show daily, circadian, or physiologic variations. **Biometrics** (the science of statistics applied to biological observations) is a rapidly expanding field that attempts to describe these variations. The selection of a group on which to base "reference groups" is another problem confronting the individual laboratory.

Traditionally, reference ranges have been defined by testing such groups as blood donors, persons who are working and "feeling healthy," medical students, student nurses, and medical technologists.[15] Many established reference ranges reported in the medical literature have questionable validity because of factors such as poor sampling techniques, questionable selection of the normal group, and questionable use of clinical methods. In developing reference values previously referred to as "normal values," the proper statistical tools of sampling, selection of the comparison group, and analysis of data must be used.

REFERENCES

1. Six Sigma: http://www.isixsigma.com/sixsigma/six_sigma.asp (retrieved October 2005).
2. Iancu DM Handy BC: The value of laboratory medicine, http://laboratorian.advanceweb.com, retrieved May 19, 2009.

3. U.S. Department of Health and Human Services: Medicare, Medicaid, and CLIA programs: regulations implementing the Clinical Laboratory Improvement Amendments of 1988 (CLIA). Final rule, Federal Register 57:7002, 1992.

4. US Department of Health and Human Services, Centers for Medicare and Medicaid Services: Laboratory requirements relating to quality systems and certain personnel qualifications. Final Rule, 42CFR Part 405 et al (16:3640), Federal Register, Jan 24, 2003.

5. Joint Commission on Accreditation of Healthcare Organizations: Periodic performance review (PPR) for laboratories, www.jcaho.org (retrieved October 2005).

6. Ford A: Labs on the brink of ISO 15189 approval, CAP News , November, 2008.

7. College of American Pathologists: Checklists, revised 10/06/2005, www.cap.org (retrieved October 2005).

8. Smith TJ: Tracking the trends, Advance for the Laboratory 33–40:344–346, 2006.

9. Astion M: Latent errors in lab services, Clin Lab News 35:15–17, 2009.

10. Becton Dickinson, Inc: Accuracy from bedside to lab, Franklin Lakes, NJ, 2003, BD Inc.

11. Institute for Quality Laboratory Medicine (IQLM): www.phppo.cdc.org (retrieved October 2005).

12. Clinical and Laboratory Standards Institute: Training and competence assessment: approved guideline, ed 2, Wayne, 2004, Pa, GP21-A2.

13. Clinical and Laboratory Standards Institute: Laboratory documents: development and control: approved guideline, ed 5, Wayne, 2006, Pa, GP2-A5.

14. Clinical and Laboratory Standards Institute: Statistical quality control for quantitative measurement: principles and definitions: approved guideline, ed 2, Wayne, 1999, Pa, C24-A2.

15. Clinical and Laboratory Standards Institute: How to define and determine reference intervals in the clinical laboratory: approved guideline, ed 2, Wayne, 2000, Pa, C28-A2.

16. Clinical and Laboratory Standards Institute: Evaluation of precision performance for clinical chemistry devices: approved guideline, ed 2, Wayne, Pa, 2004, EP5-A2.

17. Levey S, Jennings ER: The use of control charts in the clinical laboratory, Am J Clin Pathol 20:1059, 1950.

18. Westgard JO, Barry PL, Hunt MR, et al: A multi-rule Shewhart chart for quality control in clinical chemistry, Clin Chem 27:493, 1981.

BIBLIOGRAPHY

Ahrq Psnet (patient safety net): http://psnet.ahrq.gov retrieved April 20, 2009.

ASQ Hospitals See Benefits of Lean and Six Sigma ASQ Releases Benchmark Study Results March 17, 2009 retrieved www.asq.org August 19, 2009.

Astion ML, Shojania KG, Hamill TR, et al: Classifying laboratory incident reports to identify problems that jeopardize safety, Am J Clin Pathol 120:18, 2003.

Boone DJ: A history of the QC gap in the clinical laboratory, Lab Med 36(10):611, 2005.

Campbell JB, Campbell JM: Laboratory mathematics: medical and biological applications, ed 5, St Louis, 1997, Mosby.

Clinical and Laboratory Standards Institute: Continuous quality improvement: essential management approaches and their use in proficiency testing: approved guideline, ed 2, Wayne, 2004, Pa, GP22-A2.

Clinical and Laboratory Standards Institute: Preliminary evaluation of quantitative clinical laboratory methods: approved guideline, ed 2, Wayne, 2002, Pa, EP10-A2.

Elston DM: Opportunities to improve quality in laboratory medicine, Clin Lab Med 28(2):173–177, 2008.

Goldschmidt HM, Lent RS: Gross errors and work flow analysis in the clinical laboratory, Klin Biochem Metab 3:131, 1995.

Lasky FD: Technology variations: strategies for assuring quality results, Lab Med 36(10):617, 2005.

Lippi G, Mattiuzzi C, Plebani M: Event reporting in laboratory medicine, www.mMed Lab Obs 41(3):23, 2009.

Westgard JO, Westgard SA: Equivalent quality testing versus equivalent QC procedures, Lab Med 36(10):626, 2005.

Wians FH: Clinical laboratory tests: Which, why, and what do the results mean? LabMed 40(2):105, 2009.

Yost J, Mattingly P: CLIA and equivalent quality control: options for the future, Lab Med 36(10):614, 2005.

Yundt-Pacheco J, Parvin CA: The impact of QC frequency on patient results, Med Lab Obs 40(9):24–26, 2008.

REVIEW QUESTIONS

Questions 1-4: Match each organization or document with its function (a to d).

1. ___ TJC

2. ___ CAP

3. ___ COLA

4. ___ CLIA
   a. Accredits hospitals and inspects clinical laboratories
   b. Accredits physician laboratories
   c. Determines waived and nonwaived categories of assays
   d. Accredits only hospital laboratories

Questions 5-7: Match examples of errors.

5. ___ **Preanalytical, (preexamination)**

6. ___ **Analytical, (examination)**

7. ___ **Postanalytical, (postexamiantion)**
   a. Accuracy in testing
   b. Patient identification
   c. Critical value reporting

Questions 8-10: Match examples of errors. A = Preanalytical (preexamination), B = Analytical (examination), C = Postanalytical (postexamiantion) (NOTE: An answer may be used more than once.)

8. ___ **Blood from the wrong patient**

9. ___ **Specimen collected in wrong tube**

10. ___ **Quality control outside of acceptable limits**

Questions 11-15: Match the terms with the definitions (a to e).

11. ___ **Accuracy**

12. ___ **Calibration**

13. ___ **Control**

14. ___ **Precision**

15. ___ Standards
    a. How close results are to one another
    b. How close a test result is to the true value
    c. Specimen is similar to patient's blood; known concentration of constituent
    d. Comparison of an instrument measure or reading to a known physical constant
    e. Highly purified substance of a known composition

Questions 16 and 17: Match the terms with the definitions (a and b).

16. ___ Sensitivity

17. ___ Specificity
    a. Cases with specific disease or condition produce a positive result.
    b. Cases without a specific disease or condition produce a negative result.

Questions 18-20: Match the terms with the definitions (a to c).

18. ___ Mean

19. ___ Median

20. ___ Mode
    a. Another term for the average
    b. Most frequently occurring number in a group of values
    c. Number that is midway between the highest and lowest values

Questions 21 and 22: Match the terms with the definitions (a and b).

21. ___ Standard deviation

22. ___ Coefficient of variation
    a. Equal to SD divided by the mean
    b. Measure of variability

Questions 23 and 24: A = True or B = False.

23. ___ Levey-Jennings plots show values on a chart.

24. ___ Westgard rules have three warning rules and three mandatory rules.

CHAPTER 9

POINT-OF-CARE TESTING

Learning Objectives

At the conclusion of this chapter, the student will be able to:

- Compare the major advantages and disadvantages of point-of-care testing.
- Identify the four categories of Clinical Laboratory Improvement Amendments (CLIA) test procedures.
- Discuss the clinical significance of tests for fecal occult blood.
- Describe common interferences in tests for fecal occult blood and special dietary considerations necessary for specimen collection.

- Explain the chemical principle of the common slide tests for fecal occult blood.
- Provide examples of handheld point-of-care testing devices.
- Identify at least six characteristics to consider when selecting a point-of-care instrument.

POINT-OF-CARE TESTING

For many years, all or the majority of laboratory testing was performed in a central laboratory. This was necessary because of the complexity of testing. With computer chip technology, testing has emerged from the laboratory to the patient's bedside, the pharmacy, the physician's office, the patient's home and other nonlaboratory sites.[1]

Point-of-care testing (POCT) is defined as laboratory assays performed near the patient, wherever that is located. This type of off-site laboratory testing is also known as *near-patient testing* or *decentralized testing*. POCT may offer the major advantage

of reduced turnaround time of test results, which can improve patient management. The major drawback is cost. Other areas of concern include maintenance of quality control (QC) and quality assurance (QA) and proper integration of data (connectivity) into the patient's medical record.

Purpose of Point-of-Care Testing

Development of new POCT assays is increasing at a phenomenal rate. It is important to assess the purpose of POCT versus traditional laboratory-based testing. Why is point-of-care testing being performed instead of routine laboratory testing? Advantages include:

- Smaller blood specimen required
- Faster turnaround time
- Reduction of length of hospital stay
- Patient convenience
- Improved patient care management

Cost of Point-of-Care Testing

Although a test may appear to be beneficial, the downside of a low volume of tests may result in concerns about the proficiency of the testing personnel and cause reagents and controls to outdate before reasonable usage, thus escalating costs. The cost of a POCT program must look at the whole process of patient care rather than just the cost of an individual point-of-care test method versus the cost of the laboratory test method. An appropriate POCT in the emergency room, for example, may prevent the admission of a patient into the hospital. Items that should be assessed include[1]:

- Cost of training the testing personnel and maintenance of competency
- Labor associated with processing and analyzing the specimen
- Labor associated with maintaining the equipment
- Annual reagent, control, maintenance, and depreciation costs
- Costs of state licensing according to volume and test complexity
- Costs of proficiency programs for testing performed

Quality Considerations

The use of instruments with stable calibration curves is important, and a QC program should be available from the manufacturer. Data computation from the analyzing instruments should be interfaced with a computer, if possible, to provide the necessary documentation of laboratory results. QC information can also be stored in the computer. The instrument should be easy to use, and because staff in many physician office laboratories have little or no laboratory training, users of the instrument should require limited training. The reagents, whether wet or dry, should be bar-coded, prepackaged, and stable for at least 6 months.

Regulations

All sites performing laboratory testing are regulated under the Clinical Laboratory Improvement Amendments of 1988 (CLIA '88) and must be licensed to perform any testing. CLIA has granted deemed status to approved accreditation organizations and exempt states and allows these entities to accredit or license testing sites.[1] State and city governments may enact mandatory regulations, including qualifications of personnel performing the test, which may be more but not less stringent than federal regulations.

A site performing only waived tests must have a "Certificate of Waiver" license but will not be routinely inspected. They must, however, adhere to manufacturers' instructions for performing the test. "Good Laboratory Practice" dictates appropriate quality testing practices as outlined in the CLIA moderate- and high-complexity test requirements. These include the training of testing personnel, competency evaluation, and performance of quality control. The Veteran's Administration, College of American Pathologists, and The Joint Commission (TJC) do not recognize the waived category. These accreditation organizations have guidelines for waived and other point-of-care testing that must be met.[1]

Waived Testing

Diagnostic testing not performed within a traditional laboratory is called *waived testing* by TJC.[2] CLIA '88 subjects all clinical laboratory testing to federal regulation and inspection. According to CLIA,[2] test procedures are grouped into one of the following four categories: waived tests, moderately complex tests, highly complex tests, or provider-performed microscopy (PPM) tests (Box 9-1).

Test complexity is determined by criteria that assess knowledge, training, reagent and material preparation, operational technique, QA/QC

BOX 9-1	
Categories of Point of Care Testing	
Category	**Characteristic**
Waived tests	Simple procedures with little chance of negative outcomes if performed inaccurately
Moderately complex tests	More complex than waived tests but usually automated, such as blood counts and routine chemistries
Highly complex tests	Usually are nonautomated or complicated tests requiring considerable judgment, such as microbiology or cross-matching of blood
Provider-performed microscopy (PPM) tests	Slide examinations of freshly collected body fluids

characteristics, maintenance and troubleshooting, and interpretation and judgment. Any over-the-counter test approved by the U.S. Food and Drug Administration (FDA) is automatically placed into the waived category. POCT falls within either the waived or the moderately complex category, except Gram staining, which is sometimes performed as POCT and classified as highly complex testing.

Evaluation of Quality

All laboratory testing must meet the same quality standards regardless of where it is performed. Waived tests do not have specific regulatory requirements other than to follow the manufacturers' instructions. For moderately complex POCT testing, in addition to the requirements listed for waived tests, instrument validation is required for each new instrument.[2]

Voluntary participation in QA programs is also available. The Centers for Disease Control and Prevention (CDC [www.cdc.gov]) recently invited providers to participate in a testing program for human immunodeficiency virus (HIV rapid-testing MPEP). This quality assessment program offers external performance evaluation for rapid tests (e.g., OraQuick Rapid HIV-1 Antibody Test). Ultimate responsibility and control of POCT reside with the CLIA-certified laboratory and require a minimum of one laboratory staff member to be responsible for each POCT program (e.g., glucose testing).

Written policies and procedures must be available for patient preparation, specimen collection and preservation, instrument calibration, quality control and remedial actions, equipment performance evaluations, test performance, and results reporting and recording. The greatest source of error is preanalytical error, especially patient identification and specimen collection. (See Chapter 8 for a complete discussion of errors.)

POCT can be performed by nonautomated as well as automated methods.

Nonautomated Methods

Nonautomated POCT may be done by manual rapid-testing methods, such as pregnancy and fecal occult blood testing. More rapid tests are being developed for the identification of infectious organisms (e.g., group A streptococci, HIV) or cardiac markers (e.g., troponin). One-Step, Rapid Tests: Instant-ViewTn (Alfa Scientific Designs) is an example of an FDA 510-k–cleared immunoassay intended for detection of cardiac markers, such as free and complex troponins (TnI), in emergency rooms, hospital settings, and POCT situations.

FECAL OCCULT BLOOD
Clinical Significance

Tests for hemoglobin in fecal specimens are often referred to as **tests for occult blood.** This is because hemoglobin may be present in the feces, as evidenced by positive chemical tests for blood, but may not be detected by the naked eye. In other words, *occult blood* is hidden blood and requires a chemical test for its detection. Occasionally, enough blood will be present in the feces to produce a tarry black or even bloody specimen. However, even bloody specimens should be tested chemically for occult blood. In such cases the outer portion is avoided, and the central portion of the formed stool is sampled. The detection of occult blood in feces is important in determining the cause of hypochromic anemias resulting from chronic loss of blood and in detecting ulcerative or neoplastic diseases of the gastrointestinal (GI) system. Blood in the feces may result from bleeding anywhere along the GI tract, from the mouth to the anus.

Tests for occult blood are especially useful for early detection and treatment of colorectal cancer. Such tests are useful because more than half of all cancers (excluding skin) are from the GI tract. Early detection results in good survival. Persons over age 50 are commonly screened annually for occult blood. They sample their own stool specimens for three consecutive collections, apply a thin film to the test slides, and mail or bring them to the laboratory for testing. Dietary considerations are important to avoid false-positive results, and special instructions are generally included with the test slides. It is now less common practice for the laboratory to receive the actual fecal specimen to be tested for occult blood.

Bleeding at any point in the GI system representing as little as 2 mL of blood lost daily may be detected by the tests for occult blood. However, false-negative results occur for unknown reasons, possibly because of inhibitors in the feces.

Implications of both false-positive and false-negative tests are important clinically. Early diagnosis and treatment of serious disease might be missed with false-negative results, resulting in poor prognosis and death. Positive results are serious and require extensive further testing to determine the cause of bleeding or to rule out false-positive reactions. Further testing is both unpleasant for the patient and expensive.

Principle and Specificity

Numerous tests have been described for the detection of hemoglobin (or blood) in both urine and feces. Most of these tests are based on the same general principles and reaction. They all make use of peroxidase activity in the heme portion of the hemoglobin molecule.

Most tests for occult blood in feces use gum guaiac, a phenolic compound that produces a blue color when oxidized. The tests require the presence of hydrogen peroxide or a suitable precursor. The peroxidase activity of the hemoglobin molecule results in the liberation of oxygen (O_2) from hydrogen peroxide (H_2O_2), and the released oxygen oxidizes gum guaiac to a blue oxidation product. The reaction is summarized as follows:

$$Hemoglobin + H_2O_2 \rightarrow Oxygen$$
(peroxidase activity)

$$Oxygen + Reduced\ gum\ guaiac \rightarrow$$
(colorless)

$$Oxidized\ gum\ guaiac + H_2O$$
(blue)

Interfering Substances and Dietary Considerations

Several interfering substances may give false-positive results for occult blood, including dietary substances with peroxidase activity, especially myoglobin and hemoglobin in red meat. Vegetable peroxidase, as found in horseradish, can also cause positive results. Several foods have been identified as causing erroneous reactions, including turnips, broccoli, bananas, black grapes, pears, plums, and melons. Cooking generally destroys these peroxidases, and therefore patients are generally instructed to eat only cooked foods. White blood cells (WBCs) and bacteria also have peroxidase activity that might result in false-positive reactions. Various drugs, including aspirin and aspirin-containing preparations and iron compounds, are known to increase GI bleeding, causing positive results. Vitamin C and other oxidants may give false-negative results.

Patients are generally instructed to eat no beef or lamb (including processed meats and liver) for 3 days before collecting the first specimen and to remain on this diet through the collection of three successive samples. They may eat well-cooked pork, poultry, and fish. They are also instructed to avoid raw fruits and vegetables, especially melons, radishes, turnips, and horseradish. Cooked fruits and vegetables are acceptable. Ingestion of high-fiber foods, such as whole-wheat bread, bran cereal, and popcorn, is encouraged. The ingestion of more than 250 mg/day of vitamin C is to be avoided because it may cause false-negative results. The mechanism of this interference is the same as for reagent strips used in urinalysis. Aspirin and other nonsteroidal antiinflammatory drugs (NSAIDs) should be avoided for 7 days before and during the test period.

Guaiac Slide Test for Occult Blood

Various commercial tests have been developed to test for the presence of hemoglobin in feces. At least eight guaiac-based tests for occult blood are available commercially. The Hemoccult II (Smith-Kline Diagnostics), which seems to have the lowest rate of false-positive results, is described here (Procedure 9-1). Other tests are similar. In all cases, the manufacturer's directions should be followed.

Hemoccult II is available as a slide test that contains filter paper uniformly impregnated with gum guaiac. The specimen is applied in a thin film in each of two boxes on the front side of the slide. This may be done by the patient or the laboratory. The specimen is applied with a wooden applicator, which is supplied with the test kit. The kit includes dietary information for the patient and instructions for collecting the specimen.

The American Cancer Society (ACS) recommends that two samples from three consecutive specimens be collected for colorectal screening. Therefore, test kits are usually supplied to patients in groups of three slides. The patient is instructed to allow the test slides to dry overnight then return them to the physician or laboratory. The slides should be properly labeled. If the slides are to be mailed, they must be placed in an approved U.S. Postal Service mailing pouch. They may not be mailed in a standard paper envelope.

When the slides are received in the laboratory, the specimen is tested on the back (opposite side) of the test slide. When the perforated window on the back of the slide is opened, two specimen windows plus positive and negative "performance monitor areas" (controls) are revealed. If the specimen is applied in the laboratory, it must air-dry before the developer solution is applied, to increase the sensitivity of the test.

The developer solution is a stabilized mixture of hydrogen peroxide and denatured alcohol, which is supplied with the test. Only reagent supplied with the test slides can be used for color development. When the fecal specimen containing occult blood is applied to the guaiac-impregnated test paper, peroxidase in the specimen comes in contact with the guaiac. When the developing solution is then applied to the test paper, a reaction between the guaiac and peroxidase results in formation of a blue color.

The reaction requires that blood cells be hemolyzed for proper release of peroxidase. This usually takes place within the GI tract. If whole, undiluted blood is applied to the test paper, the red cells may not hemolyze, and the reaction may be weak or atypical. The test is significantly more sensitive to the presence of occult blood if the specimen is allowed to dry on the slide before the developing solution is applied. The ACS recommends that

Testing for Fecal Occult Blood: Hemoccult II

SENSA^{ELITE} METHOD

PRINCIPLE

This procedure is based on the oxidation of guaiac, a natural resin extracted from the wood of *Guaiacum officinale*, by hydrogen peroxide to a blue-colored compound if heme is present in a fecal specimen. The heme portion of hemoglobin has peroxidase activity, which catalyzes the oxidation of alpha-guaiaconic acid (active component of the guaiac paper) by hydrogen peroxide (active component of the developer) to form a highly conjugated, blue quinine compound.

Specimen

Patient Preparation and Instructions:
- General: Patients may ingest pork, chicken, turkey and fish; fruits and vegetables; high-fiber foods; and acetaminophen.
- Avoid 7 days before specimen collection and during specimen collection: No more than one adult aspirin (325 mg) a day; no other nonsteroidal antiinflammatory drugs (e.g., ibuprofen).
- Avoid 3 days before specimen collection: No red meat (e.g., beef, lamb, liver); no more than 250 mg vitamin C a day from supplements, citrus fruits, and juices. An average orange contains approximately 70 to 75 mg vitamin C; 100% of recommended daily allowance of vitamin C is 60 mg.

Specimen Collection:
- The patient should write his or her name and the physician's name on the front of the test card. Fill in Day 1 collection date. Open Day 1 flap.
- Patients should be advised to place plastic wrap on the toilet seat and to defecate onto the plastic. Obtain a small stool sample with provided applicator stick. Apply thin smear in box A. Reuse applicator stick to obtain a second sample from a different part of the stool specimen. Apply thin smear in box B. Discard specimen and supplies. Close flap. Store test card in the patient kit envelope. Let dry. Do not store smeared test card in any moisture-proof material (e.g., plastic bag).
- Repeat the previous steps for Day 2 and Day 3.
- Insert completed and overnight air-dried test card into enclosed U.S. Postal Service–approved mailing pouch. Peel tape from flap. Fold flap over. Press firmly to seal.
- Deliver or mail sealed mailing pouch to the physician or laboratory within 10 days of Day 1 collection date.

Materials and Reagents
- Hemoccult II SENSA^{elite} slides (test cards)
- Hemoccult II SENSA^{elite} developer. Stabilized mixture of less then 4.2% hydrogen peroxide, 80% denatured ethyl alcohol, and enhancer in an aqueous solution; consult material safety data sheet (MSDS) for additional information. Do not use in eyes; avoid contact with skin.
- Applicator sticks
- Patient screening kit with dispensing envelopes and patient instructions
- Flushable collection tissue or plastic wrap
- Mailing pouches (for return of test cards)
- Hemoccult II SENSA^{elite} product instructions

Storage and Stability
- Store test cards and developer at controlled room temperature (15°C to 30°C) in original packaging. Do not refrigerate or freeze. Protect from heat and light. Do not store with volatile chemicals such as ammonia, bleach, bromine, iodine, and household cleaners.
- When stored as recommended, the slides and developer will remain stable until the expiration dates that appear on each slide and developer bottle.

Quality Control

The positive and negative "performance monitor area," an internal control, is located under the sample area. The positive area turns blue; the negative area remains colorless.

PROCEDURE **9-1** (Continued)

PROCEDURE

Color Development (Performed in Laboratory):
1. Open the perforated window on the back of the slide.
2. Apply 2 drops of the peroxide solution (developer) to guaiac paper directly over each smear.
3. Read the results within 60 seconds. Any trace of blue on or at the edge of the fecal smear is positive.
4. Develop on slide performance monitor areas (controls): Apply 1 drop only of the peroxide solution between the positive and negative performance areas. Always test the specimen and read and interpret the results before developing the controls. A blue color from the positive control might spread into the specimen and cause confusion or a false-positive reaction. Read the results within 10 seconds. A blue color will appear in the positive performance monitor area and no color in the negative performance monitor area if the slides and developer are reacting according to product specifications.

Reporting Results

Any trace of blue color is positive, whether the intensity of color development is weak or strong. Reagent paper that has turned blue or blue-green before use should be discarded. If discolored test paper has been used by the patient, the test should be repeated if there is any question in interpretation.

False-Positive Results

Substances that can cause false-positive test results:
- Red meat (beef, lamb, liver)
- Aspirin (>325 mg/day) and other nonsteroidal antiinflammatory drugs (e.g., ibuprofen, naproxen)
- Corticosteroids, phenylbutazone, reserpine, anticoagulants, antimetabolites, and cancer chemotherapeutic drugs
- Alcohol in excess
- Application of antiseptic preparations containing iodine (e.g., povidone-iodine mixture)

False-Negative Results

Substances that can cause false-negative results:
- Ascorbic acid (vitamin C) in excess of 250 mg/day
- Excessive amounts of vitamin C–enriched foods, citrus fruits, and juices
- Iron supplements that contain quantities of vitamin C in excess of 250 mg/day

Limitations

Bowel lesions may not bleed at all or may bleed intermittently. Blood, if present, may not be distributed uniformly in the specimen. Consequently, a test result may be negative even when disease is present.

Clinical Applications

The Hemoccult II SENSA^elite is a rapid qualitative method for detecting fecal occult blood, which may be indicative of gastrointestinal disease. It is recommended for professional use as a diagnostic aid during routine physical examinations; to monitor hospital patients for gastrointestinal bleeding (e.g., iron deficiency anemia, recuperating from surgery); to follow patients with peptic ulcer, ulcerative colitis, and other conditions; and in screening programs of asymptomatic patients for colorectal cancer.

---

slides be tested within 6 days of preparation and that the slides not be rehydrated. Also, a single positive smear should be considered a positive test result, even in the absence of dietary restriction.

HANDHELD EQUIPMENT

Microprocessors in small and often handheld instruments provide automated, easy-to-perform testing with calibration and on-board quality control (Table 9-1). Most instruments use whole blood. Both handheld and small instruments may be used for testing (e.g., glucose meters).

The first handheld chemistry device used by patients at home, as well as at the patient bedside in an emergency room or other facility, was for testing glucose (Fig. 9-1). Glucose testing with a portable analyzer is based on electrochemical measurement protocols that have been shown to be reliable and affected by variability in hemoglobin

TABLE 9-1 Examples of Handheld and Small Automated Point-of-Care Equipment Using a Blood Specimen

Chemistry Analysis	Assay Principle	Format	Representative Product or System (Manufacturer)
Glucose	Photometry: transmittance	Disposable individual microcuvette	HemoCue (www.hemocue.com)
Glucose	Potentiometry: electrochemistry	Biosensor strips: single test	Accu-Chek (Roche) (ww.accu-chek.com)
Glucose and hemoglobin	Photometry: transmittance	Dry reagent cartridge: single test	Careside (Careside) (www.Careside.com)
Glucose and hemoglobin	Photometry: transmittance	Dry reagent cartridge: single test	Careside (Careside) (www.Careside.com)
Chemistry and drugs	Photometry: transmittance	Wet reagent cartridges: single test	Vision (Abbott) (www.abbottdiagnostics.com)
Cardiac markers Creatine kinase-MB (CK-MB), myoglobin, and troponin I	Fluorometric enzyme immunoassay	Solid-phase radial partition immunoassay technology	Stratus CS (SCS; Dade Behring) (www.dadebehring.com)
Cardiac markers Creatine kinase-MB (CK-MB), myoglobin, and troponin I	Fluorescence immunoassay	Murine monoclonal and polyclonal antibodies against CK-MB, murine monoclonal and polyclonal antibodies against myoglobin, murine monoclonal and goat polyclonal antibodies against troponin I labeled with a fluorescent dye and immobilized on the solid phase, and stabilizers	Triage (Biosite) (www.biosite.com)
β-Type natriuretic peptide (BNP)	Fluorescence immunoassay	Murine monoclonal and polyclonal antibodies against BNP, labeled with a fluorescent dye and immobilized on the solid phase, and stabilizers	Triage BNP (Biosite) (www.biosite.com)
Blood gases and electrolytes	Electrochemical	Wet reagent cartridges	iSTAT (Abbott) (www.abbottdiagnostics.com)
Hemoglobin A_{1c}	Coulometric biosensor technology	Test strip	Precision PCT (Abbott) (www.abbottdiagnostics.com)
Blood Coagulation Analyzers			
Sysmex	Detection methods: clotting, chromogenic and immunologic	Multiple reagents	Systemic CA-500 (www.medicalsiemens.com)
Prothrombin time with INR	Reflectance Photometry	Single-use cartridge	CoaguChek S (www.rochediagnostics.com)
Prothrombin time with INR, activated partial thromboplastin time, activated clotting time	Optical motion detection	Single-use tube containing an activator and a magnet	Hemochron Response 401/801* CoaguChek Pro (www.rochediagnostics.com)
Prothrombin time (PT)/INRatio Monitor	Platelet aggregation thromboelastography	Electrochemical test strip	HemoSense (www.hemosense.com)

INR, International normalized ratio.

*Three different types of activator tubes are available. Equipment is able to perform thrombin time, heparin-neutralized thrombin time, high-dose thrombin time, fibrinogen, and protamine dose assay.

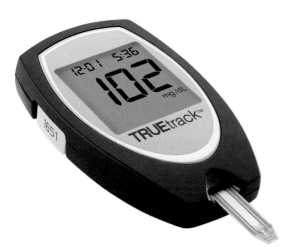

FIGURE 9-1 **Glucometer.** (Courtesy TRUEtrack Smart System, Home Diagnostics, Inc.)

level. Handheld automated equipment has been developed for many applications, including blood coagulation and blood gases. These devices use a very small quantity of blood.

For handheld devices, the blood specimen is placed directly into the device. Handheld or small analyzers are frequently located in the intensive care unit, emergency department, or surgery. Measurements can include:

- Electrolytes (Na^+, K^+, Ca^{++}, Mg^{++})
- Prothrombin time
- Partial thromboplastin time
- Activated clotting time
- Hematocrit
- Blood gases
- Urea
- Glucose

Handheld devices use a small amount of blood specimen, require minimal routine and preventive maintenance, and automate or eliminate calibration functions. This type of automation requires minimal technical support and is relatively maintenance free and easy to use. Automatic lockouts of users who are either not authorized or who do not adhere to QC procedures are a common feature of the software. Current technology uses reflectance photometry or biosensors. Some instruments use new analytical concepts such as optodes, paramagnetism, and optical immunoassays.

Compatibility with laboratory information systems is desirable. Output data are visually displayed and stored in the unit for transfer to the LIS. Vari-

ous forms of data output are used with POCT systems, including visual readings, display screen, printer, and various means of electronic transmission by RS232 ports, Ethernet ports, infrared beams, wireless radio signals, or modems.

Important characteristics of POCT devices include:

- Small blood sample
- Rapid turnaround time
- Easy portability with single-use disposable reagent cartridges or test strips
- Easy-to-perform protocol with one or two steps
- Accuracy and precision of results comparable with central laboratory analyzers
- Minimal QC tracking
- Storage at ambient temperature for reagents
- Bar-code technology for test packs, controls, and specimens
- Economical cost and maintenance free
- Software for automatic calibration, system lockouts, and data management
- Hard copy or electronic data output that interfaces with an LIS or other tracking software

REFERENCES

1. Washington State Clinical Laboratory Advisory Council: Point-of-care testing guidelines, Originally published October 2000, reviewed/revised March 2005/March 2009, retrieved July 30, 2009.
2. Department of Health and Human Services: Health Care Financing Administration: Clinical Laboratory Improvement Amendments of 1988, Federal Register 60(78), 1995, Final rules with comment period.

BIBLIOGRAPHY

Altinier S, Mion M, Cappelletti A, et al: Rapid measurement of cardiac markers on Stratus CS, Clin Chem 46:991, 2000.

Burtis CA, Ashwood ER, Bruns DE: Tietz fundamentals of clinical chemistry, ed 6, Philadelphia, 2008, Saunders.

Joint Commission on Accreditation of Healthcare Organizations: 2005-2006 Comprehensive accreditation manual for laboratory and point-of-care testing, Oak Brook Terrace, Ill, 2005, Department of Communications Laboratory Accreditation Program.

Kaplan LA, Pesce AJ: Clinical chemistry: theory, analysis, correlation, ed 5, St Louis, 2010, Mosby.

Katz B, Marques MB: Point-of-care testing in oral anticoagulation: what is the point? MLO Med Lab Obs 36:30–35, 2004, www.mlo-online.com (retrieved July 2005).

Turgeon ML: Immunology and serology in laboratory medicine, ed 4, St Louis, 2008, Mosby.

Verne B: Size up this critical medical laboratory automation, MLO Med Lab Obs 37:22,24,26,28, 2005, www.mlo-online.com (retrieved August 2005).

REVIEW QUESTIONS

1. **A major advantage of POCT is:**
   a. faster turnaround time.
   b. lower cost.
   c. ease of use.
   d. both a and b.

2. **POCT assays are usually in which CLIA category?**
   a. Waived
   b. Provider-performed microscopy
   c. Moderately complex
   d. Highly complex

3. **Over-the-counter test kits are in which CLIA category?**
   a. Waived
   b. Provider-performed microscopy
   c. Moderately complex
   d. Highly complex

Questions 4-7: A = True or B = False.
Important characteristics to be considered when selecting POCT instruments are:

4. ___ **rapid turnaround time.**

5. ___ **easy-to-perform protocol.**

6. ___ **refrigerated storage of reagents.**

7. ___ **bar code for test packs and controls.**

8. **Tests for fecal occult blood are in general use as a screening test for which of the following?**
   a. Breast cancer
   b. Colorectal cancer
   c. Enteric infection of the colon
   d. Malabsorption syndrome

Questions 9-15: Indicate whether the following statements concerning tests for fecal occult blood are A = True or B = False.

9. ___ Aspirin and nonsteroidal antiinflammatory drugs should be avoided to prevent gastrointestinal bleeding.

10. ___ False-positive reactions are often caused by peroxidase activity.

11. ___ Most tests are slide tests that involve the reduction of gum guaiac from a colorless to a colored compound.

12. ___ Tests are based on the peroxidase activity of heme.

13. ___ The presence of large amounts of ascorbic acid may cause false-positive results.

14. ___ To minimize false-positive reactions, patients should be instructed to eat only raw fruits and vegetables.

15. ___ To minimize false-positive reactions, patients need to be on a special diet for 3 days before specimen collection begins and for the duration of collection.

CHAPTER 10

LABORATORY INFORMATION SYSTEMS AND AUTOMATION

Learning Objectives

At the conclusion of this chapter, the student will be able to:

- Describe overall product and functions of laboratory information systems.
- List and describe components of a computer system.
- Define the abbreviations *LAN* and *WAN*.
- Define and give examples of preanalytical, analytical, and postanalytical testing.
- Define the abbreviation *HIPAA*, and explain the major points of the legislation.
- Identify and describe five Clinical and Laboratory Standards Institute (CLSI) standards for design, compatibility, and integration of automated clinical laboratory systems.
- State the percentage of data generated by a laboratory that is used to establish a diagnosis or monitor treatment effectiveness.

- Explain the major benefits of laboratory automation.
- Describe the five steps in automated analysis.
- Briefly describe the principle used by representative clinical chemistry analyzers to measure the concentration of substances.
- Explain the two types of technology used to count blood cells.
- Identify methods for performing automated cell differentials.
- Define the test principles used by automated instruments in urine chemical testing and microscopic analysis.

OVERVIEW OF LABORATORY INFORMATION MANAGEMENT SYSTEMS

Information is the ultimate product of the laboratory, and the ultimate goal of the laboratory is to provide accurate information in a timely manner to clinicians. To achieve these goals, laboratory information systems have become the foundation in virtually all health care environments. A **laboratory information management system (LIMS)** represents a more frequently used way of managing the modern clinical laboratory. LIMS are used because of their ability to routinely integrate automation and data handling, provide uniform methodology with complete visibility, and lead to increased productivity and process integrity.

The essential requirements of a LIMS include secure login, flexibility to add-ons and software upgrades, and most importantly, data management. The number of laboratory tests has increased as a result of the development of new diagnostic assays and the increased use of automated, high-volume instruments and handheld devices. Because the number of assays performed in the clinical laboratory and by point-of-care testing has grown so dramatically over the years, and because these assays have produced so much analytical information, the ability to process this information efficiently and accurately has become essential.

The **laboratory information system (LIS)** is the tool for delivery of this data. LIS is the integration of computers through a common database via various communication networks. When automated instruments are interfaced or point-of-care equipment connected to an LIS, productivity improves and the risk of errors decreases because the data are delivered directly to a patient's record for physician review, as well as to other departments such as medical records and billing.

Computer technology is not limited to testing. Even the most basic systems can promote a paperless laboratory and reduce time spent on manual processes. Systems can be applied to many laboratory-related preanalytical, analytical, and postanalytical functions: specimen processing, inventory control, quality control (QC), online monitoring, data entry on patients' charts, and data interpretation. Advances in functionality of LIS with new technology is changing the approach to some of the laboratory's fundamental tasks. Technology-driven enhancements include:

- QC storage and functionality
- Support of comprehensive analyzer interface, including calculations
- Tools to aid in compliance with regulations for laboratory procedures
- Capability to share data with third-party vendors

- Automated result report dissemination to support workflow models
- Rules-based logic for decision-making support[1]

Many LIMS vendors (Box 10-1) have developed systems for large and small clinical laboratories as well as off-site locations. Every November, the College of American Pathologists (CAP) publishes a detailed survey of more than 35 LIMS (www.cap.org). Software products use process automation, robust interfaces, and rules-based technology to address regulatory issues, improve efficiency, reduce errors, and increase reimbursements.

It is not possible to discuss LIMS without discussing automation. Automation describes an instrumental system that involves the mechanization of discrete processes and is "non-interventional" of self-regulating and self-timing. Many automated techniques make use of robotized units, and these are commonly seen in a QC laboratory for procedures that are susceptible to gross methodological errors. *Robotics* describes the use of instrument management systems and the way in which information is handled. More recent revisions have produced automated robotized systems capable of handling multiple-channel information sources and simultaneously running selected apparatus.

COMPONENTS OF A COMPUTER SYSTEM

A computer system consists of both hardware and software components. **Hardware** is the physical or "hard" parts of the computer, and **software** programs contain the instructions that direct computer processes or functions.

Hardware includes the physical computer itself as well as the LIS server or personal computers plus the monitors, keyboards, drives, and internal circuit boards containing silicon chips. Different chips may have different functions, including memory. Computer hardware for every LIS server and personal computer can be divided into the:

1. Central processing unit (CPU)
2. Random-access memory (RAM)
3. Peripheral devices external to the CPU

Central Processing Unit

The main chip in a small computer is called the microprocessor or **central processing unit (CPU),** which is the primary component of the computer. This hardware component is responsible for executing software instructions. The CPU is made up of a control unit, an arithmetic logic unit (ALU), and the central memory. The CPU carries out the application software instructions with choices selected by the user.

BOX 10-1

Examples of Large Laboratory and Hospital Information Systems*

Vendor	Web Address
Antek Healthware	www.antekhealthware.com
Cerner Corp.	www.cerner.com
Computer Service & Support, Inc. (LIS Systems)	www.csslis.com
Cove Laboratory Software	www.covelab.com
Dawning Technologies, Inc.	www.dawning.com
LabSoft, Inc.	www.labsoftweb.com
Meditech	www.meditech.com
Orchard Software	Orchardsoft.com
Psyche Systems Corporation	www.psychesystems.com
Sunquest Systems	www.sunquestinfo.com
Sysmex America, Inc.	www.sysmex.com/usa/

Partial listing of information systems from Medical Laboratory Observer. Clinical Laboratory Reference 2009-2010, Laboratory Information Systems.

Random-Access Memory

Random-access memory (RAM) is analogous to short-term memory in humans. When a program is run, the executable file is read from magnetic or optical storage media into the computer's main memory, RAM, from where the CPU obtains the instructions to be executed.

Peripheral Devices

Peripheral devices transfer information into and from the CPU (input/output [I/O] devices), store data and programs for use by the CPU (storage devices), and communicate with other computers (communication and network devices, discussed separately under main heading).

Input Devices

One of the most common peripheral I/O devices is the video display monitor. Monitors are usually cathode-ray tube (CRT) or liquid crystal display (LCD) screens; important attributes include the diagonal dimension, the number of pixels (picture elements), resolution, and inclusion of a touch-sensitive surface. Touch screens allow interaction with the software application and CPU through a menu. **Menus** are lists of programs, functions, or other options offered by the system. A cursor is moved to the point on the list, such as a list of tests, that is the option of choice and placed on the test desired. The position of touch on the screen determines the choice. A stylus, the operator's finger, or a mouse can be used to interact with a touch-sensitive screen to indicate a menu choice.

Bar Codes

Computer technology is applied to phlebotomy through **bar codes** verifying both the patient and the ordered tests. One system, MediCopia (Lattice Inc.), indicates the tests, appropriate tubes, and quantity of tubes required for the patient and generates bar-coded laboratory labels for tube identification at the patient's bedside. This eliminates mislabeling because the only labels available are the ones printed for that particular patient. MediCopia automatically time-stamps operations, providing physicians with valuable information on when samples were drawn. All completed draws are sent via the handheld computer back to the LIS for reconciliation. MediCopia's integrated wireless radio technology allows the caregiver to receive "non-sweep" and "stat" test orders on the handheld unit without having to return to the docking station. Some software triggers the generation of specimen labels and prints those needed for the collection process. The patient demographic information will be printed on the labels (see Fig. 10-1), along with special accession numbers in some institutions. These accession numbers will be represented in the bar-coding format for each of the patient's specimen labels. Bar coding greatly limits errors in specimen handling and improves productivity. For the greatest benefit, specimen bar coding is also coordinated with the automated instruments used for testing, in which case the sampling is done directly from the primary collection tube.

After the specimen has been collected, it is sent to the laboratory for analysis. After testing is completed, a computerized system can be used for managing specimen storage and retrieval. An example of such a system is SpecTrack (Siemens

Healthcare Diagnostics), an informatics software product enabling quick and easy storage and retrieval of specimens for the laboratory. With SpecTrack, users can find the exact storage location of any specimen from all laboratories in their network, eliminating time-consuming searches in the refrigerator or cold room.

One-dimensional (1D) bar codes are linear and consist of a series of parallel lines of varying widths. The parallel lines encode data and are read by a laser optical device known as a *scanner* or *reader*. Today, bar-code labels are critical to laboratory operations where essential patient accessioning, clinical testing, or research functions occur. Bar-code readers may be used attached as input devices. They use either manually operated light pens or laser devices that read the bars on a label and convert these data to a sequence of numbers representing specific information (Fig. 10-1). This information can be patient identification, tests requested, or identification of a reagent for a test. Bar codes are being used on identification wristbands, allowing for better control of accuracy with patient identification, and on labels for specimen containers and test requests.

The newest development in bar codes is the growing popularity of two-dimensional (2D) bar codes in the United States and Japan. A 2D bar code is nonlinear and consists of black-and-white "cells" or "modules" arranged in a matrix pattern—typically a square—which in turn encapsulates a "finder" pattern and a "reader" pattern. These 2D symbols are omnidirectionally scannable—upside down, backward or forward, and even diagonally.

A 2D bar code can store every bit of patient information in a tiny symbol that is 2 to 3 mm square, because 2D bar codes can store thousands of characters. The symbology of 2D bar codes is not as susceptible to printing defects or errors as traditional 1D bar codes. The coding pattern has a high level of redundancy, with the data dispersed in several locations throughout the symbology. This enables the bar code to be scanned correctly even if a portion of it has printed lightly or is missing altogether.

Specialized equipment is required to print 2D bar codes. The best printer for 2D labels is a direct thermal or thermal transfer printer. In addition, 2D bar codes cannot be read by a laser scanner; they must be scanned by an image-based scanner employing a charge-coupled device, (CCD) or some other digital-camera sensor technology.[2]

Radio Frequency Identification Devices

Radio Frequency Identification Devices (RFIDs)[3] are an automatic identification method that involves storing and retrieving data via tags or transponders (e.g., electronic toll collection on highways). Small RFIS tags can be attached to products. They contain silicon chips and antennas that enable the tags to receive and respond to radiofrequency queries from an RFID transceiver. Two kinds of RFID devices exist: passive and active. Active RFIDs provide real-time location for tracking and workflow improvement. RFID is being implemented in blood transfusion applications. RFID and bar codes can be viewed as complimentary to each other. The choice of technology will depend on the specific application.

Output Devices

Output is any information a computer generates as a result of its calculations or processing. The monitor, printers, and on-board instrument displays all can function as output devices. The computer directs the needed data from its central memory or from a storage device to the specific output device. An electronic chart or intermediate data may be displayed on a monitor. A printer is used for the production of hard copy and longer-lasting paper-printed records. Another specific output function of the printer is generating printed labels for specimen containers at the time of order entry for a test.

Data Storage Devices

An important LIS component is the data, or memory, storage section. This contains all the necessary instructions and data needed to operate the computer system. Any short-term information, such as patient records and laboratory data, may also be stored temporarily in the memory. In addition to central memory, magnetic or optical media are used to store less-frequently accessed data. These require more time for data retrieval but are considerably less expensive than central memory. The CAP accreditation standards require that laboratories establish methods for communication of needed information to ensure prompt, reliable

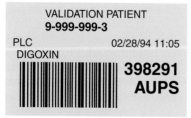

FIGURE 10-1 **Example of bar-coded specimen label.** The six-digit specimen number (398291) is bar-coded. The patient number, patient demographics, time/date, and test are written in normal readable letters. (From Kaplan LA, Pesce AJ: Clinical chemistry: theory, analysis, and correlation, ed 5, St Louis, 2010, Mosby.)

reporting of results and that they have appropriate data storage and retrieval capacity.[4]

Hard drives are revolving disks with a magnetic surface that can be easily accessed. Other forms of data storage are optical storage disks (e.g., CDs, DVDs).

Software

Software consists of the encoded instructions for the operation of a computer. Software programs that supply basic functions of the computer are called **operating systems (OS) programs,** such as Microsoft Windows. Software programs are stored on various forms of media (e.g., hard drives) for operating the program and optical disks (CD/DVD-ROMs) for distribution. Those that supply special functions for the users are called **application programs.**

Middleware

Middleware is computer software that connects software components or applications.[1] Middleware sits "in the middle" between application software that may be working on different operating systems. This newer adaptation makes a distinction between the operating system and middleware functionality but is, to some extent, arbitrary.

Automation enhancements have emerged as the result of middleware. Middleware can boost workflow productivity and efficiency and can offer function not even possible without it. When is middleware needed? It can be used to:

- Process specimens from multiple locations
- Automate algorithms
- Initiate repeat testing
- Implement autoverification and QC monitoring
- Detect patient misidentification errors
- Provide alerts for critical values

COMMUNICATION AND NETWORK DEVICES

For interaction with users, a LIS uses personal computers directly connected to the server for the LIS. Most laboratories connect microcomputers together using routers to form a **local area network (LAN)** that can access the LIS server or the **hospital information system (HIS).** Not only can microcomputers be networked to the main server (LAN) to facilitate network communications, but software is equally adept for use in **wide area networks (WANs).** A WAN connects multisite facilities into a single network. .

In most health care venues, multiple software products are employed between various departments. The exchange of information between the computer and the user is called *interfacing.* The use of an interface allows data from one or more systems to be automatically captured by the other systems. Interfacing is accomplished through several types of devices.

Most current systems use the **Health Level 7 (HL7) standard** for their interfaces. The goal of using this standard is to prevent misunderstandings between the computers by defining messages and their content. The HL7 standard is primarily used for financial and medical record information. It does not address many types of clinical information or other data, such as raw data from instrument interfaces.

For laboratory use, the interface specification should include what data will be transferred, where data will be transferred, when data will be transferred, and security and encryption considerations. Interfaces are important to the laboratory because they contribute to the overall effectiveness of the computer support of laboratory operations. It is critical to remember that interfaces pass patient information between computers without direct human intervention.

Interfacing of the laboratory computer with the analytical testing instrument allows the test result to be entered directly into the computer information system or LIS and saves laboratory time. The test result data are transferred directly over a single wired or wireless interface. A unidirectional interface transmits or uploads results; a bidirectional interface allows for simultaneous transmission or downloading of information and for the reception of uploaded information from an instrument.

With the Lifescan Accu-Chek, for example, a host RS232C bidirectional interface allows transmission of results to a personal computer from the Clinitek Status. Lifescan offers patients OneTouch Diabetes management of test results to a personal computer with a 9-pin or 25-pin serial port or USB port. Accu-Chek allows diabetic patients to download glucose information to a personal computer or to beam the information, through infrared technology, into a personal digital assistant (PDA).

A LIS is often interfaced with other information systems, most often the HIS; interfacing allows electronic communication between two computers. The HIS manages patient census information and demographics and systems for billing, and the more complex systems process and store patient medical information. The interfacing of the HIS and the laboratory computer facilitates the exchange of test request orders, return of analytical results (the laboratory report), and charges for the tests ordered and reported. When the data are verified, nurses or physicians in the patient care areas can retrieve results through terminals and printers.

This linking of hospital and laboratory computer systems is not easy, and totally integrated systems require an institutional commitment to the process. A well-designed, easily accessible HIS-LIS database offers significant improvements in medical record keeping, patient care planning, budget planning, and general operations management tasks (Fig. 10-2).

Transmitting data is the primary productivity goal that any LIS system should achieve. Most systems are capable of network printing to multiple locations or producing a fax transmission of patient results. New systems also employ the Internet to transmit information.

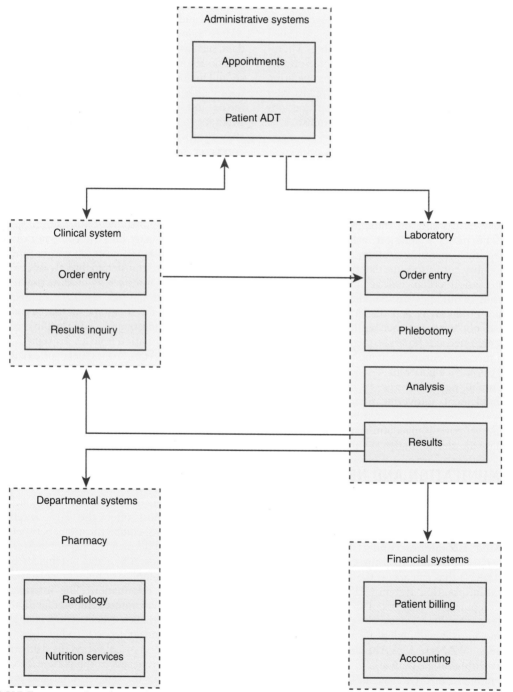

FIGURE 10-2 **Interchange of information between systems.** (From Kaplan LA, Pesce AJ: Clinical chemistry: theory, analysis, and correlation, ed 5, St Louis, 2010, Mosby.)

COMPUTER APPLICATIONS

The applications of the LIS has grown from being exclusive to high-volume chemistry and hematology instrumentation to all the other sections of the laboratory and off-site locations. General functions of the LIS can include patient identification, patient demographics, test ordering, specimen collection, specimen analysis, test results, and test interpretation. Coding systems for diagnosis, such as the CAP Systematized Nomenclature of Human and Veterinary Medicine (SNOMED), can also be managed by the LIS.

Most vendors separate the LIS into separate modules for various functions by department, such as specimen processing or high-volume hematology and chemistry testing. For example, a general laboratory system can fully automate clinical, financial, and managerial processes associated with the chemistry, hematology, coagulation, urinalysis, immunology/serology, and toxicology sections of the clinical laboratory. Software can support all aspects of departmental workflow, including QC, instrument interfaces, result entry and review functions, autoverification, worksheets for the manual areas, and result inquiry. In addition, management report options are available to provide the laboratory manager with information necessary for the optimal operation of the laboratory.

The functions of LIS can be grouped into three categories: preanalytical, analytical, and postanalytical (Box 10-2).

Preanalytical (Preexamination) Functions

Using handheld technology reduces costs, improves workflow, and eliminates preventable medical errors. If data are collected and printed or transmitted directly, it is more efficient and accurate than manual recording.

Identifying and defining the patient in the computer system must take place before any testing is done. Most health care institutions assign a unique identification number to each patient and also enter other demographic information about the patient in the information database (e.g., name, gender, age or birth date, referring or attending physician). These data are known as the **patient demographics.** This information is collected at admission to the facility and entered into the HIS. The information is then transferred electronically from the HIS to the LIS.

Test ordering, or **order entry,** is an important first step in use of the LIS. Specific data are needed during the order entry process: a patient number and a patient name, name of ordering physician(s), name of physician(s) to receive the report, test request time and date, time the specimen was or will be collected, name of person entering the request, tests to be performed, priority of the test request (e.g., "stat" or routine), and any other specimen comments pertaining to the request.

Orders can be received most efficiently by the LIS through a network with the HIS. The laboratory can also receive a paper copy of the tests requested—the test request form or requisition from which laboratory personnel enter the test request into the LIS. The same data are needed on the paper form as are needed on the electronic order. The computer will generate collection lists, work lists, or logs with patient demographics and any necessary collection or analysis information. For example, work lists generated may include a loading list for a particular analyzer. The LIS has numerous checks and balances built into it as a part of the order entry process.

Analytical (Examination) Functions

An automated analyzer must link each specimen to its specific test request. This is best done automatically through the use of bar codes on the specimen

---

BOX 10-2

Examples of Laboratory Information System Functionality

Preanalytical (Preexamination)

Reduction of manual tasks such as test ordering, specimen accessioning
Specimen labels
Specimen tracking between work stations
Centrifugation and cap removal
Error reduction, such as in correct specimen identification
Validation, such as the right assay being performed on the right tube type
Specimen integrity, such as correct volume of specimen, absence of interference from hemolysis, lipemia

Analytical (Examination)

Automated results entry
Manual results entry
Quality control
Validation of results
Output data processing
Network to laboratory automation systems

Postanalytical (Postexamination)

Archive of patient cumulative reports
Archive of specimens, such as frozen storage
Disposal of individual tubes
Workload recording
Billing
Network to other systems

Modified from Galloway T, Olson E: A few remarks on analyzers: which end is up? MLO Med Lab Obs 41:18, 2009.

label but can be done manually by the laboratory staff, who can link the sample at the instrument to the specimen number in the computer.

Molecular and Genetic Data

Molecular testing, including cytogenetics and molecular detection, is being supported by information systems today.[5] It is early in the software development cycle, and linkage of databases of relevant genetic information continues as a work in progress. Today, modules exist that can support karyotype results entry and fluorescent in situ hybridization (FISH) data. Flow cytometry and cytogenetics are supported by vendors such as Millennium Helix (Cerner Corp.), where a unique karyotype editor that promotes compliance with ISCN and paring karyotypes into easily searchable and coded concepts has been developed. Cerner's Clinical Bioinformatics Ontology (CBO) standardizes molecular findings to promote extensive analytical capabilities. The CBO has nearly 12,000 unique concepts. This promotes the comparison of results between patients, which supports family member comparisons.

The Millennium Helix also provides context-sensitive links to Online Mendelian Inheritance in Man (OMIM), a database of information and references about human genes and genetic disorders, and the National Center for Biotechnology information (NCBI). Established in 1988 as a national resource for molecular biology information, NCBI creates public databases, conducts research in computational biology, develops software tools for analyzing genome data, and disseminates biomedical information—all for the better understanding of molecular processes affecting human health and disease.

Another company offering modality-specific modules for cytogenetics, flow cytometry, and molecular testing is SCC Soft Computer. The cytogenetics module interfaces with flow cytometry instruments. Functionality includes data capture and scatterplot images.

Autoverification

Any results generated must be **verified** (approved or reviewed) by the laboratory staff before the data are released to the patient report. *Autoverification*[6,7] is a process where computer-based algorithms automatically perform actions on a defined subset of laboratory results without the need for manual intervention. Useful data for autoverification can include the display of "flags" signifying results that are outside the reference range values, the presence of **critical values** or **panic values** (possible life-threatening values), values out of the technical

range for the analyzer, or results that fail other checks and balances built into the system.

Autoverification can be of three kinds:
1. Rules-based systems
2. Neural networks
3. Pattern recognition

Rules-based systems are the most traditional. Pattern recognition is the most complex of the systems. Neural networks are midway between the two other types. The type of system selected depends on an analysis of how many tests the laboratory offers, the expected turnaround time, and the complexity of test results. Rules-based systems are the most common and the easiest to implement. Many newer automated instruments include autoverification systems. In a simple laboratory operation such as a satellite lab, the systems are inexpensive.

Autoverification of Clinical Laboratory Results (Clinical and Laboratory Standards Institute [CLSI] Approved Guideline AUTO-10A8[7]) provides a general outline that allows each laboratory to design, implement, validate, and customize rules for autoverification based on the needs of its patient population.

Quality assurance procedures, including the use of QC solutions, are part of the analytical functions of the analyzer and its interfaced computer. The Clinical Laboratory Improvement Amendments of 1988 (CLIA '88) require documentation of all QC data associated with any test results reported.

Postanalytical (Postexamination) Functions

The end product of the work done by the clinical laboratory consists of the testing results produced by the particular methodology used, which are provided in the **laboratory report.** The data can be electronically transmitted to printers, computer terminals, or handheld pager terminals, giving rapid access to the test information for the user.

Laboratory Report

An important use for the laboratory computer is to provide a comprehensive laboratory report that contains all the test information generated by the various laboratories that have performed analyses for a single patient. A paper report is still required by most accreditation agencies and by current medical practice. CLIA '88 regulations require that every LIS has the capacity to print or reprint reports easily when needed. The format of the report should be such that the test results are clear and unambiguous. Many questions need answering to establish or rule out a particular diagnosis, and the report should facilitate this process. The report should indicate any abnormality and answer these questions: What is the predictive value of the test for the disease in question? Is the result meaningful? What other factors could produce the result? What should be done next?

If the diagnosis has already been made, the information on the report form can be used for other purposes, such as managing the patient's treatment plan. The physician must know the result of the most recent laboratory test, what clinically significant changes have occurred since the last test (through the retrieval of current and historical data), whether changes in therapy are indicated, and when the test should be performed next. This information constitutes an **interpretive report.**

An interpretive report form should give information about the range of reference values, flag any abnormal values, and provide these data in a readily accessible format to support laboratories in the interpretation of clinical results in specific diagnostic areas such as cerebrospinal fluid (CSF) testing, urine assessment, and protein profiling. Besides the graphical presentation of patient results and the calculation of formulas, this program provides suggestions for the clinical interpretation of specific protein results.

Critical Patient Results

Critical patient results must be communicated immediately. The traditional way is by phone contact with the primary care provider. With automated LIS, it is essential to achieve electronic line of sight from the test order to the receipt and acknowledgment of the critical result to the appropriate health care professional. An automated process that supports critical result reporting with a manual call center backup system error-proofs critical laboratory assay communication and improves the quality of patient care and laboratory staff productivity.

PRIVACY OF INDIVIDUALLY IDENTIFIABLE HEALTH INFORMATION

With the passage of the **Health Insurance Portability and Accountability Act (HIPAA)** by the U.S. Congress in 1996, LIS security has taken on new emphasis. Communications from the LIS should meet HIPAA compliance for encryption and methodology. Users should be prompted to log on and off the software to ensure that unauthorized access is prevented. The LIS should have full transaction capture, indicating any manipulation of patient results data.

HIPAA (Public Law 104-191) establishes a minimum standard for security of electronic health information to protect the confidentiality, integrity, and availability of protected patient information. The Department of Health and Human Services (HHS) published the **Privacy Rule** on December 28, 2000, and adopted modifications on August 14, 2002. This rule set national standards for the protection of health information by health plans, health care clearinghouses, and health care providers who conduct certain transactions electronically. The HIPAA Privacy Rule establishes, for the first time, a foundation of federal protections for the privacy of protected health information. The rule does not replace federal, state, or other laws that grant individuals even greater privacy protections, and covered entities are free to retain or adopt more protective policies or practices.

Most portions of HIPAA are relevant to electronic information and the electronic interchange of information. HIPAA rules apply to any health information that can be linked to a person by name, social security number, employee number, hospital identification number, or other identifier. These provisions cover protected health information, regardless of whether it is or has been in electronic form or relates to any past, present, or future health care or payments. HIPAA legislation has a direct effect on the LIS. It includes requirements for the laboratory to collect diagnosis codes from the ordering provider on outpatient testing reimbursed by Medicare, a requirement under the Balanced Budget Act of 1997.

In addition, CLIA '88 has led to major changes in clinical laboratory data storage requirements. Records of test requests and results must be retained in a conveniently retrievable manner for 10 years for anatomic pathology and cytology results, 5 years for blood bank and immunohematology (HLA typing) results, and 2 years for all other results.

Voluntary accreditation agencies (e.g., CAP, The Joint Commission [TJC]) often act as initial reviewers for compliance with federal and state regulations. These requirements for data processing include user procedures for documenting and validating software, documenting software and hardware maintenance, and communicating standard operating procedures. CAP laboratory inspection checklists have added requirements for review of computerized verification of results, security, and privacy procedures.

FUTURE CONSIDERATIONS

Future challenges for the clinical laboratory include interfacing and integration of information exchanged, handling of patient data through HL7 output, and validation of error-free software. Integration of information and connectivity issues continue to increase as point-of-care testing increases. Although the industry has developed many standards for information interchange, a multiplicity of different information systems can still present a management and operational challenge. In addition, ensuring that the software supplied is error free and performs as specified is a crucial activity, both in the initial LIS implementation and in the installation of subsequent software releases. Most LIS vendors today utilize current Good Manufacturing Practices (cGMP) and are ISO 9000 certified. The laboratory should insist that their vendor follow the guidelines and procedures for software quality assurance.

To guide the laboratory in future information technology, the CLSI has developed interrelated standards addressing the design, compatibility, and integration of automated clinical laboratory systems worldwide,[8] including:

1. *Laboratory automation: specimen container/ specimen carrier* provides standards for designing and manufacturing specimen containers and carriers used for collecting and processing liquid samples, such as blood and urine, for clinical testing in laboratory automation systems.

2. *Laboratory automation: bar codes for specimen container identification* provides specifications for using linear bar codes on specimen container tubes in the clinical laboratory and on laboratory automation systems.

3. *Laboratory automation: communications with automated clinical laboratory systems, instruments, devices, and information systems* provides standards to facilitate the accurate and timely electronic exchange of data and information between the automated laboratory elements.

4. *Laboratory automation: systems operational requirements, characteristics, and information elements* describes the operational requirements, characteristics, and required information elements of clinical laboratory automation systems.

5. *Laboratory automation: electromechanical interfaces* provides guidance for developing a standard electromechanical interface between instruments and specimen-processing and specimen-handling devices used in automated laboratory testing procedures.

Thirteen additional CLSI documents[8-26] have been developed to address various aspects of automation and informatics. These guidelines are helpful as informational technology applications expand to include:

- **Providing primary care provider order entry.** The newest hospital information systems access laboratory information and patient results through a laboratory web page. A newer postanalytical function of the LIS is retrieval of patient laboratory results by handheld devices. With password entry, primary care providers can order assays or retrieve results remotely.

- **Integrating total automation of laboratory systems.** New LISs and robotics are adapted for and integrated into total automated laboratory systems.

- **Monitoring the quality of laboratory results.** Use of automatic Westgard rules in QC analysis conveys appropriate warning to laboratory staff. In addition, Delta checking of current and previous patient results and flagging of abnormal and questionable results are being integrated into LIS operation.

- **Interfacing of HIS and LIS.** The ability of the laboratory to retrieve data from medical records, including patient diagnosis, pharmacy data, and diagnostic imaging information, can contribute to overall quality of care.

OVERVIEW OF AUTOMATION

Aging of the population and development of more laboratory assays have resulted in an increasing number of laboratory tests done every year. The Commission estimates that clinical laboratories generate up to 80% of the information physicians rely on to make crucial treatment decisions.[27]

In addition, patients and physicians, especially emergency department staff, expect that accurate test results will be available quickly. The expectation of fast turnaround time has affected the development of both central laboratory equipment and point-of-care testing instruments. Major advances in clinical laboratory testing include miniaturization of test equipment and linking patients, specimens, and automated instruments of all sizes to robotics and information technology systems. With an impending shortage of skilled laboratory staff and economic forces creating more intense competition, clinical laboratories see automation as a key to survival.

Benefits of Automation

The major benefits of laboratory automation are:
- Reduction of medical errors
- Reduced specimen sample volume
- Increased accuracy and precision (reduced coefficient of variation)
- Improved safety for laboratory staff (e.g., stopper removal or piercing)
- Faster turnaround time of results
- Partially alleviating the impending shortage of skilled laboratory staff

According to a U.S. Institute of Medicine report,[28] medical errors in the United States may contribute to up to 98,000 deaths and more than 1 million injuries each year. New TJC guidelines highlight the importance of proper identification of patient samples; a mistake in labeling or misidentification can lead to critical medical errors such as transfusion of blood products or medication to the wrong patient. The report identified several critical errors concerning laboratory processes, including delay in diagnosis.

Patient-safety benefits from automation include workflow standardization for more precise, consistently reliable test results and improved test turnaround time for faster diagnosis and better patient care. Automated specimen processing and testing also improve safety for laboratory technologists. Because they are now handling blood samples less frequently, the technologists' exposure to pathogens and sharps injuries is reduced dramatically.

In addition to alleviating the impending shortage of laboratory staff, automation can produce a more dynamic and robust laboratory. Clinical laboratory professionals can spend more time on difficult cases while automated instruments handle routine work.

Process of Automation

The CLSI has developed interrelated standards addressing the design, compatibility, and integration of automated clinical laboratory systems worldwide. Automation can be applied to any or all of the steps used to perform a manual assay.

Automated systems include:
1. Some type of device for sampling the patient's specimen or other samples to be tested (e.g., blanks, controls, standard solutions)
2. A mechanism to add the specimen to reagents in the proper sequence
3. Incubation modules when needed for the specific reaction
4. A measuring device (e.g., photometric technology) to quantitate the extent of the reaction
5. A recording mechanism to provide the final reading or permanent record of the analytical result

Most analyzers are capable of processing a variety of specimens. To increase efficiency, it is generally advisable to perform as many steps as possible without manual intervention. Full automation reduces the possibility of human errors that arise from repetitive and boring manipulations done by laboratory staff, such as pipetting errors in routine procedures.

Steps in Automated Analysis

The major steps designed by manufacturers to mimic manual techniques are:
1. Specimen collection and processing
2. Specimen and reagent measurement and delivery

3. Chemical reaction phase
4. Measurement phase
5. Signal processing and data handling

Specimen Collection and Processing

The specimen must be collected properly, labeled, and transported to the laboratory for analysis. Specimen handling and processing are vital steps in the total analytical process (see Chapter 3). To eliminate problems associated with manually handling specimens, systems have been developed to automate this process. Automation of specimen preparation steps can include the use of bar-coded labels on samples, which allow electronic identification of the samples and the tests requested. Bar coding can identify a sample and the reagents or analyses needed and relay this information to the automated analyzer. This can prevent clerical errors that could result in improperly entering patient data for analysis. In addition, bar coding allows for automated specimen storage and retrieval.

If whole blood is used, specimen preparation time is eliminated. Whole blood may also be applied manually or by automated techniques to dry reagent cartridges or test strips containing reagents for visual observations or instrument readings of a quantitative change.

Specimen and Reagent Measurement and Delivery

Automated instruments combine reagents and a measured amount of specimen in a prescribed manner to yield a specific final concentration. This combination of predetermined amounts of reagent and sample is termed **proportioning.** It is important that reagents be introduced to the sample in the proper amounts and in specific sequences for the analysis to be carried through correctly.

The most common configuration for specimen testing with large automated equipment is the **random-access analyzer.** Random-access analysis assays are performed on a collection of specimens sequentially, with each specimen analyzed for a different selection of tests. Assays are selected through the use of different containers of liquid reagents, reagent packs, or reagent tables, depending on the analyzer. The random-access analyzer does all the selected determinations on a patient sample before it goes on to the next sample. These analyzers can process different assay combinations for individual specimens. The microprocessor enables the analyzer to perform up to 30 determinations. The selected tests are ordered from the menu, and the testing is begun with the unordered tests left undone. A sampling device begins the process by measuring the exact amount of sample into the required cells. The microprocessor controls the addition of the necessary diluents and reagents to each cell. After the proper reacting period, the microprocessor begins the spectrophotometric measurements of the various cells, the reaction results are calculated, control values are checked, and the results are reported. Some analyzers of this type have a circular configuration utilizing an analytical turntable device for the various cells. Other random-access analyzers have a parallel configuration.

Chemical Reaction Phase

Reagents may be classified as *liquid* or *dry* systems for use with automated analyzers. Reagent handling varies according to instrument capabilities and methodologies. Special test packets may be inserted into an instrument. The Vitros brand of analyzer uses slides to contain the entire reagent chemistry system. Multiple layers on the slide are backed by a clear polyester support. The coating is sandwiched in a plastic mount.

The chemical reaction phase consists of mixing, separation, incubation, and reaction time. In continuous-flow analyzers, when the sample probe rises from the cup, air is aspirated for a specified time to produce a bubble between the sample and reagent plugs of liquid. In most discrete analyzers, the chemical reactants are held in individual moving containers that are either reusable or disposable. These reaction containers also function as cuvettes for optical analysis (e.g., ADVIA), or the reactants may be placed in a stationary reaction chamber in which a flow-through process or reaction mixture occurs before and after the optical reading. In continuous-flow systems, flow-through cuvettes are used and optical readings taken during the flow of reactant fluids.

In automated analyzers, incubation is simply a waiting period in which the test mixture is allowed time to react. This is done at a specified, constant temperature controlled by the analyzer.

Measurement Phase

Traditionally, automated chemistry analyzers have relied on photometers and spectrophotometry (see Chapter 6) for measurement of absorbance. Alternative measurement methods include nephelometry, chemiluminescence, enzyme immunoassay (EIA [see Chapter 6]), and ion-selective electrodes (see Chapter 11).

To ensure the accuracy of results obtained with automated systems, there must be frequent standardization of methods. Once the standardization has been done, a well-designed automated system maintains or reproduces the prescribed conditions with great precision. Frequent standardization

and running of control specimens are essential to ensure this accuracy and precision. CLIA '88 mandated regulations in the use of control specimens for certain tests. For laboratories doing moderately complex or highly complex testing using automated analyzers, a minimum of two control specimens (negative or normal and positive or increased) must be run once every 8 hours of operation or once per shift when patient specimens are being run[27] (see Chapter 8).

Signal Processing and Data Handling

The simplest method of reading results is visual instrument readout using **light-emitting diodes (LEDs)** or a monitor. Results can be converted to hard copy, or the readout can be transmitted electronically with verified results.

Most data management devices are computer-based modules with manufacturers' proprietary software that interfaces with one or more analyzers and the host LIS. These software programs offer automated QC data management, with storage and evaluation of QC results against the laboratory's predefined acceptable limits. Every LIS has the capability for data autoverification, the process in which the computer performs the initial review and verification of test results. Data that fall within a set of predefined parameters or rules established by the laboratory are automatically verified in the LIS and the patient's files. The LIS may transmit results directly to a server or wireless pager. Laboratory staff must review all the data that falls outside the set of parameters or rules.

AUTOMATED ANALYZERS

Many different analyzers continue to be manufactured for use in the central clinical laboratory and for off-site testing. The choice of instrument depends on several factors: the volume of determinations done in the laboratory, type of data profile to be generated, level of staffing, initial cost of the instrument, its maintenance and operation costs, and time required for each analysis.

Automated instruments have been designed to perform the most frequently ordered tests, because 6 tests make up 50% of the workload of the average chemistry laboratory and another 14 tests make up an additional 40%.[28] Versatility and flexibility are often just as important as high volume and speed of testing, but automation is also desirable for less-frequently ordered tests.

In the case of large-volume hospital and reference laboratories, a **completely automated laboratory system (CALS)** may be used. Each automated instrument can operate separately as well as being integrated with other laboratory instruments.

Instruments can be linked into a single continuous operation that can include robotic specimen processing.

The three most highly automated or semiautomated clinical laboratory specialties are clinical chemistry, hematology, and more recently, urinalysis. Automated or semiautomated testing is less frequently used in blood banking and microbiology, although automated systems for testing and screening donated blood and identification of biochemical reactions of bacteria are becoming more common.

Clinical Chemistry and Immunochemistry Analyzers

The earliest automated testing occurred in clinical chemistry. Manufacturers continue to develop new assays for large-volume testing using clinical chemistry analyzers (Table 10-1). Many of the methods replicate standard manual reactions (see Chapter 6). Unique methods such as chemiluminescence have been developed for immunoassays performed by automated analyzers (Table 10-2).

Hematology Instrumentation

Automated cell counters in hematology range from high-volume instruments (Table 10-3) to simple instruments that can count red blood cells (RBCs), white blood cells (WBCs), and platelets. In more sophisticated instruments (see Evolve site), the types of WBCs can be identified and counted.

Principles of Cell Counting

Most automated cell counters can be classified as one of two types: those using electrical resistance and those using optical methods with focused laser beams, in which cells cause a change in the deflection of a beam of light. In cell counters using optical methods, deflections are converted to measurable pulses by a photo multiplier tube. In electrical resistance cell counters, blood cells passing through an aperture through which a current is flowing cause a change in electrical resistance that is counted as voltage pulses. The voltage pulses are amplified and can be displayed on an oscilloscope screen. Each spike indicates a cell. Both types of instruments count thousands of cells in a few seconds, and both increase the precision of cell counts compared with manual methods.

Hemoglobin Measurement

Hemoglobin is measured by the traditional cyanmethemoglobin flow cell method at 525 and 546 nm, depending on the instrument manufacturer. Many instruments also count immature erythrocytes (reticulocytes). Because models and features of instrumentation change rapidly, the reader is advised to refer to the respective manufacturer's website.

Examples of Automated Hematology Instruments

The Abbott Cell-Dyn Series uses multiangle polarized scatter separation (MAPSS) flow cytometry with hydrodynamic focusing of the cell stream (see Chapter 6). It features dual leukocyte counting methods. The leukocyte differential is accomplished by light scatter with 0, 90, 10, 90 (depolarized) degrees and nuclear optical count by light scatter at 0 and 10 degrees. Erythrocytes and platelets are counted by light scatter at 0 and 10 degrees. A unique feature is cyanide-free hemoglobinometry. One system, the Cell-Dyn 4000, features three independent measurements and focused flow impedance. Multidimensional light scatter and fluorescent detection are used as well.

The Siemens Diagnostics Healthcare System's ADVIA Series uses unifluidics, a darkfield optical method. Dual leukocyte methods of peroxidase staining and basophil lobularity are used.

TABLE 10-1

Summary of Features of Representative Large-Volume Clinical Chemistry Analyzers			
Manufacturer	Instrument Series	Type	Test Principle
Abbott (www.abbott.com)	Architect c8000	Random access	Photometry, potentiometry*
Beckman-Coulter (www.beckman coulter.com)	Synchron Series	Random access	Photometry, potentiometry, various types of turbidimetry, enzyme immunoassay (EIA)
Ortho Clinical Diagnostics (www.orthoclinical.com)	Vitros Series	Random access	Potentiometry, colorimetry
Roche (www.roche-diagnostics.us)	Integra Cobra	Random access discrete	Photometry, potentiometry
Siemens Diagnostics Healthcare System (www.medical.siemens.com)	ADVIA	Random access batch	Photometry, potentiometry, turbidimetry

*Potentiometry: ion-selective electrode and electrochemiluminescence.

TABLE 10-2

Summary of Features of Representative Immunochemistry Analyzers				
Manufacturer	Instrument Series	Test Principle	Type	Test Menus
Abbott	AxSYM	Chemiluminescence	Random access	Hormones, tumor markers, cardiac markers, toxicology, fertility/pregnancy, hepatitis markers, therapeutic drug monitoring (TDM)
Beckman-Coulter	ACCESS	Chemiluminescence	Random access	Hormones, tumor markers, cardiac markers, anemia profile, some therapeutic drugs, infectious disease markers
BioMerieux Biomerieux-usa.com	VIDAS	Fluorescent enzyme-linked assay	Batch	Hormones, some TDM, infectious disease markers, D-dimer assay
Roche	ELECSYS	Electrochemiluminescence	Random access	Hormones, tumor markers, cardiac markers, anemia profile, hepatitis markers
Siemens Diagnostics Healthcare Systems	ADVIA Centaur	Chemiluminescence	Random access	Hormones, tumor markers, cardiac markers, therapeutic drug monitoring, anemia profile

TABLE 10-3

Examples of Automated Hematology Instruments*		
Manufacturer	url	Series
Abbott Diagnostics	www.abbott.com	CELL-DYN
Beckman Coulter, Inc.	www.beckmancoulter.com	Coulter HmX, LH, and Ac. Tdiff Family
Cella Vision	www.cellavision.com	DM
Horiba ABX Diagnostics	www.abx.com	Pentra
Siemens Healthcare Diagnosticss	www.medical.siemens.com	ADVIA
Sysmex	www.sysmex.com	XE

*See Evolve for a comprehensive listing of current hematology instruments with features.

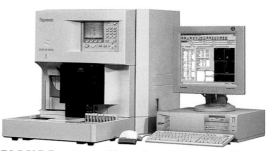

FIGURE 10-3 Hematology Automation; Sysmex XE-2100. (Courtesy Sysmex Inc., Mundelein, Ill.)

Erythrocytes and platelets are counted by flow cytometry. Hemoglobin has dual readings and colorimetric or cyanmethemoglobin and corpuscular hemoglobin mean concentration.

A third choice is the Beckman-Coulter Z1 Series. This instrument uses electrical impedance to measure the volume of the cells by direct current. Radio frequency (RF) or conductivity is used to gather information related to cell size and internal structure. Scatter or laser light is used to obtain information about cellular granularity and cell surface structure. Opacity is monitored to delineate internal structure, including nuclear size, density, and nuclear/cytoplasmic ratio. A three-dimensional analysis is the output.

With Sysmex systems (Fig. 10-3), erythrocytes and platelets are analyzed by hydrodynamic focusing, direct current (DC), and automatic discrimination. The leukocyte count is analyzed by the DC detection method and automatic discrimination. A five-part differential is produced for leukocytes by a differential detector channel (analyzed by RF and DC). A differential scattergram and an IMI scattergram are produced.

Automated Leukocyte Differentiation

In an environment of cost containment and shortage of laboratory personnel, together with increasingly sophisticated instrumentation, the so-called routine hematologic examination (complete blood count) often uses an automated rather than a manual leukocyte differential. Automated differentials can provide a great amount of useful, cost-efficient information when interpreted by an experienced laboratory staff member, especially when a manual leukocyte differential or review of the blood film is performed on abnormal results, as determined by the laboratory.

Automated three-part differentials consist of a size-distributed histogram of WBCs. In most of these instruments, three subpopulations of WBCs are counted: lymphocytes, other mononuclear cells, and granulocytes. A computer calculates the number of particles in each area as a percentage of the total WBC histogram. Any abnormal histograms are flagged for review.

Many of the multiparameter hematology analyzers provide differentiation of leukocytes, and many instruments that provide five-cell differentials are available. The major advantage of automated differentiation of leukocytes is that many thousands of cells are analyzed rapidly. New cell identification systems (e.g., CellaVision) use digital imaging to identify cells and store images (Fig. 10-4).

The multiparameter analyzers differ in the principle by which leukocytes are differentiated. In general, they can employ:

1. Impedance-related, conductivity, light-scattering measurements of cell volume
2. Automated continuous-flow systems that use cytochemical and light-scattering measurements
3. Automated computer image analysis of a blood film prepared by an instrument

The Coulter principle is used to construct a size-distributed histogram of leukocytes. These methods are combined and the electrical signals are further manipulated with computer-assisted synthesis and derivations. Several instruments are available, and none is clearly superior to the others.

Other technologies for differentiating leukocytes in particular include the CellaVision digital microscope system (see Chapter 5) as well as immunophenotyping using flow cytometry. These instruments are known as *flow cytometers*. Flow cell technology differentiates various cell populations through the use of fluorescently tagged cluster designation markers (see Chapter 12). Immunofluorescent cytoflow technology produces unique scattergrams and histograms.

Urinalysis

Instruments are available to semiautomate or totally automate the routine chemical testing in urinalysis (UA) and in some cases, microscopic examination (Table 10-4). These systems use reflectance photometers for reading their respective reagent strips. Once the strip is placed in the analyzer, the microprocessor mechanically moves the strip into the reflectometer, turns on the light source needed, records the reflectance data, calculates the results, and removes the strip for disposal.

In fully automated chemical analyses of glucose, ketones, proteins, and other constituents, the specimen is aspirated from the sample tube and added to a strip containing nine reactive reagent pads (for chemical and physicochemical tests) and

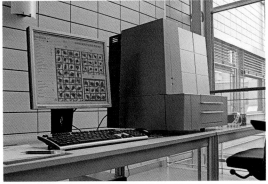

FIGURE 10-4 Hematology CellaVision DM96. (Courtesy CellaVision Inc., Jupiter, Fla.)

one nonreactive pad (for color) per specimen, supplied on a roll of plastic film to which are affixed 490 reagent strips. Use of this reflectance spectrophotometric instrument eliminates the need for "dipping" the reagent strip into the patient's urine specimen. It measures clarity, color, and specific gravity by refractive index. Samples are identified by bar code, and results may be interfaced to the laboratory computer for reporting.

MOLECULAR TESTING

Polymerase chain reaction (PCR) is an in vitro method that amplifies low levels of specific deoxyribonucleic acid (DNA) sequences in a sample to higher quantities suitable for further analysis. To use this technology, the target sequence to be amplified must be known. Each cycle of amplification theoretically doubles the amount of specific DNA sequence present and results in an exponential accumulation of the DNA fragment being amplified (amplicons). The three important applications of PCR are amplification of DNA, identification of a target sequence, and synthesis of a labeled antisense probe. PCR analysis can lead to the detection of gene mutations that signify the early development of cancer, identification of viral DNA associated with specific cancers such as human papilloma virus (HPV), a causative agent in cervical cancer, or detection of genetic mutations associated with a wide variety of diseases (e.g., coronary artery disease, associated with mutations of the gene that encodes for the low-density lipoprotein receptor [LDLR]).

Other molecular methods are the **Southern blot** and **Western blot** techniques. Single-base mutations that can be determined by Southern blot include sickle cell anemia and hemophilia A. Western blot is a technique in which proteins are separated electrophoretically, transferred to membranes, and identified through the use of labeled antibodies specific for the protein of interest.

TABLE 10-4

Representative Semiautomated Urine Analyzers				
Manufacturer	Instrument	Test Principle	Chemical Measurements*	Microscopy Analyzer
Siemens Diagnostics Healthcare	Clinitek Status + Analyzer	Reflectance photometer	Albumin, bilirubin, occult blood, creatinine, glucose, ketone, leukocytes, nitrite, pH, protein, specific gravity, urobilinogen	No
Iris (Quidel Corp.) (www.proiris.com)	AUTION Max AX-4280	Reflectance photometer	Glucose, bilirubin, ketones, occult blood, protein, nitrite, leukocytes, pH, urobilinogen	No
	iQ200 Sprint	N/A	RBCs, WBCs, hyaline casts, pathologic casts, crystals, squamous and nonsquamous epithelial cells, yeast, WBC clumps, sperm, mucus	No
Roche (www.roche.com)	Urisys 1100	Reflectance photometer	Glucose, bilirubin, ketones, occult blood, protein, nitrite, leukocytes	No
Sysmex (www.sysmex.com/us)	Sysmex UF-1000	Fluorescent flow cytometry and cluster analysis, forward scatter and impedance technologies	Albumin, bilirubin, occult blood, creatinine, glucose, ketone, leukocytes, nitrite, pH, protein, specific gravity, urobilinogen	Yes
HemoCue (www.hemocue.com)	Urine Albumin	Immunoturbidimetric reaction in microcuvettes read by photometer	Low levels of urinary albumin	No

N/A, Not applicable; *RBCs*, red blood cells; *WBCs*, white blood cells.
*The number of chemical measurements will vary depending on the number of tests impregnated on the test strip.

Microarrays (DNA chips) are another new technology of interest. DNA chips are basically the product of bonding or direct synthesis of numerous specific DNA probes on a stationary, often silicon-based support. Microarrays are miniature gene fragments attached to glass chips. These chips are used to examine gene activity of thousands or tens of thousands of gene fragments and to identify genetic mutations. Applications of microarrays in clinical medicine include analysis of gene expression in malignancies (e.g., mutations in *BRCA1*, mutations of tumor suppressor gene p53), genetic disease testing, and viral resistance mutation detection.

REFERENCES

1. Kasoff J: Advances in LIS functionality, Adv Med Lab Professionals 20, no.16:pp 16–19, August 11, 2008.
2. Hattie M: Bar coding: Labs go 2D, www.mlo-online.com, September 2009.
3. Smith TJ: Barcode: meet your match, Adv Med Lab Professionals 18, no:12–13, Dec 4, 2006.
4. College of American Pathologists Accreditation Standards: (www.cap.org) retrieved Oct. 7, 2009.
5. Winsten D: Molecular, Genetic Data and the LIS, Adv Med Lab Professionals 20, no. 15:22–25, July 28, 2008.
6. Lehman C, Burgnener R, Munoz O: Autoverification and laboratory quality critical values Vol. 2, No. 4:24–27, Oct 2009.
7. Graham. KJ: Lab limelight: autoverification, Adv Med Lab Professionals 19, no. 1:22, Jan 2007.
8. Clinical and Laboratory Standards Institute: Autoverification of clinical laboratory test results auto 10 A, approved standard, Wayne, Pa, 2006.
9. Clinical and Laboratory Standards Institute: Laboratory automation: specimen container/specimen carrier: approved standard, Wayne, Pa, 2000, AUTO 01-A.
10. Clinical and Laboratory Standards Institute: Laboratory automation: bar codes for specimen container identification: approved standard, Wayne, Pa, 2006, AUTO 02-A2.2ed.
11. Clinical and Laboratory Standards Institute: Laboratory automation: communications with automated clinical laboratory systems, instruments, devices, and information systems: approved standard, Wayne, Pa, 2009, AUTO 03-A2.
12. Clinical and Laboratory Standards Institute: Laboratory automation: systems operational requirements, characteristics, and information elements: approved standard, Wayne, Pa, 2001, AUTO 04-A.
13. Clinical and Laboratory Standards Institute: Laboratory automation: electromechanical interfaces: approved standard, Wayne, Pa, 2001 AUTO 05-A.
14. Clinical and Laboratory Standards Institute: Laboratory automation: data content for specimen identification: approved standard, Wayne, Pa, 2004, AUTO 07-A.
15. Clinical and Laboratory Standards Institute: Protocols to validate laboratory information systems: proposed guideline, Wayne, Pa, 2006, AUTO 08-A.
16. Clinical and Laboratory Standards Institute: Remote access to clinical laboratory diagnostic devices via the Internet: proposed standard, Wayne, Pa, 2006, AUTO 09-A.

17. Clinical and Laboratory Standards Institute: Laboratory instruments and data management systems: design of software user interfaces and end-user software systems validation, operation, and monitoring: approved guideline, ed 2, Wayne, Pa, 2003, GP19-A2.

18. Clinical and Laboratory Standards Institute: Standard specification for low-level protocol to transfer messages between clinical laboratory instruments and computer systems, Wayne, Pa, 2008, LIS 01-A2.

19. Clinical and Laboratory Standards Institute: Specification for transferring information between clinical laboratory instruments and information systems: approved standard, ed 2, Wayne, Pa, 2004, LIS 02-A2.

20. Clinical and Laboratory Standards Institute: Standard guide for selection of a clinical laboratory information management system, Wayne, Pa, 2003, LIS 03-A.

21. Clinical and Laboratory Standards Institute: Standard guide for documentation of clinical laboratory computer systems, Wayne, Pa, 2003, LIS 04-A.

22. Clinical and Laboratory Standards Institute: Standard specification for transferring clinical observations between independent computer systems, Wayne, Pa, 2003, LIS 05-A.

23. Clinical and Laboratory Standards Institute: Standard practice for reporting reliability of clinical laboratory information systems, Wayne, Pa, 2003, LIS 06-A.

24. Clinical and Laboratory Standards Institute: Standard specification for use of bar codes on specimen tubes in the clinical laboratory, Wayne, Pa, 2003, LIS 07-A.

25. Clinical and Laboratory Standards Institute: Standard guide for functional requirements of clinical laboratory information management systems, Wayne, Pa, 2003, LIS 08-A.

26. Clinical and Laboratory Standards Institute: Standard guide for coordination of clinical laboratory services within the electronic health record environment and networked architectures, Wayne, Pa, 2003, LIS 09-A.

27. Beckman-Coulter Conference: Lab automation, Palm Springs, Calif, 2003.

28. US Institute of Medicine: To err is human, Washington, DC, 1999, US Government Printing Office.

BIBLIOGRAPHY

Accu-Chek Products: www.accu-chek.com (retrieved August 2005).

Brown SM: Bioinformatics: a biologist's guide to biocomputing and the Internet, New York, 2000, Eaton.

Burtis CA, Ashwood ER, Bruns DE: Tietz fundamentals of clinical chemistry, ed 6, St Louis, 2008, Saunders.

Cerner Corporation: www.cerner.com (retrieved October, 2009).

Clin Lab: www.clinlabinc.com (retrieved July 2005).

Jefferson R: LIS selection guide: research your unique requirements before purchasing or upgrading your LIS, Adv Med Lab Professionals 14(13):14, 2002.

Jefferson R: POL connectivity: LIS to reference lab and beyond, Adv Med Lab Professionals 15(4):13, 2003.

Kaplan LA, Pesce AJ: Clinical chemistry: theory, analysis, and correlation, ed 5, St Louis, 2010, Mosby.

McMahan J: HIPAA and the Lab Information System Act will have direct effect on use of LIS, Adv Med Lab Professionals 14(3):8, 2002.

McMahan J: Primer on LIS interfaces, Adv Med Lab Professionals 14(20):8, 2002.

McMahan J: Necessary evils of information technology, Adv Med Lab Professionals 17(9):14, 2005.

Medical Automation Systems: www.medicalautomation.com (retrieved August 2005).

Sarker, D.K. Quality systems and control for pharmaceuticals, West Sussex, England, 2008, Wiley.

Siemens Healthcare Solutions. SpecTrack and Lab Link (retrieved October 2009).

Smith T: Making IT work: relieving the IS headache, Adv Med Lab Professionals 14(2):24, 2002.

Terese SC, Edborg M: Clinical laboratory automation, Healthcare Informatics On-Line, June 2005 (retrieved August 2005).

Turgeon ML: Immunology and serology in laboratory medicine, ed 4, St Louis, 2009, Mosby.

US Department of Health and Human Services: Standards for privacy of individually identifiable health information, 45 CFR Parts 160 and 164, Washington, DC, April 2003.

Verne B: Size up this critical medical laboratory automation, ML-OnLine, July 2005, www.mlo-online.com (retrieved August 2005).

Zakowski J, Powell D: The future of automation in clinical laboratories, IVDT :48, July 1999, www.devicelink.com (retrieved August 2005).

REVIEW QUESTIONS

1. **What is the ultimate goal of the laboratory?**
   a. Perform more tests
   b. Hire less staff
   c. Quickly produce results
   d. Produce accurate information in a timely manner

Questions 2-5: A = *True or B = False.*

Computer technology can be used for:

2. ___ **Specimen processing**

3. ___ **Inventory control**

4. ___ **Ordering tests**

5. ___ **Monitoring patient results**

Questions 6-10: Match the component with the function (a to e).

6. ___ **CPU**

7. ___ **RAM**

8. ___ **Input device**

9. ___ **Output device**

10. ___ **Interface**
    a. Short-term memory
    b. Executes software instructions
    c. Exchange of information
    d. A printer
    e. Bar code reader

11. **The Health Insurance Portability and Accountability Act (HIPAA):**
    a. sets minimum standards for security of only electronic health information.
    b. replaces federal and state laws on privacy of health information.
    c. requires laboratories to collect diagnostic codes.
    d. both a and c.

12. **The Joint Commission estimates that ___% of the information that physicians rely on is generated by the laboratory.**
    a. 20
    b. 40
    c. 80
    d. 100

13. **The major benefit(s) of laboratory automation is (are):**
    a. reduction in medical errors.
    b. improved safety for laboratory staff.
    c. faster turnaround time.
    d. all of the above.

14. **Steps in automation designed to mimic manual techniques include:**
    a. pipetting of specimen.
    b. pipetting of reagents.
    c. measurement of chemical reactions.
    d. all of the above.

15. **What is a common principle applied in immunochemistry?**
    a. Photometry
    b. Enzyme immunoassay
    c. Chemiluminescence
    d. Ion-selective electrodes

16. **When hematology cell counters detect voltage pulses, what principle is being applied?**
    a. Electrical resistance
    b. Optical deflection
    c. Photometry
    d. Turbidimetry

17. **A three-part blood cell differential separates:**
    a. erythrocytes, leukocytes, and platelets.
    b. monocytes, granulocytes, and lymphocytes.
    c. mononuclear cells, granulocytes, and lymphocytes.
    d. segmented neutrophils, eosinophils, and basophils.

18. **Semiautomated routine chemical screening of urine uses what test principle?**
    a. Ion-selective electrodes
    b. Reflectance photometry
    c. Potentiometry
    d. Turbidimetry

19. **PCR testing is useful in:**
    a. forensic testing.
    b. genetic testing.
    c. disease diagnosis.
    d. all of the above.

PART II

Clinical Laboratory Specializations

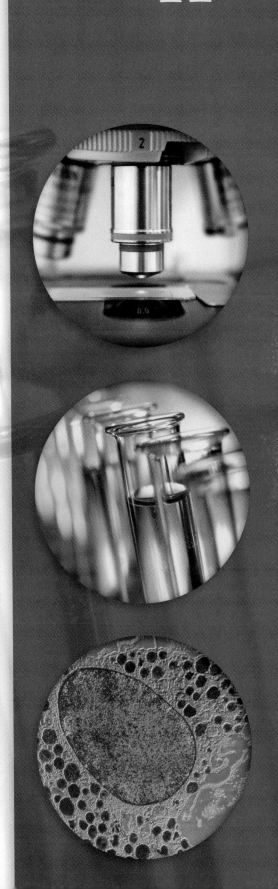

CHAPTER 11

INTRODUCTION TO CLINICAL CHEMISTRY

At the conclusion of this chapter, the student will be able to:

- Describe the normal physiology of glucose metabolism including glycogenesis, gluconeogenesis, lipogenesis, and glycolysis.
- Compare and contrast the pathophysiology of types 1 and 2 diabetes.
- Describe the symptoms of diabetes.
- Compare the conditions of hyperglycemia and hypoglycemia.
- Describe the collection procedures and various types of blood specimens for glucose analysis.
- Compare point-of-care testing to traditional testing methods for glucose.
- Describe the methods for qualitative and semiquantitative determination of glucose.
- Explain the significance of glycosylated hemoglobin in the management of diabetes.
- Identify and describe the function of electrolytes found in blood and body fluids.
- Calculate osmolality and osmolal gap, and apply them to clinical situations.
- Calculate an anion gap, and apply it to clinical situations.
- Explain the role and alterations of acid-base balance and blood gases in the body.

- Compare and contrast renal function assays.
- Describe the methodology and interpret the clinical significance of uric acid analysis.
- Compare the biochemical and physiologic characteristics of cholesterol, triglycerides, and lipoprotein.
- Compare and contrast at least three cardiac markers of acute myocardial infarction.
- Name liver and pancreatic assays, and explain their clinical significance.
- Describe the physiology of bilirubin formation and associated abnormal conditions.
- Differentiate between different forms of bilirubin, and understand the clinical significance of various forms.
- Describe at least two hormone assays and the clinical applications.
- Compare and contrast the clinical significance of various types of tumor markers.
- Describe therapeutic drug assays, and identify drugs of abuse.
- Relate the findings of laboratory assays to case study presentations.

Chemistry is an area in which changes continue to occur because of the introduction of new methodologies and increasingly sophisticated instrumentation. This chapter describes selected classic manual methods as well as analytical approaches in common use today. An understanding of both classic and current methods is helpful in mastering the basics of manual testing and automated testing. Groups of clinically related procedures and major clinical applications are discussed in this chapter.

GLUCOSE AND GLUCOSE METABOLISM

One of the most frequently performed determinations in the clinical chemistry laboratory is blood glucose. *Glucose* (Fig. 11-1) is a simple sugar, or monosaccharide, derived from the breakdown of dietary carbohydrates. Intestinal absorption of carbohydrates occurs in the small intestine, where monosaccharides, the single-sugar units of carbohydrates, are absorbed. Nonglucose monosaccharides,

including galactose and fructose, are converted to glucose by the liver.

At any given time, the blood glucose level is under the control of a number of hormones.

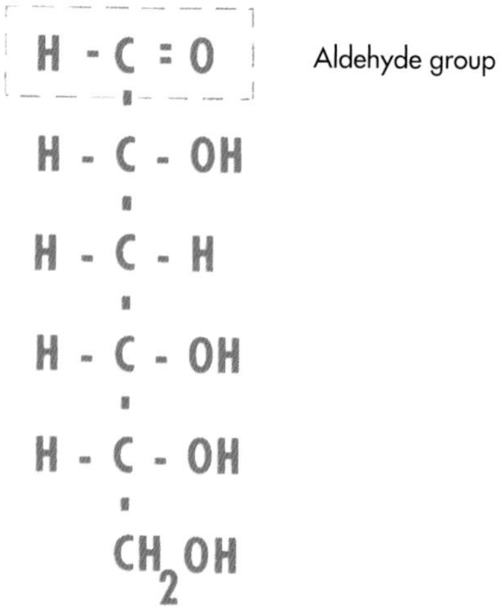

FIGURE 11-1 Glucose molecule.

Insulin, a hormone secreted by the pancreas after a meal, responds to high glucose levels, promoting glucose entry into cells (Fig. 11-2). Glucose may also be converted, under the action of insulin, to protein and fat **(lipogenesis),** with the latter stored as fat (adipose) tissue. Most body cells have limited glycogen stores, but the liver and skeletal muscles store larger amounts of glycogen. Glycogen constitutes 10% of the total weight of the liver.

Depending on the cell's needs, glucose may undergo anaerobic and aerobic metabolism to yield energy as adenosine triphosphate (ATP). **Gluconeogenesis,** the formation of glucose from lactate or amino acids, is stimulated by the hormones glucagon, cortisol, and thyroxine. Alternatively, glucose may be biochemically converted to and stored as glycogen **(glycogenesis).**

Glucose is the primary source of energy for most body cells. Insulin regulates the concentration of blood glucose by promoting its entry into the cell, followed by a number of possible metabolic fates: glycolysis, glycogenesis, lipogenesis, and protein synthesis. Several hormones have the effect of maintaining the blood glucose concentration during the fasting state. These hormones have varied cellular effects, but all oppose the action of insulin by raising the blood glucose level. **Glucagon,** secreted by the alpha (α) cells of the pancreas, is the major hormone that opposes the action of insulin, increasing blood glucose by stimulating the breakdown of glycogen **(glycogenolysis)** by the liver. A number of other hormones, some secondary to pituitary hormone release, also promote glycogenolysis, the degradation of glycogen to form glucose.

The common reference range for fasting serum plasma glucose level has traditionally been between 70 and 110 mg/dL, depending on the method of analysis.[1] Normal fasting plasma glucose level was recently defined in young men as less than 100 mg/dL.[2] The plasma glucose level increases rapidly after a carbohydrate-rich meal, returning to normal 1½ to 2 hours after eating (**postprandial** level).

Many diseases alter normal glucose metabolism. The most frequent cause of an increase in blood glucose, or **hyperglycemia,** is diabetes.

Hypoglycemia, defined as a blood glucose level less than 50 mg/dL, may have severe consequences. One cause of hypoglycemia in diabetic patients is an excessive dose of insulin. The body secretes a number of hormones that increase blood glucose levels, but only insulin lowers blood sugar.

DIABETES

Diabetes poses a significant public health challenge for the United States. Currently, 10.5 million persons have been diagnosed with diabetes, and 5.5 million persons are estimated to have the disease but are undiagnosed. Over the past decade, the number of persons with diabetes has increased steadily. During this same time period, diabetes has

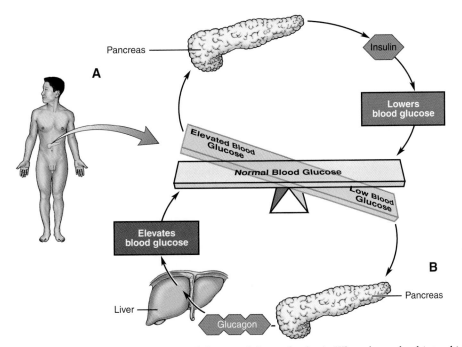

FIGURE 11-2 Glucose balance. Homeostatic balancing of glucose levels. A, When glucose level is too high, insulin lowers it to normal. B, When glucose level is too low, glucagon raises it to normal. (From Herlihy M: The human body in health and illness, ed 2, Philadelphia, 2003, Saunders.)

remained the seventh leading cause of death in the United States, primarily from diabetes-associated cardiovascular disease.[3]

The classification of diabetes includes four clinical classes[3]:

- Type 1 diabetes (results from β-cell destruction, usually leading to absolute insulin deficiency)
- Type 2 diabetes (results from a progressive insulin secretory defect on the background of insulin resistance)
- Gestational diabetes mellitus (GDM), diagnosed during pregnancy
- Other specific types of diabetes due to other causes (e.g., genetic defects in β-cell function, genetic defects in insulin action, diseases of the exocrine pancreas [e.g., cystic fibrosis], and drug or chemically induced [e.g., treatment of AIDS or after organ transplantation])

Type 1 Diabetes

Type 1 diabetes, or *insulin-dependent diabetes*, is usually diagnosed in children and young adults and was previously called *juvenile diabetes*[3] (Box 11-1). Both type 1 and type 2 diabetes have a significant genetic component. For type 1 diabetes, genetic markers that indicate a greater risk for this condition have been identified; they are sensitive but not specific.[3]

Type 1 diabetes results from the lack of insulin caused by cell-mediated autoimmune destruction of insulin-secreting pancreatic beta (β) cells. The autoimmune process leading to type 1 diabetes begins years before manifestation of clinical signs and symptoms. An estimated 80% to 90% reduction in the number of β cells is required to induce symptomatic type 1 diabetes. Children have a more rapid rate of islet cell destruction than adults. Circulating antibodies can be demonstrated in the serum of individuals with type 1 diabetes. Indicators of autoimmune destruction of the pancreas include islet cell antibodies and insulin antibodies.

The breakdown of fat (lipolysis) from adipose tissue to supply energy in diabetes can be life threatening. Increased lipolysis results in increased concentrations of ketone bodies, which can lead to ketoacidosis, particularly in type 1 diabetic patients with absolute insulin deficiency. As a consequence, a dangerous decrease in blood pH, or acidosis, may occur.

Type 2 Diabetes

The incidence of type 2 diabetes, or *non–insulin-dependent diabetes*, may be as high as 7% among adults in the United States, with as many as half the cases going undiagnosed. Type 2 diabetes occurs later in life with a gradual onset, usually after 40 years of age. This form of the disease is also called *adult-onset diabetes*.

Type 2 diabetes is characterized by insulin resistance and progressive hyperglycemia. Type 2 diabetic patients can develop complications similar to those noted in type 1 diabetes, but ketoacidosis is less likely to occur. Type 2 diabetes is also associated with the development of atherosclerosis, with an increased risk of coronary artery disease and stroke.

Higher fasting plasma glucose concentrations within the normoglycemic range constitute an independent risk factor for type 2 diabetes among young men. Such levels, along with body mass index and triglyceride levels, may help identify apparently healthy men at increased risk for developing type 2 diabetes (Box 11-2).[4]

Symptoms of Diabetes

The primary symptoms of diabetes are excessive urination **(polyuria),** abnormally high blood glucose (hyperglycemia) and urine glucose **(glycosuria),** excessive thirst **(polydipsia),** constant hunger **(polyphagia),** and sudden weight loss. During acute episodes of the disease, excessive blood ketones **(ketonemia)** and urinary ketones **(ketonuria)** may be detected. These symptoms are all caused by the body's inability to metabolize glucose and the resulting consequences of high glucose levels. **Glucosuria** is a consequence of hyperglycemia. When the blood glucose exceeds 160 to 170 mg/dL (the renal threshold for glucose), glucose appears in the urine. The actual diagnosis of diabetes is established by determining blood glucose levels (Table 11-1).

Gestational Diabetes Mellitus

Gestational diabetes mellitus is defined as glucose intolerance that is first recognized during pregnancy. In March, 2010, the International Association of Diabetes and Pregnancy Study Groups (IADPSG) released recommendations[5] for diagnosing gestation diabetes as well as overt diabetes in prgnancy (Tables 11-2 and 11-3). Under the IADPSG recommendations, all pregnant women would undergo

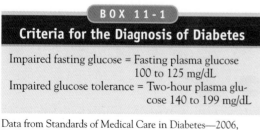

BOX 11-1
Criteria for the Diagnosis of Diabetes

Impaired fasting glucose = Fasting plasma glucose 100 to 125 mg/dL
Impaired glucose tolerance = Two-hour plasma glucose 140 to 199 mg/dL

Data from Standards of Medical Care in Diabetes—2006, Diabetes Care 29:S4-S42, 2006.

a three-step process of fasting, 1-hour and 2-hour plasma glucose tests. New recommendations are hoped to lead to one world-wide standard, optimal glycemic treatment targets, and apprpropriate postnatal follow-up of mothers and children.

BOX 11-2
Criteria for Testing for Diabetes in Asymptomatic Adult Individuals

1. Testing for diabetes should be considered in all individuals at age 45 years and older, particularly in those with a body mass index (BMI) of 25 kg/m2*; if normal, testing should be repeated at 3-year intervals.
   Testing should be considered at a younger age or be carried out more frequently in individuals who are overweight (BMI 25 kg/m2*) and have additional risk factors.

2. Additional risk factors:
   * Family history of diabetes in a first-degree relative
   * Habitually inactive
   * Membership in a high-risk minority population (e.g., African American, Latino, Native American, Asian American, Pacific Islander)
   * History of gestational diabetes or delivering a baby heavier than 9 pounds
   * Hypertension (>140/90 mm Hg)
   * Low concentration (<35 mg/dL) of high-density lipoprotein (HDL) cholesterol and/or elevated triglyceride concentrations (>250 mg/dL)
   * History of impaired fasting glucose or impaired glucose tolerance
   * Diagnosis of polycystic ovary syndrome (PCOS)
   * Diagnosis of other clinical conditions associated with insulin resistance
   * History of vascular disease

Data from Standards of Medical Care in Diabetes—2006, Diabetes Care 29:S4–S42, 2006.
*Factors may not be correct for all ethnic groups.

The metabolic and hormonal changes experienced during pregnancy contribute to this form of diabetes. Treatment of GDM reduces serious perinatal morbidity and may also improve the pregnant woman's health-related quality of life. Although most women return to normal after childbirth, studies have shown that a significant number of GDM patients will develop type 2 diabetes decades after delivery.

Other Causes of Hyperglycemia

In some cases, high blood glucose values are caused by conditions other than diabetes. Hyperglycemia can be secondary to traumatic brain injury; febrile disease; certain liver diseases; and overactivity of the adrenal, pituitary, or thyroid glands. Often, hyperglycemic patients have impaired glucose tolerance when the fasting glucose or 2-hour postprandial glucose level is elevated above normal.

Stress-induced hyperglycemia is a condition encountered in nondiabetic persons as well as diabetic patients and is common in patients with severe illness. It is standard procedure for hospitalized patients in intensive care to have their blood glucose levels monitored frequently. Maintenance of the blood sugar at close to normal limits, referred to as *tight glycemic control*, is accomplished by infusion of intravenous insulin. Bedside testing for blood glucose has made this possible. This procedure has been shown to significantly reduce morbidity, including renal dysfunction, and mortality in critically ill patients with stress-induced hyperglycemia.[6]

Hypoglycemia

Hypoglycemia is a blood glucose concentration below the fasting value, with a transient decline in blood sugar 1½ to 2 hours after a meal. *Glycogen storage disease*, associated with impaired breakdown of stored glycogen in the liver, causes hypoglycemia.

TABLE 11-1

Diagnosis of Diabetes and Prediabetes		
Time of Specimen Collection for Plasma Glucose Testing	Laboratory Results	Plasma Reference(Normal) Values
Fasting	≥126 mg/dL (7.0 mmol/L) occurring on two occasions	<100 g/dL (5.6 mmol/L)
Random	≥200 mg/dL (11.1 mmol/L)	<140 g/dL (7.8 mmol/L)
2-hour post glucose (75 gram glucose load)	≥200 mg/dL	< 140 g/dL (7.8 mmol/L)
Prediabetes Impaired fasting glucose	100-125 mg/dL 5.6-6.9 mmol/L	<100 g/dL (5.6 mmol/L)
Prediabetes Impaired glucose tolerance	140-199 mg/dL 7.8-11.0 mmol/L	<100 g/dL (5.6 mmol/L)

From McPherson RA, Pincus MR: Henry's clinical diagnosis and management by laboratory methods, ed 21, Philadelphia, 2006, Saunders, pp 185, 189.

TABLE 11-2

Proposed Diagnostic Thresholds		
Gestational Diabetes		
Screening Time	Glucose Threshold mmol/L	Glucose Threshold mg/dL
Fasting plasma glucose	5.1	92
1-hour plasma glucose	10.0	180
2-hour plasma glucose	8.5	153

From Metzger BE: Diagnosis and classification of hyperglycemia in pregnancy, consensus panel, Diabetes Care, 33:676–682, 2010.

TABLE 11-3

Proposed Diagnostic Thresholds		
Overt Diabetes in Pregnancy		
	mmol/L	mg/dL
Fasting plasma glucose	≥ 7.0	≥ 126
HbA1c	≥ 6.5%	
Random plasma glucose	≥ 11.1	≥ 200 + confirmation

From Metzger BE: Diagnosis and classification of hyperglycemia in pregnancy, consensus panel, Diabetes Care 33:676–682, 2010.

Other causes of low blood glucose include *islet cell hyperplasia* and *insulinoma*. Both these conditions result in an increased concentration of insulin in the blood (*hyperinsulinemia*). A decrease in blood glucose is life threatening because the brain and cardiac cells depend on glucose in the blood and interstitial fluids.

Hypoglycemia can lead to nausea and vomiting, muscle spasms, unconsciousness, and death. The most common causes of hypoglycemia in neonates are prematurity, maternal diabetes, GDM, and maternal toxemia. These conditions are usually transient. If the onset of hypoglycemia is in early infancy, it is usually less transitory and may be caused by an inborn error of metabolism or *ketotic hypoglycemia*, a type of hypoglycemia that usually develops after fasting or a febrile illness.

Collection of Blood Specimens for Glucose

Capillary Blood Specimens

An advantage of using whole blood is the convenience of measuring glucose directly with capillary blood, as for infants in mass screening programs for the detection of diabetes and in the home monitoring done by many diabetic patients. Capillary

blood must be thought of as essentially *arterial* rather than venous. In the fasting state, the arterial (capillary) blood glucose concentration is 5 mg/dL higher than the venous concentration.

Venous Blood Specimens

Whole blood, plasma, or serum from a fasting patient can be used for a glucose assay. An evacuated (gray-top) tube containing the preservative *sodium fluoride* is often used for the collection of blood for glucose testing. Fluoride inhibits glucose metabolism by the cells in the sample, allowing for an accurate glucose determination if a number of hours will elapse before analysis. Glycolysis decreases serum glucose by approximately 5% to 7% per hour (5 to 10 mg/dL) in normal, uncentrifuged coagulated blood at room temperature.[7]

Use of serum or plasma separator gel tubes, processed as quickly as possible (within 30 minutes) is another method of collection.

Types of Blood Specimens

Because the amount of glucose in the blood increases after a meal, it is important that assays to monitor glucose metabolism be done on fasting blood specimens or on specimens drawn 2 hours after a meal (2-hour postprandial). A random sample of blood is of limited value for a glucose determination. The term *fasting* means that the patient has had no food or drink for 8 to 12 hours. A strict fast is necessary, including no coffee, tea, or other caffeinated drink and no drugs that might affect the blood glucose level. Patients also should avoid emotional disturbances that might cause liberation of glucose into the blood.

For nonpregnant women, the fasting serum or plasma glucose concentration should normally be less than 110 mg/dL and a postprandial serum or plasma specimen less than 126 mg/dL.

In the detection and treatment of diabetes, it is sometimes necessary to have more information than can be obtained from only testing the fasting specimen for glucose. Patients with mild or diet-controlled diabetes may have fasting serum or plasma glucose levels within the normal range, but they may be unable to produce sufficient insulin for prompt metabolism of ingested carbohydrates. As a result, the serum or plasma glucose rises to abnormally high levels, and the return to normal levels is delayed. Such a pattern will be noted with an *oral glucose tolerance test* (Fig. 11-3).

Other Body Fluids

Glucose testing may be requested on other body fluids, such as cerebrospinal fluid (CSF) and urine. CSF should be analyzed for glucose immediately

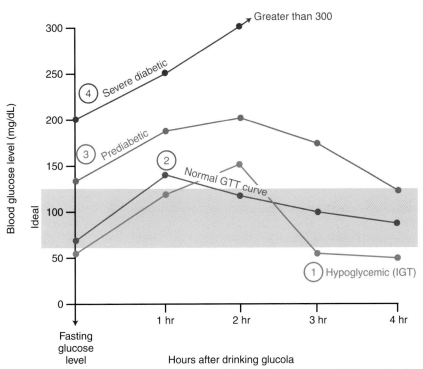

FIGURE 11-3 Glucose curve. Comparative patterns of glucose tolerance testing (GTT) results. Compare the blood glucose levels for each condition during the initial fasting test, then the subsequent levels for each hourly test after consumption of the glucose drink. (From Garrels M, Oatis CS: Laboratory testing for ambulatory settings: a guide for health care professionals, Philadelphia, 2006, Saunders.)

because contamination with bacteria will quickly reduce the level of glucose. If a delay in measurement is unavoidable, the specimen should be centrifuged and stored at 4°C or −20°C.[8]

In a 24-hour collection of urine, glucose may be stabilized by the addition of a preservative. Urine specimens should be stored at 4°C during collection because they can lose up to 40% of the glucose concentration after 24 hours at room temperature.

Point-of-Care Testing for Glucose

Many patients regularly monitor their own blood glucose concentrations. The Standards of Medical Care in Diabetes—2006 indicates that patients who maintain normal blood glucose levels by intensive monitoring significantly reduce their risk of developing diabetic complications.[4]

Recent advances in capillary blood glucose meters have made it possible for almost all diabetic patients to test themselves with these easy-to-use instruments. However, blood glucose meters, as consumer products, do differ from traditional laboratory methods for measuring glucose. For manufacturers of point-of-care instruments, they must balance accuracy with many other factors to assure that these meters perform in the hands of patients (Table 11-4).

The specimen used for this point-of-care test is generally capillary blood obtained by finger puncture. Products[8] using reagent test strips for monitoring blood glucose include OneTouch (LifeScan [Fig. 11-4]), Accu-Chek Easy (Boehringer Mannheim), and Glucometer Elite (Bayer). The strips used for these tests are impregnated with the enzyme glucose oxidase. Any glucose present in the blood is converted to gluconic acid and hydrogen peroxide, with the glucose oxidase used to catalyze the reaction. A second enzyme, peroxidase, is also present on the strip. The peroxidase uses the hydrogen peroxide formed in the first reaction to oxidize an indicator also present on the strip to give a detectable color change. The color change can be read on a reflectance meter, where the result (in mg/dL) is visualized. Although whole blood is tested, results are converted to plasma glucose values by the instrument.

Another product, HemoCue Glucose, utilizes transmittance photometry and single-test cartridges. The cartridge is inserted into a microcuvette that draws up 5 mL into the photometer, where the analysis takes place and the result is displayed. The reaction is based on the glucose dehydrogenase method. The cartridge/microcuvette is the unique part to this system; it is a self-filling, disposable cuvette and serves as a pipette, test tube, and measuring vessel. The reagent is contained in the tip of the microcuvette, where the chemical reaction takes place.

TABLE 11-4

Point-of-Care Meters versus Laboratory Instruments	
Glucose Meter	Laboratory Instruments
No standard reference controls	Standard reference controls
No hematocrit effect by analysis of serum or plasma	Hematocrit effect mitigated by measurement or algorithms
Can cost > $10,000	Costs < $100
Maintenance costs are >$1000 a year	No maintenance required
Trained laboratory personnel performs test	Patient performs test
Calibration many times each day	No user calibration
Controlled environment	Variables include temperature, altitude, etc.
Controls tested frequently	Control solution use limited
Large piece of equipment, sensitive to vibrations and shock	Small, portable, resistant to vibrations and shock
≥ 5mL specimen	≤1µL specimen
≥ 60 second throughput	≤10 second throughput
± 4% to ±10% inaccuracy	Inaccuracy is generally ≥2× reference method (laboratory instrument)

From Malone B: Blood glucose meters, glucose analysis: Lab instruments versus points-of care meters, AdvaMed Clinical Laboratory News 36(5):3, 2010.

The majority of point-of-care testing (POCT) and training is overseen by the laboratory, but nonlaboratory personnel perform the testing. It is important that users of these bedside or home-monitoring methodologies be fully instructed in and informed about their proper use. The instruments must be calibrated with either control solutions of glucose of a known concentration or with a calibration strip or cartridge supplied with each lot of test strips or cartridges. The procedure supplied by the manufacturer must always be followed when any of these products is used.

Methods for Qualitative and Semiquantitative Determination of Glucose

Qualitative laboratory testing provides a semi-quantitative estimation of the amount of glucose present in a specimen (e.g., urine). Glucose methods once relied on the reducing ability of glucose as demonstrated by the classic Benedict's reaction. A reducing sugar, such as glucose, converts Cu^{2+} ions in alkaline solution to Cu^+ ions, producing a color

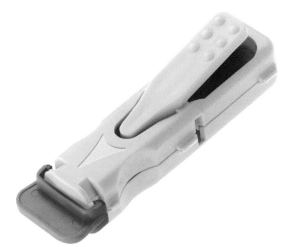

FIGURE 11-4 OneTouch lancing device. (Courtesy LifeScan Inc., Milpitas, Calif.)

change. This reaction is the basis for Clinitest tablets, which react with urinary reducing substances, but the test detects reducing sugars that are not specifically glucose. Urine dipstick methods for glucose determination use test strips impregnated with enzyme reagent (see Chapter 14).

Methods for Quantitative Determination of Glucose

The most common quantitative methods for glucose determination use the enzymes glucose oxidase and hexokinase.

Glucose Oxidase

As previously mentioned, glucose oxidase catalyzes the oxidation of glucose to gluconic acid and hydrogen peroxide. The enzyme is specific for β-D-glucose, the form of glucose in the blood. In some methods, the amount of hydrogen peroxide produced or oxygen consumed is measured by an electrode. In other methods, a second enzyme, peroxidase, catalyzes the oxidation of a chromogen to a colored product. In this case, the color formed is proportional to the amount of glucose present. When peroxidase is used in these procedures, the test is subject to interference from reducing agents such as ascorbic acid, which react with hydrogen peroxide, resulting in falsely low results.

GLUCOSE OXIDASE REACTION

$$\beta\text{-D-glucose } H_2O \xrightarrow{\text{glucose oxidase}} \text{D-gluconic acid} + H_2O_2$$

$$2H_2O_2 + 4 \text{ Aminopyrine} + 1,7\text{-Dehydroxynapthylene} \xrightarrow{\text{peroxidase}} \text{A red dye} + H_2O$$

The glucose oxidase procedure has been adapted to a wide range of automated instruments. Vitros Clinical Chemistry Analyzers (Johnson & Johnson) employ dry chemical reagents in either strip or film form. In these instruments, the oxidation of an indicator dye is used to form a colored compound that results from the action of hydrogen peroxide and peroxidase. The specimen is deposited on the Vitros Clinical Chemistry Slide and is evenly distributed by the spreading layer. Water and any nonprotein components, including glucose, move to the underlying reagent layer. After a fixed incubation period, the reflectance density of the red dye formed in the reaction is measured by the spectrophotometer through the transparent polyester support. The result is obtained in about 5 minutes.

Glucose oxidase methods can be used to measure glucose in CSF. These methods should not be used for urine unless the urine is pretreated, because urine contains a high concentration of substances that interfere with the peroxidase reaction.

Hexokinase

The hexokinase method is the one used most often in automated chemistry analyzers. Hexokinase methods are less subject to interference than the glucose oxidase–peroxidase methods. The DuPont ACA instrument uses the hexokinase method based on the formation of glucose-6-phosphate from glucose. In the reaction, adenosine triphosphate (ATP) is simultaneously converted to adenosine diphosphate (ADP). The glucose-6-phosphate formed becomes the substrate for a second enzymatic reaction in which the coenzyme nicotinamide adenine dinucleotide phosphate (NADP) is reduced to NADPH, with 6-phosphogluconate being formed.

HEXOKINASE REACTION

$$\text{Glucose} + \text{ATP} \xrightarrow{\text{hexokinase}} \text{Glucose-6-phosphate} + \text{ADP}$$

$$\text{Glucose-6-phosphate} + \text{NADP} \xrightarrow[\text{dehydrogenase}]{\text{glucose-6-phosphate}} \text{6-Phosphogluconate} + \text{NADPH} + \text{H}^+$$

The formation of NADPH can be followed by an increase in absorbance at 340 nm, which is proportional to the amount of glucose present in the original specimen. Although other hexoses (six carbon sugars) can also react in the hexokinase procedure, they are not normally encountered in the blood. If plasma is to be used with this procedure, fluoride, heparin, oxalate, and ethylenediaminetetraacetic acid (EDTA) are acceptable anticoagulants.

The hexokinase method is also an excellent test to determine glucose in urine and other biological fluids. This method has been proposed as a basis-of-reference method because of its accuracy and precision.

Glucose Reference Values[9]

Reference values for the individual glucose methods can vary significantly. Each laboratory must determine and evaluate the reference range for its particular facility.

There is no significant difference in serum or plasma glucose concentration between males and females or between races. In normal CSF, the glucose concentration is about two-thirds of the plasma level. It is important to measure the blood glucose concentration simultaneously when CSF glucose is tested so that the CSF glucose results can be evaluated appropriately. There is normally no detectable glucose in urine.

Values in parentheses are in SI units.

Glucose, fasting, serum:

Child	70-105 mg/dL (3.89-5.83 mmol/L)
Adult	70-110 mg/dL (3.89-6.1 mmol/L)

Glucose, fasting, whole blood:

Adult	60-95 mg/dL (3.33-5.27 mmol/L)

Glycated hemoglobin, total, blood:

5.3%-7.5% total blood hemoglobin

Glucose, CSF:

Infant, child	60-80 mg/dL (3.33-4.44 mmol/L)
Adult	40-70 mg/dL (2.22-3.9 mmol/L)

Laboratory Tests for Diabetic Management

In addition to blood glucose, a number of other tests are used to manage diabetic patients. These include glycosylated hemoglobin, ketones, and microalbumin.

Glycosylated Hemoglobin

Long-term estimation of glucose concentration can be followed by measuring glycosylated hemoglobin (Hb A_{1c}). Hemoglobin A (Hb A) is formed when glucose binds to an amino group that is part of the Hb A protein. The reaction occurs at the N-terminal valine of the hemoglobin beta chains (see Chapter 12, Fig. 12-10). Formation of Hb A_{1c} is nonenzymatic and occurs over the life span (average 120 days) of the red blood cell. Because these cells are freely permeable to blood glucose, the amount of total Hb A_{1c} is related to the time-averaged glucose concentration over the 4 to 6 weeks before the measurement. A level of 8% or less is considered "good" glycemic control. The test is not used to diagnose diabetes.

Common automated chemistry analyzers can use an enzymatic assay: Diazyme A_{1c} (Hitachi 7170). Glycosylated hemoglobin methods also include electrophoresis, ion-exchange chromatography, and high-performance liquid chromatography.

Ketone Bodies

During carbohydrate deprivation caused by decreased carbohydrate utilization (e.g., diabetes, starvation or fasting, prolonged vomiting), blood levels of ketones derived from lipid breakdown increase to meet energy needs. The three ketone bodies are:
- Acetone (2%)
- Acetoacetic acid (20%)
- 3-β-Hydroxybutyric acid (78%)

Ketonemia refers to the accumulation of ketones in blood, and *ketonuria* refers to accumulation of ketones in urine. Measurement of ketones is recommended for patients with type 1 diabetes during acute illness, as well as in other conditions, including stress, pregnancy, and extremely elevated blood glucose levels, or if signs of ketoacidosis are present.

A common method for screening for ketones uses sodium nitroprusside in the urine reagent strip test and Acetest tablets. Sodium nitroprusside reacts with acetoacetic acid in an alkaline pH to form a purple color. An enzymatic method employed by some automated instruments uses the enzyme β-hydroxybutyrate dehydrogenase to detect either β-hydroxybutyric acid or acetoacetic acid, depending on the pH of the solution used.

Microalbumin

Diabetes causes progressive changes in renal tissue, resulting in diabetic nephropathy. This complication develops over many years. An early sign of degeneration is an increase in urinary albumin. *Microalbuminuria* is a powerful predictor for the future development of diabetic nephropathy.

The use of a random spot collection for the measurement of an microalbumin-to-creatinine ratio is the preferred method. Microalbuminuria is confirmed when two specimens collected within a 6-month period are elevated. Chemistry and immunoassay integrated analyzers (e.g., ci8200, Abbott Laboratories) perform microalbumin analysis. POCT for microalbuminuria screening also is available (e.g., HemoCue Urine Albumin System).

ELECTROLYTES

Electrolytes are substances that form or exist as ions or charged particles when dissolved in water. Electrolytes are either negatively charged *anions* or positively charged *cations*. Cations move toward the cathode and anions toward the anode in an electrical field. Electrolytes include sodium (Na^+), potassium (K^+), calcium (Ca^{2+}), magnesium (Mg^{2+}), chloride (Cl^-), bicarbonate (HCO_3^-), sulfate (SO_4^{2-}), and phosphate (HPO_4^{2-}).

The chief positively charged constituents (cations) are *sodium* (Na^+) and *potassium* (K^+). The chief negatively charged constituents (anions) are *chloride* (Cl^-) and *bicarbonate* (HCO_3^-). Because sodium, potassium, chloride, and bicarbonate represent the major electrolytes, they are most likely to show variation when an electrolyte problem exists. These four electrolytes are discussed together because changes in the concentration of one are almost always accompanied by changes in the concentration of one or more of the others. Although these electrolytes are found throughout the body, their concentrations or activities vary from one body compartment to another. Assays are usually done on plasma or serum.

It is essential that the positively charged particles balance, or electrically neutralize, the negatively charged particles. The kidneys and lungs are the organs that exert the most control over electrolyte concentration. If the body is unable to maintain normal control over acceptable concentrations of electrolytes, either by excretion or conservation, an *electrolyte imbalance* occurs. Having an abnormal concentration of one or more of the electrolyte constituents is extremely harmful to the patient and can be fatal because most of the body's essential metabolic processes are affected by or dependent on electrolyte balance.

Sodium

Sodium (Na^+) is the major cation, or positively charged particle, and is found in the highest concentration in extracellular fluid. It is important in maintaining the osmotic pressure and in electrolyte balance. Sodium is associated with the levels of chloride and bicarbonate ions and therefore has a major role in maintaining the acid-base balance of the body cells. A low serum sodium level is called **hyponatremia.** Low sodium levels are found in a variety of conditions, including severe polyuria, metabolic acidosis, Addison's disease, diarrhea, and some renal tubular diseases. A high level of sodium is called **hypernatremia.** Clinical conditions resulting in excess body sodium include cardiac failure (congestive heart failure), liver disease (ascites), and renal disease (nephritic syndrome).

BOX 11-3
Osmolality of Plasma

$$\text{Osmolality (osmol/kg } H_2O) = 1.86(Na^+) + \frac{(glucose)}{18} + \frac{BUN}{2.8}$$

Note:
1.86 = Used because each sodium ion is balanced by an anion, but dissociation is not perfect.
18 = Molecular weight of glucose is 180; factor of 18 converts mg/dL to mmol/L. This is the unit used to express osmolality.
2.8 = Represents the molecular weight of blood urea nitrogen (BUN) is 28; therefore 2.8 is used.

BOX 11-4
Case Study of Plasma Osmolality

A 40-year old women suffering from vomiting and diarrhea had the following laboratory values: Na^+ 145 mmol/L, glucose 750 mg/dL, BUN 25 mg/dL.

$$\text{Osmolality (osmol/kg } H_2O) = 1.86(Na^+) + \frac{(glucose)}{18} + \frac{BUN}{2.8}$$

Calculation:

$$\text{Osmolality (Osmol/kg } H_2O) = 1.86(145) + \frac{750}{18} + \frac{25}{2.8}$$

$$= 270 + 41.7 + 8.9$$

$$= 321 \text{ mOsm/kg } H_2O$$

An increased sodium level is found in Cushing's syndrome (in which there is hyperactivity of the adrenal cortex and more hormones than normal are produced), severe dehydration caused by primary water loss, certain types of brain injury, and diabetic coma after therapy with insulin, as well as after excess treatment with sodium salts. The kidneys can conserve or excrete large concentrations of sodium depending on the Na^+ concentration of the extracellular fluids and the blood volume.

Osmolality

Osmolality is based on the number of dissolved particles in a solution. Osmolality measures the total concentration of all of the ions and molecules present in serum or urine. Sodium, glucose, and urea are major contributors to the total osmolality of serum (Boxes 11-3 and 11-4). The reference range of osmolality for adults is 275 to 295 mOsm/Kg. In contrast, in the calculation of the osmolal gap (Box 11-5), the difference between the calculated osmolality and the measured osmolality, elevation in the gap is usually due to factors other than Na^+, glucose, or BUN. Clinically, the

BOX 11-5
Case Study of Osmolal Gap

What is the osmolal gap? The patient is a 22-year-old intoxicated male with Na^+ 142 mmol/L, glucose 105 mg/dL, and BUN 12 mg/dL. His measured plasma osmolality is 320 mOsm/Kg. His calculated osmolality is 274 mOsm/Kg.

$$\text{Osmolal gap} = \text{Calculated osmolality} - \text{Measured plasma osmolality}$$

$$= 320 - 274 \text{ mOsm/kg}$$

$$= 46 \text{ mOsm/kg}$$

Average reference range osmolal gap = 0-10 mOsm/kg H_2O.

presence of ketones or alcohol in the plasma can elevate the osmolal gap. The average osmolal gap is 0 to 10 mOsm/Kg H_2O.

Osmolality is important because it is the condition to which the hypothalamus responds. If a calculated osmolality is elevated above the reference range, the patient is suffering from dehydration. The regulation of osmolality affects the Na^+ concentration in plasma mainly because Na^+ and associated anions account for approximately 90% of the osmotic activity in plasma.

Regulation of Plasma Na+

The following three processes are important to the regulation of plasma Na^+ concentration:
- Intake of water in response to thirst, which is stimulated or suppressed by plasma osmolality
- Excretion of water, which is primarily influenced by antidiuretic hormone released in response to changes in either blood volume or osmolality
- Regulation of blood volume, which affects sodium excretion through aldosterone, angiotensin II, and atrial natriuretic peptide

Potassium

Potassium (K^+) is the major intracellular cation, but it is also found extracellularly (see Special Considerations for Specimens). Potassium has an important influence on the muscle activity of the heart. Abnormally low potassium levels, **hypokalemia,** can result from prolonged diarrhea or vomiting or from inadequate intake of dietary potassium. Even in conditions of potassium deficiency, the kidney continues to excrete potassium. The body has no effective mechanism to protect itself from excessive loss of potassium, so a regular daily intake of potassium is essential.

An elevated potassium level in serum is called **hyperkalemia.** Because potassium is primarily excreted by the kidney, it becomes elevated in kidney dysfunction or urinary obstruction. As with sodium, potassium is influenced by the presence of the adrenocortical hormones and is associated with acid-base balance. In renal tubular acidosis, there is increased retention of potassium in the serum. One important purpose of renal dialysis is the removal of accumulated potassium from the plasma.

Sodium and Potassium in Body Fluids

Urinary Na^+ excretion varies with dietary intake, but for individuals on an average diet containing 8 to 15 g/day, a range of 40 to 220 mmol/day is typical. Diurnal variation exists in Na^+ excretion, with reduced levels at night.

After K^+ is absorbed by the gastrointestinal tract, it is rapidly distributed, with most excreted by the kidneys. K^+ filtered through the glomeruli is reabsorbed almost completely in the proximal tubules and then secreted in the distal tubules in exchange for Na^+ under the influence of aldosterone.

Factors that regulate distal tubular secretion of K^+ include the following:
- Na^+ and K^+ intake
- Water flow rate in the distal tubules
- Plasma level of mineralocorticoids
- Acid-base balance

Renal regulation of K^+ excretion is influenced by renal tubular acidosis and by metabolic and respiratory acidosis and alkalosis. Retention of K^+ is present in patients with chronic renal failure.

The Na^+ concentration of CSF is 138 to 150 mmol/L. Mean fecal Na^+ excretion generally is considered to be less than 10 mmol/day. In cases of severe diarrhea, fecal loss of K^+ may be as much as 60 mmol/day.

CSF values for K^+ are approximately 70% of plasma values. Urinary excretion of K^+ varies with dietary intake but typically ranges from 25 to 125 mmol/day.

Chloride

Chloride is found in serum, plasma, CSF, tissue fluid, and urine. Physiologically, only the concentration of chloride in the extracellular fluid is important.

The chief extracellular anions are chloride and bicarbonate, and there is a reciprocal relationship between them: a decrease in the amount of one produces an increase in the amount of the other. The chloride ion (Cl^-) is the most important anion of the extracellular fluids in the body. It is the major anion that counterbalances the major cation, sodium. This means that the sum of all the cations equals the sum of all the anions.

In the blood, two-thirds of chloride is found in the plasma and one-third in the red blood cells (RBCs). Because of the difference in chloride concentration between the RBCs and the plasma, the test for chloride is routinely performed on plasma (or serum) and not on whole blood.

Chloride has an important role in two main functions in the body: (1) determining the osmotic pressure, which controls the distribution of water among cells, plasma, and interstitial fluid, and (2) maintaining electrical neutrality.

Chloride plays an important role in the buffering action when carbon dioxide exchange takes place in the RBCs. This activity is known as the **chloride shift.** When blood is oxygenated, chloride travels from the RBCs to the plasma, and at the same time, bicarbonate leaves the plasma and enters the RBCs. An example of the chloride shift in the laboratory is the replacement action that occurs when a specimen for a chloride determination is allowed to stand for a time before the cells and plasma are separated. When whole blood comes into contact with air, carbon dioxide (and thus bicarbonate) escapes from the blood. As carbon dioxide leaves the plasma, chloride diffuses (or shifts) out of the RBCs to replace bicarbonate, which is reentering the cell to maintain equilibrium. The contact between whole blood and air has the effect of lowering the plasma carbon dioxide and raising the plasma chloride. Specimens of whole blood left in contact with air can produce falsely high plasma or serum chloride values. The cells must be removed from the plasma by centrifugation as quickly as possible. Once separated from the cells, the serum or plasma has a very stable chloride concentration.

Another important function of chloride is to regulate the fluid content of the body and its influence on the kidney. The kidney maintains the electrolyte concentration of the plasma within very narrow limits. Renal function is set to regulate the composition of the extracellular fluid first and then the volume. Consequently, if the body loses salt (sodium chloride), water is lost.

High serum or plasma chloride values are seen in dehydration and conditions that cause decreased renal blood flow, such as congestive heart failure. Excessive treatment with or dietary intake of Cl^- also results in high serum levels. Low serum or plasma Cl^- values may be seen when salt is lost, such as in chronic pyelonephritis. A low Cl^- value may also be seen in metabolic acidotic conditions that are caused by excessive production or diminished excretion of acids, such as diabetic acidosis and renal failure. Prolonged vomiting from any cause may ultimately result in a decrease in serum and body chloride levels.

Bicarbonate

Bicarbonate (HCO_3^-), after chloride, is the other major extracellular anion in body fluids. As the blood perfuses the lungs, carbon dioxide (CO_2) and H_2O are formed. During the metabolic processes, carbonic acid (H_2CO_3) dissociates and forms bicarbonate. This is a reversible reaction, and depending on body tissue requirements, bicarbonate may be reconverted to H_2CO_3, followed by the formation of H_2O and CO_2. The reactions are:

$$CO_2 \text{ (gas)} \leftrightarrow CO_2 \text{ (dissolved)} + H_2O \leftrightarrow$$

$$H_2CO_3 \leftrightarrow H^+ + HCO_3^-$$

Bicarbonate is filtered by the kidney, but little or no bicarbonate is found in the urine. The proximal tubules reabsorb 85% of HCO_3^-, and the remaining 15% are reabsorbed by the distal tubules. Bicarbonate is most often measured with other combined forms of CO_2 (CO_2, HCO_3^-, carbamino groups) as total CO_2. Because about 90% of all the CO_2 in serum is in the form of bicarbonate, this combined form approximates the actual bicarbonate concentration very closely. Total CO_2 is the total of H_2CO_3, dissolved CO_2 gas, and HCO_3^-. Assay methods for bicarbonate are actually a measure of total CO_2.

Along with pH and carbon dioxide pressure (P_{CO_2}) determinations, the total CO_2 concentration is a useful measurement in evaluating acid-base disorders. The bicarbonate or carbon dioxide value in itself is not as significant as the value in the context of the other electrolytes assayed. Assays for total CO_2 are performed by using a P_{CO_2} electrode to measure the rate of released CO_2 being formed.

Anion Gap

The calculation of the mathematical difference between the anions (Cl^- and HCO_3^-) and the cations (Na^+ and K^+) is known as the **anion gap** (Boxes 11-6 and 11-7). If Cl^- and HCO_3^- are summed and subtracted from the sum of Na^+ and K^+ concentrations, the difference should be less than 16 mmol/L, with a range of 10 to 20 mmol/L. If the anion gap exceeds 16 mmol/L, this is usually an indication of increased concentrations of the unmeasured anions (PO_4^{3-}, SO_4^{2-}, protein ions). Increased anion gaps can also result from ketotic states, lactic acidosis, salicylate and methanol ingestion, uremia, or increased plasma proteins. Decreased anion gaps of less than 10 mmol/L can result from either an increase in unmeasured cations (Ca^{2+}, Mg^{2+}) or a decrease in the unmeasured anions.

The anion gap is also useful as a quality control measure for electrolyte results. If an increased

BOX 11-7

Renal Function Panel

Assay	Type of Specimen
Albumin	Serum or plasma
Calcium	Serum or plasma
Carbon dioxide	Serum or plasma
Creatinine	Serum or plasma
Chloride	Serum or plasma
Glucose	Serum or plasma
Phosphorous, inorganic	Serum or plasma
Potassium	Serum or plasma
Sodium	Serum or plasma
Urea nitrogen	Serum or plasma

From www.aruplab.com. Accessed June 6, 2009.

anion gap is found for electrolytes in a healthy person, one or more of the test results may be erroneous, and the tests should be repeated.

Special Considerations for Specimens

Plasma can be assayed for electrolyte concentration after use of lithium or sodium heparin as the anticoagulant, except in testing for sodium, in which case sodium heparin cannot be used. Electrolyte testing can also be done on serum. Capillary samples can be collected into microcontainers or capillary tubes. Centrifugation should be done using the unopened primary collection tubes, and the plasma or serum should be separated from the RBCs promptly. Each assay has specific requirements and technical factors relating to the specimen collection and handling.

Sodium

Lithium heparinized plasma, serum, urine, and other body fluids are suitable specimens. Sodium heparin should not be used, as already noted, because the presence of sodium will interfere with the assay for sodium. Cells must be separated from serum or plasma as soon as possible.

Sodium is stable in serum for at least 1 week at room or refrigerator temperature, or it can be frozen for up to 1 year. Sodium can be measured in 24-hour urine specimens and in CSF.

Potassium

Lithium or sodium heparin is the preferred anticoagulant for plasma specimens; an anticoagulant containing potassium cannot be used. Serum can also be tested. The collection of blood for potassium studies requires special attention and technique. Because the concentration of potassium in the RBC is about 20 times that in serum or plasma, hemolysis must be avoided. Technical errors that can contribute to an elevation in K^+ are:

- Recentrifugation of specimens in gel tubes
- Inadequate centrifugation
- Centrifuging blood specimen tubes with the stoppers removed
- Pouring blood from one tube to another
- Delayed centrifugation
- Refrigerating a specimen before K^+ analysis
- Improper venipuncture technique (e.g., IV fluid contamination)

To avoid a shift of potassium from the RBCs to the plasma or serum, it is important to separate the cells from the plasma or serum within 3 hours of collection. When blood is collected for a potassium test, the patient should not open and close the fist before venipuncture; this muscle action can increase plasma potassium levels by 10% to 20%. Potassium levels in plasma are about 0.1 to 0.2 mmol/L lower than those in serum because of the release of potassium from ruptured platelets during the coagulation process.

Potassium in serum promptly separated from the blood clot is stable for at least 1 week at room or refrigerator temperature. Specimens may be frozen for up to 1 year. Potassium levels in urine vary with dietary intake and are measured in a 24-hour collection.

Chloride

The anticoagulant used most frequently for chloride is lithium or sodium heparin. Serum separator gel tubes are also often used for specimens in chloride testing. Chloride is assayed in serum, plasma, urine, or sweat and in other body fluids. Moderate hemolysis does not significantly affect Cl^- concentration in the serum.

Bicarbonate

Lithium or sodium heparinized plasma or serum may be used for the bicarbonate assay. Arterial blood is generally collected. The pH and bicarbonate concentrations are most accurately determined immediately when the tube is opened and as quickly as possible after collection and centrifugation of the unopened tube. A specimen to be assayed for total CO_2 must be handled anaerobically to minimize losses of CO_2 and HCO_3^- (converted to CO_2) into the atmosphere. A falsely low total CO_2 would result if this loss has occurred. In the laboratory, the specimen can be protected by placing a stopper on the container.

Methods for Quantitative Measurement

Four electrolytes—sodium, potassium, chloride, and bicarbonate—are generally grouped together for testing, called an *electrolyte profile*.

Sodium and Potassium

Ion-selective electrode (ISE) potentiometry uses a glass ion-exchange membrane for sodium assay and a valinomycin neutral-carrier membrane for potassium assay and has been incorporated into many automated chemistry analyzers. ISE methods measure the activity of an ion in the water-volume fraction in which it is dissolved. Generally, two types of ISE measurements are made on biological samples: direct and indirect. Direct measurements are becoming more common. *Direct* measurement is done on undiluted samples; *indirect* measurement requires prediluted samples for measurement of ion activity. Lipemia and protein cause a false decrease in indirect ISE measurements because they occupy plasma volume.

The Vitros Clinical Chemistry Analyzer uses the ISE method. This instrument uses a dry multi-layered slide with a self-contained analytical element coated on a polyester support. Each slide contains a pair of ISEs; one is used as a reference electrode and the other as a measuring electrode. Depending on which slide electrode is selected, the instrument can assay sodium or potassium. Another ISE is also available for chloride assay using this same instrument. In this method, 10 mL of specimen and reference standard is applied to the appropriate Vitros Clinical Chemistry Slide, and the slide is introduced into the instrument. An electrometer in the instrument measures the potential difference between the two half-cells of the reference and the sample, and the result is calculated.

Chloride

The most common methods for chloride assays now use ISE-based technology. The sensing element is usually silver–silver chloride or silver sulfide.

Another common method for chloride assay employs a quantitative displacement of thiocyanate by chloride from mercuric thiocyanate and formation of a red ferric thiocyanate complex. The amount of the colored compound, as measured with a spectrophotometer, is proportional to the concentration of chloride present in the specimen. In this method, chloride first combines with free mercury ions to form a colorless compound, then displaces any thiocyanate from mercuric thiocyanate. The free thiocyanate ions react with iron to produce the red-colored end product.

SWEAT CHLORIDE

The chloride content of sweat is useful in diagnosing cystic fibrosis, a disease of the exocrine glands. A sweat sample is collected by forearm stimulation with the use of pilocarpine nitrate in a process referred to as iontophoresis. Chloride concentration can then be measured directly with the use of ISEs.

Affected infants usually have concentrations of sweat chloride greater than 60 mmol/L, and affected adults, concentrations greater than 70 mmol/L (reference values average about 40 mol/L). In 98% of patients with cystic fibrosis, the secretion of chloride in sweat is two to five times normal. The chloride content of normal sweat varies with age.

Bicarbonate

The routine bicarbonate (determined as total CO_2) assay is automated. The first step in automated methods in general is the acidification of the sample to convert the various forms of bicarbonate present to gaseous CO_2. To keep automated methods in control, another important consideration for bicarbonate assays is the need to include several standard solutions with the assay of the unknowns.

Other Electrolytes

Calcium

Calcium (Ca^{2+}) is essential for myocardial contraction. A decreased level of ionized calcium impairs cardiac function and produces irregular muscle spasms (tetany). Three hormones—parathyroid hormone, vitamin D, and calcitonin—regulate serum calcium.

Most calcium in the body is part of bone. Only 1% is in the blood and other extracellular fluids. Calcium in blood exists as free calcium ions or ionized calcium (45%) or is bound to protein or anions. If a patient has **hypocalcemia,** neuromuscular irritability and cardiac irregularities are

the primary symptoms. **Hypercalcemia** results from primary hyperparathyroidism or various types of malignancy. Mild hypercalcemia is often asymptomatic.

The preferred specimen for total calcium determinations is serum. The two commonly used methods for total calcium analysis are o-cresolphthalein complex I (CPC) and arsenazo III, forming a colored complex with calcium, which is measured spectrophotometrically. Commercial analyzers that measure ionized free calcium use ISEs for measurements. It is important that a serum specimen for ionized calcium remain *uncapped* until immediately before analysis, because loss of CO_2 produces an increase in pH and altered protein binding.

Magnesium

Magnesium (Mg^{2+}) is the fourth most abundant cation in the body and second most abundant intracellular ion. High concentrations of magnesium are found in bone and muscle. Less than 1% is present in serum and erythrocytes. Two thirds of Mg^{2+} present in serum is free or ionized magnesium. Magnesium has many functions in the body and is an essential cofactor of more than 300 enzymes. Measurement of Mg^{2+} is useful in cardiovascular, metabolic, and neuromuscular disorders. Serum levels are useful in determining acute changes in the ion.

Hypomagnesemia is most frequently observed in hospitalized patients in intensive care units (ICUs) or patients receiving diuretics or digitalis therapy. Hypomagnesemia is rare in nonhospitalized patients. **Hypermagnesemia** is seen less frequently than hypomagnesemia.

Symptoms do not usually occur until serum Mg^{2+} levels fall below 0.5 mmol/L. Manifestations of hypomagnesemia most often involve the cardiovascular and neuromuscular systems. Metabolic conditions (e.g., hyponatremia, hypokalemia, hypocalcemia, hypophosphatemia) or psychiatric symptoms (e.g., depression, agitation, psychosis) can also occur. Severe elevations of magnesium level usually result from decreased renal function and an intake of commonly prescribed magnesium-containing medications (e.g., antacids).

Nonhemolyzed serum or lithium heparin plasma may be analyzed. Hemolysis must be avoided because the concentration of Mg^{2+} inside of an erythrocyte is 10 times greater than in the extracellular fluid. Citrate and EDTA anticoagulants are unacceptable because they will bind with magnesium.

The three most common methods for measuring total serum magnesium are colorimetric: calmagite, formazan dye, and methylthymol blue. One limitation in the measurement of total magnesium concentrations in serum is that approximately 25% of magnesium is protein bound. Total magnesium may not reflect the physiologically active, free ionized magnesium. Because magnesium is primarily an intracellular ion, serum concentrations will not necessarily reflect the status of intracellular magnesium. As much as a 20% depletion of tissue or cellular magnesium may not be reflected in the serum magnesium concentrations.

Reference Values[7,9]

Reference values are generally instrument specific. Manufacturers' manuals must be consulted for specific reference values for a particular instrument and specimen type.

Sodium:

136-142 mmol/L	Serum or plasma (infancy through adulthood)
40-220 mmol/24 hr	Urine (on an average diet; sodium varies with dietary intake)
70% of value determined simultaneously for plasma or serum sodium	CSF
10-40 mmol/L	Sweat
>70 mmol/L	Sweat (suggests cystic fibrosis)

Potassium:

3.5-5.1 mmol/L	Serum, adults
3.7-5.9 mmol/L	Newborns (serum values for newborns are higher than for adults)
3.5-4.5 mmol/L	Plasma, adults
25-125 mmol/24 hr	Urine, on average diet (urinary potassium varies with dietary intake)

Chloride:

98-107 mmol/L	Serum or plasma, adult (upper limit to 110 mmol/L for both full-term and premature neonates)
118-132 mmol/L	CSF
110-250 mmol/ 24 hr	Urine (varies with dietary intake)
5-35 mmol/L	Sweat, normal adult
30-70 mmol/L	Sweat, marginal
60-200 mmol/L	Sweat, cystic fibrosis (>60 mmol/L for 98% of persons with cystic fibrosis)

Bicarbonate:

22-29 mmol/L	Serum, venous, adults (values for newborns and infants are lower)
21-28 mmol/L	Arterial, adults

Calcium:

2.15-2.65 mmol/L	Children
2.15-2.50 mmol/L	Adults

Calcium (ionized):

1.20-1.48 mmol/L	Neonates (4.8-5.9 mg/dL)
1.20-1.38 mmol/L	Children
1.16-1.32 mmol/L	Adults (4.6-5.3 mg/dL)

Magnesium:

0.63-1.0 mmol/L	Serum, plasma

ACID-BASE BALANCE AND BLOOD GASES

Many abnormal conditions are accompanied by disturbances of acid-base balance and electrolyte composition. These changes are usually apparent in the acid-base pattern and anion-cation composition of extracellular fluid (e.g., blood plasma).

A description of acid-base balance involves an accounting of the carbonic (H_2CO_3, HCO^-_3, CO^{2-}_3, CO_2) and noncarbonic acids and conjugate bases in terms of input (intake plus metabolic production) and output (excretion plus metabolic conversion) over a given time interval. The acid-base status of the body fluids is typically assessed by measurements of total CO_2, plasma pH, and PCO_2, because the bicarbonate/carbonic acid system is the most important buffering system of the plasma.[7]

The normal hydrogen ion concentration [H^+] in extracellular body fluid ranges from pH 7.34 to pH 7.44. Through mechanisms that involve the lungs and kidneys, the body controls and excretes H^+ to maintain pH homeostasis. The body's first line of defense against extreme changes in [H^+] is the buffer systems present in all body fluids. All buffers consist of a weak acid, such as carbonic acid, and its salt or conjugate base, such as bicarbonate, for the bicarbonate–carbonic acid buffer system. Other buffers include the phosphate buffer system.

The role of the lungs and kidneys in maintaining pH is depicted with the **Henderson-Hasselbalch equation.** The numerator (HCO_3^-) denotes kidney functions, and the denominator (PCO_2) denotes lung function.

$$pH = pK' + \log \frac{HCO_3^-}{\alpha \times PCO_2}$$

This equation can also be written as:

$$pH = 6.1 + \log (c\, HCO_3^- / cdCO_2)$$

The average normal ratio of the concentrations of bicarbonate and dissolved CO_2 in plasma is 25 (mmol)/1.25 (mmol/L) = 20/1. Any change in the concentration of either bicarbonate or dissolved CO_2 is accompanied by a change in pH. The change in the ratio can occur because of a change in either the numerator (renal component) or the denominator (respiratory component).

Clinical terms are used to describe the acid-base status of a patient. *Acidemia* is defined as an arterial blood pH less than 7.35, and *alkalemia* is defined as an arterial blood pH greater than 7.45. The terms *acidosis* and *alkalosis* refer to pathologic states that lead to acidemia or alkalemia. If an acid-base disorder is caused by ventilatory (lung) dysfunction, it is called *respiratory*. If the renal or metabolic system is involved, it is called *metabolic*.

Acid-base disorders are traditionally classified as:

1. Metabolic acidosis
2. Metabolic alkalosis
3. Respiratory acidosis
4. Respiratory alkalosis

Metabolic acidosis is detected by decreased plasma bicarbonate. Bicarbonate is lost in the buffering of excess acid. Causes of this disturbance include:

1. Production of organic acids that exceed the rate of elimination (e.g., diabetic acidosis)
2. Reduced excretion of acids (H^+), with an accumulation of acid that consumes bicarbonate (e.g., renal failure)
3. Excessive loss of bicarbonate, such as with increased renal excretion or excessive loss of duodenal fluid (e.g., severe diarrhea)

Metabolic alkalosis occurs when either excess base is added to the system, base elimination is decreased, or acid-rich fluids are lost. Conditions leading to metabolic alkalosis are numerous and include prolonged vomiting, upper duodenal obstruction, or Cushing syndrome.

Respiratory acidosis is a condition of decreased elimination of CO_2. Causes of decreased elimination include chronic obstructive pulmonary disease (COPD), which is the most common cause, drugs such as narcotics and barbiturates, infections of the central nervous system (e.g., meningitis, encephalitis), coma caused by intracranial hemorrhage, and sleep apnea.

Respiratory alkalosis is a condition caused by increased rate or depth of respiration, or both, and produces excess elimination of acid via the respiratory system. Factors that can cause respiratory alkalosis include anxiety or hysteria, febrile states, and asthma.

TABLE 11-5

Classification and Characteristics of Simple Acid-Base Disorders		
	Primary Change	Compensatory Response
Metabolic		
Acidosis	↓ $cHCO_3^-$,	↓ PCO_2
Alkalosis	↑ $cHCO_3^-$,	↑ PCO_2
Respiratory		
Acidosis	↑ PCO_2	↑ $cHCO_3^-$
Alkalosis	↓ PCO_2	↓ $cHCO_3^-$

Modified from Burtis CA, Ashwood ER, Bruns DE: Tietz fundamentals of clinical chemistry, ed 6, St Louis, 2008, Saunders, p 668.
$cHCO_3^-$, Cytoplasmic bicarbonate; PCO_2, partial pressure carbon dioxide.

If a patient has a straightforward acid-base disorder, laboratory results are classic (Table 11-5). However, most cases of acid-base imbalance deviate from being a simple disorder because of compensatory responses by the respiratory and renal systems attempting to correct the imbalance in this dynamic situation.

RENAL FUNCTION

Kidney disease affects at least 8 million Americans. More people die annually from kidney failure than from colon cancer, breast cancer, or prostate cancer. Chronic kidney disease or kidney failure significantly increase a patient's risk of cardiovascular disease.

A variety of laboratory assays (see Box 11-7) can be performed to support a diagnosis of renal disease or dysfunction. Additional renal function markers (Table 11-6) may be of value.

Nitrogen (N) exists in the body in many forms, mostly in components of complex substances. Nitrogen-containing substances are classified into two main groups: *protein nitrogen* (protein substances containing nitrogen) and *nonprotein nitrogen* (NPN). **Urea** is the major NPN constituent and accounts for more than 75% of the total NPN excreted by the body; other NPNs are amino acids, uric acid, creatinine, creatine, and ammonia, listed in the order of their quantitative importance.

Normally, more than 90% of the urea is excreted through the kidneys. Urea nitrogen, uric acid, and creatinine occur in increased levels as a consequence of decreased renal function. Increased concentrations of several of the major constituents of NPN are used as indicators of diminished renal function. Most laboratories perform serum urea nitrogen measurements in conjunction with creatinine tests when tests for renal function are

TABLE 11-6

Renal Function Markers		
Test Name	Type of Specimen	Recommended Use
Alpha-1-microglobulin	Urine	May indicate renal involvement in patients with urinary tract infections or diabetes mellitus
Beta-2 microglobulin	Urine	May indicate renal involvement in patients with diabetic nephropathy, cadmium toxicity, or progressing idiopathic membranous nephropathy
Glomerular filtration rate, estimated	Calculation	Monitor renal function (Test reports serum creatinine reference intervals.)
Alpha-2-macroglobulin	Urine	May be used as a marker of membrane permeability in serum and fluids. May be used as a screening test
Microalbumin	Urine	Useful in monitoring diabetic nephropathy in insulin-dependent diabetes mellitus
Cystatin C	Serum	May be a marker of renal disease; however, test lacks specificity

From www.aruplab.com. Accessed June 6, 2009.

needed, because as combined assays they are more specific indicators of renal function disorders. The usefulness of the serum urea nitrogen test alone to determine kidney function is limited because of its variable blood levels, which result from nonrenal factors. It is common practice to calculate a **urea nitrogen/creatinine ratio:**

$$\frac{\text{Serum urea nitrogen (mg/dL)}}{\text{Serum creatinine (mg/dL)}}$$

The normal ratio for a person on a normal diet is between 12 and 20. Significantly lower ratios indicate acute tubular necrosis, low protein intake, starvation, or severe liver disease. High ratios with normal creatinine values indicate tissue breakdown, prerenal azotemia, or high protein intake. High ratios with increased creatinine may indicate a postrenal obstruction or prerenal azotemia associated with a renal disease.

Urea/Urea Nitrogen

Urea (urea nitrogen) is the chief component of the NPN material in the blood; it is distributed throughout the body water, and it is equal in concentration in intracellular and extracellular fluid. Gross alterations in NPN usually reflect a change in the concentration of urea. The liver is the sole site of urea formation. As protein breaks down (e.g., as amino acids undergo deamination), *ammonia* is formed in increased amounts. This potentially toxic substance is removed in the liver, where the ammonia combines with other amino acids and is converted to urea by enzymes present in the liver. Urea is a waste product of protein metabolism, which is normally removed from the blood in the kidneys. The amount of urea in the blood is determined by the amount of dietary protein and

by the kidney's ability to excrete urea. If the kidney is impaired, urea is not removed from the blood and accumulates in the blood. An increased concentration of serum or plasma urea may indicate a flaw in the filtering system of the kidneys.

In the past, it was common practice in the laboratory to determine urea as urea nitrogen, using whole blood; this determination was called *blood urea nitrogen,* or BUN.[10] Methodologies used by automated instruments can measure urea directly using serum or plasma. The terms *blood urea nitrogen* (BUN), *urea nitrogen,* and *urea* are still used interchangeably. The chemical formula for urea is NH_2CONH_2. Because urea nitrogen is a measure of nitrogen, not urea, one can convert milligrams of urea nitrogen to milligrams of urea by multiplying the urea nitrogen value by 2.14, or 60/28. The molecular weight of urea is 60, and it contains two nitrogen atoms with a combined weight of 28.

Assays for urea/urea nitrogen and creatinine are performed concurrently because creatinine is considered to be a better single test for kidney function than urea nitrogen alone.

Clinical Significance

The assay for urea is only a rough estimate of renal function and will not show any significant level of increased concentration until the glomerular filtration rate is decreased by at least 50%. A more reliable single index of renal function is the test for serum creatinine. Contrary to urea concentration, creatinine concentration is relatively independent of protein intake (from the diet), degree of hydration, and protein metabolism.

The amount of urea in the blood is determined by the dietary protein and the kidney's ability to excrete urea. If the kidney is impaired, the urea is not removed from the blood, and as it accumulates, the urea level increases. The urea concentration is also influenced by diet; people who are undernourished or who are on low-protein diets may have urea levels that are not accurate indications of kidney function. Because the concentration of urea is directly related to protein metabolism, the protein content of the diet will affect the amount of urea in the blood. The ability of the kidneys to remove urea from the blood will also affect the urea content. Urea concentration is primarily influenced by the protein intake. In the normal kidney, urea is removed from the blood and excreted in the urine. If kidney function is impaired, urea will not be removed from the blood, resulting in a high urea concentration in the blood. Considerable deterioration must usually be present before the urea level rises above the reference range.

The condition of abnormally high urea nitrogen in the blood is called **uremia.** A significant increase in the plasma concentrations of urea and creatinine, in kidney insufficiency, is known as **azotemia.** Decreased levels are usually not clinically significant unless liver damage is suspected. During pregnancy, lower-than-normal urea levels are often seen. Azotemia can result from prenal, renal, or postrenal causes:

- **Prerenal azotemia** is the result of poor perfusion of the kidneys and therefore diminished glomerular filtration. The kidneys are otherwise normal in their functioning capabilities. Poor perfusion can result from dehydration, shock, diminished blood volume, or congestive heart failure. Another cause of prerenal azotemia is increased protein breakdown, as in fever, stress, or severe burns.
- **Renal azotemia** is caused primarily by diminished glomerular filtration as a consequence of acute or chronic renal disease. Such diseases include acute glomerulonephritis, chronic glomerulonephritis, polycystic kidney disease, and nephrosclerosis.
- **Postrenal azotemia** is usually the result of any type of obstruction in which urea is reabsorbed into the circulation. Obstruction can be caused by stones, an enlarged prostate gland, or tumors.

Specimens

Urea may be determined directly from serum, heparinized (sodium or lithium heparin) plasma, urine, or other biological specimens. Anticoagulants containing fluoride (gray-top evacuated tubes) will also interfere with methods using urease because fluoride inhibits the urease reaction. Urea can be lost through bacterial action, so the specimen should be analyzed within a few hours after collection or should be preserved by refrigeration. Refrigeration at 4°C to 8°C preserves the urea without measurable change for up to 72 hours.

Urine urea is particularly susceptible to bacterial action, so in addition to refrigerating the urine specimen at 4°C to 8°C, the pH can be maintained at less than 4 to help reduce the loss of urea.

Methods for Quantitative Determination

The oldest method for urea assay was the addition of the enzyme urease to whole blood, serum, or plasma. During incubation with urease, urea is converted to ammonium carbonate ($[NH_4]_2CO_3$) by the urease. The ammonia in the ammonium carbonate is analyzed in one of several ways. One classic manual method, devised by Gentzkow,[10] measures the amount of ammonium carbonate formed by having it react with Nessler's solution.

The most common automated methods in use today are indirect methods based on a preliminary hydrolysis step in which the urea present is converted to ammonia (NH_3) by the enzyme urease. The measurement of ammonia differs according to specific instrumentation. In one commonly used analyzer, an enzymatic measurement of the NH_3 formed is accomplished by an indicator reaction using glutamate dehydrogenase (GLDH) to oxidize NADH to NAD^+. The disappearance of NADPH is measured at 340 nm. It is a very specific, rapid test for urea. The reaction follows:

$$Urea + H_2O \xrightarrow{\text{urease}} (NH_4)_2CO_3$$
$$NH_4^+ + \alpha\text{-Ketoglutaric acid} + NADH \xrightarrow{\text{GLDH}}$$
$$ADP + H^+ + NAD^+ + Glutamic\ acid$$

The kidneys and lungs are the organs that exert the most control over electrolyte concentration.

Potentiometric methods using an ammonia ISE are available. Urea may be measured by condensation with diacetyl monoxime in the presence of strong acid and an oxidizing agent to form a yellow diazine derivative. Iron (III) and thiosemicarbizide are added to the reaction mixture to stabilize the color.

Reference Values

Values in parentheses are in SI units.[7]

Urea nitrogen, serum:

Adult	7-18 mg/dL	(2.5-6.4 mmol urea/L)
>60 yr	8-21 mg/dL	(2.9-7.5 mmol urea/L)
Infant/child	5-18 mg/dL	(1.8-6.4 mmol urea/L)

Urea, serum:

Adult	5-39 mg/dL	(2.5-6.4 mmol/L)

Urea nitrogen, urine:

12-20 g/24 hr (428-714 mmol urea/24 hr)

Creatinine

Creatinine in the blood results from the spontaneous formation of creatinine from creatine and creatine phosphate. Its formation and release into the body fluids occur at a constant rate and have a direct relationship to muscle mass. Therefore, creatinine concentration varies with age and gender. The clearance of creatinine from the plasma by the kidney is measured as an indicator of the glomerular filtration rate. Serum or plasma specimens are preferred over whole blood because considerable noncreatinine chromogens are present in RBCs, which can cause falsely elevated creatinine assay results.

Specimens

Serum, heparinized plasma, or diluted urine can be assayed for creatinine. Ammonium heparinized plasma should not be used for methods that measure ammonia production to quantify creatinine. Usually urine is diluted 1:100 or 1:200. Creatinine is stable in serum or plasma for up to 1 week if the specimen has been refrigerated. It is important to separate the cells promptly to prevent hemolysis and to minimize ammonia production. Hemolysis causes falsely elevated creatinine values.

Methods for Quantitative Determination

Most methods for creatinine employ the Jaffe reaction,[11] the oldest clinical chemistry method still in use. Creatinine reacts with alkaline picrate to form an orange-red solution that is measured in the spectrophotometer. To improve the specificity of the reaction and to eliminate interference from the many noncreatinine substances in blood that can also react with the alkaline picrate solution and yield falsely elevated values, an acidification step is added. These noncreatinine Jaffe-reacting chromogens include proteins, glucose, ascorbic acid, and pyruvate. The color from true creatinine is less resistant to acidification than the color from the noncreatinine substances. The difference between the two colors is measured photometrically.

Kinetic alkaline picrate methods and enzymatic creatinine methods are often used in automated analyzers. Kinetic methods have reduced some of the interferences caused by noncreatinine chromogens. A kinetic Jaffe method measures the rate of color change, with the interference by slower-reacting chromogens minimized. Another approach to the analysis of creatinine is the measurement of the color formed when creatinine reacts with 3,5-dinitrobenzoate. This method has been successfully adapted to a reagent strip, but the color is less stable than that of the classic Jaffe chromogen assay.

Enzymatic methods, such as creatinine aminohydrolase (creatinine deaminase) or creatininase (creatinine amidohydrolase), make the reaction more specific and sensitive for creatinine than the colorimetric methods.

Reference Values

Values in parentheses are in SI units.[9]

Creatinine, serum or plasma (Jaffe kinetic or enzymatic method):

Adult men	0.7-1.3 mg/dL (62-115 µmol/L)
Adult women	0.6-1.1 mg/dL (53-97 µmol/L)

Creatinine, urine:

Adult men	14-26 mg/kg/24 hr (124-230 µmol/kg/24 hr)
Adult women	11-20 mg/kg/24 hr (97-177 µmol/kg/24 hr)

Creatinine excretion decreases with age.

Creatinine clearance:

Male (<40 yr)	90-139 mL/min/1.73 m^2
Female (<40 yr)	80-125 mL/min/1.73 m^2

Clinical Significance

Creatinine in the blood results from creatine originating in the muscles of the body. Creatinine is freely filtered by the glomeruli of the kidney, with a small percentage secreted by the renal tubules, but it is not reabsorbed under normal circumstances. There is a relatively constant excretion of creatinine in the urine that parallels creatinine production. In renal disease, the creatinine excretion is impaired, as reflected by increased creatinine in the blood.

The serum creatinine concentration is relatively constant and is somewhat higher in males than in females. The constancy of concentration and excretion makes creatinine a good measure of renal function, especially of glomerular filtration. The concentration of creatinine is not affected by dietary intake, degree of dehydration in the body, or protein metabolism, which makes the assay a more reliable single screening index of renal function than the urea assay.

A useful index relates creatinine excretion to muscle mass or lean body weight, taking into consideration variables in individual body sizes. This index is known as the **creatinine clearance.**

CREATININE CLEARANCE

Creatinine clearance is defined as milliliters of plasma cleared of creatinine by the kidneys per minute. The result is normalized to a standard person's surface area by using the height and weight of the patient. Creatinine clearance is an indirect method used to assess the glomerular filtration functioning capabilities of the kidneys.

To perform this test for creatinine clearance, timed specimens of both blood and urine must be collected. All voided urine must be carefully collected for 24 hours. The urine specimen is preserved by refrigeration as successive additions are made to the total collection. Blood is collected at about 12 hours into the urine collection period. Creatinine is measured in the blood (serum or plasma) and in the timed urine specimen (24 hour). The creatinine clearance is calculated as follows:

$$U/P \times V \times 1.73/A = \text{Plasma cleared (mL)/min}$$

where U is the urine creatinine concentration (mg/dL), P is the plasma creatinine concentration (mg/dL), V is the volume in milliliters of urine excreted per minute, A is the patient's body surface area in square meters, and 1.73 is the standard body surface area in square meters. A nomogram is used to find the patient's body surface area. Most automated analyzers have calculating capabilities for this value if the specific patient height and weight data are entered into the system.

Glomerular Filtration Rate

No direct method is available to measure **glomerular filtration rate (GFR),** or the quantity of glomerular filtrate formed per unit time in all nephrons of both kidneys. Various substances in plasma and urine can be used to estimate the GFR, however, by measuring a plasma or serum marker of GFR or by using an estimation equation for GFR. To be used in the measurement of GFR by urinary clearance, exogenous substances should have the following characteristics:
- Should be physiologically inert
- Should be freely filtered and not bound to protein
- Should not be reabsorbed, secreted, synthesized, or metabolized by renal tubules

The amount of the substance filtered from the blood (plasma concentration, or Px) by the kidneys should equal the amount excreted in the urine (urine concentration, or Ux). V is the urine flow. The equation for calculation follows:

$$GFR \times Px = Ux \times V$$

Inulin has historically been the gold standard for measurement of GFR. An alternative to inulin clearance is the measurement of radiolabeled substances, such as iothalamate. The determination of GFR with these compounds is rarely done because of cost and inconvenience to the patient.

Prediction Equations

The National Kidney Disease Education Program and National Kidney Foundation recommend that laboratories use prediction equations to estimate GFR from serum creatinine (S_{CR}) for patients with chronic kidney disease and for patients at risk for developing chronic kidney disease. Some groups advocate use of the Cockcroft-Gault Modification of Diet in Renal Disease Study (MDRD) equation as a prediction equation. The MDRD equation is considered to be more accurate because it factors in ethnicity, age, and gender. The MDRD equation has gained widespread use for the estimation of creatinine clearance (C_{CR}) because of its enhanced accuracy in the estimation of GFR.

$$C_{CR}\,(\text{mL/min}) = \frac{(140 - \text{Age}) \times \text{Weight}}{72 \times S_{CR}} \times (0.85\,\text{if female})$$

The Cockcroft-Gault formula[12] is used for medical decision making. The importance of an accurate estimation of the GFR, as provided by this equation, is exemplified by the following uses of GFR:
1. Detect the onset of renal insufficiency
2. Adjust drug dosages for drugs excreted by the kidney
3. Evaluate therapies instituted for patients with chronic renal disease
4. Document eligibility for Medicare reimbursement in end-stage renal disease
5. Accrue points for patients awaiting cadaveric kidney transplants

ABBREVIATED MDRD EQUATION

$$GFR\,(\text{mL/min}/1.73\,\text{m}^2) = 186 \times S_{CR}^{-1.154} \times \text{Age}^{-0.203} \times (0.743\,\text{if female}) \times (1.21\,\text{if African American})$$

Creatinine clearance values decrease approximately 6.5 mL/min/1.73 m² per decade.

Cystatin C

Cystatin C has been identified as a superior marker to serum creatinine for GFR assessment. Cystatin is a low-molecular-weight part of the cystatin superfamily of cysteine proteinase inhibitors that is thought to be a potentially more reliable marker for GFR. A significant advantage of cystatin is that it is present in constant amounts in all body cells and is not influenced by muscle mass. Cystatin C can be measured by either particle-enhanced turbidimetry or particle-enhanced nephelometry. Both immunoassay methods produce rapid and precise measurements.

GFR is inversely proportional to cystatin C concentration: if GFR is elevated, cystatin C concentration is decreased, and vice versa.

Reference Value

A common reference interval in women and men was calculated to be 0.54-1.21 mg/L (median 0.85 mg/L, range 0.42 to 1.39 mg/L).[13]

Clinical Significance

This novel serum marker of the glomerular filtration rate (GFR) is a critical measure of normal kidney function. It is at least as good as serum creatinine for detecting renal dysfunction.

Creatine

Creatine is synthesized primarily in the liver and then transported to other tissue (e.g., muscle), where it serves as high-energy source to drive metabolic reactions. Creatine phosphate loses phosphoric acid and creatine loses water to form creatinine, which passes into the plasma. Creatine can increase the performance of athletes in activities that require quick bursts of energy, such as sprinting, and can help athletes to recover faster after expending bursts of energy.

Clinical Significance

Elevated levels of creatine are found in muscular diseases or injury (e.g., muscular dystrophy or trauma). Creatine testing is rarely performed.

URIC ACID

Uric acid is the final breakdown product of purine nucleoside metabolism. Three major disease states associated with elevated plasma uric acid are gout, increased catabolism of nucleic acids, and renal disease. Both renal damage and increased nuclear catabolism resulting from chemotherapy contribute to increased serum uric acid levels.

Uric acid can be measured in heparinized plasma, serum, or urine. Serum should be removed from cells as quickly as possible to prevent dilution by intracellular contents. Diet can affect uric acid concentrations. Uric acid is stable in plasma or serum after RBCs have been removed. Serum samples may be stored refrigerated for 3 to 5 days.[14]

Methods of analysis for uric acid include enzymatic methods such as uricase, chemical methods such as phosphotungstic acid (PTA), and high-performance liquid chromatography (HPLC). The PTA method is based on the development of a blue reaction as PTA is reduced by urate in alkaline medium. The color is read at 650 to 700 nm. HPLC using ion-exchange or reversed-phase columns is used to separate and quantify uric acid.

Uricase is a reaction measured in either the kinetic or the equilibrium mode. The decrease of absorbance as urate is converted has been measured at wavelengths varying from 282 to 292 nm. Most current enzymatic assays for uric acid in serum involve a peroxidase system coupled with one of several oxygen acceptors to produce a chromogen:

$$\text{Uric acid} \xrightarrow{\text{uricase}} \text{Allantoin} + H_2O_2 + CO_2$$

Reference Values[9]

Uric acid (uricase method):

Adult, female, plasma, serum	2.6-6.0 mg/dL
Adult, male	0.5-7.2 mg/dL
Child	2.0-5.5 mg/dL
Urine, 24 hour	250-750 mg/day

Clinical Significance

Plasma levels of uric acid are variable and higher in males than in females. Plasma urate is completely filterable, and both proximal tubular resorption and distal tubular secretion occur. With advanced chronic renal failure, the plasma uric acid level progressively increases.[14] With progressive renal failure, uric acid is retained. Uric acid concentration in the blood increases in advanced chronic renal failure, but this rarely results in classic gout. Uric acid is elevated in about 40% of patients with essential hypertension. Uric acid levels may also be elevated by thiazide diuretics, leading to gout in some cases.[15]

AMMONIA

Ammonia arises from the breakdown of amino acids, and high concentrations are neurotoxic. Clinical conditions in which blood ammonia levels are useful include hepatic failure, Reye syndrome, and inherited deficiencies of urea cycle enzymes. Liver disease is the most common cause of abnormal ammonia metabolism. Ammonia is used to monitor the progress of disease severity.

Careful specimen handling is extremely important for plasma ammonia assays. Whole-blood ammonia concentration rises rapidly after specimen collection because of in vitro amino acid breakdown. Heparin and EDTA are suitable anticoagulants. Samples should be centrifuged at 0°C to 4°C within 20 minutes of collection and the plasma or serum removed. Specimens should be assayed as soon as possible or frozen.

Methods of measurement include ISEs, which measure the change in pH of a solution of ammonium chloride as ammonia diffuses across a semipermeable membrane, and an enzymatic assay using glutamate dehydrogenase.

Reference Values[16]

0-1 day:	64-107 μmol/L
2-14 days:	56-92 μmol/L
15 days-17 years:	21-50 μmol/L
18 years and older:	0-27 μmol/L

Clinical Significance

Significant hyperammonemia during childhood can be observed with urea cycle defects, many of the organic acidemias, transient hyperammonemia of the newborn (THAN), and fatty acid oxidation defects. In these cases, ammonia levels are markedly elevated and frequently exceed 1000 μmol/L. Hyperammonemia can also be seen in conditions associated with liver dysfunction or renal failure, but ammonia levels in these cases of liver disease rarely exceed 500 μmol/L. Mild transient hyperammonemia is relatively common in newborns, can reach levels that are twice normal, and is usually asymptomatic.

LIPIDS

Lipids are a class of biochemical compounds. The **major plasma lipids,** including cholesterol (or total cholesterol [TC]) and the triglycerides, do not circulate freely in solution in plasma but are bound to proteins and transported as macromolecular complexes called *lipoproteins.*

Lipids play an important role in many metabolic processes. They act as:

- Hormone or hormone precursors
- Energy storage and metabolic fuels
- Structural and functional components in cell membranes
- Insulation to allow conduction of nerve impulses or heat loss

Lipids are important because a clear relationship has been demonstrated between plasma lipids and lipoproteins and atherosclerosis. **Atherosclerosis,** a condition of deposition of plaques in the blood vessels, has been proven to lead to coronary artery disease. According to the recommendations of the National Cholesterol Education Program (NCEP),[17,18] a lipid profile is useful in the evaluation of risk status for *coronary heart disease* (CHD).

Cholesterol

Cholesterol is found in animal fats. Only a portion of the body's cholesterol is derived from dietary intake; about 70% of the daily production of cholesterol production comes from the liver. Although increases in cholesterol have been implicated in increased atherosclerotic diseases, cholesterol is also an essential component for normal biological functions. It serves as an essential structural component of animal cell membranes and subcellular particles and as a precursor of bile acids and all steroid hormones, including sex and adrenal hormones.

MEASUREMENT OF CHOLESTEROL SPECIMEN

A serum specimen collected in a serum separator evacuated tube from a patient who has been fasting for 12 to 15 hours is the preferred lipid-testing specimen. If a serum separator collection tube is not used, serum for analysis must be separated from red blood cells to prevent an exchange of cholesterol between RBC membranes and the serum or plasma. If analysis must be delayed, the serum can be refrigerated at 4°C for several days.

TOTAL CHOLESTEROL

In routine laboratories, the most common methodology used to determine cholesterol is by enzymatic assay. In most automated methods, the enzyme cholesterol esterase hydrolyzes cholesterol esters to free cholesterol. The free cholesterol produced, along with free cholesterol that was initially present in the sample, is then oxidized in a reaction catalyzed by cholesterol oxidase. The hydrogen peroxide (H_2O_2) formed oxidizes various compounds to form a colored product that is measured photometrically; the magnitude of the colored compound formed is proportional to the amount of cholesterol present in the sample. Some interferences are noted with lipemic samples when direct methods are used.

Triglycerides

The fat found in food is composed mainly of **triglycerides.** A very small proportion of the lipids, about 1% to 2%, includes cholesterol and other fats. Lipids constitute 95% of tissue storage fat and are transported to and from body tissues in lipoprotein complexes.

Triglycerides are digested by the action of pancreatic and intestinal lipases. After absorption, triglycerides are resynthesized in the intestinal epithelial cells and combined with cholesterol and apolipoprotein B48 to form chylomicrons. **Chylomicrons** give serum its characteristic milky appearance (lipemia) when blood is drawn after a meal.

Measurement of Triglycerides

The appearance of the plasma or serum can be observed and noted after a minimum 12-hour fast. If the plasma is clear, the triglyceride level is probably less than 200 mg/dL. When the plasma appears hazy or turbid, the triglyceride level has increased to greater than 300 mg/dL, and if the specimen appears opaque and milky (lipemic, from chylomicrons), the triglyceride level is probably greater than 600 mg/dL.

Triglyceride methods are usually enzymatic. In most automated enzymatic methods, hydrolysis of the triglyceride present in the sample is usually achieved by lipase (triacylglycerol acylhydrolase). The resulting glycerol produced is assayed by various coupled-enzyme methods. The presence of free glycerol in the samples can interfere with the analysis; assays adjust for this positive interference. Reagents must be carefully checked in automated methodologies because some reagents have a short period of stability after reconstitution.

Lipoproteins

Lipids are transported in the plasma to various body tissues by lipoproteins. **Lipoproteins** are particles with triglycerides and cholesterol esters in their core and phospholipids and free cholesterol near the surface. Lipoproteins also contain one or more specific proteins, apolipoproteins, located on the surface of the particle.

The **major lipoprotein classes**—chylomicrons, very low-density (pre-β) lipoproteins (VLDL), low-density (β-) lipoproteins (LDL), and high-density (α-) lipoproteins (HDL)—although closely interrelated, are usually classified in terms of physicochemical properties. Based on differences in their hydrated densities, lipoproteins can be separated by ultracentrifugation into the following:

- Chylomicrons
- VLDL (very low-density lipoprotein)
- IDL (intermediate-density lipoprotein)
- LDL (low-density lipoprotein), which carries about 70% of total plasma cholesterol
- HDL (high-density lipoprotein), including HDL2 and HDL3

In a fasting state, most plasma triglycerides are present in VLDL. In a nonfasting state, chylomicrons appear transiently and contribute significantly to the total plasma triglyceride levels.

Apolipoprotein E (apo E) is present on plasma lipoproteins, including chylomicrons, VLDL, and HDL. Apo E plays an important role in lipoprotein metabolism as the ligand for lipoprotein receptors. Apo E may also be involved in nerve regeneration, the immune response, and the differentiation of nerve and muscle cells.

Clinical Significance[16-18]

The major plasma lipids of interest are total cholesterol and the triglycerides. When an elevation of these plasma lipids is observed, the condition is called **hyperlipidemia.** Cholesterol and triglycerides can be used to detect numerous types of hyperlipidemia.[19]

For patients without clinical evidence of coronary or other atherosclerotic vascular disease, the NCEP recommends **health screening,** including measurement of TC and HDL cholesterol, at least once every 5 years. **Further evaluation** is performed for those patients with a high TC, low HDL cholesterol (<35 mg/dL), or borderline TC who have at least two CAD risk factors (age > 45 for men, > 55 for women or postmenopausal state without estrogen replacement, high blood pressure, smoking, diabetes, HDL < 35 mg/dL, or a family history of CAD before age 55 in a male first-degree relative or before age 65 in a female first-degree relative).

This evaluation should include fasting levels of TC, triglyceride, and HDL. LDL is then calculated by applying the following formula:

$$\text{LDL cholesterol} = \frac{\text{TC} - \text{HDL cholesterol} - \text{triglyceride}}{5}$$

(This formula is valid only when triglyceride is <400 mg/dL. A high HDL level [>60 mg/dL] is considered a negative risk factor and reduces the number of risk factors by one.)

The NCEP recommends that treatment decisions be based on the calculated level of LDL. For patients with an elevated LDL (≥160 mg/dL) who have fewer than two risk factors in addition to elevated LDL and who do not have clinical evidence of atherosclerotic disease, the goal of treatment is an LDL level less than 160 mg/dL. For those who have at least two other risk factors, the goal of treatment is an LDL level less than 130 mg/dL. When LDL levels remain higher than 160 mg/dL despite dietary measures, and the patient has two or more risk factors (in addition to high LDL), or when LDL levels remain higher than 190 mg/dL even without added risk factors, the addition of drug treatment should be considered.

For those with CAD, peripheral vascular disease, or cerebrovascular disease, the goal of treatment is an LDL less than 100 mg/dL.

All patients with clinical evidence of coronary or other atherosclerotic disease should be evaluated with a fasting blood sample for measurement of TC, triglyceride, and HDL. LDL is calculated.

In contrast to plasma TC, it is unclear whether plasma triglycerides are independent risk variables. A triglyceride level of less than 200 mg/dL is considered normal, 200 to 400 mg/dL is borderline high, and greater than 400 mg/dL is high. Hypertriglyceridemia has been associated with diabetes, hyperuricemia, and pancreatitis (when levels are > 600 mg/dL).

Types of Hyperlipidemia

The types of hyperlipidemia are listed in Table 11-7.

TABLE 11-7

		Types of Hyperlipidemia	
Type	Name	Characterists	Etiology
Type I	Exogenous hypertri- glyceridemia; familial fat-induced lipemia; hyperchylomicronemia	Relatively rare inherited deficiency of either lipoprotein lipase activity or the lipase-activating protein, apo C-II, causing inability to effectively remove chylomicrons and VLDL triglycerides from blood	Manifested in children or young adults; symptoms and signs exacerbated by increased dietary fat that accumu- lates in circulation as chylomicrons No evidence that type I hyperlipopro- teinemia predisposes to atheroscle- rosis
Type II	Hyperlipoproteinemia	Elevation of low-density lipoprotein (LDL)	May be primary or secondary Primary type II includes genetic conditions that lead to elevation of LDL-familial hypercholesterolemia, familial combined hyperlipidemia, familial defective apolipoprotein B, and polygenic hypercholester- olemia
Type III	Hyperlipoproteinemia (also called *familial dysbetalipo- proteinemia*)	Characterized by accumulation in plasma of a β migrating VLDL, which is rich in triglycerides and TC	Less common familial disorder
Type IV	Hyperlipoproteinemia endogenous hypertriglyc- eridemia; hyperprebetali- poproteinemia	Characterized by variable elevations of plasma triglyceride contained predominantly in very low-density (pre-β) lipoproteins	Common disorder often associated with a familial distribution; possible predisposition to atherosclerosis
Type V	Hyperlipoproteinemia (mixed hypertriglyceride- mia, mixed hyperlipemia, hyperprebetalipoprotein- emia with chylomicrons)	Associated with defective clearance of exogenous and endogenous triglycerides Plasma triglyceride levels usually markedly elevated, with only mod- est rises in TC	Uncommon disorder, sometimes familial, associated with risk of life- threatening pancreatitis

Secondary Elevations of Low-Density Lipoproteins

In North America and Europe, dietary cholesterol and saturated fats are the most common causes of mild to moderate elevations of LDL. Hypercholes-terolemia is common in **biliary cirrhosis,** as is a marked increase in the serum phospholipids and an elevated free cholesterol/cholesterol ester ratio (>0.2).

Hypercholesterolemia resulting from increased LDL levels may be associated with various disorders:

- **Endocrinopathies** such as hypothyroidism and diabetes mellitus; hypercholesterolemia usually reversed by hormone therapy
- Hypoproteinemias, as in **nephrotic syndrome**
- Metabolic aberrations such as **acute porphyria**
- Dietary excesses with cholesterol-rich foods, producing elevated LDL levels
- Menopause without estrogen replacement therapy
- Secondary to increased HDL levels in post-menopausal women or in younger women who take oral contraceptives or hormone replace-ment therapy, which contains primarily estrogen

Secondary Hypertriglyceridemia

The most common forms of hypertriglyceride-mia seen in clinical practice are those secondary to alcohol and drug consumption and with disor-ders such as chronic, severe, uncontrolled diabetes mellitus.

Familial Lecithin Cholesterol Acyltransferase Deficiency

Familial lecithin cholesterol acyltransferase deficiency is a rare disorder inherited as a reces-sive trait. It is characterized by lack of the enzyme that normally esterifies cholesterol in the plasma. The disorder is manifested by marked hyper-cholesterolemia and hyperphospholipidemia (free cholesterol and lecithin) together with hypertriglyceridemia.

Renal and liver failure, anemia, and lens opaci-ties are common in familial lecithin cholesterol acyltransferase deficiency. Treatment with a fat-restricted diet reduces the concentration of lipo-protein complexes in plasma and may help prevent kidney damage. Kidney transplantation has been successful for renal failure.

Reference Values[7,9]

Values in parentheses are in SI Units.

Cholesterol, serum, adults (NCEP guideline recommendations for adults in terms of risk for CHD[15]):

Desirable	<200 mg/dL (<5.18 mmol/L)
Borderline/moderate risk	200-239 mg/dL (5.18-6.19 mmol/L)
High risk	>240 mg/dL (>6.22 mmol/L)

Triglycerides, serum (recommended desirable levels for adults, after a 12-hour fast):

Male	40-160 mg/dL
Female	35-135 mg/dL

Note: Reference values for triglycerides vary for females and males, with females having values slightly lower. Specific age-related reference value tables are available in clinical chemistry textbooks, if needed. Triglyceride values increase with age until age 60, when they decrease slightly. Levels for blacks are 10 to 20 mg/dL lower than for whites. The NCEP recommendations have eliminated the use of reference values for triglycerides but include a few cutoff values (as used for total cholesterol) to simplify the decision-making process.

HDL cholesterol:

Negative risk factor for CHD	>60 mg/dL
Positive risk factor for CHD	<35 mg/dL

Adult Values
Cholesterol:

Desirable	199 mg/dL or less
Borderline	200-239 mg/dL
Higher risk	240 mg/dL or greater

Triglycerides:

Desirable	149 mg/dL or less
Borderline	150-199 mg/dL
Higher risk	200-499 mg/dL

HDL cholesterol:

Desirable	40 mg/dL or greater
Higher risk	39 mg/dL or less

LDL cholesterol (measured):

Desirable if patient has CHD	99 mg/dL or less
Desirable	129 mg/dL or less
Borderline	130-159 mg/dL
Higher risk	160 mg/dL or greater

VLDL cholesterol (calculated):

Desirable	30 mg/dL or less

Children and adolescents, 0-19 years
Total cholesterol:

Desirable	169 mg/dL or less
Borderline	170-199 mg/dL
Higher risk	200 mg/dL or greater

LDL cholesterol (measured):

Desirable	109 mg/dL or less
Borderline	110-129 mg/dL
Higher risk	130 mg/dL or greater

LDL cholesterol, direct:

0-19 years	0-110 mg/dL
>20 years	0-130 mg/dL

Adults, 20 years and older

Desirable if patient has CHD	99 mg/dL or less
Desirable	129 mg/dL or less
Borderline	130-159 mg/dL
Higher risk	160 mg/dL or greater

Children and adolescents, 0-19 years

Desirable	109 mg/dL or less
Borderline	110-129 mg/dL
Higher risk	130 mg/dL or greater

Interpretive Data

Men older than 45 and women older than 55 or affected by premature menopause without estrogen replacement therapy:

- +1 Family history of premature CHD
- +1 Current smoker
- +1 Hypertension
- +1 Diabetes mellitus
- +1 Low HDL cholesterol: 39 mg/dL or less
- −1 High HDL cholesterol: 60 mg/dL or greater

LDL cholesterol (measured), therapeutic goal:
- 100 mg/dL or less if CHD is present
- 129 mg/dL or less if no CHD and two or more risk factors
- 159 mg/dL or less if no CHD

CARDIAC DISEASE

Serial Sampling for Cardiac Markers

After the onset of symptoms of a myocardial infarction (MI), such as chest pain, there is a time window during which the cardiac markers released from myocardial tissue have elevated values in blood. Although the pattern varies somewhat among individuals, a typical pattern is defined for each marker (Fig. 11-5). Some studies have recommended sampling a sequence of blood specimens collected on admission and at 2 to 4 hours, 6 to 8 hours, and 12 hours after MI is suspected. The European Society of Cardiology and American College of Cardiology consensus report[19] stressed the importance of serial sampling for cardiac markers, recommending sampling on presentation, at 6 to 9 hours, and again at 12 to 24 hours if earlier specimens were negative and

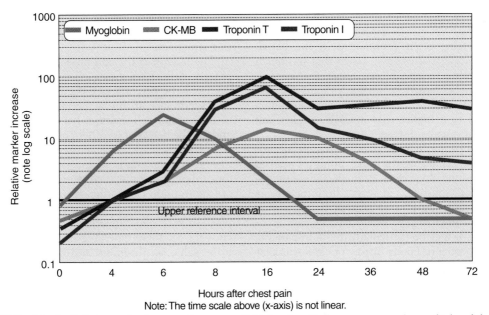

FIGURE 11-5 Relative marker increase after myocardial infarction. Markers are expressed as multiples of the upper limit of the reference interval. Therefore the relative increase varies depending on the normal reference interval used. The time scale (x axis) is not linear. (Modified from Wu A: Cardiac markers, Totowa, NJ, 1998, Humana Press.)

clinical suspicion of MI is high. Point-of-care testing or central laboratory testing must be available 24 hours a day.

Before the introduction of current cardiac markers, physicians used *total creatine kinase* (CK) and *lactate dehydrogenase* (LDH) isoenzymes to diagnose and assess myocardial damage. In addition to the elimination of these markers, the traditional standard of laboratory diagnosis of acute MI, the MB *isoform of creatine kinase* (CK-MB), is requested less frequently. More than two decades ago, monoclonal antibody–based assays for *cardiac-specific troponin T* (cTnT) and *cardiac-specific troponin I* (cTnI) isoforms were introduced as cardiac markers.

The current marker assay combination for diagnosis of acute MI and myocardial injury is:
- Myoglobin
- Troponins
- CK isoenzyme (CK-MB)

Myoglobin

A heme protein found in striated skeletal and cardiac muscles, **myoglobin** is an early marker of injury to muscle tissue. A rise in myoglobin concentration is detectable in blood as early as 1 to 3 hours after the onset of MI symptoms and can be used to rule out the diagnosis in the 2- to 6-hour period after the onset of symptoms. The disadvantage of myoglobin is that it is not cardiac specific. It can be increased in trauma, diseases of the skeletal muscle, and renal failure. Myoglobin concentrations for adult men range from 30 to

90 ng/dL; women typically demonstrate concentrations of less than 50 ng/mL.

Myoglobin can be measured by latex agglutination, enzyme-linked immunosorbent assay (ELISA), immunonephelometry, and fluoroimmunoassay. A spot test using immunochromatography is also available.

Troponins

Cardiac troponin (cTn) is currently acknowledged as the "gold standard" of cardiac biomarkers. **Troponin** is a complex of three proteins that bind to the thin filaments of striated cardiac or skeletal muscle and regulate muscle contraction. The complex consists of:
- Troponin T (TnT)
- Troponin I (TnI)
- Troponin C (TnC)

The largest portion of TnI released into the blood circulation after damage to myocardial tissue is in the form of a complex with cardiac-specific TnC (cTnC). Troponins remain elevated in blood for 4 to 10 days after MI and thus are valuable for late-presenting patients.

Creatine Kinase MB

CK-MB can become elevated after tissue injury. An increased ratio of MB_2/MB_1 is sensitive for early diagnosis of myocardial cell death. CK-MB is relatively cardiospecific because of excellent sensitivity within 4 to 6 hours after onset of symptoms in MI patients.

Homocysteine

Homocysteine is an amino acid in the blood. Epidemiologic studies have shown that too much homocysteine in the blood, hyperhomocysteinemia, can be caused by folate, vitamin B_6, and vitamin B_{12} deficiencies. Hyperhomocysteinemia is related to a higher risk of CHD, stroke, and peripheral vascular disease.

Homocysteine may have an effect on atherosclerosis by damaging the inner lining of arteries and promoting blood clots. A direct causal link has not been established, but recent findings suggest that laboratory testing for plasma homocysteine levels can improve the assessment of cardiovascular risk. It may be particularly useful in patients with a personal or family history of cardiovascular disease, but in whom the well-established risk factors (smoking, high blood cholesterol, high blood pressure) do not exist.

C-Reactive Protein

Cardiovascular disease is now considered a process with a low-level inflammatory component. **C-reactive protein (CRP)** is an inflammation-sensitive protein that can be measured by immunoassays. It is being used as an indicator of risk for cardiovascular disease.

CRP appears to be one of the most sensitive acute-phase indicators of inflammation in certain populations of patients, especially middle-aged and elderly healthy individuals. There are two forms of this test: (1) monitoring the "traditional" inflammatory processes and (2) performing the highly-sensitive CRP (hsCRP), also referred to as *cardioCRP*. The hsCRP detects the same protein as the traditional CRP but can detect small changes at much lower levels. Patients with high CRP values cannot benefit from the hsCRP, because elevated CRP masks the smaller changes.

Natriuretic Peptides

B-type natriuretic peptide (BNP), formerly known as *brain natriuretic peptide*, is used to differentiate dyspnea due to heart failure from pulmonary disease. The heart is the major source of circulating BNP and releases this polypeptide in response to both ventricle volume expansion and pressure overload. As such, BNP is used as a diagnostic tool for heart failure.

Miscellaneous Markers

As with CRP, *fibrinogen* is an acute-phase protein produced in response to inflammation. Including measurement of fibrinogen in screening for cardiovascular risk may be valuable in identifying patients who need aggressive heart disease prevention strategies.

The *D-dimer* is the end product of the ongoing process of thrombus formation and dissolution that occurs at the site of active plaques in acute coronary syndromes. It can be used for early detection of myocardial cell damage, but it is not specific and can be detected in other conditions in which plaque forms.

Microalbuminuria is an independent risk factor for cardiovascular disease in patients with diabetes or hypertension (see earlier discussion).

Although many biomarkers have been proposed as potential biomarkers of cardiac ischemia (Box 11-8), these emerging markers have added little value to diagnosis and risk stratification. There is a continuum from vascular inflammation to myocardial dysfunction along with associated biomarkers with each stage of acute coronary syndrome (ACS). The biochemical profile markers associated with the various stages of ACS[20] are:

- Proinflmmatory Cytokines
- Plaque Destabilization
- Plaque Rupture
- Acute Phase Reactants (e.g., C-RP)
- Ischemia
- Necrosis (e.g., cTnT and CTnI), and
- Myocardial Dysfunction (e.g., BNP and NT-proBNP)

The search continues for the next superstar cardiac biomarker to identify a circulating blood abnormality before a cardiac event occurs, (e.g., MI).

Box 11-8

Proposed Biomarkers of Cardiac Ischemia

- Adhesion molecules
- CD40 ligand
- Choline
- C-reactive protein (C-RP)
- Cytokines
- Fatty acid binding protein
- Glycogenphosphorylase-BB
- Ischemia-modified albumin
- Isopentanes
- Monocyte chemotactic protein
- Myoglobin
- Natriuretic peptides
- Oxidized LDL
- Phospholipase A2
- Placental growth factor
- Pregnancy-associated plasma protein A
- Serum amyloid
- Unbound free fatty acids

From Apple FS: Cl Lab News, Cardiac Ischemia 35(9):9, 2009.

LIVER AND PANCREATIC TESTING

Laboratory assays are best used in groups as a battery of tests to assess liver disease. If abnormal, biochemical tests of liver function (Table 11-8) suggest a category of liver disease:

- Hepatocellular damage
- Cholestasis
- Excretory function
- Biosynthetic function

Bilirubin

A frequently used assay for assessing liver excretory function is the measurement of serum bilirubin concentration. **Bilirubin** is derived from the iron-containing heme portion of hemoglobin, which is released from the breakdown of RBCs. Bilirubin complexed to albumin, called **unconjugated bilirubin,** is transported to the liver, where it is processed into **conjugated bilirubin** by the liver cells. In this form, bilirubin enters the bile fluid for transport to the small intestine. In the small intestine, most of the conjugated bilirubin is converted to urobilinogens (see Chapter 14). At least four bilirubin fractions can be separated and identified by liquid chromatography, the least understood being the delta fraction (B delta), which apparently is covalently bound to albumin.

Clinical Significance: Jaundice

Jaundice, or **icterus,** the yellow discoloration of plasma, skin, and mucous membranes, is caused by the abnormal metabolism, accumulation, or retention of bilirubin. There are three types of jaundice:

1. Prehepatic
2. Hepatic
3. Posthepatic

Increased hemolysis of RBCs (e.g., hemolytic anemia) can result in prehepatic jaundice. Hepatitis and cirrhosis of the liver can result in hepatic

TABLE 11-8

Laboratory Assays to Assess Liver Disease		
Category	Laboratory Assay	Comments
Hepatocellular damage	Aspartate aminotransferase (AST)	Found in numerous tissues including liver, cardiac muscle, skeletal muscle, kidneys, brain, and pancreas
	Alanine aminotransferase (ALT)	Found primarily in liver; considered best laboratory test for liver injury
Cholestasis	Alkaline phosphatase (ALP)	Usually increased during periods of growth (e.g., children, teenagers) and during pregnancy
	Gammaglutamyl transferase (GGT)	Very sensitive to small liver insults (e.g., alcohol consumption) May be elevated in hepatocellular disease
	5′ nucleotidase (5′ NT)	Very sensitive and specific for hepatobiliary disease
Liver excretory function	Serum bilirubin	Heme product from catalysis and conjugation with glucuronic acid Three fractions: conjugated, unconjugated, and delta bilirubin (albumin-bound) Causes jaundice when concentrations exceed 1.5 mg/dL
	Urine bilirubin	Performed qualitatively using a urine dipstick
	Blood ammonia	Liver converts ammonia to urea Significant liver dysfunction results in elevated serum ammonia Poor correlation between ammonia level and degree of liver disease
Assays of biosynthetic function	Total protein, albumin, and globulins	Altered ratio of albumin to globulin in liver disease
	Coagulation factors	All factors produced in liver Factors II, VII, IX, and X are vitamin K sensitive (meaning they require adequate quantities of vitamin K for production) Prothrombin time (PT) is a collective measure of factors II, V, VII, and X Elevated PT unresponsive to vitamin K supplementation suggests poor liver functionality

Modified from www.aruplab.com. Accessed June 7, 2009.

jaundice. Obstruction of the biliary tract caused by strictures, neoplasms, or stones can also result in jaundice.

The clinical finding of jaundice is nonspecific and can result from a variety of disorders. Specific disorders involving bilirubin metabolism represent specific defects in the way the liver processes the bilirubin. These can be transport defects, impairment in the conjugation step in the liver itself (hepatic function), or a defect in the excretory function of transporting the conjugated bilirubin from the liver cells into bile fluid.

NEONATAL JAUNDICE

Elevations in serum bilirubin occur in some infants, especially premature babies in the first few days of life. This is an example of **physiologic jaundice** and may involve a deficiency of the enzyme that transfers glucuronate groups onto bilirubin or may signal liver immaturity. Some infants lack glucuronosyltransferase, the enzyme necessary for conjugation of bilirubin glucuronide, and this results in a rapid buildup of unconjugated bilirubin. The unconjugated bilirubin readily passes into the brain and nerve cells and is deposited in the nuclei of these cells. This condition is called **kernicterus** and can result in cell damage leading to mental impairment or death.

Neonatal jaundice can persist until glucuronosyltransferase is produced by the liver of the newborn, usually within 3 to 5 days. All newborns have serum unconjugated bilirubin values greater than the reference values in a healthy adult, and 50% of newborns will be clinically jaundiced during the first few days of life.

Normal, healthy, full-term neonates can have unconjugated bilirubin values up to 4 to 5 mg/dL, and in a small percentage of newborns, this value can be as high as 10 mg/dL. These elevated values usually decrease to normal levels in 7 to 10 days. If toxic levels do occur (exceeding 20 to 25 mg/dL), treatment must be rapidly initiated. Infants with physiologic jaundice can be treated with phototherapy.

Specimens

Bilirubin analyses may be done on serum or plasma, although serum is preferred. The blood should be drawn when the patient is in a fasting state to avoid alimentary lipemia, which can result in falsely increased bilirubin values because of the turbidity of the specimen. Exposure of serum to heat and light results in oxidation of bilirubin. For this reason, specimens for bilirubin assays must be protected from the light. The procedure should be carried out as soon as possible, at least within 2 or 3 hours after the blood has clotted. Specimens

can be stored in the dark in a refrigerator for up to 1 week or in the freezer for 3 months without significant loss of bilirubin.

Methods for Quantitative Determination of Bilirubin

Most assays for serum bilirubin are based on a diazo reaction. In this procedure, bilirubin reacts with diazotized sulfanilic acid to form azobilirubin, which has a red-purple color. This basic reaction was modified by van den Bergh and Muller by the addition of alcohol, usually methanol, which accelerates the reaction of unconjugated bilirubin, called *indirect bilirubin*. The reacting substance, in the absence of alcohol, is the direct fraction of bilirubin, or conjugated bilirubin. Total bilirubin is the combination of conjugated and unconjugated bilirubin.

Many procedures involve a modification of the original Malloy-Evelyn technique, which uses a diazo reaction with methanol added.[21] Another common procedure is the Jendrassik-Grof modification, which is carried out in an alkaline solution.[22] Both the Malloy-Evelyn and the Jendrassik-Grof modifications have been automated and are currently used to perform bilirubin assays.

Automated Bilirubin Assays

In the Vitros Clinical Chemistry Analyzers, bilirubin is separated from the protein matrix by means of thin-film technology. Dry reagents are within the multilayered slides, and the reaction occurs within the layers as the serum passes through them. Total bilirubin is determined by diazotization after unconjugated bilirubin and conjugated bilirubin have been dissociated from albumin. The bilirubin diffuses into a polymer layer that complexes with the bilirubin. The reaction is monitored with a reflectance spectrophotometer. This method provides for the measurement of direct bilirubin.

Reference Values[7,9]

Total serum bilirubin, adult: 0.3-1.2 mg/dL
Direct (conjugated) serum bilirubin: 0-0.2 mg/dL
Total serum bilirubin in infants:

Age	Premature	Full Term
Cord	<2.0 mg/dL	<2.0 mg/dL
0-1 day	<8.0 mg/dL	2.0-6.0 mg/dL
1-2 days	<12.0 mg/dL	6.0-10.0 mg/dL
3-5 days	<16.0 mg/dL	1.5-12.0 mg/dL

Conjugated bilirubin levels up to 2 mg/dL are found in infants by 1 month of age, and this level remains through adulthood.

Enzymes

Tests for several serum enzymes are used in the differential diagnosis of liver disease. These tests include alkaline phosphatase, gamma-glutamyltransferase, lactate dehydrogenase, aspartate aminotransferase and alanine aminotransferase, and 5′ nucleotidase. Bile acids, triglycerides, cholesterol, serum proteins, coagulation proteins, and urea and ammonia assays are also used in the diagnosis of liver disease.

Aspartate Aminotransferase and Alanine Aminotransferase

These transaminase enzymes catalyze the conversion of aspartate and alanine to oxaloacetate and pyruvate, respectively. The highest level of alanine aminotransferase (ALT) is found primarily in the liver. Aspartate aminotransferase (AST) is found in the liver, heart, kidney, and muscle tissue. Acute destruction of tissue in any of these areas with damage at the cellular level results in rapid release of the enzymes into the serum. ALT and AST are elevated at the onset of viral jaundice and in chronic active hepatitis. With the onset of acute liver necrosis, both enzymes also are increased, but the increase in ALT is higher.

Gamma-Glutamyltransferase

Gamma-glutamyltransferase (GGT) is normally in highest concentration in the renal tissue, but it is also generally elevated in liver disease. Serum GGT is usually elevated earlier than the other liver enzymes in diseases such as acute cholecystitis, acute pancreatitis, acute and subacute liver necrosis, and neoplasms of sites where liver metastases are present. Increased levels of GGT are found in the blood when there is obstruction to bile flow, or cholestasis. Elevation of GGT is seen in chronic alcoholism.

Alkaline Phosphatase

Alkaline phosphatase can be present in many tissues. It is generally localized in the membranes of cells. Alkaline phosphatase is found in the highest activity in the liver, bone, intestine, kidney, and placenta. The enzyme appears to facilitate the transfer of metabolites across cell membranes and is associated with lipid transport and the calcification process in bone synthesis. Increased blood levels are found when cholestasis or bone degeneration is present.

Proteins

Hypoproteinemia is a condition involving a total protein level less than the reference interval. It can be caused by an excessive loss of protein in the urine in renal disease, leakage into the gastrointestinal tract in inflammatory conditions, loss of blood, and severe burns. A dietary deficiency and intestinal malabsorption may be other causes. Decreased protein synthesis is observed in liver disease. **Hyperproteinemia** is not seen as often as hypoproteinemia. Dehydration is one condition that would contribute to an increased level of total serum protein.

Albumin is the major protein synthesized by the liver and present in the circulating blood. When the liver has been chronically damaged (e.g., cirrhosis), the albumin level may be low (**hypoalbuminemia**). Malnutrition can also cause a low albumin level, with no associated liver disease.

Serum is the most frequently analyzed specimen for total protein or protein fractions, including albumin and globulin. The reference interval for total protein is 6.5 to 8.3 g/dL for ambulatory adults. The reference range for albumin is 3.5 to 5.5 g/dL.

The classic colorimetric method for the measurement of total protein and albumin is the Biuret method. In this reaction, cupric ions (Cu^{2+}) complex with the groups involved in the peptide bond. In an alkaline medium and in the presence of at least two peptide bonds, a violet-colored chelate is formed. Biuret reagent also contains sodium-potassium tartrate, which complexes cupric ions to prevent their precipitation in the alkaline solution, and potassium iodide, which acts as an antioxidant. The test solution is measured photometrically; the darker the solution, the higher the concentration of protein. A handheld refractometer can also be used.

Dye-binding methods can also be used to measure total proteins and are the most frequently used methods for determining albumin. This methodology is based on the ability of most proteins in serum to bind to dyes such as bromphenol blue. Coomassie brilliant blue 250 bound to protein is used in a spectrophotometric method, but dye-binding methods are frequently used to stain protein bands after electrophoresis.

In normal, healthy individuals, the various plasma proteins are present in delicately balanced concentrations, with a normal ratio of albumin to globulin (A/G ratio) of 2:1. A reversal in this ratio can be observed in disease of the kidney and liver. Chronic infections also produce a decrease in the albumin concentration.

Serum Protein Electrophoresis

Electrophoresis separates proteins on the basis of their electrical charge densities (Fig. 11-6). The direction of movement depends on whether the charge is positive or negative; cations (positive net charge) migrate to the cathode (negative terminal), and anions (negative net charge) migrate to the anode (positive terminal) (Fig. 11-7). The speed of the migration depends on the degree of ionization of the protein at the pH of the buffer solution. In addition to the charge density, the velocity of movement also depends on the electrical field strength, size and shape of the molecule, temperature, and characteristics of the buffer.

Cellulose acetate is the support medium typically used. Proteins can be separated into five distinct protein zones, which constitute many individual proteins:

1. Albumin
2. Alpha-1 (α_1) globulin
3. Alpha-2 (α_2) globulin

4. Beta (β) globulins
5. Gamma (γ) globulins

This method of analysis is useful for evaluation of patients who have abnormal liver function tests, because it allows a direct quantification of multiple serum proteins.

By modifying the standard electrophoretic technique, high-resolution protein electrophoresis, the five major fractions (see Fig. 6-14) can be further separated.[22] The technique is usually performed with an agarose gel support medium.

Zone	Serum Proteins Found in Zones	
1.	Prealbumin zone	Prealbumin
2.	Albumin zone	Albumin

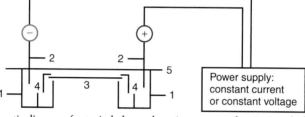

FIGURE 11-6 Schematic diagram of a typical electrophoresis apparatus showing two buffer boxes with baffle plates. *1,* electrodes; *2,* electrophoretic support; *3,* wicks; *4,* cover; *5,* power supply. (From Burtis CA, Ashwood ER, Bruns DE: Tietz fundamentals of clinical chemistry, ed 6, St Louis, 2008, Saunders.)

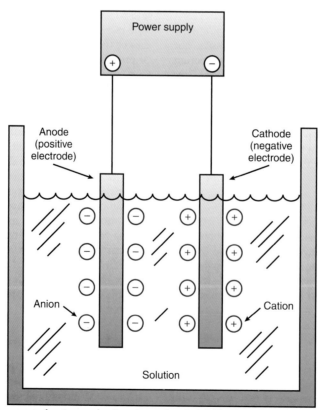

FIGURE 11-7 Movement of cations and anions in an electrical field. (From Burtis CA, Ashwood ER, Bruns DE: Tietz fundamentals of clinical chemistry, ed 6, St Louis, 2008, Saunders.)

Zone	Serum Proteins	Found in Zones
3.	Albumin-α_1 interzone	α-Lipoprotein, α-fetoprotein
4.	α_1 zone	α_1-Antitrypsin, α_1-acid-glycoprotein
5.	α_1-α_2 interzone	Gc-globulin, inter-α-trypsin inhibitor, α_1-antichymotrypsin
6.	α_2 zone	α_2-Macroglobulin, haptoglobin
7.	α_2-β_1 interzone	Cold insoluble globulin, hemoglobin
8.	β_1 zone	Transferrin
9.	β_2-β_1 interzone	β-Lipoprotein
10.	β_2 zone	C3
11.	γ_1 zone	IgA (fibrinogen), IgM (monoclonal Igs, light chains)
12.	γ_2 zone	IgM (C-reactive protein), IgM monoclonal Igs, light chains

The most significant finding from an electrophoretic pattern is monoclonal immunoglobulin (Ig) disease. A spike in the α, β, or α_2 indicates a need for further consideration of a monoclonal disorder. A deficiency of immunoglobulin G (IgG) suggests an immunodeficiency disorder or nephrotic syndrome.

Proteins in Other Body Fluids

Urine and CSF are the most frequently analyzed body fluids for protein concentration. Increases in protein in the urine result from either glomerular or tubular dysfunction. Abnormally increased total CSF proteins may be found in conditions where there is an increased permeability of the capillary endothelial barrier through which ultrafiltration occurs (e.g., meningitis, multiple sclerosis, cerebral infarction). The degree of permeability can be evaluated by measuring the CSF albumin and comparing it with the serum albumin. Diagnosis of specific disorders frequently requires measurement of individual protein fractions.

Coagulation: Prothrombin Time

Another measure of hepatic synthetic function is the **prothrombin time (PT).** The serum proteins are associated with the incorporation of vitamin K metabolites into a protein that allows normal coagulation (clotting of blood). If a patient has a prolonged PT, liver disease may be present, but a prolonged PT is not a specific test for liver disease. Diseases such as malnutrition, in which decreased vitamin K ingestion is present, may result in prolonged PT.

Pancreatic Function

The pancreas is a large gland involved in the digestive process as well as a gland that produces insulin and glucagons. Both these hormones are involved in carbohydrate metabolism. Other than trauma, three diseases cause most cases of pancreatic disease:

- Cystic fibrosis
- Pancreatitis
- Pancreatic carcinoma

Cystic fibrosis (CF) is an inherited autosomal recessive disorder that causes the small and large ducts and the acini (grapelike clusters lining the ducts) to dilate and change into small cysts filled with mucus. This eventually results in pancreatic secretions not reaching the digestive tract, possibly leading to an obstruction. The chloride content of sweat is useful in diagnosing CF, a disease of the exocrine glands. Affected infants usually have concentrations of sweat chloride greater than 60 mmol/L; adult values are typically greater than 70 mmol/L (reference values average about 40 mol/L). In 98% of CF patients, the secretion of chloride in sweat is two to five times normal. The determination of increased chloride in sweat, as well as an increase of other electrolytes, is useful in the diagnosis of CF. The chloride content of normal sweat varies with age. To collect the sample, the patient is induced to sweat, and the sweat can be measured directly by use of ISEs.

Pancreatitis, inflammation of the pancreas, is caused by autodigestion of the pancreas from reflux of bile or duodenal contents into the pancreatic duct. It may be acute, chronic, or relapsing and recurrent. Pancreatic carcinoma is the fifth most frequent form of fatal cancer in the United States.

Laboratory assays of pancreatic function include assays for the enzymes amylase and lipase. In addition, assessment of extrahepatic obstruction (e.g., bilirubin) and endocrine-related tests (e.g., glucose) can reflect changes in the endocrine cells of the pancreas. Stool specimens can also be analyzed for excess fat, as well as the enzymes trypsin and chymotrypsin.

Amylase is an enzyme that catalyzes the breakdown of starch and glycogen. The islet cells of the pancreas and salivary glands are the major tissue of serum amylase. Amylase is the major digestive enzyme of starches. The clinical significance of serum and urine amylase is in the diagnosis of acute pancreatitis. Amylase begins to increase in concentration in the blood 2 to 12 hours after onset of an attack and peaks at 24 hours.

Lipase is an enzyme that hydrolyzes the ester linkage of fats to produce alcohols and fatty acids. Lipase is found primarily in the pancreas. Clinical assays of serum lipase are limited almost exclusively to the diagnosis of acute pancreatitis.

HORMONE ASSAYS

A *hormone* is defined as a chemical substance produced by a specialized gland in one part of the body and carried to a distant target organ where a regulatory response is elicited. Hormones may also be secreted by nonglandular tissues in more than one site and transported by mechanisms other than the blood circulation. A frequently performed hormone assay is measurement of thyroid hormone.

Thyroid

The thyroid is one of the largest endocrine glands in the body. This hormone-producing gland is found in the front at the base of the neck. The trace mineral, iodine, is essential for the production of thyroid hormones. In some parts of the world, iodine deficiency is common, but the addition of iodine to table salt has virtually eliminated this problem in the United States. In areas of the world where iodine is lacking in the diet, the thyroid gland can be considerably enlarged, resulting in the development of a goiter. The thyroid gland is sensitive to the effects of various radioactive isotopes of iodine produced by nuclear fission. In the event of large accidental releases of such material into the environment (e.g., the Chernobyl disaster), the uptake of radioactive iodine isotopes by the thyroid can result in an increase in thyroid cancer in children. Theoretically, the selective uptake of radioactive isotopes of iodine can be blocked by saturating the uptake mechanism with a large surplus of nonradioactive iodine taken in the form of potassium iodide tablets.

The thyroid secretes hormones, principally thyroxine (T_4) and triiodothyronine (T_3). The amount of thyroid hormone secreted from the gland is about 90% T_4 and about 10% T_3. The function of thyroid hormones is to control metabolism (the rate at which the body uses fats and carbohydrates), help control body temperature, influence heart rate, and help regulate the production of protein.

The rate at which T_4 and T_3 are released is controlled by the pituitary gland and the hypothalamus. The hypothalamus signals the pituitary gland to make the hormone, thyroid-stimulating hormone (TSH). The pituitary gland then releases TSH; the concentration of TSH depends on how much T_4 and T_3 are in the blood. The thyroid gland also regulates its production of hormones based on the amount of TSH it receives.

Calcitonin is another hormone produced by the thyroid gland. It participates in regulating the amount of calcium in the blood and maintaining calcium homeostasis.

Hypothyroidism

The thyroid's hormone secretion process usually works well, but it sometimes fails to produce enough hormones, a condition called *hypothyroidism*. The autoimmune disease referred to as *Hashimoto thyroiditis* is the most common cause of hypothyroidism. Exogenous factors that contribute to hypothyroidism are radiation therapy, thyroidectomy, or medications such as lithium.

Some women develop hypothyroidism during or after pregnancy, a condition known as *postpartum hypothyroidism*. If untreated during pregnancy, hypothyroidism increases the risk of miscarriage, premature delivery, and preeclampsia. It can also adversely affect the developing fetus and can cause fetal death or a low IQ in liveborn (endemic cretinism) infants.

Women are 5 to 8 times more likely than men to suffer from hypothyroidism. Women in the age group of 40 to 60 years are more likely to experience hypothyroidism. Although hypothyroidism most often affects middle-aged women, anyone can develop hypothyroidism, including infants and teenagers.

Hyperthyroidism

In hyperthyroidism, a condition resulting from an overactive thyroid, too much T_4 is produced. Graves' disease, an autoimmune disorder in which antibodies produced by the immune system stimulate the thyroid to produce too much T_4, is the most common cause of hyperthyroidism.

Hyperthyroidism can significantly accelerate the body's metabolism, causing sudden weight loss, a rapid or irregular heartbeat, sweating, and nervousness or irritability.

Table 11-9 compares the features of hypothyroidism and hyperthyroidism.

Laboratory Diagnosis

A wide variety of laboratory assays (Table 11-10) are available for thyroid disease testing. If hypothyroidism is suspected, initial evaluation should include TSH, free T_4, and thyroid antibodies. Some common medicines can interfere with assay results (Table 11-11).

TUMOR MARKERS

In tumor immunology, a fundamental tenet is that when a normal cell is transformed into a malignant cell, it develops unique antigens not normally present on the mature normal cell. A tumor marker (e.g., hormone, enzyme) is a substance present in or produced by a tumor itself, or produced by the host in response to a tumor, that can be used to differentiate a tumor from normal tissue or to determine the presence of a tumor. Nonneoplastic conditions can also exhibit tumor marker activity. Some tumor markers are used to screen for cancer, but markers are used more often to monitor recurrence of cancer or to determine the degree of tumor burden in the patient. To be of any practical use, the tumor marker must be able to reveal the presence of the tumor while it is still susceptible to destructive treatment by surgical or other means. Tumor markers can be measured quantitatively in tissues and body fluids using biochemical, immunochemical, or molecular tests.

TABLE 11-9

Comparison of Hypothyroidism and Hyperthyroidism		
Diagnosis	Thyroid Stimulating Hormone	Free T_4 (FT4)
Hypothyroidism	Increased	Decreased
Hyperthyroidism	Decreased	Increased

TABLE 11-10

Thyroid Laboratory Assays	
Assay Name	Recommended Use
Thyroid-stimulating hormone (TSH)	Initial screening test for suspected hypothyroidism and hyperthyroidism.
Thyroid stimulating hormone	TSH falls and may be below lower adult reference limit in 20% of pregnancies Most reliable marker of thyroid function when illness is suspected Reference intervals for free T_4 have not been well established in pregnant patients; some advocate use of total T_4 in place of free T_4 during pregnancy
Thyroxine, free (free T_4)	In 2% of pregnancies, T_4 is supranormal around 10-12 weeks, because hCG is at its peak and TSH is at its nadir.
Thyroid antibodies	Detect antibodies for diagnosing autoimmune disease Test includes thyroid peroxidase (TPO) and thyroglobulin antibodies
Thyroxine	Some advocate using total T_4 in place of free T_4 during pregnancy.
Thyroid stimulating immunoglobulin	Detect thyroid antibodies for diagnosing autoimmune disease (Graves' disease)
Thyroid peroxidase (TPO) antibody	Detect antibodies for diagnosing autoimmune disease
Thyroid stimulating hormone receptor antibody (TRAb)	Detect antibodies for diagnosing autoimmune disease
Thyroglobulin antibody	Detect antibodies for diagnosing autoimmune disease Test is part of thyroid antibody panel

Reference modified from aruplab.com. Accessed July 29, 2009.
Note: Serum is the preferred specimen used in the measurement of T_4, but plasma EDTA or heparin is also used. Storage of serum specimens at room temperature up to 7 days results in no significant loss of T_4.

TABLE 11-11

Examples of Drugs That May Alter Thyroid Function Assays					
Drugs That May Alter Thyroid Function Tests					
Drug	TSH	T_3		T_4		Mechanism
		Total	Free	Total	Free	
Androgens	Normal	Reduced	Normal	Reduced	Normal	Reduced TBG synthesis
Aspirin	Normal	Increased	Normal	Increased	Normal	Reduced TBG binding
Estrogens	Normal	Increased	Normal	Increased	Normal	Increased TBG synthesis
Lithium	Increased	Reduced	Reduced	Reduced	Reduced	T_3 and T_4 release inhibition
Neuroleptics	Normal	Increased	Normal	Increased	Normal	Increased TBG synthesis

Modified from Dominguez LJ, Bevilacqua M, Dibella G, et al: Diagnosing and managing thyroid disease in the nursing home, J Am Med Dir Assoc 9:11, 2008.
T_3, Triiodothyronine; T_4, thyroxine; *TBG*, thyroxine binding globulin.

Tumor markers play an especially important role in the diagnosis and monitoring of patients with prostate, breast, and bladder cancers. At Memorial Sloan-Kettering Cancer Center in New York, the three tumor markers with the most remarkable increase in volume of testing are carcinoembryonic antigen, prostate-specific antigen, and CA 15-3.

Older, well-established markers include alkaline phosphatase and collagen-type markers in bone cancer, immunoglobulins in myeloma, catecholamines and their derivatives in neuroblastoma and pheochromocytoma, and serotonin metabolites in carcinoid. In addition, there are many breast tissue prognostic markers, including hormone receptors, cathepsin D, HER/neu oncogenes, and plasminogen receptors and inhibitors. The list of Food and Drug Administration (FDA)–approved tumor markers continues to grow. Multiple marker combinations may also be useful in the management of some types of cancer.

Specific Markers[22]

Specific tumor markers include:
- Alpha-fetoprotein
- Beta subunit of human chorionic gonadotropin (βhCG)
- CA 15-3
- CA 19-9
- CA 27.29
- CA 125
- Carcinoembryonic antigen
- Prostate-specific antigen and prostatic acid phosphatase
- Miscellaneous enzyme markers
- Miscellaneous hormone markers

Alpha-Fetoprotein

Alpha-fetoprotein (AFP) is normally synthesized by the fetal liver and yolk sac. It is secreted in the serum in nanogram to milligram quantities in these conditions: hepatocarcinoma, endodermal sinus tumors, nonseminomatous testicular cancer, teratocarcinoma of the testis or ovary, and malignant tumors of the mediastinum and sacrococcyx. In addition, a small percentage of patients with gastric and pancreatic cancer with liver metastasis may have elevated AFP levels. Both AFP and βhCG should be quantitated initially in all patients with teratocarcinoma, because one or both markers may be secreted in 85% of patients (see Chapter 17). The concentration of AFP may be elevated in nonneoplastic conditions such as hepatitis and cystic fibrosis.

AFP is a very reliable marker for following a patient's response to chemotherapy and radiation therapy. Levels should be obtained every 2 to 4 weeks (metabolic half-life in vivo is 4 days).

Beta Subunit of Human Chorionic Gonadotropin

βhCG, an ectopic protein, is a sensitive tumor marker with a metabolic half-life in vivo of 16 hours. A serum level of βhCG greater than 1 ng/mL is strongly suggestive of pregnancy or a malignant tumor such as endodermal sinus tumor, teratocarcinoma, choriocarcinoma, molar pregnancy, testicular embryonal carcinoma, or oat cell carcinoma of the lung.

CA 15-3

CA 15-3 is a high-molecular-weight glycoprotein coded by the MUC-II gene and expressed on the ductal cell surface of most glandular epithelial cells. The main purpose of the assay is to monitor breast cancer patients after mastectomy. CA 15-3 is positive in patients with other conditions, including liver disease, some inflammatory conditions, and other carcinomas. A change in the CA 15-3 concentration is more predictive than the absolute concentration. Changes in tumor burden are reflected by changes in the tumor marker concentration.

CA 27.29

The CA 27.29 tumor marker may be useful in conjunction with other clinical methods for detecting early recurrence of breast cancer. It is not recommended as an assay for breast cancer screening. Increased levels of CA 27.29 (>38 U/mL) may indicate recurrent disease in a woman with threatened breast carcinoma and may indicate the need for additional testing or procedures.

CA 19-9

CA 19-9 levels are elevated in patients with pancreatic, hepatobiliary, colorectal, gastric, hepatocellular, pancreatic and breast cancers. Its main use is as a marker for colorectal and pancreatic carcinoma.

CA 125

CA 125 is elevated in carcinomas and benign disease of various organs, including pelvic inflammatory disease (PID) and endometriosis, but it is most useful in ovarian and endometrial carcinomas.

Carcinoembryonic Antigen

Carcinoembryonic antigen (CEA) plasma levels greater than 12 ng/mL are strongly correlated with malignancy. Elevated neoplastic states frequently associated with an increased CEA level are endo-dermally derived gastrointestinal neoplasms and neck and breast carcinomas. Also, 20% of smokers and 7% of former smokers have elevated CEA levels.

CEA is used clinically to monitor tumor progress in patients who have diagnosed cancer with a high blood CEA level. If treatment leads to a decline to normal levels (<2.5 ng/mL), an increase in CEA may indicate cancer recurrence. A persistent elevation is indicative of residual disease or poor therapeutic response. In patients who have undergone colon cancer resection surgery, the rate of clearance of CEA levels usually returns to normal within 1 month but may take as long as 4 months. Blood specimens should be obtained 2 to 4 weeks apart to detect a trend.

Prostate-Specific Antigen

Prostate-specific antigen (PSA) is a marker specific for prostate tissue but not for prostate cancer. It is a highly debated marker in the diagnosis of prostate cancer. Blood levels of PSA are increased when normal glandular structure is disrupted by benign or malignant tumor inflammation. Serum PSA is directly proportional to tumor volume, with a greater increase per unit volume of cancer compared with benign hyperplasia. Free PSA assists in distinguishing cancer of the prostate from benign prostatic hypertrophy. PSA levels appear useful for monitoring progression and response to treatment among patients with prostate cancer.

Miscellaneous Enzyme Markers

Lactate dehydrogenase (LDH) is elevated in a wide variety of malignancies and other medical disorders. The level of LDH has been shown to correlate to tumor mass in solid tumors, so it can be used to monitor progression of these tumors.

Neuron-specific enolase has been detected in neuroblastoma, pheochromocytoma, oat cell carcinomas, medullary thyroid and C cell parathyroid carcinomas, and other neural crest–derived cancers.

Placental *alkaline phosphatase* can be detected during pregnancy. It is also associated with the neoplastic conditions of seminoma and ovarian cancer.

Miscellaneous Hormone Markers

Elevated or inappropriate serum levels of hormones can function as tumor markers. Adrenocorticotropic hormone (ACTH), calcitonin, and catecholamines may be secreted by differentiated tumors of endocrine organs and squamous cell lung tumors. Oat cell carcinomas may produce βhCG, antidiuretic hormone (ADH), serotonin, calcitonin, parathyroid hormone, and ACTH. These hormones can be used to follow a patient's response to therapy.

In addition, some breast cancers demonstrate progesterone and estradiol (estrogen) receptors, which are strongly correlated with a positive response to antihormone therapy. Patients with neuroblastomas and pheochromocytomas secrete catecholamine metabolites that can be detected in the urine. Neuroblastomas also release neuron-specific enolase and ferritin; these markers can be used for diagnosis and prognosis.

Breast, Ovarian, and Cervical Cancer Markers

For more than a decade, cancer antigens have been used to monitor therapy and evaluate recurrence of cancer. Estrogen and progesterone receptors are universally accepted as both prognostic markers and therapeutic choice indicators. A relatively new approach has been the use of the oncogene HER2/neu as a prognostic indicator and a marker related to the choice of therapy. This is particularly useful since the introduction of Herceptin as a chemotherapeutic agent that targets the HER2/neu receptor. Breast cancer patients who express HER2/neu in their cancers have a poor prognosis with shorter disease-free and overall survival than patients who do not express HER2/neu. HER2/neu in serum may be used to detect early recurrence, and elevated serum levels of HER2/neu correlate with the presence of metastatic disease and suggest a poor prognosis. Combining HER2/neu serum measurements with other markers (e.g., CEA, CA 15-3) may improve the sensitivity of detection of recurrence.

THERAPEUTIC DRUG MONITORING

Therapeutic drug monitoring (TDM) is the process by which the concentration of a chemical substance administered therapeutically or diagnostically is measured. TDM is only of value for a limited number of drugs. For it to be clinically worthwhile, the following criteria should be met:

1. An established relationship between plasma drug concentration and therapeutic response and/or toxicity
2. A poor relationship between plasma concentration and drug dosage
3. A good clinical indication for the assay (e.g., no response to treatment, suspected noncompliance, signs of toxicity)

TABLE 11-12

Sampling Times and Target Ranges for TDM Assays				
Drug	Minimum Plasma/ Serum Volume (mL)	Approximate Time to Steady State (Days)	Recommended Sampling Time	Target Range
Amitriptyline (+ nortriptyline)	2.0	7-10	Predose	100-250 µg/L
Caffeine	0.2	2	1-2 h Postdose	12-36 mg/L
Carbamazepine	0.5	2-4	Predose	4-12 mg/L
Clomipramine (+ norclomip- ramine)	2.0	28-42	Predose	150-800 µg/L
Desipramine	2.0	10-14	Predose	100-250 µg/L
Digoxin	0.5	5-7	6-24 h Postdose	0.8-2.0 µg/L
Dothiepin (+ nordothiepin)	2.0	7	Predose	100-300 µg/L
Ethosuximide	0.5	7-14	Predose*	40-100 mg/L
Fluoxetine (+ norfluoxetine)	2.0	28-42	Predose	150-800 µg/L
Gabapentin	0.5	1-2	Predose	2-20 mg/L
Imipramine (+ desipramine)	2.0	7	Predose	150-300 µg/L
Lamotrigine	0.5	4-6	Predose	1-4 mg/L
Nortriptyline	2.0	10-14	Pre-dose	50-150 µg/L
Phenobarbitone	0.5	10-20	Predose*	15-40 mg/L
Phenytoin	0.5	7-35	Predose*	10-20 mg/L
Theophylline, adults (1)	0.5	2	2-4 h Postdose	10-20 mg/L
Theophylline, neonates (2)	0.5	2	2-4 h Postdose	5-10 mg/L
Valproic acid (3)	0.5	2-3	Predose	Up to 100 mg/L
Vigabatrin	0.5	5-10	Predose	5-35 µg/L

Adapted from www.toxlab.co.uk/tdm.htm. Accessed July 15, 2009.

*Pre-dose collection time unimportant because of the long half-life of the drug; however, for consistency, a predose measurement is preferred.
(1) Theophylline used to treat asthma in adults.
(2) Theophylline used to treat neonatal apnea.
(3) For valproic acid, there is no established target range. If the predose concentration is greater than 100 mg/L with no clear therapeutic effect, further increases in dose are unlikely to be beneficial.

4. Appropriately timed peak/trough specimens with proper patient information
5. An adequate amount of clinical information to allow the interpretation of laboratory assay results

Peak and Trough

For many drugs, a relationship exists between the drug concentration in plasma and the clinical effects of the drug. Any concentration larger than the minimum may be toxic, but a minimum concentration is needed for effectiveness to achieve the desired pharmacologic effect. The therapeutic range of a drug is a concentration somewhere in the middle of the concentration/response curve.

Initially, a greater proportion of drug is absorbed than is distributed, metabolized, and eliminated; this is the **peak** concentration. Most drugs are administered in a series of doses. Depending on

the drug half-life in the normal population sample, this time ranges from less than a day to more than 3 months. For drugs with a long half-life compared to the dosing interval, drug accumulation can be very dramatic (i.e., drug concentrations following the first dose are much lower than drug concentrations at steady state). The goal of therapy is to have the drug accumulate until a steady state is achieved, or equal drug input and output. In general, a blood specimen should **not** be taken until "steady-state" has been achieved (approximately five times the drug's half-life). The peak concentration and **trough** concentration, or minimum steady-state concentration, oscillate after each dose within a certain range. The goal is to achieve the therapeutic range.

Drugs in various categories can be monitored. These include:

- Aminoglycoside antibiotics such as gentamicin
- Glycopeptide antibiotics such as vancomycin

TABLE 11-13

Therapeutic Ranges of Drugs	
Drug	Therapeutic Range (mg/L)
Digoxin	0.5 - 2.1*
Amiodarone	1.0 - 2.5
Lignocaine	2.0 - 5.0
Quinidine	2.0 - 5.0
Flecainide	0.2 - 0.9
Mexiletine	0.5 - 2.5
Salicylate	150 - 300
Perhexiline	0.15 - 0.6
Theophylline	10 - 20
Phenytoin	10 - 20
Carbamazepine	5.0 - 12
Sodium valproate	50 - 100
Phenobarbitone	15 - 40
Gentamicin, tobramycin, netilmicin	Trough < 2[†]; peak > 5
Amikacin	Trough < 5[†]; peak > 15
Vancomycin	Trough < 10; peak 20-40
Lithium	0.6-1.2[‡]

From www.australianprescriber.com. Accessed July 15, 2009.
*Microgram/L.
[†]For 8-hourly dosing.
[‡]mmol/L.

- Anticonvulsant (antiepileptic) drugs such as carbamazepine, phenytoin, ethosuximide, phenobarbitone, valproic acid
- Cardioactive drugs such as digoxin
- Respiratory stimulants such as theophylline
- Tricyclic antidepressants such as amitriptyline, clomipramine, desipramine, dothiepin, imipramine, nortriptyline
- SSRI antidepressants such as fluoxetine (Prozac)
- Mood stabilizers, especially lithium citrate

It is important to record the exact time and date of the specimen in relation to the last dose of the drug (Table 11-12), with a note of all other drugs prescribed. Effective and safe therapeutic plasma concentrations of drugs vary (Table 11-13).

DRUGS OF ABUSE

Assessment of drugs of abuse or overdose can occur with prescription, over-the-counter, or illicit drugs. Testing for drugs of abuse can be performed by various methods. Rapid point-of-care testing is simple and of immediate value to a primary care provider. Drugs of abuse include alcohol, marijuana, cocaine, benzodiazepines, barbiturates, opiates, and amphetamines.

CASE STUDIES

CASE STUDY 11-1

A 35-year-old man (height 67 inches, weight 73.3 kg) with known chronic renal disease for 6 months has blood drawn for serum creatinine and urea tests. Urine is collected for a 24-hour quantitative creatinine test; the total volume of urine collected is 1139 mL. The following laboratory results are obtained for the testing done:

Urine creatinine: 56 mg/dL

Serum creatinine: 9.6 mg/dL

Serum urea: 75 mg/dL

1. Given these data, what is this patient's standardized creatinine clearance?
   a. 4.3 mL/min
   b. 4.6 mL/min
   c. 6.2 mL/min
   d. 5.8 mL/min

2. What is the normal range for creatinine clearance for this patient?

CASE STUDY 11-2

As part of a lipid-screening profile, the following results were obtained for a blood specimen drawn from a 30-year-old woman immediately after she had eaten breakfast:

Triglycerides: 200 mg/dL

Cholesterol: 180 mg/dL

Which of the following would be a reasonable explanation for these results?

a. The results fall within the reference values for the two tests; they are not affected by the recent meal.

b. The cholesterol is normal, but the triglyceride test is elevated; retest using a 12-hour fasting specimen, because the triglyceride test is affected by the recent meal.

c. The results are elevated for the two tests; retest for both using a 12-hour fasting specimen, because both the cholesterol and the triglyceride test are affected by the recent meal.

d. The results for both tests are below the normal reference values despite the recent meal.

CASE STUDY 11-3

An adult male patient with jaundice complains of fatigue. He has a decreased blood hemoglobin level (he is anemic) and an elevated serum bilirubin value, most of which represents unconjugated bilirubin. His liver enzyme tests are within the normal reference ranges.

The most likely disease process for this patient is:

a. a gallstone obstructing the common bile duct.

b. hemolytic anemia in which his red blood cells are being destroyed.

c. infectious (viral) hepatitis.

d. cirrhosis of the liver.

CASE STUDY 11-4

An 8-year-old boy comes to see his family physician with his mother. He has been urinating excessively and has also has been drinking an excessive quantity of water. He recently recovered from a viral upper respiratory infection; he has lost some weight since his last visit to the clinic 6 months ago; and he has a slight fever (100°F). Laboratory tests are ordered, fasting blood is drawn for testing, and a urinalysis is done. The following laboratory results are reported:

Serum creatinine: 0.8 mg/dL

Serum glucose: 180 mg/dL

White blood count: 15×10^9/L

Hemoglobin: 14.0 g/dL

Urinalysis

Specific gravity: 1.025

Glucose: 1000 mg/dL

Ketones: Moderate

Protein, nitrite, blood: Negative

Sediment: No abnormal findings

On the basis of the case history and the laboratory findings, what is a likely diagnosis of this patient's disease?

a. Diabetes mellitus

b. Hyperthyroidism

c. Acute glomerulonephritis

d. Recurring upper respiratory infection

CASE STUDY 11-5

A 40-year-old woman with nausea, vomiting, and jaundice is seen in the clinic. Laboratory tests are ordered on blood and urine. The following laboratory results are reported:

Hemoglobin: Normal

White blood cell count: Normal

Serum Bilirubin

Total: 6.5 mg/dL

Conjugated (direct): 5.0 mg/dL

Serum Enzymes

Aspartate aminotransferase (AST): 300 U/L (normal: 0-45 U/L)

Gamma-glutamyltransferase (GGT): 70 U/L (normal: 0-45 U/L)

Alkaline phosphatase: 180 U/L (normal: 0-150 U/L)

Urine (appearance is dark brown)

Urobilinogen: Normal/decreased

Bilirubin: Positive

These results can best be interpreted as representing which of the following?

a. Unconjugated hyperbilirubinemia, probably from hemolysis

b. Unconjugated hyperbilirubinemia, probably from an injury to the liver cells

c. Conjugated hyperbilirubinemia, probably from biliary tract disease

d. Conjugated hyperbilirubinemia, probably from an obstruction such as gallstones

CASE STUDY 11-6

A 35-year-old man is admitted to the ER with chest pain; past history reveals other episodes of this same pain but of a shorter duration. Inquiry into his personal habits reveals that he is a cigarette smoker and that he follows a modified low-fat diet and engages in some regular exercise. His father died of ischemic heart disease at age 45, and other members of his family have had lipid-related disorders. Fasting blood is drawn for chemistry and hematology tests, and urine is collected for examination. Laboratory results are:

Hemoglobin: 15.0 g/dL

White blood cell count: Mildly elevated

Serum glucose: 120 mg/dL

Serum triglycerides: 300 mg/dL

Serum LDL cholesterol: 150 mg/dL

Serum total cholesterol: 275 mg/dL

Serum enzymes[*]: All mildly increased

Urinalysis: Normal findings

1. Which of the information in the history and laboratory findings is considered the most important risk factor influencing the development of life-threatening coronary heart disease in this patient?

a. LDL cholesterol level

b. Triglyceride level

c. Family history

d. Cigarette smoking

2. Treatment focuses on which of the risk factors noted in this patient?

a. Lowering the LDL cholesterol

b. Lowering the total cholesterol

c. Giving up smoking cigarettes

d. Engaging in a more strenuous exercise program

---

[*]For assessing damage to heart muscle.

REFERENCES

1. Glucose clinical laboratory reference: 2005-2006, MLO Med Lab Obs 37(13):6, 2005.
2. Tirosh A, et al: Normal fasting plasma glucose levels and type 2 diabetes in young men, N Engl J Med 353:14, Oct 6, 2005.
3. US Department of Health and Human Services: Healthy People 2010, vol 1, ed 2, Chapter 5, Nov 2000.
4. Standards of Medical Care in Diabetes—2006, Diabetes Care 29:S4–S42, 2006.
5. American Diabetes Association Postion Statement: Diagnosis and Classification of Diabetes Mellitus, Diabetes Care 676–682, 2010.
6. Krinsley JD: Effect of an intensive glucose management protocol in the mortality of critically ill adult patients, Mayo Clin Proc 79:9992, 2004.
7. Burtis CA, Ashwood ER, editors: Tietz fundamentals of clinical chemistry, ed 4, Philadelphia, 1996, Saunders.
8. Clinical Laboratory Buyers Guide and Annual Report: Clinical laboratory reference, 2005–2006, Adv Admin Lab vol. 14, Dec 2005:no 12.
9. Bishop ML, Fody EP: Reference values for frequently assayed clinical chemistry analytes. Clinical chemistry: principles, procedures, correlations, ed 5, Philadelphia, 2005, Lippincott, Williams & Wilkins.
10. Gentzkow CJ: Accurate method for determination of blood urea nitrogen by direct nesslerization, J Biol Chem 143:531, 1942.
11. Jaffe M: Uber den Niederschlag welchen Pikrinsaure in normalen Harn erzeugt und uber eine neue Reaktion des Kreatininins, Z Physiol Chem 10:391, 1886.
12. Levey AS, Bosch JP, Lewis JB, et al: A more accurate method to estimate glomerular filtration rate from serum creatinine: a new prediction equation, Ann Intern Med 130:461, 1999.
13. Erlandsen EJ, Randers E, Kristensen JH: Reference intervals for serum cystatin C and serum creatinine in adults, Clin Chem Lab Med 36:393–397, 1998.
14. Bishop ML, Fody EP: Clinical chemistry: principles, procedures, correlations, ed 5, Philadelphia, 2005, Lippincott Williams & Wilkins, pp 230, 484.
15. Kaplan LA, Pesce AJ, Kazmierczak SC: Clinical chemistry: theory, analysis, and correlation, ed 4, St Louis, 2003, Mosby.
16. Tolman KG, Raj R: Liver function. In Burtis CA, Ashwood ER, editors: Tietz textbook of clinical chemistry, ed 3, Philadelphia, 1999, Saunders.
17. Report of the National Cholesterol Education Program Expert Panel on Detection: Evaluation, and Treatment of High Blood Cholesterol in Adults, Arch Intern Med 148:36, 1988.
18. Summary of the Second Report of the National Cholesterol Education Program (NCEP) Expert Panel on Detection: Evaluation, and Treatment of High Blood Cholesterol in Adults (Adult Treatment Panel II), JAMA 269(23):1421, 3015, 1993.
19. Myocardial infarction redefined: a consensus document of the Joint European Society of Cardiology/American College of Cardiology Committee for the Redefinition of Myocardial Infarction, J Am Coll Cardiol 36(3):959, 2000.
20. Apple FS: Cl Lab News, Cardiac Ischemia 35(9):9, 2009.
21. Malloy HT, Evelyn KA: The determination of bilirubin with the photoelectric colorimeter, J Biol Chem 119:481, 1937.
22. Turgeon ML: Immunology and serology in laboratory medicine, ed 4, St Louis, 2009, Elsevier.

BIBLIOGRAPHY

Atkinson MA, Maclaren JK: The pathogenesis of insulin-dependent diabetes mellitus, N Engl J Med 331(21):1428, 1994.

Bodor GS: Cardiac troponins, Clin Lab News :p 10, May 2003.

Clinical and Laboratory Standards Institute: Glucose testing in settings without laboratory support: approved guideline, ed 2, Wayne, 2005, Pa, AST4-A2.

Clinical and Laboratory Standards Institute: Standardization of Sodium and Potassium Ion-Selective Electrode Systems to the Flame Photometric Reference Method: approved standard, ed 2, Wayne, Pa, 2000, reaffirmed June, 2003, C29-A2.

Clinical and Laboratory Standards Institute: Sweat testing: sample collection and quantitative analysis: approved guideline, ed 2, Wayne, 2000, Pa, C34-A2.

Clinical and Laboratory Standards Institute: Point-of-Care blood glucose testing in acute and chronic care facilities: approved guideline, ed 2, Wayne, 2002, Pa, C30-A2.

Elefano EC, et al: Analytical evaluation of HgbA1c, microalbumin, CRP, and RF on Architect ci8200 integrated system and workflow computer simulation. Abstract 24. Pushing the Technology Envelope II: an Exploration of the Future of Clinical Laboratory Testing, 2005 Oak Ridge Conference, April 2005:Baltimore.

Helmersson JB, Vessby A, Larson A, et al: Association of type 2 diabetes with cyclooxygenase-mediated inflammation and oxidative stress in an elderly population, Circulation 109:1729, 2004.

Larson TS: Lab estimation of GFR, Clin Lab News 30(6):8, 2004.

Maylin R, et al: Development of an automated enzymatic assay for detection of HbA1c in human whole blood. Abstract 16. Pushing the Technology Envelope II: an Exploration of the Future of Clinical Laboratory Testing, 2005 Oak Ridge Conference, April 2005:Baltimore.

Pizzi R: NACB presents draft of LMPG for tumor markers, Clin Lab News 31(10):16, 2005.

Rezendes DA, Faix JD: The role of the clinical laboratory in the new approach to diabetes, Clin Lab News 23(7):1, 1997.

Tracey RP: C-reactive protein and cardiovascular disease, Clin Lab News 24(8):14, 1998.

Woeste S: Diagnosing prostate cancer, Lab Med 36(7):399, 2005.

REVIEW QUESTIONS

1. **One of the major hormones that controls high glucose levels after a meal is:**
   a. insulin.
   b. thyroxine.
   c. glucagon.
   d. lipase.

2. **In a person with normal glucose metabolism, the blood glucose level usually increases rapidly after carbohydrates are ingested but returns to a normal level after:**
   a. 30 minutes.
   b. 60 minutes.
   c. 90 minutes.
   d. 120 minutes.

3. **Which of the following organs uses glucose from digested carbohydrates and stores it as glycogen for later use as a source of immediate energy by the muscles?**
   a. Kidneys
   b. Liver
   c. Pancreas
   d. Thyroid

4. **In a person with impaired glucose metabolism, such as in type 1 diabetes, what is true about the blood glucose level?**
   a. It increases rapidly after carbohydrates are ingested but returns to a normal level after 120 minutes.
   b. It increases rapidly after carbohydrates are ingested and stays greatly elevated even after 120 minutes.
   c. It does not increase after carbohydrates are ingested and stays at a low level until the next meal.
   d. It increases rapidly after carbohydrates are ingested but returns to a normal level after 30 minutes.

5. **Which of the following is not a classic symptom of type 1 diabetes?**
   a. Polyuria
   b. Polydipsia
   c. Polyphagia
   d. Proteinuria

6. **Which of the following statements is true about type 1 diabetes mellitus?**
   a. It is associated with an insufficient amount of insulin secreted by the pancreas.
   b. It is associated with inefficient activity of the insulin secreted by the pancreas.
   c. It is a more frequent type of diabetes than the non–insulin-dependent type (type 2).
   d. Good control of this disease will eliminate complications in the future.

7. **What can be the result of uncontrolled elevated blood glucose?**
   a. Coma from insulin shock
   b. Diabetic coma
   c. Ketones in the urine
   d. Both b and c

8. **Gestational diabetes can occur during pregnancy in some women. Which of the following can occur for a significant number of these women?**
   a. Can develop type 1 diabetes at a later date
   b. Can develop type 2 diabetes at a later date
   c. Continue to manifest signs of diabetes after delivery
   d. No effect

9. **The level of glycosylated hemoglobin in a diabetic patient reflects which of the following?**
   a. Blood glucose concentration at the time blood was collected
   b. Average blood glucose concentration over the past week
   c. Average blood glucose concentration over the past 2 to 3 months (life span of a red cell)
   d. More than one of the above

10. **A sweat chloride result of 50 mmol/L is obtained for an adult patient who has a history of respiratory problems. What would be the best interpretation of these results, based on known reference values?**
    a. Normal sweat chloride, not consistent with cystic fibrosis
    b. Marginally elevated results, borderline for cystic fibrosis
    c. Elevated results, diagnostic of cystic fibrosis

11. **Which of the following electrolytes is the chief cation in the plasma, is found in the highest concentration in the extravascular fluid, and has the main function of maintaining osmotic pressure?**
    a. Potassium
    b. Sodium
    c. Calcium
    d. Magnesium

12. **Analysis of a serum specimen gives a potassium result of 6.0 mmol/L. Before the result is reported to the physician, what additional step should be taken?**
    a. The serum should be observed for hemolysis; hemolysis of the red cells will shift potassium from the cells into the serum, resulting in a falsely elevated potassium value.
    b. The serum should be observed for evidence of jaundice; jaundiced serum will result in a falsely elevated potassium value.
    c. The test should be run again on the same specimen.
    d. Nothing needs to be done; simply report the result.

13. **The anion gap can be increased in patients with:**
    a. lactic acidosis.
    b. toxin ingestion.
    c. uremia.
    d. more than one of the above.

14. Calculation of the anion gap is useful for quality control for:
    a. calcium.
    b. tests in the electrolyte profile (sodium, potassium, chloride, and bicarbonate).
    c. phosphorus.
    d. magnesium.

15. Ninety percent of the carbon dioxide present in the blood is in the form of:
    a. bicarbonate ions.
    b. carbonate.
    c. dissolved CO_2.
    d. carbonic acid.

Questions 16-19: Match the following lab findings (a to d) with the corresponding acid-base disorder.

16. ___ Metabolic acidosis

17. ___ Metabolic alkalosis

18. ___ Respiratory acidosis

19. ___ Respiratory alkalosis

Key: $cHCO^-_3$, Cytoplasmic bicarbonate; PCO_2, partial pressure carbon dioxide.
    a. ↓ $cHCO^-_3$
    b. ↑ $cHCO^-_3$
    c. ↑ PCO_2
    d. ↓ PCO_2

20. Nitrogen is excreted principally in the form of:
    a. creatinine.
    b. creatine.
    c. uric acid.
    d. urea.

21. The main waste product of protein metabolism is:
    a. creatinine.
    b. creatine.
    c. uric acid.
    d. urea.

22. The protein content of the diet will affect primarily the test results for:
    a. creatinine.
    b. creatine.
    c. uric acid.
    d. urea or urea nitrogen.

23. Creatinine concentration in the blood has a direct relationship to:
    a. muscle mass.
    b. dietary protein intake.
    c. age and gender.
    d. more than one of the above.

24. In the Jaffe reaction, a red-orange chromogen is formed when creatinine reacts with:
    a. picric acid.
    b. Biuret reagent.
    c. diacetyl monoxime.
    d. both a and b.

25. Creatinine clearance is used to assess the:
    a. glomerular filtration capabilities of the kidneys.
    b. tubular secretion of creatinine.
    c. dietary intake of protein.
    d. glomerular and tubular mass.

26. Expected creatinine clearance for a patient with chronic renal disease would be:
    a. very low; renal glomerular filtration is functioning normally.
    b. normal; renal glomerular filtration is functioning normally.
    c. very high; renal glomerular filtration is not functioning normally.
    d. very low; renal glomerular filtration is not functioning normally.

27. A serum creatinine result of 6.6 mg/dL is most likely to be found in conjunction with which of the following other laboratory results?
    a. Urea, 15 mg/dL
    b. Urea, 85 mg/dL
    c. Urea nitrogen, 10 mg/dL
    d. Urea nitrogen/creatinine ratio, 15

28. A urea nitrogen result for a serum sample is reported as 10 mg/dL. Calculate the concentration of urea for this sample, using the following information: the chemical formula for urea is NH_2CONH_2 (atomic weights: carbon 12, oxygen 16, nitrogen 14, hydrogen 1). The urea concentration for this sample is:
    a. 28 mg/dL.
    b. 21 mg/dL.
    c. 92 mg/dL.
    d. 43 mg/dL.

29. Testing blood from a patient with acute glomerulonephritis would most likely result in which of the following laboratory findings?
    a. Decreased creatinine
    b. Decreased urea
    c. Increased glucose
    d. Increased creatinine

30. Uric acid is the final breakdown product of which type of metabolism?
    a. Urea
    b. Glucose
    c. Purine
    d. Bilirubin

31. Which of the following lipid results would be expected to be falsely elevated in a blood specimen drawn from a nonfasting patient?
    a. Total cholesterol
    b. Triglycerides
    c. HDL cholesterol
    d. More than one of the above

32. Blood is collected from a patient who has been fasting since midnight; the collection time is 7 AM. Which of the following tests would not give a valid test result?
    a. Cholesterol
    b. Triglycerides
    c. Total bilirubin
    d. Potassium

33. Which of the following laboratory values is considered a positive risk factor for the occurrence of coronary heart disease?
    a. HDL cholesterol > 60 mg/dL
    b. HDL cholesterol < 35 mg/dL
    c. LDL cholesterol < 130 mg/dL
    d. Total cholesterol < 200 mg/dL

34. Noting the appearance of plasma or serum can give important preliminary findings about lipid levels in the blood when it is collected from a fasting patient. When the specimen appears opaque and milky (lipemic), what is the approximate expected level of triglycerides in the sample?
    a. Within the normal range; test is unaffected by meals.
    b. From 200 to 300 mg/dL
    c. Greater than 600 mg/dL
    d. No preliminary findings can be made from observation of the serum.

35. Which of the following is considered a primary risk factor for the development of coronary heart disease later in life?
    a. Cigarette smoking
    b. Stress
    c. Diabetes mellitus
    d. Lack of exercise

36. Which of the following is considered a secondary risk factor for the development of coronary heart disease later in life?
    a. Cigarette smoking
    b. Increased HDL cholesterol
    c. Decreased HDL cholesterol
    d. Obesity

37. When a hyperlipidemic condition exists for a sufficient length of time, it may be associated with the development of which of the following conditions?
    a. Obesity
    b. Diabetes mellitus

c. Atherosclerosis
d. Viral hepatitis

38. In what major organ of the body is the majority of the body's cholesterol synthesized?
    a. Heart
    b. Pancreas
    c. Gallbladder
    d. Liver

39. The National Cholesterol Education Program (NCEP) has established cutoffs for total cholesterol and LDL cholesterol to define persons at high risk for coronary heart disease later in life. What is the cutoff for a desirable LDL cholesterol concentration?
    a. <130 mg/dL
    b. <160 mg/dL
    c. <200 mg/dL
    c. >130 mg/dL

40. Which of the following enzymes is found primarily in the liver?
    a. Aspartate aminotransferase
    b. Alkaline phosphatase
    c. Alanine aminotransferase
    d. Gamma-glutamyltransferase

41. Elevated concentrations of serum amylase and lipase are often seen in:
    a. acid reflux disease.
    b. gallstones.
    c. acute pancreatitis.
    d. acute pharyngitis.

42. What is the classic symptom or manifestation of liver disease?
    a. Hemolysis of red cells
    b. Jaundice
    c. Kernicterus
    d. Formation of gallstones

43. In an adult, if the total bilirubin value is 3.1 mg/dL and the conjugated bilirubin is 1.1 mg/dL, what is the unconjugated bilirubin value?
    a. 2.0 mg/dL
    b. 4.2 mg/dL
    c. 1.0 mg/dL
    d. 3.4 mg/dL

44. A rapid buildup of unconjugated bilirubin in a newborn can result in kernicterus, which is an accumulation of bilirubin in the:
    a. heart tissue.
    b. liver cells.
    c. brain tissue.
    d. kidney tissue.

Questions 45-47: *Match each of the following defects of bilirubin metabolism with the corresponding type of jaundice (a to c).*

45. ___ Impairment of conjugation of bilirubin by the liver cells.

46. ___ Transport defects involving release of the bilirubin bound to plasma albumin to the liver cell for conjugation with glucuronide.

47. ___ Defect in transporting the conjugated bilirubin out of the liver cells and into the bile fluid.
   a. Prehepatic jaundice
   b. Hepatic jaundice
   c. Posthepatic jaundice

48. In which of the following conditions resulting in jaundice is there an increase in both conjugated and unconjugated bilirubin?
   a. Hemolysis of red cells
   b. Viral hepatitis
   c. Obstruction from gallstones
   d. Constriction of the biliary tract from a neoplasm

49. In which of the following conditions resulting in jaundice is there an increase primarily in unconjugated bilirubin?
   a. Increased hemolysis of red cells
   b. Viral hepatitis
   c. Biliary obstruction
   d. Cirrhosis of the liver

50. In a premature newborn, a deficiency of what enzyme can affect the conjugation of bilirubin glucuronide in the liver?
   a. Glucuronosyltransferase
   b. Aspartate aminotransferase
   c. Alanine aminotransferase
   d. Gamma-glutamyltransferase

51. Which of the following types of bilirubin is water soluble?
   a. Unconjugated bilirubin
   b. Conjugated bilirubin (bilirubin glucuronide)

CHAPTER 12

PRINCIPLES AND PRACTICE OF CLINICAL HEMATOLOGY

Learning Objectives

At the conclusion of this chapter, the student will be able to:

- Summarize the process of hematopoiesis.
- Describe the formation of erythrocytes, leukocytes, and thrombocytes.
- Discuss the mode and use for the three types of anticoagulants used for hematology assays.
- Explain the proper processing and testing of specimens.
- Identify at least three types of unsuitable blood specimens and the effect of each on test results.
- Compare the effects of isotonic, hypotonic, and hypertonic solutions on blood cells.
- Apply the principle of osmotic pressure to the study of red cell membrane defects in the osmotic fragility test.
- Identify the types of mature leukocytes found in circulating blood, and describe the characteristics of each.
- Describe hemoglobin synthesis and normal and abnormal types of hemoglobin.
- Briefly explain the hemoglobin procedures for normal hemoglobin and for abnormal hemoglobin S.

- Describe the principle and procedure of the microhematocrit determination.
- Define and calculate red blood cell indices of mean corpuscular volume (MCV), mean corpuscular hemoglobin (MCH), and mean corpuscular hemoglobin concentration (MCHC).
- Explain the formula and application of the red cell distribution width (RDW).
- Describe the procedure for counting and calculating erythrocytes, leukocytes, and platelets.
- Explain the proper preparation and examination of a peripheral blood film.
- Calculate a corrected white cell count.
- Compare the three categories of anemia, based on morphology.
- Identify and describe the morphologic alterations of size, shape, color, inclusions, and abnormal distribution patterns in erythrocytes.
- Identify and describe leukocyte alterations.
- Describe the performance, calculations, and applications of a reticulocyte count.
- Describe the performance and application of the erythrocyte sedimentation rate (ESR).

INTRODUCTION TO HEMATOLOGY

The total volume of blood in an average adult is about 6 L, or 7% to 8% of the body weight. About 45% of this amount is composed of red blood cells (erythrocytes), white blood cells (leukocytes), and platelets (thrombocytes); the remaining 55% is the liquid fraction, **plasma.** The formed elements of whole blood are suspended in plasma. Approximately 90% of the composition of plasma is water; the remaining 10% consists of soluble biochemicals including proteins, carbohydrates, vitamins, hormones, enzymes, lipids, salts, and trace metals.

Overall Blood Cell Maturation and Function

Hematopoiesis

Blood cell production, or **hematopoiesis**, begins in embryonic development. In the embryo, self-renewing hematopoietic stem cells develop initially in the primitive yolk sac and then migrate to the fetal liver. Beginning in the fetal liver and later in bone marrow, these pluripotential, CD34+, hematopoietic stem cells give rise to the earliest myeloid and lymphoid progenitors (Fig. 12-1). Less

than 1% of the marrow consists of stem cells. They have the ability to repopulate the bone marrow after injury or lethal radiation, which is the basis of bone marrow transplantation.

Until age 5 years, the marrow in all the bones is red and cellular and actively produces cells. Between 5 and 7 years of age, the long bones become inactive, and fat cells appear to replace the active marrow. Through the maturing years, *red marrow* is gradually displaced by fat cells in the other bones and transformed into *yellow marrow.* After age 18 to 20 years, red marrow remains only in the vertebrae, ribs, sternum, skull, and partially in the femur and humerus.

Blood cell differentiation and maturation occur primarily in bone marrow, where the environment is well organized and complex. Mature cells must migrate across the sinusoidal endothelia of the marrow capillaries to enter the peripheral circulation. The endothelial membrane allows passage of the more deformable mature cells and holds back the immature cells, which are more rigid and less motile. Pathologic processes can facilitate the release of more immature cells by affecting the cellular composition of the sinusoidal endothelia.

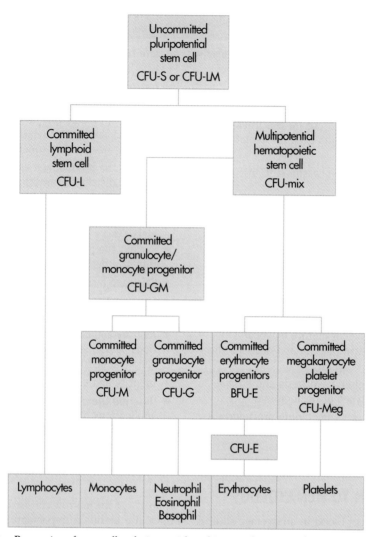

FIGURE 12-1 Progression of stem cells: pluripotential, multipotential, committed progenitor, and mature cell forms. Intermediate stages are not shown. *CFU,* Colony-forming unit; *S,* spleen; *LM,* lymphoid-myeloid; *GM,* granulocyte-monocyte; *E,* erythroid; *BFU-E,* burst-erythroid.

Myeloid progenitors differentiate into colony-forming cells of the erythroid and myeloid lineages and cells that give rise to megakaryocytes, eosinophils, and basophils (Fig. 12-2).

Lymphoid progenitors give rise to natural killer (NK) cells, T lymphocytes, and B lymphocytes. *B lymphocytes* (B cells) differentiate further in the bone marrow and further still on encountering an antigen. *T lymphocytes* (T cells) differentiate and acquire antigen specificity, principally in the thymus and in some cases other lymphoid organs (e.g., gut). If productive gene rearrangement does not occur as the result of antigen exposure, the lymphocytes will die. T cells develop in the thymus and extrathymic tissues from a lymphoid precursor.

Lymphocytes circulate in the peripheral blood and lymphatic tissues and through secondary lymphoid organs (e.g., lymph nodes, spleen). B cells develop from lymphoid progenitors in the bone marrow and at sites at which the B cell encounters antigen (e.g., secondary lymphoid organs).[1]

All stages in the maturation process are gradual, and it is often impossible to identify an exact stage with certainty. The most immature forms of all cell types appear very similar morphologically, and their identification is often based on surrounding cell types in various stages of development.

Erythrocyte Maturation and Function

Red blood cells (RBCs, erythrocytes) are normally produced in the bone marrow. Their maturation takes 3 to 5 days, and 6 stages of development have been described. Several systems of nomenclature have been used to describe these stages, two of which are discussed here. The stages of erythrocyte maturation from the youngest to the mature cell are (1) pronormoblast (rubriblast), (2) basophilic

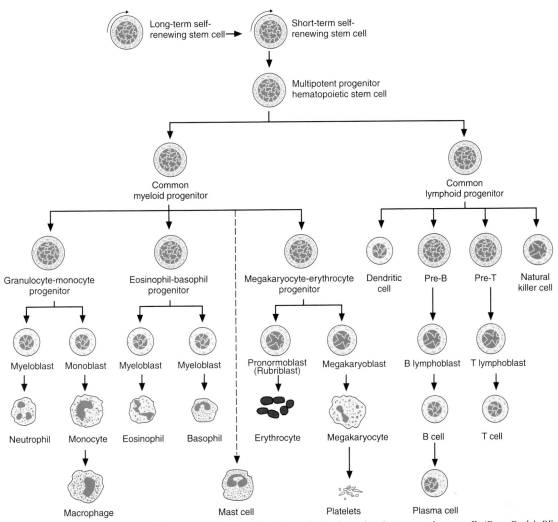

FIGURE 12-2 **Diagram of hematopoiesis shows derivation of cells from the pluripotential stem cell.** (From Rodak BF, Fritsma GA, Keohane EM: Hematology: clinical principles and applications, ed 4, St Louis, 2012, Saunders.)

normoblast (prorubricyte), (3) polychromatophilic normoblast (rubricyte), (4) orthochromic normoblast (metarubricyte), (5) reticulocyte (diffusely basophilic erythrocyte), and (6) mature erythrocyte (Table 12-1 and Fig. 12-3).

Red blood cells gradually progress from one stage to another, steadily decreasing in size. On staining, a decrease in intensity of blue color results from the erythrocytes' loss of ribonucleic acid (RNA). An increase in red color is caused by increased hemoglobin concentration. There are no granules in the cytoplasm in the mature erythrocyte.

The nucleus is generally round and in the center of the cell. In the early stages, the chromatin is fine and lacelike. As the cell matures and the nucleus becomes smaller, the chromatin becomes coarse and more condensed. Finally, the nucleus degenerates into clumps or a solid pyknotic mass, which is eventually released (or *extruded*) from the cell. At the same time, the color of the nucleus

changes from purplish red to dark blue. When the nucleus is extruded, it is phagocytosed and digested by marrow macrophages. The *reticulocyte,* or early nonnucleated erythrocyte, then squeezes through an opening in the endothelial lining of the marrow cavity and enters the peripheral circulatory system.

The earliest normoblast (*pronormoblast*) appears morphologically similar to other blasts (e.g., myeloblasts, lymphoblast), but cells of the erythrocyte series tend to stain more intensely blue than blasts cells related to other cell lines. The intensity of the blue color results from the combination of hemoglobin and RNA in the cytoplasm. The stages are described in terms of the staining reaction of the cytoplasm as it gains in hemoglobin concentration: *basophilic* cytoplasm is blue, *polychromatophilic* cytoplasm shows shades of blue and gray as hemoglobin increases, and *orthochromic* cytoplasm is orange red.

TABLE 12-1

						Erythrocyte Development	
Nomenclature Rubriblastic	Alternate Nomenclature Normoblastic	Percent in Bone Marrow	Hours in Bone Marrow	Overall Size	N/C Ratio	Nucleus	Cytoplasm
Rubriblast	Pronormoblast	1	12	12-20	8:1	Round to oval shape with 1 or 2 nucleoli; chromatin has fine clumps	Intensely blue
Prorubricyte	Basophilic normoblast	1-4	20	10-15	6:1	Some chromatin clumping, no (or 1) nucleoli	Deeper, richer blue than blast
Rubricyte	Polychromatic normoblast	10-20	30	10-12	4:1	No nucleoli, clumpy chromatin	Murky gray blue
Metarubricyte	Orthochromic normoblast	5-10	48	8-10	1:2	Nucleus is almost or completely pyknotic; incapable of DNA synthesis	Pink-orange; slightly bluish hue
Reticulocyte	Reticulocyte	1	48-72	8-10	—	No nucleus	Bluish hue
Reticulocyte*	Reticulocyte	—	24-48	8-8.5	—	No nucleus	—

N/C, Nuclear/cytoplasmic; DNA, deoxyribonucleic acid.
*Note circulating peripheral blood.

RBCs have a total life span of about 120 days, and the body releases new red cells into the circulatory system every day. Worn-out RBCs are removed from the blood circulation by the **mononuclear phagocytic system,** which is composed of connective tissue cells that carry on **phagocytosis,** a process in which a cell engulfs and digests foreign material (see Chapter 17). These cells are located in the blood sinusoids (tiny blood vessels) in the liver, spleen, and bone marrow and in the lining of the lymph channels in the lymph nodes.

Many cellular components are reusable, including iron (from the *heme* portion of the hemoglobin molecule) and protein (from the *globin* portion of the hemoglobin molecule). The remaining heme portion of the hemoglobin molecule (with iron removed) is converted to bilirubin, concentrated in the bile, and eliminated from the body in feces, and to a much smaller extent in urine, as urobilin and urobilinogen. The metabolism and elimination of bilirubin are described in Chapters 11 and 14. Fig. 12-4 shows a schematic representation of the RBC formation and destruction process.

The main function of the RBC is to carry oxygen to the cells of the body. Oxygen is transported in a chemical combination with *hemoglobin.* The concentration of hemoglobin in the blood is a measure of its capacity to carry oxygen, on which all cells are absolutely dependent for energy and therefore life. In the tissues, oxygen is exchanged for carbon dioxide, which is carried to the lungs for excretion in exchange for oxygen. To combine with and therefore transport oxygen, the hemoglobin molecule must have a certain combination of heme (which contains iron) and globin. Deficiencies in the presence or metabolism of these substances will result in a decrease in hemoglobin- and oxygen-carrying capacity.

Granulocyte Maturation and Function

Neutrophils normally mature in the bone marrow in the following stages, from the youngest to the most mature: myeloblast, promyelocyte (progranulocyte), myelocyte, metamyelocyte, band, and segmented neutrophils. These maturation stages are similar for all granulocytes (Table 12-2).

Cells of the neutrophil series are generally round with smooth margins or edges. As the cells mature, they become progressively smaller. Most immature cells have cytoplasm that stains dark blue and becomes light pink as the cells mature. As the cells mature from the myeloblast to the promyelocyte stage, nonspecific granules that stain blue to reddish purple appear in the cytoplasm. Eventually, these nonspecific granules are replaced by specific neutrophilic granules. Both types of granules are not produced at the same time, but they may both be seen in the promyelocyte and myelocyte stages.

Nuclear changes also occur as the cells mature. In the *myeloblast,* the nucleus is round or oval and very large in proportion to the rest of the cell. As the cell matures, the nucleus decreases in relative size and begins to contort or form lobes. At the same time, the nuclear chromatin changes from a fine, delicate pattern to the more clumped pattern characteristic of the mature cell. The staining of the nucleus also changes from reddish purple to

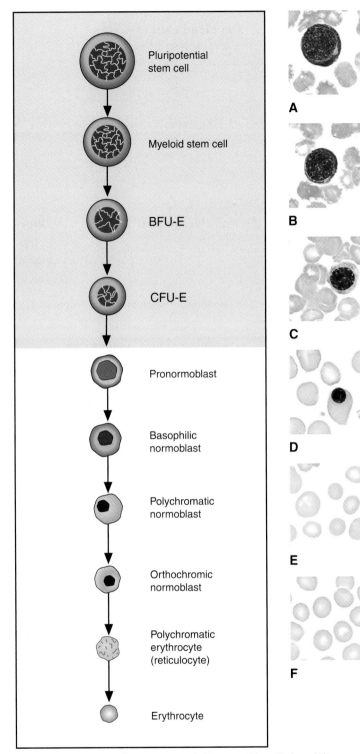

FIGURE 12-3 Maturation of the erythrocyte series. A, Pronormoblast; B, basophilic normoblast; C, polychromatic normoblast; D, orthochromic normoblast; E, polychromatic erythrocyte; F, erythrocyte. (From Carr JH, Rodak BF: Clinical hematology atlas, ed 3, St Louis, 2009, Saunders.)

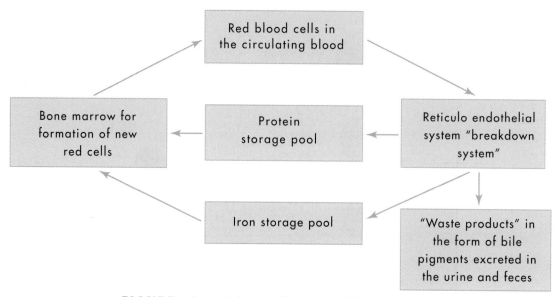

FIGURE 12-4   Red blood cell formation and destructive process.

TABLE 12-2

Granulocytic Leukocyte Development				
Nomenclature	Overall Size (μm)	N/C Ratio	Nuclear Characteristics	Cytoplasmic Characteristics
Myeloblast	10-18	4:1	Oval or round shape, 1 to 5 nucleoli	Auer rods can be present, no granules
Promyelocyte	14-20	3:1	Oval or round shape, 1 to 5 nucleoli	Heavy granulation
Myelocyte	12-18	2:1-1:1	Oval or indented	Specific blue-pink granules
Metamyelocyte	10-18	1:1	Indented	Specific blue-pink granules
Band	10-16	1:1	Elongated, curved	Specific blue-pink granules
Segmented neutrophil	10-16	1:1	Distinct lobes	Specific blue-pink granules
Mature basophil	10-16	1:1	Distinct lobes	Blue-black granules
Mature eosinophil	10-16	1:1	Distinct lobes	Orange granules

bluish purple as the cell matures. Nucleoli may be apparent in the early forms but gradually disappear as the chromatin thickens and the cell matures.

The term **shift to the left** refers to the release into the peripheral blood of immature cell forms normally present only in bone marrow. It is derived from the diagrammatic representation of cell maturation, in which the more immature forms are shown on the left side (Fig. 12-5).

Neutrophils exist in the peripheral blood for about 10 hours after they are released from the marrow. During this time, they move back and forth between the general blood circulation and the walls of the blood vessels, where they accumulate. They also leave the blood and enter the tissues, where they carry out their primary functions. In the tissues, neutrophils are used to fight bacterial infections and are then destroyed or eliminated from the body by the excretory system (intestinal tract, urine, lungs, or saliva).

Metabolically, neutrophils are very active and can carry out both anaerobic and aerobic glycolysis. The neutrophilic granules contain several digestive enzymes that are able to destroy many types of bacteria. The cells are capable of random locomotion and can be directed to an area of infection by the process of chemotaxis. Once in the tissues, the neutrophils destroy bacteria by engulfing them and releasing digestive enzymes into the phagocytic vacuole thus formed.

The first recognizable precursor of *eosinophils* is the eosinophil myelocyte. Culture studies show that there is a separate eosinophilic-committed progenitor cell (colony-forming unit, eosinophil [CFU-Eo]). Eosinophil myeloblasts cannot be recognized microscopically from the neutrophilic myeloblast. Eosinophils exist in the peripheral blood for less than 8 hours after release from the marrow and have a short survival time in the tissues. The function of eosinophils is not completely

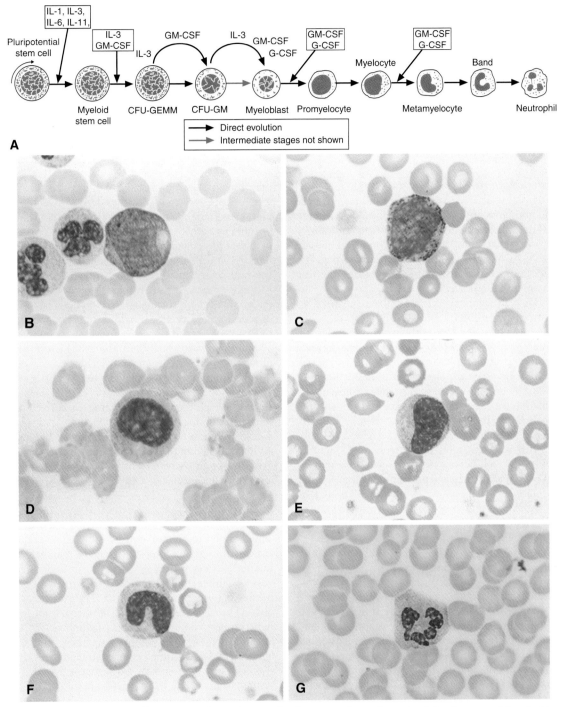

FIGURE 12-5 A, Differentiation of granulocytes showing appropriate colony-stimulating factors and interleukins (ILs). CSF, Colony-stimulating factors; CFU-GEMM, colony-forming unit, granulocyte-erythrocyte-monocyte/macrophage-megakaryocyte; CFU-GM, colony-forming unit, granulocyte-monocyte; GM-CSF, granulocyte-macrophage colony-stimulating factor. B, Myeloblast showing delicate chromatin, multiple nucleoli, and nongranular cytoplasm. C, Promyelocyte with a concentration of primary granules. D, Neutrophilic myelocyte with secondary granules, no nucleoli and the beginning condensation of chromatin in the nucleus. E, Metamyelocyte with the classic kidney bean–shaped nucleus. F, Band form with a nucleus whose indentation is greater than 50% of the width of the nucleus. Remaining primary granules are a lighter blue. G, Polymorphonuclear (PMN) cell with a typically twisted and segmented nucleus. (Modified from Rodak BF, Fritsma GA, Doig K: Hematology: clinical principles and applications, ed 3, St Louis, 2007, Saunders.)

TABLE 12-3

Monocytic Leukocyte Development				
Nomenclature	Overall Size (µm)	N/C Ratio	Nuclear Characteristics	Cytoplasmic Characteristics
Monoblast	12-20	4:1	Oval or folded shape; 1, 2, or more nucleoli	Vacuoles variable, irregularly shaped
Promonocyte	12-20	3:1-2:1	Elongated, folded, 0 to 2 nucleoli	Blue-gray, abundant, vacuoles variable
Mature monocyte	12-18	2:1-1:1	Horseshoe-shaped, folded, lacelike chromatin	Vacuoles common, blue-gray, abundant

understood. They do leave the peripheral blood when adrenal corticosteroid hormones increase and proliferate in response to immunologic stimuli. Eosinophils are capable of locomotion and phagocytosis and respond to foreign proteins. They are active in allergic reactions and certain parasitic infections, especially those involving parasitic invasion of the tissues.

Basophils occur in very low numbers (mean 0.6%) in normal peripheral blood. The first recognizable basophilic cell type is the basophil myelocyte, which contains basophilic granules. Their life span in blood is similar to that of neutrophils and eosinophils, and they are capable of sluggish locomotion. The granules contain histamine, heparin or a heparin-like substance, and peroxidase. The rapid release of mediators from immunoglobulin E (IgE)–primed basophils and mast cells activated by exposure to parasite-associated antigens is thought to contribute significantly to the local inflammation associated with IgE-dependent immune responses to parasites. If the same events are triggered by antigens from pollen, food, drugs, or insect venom, the result is a disorder of immediate hypersensitivity[1] (see Chapter 17).

Monocyte Maturation and Function

Monocytes, as with granulocytes, are produced mainly in the bone marrow. The stages of development are myelomonoblast, promonocyte, and monocyte (Table 12-3). The myelomonoblast looks very similar to the myeloblast or the lymphoblast, and it may be impossible to distinguish myelomonoblasts morphologically on films prepared with Wright's stain. In such cases, the term *blast* is used. It may be necessary to classify the type of blast present on the basis of other cell types in the area.

Monocytes remain in the peripheral blood for hours to days after leaving the bone marrow, depending on the reference cited. They are very motile phagocytic cells, but unlike neutrophils, monocytes do not die after they engage in phagocytic activity. Instead, after 1 to 3 days in the peripheral blood, monocytes move into the body tissues and are transformed into **macrophages;** they

may remain for months, depending on location. Macrophages are thought to be derived from both monocytes and histiocytic cells. Cells that have become free are known as **histiocytes,** and a histiocyte that has begun to phagocytose is called a *macrophage.* The macrophage is the final mature form of the monocyte when it travels through the tissues. Monohistiocytic cells (histiocytes, monocytes, and macrophages) are considered to be related in terms of function and origin. In addition to phagocytosing bacteria, macrophages interact with lymphocytes in the synthesis of antibodies. Macrophages process and present antigens to T cells.

The mononuclear **phagocytes** (monocytes and macrophages) are important in the defense against microorganisms, including mycobacteria, fungi, bacteria, protozoa, and viruses. They play a role in immune response, phagocytic defense, and the inflammatory response. They also secrete cytokines, remove senescent blood cells, and have antitumor activity.

Lymphocyte Maturation and Function

The lymphatic system consists of a network of vessels throughout most of the body tissues. The smaller vessels unite to form larger and larger vessels, which finally come together in two main trunks, the right lymphatic duct and the thoracic duct. The ducts empty into the circulatory system through veins in the neck. Lymph nodes are located all along the lymphatic vessels, and the lymph (fluid within the system) circulates through the nodes as it progresses through the lymphatic system. Many of the lymphocytes are formed in the lymph nodes and circulate back and forth between the blood, the organs, and the lymphatic tissues. Functionally, there are two types of lymphocytes, T cells, or T lymphocytes, and B cells, or B lymphocytes.

T cells arise in the thymus from fetal liver or bone marrow precursors that seed the thymus during embryonic development. These CD34+ progenitor cells develop in the thymic cortex. B lymphocytes are derived from hematopoietic stem cells by a complex series of differentiation events

TABLE 12-4

Lymphocyte Development				
Nomenclature	Overall Size (μm)	N/C Ratio	Nuclear Characteristics	Cytoplasmic Characteristics
Lymphoblast	15-20	4:1	Round or oval, 1 or 2 nucleoli	Medium blue
Prolymphocyte	15-18	4:1 to 3:1	Oval, slightly indented	Medium blue; may have few azurophilic granules
Mature lymphocyte	Small: 6-9 Large: 17-20	Small: 4:1-3:1 Large: 2:1	Round or oval	Light blue; few azurophilic granules may be present

that occur in the fetal liver and, in adult life, in the bone marrow. B-lymphocyte differentiation is complex and proceeds through both an antigen-independent and antigen-dependent state, culminating in the generation of mature, end-stage, nonmotile cells called *plasma cells*. Some activated B cells differentiate into memory B cells, long-lived cells that circulate in the blood.

The stages of development are lymphoid stem cell, lymphoblast, pre–T cell or pre–B cell, and T lymphocyte or B lymphocyte (Table 12-4). The number of precursor stages that exist from the lymphoid stem cell to the first identifiable B lymphocytes and T lymphocytes is not known. Lymphoid stem cells are indistinguishable from other undifferentiated stem cells. These stem cells are also called *lymphoblasts* by many hematologists. Lymphoid stem cells, or lymphoblasts, look very similar to myeloblasts.

Lymphocytes act to direct the immune response system of the body. Maturation of lymphocytes in the bone marrow or thymus results in cells that are immunocompetent. The cells are able to respond to antigenic challenges by directing the immune responses of the host defense. They migrate to various sites in the body to await antigenic stimulus and activation. Only when immunologic studies are performed can these cells be identified as belonging to specific subsets of lymphocytes. As lymphocytes mature, their identity and function are specified by the antigenic structures on their external membrane surface.

T lymphocytes mature in the thymus, an organ found in the anterior mediastinum, and function in cell-mediated immune responses such as delayed hypersensitivity, graft-versus-host reactions, and allograft rejection. T cells make up the majority of the lymphocytes circulating in the peripheral blood. In the periphery of the thymus, they further differentiate into multiple different T-cell subpopulations with different functions, including cytotoxicity and the secretion of soluble factors, termed *cytokines*. Many different cytokines have been identified, including 25 interleukin molecules and more than 40 chemokines; their functions include growth promotion, differentiation, chemotaxis, and cell stimulation.

B lymphocytes most likely mature in the bone marrow and function primarily in antibody production or the formation of immunoglobulins. B cells constitute about 10% to 30% of the blood lymphocytes. Memory B cells may live for years, but mature B cells that are not activated only live for days.

Platelet (Thrombocyte) Maturation and Function

Another formed element of the blood is the platelet, or **thrombocyte.** Platelets are produced in the bone marrow by cells called *megakaryocytes,* which are large and multinucleated. Platelets do not have a nucleus and are not actually cells; they are portions of cytoplasm pinched off from megakaryocytes and released into the bloodstream (Table 12-5).

Mature platelets are small, colorless bodies 1.5 to 4 μm in diameter. Platelets are generally round or ovoid, although they may have projections called *pseudopods*. Platelets have a colorless to pale-blue background substance containing centrally located, purplish red granules.

In the bloodstream, platelets are an essential part of the blood-clotting mechanism. They act to maintain the structure or integrity of the endothelial cells lining the vascular system by plugging any gaps in the lining. They also function in the clotting process by (1) acting as plugs around the opening of a wound and (2) releasing certain factors necessary for the formation of a blood clot.

BLOOD CELL DEVELOPMENT
Red Blood Cells (Erythrocytes)

In adults, erythrocytes are formed in the bone marrow. The mature RBC is often described as a biconcave disk that lacks a nucleus (Fig. 12-6). The cell is about 7 to 8 μm in diameter.

TABLE 12-5

Development of Platelets				
Nomenclature	Overall Size (μm)	N/C Ratio	Nuclear Characteristics	Cytoplasmic Characteristics
Megakaryocyte	30-160	1:1-1:12	Lobulated	Pinkish blue, abundant
Platelet	2-4	—	Anuclear	Light-blue fragments

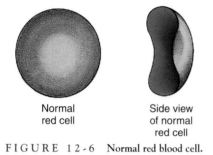

Normal red cell

Side view of normal red cell

FIGURE 12-6 **Normal red blood cell.**

The RBC begins as a nucleated cell within the bone marrow. As the cell matures in the bone marrow, its diameter decreases, and the nucleus becomes denser and smaller and is finally released from the cell (extruded). While this occurs, the concentration of hemoglobin increases. This is seen as a progressive change in color of the cytoplasm from blue to orange on a Wright-stained blood film. The whole sequence of maturation from an early cell precursor to a circulating red cell takes 3 to 5 days (see Table 12-1).

Reticulocytes

The young RBC that has just extruded its nucleus is referred to as a **reticulocyte.** It is about the same size as or slightly larger than a mature RBC. Reticulocytes differ morphologically from mature RBCs because they contain a fine basophilic reticulum or network of RNA (ribonucleic acid), a cytoplasmic remnant that decreases as the cell matures.

Under normal conditions, reticulocytes remain and mature further in the bone marrow for a day or two before they are released into the peripheral blood. RBCs are released into the peripheral blood as reticulocytes by squeezing (or insinuating) through openings in the endothelial cells lining the marrow cavity. These reticulocytes become fully mature and lose all RNA within a day or two. The number of reticulocytes in the peripheral blood is an indication of the degree of RBC production by the marrow.

With Wright's stain, reticulocytes appear pink-gray or pale purple; they have a slight bluish tinge. This **polychromasia** or **polychromatophilia** (many colors) represents the presence of RNA within the cell. With special supervital stains, such as brilliant cresyl blue or new methylene blue, the basophilic reticulum of RNA appears blue. Normally about 1% of the circulating RBCs are reticulocytes.

White Blood Cells (Leukocytes)

Formed elements of the blood go through a series of developmental stages. Normally only mature cells are seen in the peripheral blood circulation. Immature cells may appear in the peripheral blood in certain disease states. Each cell type has a normal life span and function (see Tables 12-2 through 12-5).

CLINICAL HEMATOLOGY

Several hematologic tests are basic to the initial evaluation and follow-up of the patient. The **complete blood count (CBC)** forms the foundation procedure performed in hematology. The CBC consists of the measurement of hemoglobin, hematocrit, red blood cell count with morphology, white blood cell count with differential, and platelet estimate. The RBC indices of mean corpuscular volume (MCV), mean corpuscular hemoglobin (MCH), and mean corpuscular hemoglobin concentration (MCHC) are now a standard part of a routine automated CBC.

The blood cells discussed in this chapter are **erythrocytes, leukocytes,** and **thrombocytes.** Laboratory tests performed in the hematology laboratory include:

- Counting the number or concentration cells
- Determining the relative distribution of various types of cells
- Measuring biochemical abnormalities of the blood
- Hemostasis and coagulation assays (see Chapter 13)

The entire range of disorders seen in hematology includes hereditary, immunologic, nutritional, metabolic, traumatic, and inflammatory conditions. Many disorders, either primarily hematologic in nature or more frequently hematologic manifestations secondary to other diseases, can produce abnormalities of the red cells, white cells and/or platelets. Additional laboratory assays can assist in detection of the primary cause of hematologic abnormalities. Physicians depend on laboratory results, in combination with the clinical history and physical examination, to determine the state of health or disease of a patient.

Anticoagulants

Three types of anticoagulants are commonly used in the hematology laboratory: tripotassium ethylenediaminetetraacetic acid (K_3 EDTA), heparin, and sodium citrate. Each of the anticoagulant types prevents the coagulation of whole blood in a specific manner. The proper proportion of anticoagulant to whole blood is important to avoid the introduction of errors into test results. The specific type of anticoagulant needed for a procedure should be stated in the laboratory procedure manual.

EDTA

Tripotassium ethylenediaminetetraacetate (**EDTA, K_3 EDTA**) is found in lavender-top evacuated tubes. EDTA is used in concentrations of 1.5 mg per 1 mL of whole blood. The mode of action of this anticoagulant is that it removes ionized calcium (Ca^{2+}) through the process of *chelation*. This process forms an insoluble calcium salt that prevents blood coagulation. EDTA is the most frequently used anticoagulant in hematology for the *complete blood cell count* (CBC) or any of its component tests (hemoglobin, packed cell volume or microhematocrit, total leukocyte count and leukocyte differential count, and platelet count). The proper ratio of EDTA to whole blood is important because some test results will be altered if the ratio is incorrect. Excessive EDTA produces shrinkage of erythrocytes, thus affecting tests such as the manually performed packed cell volume (microhematocrit).

Heparin

Heparin is used as an in vitro and in vivo anticoagulant. It is found in green-top evacuated tubes. In BD Vacutainer Blood Collection Tubes, the heparin concentration is 14 to 17 U/mL. Heparin acts as an *antithrombin*, or substance that inactivates the blood-clotting factor thrombin. This inactivation of thrombin is caused by the complexing of heparin with the antithrombin III (AT III) molecule and catalyzing the inhibition of thrombin. BD also manufactures the Vacutainer Plus plastic citrate tube. Its innovative tube geometry minimizes tube headspace and associated platelet activation to optimize *activated partial thromboplastin time* (aPTT) monitoring of patients receiving unfractionated heparin. The in vitro formation of fibrin in heparinized plasma opposes the anticoagulation action of heparin and can result in the subsequent formation of fibrin in the plasma. BD Vacutainer Systems recommends several specimen-processing steps to help ensure a good-quality heparinized plasma sample to aid in minimizing the formation of latent fibrin. Heparin is the preferred anticoagulant for the osmotic fragility test and is used to coat "micro" (capillary blood) collection tubes. However, heparin is an inappropriate anticoagulant for many hematologic tests, including Wright-stained blood smears, because the smear will stain too blue.

Sodium Citrate

Sodium citrate in the concentration of a 3.2% solution, found in a blue-top evacuated tube, has been adopted as the appropriate concentration by the International Committee for Standardization in Hematology and the International Society for Thrombosis and Hemostasis. It also appears in the College of American Pathologists (CAP) revised checklist section for hematology and coagulation as the appropriate concentration.

Sodium citrate removes calcium from the coagulation system by precipitating it into an unusable form. Sodium citrate is effective as an anticoagulant because of its mild calcium-chelating properties. This anticoagulant is used for the Westergren erythrocyte sedimentation rate (ESR; see later section). The correct ratio of one part anticoagulant to nine parts of whole blood in blood collection tubes is critical. An excess of anticoagulant can alter the expected dilution of blood and produce errors in the results.

Processing and Testing the Specimen

After the blood specimen has been collected from the patient, it must be transported to the laboratory for analysis. Assuming the specimen was properly labeled when it was drawn and that it has been handled properly, it is examined in the laboratory as quickly as possible to prevent deterioration. Laboratory tests are done on fresh specimens whenever possible. White cell counts, microhematocrit, platelet counts, and sedimentation rates can be determined up to 24 hours after blood is collected in EDTA if it is refrigerated at 4°C.

Immediately after the blood has been properly drawn and placed in the tube containing the anticoagulant, it should be gently mixed by gentle inversion 5 to 10 times. This is necessary to ensure thorough contact with the anticoagulant. Clotted specimens are absolutely unacceptable for most tests done in the hematology laboratory, especially cell counts. If there is even a tiny clot in a specimen, the cell count will be grossly inaccurate. To comply with Standard Precautions, gloves must be worn during all laboratory handling and testing using blood specimens. All samples are to be considered as potentially infectious, and the proper use of barrier-protective apparel and devices is essential.

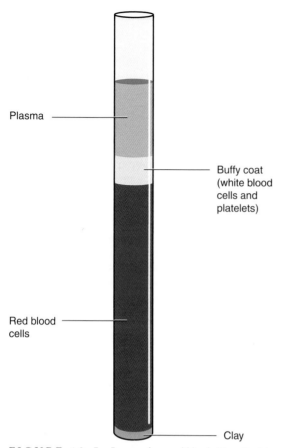

Plasma

Buffy coat
(white blood
cells and
platelets)

Red blood
cells

Clay

FIGURE 12-7 **Layers of normal blood.** (From Rodak
BF, Fritsma GA, Doig K: Hematology: clinical principles and
applications, ed 3, St Louis, 2007, Saunders.)

When a preserved blood specimen is allowed to
stand for a time, the components will settle into
the following three distinct layers (Fig. 12-7):
1. *Plasma,* the top layer
2. *Buffy coat,* a grayish white cellular layer
   composed of white blood cells (WBCs) and
   platelets
3. *Red blood cells* (RBCs), the bottom layer
   Some hematologic procedures are based on the
ability of the blood specimen to settle into layers
when it has been preserved by use of an anticoagulant. Immediately before a test is performed
on a blood specimen, the blood sample must be
mixed by repeated gentle inversion at least 15
times. This can be accomplished by hand or with
a mechanical tube inverter. If the blood sample
has stood for a few minutes, it should be mixed
again.

Appearance of Specimens

When the blood specimen has been properly drawn
and processed, plasma will have a light-yellow
or straw color. Occasionally, the plasma may have
an altered color because of a disease process or as
the result of improper collection technique or handling of the specimen.

Hemolysis

The breakup or rupturing of RBCs, **hemolysis,** can
produce red-colored plasma. Hemolysis is one of
the changes resulting from alterations in osmotic
pressure in the solution surrounding the red cells.
Hemolysis can occur when the membrane surrounding the RBCs has been mechanically ruptured either in vivo, as the result of a disease
process, or in vitro, as the result of difficult collection of poor handling.

Unsuitable Hematologic Specimens

Two types of blood samples are unsuitable for
hematology tests: *clotted samples* and *hemolyzed
samples*. Clotted specimens are unsuitable for cell
counts because the cells trapped in the clot are
not counted. A cell count on a clotted sample
will be falsely low. In hemolyzed specimens, the
RBCs are no longer intact and will yield falsely
decreased results. Although hemolyzed specimens are generally considered unacceptable for
testing, in certain cases of intravascular hemolysis, hemolysis is a clinically significant finding
and not cause for rejection of the specimen for
testing.

Homeostasis

All the fluid and cellular elements that make up
the blood are in a constant state of exchange. The
overall effect is a state of equilibrium in which
the supply is equal to the demand for normal
body function. This state of equilibrium is termed
homeostasis, and various tests done on blood
measure the overall state of homeostasis within
the body. Many of the constituents of plasma (or
serum, if the blood is allowed to clot) are measured in the clinical chemistry laboratory (see
Chapter 11).

Osmosis and Osmotic Pressure

The principle of osmotic pressure and osmosis is
important whenever a solution or diluent is used
as part of a hematologic procedure. In simple
terms, **osmosis** is the passage of a solvent through
a membrane from a dilute solution into a more
concentrated one. The difference in concentration
between the solutions on either side of the membrane causes the phenomenon called **osmotic pressure.** If the concentrations of these solutions are
the same, there will be no pressure.

Isotonic, Hypotonic, and Hypertonic Solutions

When the concentration is the same in the diluent solution as it is inside the RBC, the diluent is called an **isotonic** solution. If the diluent is less concentrated than the inside of the RBC, the solution is called **hypotonic.** From the definition of osmosis, it can be seen that in the case of a hypotonic (dilute) solution, the passage of diluent will be from outside the RBC into the RBC, causing the cell to swell and eventually to rupture, or hemolyze.

If the solution outside the RBC is more concentrated than that inside it, the outside solution is called *hypertonic.* In the case of a hypertonic solution, the osmosis of the solvent is from the inside of the red cell to the surrounding solution. When this happens, the RBC will shrink from loss of liquid and will become crenated.

When in plasma, the RBCs are in an isotonic solution. For this reason, any diluent used to dilute blood for hematology tests must have the same ionic concentration as plasma. When a solution has the same concentration or is isotonic with plasma, it is called a **physiologic solution.** One common physiologic solution is isotonic saline solution, a 0.85-g/dL solution of sodium chloride (NaCl). If RBCs are placed in an isotonic saline solution, their size is preserved. Hypotonic and hypertonic solutions are unsatisfactory as diluents for hematologic studies.

HEMOGLOBIN

The determination of **hemoglobin (Hb)** can be performed separately or as part of a routine CBC. Although the meaning of the CBC will vary somewhat from institution to institution, a hemoglobin measurement is standard and is part of the automated instrumentation that includes cells counts and a calculated hematocrit. The measurement of hemoglobin is relatively simple and can be done quickly by the laboratory. Single-analyte systems (e.g., HemoCue) are available and are waived under the **Clinical Laboratory Improvement Amendments of 1988 (CLIA '88).**

Hemoglobin Synthesis and Structure

Hemoglobin synthesis is a complex process, starting in the bone marrow with the production of the erythrocytes. The **heme** (iron-containing) portion of the molecule combines with **globin** (the protein portion) and forms an activated form of hemoglobin that is ready to transport oxygen. Each hemoglobin molecule consists of four heme groups and a globin moiety, which is composed of four polypeptide chains.

Heme

The heme group is an iron complex containing one iron atom. Iron is essential for the primary function of the hemoglobin molecule: carrying oxygen to the tissues. If iron is lacking because of either inadequate dietary intake or increased loss from the body, anemia results because hemoglobin is not formed in sufficient quantity. When reduced hemoglobin is exposed to oxygen at increased pressure, oxygen is taken up at the iron atom until each molecule of hemoglobin has bound four oxygen molecules, with one molecule at each iron atom. This is not a true oxidation-reduction (redox) reaction, so the hemoglobin molecule carrying oxygen is said to be oxygenated. The molecule fully saturated with oxygen (four oxygen molecules per hemoglobin) is called **oxyhemoglobin.** It contains 1.34 mL of oxygen per gram of hemoglobin. Oxyhemoglobin carries oxygen from the lungs to the tissues of the body. Hemoglobin returning to the lungs with carbon dioxide from the tissues is known as **reduced hemoglobin.**

Heme is itself a complex molecule. It is made up of a series of tetrapyrrole rings, terminating in protoporphyrin, with a central iron (Fig. 12-8, A). Because the heme molecule is a porphyrin, a group of diseases called the *porphyrias* result from certain disorders of heme synthesis. Normally, heme is excreted from the body as bilirubin, which is eventually converted to the various bile salts and pigments. Iron is normally removed and retained by the mononuclear phagocytic system, stored, and reused in the production of new hemoglobin.

Globin

The globin portion of the hemoglobin molecule is a protein substance that consists of four chains of amino acids (polypeptides). Each of the four globin chains is attached to a heme portion to form a single hemoglobin molecule (see Fig. 12-8, B).

Hemoglobin Variants

Different structural forms of hemoglobin may occur in the red cells. These **hemoglobin variants** differ in the content and sequence of amino acids in the globin chains. The alpha chain is composed of 141 amino acids in a specific sequence, and the beta chain contains 146 amino acids of a specific sequence. Other polypeptide globin chains that may be encountered include gamma, delta, and possibly epsilon.

Normal Adult Hemoglobins: A and A2

The principal adult hemoglobin, Hb A, contains two alpha (α) and two beta (β) globin chains. In another form of adult hemoglobin (Hb A_2), the

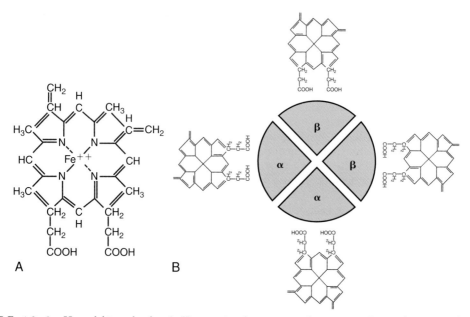

FIGURE 12-8 Hemoglobin molecules. A, Heme moiety (one protoporphyrin ring with a single iron atom). B, Hemoglobin A molecule (four heme groups with their appropriate globin chains: two alpha, two beta).

alpha chains are paired with two delta polypeptide chains. The delta chains are related to beta chains, but 10 amino acids have been substituted. These are the major normal forms of adult hemoglobin. Other genetically determined forms of hemoglobin may be demonstrated by means of electrophoresis. Many abnormal forms of hemoglobin lead to clinical illness because they interfere with the blood's oxygen-carrying capacity.

The combination of Hb A and Hb A_2 should normally make up 95% of the hemoglobin in an adult, with Hb F making up 5% or less.

Hemoglobin F

Hemoglobin F is the major form found during intrauterine life and at birth. In fetal hemoglobin (Hb F), the two alpha globin chains are paired with two gamma chains. Adult hemoglobin (Hb A) is formed in small amounts by the fetus and rapidly increases after birth.

Abnormal Hemoglobin Variants

Disorders in which the presence of structurally abnormal hemoglobins is considered to play an important role pathologically are called **hemoglobinopathies.** In some hemoglobinopathies, all the hemoglobin is in one abnormal form. In other types, two abnormal forms may be present, or some normal forms and some abnormal forms are present. The structurally abnormal hemoglobins usually consist of polypeptide chains with a normal number of amino acids but with a single amino acid substitution. These substitutions are under genetic control, and the hemoglobinopathies may be either inherited or the result of genetic mutations. In clinically significant disease, either the alpha or the beta chain may be affected; however, most of the hemoglobinopathies are the result of beta-chain abnormalities.

The four clinically important abnormal hemoglobins are Hb S, Hb C, Hb D, and Hb E. These are all genetic disorders that affect the protein portion of the hemoglobin molecule by altering the structure of the polypeptide chain. These abnormal hemoglobins as well as the normal ones can be distinguished from one another by various methods, including high-performance liquid chromatography (HPLC) and electrophoresis.

HEMOGLOBIN S

The most common abnormal hemoglobin is Hb S. It is predominantly found in the black population and is responsible for *sickle cell anemia.* Hemoglobin S has an amino acid substitution in the beta chain, where valine is substituted for glutamic acid at the sixth position in the normal beta chain. It causes sickling of the RBCs under conditions of reduced oxygen concentration, resulting in sickle cell anemia when present in the homozygous state.

HEMOGLOBIN C

Hemoglobin C results from an amino acid substitution of lysine for glutamic acid on the sixth position of the beta chain. It may be inherited in combination with Hb S and may occur in a homozygous or heterozygous state. The RBCs may appear as target cells when Hb C is present; less frequently, crystals of precipitated Hb C may be seen in the RBCs.

Hemoglobin Derivatives

Circulating blood carries a composite of derivatives of hemoglobin. Most of the hemoglobin in circulating blood is oxyhemoglobin and reduced hemoglobin. Other hemoglobin derivatives found in normal circulating blood include carboxyhemoglobin (hemoglobin combined with carbon monoxide), methemoglobin (or hemiglobin), which is oxidized hemoglobin, and minor amounts of other derivatives. When iron in the hemoglobin molecule is converted from the 2+ to the ferric 3+ state, it can combine with other substances besides oxygen and is no longer capable of oxygen transport. When sufficient quantities of these hemoglobin derivatives are present in circulating blood, **hypoxia** (lack of oxygen) or **cyanosis** (bluish discoloration of the skin and mucous membranes) will be seen clinically.

Oxyhemoglobin and Reduced Hemoglobin

Oxyhemoglobin and reduced hemoglobin are the major forms of circulating hemoglobin. The main function of hemoglobin is to transport oxygen from the lungs, where oxygen tension is high, to the tissues, where it is low. At an increased oxygen tension (100 mm Hg), hemoglobin is oxygenated by the reversible association of an oxygen molecule at each iron atom, forming oxyhemoglobin (HbO_2). At the reduced oxygen tension of the tissues (down to 20 mm Hg), oxygen is dissociated from the iron in each heme group and replaced by carbon dioxide. This is called *reduced hemoglobin* (Hb). This is not an oxidation-reduction reaction, because iron is in the ferrous state in both HbO_2 and Hb.

Carboxyhemoglobin

The hemoglobin molecule has a much greater affinity for carbon monoxide (CO) than for oxygen and will readily combine with CO if it is present even in low concentration. The affinity of CO for hemoglobin is 200 times greater than the affinity of oxygen. Carboxyhemoglobin (HbCO) cannot bind to and carry oxygen and will result in carbon monoxide poisoning even at relatively low CO concentrations. The formation of HbCO is reversible, and if CO is removed, the hemoglobin will once again combine with oxygen. Clinically, with sufficient HbCO levels, the skin will turn bright cherry red, and at high levels (>50% to 70% of total hemoglobin), the individual can be asphyxiated. Carboxyhemoglobin is found normally in small amounts, especially in the blood of smokers, where concentrations range from 1% to 10% of circulating hemoglobin.

Methemoglobin

Methemoglobin, also referred to as *hemiglobin* (Hi), is a hemoglobin derivative in which the iron has been oxidized from the ferrous to the ferric state and is therefore incapable of combining reversibly with oxygen. The formation of methemoglobin is usually an acquired condition resulting from the presence of certain chemicals or drugs, and is reversible. An inherited methemoglobinemia may result from a structurally abnormal globin chain or an RBC enzyme defect. Up to 1.5% of circulating hemoglobin is normally methemoglobin.

The formation of methemoglobin is used as an intermediary in the cyanmethemoglobin (or hemiglobincyanide) method for the quantitation of whole-blood hemoglobin.

Hemiglobincyanide (Cyanmethemoglobin)

To measure total hemoglobin concentration in blood, it is necessary to prepare a stable derivative containing all the hemoglobin forms that are present. All forms of circulating hemoglobin are readily converted to hemiglobincyanide (HiCN), except for sulfhemoglobin, which is rarely present in significant amounts. For this reason, the hemiglobincyanide, or cyanmethemoglobin, method is the standard method for the determination of hemoglobin.

Sulfhemoglobin

Another abnormal hemoglobin derivative is sulfhemoglobin. The formation of sulfhemoglobin is irreversible, and it remains in the RBC for the cell's entire 120-day lifespan. Its exact nature is unclear, but sulfhemoglobulin is thought to be formed by the action of some drugs and chemicals, such as sulfonamides. Although sulfhemoglobin is incapable of transporting oxygen and cannot be converted back to normally functioning hemoglobin, it rarely exceeds 10% of the total hemoglobin. This is not a life-threatening level, although sulfhemoglobinemia may be seen clinically as cyanosis.

Variations in Reference Values

The reference (or normal) values for hemoglobin in peripheral blood vary with the age and gender of the individual. Altitude also affects the hemoglobin measurement in that the normal hemoglobin concentration is higher at high altitudes than at sea level. At 1 to 2 days of age, hemoglobin concentration is normally 14.5 to 22.5 g/dL. It decreases to 9.5 to 13.5 g/dL by about 3 to 6 months of age.

By 6 years of age, a normal hemoglobin value is 11.5 to 15.5 g/dL. Adult values range from 12 to 16 g/dL in women and 13.5 to 17.5 g/dL in men. There may be a slight decrease in the hemoglobin level after 50 years of age.

When the hemoglobin value is below normal, the patient is said to be *anemic.* Anemia is a very common condition and frequently a complication of other diseases (see Erythrocyte Alterations). In this condition, circulating erythrocytes may be deficient in number, in total hemoglobin content per unit of blood volume, or both. A decrease in hemoglobin can result from bleeding conditions in which the patient loses erythrocytes. An increase in hemoglobin, usually due to an increase in the number of erythrocytes (erythrocytosis), is seen in polycythemia and newborn infants.

Hemoglobin Measurement in the Laboratory

Hemoglobin is determined in grams per deciliter (g/dL). The hemiglobincyanide (HiCN), or cyanmethemoglobin, method is the internationally recognized method of choice. All forms of circulating hemoglobin, except for sulfhemoglobin, are readily converted to cyanmethemoglobin.

Hemiglobincyanide (Cyanmethemoglobin) Method

The HiCN, or cyanmethemoglobin, method uses a modified Drabkin's reagent that contains potassium cyanide, potassium ferricyanide, dihydrogen potassium phosphate (KH_2PO_4), which shortens the conversion time to 3 minutes, and a nonionic detergent that minimizes turbidity and enhances RBC lysis. When the cyanmethemoglobin reagent is mixed with the blood specimen, the stable pigment HiCN is formed and can be measured quantitatively in a spectrophotometer.

Automated Hemoglobinometry

Various automated and semiautomated techniques measure hemoglobin as well as determine the white cell count, red cell count, hematocrit, and red cell indices. Hemoglobin determinations done by an automated instrument generally use the cyanmethemoglobin method. The sample is lysed by using the detergent-modified Drabkin's reagent, and light absorbance is measured at 540 nm.

Specimens

The test for hemoglobin can be done on freeflowing capillary blood obtained from a finger puncture or on venous blood preserved with an anticoagulant. The anticoagulant of choice for hematologic studies, including hemoglobin determinations, is EDTA. The hemoglobin content of blood remains unchanged for several days when the blood is properly anticoagulated and refrigerated at 4°C.

Point-of-Care Hemoglobin Assay

The HemoCue method is an example of a singlepurpose, self-contained instrument that measures hemoglobin only. This method of hemoglobin determination is waivered under CLIA '88. It gives a reliable quantitative value and can be performed within 45 seconds. The instrument uses a microcuvette that serves as a sampling device, a test tube, and a measuring device. It automatically measures precisely 10 μL of blood from a capillary puncture or from a tube of anticoagulated blood collected by venipuncture. The microcuvette does not require mixing or dispensing of reagents. It contains an exact quantity of a dry reagent that yields a reaction when contact is made with the measured blood sample. Once the blood is sampled, the microcuvette is placed into the HemoCue photometer, and the hemoglobin concentration is displayed in g/dL.

PRINCIPLE: HEMOGLOBIN DETERMINATION: HEMOCUE METHOD

This point-of-care testing assay for hemoglobin is based on a modified azidemethemoglobin reaction. Erythrocyte membranes are disintegrated by sodium deoxycholate, releasing the hemoglobin from the cells. Sodium nitrite converts the hemoglobin iron from the ferrous to the ferric state to form methemoglobin, which then combines with azide to form azidemethemoglobin. The concentration of azidemethemoglobin is measured optically to determine the concentration of hemoglobin in the patient's blood (see procedure at http://evolve.elsevier.com/Turgeon/clinicallab).

Reference Values[2] (SI Units)

Adult male, 13.5-17.5 g/dL
Adult female, 12.0-16.0 g/dL
3-6-month-old infant, 9.5-13.5 g/dL
6-12-year-old child, 11.5-15.5 g/dL
The mean hemoglobin level of blacks of both genders and all ages is reported to be 0.5 to 1.0 g/dL below the mean for comparable whites.

HEMATOCRIT (PACKED CELL VOLUME)

The **hematocrit (Hct),** or **packed cell volume,** is a macroscopic observation of volume of the packed RBCs in a sample of whole blood, if measured by

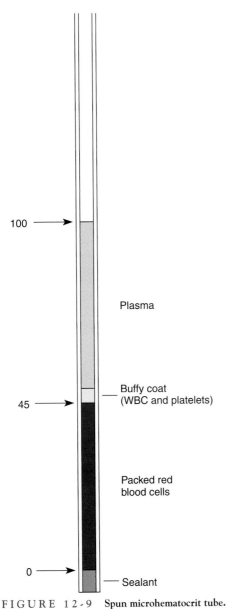

100 →

Plasma

45 →

Buffy coat
(WBC and platelets)

Packed red
blood cells

0 →

Sealant

F I G U R E 1 2 - 9   **Spun microhematocrit tube.**

Automated hematology instruments give a calculated hematocrit value and have generally replaced the manual methods.

A quick quality control check of hemoglobin results (in g/dL) in healthy patients (normochromic, normocytic) is done by comparing the hemoglobin with the hematocrit results (in % units), using the following formula:

$$Hb \times 3 = Hct \pm 3 \text{ units}$$

Methods for Measurement

The **spun microhematocrit method** can be done with either free-flowing capillary blood from a skin puncture or EDTA-anticoagulated venous blood (Procedure 12-1). Only a very small amount of blood is needed. The test uses a high-speed centrifuge with a relatively short centrifugation time.

An **automated hematocrit** result is obtained when multiparameter instruments are used. This result is computed from individual red cell volumes (MCV) and the red cell count and is not affected by the trapped plasma that is left in the RBC column for the manual methods. Hematocrit value obtained with the automated instruments is slightly lower than the value obtained by the centrifugation methods.

Specimens

Again, for the spun microhematocrit method, either venous blood anticoagulated with EDTA or freely flowing capillary blood may be used. With capillary blood, microhematocrit tubes coated with heparin are used. With venous blood, plain uncoated microhematocrit tubes must be used. Blood that has been properly anticoagulated with EDTA is used for automated analysis.

Equipment for Microhematocrit

Capillary Tubes

Special nongraduated capillary tubes are used. These tubes are 1 mm in diameter and 7 cm long. They can be purchased (1) lined with dried heparin for use with capillary blood or (2) plain (without heparin) for use with previously anticoagulated venous blood. Some type of seal is needed for one end of the tube before it can be centrifuged. A special sealing compound (similar to modeling clay) can be used for this purpose. Also, tubes are available that have a self-sealing plug and a multilayered Mylar wrap to ensure safer blood handling by preventing breakage during collection and centrifugation and resulting contamination of the sealant.

manual technique. The manual procedure is relatively simple and reliable. A hematocrit is used in evaluating and classifying the various types of anemias according to red cell indices.

When whole blood is centrifuged, the heavier particles fall to the bottom of the tube, and the lighter particles settle on top of the heavier cells. The hematocrit is the percentage of RBCs in a volume of whole blood. It is expressed as units of percent or as a ratio in the SI system.

When the hematocrit result is read, it is important to take the reading at the top of the RBC layer, particularly when there is an extremely elevated white cell or platelet count. The buffy coat should not be included in the measurement of red cell volume for the hematocrit result (Fig. 12-9).

Packed Cell Volume of Whole Blood (Hematocrit): Centrifugation Method

PRINCIPLE

The packed cell volume (PCV), hematocrit, is a measurement of the ratio of the volume occupied by the red blood cells (RBCs) to the volume of whole blood after centrifugation in a sample of capillary or venous blood expressed as a percentage. Clinically, the hematocrit is used to screen for anemia or other red cell volume alterations. In conjunction with an erythrocyte count, the hematocrit is used to calculate the mean corpuscular volume (MCV). The hematocrit is also used in conjunction with the hemoglobin concentration to calculate the mean corpuscular hemoglobin concentration (MCHC).

SPECIMEN

Anticoagulated venous blood or capillary blood collected directly into heparinized capillary tubes can be used. Specimens should be centrifuged within 6 hours of collecting. Hemolyzed specimens cannot be used for testing.

REAGENTS, SUPPLIES, AND EQUIPMENT

- Capillary tubes, either plain or heparin-coated
- Clay-type tube sealant
- Microhematocrit centrifuge
- Microhematocrit reading device

CALIBRATION

The calibration of the centrifuge should be checked regularly for timer accuracy, speed, and maximal packing of cells.

QUALITY CONTROL

Commercially available whole blood can be used to check the accuracy of normal and abnormal levels.

PROCEDURE

1. Well-mixed anticoagulant blood should be drawn into two microhematocrit tubes by capillary action. Free-flowing capillary specimens should be collected directly into heparinized capillary tubes. The tubes should be filled to about three-fourths of their length. Wipe off the outside of the tubes with a suitable wipe.
2. Seal one end of each tube with a small amount of claylike material by placing the dry end of the tube into the sealant, holding the index finger over the opposite end to prevent blood from leaking out of the tube onto the sealant.
3. Place the filled and sealed capillary tubes into the centrifuge. The sealed ends should point toward the outside of the centrifuge. The duplicate samples should be placed opposite the other to balance the centrifuge. Record the position number of each specimen.
4. Securely fasten the flat lid on top of the capillary tubes. Close the centrifuge top and secure the latch. Set the timer for 5 minutes. The fixed speed of centrifugation should be 10,000 to 15,000 rpm.
5. After the centrifuge has stopped, open the top and remove the cover plate. Within 10 minutes, read the microhematocrit on a reader. Measure the microhematocrit by adjusting the top of the clay sealant to the 0 mark and reading the top of the red cell column. Do not include the buffy coat in reading the packed erythrocyte column. A capillary tube reader with an ocular that has cross-markings produces the most accurate reading.

REPORTING RESULTS

The microhematocrit is preferentially expressed as a decimal fraction, such as 0.45 L/L, rather than as 45%. In current practice, the percentage expression is most commonly used.
Reference values:

Males, range 41.5%-50.4%
Females, range 36.0%-45.0%

P R O C E D U R E **12-1** (Continued)

PROCEDURE NOTES

Sources of Error

Erroneous results can be caused by inclusion of the buffy coat in reading the packed column, hemolysis of the specimen, and inadequate mixing. If the centrifugation time is too short or the speed is too low, an increase in trapped plasma (1%-3%) will occur in normal blood. Increased amounts of trapped plasma can produce errors in patients with an erythrocyte abnormality, such as sickle cell anemia. Do not allow the tubes to remain in the centrifuge for more than 10 minutes after the end of centrifugation because the interface between the plasma and the cells will become slanted, and an inaccurate reading will result.

Clinical Applications

The microhematocrit is used for detecting anemia, polycythemia, hemodilution, or hemoconcentration.

REFERENCES

Clinical and Laboratory Standards Institute: Procedure for determining packed cell volume by the microhematocrit method: approved standard, ed 3, Wayne, PA, 2000, H7-A3.
Turgeon M: Clinical hematology, ed 4, Philadelphia, 2005, Lippincott Williams & Wilkins.

Centrifuge

A special microhematocrit centrifuge is used, capable of producing centrifugal fields up to 10,000 g (Fig. 12-10).

Reading Device

Because capillary tubes are not graduated, a special reading device is used to measure the percentage of packed RBCs after centrifugation.

Results

In current laboratory practice, hematocrit values are generally expressed as a percentage. With the SI system, however, packed cell volume is preferably expressed as a decimal; the units are undesignated, but units of liter per liter (L/L) are implied, so a 45% result is reported as 0.45.

Precautions and Technical Factors

The blood sample must be properly collected and preserved. Anticoagulated blood samples using EDTA should be centrifuged within 6 hours of collection. EDTA is the anticoagulant of choice. The blood must not be clotted or hemolyzed for any hematocrit test. If clotted blood is used, there will be false packing of the RBCs, and the true packing in the tube will not be noted (a falsely high result will be observed). In a hemolyzed specimen, some RBCs have been destroyed, so again the RBC packing will not be true (a falsely low result will be observed). Centrifugation must be sufficient to yield maximum packing of the red cells.

The hematocrit value is frequently accompanied by a hemoglobin determination. Again, there should be a correlation between the two results: the hematocrit result in percent units should be approximately three times the hemoglobin result, assuming the red cells are of normal size and color.

Any capillary blood samples collected should be freely flowing. The capillary tubes must be properly sealed so that no leakage occurs. These tubes are not calibrated, so the level of packed RBCs and the total volume of the cells and plasma must be accurately measured by some convenient reading device. The buffy coat layer is not included in the reading for the hematocrit.

Even with adequate centrifugation, providing tightly packed RBCs, a small amount of plasma remains trapped around the cells. This is unavoidable, and in normal blood, with normally shaped and sized RBCs, this trapped plasma accounts for 1.5% to 3% of the height of the red cell column in a microhematocrit tube. When the RBCs have an irregular shape or size, there will be an increase in the amount of plasma being trapped.

When hematocrits are determined by use of automated hematology analyzers, the hematocrit is determined indirectly by determining the average size of the RBC population (the mean corpuscular volume, or MCV) and multiplying it by the total RBC count. The hematocrit value as determined by automation is therefore consistently lower than that done by the spun microhematocrit method.

Unique to the microhematocrit is the error caused by excess EDTA (inadequate blood for the fixed amount of EDTA in the blood collection tube). The microhematocrit will be falsely

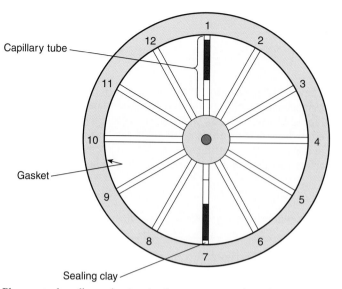

Capillary tube

Gasket

Sealing clay

FIGURE 12-10 Placement of capillary tubes in microhematocrit centrifuge. Centrifuge must be balanced by placing tubes directly across from each other, as shown for places 1 and 7.

low because of cell shrinkage. Thus, heparinized capillary tubes must not be used with anticoagulated blood samples.

With good technique, the precision of the hematocrit is 1%. Inadequate centrifugation will give falsely high results. If the tubes are not sealed properly, falsely low results will be obtained because more RBCs will be lost than plasma.

Reference Values[2]

Reference values for hematocrit (Hct, packed cell volume) are influenced by age, gender, and altitude and vary among authors (see Hemoglobin).

Generally accepted values at sea level are:
Adult male, 41.5%-50.4%
Adult female, 36%-45%

RED BLOOD CELL INDICES

In the classification of anemias, quantitative measurements of the average size, hemoglobin content, and hemoglobin concentration of RBCs are especially useful (see Erythrocyte Alterations). These can be calculated from red cell count, hemoglobin concentration, and hematocrit. The indices are the *mean corpuscular* (cell) *volume* (MCV), the *mean corpuscular* (cell) *hemoglobin* (MCH), and the *mean corpuscular* (cell) *hemoglobin concentration* (MCHC).

The MCV represents the volume or size of the average RBC, the MCH represents the weight of hemoglobin in the average RBC, and the MCHC represents the hemoglobin concentration or color of the average RBC. A derived measurement determined electronically is the *red cell distribution width*

(RDW). This is a measurement of the degree of variability in RBC size. Determination of these indices has become routine with the use of automated multiparameter instruments. These instruments measure the hemoglobin, MCV, and RBC count, then automatically calculate the Hct, MCH, and MCHC.

When the indices are calculated from manually determined values for hemoglobin, hematocrit, and red cell count, the greatest inaccuracy results from errors associated with the RBC count. By electronic counting of the number of RBCs, this error is significantly reduced. Indices calculated by electronic methods have been found to be more accurate. It is important to verify all indices against observations of stained blood films. When the RBC indices are used in conjunction with an examination of the stained blood film, a clear picture of RBC morphology is obtained.

Because an RBC is very small and the amount of hemoglobin in a single cell is minute, the units in which the RBCs are measured and recorded are *micrometers* (μm) and *picograms* (pg). With automated hematology instrumentation, reporting the red cell indices is routine, and the data are considered highly reliable. Red cell indices are calculated from the following hematology data (with abbreviations) in units as indicated:

Test Name	Abbreviation	Units
Hematocrit	Hct	%
Packed cell volume	PCV	L/L
Red cell count	RBC	$\times 10^{12}$/L
Hemoglobin	Hb	g/dL

Mean Corpuscular Volume

The MCV is the average volume of an RBC in *femtoliters* (fL). One fL = 10^{-15} L = one cubic micrometer (μm^3). The MCV is calculated manually by dividing the volume of packed red cells (hematocrit) by the number of red cells, using the formula:

$$\text{MCV (fL)} = \frac{\text{Hct} \times 1}{\text{RBC}}$$

The factor 10 is introduced to convert the hematocrit reading (in %) from volume of packed red cells per 100 mL to volume per liter. Example: If the Hct is 45% and the red cell count is 5×10^{12} cells per liter:

$$\text{MCV} = \frac{45 \times 10}{5} = 90 \text{ fL}$$

The MCV in normal adults is between 80 and 96 fL.

The MCV indicates whether the RBCs will appear small (*microcytic*), normal (*normocytic*), or large (*macrocytic*). If the MCV is less than 80 fL, the RBCs will be microcytic. If it is greater than 100 fL, the RBCs will be macrocytic. If it is within the normal range, the RBCs will be normocytic. In some macrocytic anemias (e.g., pernicious anemia) the MCV may be as high as 150 fL. In microcytic anemia with marked iron deficiency, it may be 60 to 70 fL. The chief source of error in the MCV is the considerable error in the manual red cell count, if used.

With automated cell counters and electronically calculated indices, the MCV is measured directly, and the hematocrit is calculated from MCV and red cell count (Hct = MCV × RBC). The MCV is now considered the most reliable automated index and is probably the most effective discriminant for the classification of anemias. Previously, the MCHC was the most reliable index because it was calculated from the two manual measurements that could be done most accurately, Hct and Hb.

Mean Corpuscular Hemoglobin

The MCH is the content (weight) of hemoglobin in the average RBC. It is measured in picograms. One picogram (pg) = 10^{-12} g = 1 micromicrogram ($\mu\mu g$). The MCH is obtained by dividing the hemoglobin by the red cell count. A simple formula can be used to calculate this value:

$$\text{MCH (pg)} = \frac{\text{Hb} \times 10}{\text{RBC}}$$

The factor 10 is used to convert the hemoglobin from grams per deciliter to grams per liter.

Example: If the hemoglobin is 15 g/dL and the RBC is 5×10^{12} cells per liter:

$$\text{MCH} = \frac{15 \times 10}{5} = 30 \text{ pg}$$

The normal range for the MCH is 27 to 33 pg. MCH should always correlate with the MCV and the MCHC. MCH may be as high as 50 pg in macrocytic anemias or as low as 20 pg or less in hypochromic microcytic anemias.

The chief source of MCH error is the RBC count, if done manually. However, when the red cell count is determined by electronic cell counters, the MCH is a reliable index.

Mean Corpuscular Hemoglobin Concentration

The MCHC is the average hemoglobin concentration in a given volume of packed red cells. It is expressed as grams per deciliter. MCHC may be calculated from the MCV and the MCH or from the hemoglobin and hematocrit values by using the following formula:

$$\text{MCHC (g/dL)} = \frac{\text{MCH}}{\text{MCV}} \times 100$$

or

$$\text{MCHC (g/dL)} = \frac{\text{Hb}}{\text{Hct}} \times 100$$

Example: If the hemoglobin concentration is 15 g/dL and the Hct is 45%:

$$\text{MCHC} = \frac{15}{45} \times 100 = 33.3 \text{ g/dL}$$

If a packed cell volume of 0.45 is used in the previous example:

$$\text{MCHC} = \frac{15}{0.45} = 33.3 \text{ g/dL}$$

Reference values range from 33 to 36 g/dL, and values below 32 g/dL indicate hypochromasia. An MCHC above 40 g/dL would indicate malfunctioning of the instrument. An impossibly high MCHC (>40 g/dL) also could indicate the presence of cold agglutinins in the specimen. An MCHC of 37 g/dL is near the upper limits for hemoglobin solubility and the physiologic upper limits for the MCHC. The MCHC typically increases only in spherocytosis. In other anemias it is decreased or normal. In true hypochromic anemias, the hemoglobin concentration is reduced, and values as low as 20 to 25 g/dL may be seen.

Red Cell Distribution Width

The RDW is a measurement of the degree of *anisocytosis* present, or the degree of variability in RBC size, in a blood sample. This measurement is derived by the automated multiparameter instruments that can directly measure the MCV. If anisocytosis is present on the peripheral blood film, and the variation in RBC size is prominent, there is an increase in the standard deviation of the MCV from the mean.

In Coulter instruments (e.g., Coulter Model S Plus) a red cell histogram is plotted, and the RDW (%) is defined as the coefficient of variation of the MCV:

$$RDW\,(\%) = \frac{\text{Standard deviation (SD) of MCV}}{\text{Mean MCV}} \times 100$$

The reference range for RDW is from 11% to 15%, but it varies with the instrument used.

Indices: Precautions, Technical Factors, and General Comments

Any manual RBC count, hematocrit, or hemoglobin concentration used in the calculations must be accurate. It is also essential to check the appearance of the RBCs in a well-stained blood film against the calculated indices. The calculations must agree with the appearance of the red cells in the blood film. For example, a corresponding decrease in hemoglobin color intensity should be observed on the blood film when there is a low MCHC (increase in amount of central pallor in RBCs), but often it is difficult to recognize hypochromasia under these circumstances. The MCHC is often below 30 g/dL before hypochromasia is observed on the blood film.

Reference Values[2]

Mean corpuscular volume (MCV): range 80-96.1 fL

Mean corpuscular hemoglobin (MCH): range 27.5-33.2 pg

Mean corpuscular hemoglobin concentration (MCHC): range 33.4-35.5 g/dL

Red cell distribution width (RDW): range 11.5%-14.5%

BLOOD CELL COUNTS

Counting the various cells found in blood is a fundamental procedure in the hematology laboratory. In modern laboratories, most cell counts are performed with automated equipment, but body fluids may be analyzed by manual methods. Electronic counting devices avoid human error, which is significant in manual cell counts, and are statistically more accurate because of sampling; these devices count many more cells than can be counted manually.

The procedures in this chapter are presented in a format consistent with the guidelines set forth by CLSI.[3]

1. Procedure title and specific method
2. Test principle, including type of reaction and clinical reasons for the test
3. Specimen collection and preparation
4. Reagents, supplies, and equipment
5. Calibration of a standard curve
6. Quality control
7. Procedure
8. Calculations
9. Reporting results (normal values)
10. Procedure notes, including sources of error, clinical applications, and limitations of the procedure
11. References

Units Reported

Because there are a great number of cells per unit volume of blood, it is necessary to dilute the blood before attempting to count them. Methods for counting cells are designed to obtain the number of cells in 1 L of whole blood; this is the unit (SI) of measurement of volume recommended by the International Council for Standardization in Haematology (ICSH).

The enumerated constituents are reported in units per liter of blood, the number of cells actually counted (platelets, RBCs, WBCs) must be converted to the number present per liter of blood. Previously, cells were counted and reported as the number of cells per cubic millimeter (mm³). This was a convenient unit of measurement because cells were counted in a hemocytometer, an accurately ruled chamber or device where cells were counted in areas of square millimeters, and results were converted to number per cubic millimeter. One cubic millimeter is essentially equal to one microliter. This is summarized as follows:

$$1\ mm^3 = 1\ \mu L = 1 \times 10^{-6} L$$

Therefore:

$$1 \times 10^6 \mu L = 1\ L$$

Specimens

Free-flowing capillary blood obtained from a skin puncture (see Chapter 3) or venous blood preserved with an anticoagulant may be used. The anticoagulant of choice is EDTA.

Before using any blood sample, it must be checked to be sure that it has been preserved with the proper anticoagulant and has been properly labeled, and that its appearance indicates a good collection technique was used. Each sample should be checked for hemolysis and small clots, known as *fibrin clots,* as soon as it is received. Clotted blood or samples with fibrin clots are unacceptable for cell counts. Standard Precautions must always be used when any blood specimen is handled.

Diluents Used

White Cell Counts

In order to count leukocytes, the diluting fluid must destroy the more numerous RBCs so WBCs may be counted more readily. (WBCs need not be eliminated when RBCs are being counted.) The principle of osmotic pressure is again employed but in a different way. A lysing agent hemolyzes the RBCs, it converts the hemoglobin released from the red cells into acid hematin, which gives the resulting solution a brown color. The intensity of the brown color is directly related to the amount of hemoglobin present in the RBCs.

Counting Red and White Blood Cells

The RBC (erythrocyte) and WBC (leukocyte) counts are basic procedures performed by automated instruments. Although generally replaced by automated cell counts, manual leukocyte counts may still be done in special circumstances (e.g., counting cells in body fluids, such as cerebrospinal fluid or synovial fluid) (see Chapter 15, Body Fluids and the procedure at http://evolve.elsevier.com/Turgeon/clinicallab).

Clinical Significance of Cell Counts

RED BLOOD CELL COUNTS

Anemia is a term generally applied to a decrease in the number of RBCs (erythrocytes). There are many types of anemias (see later discussion). Anemia can be caused by excessive blood loss or blood destruction (hemolytic anemia). Anemias caused by decreased blood cell or hemoglobin formation include pernicious anemia, bone marrow failure anemia, and iron-deficiency anemia. Polycythemia is a condition in which the number of erythrocytes is increased.

WHITE BLOOD CELL COUNTS

The normal WBC count for adults varies from 4.5 to 11.3 × 10^9/L. An increase in the WBC (leukocyte) count above the normal upper limit is termed **leukocytosis.** A decrease below the normal lower limit is termed **leukopenia.** Leukopenia may occur with certain viral infections, with typhoid fever and malaria, after radiation therapy, after the administration of certain drugs, and in pernicious anemia. Leukocytosis may occur in many acute infections, especially bacterial infections, in severe malaria, after hemorrhage, during pregnancy, postoperatively, in some forms of anemia, in some carcinomas, and in leukemia.

Leukemia is characterized by uncontrolled proliferation of one or more of the various hematopoietic cells and is associated with many changes in the circulating cells of the blood. Blood films prepared from patients with leukemia should be examined only by a qualified person—a pathologist or an experienced clinical laboratory scientist. There are two main classifications of leukemia, *lymphocytic* and *myelocytic,* according to the predominant type of leukocyte seen. Leukemias are further divided into the subclassifications acute and chronic. In the *acute* condition, the disease progresses rapidly, and morphologic changes are marked. In the *chronic* condition, the changes are neither as rapid nor as marked.

The normal WBC count varies with age. The white cell count of a newborn baby is 9 to 30 × 10^9/L at birth and drops to 6.0-17.5 × 10^9/L at 6 months of age.

As mentioned earlier, the white count is used to indicate the presence of infection and follow the progress of certain diseases. It may be elevated in acute bacterial infections, appendicitis, pregnancy, hemolytic disease of the newborn, uremia, and ulcers. It may be decreased in hepatitis, rheumatoid arthritis, cirrhosis of the liver, and systemic lupus erythematosus. A child's leukocyte count usually shows a much greater variation during disease than an adult's count. An individual's leukocyte count is subject to some variation during a normal day, being slightly higher in the afternoon than in the morning. There is also an increase in the WBC count after strenuous exercise, emotional stress, and anxiety.

Platelet Counts

Platelets, or thrombocytes, function in blood coagulation and are therefore associated with the bleeding and clotting, or *hemostatic,* mechanism of the body. Platelets are formed in the bone marrow from megakaryocytes. They are difficult to count accurately for several reasons; platelets are small and difficult to discern, and they have an adhesive character and become attached to surfaces or to particles of debris in the diluting fluid. They disintegrate easily and are difficult to distinguish from debris. Because of their sticky nature, platelets clump easily and tend to adhere to other platelets in clumps. The clumping tendency of platelets is decreased if EDTA is used as an anticoagulant.

Specimens

Capillary blood from a finger puncture can be used, but venous blood generally gives more satisfactory results. Platelet counts on capillary blood are generally lower than those on venous blood because of immediate platelet clumping at the puncture site. Again, EDTA is the anticoagulant of choice for platelet counts because it lessens the tendency for platelet clumping.

Methods Used to Count Platelets

Most platelet counts are performed using automated instruments. The quantitative platelet count is correlated with a semi-quantitative estimate from a stained peripheral blood smear. If the instrument count and the blood smear do not match, a manual platelet count is performed (see procedure at http://evolve.elsevier.com/Turgeon/clinicallab). This rare situation typically happens when the platelet count is very low and the patient has a moderate number of schistocytes.

Clinical Significance of Platelet Count

The normal number of platelets, depending in part on the method employed for their enumeration, ranges from 150 to 450 × 10^9/L whole blood. A count lower than normal may be associated with a generalized bleeding tendency and a prolonged bleeding time. A count higher than normal may be associated with a tendency toward thrombosis. There are several diseases in which a high or low platelet count can result.

Thrombocytopenia, or a decrease in platelets, is found in thrombocytopenic purpura, in some infectious diseases, in some acute leukemias, in some anemias (aplastic and pernicious), and when the patient is undergoing radiation treatment or chemotherapy.

Thrombocytosis, or an increase in platelets, can be found in rheumatic fever, in asphyxiation, after surgical treatment, after splenectomy, with acute blood loss, and with some types of chemotherapy used in the treatment of leukemia.

Automated Cell-Counting Methods

Instruments for cell counting and automated differential analysis are now routinely found in most laboratories. Because automated instruments count a much larger numbers of cells than manual counting methods, there is greater precision. Thousands of particles pass through the instrument's aperture

in a few seconds. Smaller analyzers are commonly used in STAT and lower volume hematology laboratories. Larger and more complex systems are used in larger clinical and research laboratories. A significant innovation is automated front-end (preanalytical [preexamination]) instrumentation/robotics and total work cells linked by a track or conveyor.

The degree of instrumental sophistication is frequently described by the number of parameters that the instrument generates. The term, **parameter,** is a statistical term that refers to any numerical value that describes an entire population. Today, the term *data point* is also used to refer to a measured output.

Counting of the cellular elements of the blood (erythrocytes, leukocytes, and platelets) can be based on one of two classic methods:
1. Electrical impedance
2. Optical detection

The Electrical Impedance Principle

In the basic Coulter counter cells passing through an aperture through which a current is flowing cause changes in electrical resistance that are counted as voltage pulses (Fig. 12-11). A reduced-pressure system operated by a vacuum unit draws the suspension through the aperture into a system of tubing following a column of mercury. The Coulter system is based on the principle that cells are poor electrical conductors compared with a saline diluent that is a good conductors.

A current flows through the aperture between the internal and external electrodes. Each cell that passes through the aperture displaces an equal volume of conductive solution, increasing the electrical resistance and creating a voltage pulse, because its

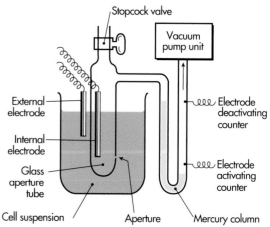

FIGURE 12-11 Schematic diagram of a cell counter based on voltage pulse–counting (Coulter principle). Cells flow through an aperture that separates two compartments. Electrical potential between electrodes changes as cells pass. Number of impulses translates to cell count, and pulse amplitude depends on cell volume that displaces conductive fluid.

resistance is much greater than that of the conductive solution. The pulses are counted. If two or more cells enter the aperture at the same time, they will be counted as one cell. This produces a *coincidence error*.

The Optical Detection Principle

In the optical or hydrodynamic focusing method of cell counting and cell sizing, laser light is used. A diluted blood specimen passes in a steady stream through which a beam of laser light is focused. As each cell passes through the sensing zone of the flow cell, it scatters the focused light. Scattered light is detected by a photodetector and converted into an electrical pulse. The number of pulses generated is directly proportional to the number of cells passing through the sensing zone in a specific period. The instrument accomplishing this task is known as a **flow cytometer**.

Light is scattered at angles proportional to the structural features of a cell as it passes through the light beam (Fig. 12-12). Most laser systems use light sensors that detect forward scatter of the beam (180 degrees from the light source) and right-angle (90-degree) scatter. Forward scatter is correlated with cell volume or density, analogous to the impedance counting of the Coulter instruments. Right-angle deflection depends on cellular contents, mainly the granularity of the cell cytoplasm. Photodetectors convert the light signals to electrical impulses that are processed by a computer. Both intrinsic and extrinsic properties of cells can be analyzed by flow cytometry. Intrinsic properties include forward- and right-angle light scatter, which correlate with size and granularity of a cell, respectively. In contrast, extrinsic properties rely on the binding of various probes to the cells. A fluorochrome dye can be employed in the cell suspension to enhance the cell identification. This dye can directly stain or tag certain cell components, such as a granule or an enzyme. The dye can be attached to an immunologic component, such as an antibody to a lymphocyte surface antigen. Different wavelengths of light excite different types of fluorochrome dyes, enabling particular tagged cells to be counted separately.

A histogram or graphic representation of output provides information about erythrocyte, leukocyte, and platelet frequency and cellular identification. The display of data (Fig. 12-13) includes cell counts, RBC indices, and white blood cell (WBC) differentials. Characteristics can be used to differentiate the various types of WBCs and to produce scatter plots with a five-part differential.

The Erythrocyte Histogram

The erythrocyte histogram reflects the native size of erythrocytes or any other particles in the erythrocyte size range. In a homogeneous cell population, the curve assumes a symmetrical bell-shaped or gaussian distribution. A wide or more flattened curve is seen when the standard deviation (SD) from the mean is increased.

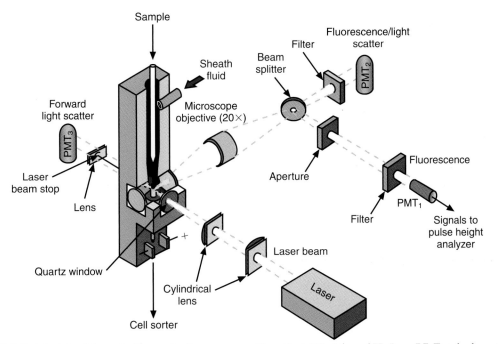

FIGURE 12-12 **Schematic diagram of a flow cytometer.** (From Burtis CA, Ashwood ER, Bruns DE: Tietz fundamentals of clinical chemistry, ed 6, St. Louis, 2008, Saunders.)

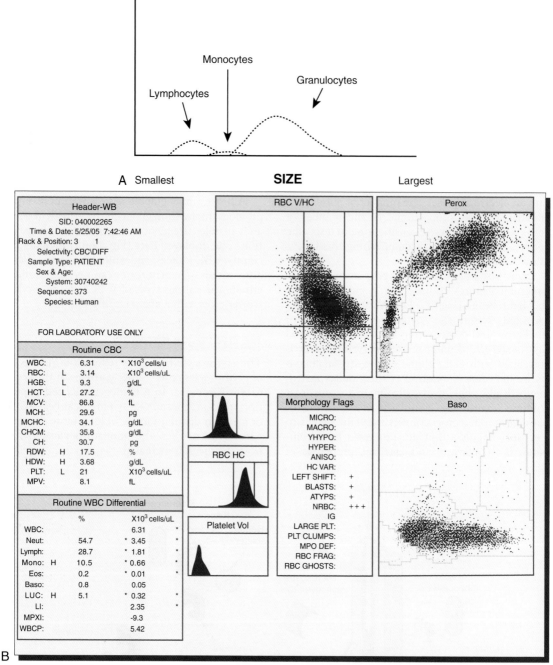

FIGURE 12-13 **A, Normal Coulter CBC readout. B, Abnormal Coulter CBC readout. (B,** From Rodak BF, Fritsma GA, Keohane EM: Hematology: clinical principles and applications, ed 4, St Louis, 2012, Saunders.)

Red Cell Distribution Width

A new parameter, the RDW, expresses the coefficient of variation of the erythrocyte volume distribution. It is calculated directly from the histogram. A portion of the curve at the extreme ends is excluded from the computation to exclude clumps of platelets, large platelets, or electrical interference on the left side of the curve. The portion of the right side of the curve that is excluded represents grouped or clumped erythrocytes.

The RDW is calculated by dividing the SD by the mean of the red cell size distribution.

$$RDW = \frac{SD}{Mean\ size} \times 100$$

The RDW is expressed numerically as the coefficient of variation percentage. The normal range is 11.5% to 14.5%. The RDW is increased above the normal limits in iron deficiency, vitamin B12 deficiency, and folic acid deficiency. In the hemoglobinopathies, the RDW is increased in proportion to the degree of anemia that accompanies the hemoglobin disorder.

The Leukocyte Histogram

Size-referenced leukocyte histograms display the classification of leukocytes according to size following lysis. It does not display the native cell size. The lytic reagent causes a cytochemical reaction. As a result of the reaction, the cytoplasm collapses around the nucleus, producing differential shrinkage. Therefore the histogram of leukocyte subpopulations reflects the sorting of these cells by their relative size, which is primarily related to their nuclear size.

The histogram differentiates lymphocytes, mononuclear cells, and granulocytes. Mononuclear cells include blasts or other immature cells, such as promyelocytes and myelocytes, as well as monocytes; however, in a normal specimen, monocytes represent the mononuclear cells.

Platelet Histograms

Platelet counting and sizing in both the electrical impedance and optical systems reflect the native cell size. In the electrical impedance method, counting and sizing take place in the RBC aperture. In the optical system, forward light scatter pattern discrimination between erythrocytes and platelets in the flow cell determines the platelet count and frequency distribution.

MEAN PLATELET VOLUME CALCULATION

The MPV is a measure of the average volume of platelets in a sample. It is derived from the same data as the platelet count. The volume increases as the platelet count decreases. Because of this inverse relationship, the MPV and the platelet count must be considered together.

PLATELET DISTRIBUTION WIDTH

The PDW is a measure of the uniformity of platelet size in a blood specimen. This parameter serves as a validity check and monitors false results. A normal PDW is less than 20%.

RADIO FREQUENCY

In this newer application, high-voltage electromagnetic current is used to detect cell size, based on the cellular density. The radio frequency (RF) pulse is directly proportional to the nuclear size and density of a cell. RF or conductivity is related to the nuclear-cytoplasmic ratio, nuclear density, and cytoplasmic granulation.

Types of Automated Cell Counting Instruments

Major types of automation are representative of the ways that blood cells can be counted, leukocytes differentiated, and other components calculated. Hemoglobin is measured by the traditional cyanmethemoglobin flow-cell method at 525 and 546 nm or with a cyanide free compound by other instrument manufacturers. Larger instruments (see Evolve submitted for chapter 10) have more detailed data output. Technology continues to deliver new automation capabilities in hematology.

Quality Control

All automated methods require the use of quality assurance measures (see Chapter 8), including the use of quality control materials to ensure that the instrument is functioning correctly and that valid results are reported.

Reference Values*

Red blood cell (RBC) count ($\times 10^{12}/L$):

1 to 2 days of age (capillary blood)	4.0-6.6 $\times 10^{12}/L$
3 to 6 months	3.1-4.5 $\times 10^{12}/L$
6-12 years	4.0-5.2 $\times 10^{12}/L$
21 years and older	
Men	4.5-5.9 $\times 10^{12}/L$
Women	4.5-5.1 $\times 10^{12}/L$

Hemoglobin

1 to 2 days of age	14.5-22.5 g/dL
3-6 months	9.5-13.5 g/dL
6-12 years	11.5-15.5 g/dL
21 years and older	
Male	13.5-17.5 g/dL
Female	12.0-16.0 g/dL

White blood cell (WBC) count ($\times 10^9/L$):

1 day of age (capillary blood) 9.4-34.0 $\times 10^9/L$
6 months 6.0-17.5 $\times 10^9/L$
10 years, 4.5-13.5 $\times 10^9/L$
21 years and older 4.4-11.3 $\times 10^9/L$

Platelet counts ($\times 10^9/L$): 150 to 450 $\times 10^9/L$

---

*Greer JP, et al: Wintrobes's clinical hematology, ed 11, Philadelphia, 2004, Lippincott Williams & Wilkins, pp 2697–2719.

EXAMINATION OF THE PERIPHERAL BLOOD FILM

Microscopic examination of the peripheral blood is done by preparing, staining, and examining a thin smear of blood on a slide. With the use of automatic counting devices that determine hemoglobin, hematocrit, and red cell, white cell, and platelet counts, together with MCV, MCH, MCHC, RDW, WBC differential, and histograms, there is a tendency to place less emphasis on the routine examination of the peripheral blood film (Procedure 12-2).

Traditionally, the microscopic examination of the peripheral blood film has been used to study the morphology of RBCs (erythrocytes), WBCs (leukocytes), and platelets. The percentage of each cell type present in a peripheral blood film can be determined by direct microscopic observation, the **white blood cell (leukocyte) differential.** An additional examination of the bone marrow may be necessary in certain cases, but this is not a routine procedure. Platelets are also routinely assessed in clinical hematologic studies by observing their number and morphology in the peripheral blood film.

Sources of Blood for the Blood Film

Fresh blood from a finger or heel puncture can be used for morphologic examination of the white and red cells. CLSI has deleted the use of the big toe as a site for collecting peripheral blood because of the lack of documentation supporting or discouraging blood collection from this site.[5]

The finger must not be squeezed excessively to obtain the drop of blood, and it must not be touched with the slide. Only the drop of blood should touch the slide. Any oils or moisture from the finger will lead to a poorly prepared film.

Most of the work in the hematology laboratory is done on venous blood. EDTA is the anticoagulant of choice. EDTA preserves the morphologic features of the white and red cells and gives a more even distribution of the platelets. If blood is collected in EDTA for morphologic studies, the film should be prepared as soon as possible, certainly within 2 hours.

PROCEDURE **12-2**

Leukocyte Differential Count

PRINCIPLE

A stained smear is examined to determine the percentage of each type of leukocyte present and assess the erythrocyte and platelet morphology. Increases in any of the normal leukocyte types or the presence of immature leukocytes or erythrocytes in peripheral blood are important diagnostically in a wide variety of inflammatory disorders and leukemias. Erythrocyte abnormalities are clinically important in various anemias. Platelet size irregularities suggest particular thrombocyte disorders.

SPECIMEN

Peripheral blood, bone marrow, and body fluid sediments, such as spinal fluid, are appropriate specimens. Whole-blood smears may be made from EDTA-anticoagulated blood or prepared from free-flowing capillary blood. Smears should be made within 1 hour of blood collection from EDTA specimens stored at room temperature to avoid distortion of cell morphology. Unstained smears can be stored for indefinite periods, but stained smears gradually fade.

REAGENTS, SUPPLIES, AND EQUIPMENT
- A manual cell counter designed for differential counts
- Microscope, immersion oil, and lens paper

QUALITY CONTROL

A set of reference slides with established parameters should be established to assess the competence of an individual to perform differential and morphologic identification of leukocytes and erythrocytes. Participation in a quality assessment program (e.g., College of American Pathologists Proficiency Testing) continues to document performance.

PROCEDURE

1. Use a correctly prepared and stained smear.
2. Focus the microscope on the 10× (low-power) objective. Scan the smear to check for cell distribution, clumping, and abnormal cells. Add a drop of immersion oil, and switch to the 100× (oil-immersion) objective.

Begin the count by determining a suitable area. Extend the examination from the area where approximately half the erythrocytes are barely overlapping to an area where the erythrocytes touch each other.

PROCEDURE **12-2** (Continued)

If an areas is too thick, cellular details such as nuclear chromatin patterns are difficult to examine. In areas that are too thin, distortion of cells makes it risky to identify a cell type.

3. Count the leukocytes using a tracking pattern. Each cell identified should be immediately recorded as a neutrophil (band) or polymorphonuclear neutrophil (PMN), lymphocyte, monocyte, eosinophil, or basophil. (See Table 12-6 and text discussion for a brief leukocyte morphology reference.)

4. Abnormalities of leukocytes, erythrocytes, and platelets should be noted. Nucleated erythrocytes are not included in the total count but are noted per 100 white blood cells (WBCs). A total of at least 100 leukocytes should be counted. Express the results as a percentage of total leukocytes counted.

REPORTING RESULTS

Reference values, particularly the band neutrophil percentage, may vary. Values for children differ from adult reference values.

Comparison of Normal Leukocyte Values in Peripheral Blood (Adult)

	Neutrophil	*Lymphocyte*	*Monocyte*	*Eosinophil*	*Basophil*
Average percentage	59%	34%	4%	2.7%	0.3%

PROCEDURE NOTES

Less than 2% of the leukocytes should be disrupted or unidentifiable forms. If a disrupted cell is clearly identifiable, include it in the differential count. Classify unidentifiable or disrupted cells as "other," and note them on the report if more than a few are observed.

PREPARATION OF BUFFY COAT SMEARS

Principle

An anticoagulated specimen is centrifuged to separate the specimen physically into three layers: plasma, leukocytes and platelets, and erythrocytes. The interface layer between the plasma and erythrocytes is referred to as the buffy coat. If this layer of concentrated cells is removed by pipetting, push wedge–type smears can subsequently be prepared and stained for microscopic examination. This technique is useful in the performance of leukocyte differential counts on patients with extremely low total leukocyte counts or in special testing procedures.

Specimen

A freshly drawn specimen of EDTA-anticoagulated whole blood is needed.

PROCEDURE

1. Centrifuge the specimen of whole anticoagulated blood for at least 5 minutes at 2000 to 2500 rpm.

2. With a Pasteur pipette, remove most of the top plasma layer and discard.

3. The interface layer, along with a small amount of plasma and a small volume of erythrocytes, can then be removed using a Pasteur pipette.

4. A drop of this suspension can be placed on a microscope slide and a push-wedge smear prepared. Air-dry and stain.

CLINICAL APPLICATIONS

Selected disorders are associated with increases in normal leukocytes. An increase in neutrophils is associated with bacterial infections, inflammation, or chronic leukemias. An increase in lymphocytes is associated with viral infections. Increased eosinophils are observed in active allergies and invasive parasites.

REFERENCES

Clinical and Laboratory Standards Institute: Reference leukocyte differential count (proportional) and evaluation of instrumental methods: approved standard, Wayne, PA, 1992, H20-A.

DeNunzio J: Preparation of buffy coats from blood samples with extremely low white cell count, Lab Med 16:497, 1985.

Turgeon M: Clinical hematology, ed 4, Philadelphia, 2005, Lippincott Williams & Wilkins.

Preparation of the Blood Film

Blood is most often examined under the microscope by preparing a thin film or smear of blood on a slide or a coverglass, fixing the blood film, then staining it with a polychromatic stain (Fig. 12-14). Smears can also be prepared by centrifugation; centrifugal force is used to spread a monolayer of blood cells over the surface of a slide.

Coverglass Blood Films

When a coverglass is used to prepare a blood film, more of the prepared film can be examined, which reduces the sampling error. With a slide, only a relatively small counting area can be examined. In addition, the leukocytes and platelets are more evenly distributed on a coverglass. The disadvantages of the coverglass method are that it is more

time consuming, more difficult to learn and perform correctly, and requires more care in handling of the preparations. Automatic staining devices are available for slides, but not for coverglasses.

Wedge Blood Films

Although the coverglass method is recommended by many hematologists, the slide (push-wedge) blood film method is much more frequently used (Fig. 12-15 and Procedure 12-3). It is the method used by CLSI for the reference leukocyte differential count to evaluate any leukocyte method.[6] The directions for the examination of the blood film can also be applied to the coverglass method. The correct interpretation of a blood film requires:
1. Correct preparation of the blood film
2. Proper staining
3. Accurate examination

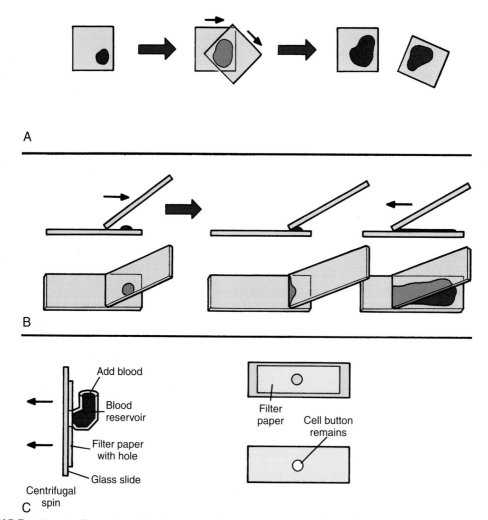

FIGURE 12-14 Preparation of blood smears. A, Coverglass preparation. Drop of blood or marrow is spread between two coverglasses as they are pulled in opposite directions. B, Wedge smear. Drop of blood is pulled across slide by another slide at an acute angle, creating a wedge-shaped smear with a decreasing cell density. C, Centrifugal smear. Drop of blood is spun from a central point, creating an evenly dispersed monolayer of cells. (Redrawn from Powers LW: Diagnostic hematology, St Louis, 1989, Mosby.)

The equipment used for making blood films must be meticulously clean. Use of a spreading device is recommended; for example, a margin-free spreader slide with ground-glass edges may be used to spread the film of blood on the clean, lint-free slide. The edges of the spreader slide must be clean and free from chips. Coverglasses held by a suitable clip or holder can also be used as spreading devices. The spreading device must be cleaned thoroughly with alcohol and dried between films, and it must be discarded when chipped or broken.

Cytocentrifuged Blood Films

With the use of a cytocentrifuge, a monolayer of cells can be prepared. These centrifuges facilitate rapid spreading of the cells across a slide from a central point by virtue of their high-torque, low-inertia motors. With a cytocentrifuged preparation, cellular destruction and artifacts present in the wedge slide method are eliminated. Only small volumes of a sample are used, and the cells are evenly distributed and less distorted, producing better conditions for critical morphologic studies. They are especially useful for other body fluids, such as cerebrospinal, pleural, or synovial fluid or urine.

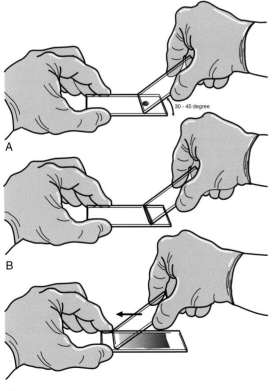

A

B

C

FIGURE 12-15 **Slide (push-wedge) technique for preparing a peripheral blood smear.** (From Rodak BF, Fritsma GA, Doig K: Hematology: clinical principles and applications, ed 3, St Louis, 2007, Saunders.)

Criteria and Precautions for a Good Blood Film

A well-made blood film (Fig. 12-16) should satisfy certain criteria when observed macroscopically:

1. The body of the blood film should be smooth and not interrupted by ridges, waves, or holes.
2. The blood smear should be thickest at the origin and gradually thin out, rather than having alternating thick and thin areas. Pushing the spreader slide with an uneven motion results in thicker and thinner areas in the body of the film.
3. A good blood film should cover half to three-fourths the length of the slide. All of the initial drop of blood should be incorporated into the film, not just part of it.
4. The thin end of the smear should have a good feather edge. The film should fade away without a defined border on the end. In some institutions, a fairly straight feather edge is sought; others prefer a more tonguelike edge.
5. A defined border at the end of a blood film indicates that most of the WBCs have piled up at the end. When this occurs, the heavier neutrophils accumulate at the end to a greater extent than the other WBC types, giving an incorrect distribution of the WBC types in the body of the smear. Platelets also tend to accumulate at the end of a smear, decreasing the number in the body of the smear. This will also result in inaccurate percentages for the cell types within the body of the film, because the relatively stickier neutrophils and platelets tend to concentrate in such tails.
6. Slides should be made in one motion. The drop of blood should be placed on the slide and the smear made immediately; drying of the blood drop will lead to uneven distribution of cells in the body of the film, and the larger WBCs will accumulate at the end. Rouleaux formation of the RBCs and platelet clumping will also occur if the blood is not spread immediately.
7. Pressing down on the spreader slide will also lead to an accumulation of WBCs and platelets at the end. This is why the spreader slide should be evenly balanced between the finger and thumb.
8. The degree of thickness or thinness of the blood film is also important. When a film is too thick, the cells pile up, making them difficult to count and obscuring their morphology. A very thin film is satisfactory for morphologic studies, but it may be tedious to examine. The thickness of the film is determined by the size of the drop of blood used, the speed of the stroke used to move the spreader slide, and the angle at which the

Making a Blood Film (Push-Wedge Slide Method)

1. Place a drop of capillary or well-mixed venous blood preserved with EDTA on one end of a slide, on the midline about 1 cm from the end. The drop should be about 2 mm in diameter (about the size of a match head), as shown in Fig. 12-22. Venous blood must be well mixed by gentle inversion at least 15 times; it should also be checked for clots. If capillary blood is used, touch the top of the drop to the slide, being careful not to let the skin touch the slide. Transfer venous blood to the slide with the aid of two wooden applicator sticks or a plain capillary pipette.

2. Lay the specimen slide on a flat surface, and hold it in position at the left end (these directions are for a right-handed person) with the middle finger or thumb and index finger of the left hand (see Figs. 12-21 and 12-22).

3. Place the smooth clean edge of the spreader slide on the specimen slide just in front (to the left of) the drop of blood (see Figs. 12-21 and 12-22).

4. Using the right hand, balance the spreader slide on one or two fingers (e.g., the middle finger or the index and middle fingers) and draw it backward into the drop of blood at an angle of approximately 45 degrees to the specimen slide.

5. Decrease the spreader slide angle to about 25 to 30 degrees, and allow the blood to flow evenly across the edge of the spreader slide (see Fig. 12-22).

6. When the blood has spread evenly across the edge of the spreader slide, quickly push the spreader slide over the entire length of the specimen slide. As the spreader is moved, a thin film of blood will be deposited behind it. The blood film should take up half to three-fourths of the slide when properly prepared (see Fig. 12-23). The goal is to achieve a wedge-shaped smear with a thin, feathery edge.

7. Turn the spreader slide over (this gives another clean edge) and prepare a second blood film, using the same procedure. Two films should always be prepared for the same blood specimen.

8. Dry the blood film immediately. If it is not dried quickly, the blood cells will shrink and appear distorted.

9. Label the film by writing the name of the patient and the date in the dried blood at the thick end of the film, using a lead pencil (see Fig. 12-23).

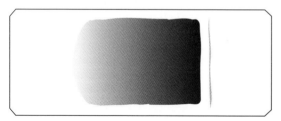

FIGURE 12-16 Well-made peripheral blood smear. (From Rodak BF, Fritsma GA, Doig K: Hematology: clinical principles and applications, ed 3, St Louis, 2007, Saunders.)

spreader slide is moved. A thick film results when the drop of blood is large, the angle is greater than 45 degrees, and the spreading motion is fast. A thin film results when the drop of blood is small, the angle is less than 30 degrees, and the motion is slow.

9. Blood films with vacuoles or bubbles result from the use of dirty slides or in some cases from an excess of fat in the specimen (e.g., specimen obtained after a fatty meal).

Only a small part of a blood film is actually examined microscopically. This part is referred to as the *examination area* or *counting area*, as shown in Fig. 12-17. The counting area must be one where the red and white cells are clearly separated and well distributed, with the RBCs barely touching each other.

Fig. 12-18 provides examples of unacceptable blood smears.

Staining the Blood Film

After a blood film has been prepared, the next step is promptly staining the blood smear. If it cannot be stained within a few hours, it should be fixed by immersion in absolute methyl alcohol (methanol) for 1 or 2 seconds and air dried. If this is not done, the slides will stain with a pale-blue background of dried plasma.

The stain most often used for the examination of blood films is **Wright's stain** or a variation, **Wright-Giemsa stain** (Procedure 12-4). Both Wright's and Wright-Giemsa stain are adaptations of polychrome Romanowsky stains. Such polychrome stains produce multiple colors when applied to cells because these stains are composed of both basic and acidic aniline dyes. Romanowsky stains contain *methylene blue* (a basic dye), *eosin* (an acidic dye), and *methylene azure* (an oxidation product of methylene blue also referred to as *polychrome methylene blue*). Variations of the Romanowsky stains differ in the way the methylene azure is produced or added to the stains.

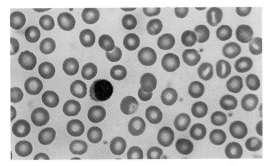

FIGURE 12-17 Stained peripheral blood smear demonstrating appropriate area in which to perform WBC differential and morphology assessment and platelet estimate. Entire field would contain 200 to 250 RBCs (×1000). (From Carr JH, Rodak BF: Clinical hematology atlas, ed 3, St Louis, 2009, Saunders.)

Polychrome stains produce multiple colors because they dye both acidic and basic cell components in an acid-base reaction. The acidic cell components, such as nuclei (nuclear DNA) and cytoplasmic RNA, are stained blue-violet by the basic methylene azure. They are called **basophilic** because they stain with the basic dye. The more basic cell components, such as hemoglobin and eosinophilic granules, are stained orange to pink and are called **acidophilic** because they stain with the acidic dye. Some structures within cells stain with both components, such as the neutrophilic granules, whereas the azurophilic granules stain with methylene azure.

The staining method for blood films fixes dead cells, as opposed to **supravital staining,** which is used with living cells. **Fixation** is the process by which the blood is made to adhere to the slide and the cellular proteins are coagulated. Wright's stain and Wright-Giemsa stain are used as methanol solutions. The blood cells are fixed by the methanol in the first step of the staining reaction, when

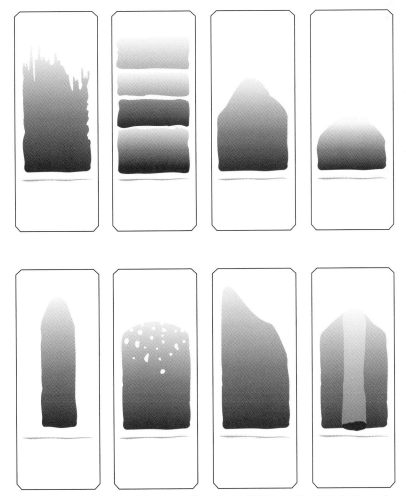

FIGURE 12-18 **Examples of unacceptable smears.** (From Rodak BF, Fritsma GA, Doig K: Hematology: clinical principles and applications, ed 3, St Louis, 2007, Saunders.)

Staining Blood Films Using Wright-Giemsa Stain

1. Place the dried blood film on a level staining rack, with the film side up and the feather edge away from you. Allow the dried film to set at least 5 minutes before staining is begun.

2. Fix the film by flooding the slide with the filtered stain. The amount of stain is important. There must be enough to avoid excessive evaporation, which would result in precipitation of stain on the slide.

3. Allow the stain to remain on the slide for 3 to 5 minutes. This is the fixation period. Determine the exact timing for each batch of stain used.

4. Without removing the Wright-Giemsa stain, add phosphate buffer, using about 1 to 1½ times as much buffer as stain on the slide so that a layer piles up but none spills off. Add the buffer drop-wise; then blow on the surface to mix the stain and buffer. A metallic greenish sheen should form on the surface when the slide is buffered adequately.

5. Allow the stain and buffer mixture to remain on the slide for 10 to 15 minutes. During this time, the staining takes place as a result of the combination of dye and buffer at the correct pH.

6. Wash the slide with a steady stream of deionized water. Precipitation of the metallic scum on the film must be avoided. This is done by first flooding the slide with water, then washing and tipping the slide simultaneously. If this is not done and the dye is poured off the slide before it is washed, the insoluble metallic scum will settle on the blood film.

7. Wipe the dye from the back of the slide when it is still wet by rubbing with a piece of moist gauze.

8. Place the slide in a vertical position to air dry, with the feather edge (thin edge) up. Never blot a blood film dry. The heaviest part of the film is at the bottom to allow precipitated stain to flow away from the edge, which will be used for examination of the blood film.

9. Do not use the slide for microscopic examination until it is dry.

the Wright's or Wright-Giemsa dye mixture is added to the blood film. Heat can also be used for fixation, but it is not necessary when the stain contains methanol. The actual polychrome staining of the blood film takes place in the second step of the procedure, when an aqueous phosphate buffer solution with a pH of 6.4 is added to the Wright-Giemsa dye.

Wright's stain or Wright-Giemsa stain can be purchased as a dry powder, which is diluted in absolute, anhydrous, acetone-free methyl alcohol (chemically pure [CP]), or as a prepared methanol solution. Both powders and solutions are certified by the Biological Stain Commission.[7] The preparation of methylene azure by oxidation of methylene blue and addition of eosin is quite complex, so Wright's stain powder may vary slightly from lot to lot. This necessitates determination of fixing and staining times for each new batch.

Rapid-Staining Methods Using a Dipping Technique

Modification of Wright's stain has been incorporated into various commercially available quick-staining methods. Blood films are prepared in the classic way, usually by the wedge method, and then

stained. Each commercial product is somewhat different, so the manufacturer's instructions must be carefully followed. The advantage of these products is that they are faster to use than the traditional Wright-staining method described earlier. Slides are usually dipped into each of the various staining reagents, with only a few seconds being taken for each step. For critical morphologic studies, the traditional Wright's stain should be used because some of the morphologic detail is lost when certain quick stains are used.

The traditional Wright-staining technique has also been adapted to a "boat" or container staining method. Slides are placed (feather edge up) in slide holders and moved at specific times to containers filled with (1) acetone-free methyl alcohol, (2) Wright-Giemsa stain, and (3) Wright's stain mixed with phosphate buffer, then rinsed by being dipped five times each in three separate containers of deionized water.

Characteristics of Properly Stained Blood Film

If the blood film has been stained properly, it will appear more pink when observed with the naked eye. When examined microscopically with the low-power (10×) objective, the film should be thin enough so that the red and white cells are clearly separated. There should not be an excessive accumulation of WBCs and platelets at the edge of the film. In addition, there should be no precipitated stain.

The RBCs should appear red-orange through the microscope. Correctly stained leukocytes should have the following colors under the microscope. The lymphocytes and neutrophils should have dark-purple nuclei, and the monocyte nuclei should be a lighter purple. The granules should be bright orange in the eosinophils and dark blue in the basophils. The appearance of the cytoplasm varies with the type of leukocyte. In monocytes the cytoplasm should be blue-gray or have a faint bluish tinge. The neutrophil cytoplasm should be light pink with lilac granules, and the lymphocyte cytoplasm should be a shade of blue, generally clear blue or robin's-egg blue. The platelets should stain violet to purple. If the blood film does not meet these criteria, it should be discarded, and a new film should be stained and examined.

Precautions and Sources of Error When Staining Blood Films

1. When the blood film is being stained, it is important that the staining rack be level so the stain is uniform throughout the film.
2. It is important that the stain and buffer be made correctly. When prepared in the laboratory, the stain should stand for 1 month before it is used. Wright's and Wright-Giemsa stains can be purchased ready to use. These reagents must be checked out carefully before being used for daily staining needs.
3. The pH of the buffer must be correct. With every new batch of stain and buffer, the fixing and staining times should be checked by staining a few slides. If staining of the cells is satisfactory, the times used for fixing and staining should be noted and used with that batch of reagents. If the pH is too acid or too alkaline, the stain will give a false color and appearance to the cells.
4. Adequate fixing time must be allowed. A minimum of 3 minutes is recommended for the initial reaction of the blood film and Wright-Giemsa stain. Inadequate fixation allows dissolution of the nuclear chromatin, so overfixation is preferable. To achieve the proper staining reactions in the cells, the correct timing must be determined for each batch of stain and buffer, and the correct staining technique must be used.
5. Properly applied Wright-Giemsa stain dyes both acidic and basic components of the blood cells. The phosphate buffer controls the pH of the staining system. If the pH is too acid, the parts of the cell taking up acidic dye will be overstained and will appear too red, whereas the parts of the cells taking up basic dye will appear pale. If the pH of the staining system is *too alkaline*, the parts of the cells taking up basic dye will be overstained, giving an overall blue effect, with dark-blue to black nuclear chromatin and bluish RBCs.

The following situations will indicate staining errors:

- A *faded or washed-out appearance* of all the cells is caused by overwashing, understaining, or underfixing; leaving water on the slide; or using improperly made stain.
- When the slide has an *excessively blue appearance* on gross examination, the RBCs will appear blue-red and the WBCs will be darker and more granular microscopically. This may result from overfixing or overstaining, inadequate washing, using a stain or buffer that is too alkaline, or using too thick a film. It may be corrected by decreasing the fixation time (time before buffer is added to dye) or increasing the time during which the buffer and stain mixture stands on the slide. Alternatively, the amount of stain used may be decreased and the amount of buffer increased. Finally, the pH of the buffer may be checked with a pH meter and readjusted to 6.4, or a new Wright-Giemsa stain may be tried.
- When the slide has an *excessively red appearance* to the naked eye, the RBCs will appear bright red, the WBCs will appear indistinct with pale-blue rather than purple nuclei, and brilliant-red eosinophilic granules will be seen microscopically. This may be caused by understaining, overwashing, or use of stain, buffer, or wash water that is too acidic. To correct this situation, the following measures may be taken. The fixation or staining time may be increased. The washing technique may be corrected so that it is adequate but not excessive. The pH of the buffer and water may be checked with a pH meter and adjusted, or a new stain or buffer may be used.
- *Large amounts of precipitated stain* on the film result from either improper washing (not washing enough to remove the metallic scum) or using an old stain that has started to precipitate. This may be corrected by using the proper washing technique—first flooding the slide with water and then tipping and washing the slide simultaneously—and making sure that the stain is filtered daily.

Examination of the Blood Film: General Comments

Accurate examination of the blood film depends on proper use of the microscope (see Chapter 5). The film is first examined with the low-power (10×) objective, with the slide being moved with the mechanical stage to position different areas into the field of view. The difference in appearance of the various areas results from the technique used in preparing the film: the film is relatively thick at the beginning and gradually thins out to a feather edge. Most of the cells seen under the low-power objective are RBCs, which appear as small, round, reddish orange bodies.

Scattered among the red-staining cells are the less numerous WBCs, which are larger and more complex in appearance than the RBCs. The WBCs consist of nuclei surrounded by cytoplasm. The nuclei stain purple, and the cytoplasms stain different colors depending on their contents. The size of the cell; the shape, size, and chromatin pattern of the nucleus; the presence of nucleoli in the nucleus; and the contents, staining reaction, and relative size of the cytoplasm are used in the identification of WBCs.

With the low-power objective, an area of the film is found where the RBCs are just touching and are not overlapping or piled on top of one another (see Fig. 12-18). This area will be found near the feather edge of the film. The color of the cells should be examined at this magnification. When this area has been found, the oil-immersion (100×) objective should be used next. The high-dry (43×) objective is not suitable for examination of blood films, because important morphologic changes cannot be seen at this magnification. To change to the oil-immersion lens, the low-power objective is moved out of position, and a drop of immersion oil is placed on the selected area of the blood film. The oil-immersion lens is moved into the oil while the viewer looks at it from the side. The oil must be in direct contact with the lens. If necessary, it can be focused with the fine adjustment. If the slide has been placed upside down on the microscope stage, it will be impossible to bring the blood cells into focus. More light will be needed with the oil-immersion lens. It can be obtained by repositioning the condenser (which should be all the way up for maximum resolution under oil immersion), opening the iris diaphragm, and increasing the intensity of the light source.

Under the oil-immersion objective, RBCs appear as round, unstructured bodies containing no nuclei, granules, or discrete material. The red color is darker at the edge of the cell than in the center. This variation is caused by the biconcave shape of the red cell, which contains less pigment (hemoglobin) in its thinner center. With oil immersion, most RBCs in a normal blood film are about the same size, averaging 7.2 μm in diameter. A normal RBC is uniformly round on a dry film, although variations in shape can be produced by poor spreading technique in the preparation of the blood film.

The blood film must first be evaluated for acceptable gross appearance and staining. It must be evaluated for acceptable WBC distribution by observing the feather edge under low power. The number of leukocytes and platelets should be estimated, and the erythrocyte and platelet morphology should be described.

Microscopic Examination of the Blood Film

After the initial preparations, manipulation of the microscope, and observations previously described, the following steps are taken in the examination of every blood film. Generally, the blood film is under low power and oil immersion. The general steps are outlined here and described in the following sections.

Low-power examination (10× objective) includes:
1. Evaluation of the overall quality of the blood film
2. Estimate of the leukocyte count
3. Scan of the blood film for abnormal cells and clumps of platelets

Oil-immersion examination (100× objective) includes:
1. Examination of the erythrocytes for alterations and variations in morphology
2. Estimation of platelet count and evaluation of morphologic changes
3. Differential count of the leukocytes
4. Examination of the leukocytes for morphologic alterations

Low-Power (10× Objective) Examination

1. *Evaluate the quality of the blood film.* The film should be thin enough that the red and white cells are clearly separated. The space between the cells should be clear. There should be no precipitated dye. The red and white cells should be properly stained, and there should be no large accumulation of WBCs at the feather edge of the blood film. If the blood film does not meet these criteria, it should not be examined further; a new film must be made.
2. *Estimate the red and white cell counts.* A rough estimate of the RBC count as increased, decreased, or normal can be made by noting the number of cells and the space between them.

Normally, fewer and fewer intercellular spaces will be seen as the observer moves into the thicker portion of the blood film. In the optimal counting area, there should be no agglutination (clumping) or rouleaux formation (cells stacked like coins). The optimal counting area is generally two to three microscope fields in from the feather edge.

To find the optimal counting area, focus on the feather edge, then begin moving into the body of the blood film. At the very thin edge of the film, about one or two microscope fields into the body of the blood film, the RBCs flatten out, appear completely filled with hemoglobin (showing no area of central pallor), and are generally distorted and show a cobblestone appearance. In the thick end of the film, the morphologic characteristics of all cell types are difficult to distinguish, and the RBCs show an apparent rouleaux formation (see Fig. 12-18).

The number of WBCs is estimated in the optimal counting area of the film. With the low-power (10×) objective and the usual 10× eyepiece (a total magnification of 100 times), five leukocytes in one low-power field are equal to approximately 1000 cells per microliter, or the number of cells per low-power field times 200 equals the number of cells per microliter. In other words, 5 WBCs in one low-power field are equal to a WBC count of approximately 1×10^9/L; thus the number of WBCs per low-power field divided by 5 is equal to the number of cells $\times 10^9$ per liter.

As a general observation, approximately 20 to 30 WBCs per field are equivalent to a WBC count of approximately 5×10^9/L. Under the same magnification, 40 to 60 WBCs per field are equivalent to a WBC count of approximately 10×10^9/L.

3. *Scan the blood film for abnormal cells and clumps of platelets.* The slide should also be examined under low power for the presence of immature or abnormal cells. With experience, the cells may be recognizable under low power; however, they are positively identified under oil immersion. If very few such abnormal cells are present, they may be overlooked if the slide is examined under oil immersion alone, in which the examination area is much smaller. Such abnormal cells should be sought especially in the feather edge and along the sides of the slide.

The optimal counting area, sides, and feather edge should also be scanned for clumps of platelets. Clumps of platelets should not be seen normally; however, when the platelet count is increased, they may be found along the sides and in the feather edge.

Oil-Immersion (100× Objective) Examination

1. *Examine the red cells for alterations and variations in morphologic features.* The normal RBC is a nonnucleated, biconcave disk containing hemoglobin. Most RBCs measure 7.2 to 7.9 μm on a stained blood film. The normal RBC is approximately 2 μm thick. The mean volume, calculated from the hematocrit and the RBC count, is 87 fL. In estimating the diameters of WBCs or other structures, it is often advantageous to use the RBC as a 7-μm measuring stick.

When normal RBCs are studied on dried and stained blood films, they are almost uniform in size, shape, and color. Such normal-appearing cells are referred to as *normocytic* (normal size) and *normochromic* (normal color).

The normal RBC appears as a disk with a rim of hemoglobin and a clear central area, referred to as *central pallor*. The area of central pallor is normally less than one-third the RBC's diameter, although there is some variation within the film. The amount of color in the cell (the staining reaction) and the corresponding amount of central pallor reflect the amount of hemoglobin in the cell. Normal RBCs are pink. The staining reaction is referred to in terms of **chromasia,** and RBCs with a normal amount of color are referred to as *normochromic* or, less frequently, *orthochromatic.* Normochromic, normocytic RBCs are shown in Fig. 12-19.

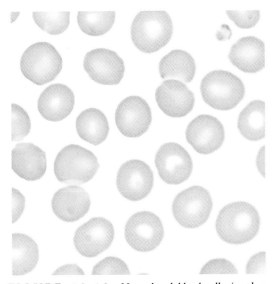

FIGURE 12-19 **Normal red blood cells (erythrocytes).** (From Carr JH, Rodak BF: Clinical hematology atlas, ed 3, St Louis, 2009, Saunders.)

It is important to observe RBC morphology only in the optimal counting area that is found by using the low-power (10×) objective. When RBCs are examined morphologically, the following characteristics must be observed and noted:

a. Variations in color
b. Variations in size (anisocytosis)
c. Variations in shape (poikilocytosis)
d. Variations in structure and inclusions
e. Presence of artifacts and abnormal distribution patterns
f. Presence of nucleated red cells

Various terms are used to describe changes in the RBC size, shape, and staining reaction. The degree of the observed RBC alteration is noted as slight, moderate, or marked. The previous morphologic alterations of erythrocytes are further described as follows:

a. *Variations in color or staining reaction.* The normal amount of hemoglobin and normal staining is referred to as **normochromia.** A decrease in color caused by reduced hemoglobin content is called **hypochromia.** Variation in staining color (pinkish blue) is called *polychromatophilia.*

b. *Alterations in size.* An overall excessive variation in cell size is referred to as **anisocytosis.** The degree of anisocytosis is reflected by the RDW. Examples of anisocytosis include:
   • Macrocytosis
   • Microcytosis

c. *Alterations in shape.* An overall abnormal variation in shape is referred to as **poikilocytosis.** Examples of poikilocytosis include:
   • Spherocytes
   • Schistocytes
   • Sickle cells, or drepanocytes
   • Ovalocytes
   • Target cells

d. *Red cell inclusions.* Several inclusions are also seen under certain conditions in the RBCs, and they must be identified. Examples include:
   • Basophilic stippling
   • Siderocytes
   • Howell-Jolly bodies

e. Abnormal red cell distribution. This includes:
   • Rouleaux formation
   • Agglutination

f. *Presence of nucleated red cells.* When nucleated metarubricytes (normoblasts) are seen on the blood film, the number of these cells per 100 WBCs is reported. It is necessary to correct the total WBC count when nucleated RBCs are present (see earlier formula for correction).

2. Estimate the platelet count and evaluate for morphologic changes. The blood film is examined with the oil-immersion objective to estimate the number of platelets and detect morphologic alterations. The platelet count is estimated as adequate, decreased, or increased.

Platelets generally vary from 2 to 5 μm in diameter. They are ovoid structures with a colorless to pale-blue background containing centrally located, reddish to violet granules. Platelets are not cells but portions of cytoplasm pinched off from megakaryocytes (giant cells of the bone marrow). Platelets are often increased in size when the blood is being actively regenerated; their size is also a function of age, with younger cells generally being larger. Bizarre forms are also noted after splenectomy and in myelofibrosis, hemorrhagic thrombocytosis, and polycythemia vera. Giant platelets are characteristic of platelet disorders associated with thrombocytopenia and the megaloblastic anemias.

Normally, 6 to 20 platelets should be seen in each oil-immersion field, representing a normal platelet count of 150 to 450 × 10^9/L. A rough estimate of the platelet count can be made by letting each platelet seen in an oil-immersion field equal approximately 20 × 10^9/L. Values as low as 3 to 5 platelets per oil-immersion field have been considered to represent a normal platelet count. The difference in normal values is probably a result of the use of specimens from different sources. The lower value is more consistent with capillary blood, where some of the platelets are utilized in the clotting mechanism, and the higher value is consistent with anticoagulated venous blood. Estimate the platelet count as adequate, decreased, or increased and report as follows:

a. Report the platelet estimate as *adequate* if 6 to 20 platelets are seen per oil-immersion field. Several fields should be checked, and the platelets may be estimated while the WBC differential is being done.

b. Report the platelets as *decreased* if the average number of platelets is less than 6, unless the blood film was prepared on capillary blood. In the latter case, 3 to 5 platelets per oil-immersion field is normal. Before reporting as decreased, scan the slide for clumps of platelets with the low-power objective, especially at the feather edge. If the blood film is well made (without aggregates at the feather edge) and platelets can be found only with great difficulty, the platelet count is below 20 × 10^9/L, and the estimate should be reported as decreased. In addition, the tube of blood should be rechecked for the presence of clots, because platelets would be utilized in the clots and the blood film value artificially decreased.

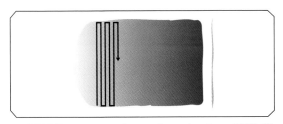

FIGURE 12-20 **Pattern for performing a WBC differential.** (From Rodak BF, Fritsma GA, Doig K: Hematology: clinical principles and applications, ed 3, St Louis, 2007, Saunders.)

c. Report the platelets as *increased* if there are more than 20 platelets per oil-immersion field. If many masses of platelets are present at the feather edge, and if platelets in the body of the film are sufficiently abundant to attract the attention of the observer, it is reasonable to assume that the platelet count is increased.

d. Observe the platelet morphology. Report the presence of large, bizarre, or atypical forms. This may be done while the leukocyte differential is being done (Fig. 12-20). This is correct.

3. *Perform the differential count of white cells.* The differential count consists of identifying and counting a minimum of 100 WBCs. After the RBCs and platelets have been examined, the WBCs are classified and counted in the optimal counting area of the blood film under oil immersion (see Procedure 12-3).

In certain situations it may be necessary to count more or fewer than 100 cells. If the relative numbers of specific types of WBCs differ greatly from the accepted normal values, it is advisable to count 200 cells or more before recording percentages. Specifically, 200 cells should be counted if more than 5% of the cells are eosinophils, if more than 2% are basophils, if more than 10% are monocytes, or if the percentage of lymphocytes is greater than 50%. If the differential for an adult with a normal WBC count shows fewer than 15 or more than 40 lymphocytes, an additional 100 cells should be counted on another blood film to rule out distribution errors.

In cases of leukopenia, if the WBC count is less than 1×10^9/L, only 50 cells need to be counted in the leukocyte differential. When such changes are made, the percentages of the different cell types must be calculated, and the number of cells actually counted in the differential must be noted on the report form—for example, "3% basophils, 200 cells counted." Occasionally the absolute number of cells of each type is of interest, although values are usually reported as percentages. To calculate the absolute value, multiply the percentage of each cell type, expressed as a decimal, by the total WBC count.

4. *Examine the leukocytes for morphologic alterations.* As the WBCs are being classified and counted, any morphologic alterations or abnormalities should be noted. A WBC cannot be skipped simply because it cannot be identified. Experience is necessary for morphologic studies of WBCs, especially when an immature or abnormal cell is seen. Persons with limited training in hematology should not attempt to identify abnormal WBCs. This should be done by a more qualified person, such as a pathologist or a clinical laboratory scientist with special hematologic training. Persons with limited training should be able to identify and classify normal WBCs but should be encouraged to seek assistance when a questionable cell is seen.

Normal Leukocyte Morphology

Five types of WBCs normally are encountered in peripheral blood: neutrophils (segmented and band), eosinophils, basophils, monocytes, and lymphocytes (Table 12-6 and Fig. 12-21). To identify leukocyte morphology, the cells should be examined for the following features:

1. Nuclear chromatin pattern
2. Nuclear shape
3. Size and number of nucleoli, when present
4. Cytoplasmic inclusions
5. Nuclear/cytoplasmic (N/C) ratio

When a blood film is stained with Wright's (a Romanowsky) stain and examined with the microscope, the majority of the cells seen will be RBCs, which appear as small, rounded, pink, or reddish orange bodies. Scattered among the red-staining cells are the less numerous leukocytes.

The leukocytes are larger and more complex in appearance than the RBCs. They consist of a nucleus surrounded by cytoplasm. Usually the nucleus is centrally located and is a prominent purple-staining body. It can be round or oval (as in the lymphocyte) or lobulated (as in the neutrophil and eosinophil). The cytoplasm, which gives the cell its shape, stains a variety of colors, depending on its contents. The size of the cell, the shape and size of the nucleus, and the staining reactions of the nucleus and the cytoplasm aid in the identification of leukocytes.

Leukocytes are categorized as granulocytes and nongranulocytes (lymphocytes). Granulocytes are leukocytes that come from the **myeloid** series of cell development. As mature cells, neutrophils, eosinophils, and basophils contain specific granulation in their cytoplasm. Monocytes are classified as myeloid cells that contain nonspecific granulation.

TABLE 12-6

Comparison of Normal Leukocytes in Peripheral Blood

Nomenclature	Nuclear Shape	Chromatin	Cytoplasmic Color	Granules	Average Percentage
Segmented neutrophil	Lobulated	Very clumped	Pink	Many, pinkish blue	56%
Band neutrophil	Curved	Moderately clumped	Blue, pink	Many, pinkish blue	3%
Lymphocyte	Round	Smooth	Light blue	Few red (azurophilic)	34%
Monocyte	Indented, folded or twisted	Lacelike	Gray	Fine, dusty blue	4%
Eosinophil	Lobulated	Very clumped	Granulated	Many, orange	2%-3%
Basophil	Lobulated	Very clumped	Granulated	Many, dark blue	0.6%

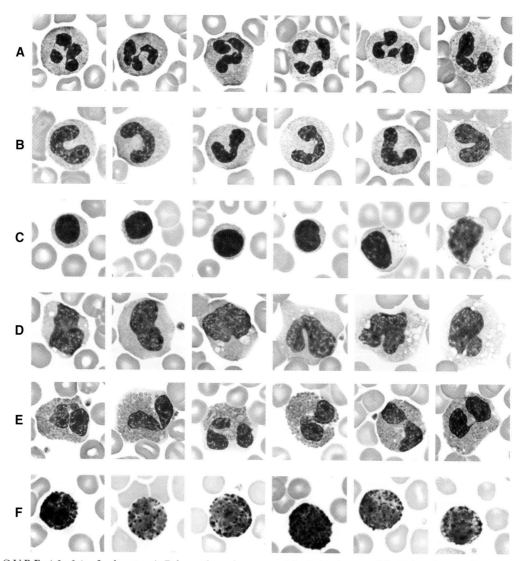

FIGURE 12-21 **Leukocytes. A, Polymorphonuclear neutrophils; B, band neutrophils; C, lymphocytes; D, monocytes; E, eosinophils; and F, basophils.** (From Carr JH, Rodak BF: Clinical hematology atlas, ed 3, St Louis, 2009, Saunders.)

Lymphocytes are cells derived from the lymphoid series of cell development. They are nongranulocytes that may contain nonspecific granulation.

Segmented Neutrophils

The most numerous of the granulocytes are polymorphonuclear neutrophil leukocytes (PMNs), or segmented neutrophil leukocytes. Neutrophils make up about 59% of the leukocytes in peripheral blood, with a range of 35% to 71%. Infants and children have fewer neutrophils and more lymphocytes.

Neutrophils are generally round cells, varying in diameter from 10 to 15 μm. The nucleus forms a relatively small part of the cell. The nucleus can assume various shapes, but it is usually lobular. That is, the nucleus is usually constricted, forming a series of lobes connected by narrow strands or filaments of chromatin; it may have two to five lobes. The nuclear chromatin is coarse and clumped and stains deep purple. These irregular chromatin masses are distinct and distinguishable from the lighter-purple parachromatin. The nuclear membrane is distinct, and no nucleoli are visible. The N/C ratio is 1:3. The abundant cytoplasm is colorless or faintly pink and contains a large number of very small, often indiscrete, lilac specific neutrophilic granules distributed irregularly throughout it. A variable number of nonspecific azurophilic granules may be present.

Band Neutrophils

The band neutrophil is a younger form of the mature neutrophil. Laboratories differ in the reporting of band neutrophils. Some classify and report band and segmented neutrophils separately; others report total neutrophils. Normal adults generally have about 3% band neutrophils in their peripheral blood. An obvious increase of band neutrophils should be reported.

Morphologically, band neutrophils resemble segmented cells except for the shape of the nucleus. In band neutrophils the nucleus may be rod or band shaped, when distinct lobes have not yet formed, or it may have begun to form lobes. In the latter case, the lobes are connected by wide strips or bands rather than by narrow threads or filaments, as in segmented neutrophils. The differentiation between band and segmented neutrophils may be difficult; if there is doubt, the cell should be classified as "segmented."

Generally, an increased WBC count (leukocytosis) results from an increase in the absolute number of neutrophils present in the blood; in this case it is called **neutrophilia.** Neutrophilia is found in acute infections (especially bacterial infections); metabolic, chemical, and drug intoxications; acute hemorrhage; postoperative states; certain noninflammatory conditions (e.g., coronary thrombosis); malignant neoplasms; and after acute hemolytic episodes. Neutrophilia is usually accompanied by a shift to the left, or an increase in the number of immature cells, and by toxic changes in the cytoplasm. An increase in the number of band forms, which may be accompanied by the presence of more immature neutrophils, is significant. Toxic changes in the neutrophil cytoplasm are indicated by the presence of deeply stained basophilic (or toxic) granules, pale-blue Döhle bodies, and vacuolization, or pyknosis. The cell size may be increased or decreased.

Neutropenia is a reduction of the absolute neutrophil count. Severe neutropenia has been called *agranulocytosis.* The risk of infection is considerably increased as the neutrophil count falls below about 1×10^9/L. For this reason, neutrophil counts are important in the care of patients undergoing chemotherapy or other conditions in which the bone marrow is suppressed.

Eosinophils

Eosinophils are granulocytes and generally make up about 3% of the circulating leukocytes. They are slightly larger than neutrophils, usually 12 to 16 μm in diameter. The nucleus occupies a relatively small part of the cell. The nucleus is usually bilobed, and occasionally three lobes are seen. The nuclear structure is similar to that of the neutrophil, but the lobes are plumper and the chromatin often stains lighter purple than in the neutrophil. The nuclear membrane is distinct, and no nucleoli are visible. The cytoplasm is usually colorless, but it may be faintly basophilic. It is crowded with spherical acidophilic granules, which stain red-orange with eosin and are larger and more distinct than neutrophilic granules. The granules are evenly distributed throughout the cytoplasm but are rarely seen overlying the nucleus. They are hard, firm bodies that are not easily damaged; they remain intact when pressed into the nucleus or even when the whole cell is damaged and the cell membrane is broken. Eosinophilic granules are also highly refractive, a feature that is often a valuable distinguishing characteristic.

Eosinophilia, an increase in the number of eosinophils above normal, is associated with a wide variety of conditions, but especially with allergic reactions, drug reactions, certain skin disorders, parasitic infestations, collagen vascular diseases, Hodgkin's disease, and myeloproliferative diseases. **Eosinopenia,** or decreased number of eosinophils, is seen with hyperadrenalism.

Basophils

Basophils, which are also granulocytes, normally constitute an average of 0.6% of the total circulating leukocytes. They are about the same size as neutrophils, 10 to 14 µm in diameter, but their nuclei usually occupy a relatively greater portion of the cell. The nucleus is often extremely irregular in shape, varying from a lobular form to a form showing indentations that are not deep enough to divide it into definite lobes. The nuclear pattern is indistinct; there appears to be a mixture of chromatin and parachromatin, and this mixture stains purple or blue and shows little structure. The nuclear membrane is fairly distinct, and no nucleoli are visible. The cytoplasm is usually colorless; it contains a variable number of deeply stained, coarse, round, or angular basophilic granules. The granules (metachromatic) stain deep purple or black; occasionally a few smaller, brownish granules may be present. They may overlie and obscure the nucleus. Because the granules are soluble in water, occasionally a few or even most of them may be dissolved during the staining procedure. When this occurs, the cell will contain vacuoles in place of granules, and the cytoplasm may appear grayish or brownish in their vicinity. The cytoplasm of a mature basophil is colorless. An immature basophil has a pale-blue cytoplasm and can be seen in myelogenous leukemias.

Basophilia, an increase in the number of basophils, can be observed in chronic myelogenous leukemia. It is also seen in allergic reactions, myeloid metaplasia, and polycythemia vera. The basophil number may increase temporarily after irradiation, and basophilia may be present in chronic hemolytic anemia and after splenectomy.

Tissue basophils, also called **mast cells,** are similar but not identical to basophilic granulocytes. They are larger and differ somewhat in their chemical makeup and function.

Monocytes

Monocytes, as with the granulocytes, are derived from the myeloid cell line. They make up about 4% to 6% of normal circulating leukocytes, ranging from 2% to 10% depending on the laboratory or author. Monocytes are the largest of the normal leukocytes, usually larger than neutrophils, measuring from 12 to 22 µm in diameter.

The nucleus is fairly large; it may be round, oval, indented, lobular, notched, or rarely even segmented, but most frequently it is indented or horseshoe shaped. The nuclear chromatin stains light purple and is delicate or lacy. Chromatin and parachromatin are sharply segregated, and the chromatin is distributed in a linear arrangement of delicate strands, which gives the nucleus a stringy

appearance. (Occasionally the nuclear pattern resembles that of a lymphocyte, and the cytoplasmic differences must be relied on for identification.) The nuclear membrane is delicate but not distinct, and nucleoli usually are not seen.

The cytoplasm is abundant, and stains gray or gray-blue. It may contain numerous small, poorly defined granules, resulting in a "ground-glass" appearance, and is often vacuolated. Extremely fine and abundant azurophilic granules are present; this granulation is called *azure dust* and is seen only in monocytes. The granules vary in color from light pink to bright purplish red. In addition, phagocytized particles may be seen in the cytoplasm.

Lymphocytes

Lymphocytes make up about 34% of the leukocytes in the normal adult. Infants and children normally have more lymphocytes and fewer neutrophils than adults, a reversed differential. Lymphocytes fall into two general groups: small (approximately 7-10 µm) and large (up to 20 µm). Most normal lymphocytes are small.

When observed microscopically, lymphocytes are described based on their size and cytoplasmic granularity. Small lymphocytes are found in the greatest numbers. The small lymphocyte is composed chiefly of nucleus and is the type of lymphocyte predominating in normal adult blood. It is about the same size as a normocytic RBC and is a useful size marker during examination of the peripheral blood film, especially in cases of megaloblastic anemia, in which all cell forms other than lymphocytes are increased in diameter. The nucleus is round or slightly notched, and the nuclear chromatin is in the form of coarse, dense, deeply staining blocks. There is relatively little parachromatin, and it is not very distinct. Almost the entire nucleus stains deep purple. The nuclear membrane is heavy and distinct, and nucleoli are not usually seen. The cytoplasm appears in the form of a narrow band that stains pale blue with few, if any, red (azure) granules.

The large lymphocyte shows a further increase in the size of the nucleus and an increase in the relative amount of cytoplasm. The nucleus contains more parachromatin and thus stains more lightly than the nuclei of the smaller forms. The chromatin is still present in clumps, without distinct outlines because of the blending of chromatin and parachromatin. The nuclear membrane is distinct, and nucleoli usually are not seen. The cytoplasm in this form can be abundant, and azure granules are frequently seen. The cytoplasm color varies from colorless to a clear light or medium blue. The cytoplasm of the large granular lymphocyte can be deeply basophilic. Mature lymphocytes include different subsets of highly specialized lymphocytes. Morphologically, B and T lymphocytes appear identical on a Wright-stained blood film.

After antigenic stimulation, small lymphocytes can undergo transformation. These transformed cells appear large (15-25 μm) on Wright-stained films, with a relatively large amount of deep-blue cytoplasm, and are called *large granular lymphocytes*. The large nucleus has a reticular appearance, with uniform chromatin and prominent nucleoli. Such cells have various names, including *reactive, atypical, variant,* and *reticular lymphocytes*.

Nucleoli are rarely seen in lymphocytes of normal blood, but they may be seen in cells that have been crushed during the spreading of the film. Blood lymphocytes may contain nucleoli, but they are normally obscured by the coarse nuclear chromatin.

It is sometimes difficult to distinguish between nucleated RBCs and small lymphocytes. The staining reaction of the parachromatin of the two cells is an important diagnostic criterion; the parachromatin of the lymphocyte is pale blue or violet, and that of the nucleated RBC is pinkish blue. The N/C ratio is much higher in lymphocytes that in nucleated red cells.

Lymphocytosis, an increase in the number of lymphocytes, is associated with viral infections. It is characteristic of certain acute infections (e.g., infectious mononucleosis; pertussis, mumps, and rubella; German measles) and of chronic infections (e.g., tuberculosis, brucellosis, infectious hepatitis). The changes seen in these diseases have been referred to as *reactive* or *atypical changes* and are particularly associated with infectious mononucleosis. The cells are called *reactive lymphocytes* because the increased amount and apparent activity of the cytoplasm indicate that it may be reacting to some sort of stimulus. CLSI recommends that these cells be referred to as **variant** forms.[4]

Plasma Cells

In addition to the five types of mature white cells that normally appear in the peripheral blood, the plasma cell (plasmacyte) rarely can occur in certain blood specimens. It is large, with a round or oval nucleus that is usually in an eccentric position. The chromatin consists of deeply stained, heavy masses that may be arranged in a radial pattern. The cytoplasm is strongly basophilic. There may be a pale, clear zone in the cytoplasm to one side of the nucleus, referred to as a *hof*. Immature forms may occasionally be seen. Plasma cells function in the synthesis of immunoglobulins. They may be found in the peripheral blood of patients with measles, chickenpox, or scarlet fever and in the malignant conditions of multiple myeloma and plasmacytic leukemia.

Reporting Leukocyte Differential Results (Relative and Absolute Counts)

The numbers and types of leukocytes counted are traditionally reported in percent numbers; cells are identified while examining and counting 100 WBCs in a systematic manner. These results are reported in **relative numbers,** or percentages. The alternative method is to report the differentials in terms of absolute numbers. Using this method, the numbers and types of cells counted are reported in number of cells $\times 10^9$/L. Increases or decreases of individual cell lines are reported individually along with the total WBC count. The absolute count provides a much more accurate measure of the actual numbers of cell types present in the peripheral blood. The absolute cell count by cell type is obtained by multiplying the relative number of WBCs (in decimal units) by the total WBC count per liter.

For example, if a patient's WBC count is 7.0×10^9/L and 70% neutrophils are identified in the leukocyte differential, the relative neutrophil count is 70%. The absolute neutrophil count is:

$$0.70 \times (7.0 \times 10^9/L)$$
$$= 4.9 \times 10^9 \, \text{neutrophils}/L \, (4900/\mu L)$$

Reference Values[2]

Adults

Cell Type	%
Neutrophils	
Band	0-3%
Segmented	40-74%
Eosinophils	1-4%
Basophils	0.5-1%
Lymphocytes	22-40%
Monocytes	2-6%

Pediatric

Birth	% Neutrophils	aver 61%
	% Lymphocyte	aver 31%
1 Year	% Neutrophils	31%
	% Lymphocyte	61%
10 Years	% Neutrophils	54%
	% Lymphocyte	38%

Absolute cell
  counts
PMNS
  1.4-6.5 $\times 10^9$/L
Band neutrophils
  0-0.7 $\times 10^9$/L
Lymphocytes
  1.2-3.4 $\times 10^9$/L

Leukocyte Differentials Provided by Hematology Analyzers

Many of the multiparameter hematology analyzers provide differentiation of leukocytes, and many instruments that provide five-cell differentials are available. The major advantage of automated differentiation of leukocytes is that many thousands of cells are analyzed rapidly. In an environment of cost containment and shortage of laboratory personnel, together with more and more sophisticated instrumentation, the complete blood count (CBC) often uses an automated rather than a manual leukocyte differential. Each laboratory needs to develop a policy for the preparation of a blood film and visual examination and counting of cells when the automated results are flagged, so that clinically significant findings will not be missed.

Automated differentials can provide a great amount of useful, cost-efficient information when interpreted by an experienced laboratorian, especially when a manual leukocyte differential or review of the blood film is performed on abnormal results, as determined by the laboratory. The multiparameter analyzers differ in the principle by which leukocytes are differentiated. In general, they employ (1) impedance-related, conductivity, light-scattering measurements of cell volume, (2) automated continuous-flow systems that use cytochemical and light-scattering measurements, and (3) automated computer image analysis of a blood film prepared by an instrument.

Newer technology, digital microscopy provides the latest method for performing a leukocyte differential count.

Blood Cell Alterations

Morphologic changes in the red and white blood cells seen on the stained blood film aid in determining the nature of many blood diseases. Certain diseases produce fairly characteristic alterations of RBCs, WBCs, and platelets, in addition to other clinical signs. All WBCs in the circulating blood should be mature. The presence of immature WBCs in the blood is considered abnormal. Immature WBCs may be differentiated from mature cells by size, the appearance of intracellular structure (e.g., presence of granules, changes in nucleoli, chromatin, or nucleus), and staining properties.

There is a progressive decrease in cell size with maturity, with the nucleus becoming smaller and the N/C ratio decreasing. In granulocytes, granules appear with maturity. In immature WBCs the nucleus is round; with age it becomes lobular or indented. Chromatin is fine and lacy in the young cell and eventually becomes coarse and clumped.

Nucleoli may be present in young cells and absent in the mature forms. The cytoplasm is basophilic (stains blue) in young granulocytes and eventually turns pink with maturity. The young nucleus stains reddish violet and becomes strongly basophilic with maturity. The granules in the cytoplasm assume specific staining qualities with increasing cell maturity.

Certain evidence of cell function is observed that is characteristic of specific developmental stages of the WBCs. Examples are the presence of nucleoli, which indicate a young cell; mitotic figures, which indicate a young cell; cytoplasmic inclusions, which are characteristic of a mature cell; phagocytosis, seen in mature cells; and hemoglobin, seen in mature RBCs.

Erythrocyte Alterations

MORPHOLOGIC ALTERATIONS IN ERYTHROCYTES

The morphologic examination of RBCs is very helpful in evaluating and determining the cause of anemia; it is important that the clinical laboratorian recognize and report changes in erythrocyte morphology so the patient can be effectively evaluated and treated. The following must be observed and noted:

1. Color or staining reaction
2. Size
3. Shape
4. Structure and inclusions
5. Artifacts and abnormal distribution pattern
6. Nucleated red cells

RBCs are described as normochromic and normocytic when they are of normal color, size, and shape.

ALTERATIONS IN ERYTHROCYTE COLOR OR HEMOGLOBIN CONTENT

Normochromic Cells

Red cells are described as **normochromic** when they contain the normal amount of hemoglobin. With Wright's stain, the RBCs show a deep orange-red color in the peripheral area, which gradually diminishes toward the center of the cell. The diameter of the pale central area (central pallor) is less than one-third the diameter of a normochromic erythrocyte.

Hypochromic Cells

RBCs that are very pale and show an increased area of central pallor (making up more than one-third that of the cell) are termed **hypochromic** (Fig. 12-22). Hypochromasia is the result of a decrease in the hemoglobin content of the cell and is often accompanied by a decrease in cell size. This is seen as a decreased MCV, or *microcytosis*, as evidenced

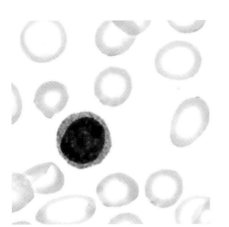

FIGURE 12-22 **Hypochromic red blood cells.** (From Carr JH, Rodak BF: Clinical hematology atlas, ed 3, St Louis, 2009, Saunders.)

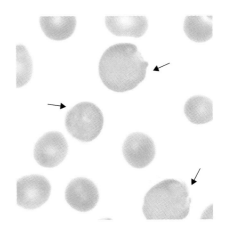

FIGURE 12-23 **Polychromatic red cells.** (From Carr JH, Rodak BF: Clinical hematology atlas, ed 3, St Louis, 2009, Saunders.)

by low MCH and MCHC values. The cells tend to flatten out on the blood film and may appear normal in size. Such RBCs are particularly characteristic of iron-deficiency anemias.

Hyperchromasia

True hyperchromasia cannot exist, because normal RBCs are filled with hemoglobin and cannot be oversaturated or the cell membrane would burst. However, certain RBCs appear to have an increased hemoglobin content. For example, cells that are larger than normal (macrocytes) are also thicker, and therefore the color intensity appears greater on the blood film. Another abnormally shaped erythrocyte, the spherocyte, which is a round cell without a depression in the center, also appears hyperchromic because it is thicker and stains equally throughout the cell.

Polychromasia

Polychromasia refers to RBCs that show a faint blue or blue-orange color with Wright's stain (Fig. 12-23). This is a mixed staining reaction, because both blue RNA and red hemoglobin are present. Polychromic cells are young cells that have just extruded their nuclei and stain diffusely basophilic because of the presence of small numbers of ribosomes (or cytoplasmic RNA). When such cells enter the bloodstream, they lack 20% of their final hemoglobin content and retain the ribosomes for hemoglobin synthesis. Polychromatophilic RBCs are generally larger than mature cells. With supravital dyes (e.g., new methylene blue) the RNA reticulum stains blue, and the cells are called *reticulocytes*. The degree of polychromasia (or an increased reticulocyte count) is an indication of increased erythrocyte formation by the marrow and is characteristically seen in the various hemolytic anemias.

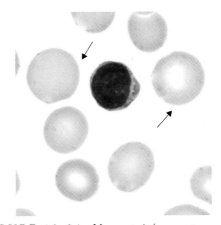

FIGURE 12-24 **Macrocytosis (macrocytes, *arrows*).** (From Carr JH, Rodak BF: Clinical hematology atlas, ed 3, St Louis, 2009, Saunders.)

ALTERATIONS IN ERYTHROCYTE SIZE

Anisocytosis

Anisocytosis is a general term indicating increased variation in the size of RBCs in the blood film. It is often accompanied by variations in hemoglobin concentration.

Macrocytosis

Macrocytes are large RBCs (Fig. 12-24). They have a mean cell diameter greater than 9 μm or an MCV greater than 100 fL. They should be differentiated from polychromatophilic erythrocytes, which are also large. Macrocytes are characteristic of the megaloblastic anemias of folic acid or vitamin B_{12} deficiency.

Microcytosis

Microcytes are small RBCs, less than 6.5 μm in diameter, with an MCV less than 78 fL. They are often associated with hypochromasia, but their decreased size may not be appreciated on the blood film because they tend to flatten out. Microcytosis is characteristic of iron-deficiency anemia, thalassemia, lead poisoning, sideroblastic anemia, idiopathic pulmonary hemosiderosis, and anemias of chronic diseases (Fig. 12-25).

ALTERATIONS IN ERYTHROCYTE SHAPE

Discocyte

When an RBC is not being subjected to external deforming processes, its normal shape is that of a smooth biconcave disk. One term used to describe a red cell with a normal shape is *discocyte*.

Poikilocytosis

Poikilocytosis is a general term indicating an increased variation in the shape of RBCs. Many different variations in shape are seen in blood films; RBCs have been described as appearing pear, oat, teardrop, or helmet shaped; triangular; or fragmented or as having various numbers and types of membrane projections. The size and hemoglobin content can vary greatly within poikilocytes. They are found in a variety of anemias and hemolytic states, and a particular shape may or may not indicate a specific type of disease.

Elliptocyte and Ovalocyte

Elliptocytes and ovalocytes are oval, or egg shaped, showing varying degrees of elliptical shaping from slightly oval to almost a cylindrical form (Fig. 12-26). Large elliptocytes, called *macro-ovalocytes*, are characteristic of megaloblastic anemias. Because of their increased size and thickness, these cells may not show an area of central pallor on the blood film. More elongated forms may occur in a variety of conditions, the most striking and least pathologic being hereditary elliptocytosis.

Sickle Cell (Drepanocyte)

Sickle cells are typically narrow and shaped like a sickle with two pointed ends (Fig. 12-27). They may also vary from crescent-shaped to bipolar spiculated forms to cells with long, irregular spicules. Sickle cells are the result of a genetic condition in which abnormal hemoglobin (Hb S) is present in a homozygous state in RBCs. Sickling of red cells is enhanced by lack of oxygen. Sickle cells may be found in sickle cell disease (Hb SS) or when Hb SC or Hg S β-thalassemia is present. Sickle cells are not found in sickle trait alone (e.g., Hb AS).

Target Cell (Codocyte)

Target cells resemble targets, showing a peripheral ring of hemoglobin, an area of pallor or clearing, and then a central area of hemoglobin (Fig. 12-28). The codocyte circulates as a bell-shaped cell but takes on the target shape when dried on

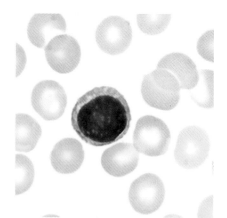

FIGURE 12-25 **Microcytosis.** (From Carr JH, Rodak BF: Clinical hematology atlas, ed 3, St Louis, 2009, Saunders.)

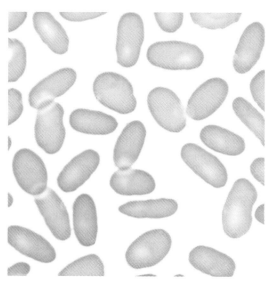

FIGURE 12-26 **Elliptocytes.** (From Carr JH, Rodak BF: Clinical hematology atlas, ed 3, St Louis, 2009, Saunders.)

a slide for morphologic examination. Target cells represent another membrane defect; they have excessive cell membrane in relation to the amount of hemoglobin. They are seen in a variety of clinical conditions, especially in various hemoglobin abnormalities and in chronic liver disease.

Spherocyte

Spherocytes are RBCs that are not biconcave; instead, they appear round or spherical because of the loss of a portion of the cell membrane (Fig. 12-29). As a result, they are small cells, usually less than 6 μm in diameter, and are often called *microspherocytes*. They appear hyperchromic, staining a uniform intense orange-red because of the lack of central pallor, a result of the round shape. Spherocytes are characteristic of certain hemolytic anemias, both hereditary (hereditary spherocytosis) and acquired (e.g., drug induced). They also

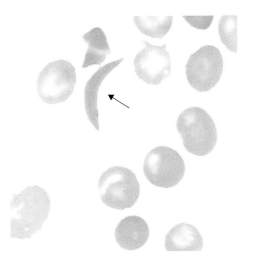

FIGURE 12-27   Sickle cell, or drepanocyte *(arrow)*. (From Carr JH, Rodak BF: Clinical hematology atlas, ed 3, St Louis, 2009, Saunders.)

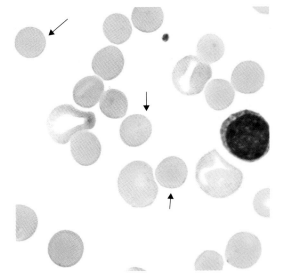

FIGURE 12-29   Spherocytes *(arrows)*. (From Carr JH, Rodak BF: Clinical hematology atlas, ed 3, St Louis, 2009, Saunders.)

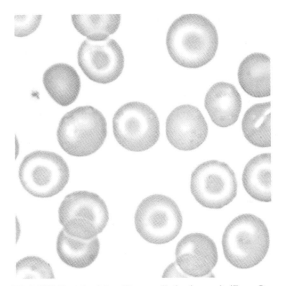

FIGURE 12-28   Target cells (codocytes). (From Carr JH, Rodak BF: Clinical hematology atlas, ed 3, St Louis, 2009, Saunders.)

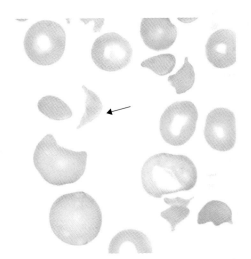

FIGURE 12-30   Schistocyte, or fragmented cell *(arrow)*, resembling sickle cell. (From Carr JH, Rodak BF: Clinical hematology atlas, ed 3, St Louis, 2009, Saunders.)

are associated with the presence of polychromasia and an increased reticulocyte count.

Stomatocyte

Stomatocytes show a slitlike or mouthlike, rather than round, area of central pallor on the blood film. They are not biconcave but bowl shaped or concave on only one side. They are often found in chronic liver disease.

Schistocyte (Fragmented Cell, Helmet Cell)

Schistocytes have a variety of names and forms, depending on what is left after the cell is physically fragmented (Fig. 12-30). Helmet cells are

small triangular cells with one or two pointed ends that resemble a helmet. *Schistocytosis* is a very serious pathologic condition. It may be the result of mechanical fracture of cells as they pass through the circulatory system, as on filaments of fibrin resulting from disseminated intravascular coagulation (DIC) or on artificial heart valves. Schistocytes are also seen in cases of severe burns. The fragmentation may also be the result of toxic or metabolic injury, as seen with certain malignancies. Schistocytes are characteristic of microangiopathic hemolytic anemias, and their presence is a danger signal requiring immediate action by the physician.

Teardrop Cell (Dacryocyte)

These pear-shaped or teardrop-shaped RBCs have an elongated point or tail at one end (Fig. 12-31). They may be the result of the cell squeezing and subsequently fracturing as it passes through the spleen.

Burr Cell, Crenated (Echinocyte)

Burr cells or echinocytes are RBCs with scalloped, spicular, or spiny projections regularly distributed around the cell membrane. They can usually revert back to normal cells. The term *crenated* is sometimes reserved for artifactual spicular cells, such as artifacts that result when the blood film is not adequately dried.

Acanthocyte (Spike Cell, Acanthoid Cell)

Acanthocytes are similar to echinocytes, but their spiny projections are irregularly distributed around the cell membrane. They are not artifacts and cannot revert to normal cells. Acanthocytes are related to and may occur with schistocytes and represent serious pathologic conditions.

Keratocyte (Horn Cell)

Keratocytes are shaped like a half-moon or spindle. They have a relatively normal cell volume but have been deformed so that they appear to have two or more spicules.

ALTERATIONS IN ERYTHROCYTE STRUCTURE AND INCLUSIONS

Basophilic Stippling

The presence of dark-blue granules evenly distributed throughout the RBC is called **basophilic stippling** (Fig. 12-32).The stippling may be very fine, dotlike, or coarse and larger. The stippled cell may resemble the polychromatophilic erythrocyte, but these are actual granules, not merely an overall blueness. Stippling does not exist in the circulating RBC but results from precipitation of ribosomes and RNA in the staining process. However, the stippling is not an artifact in the clinical sense because it may indicate abnormal erythrocyte formation in the marrow, as in thalassemia minor, megaloblastic anemia, and lead poisoning.

Siderocyte (Pappenheimer Body)

Siderocytes contain small, dense, blue-purple granules of free iron uncombined with hemoglobin (Fig. 12-33). Usually only one or two of these granules are present in a cell, and they are located in the cell periphery. Siderocytes may be confused with Howell-Jolly bodies and can be distinguished and seen better with a specific stain for iron, such as Prussian blue. When siderocytes, or siderosomes, are Wright-stained, they are sometimes called *Pappenheimer bodies*. They are rarely seen in peripheral blood except after removal of the spleen.

Howell-Jolly Body

Howell-Jolly bodies are round, densely staining purple granules that stain similar to dense nuclear chromatin (Fig. 12-34). Usually, only one or two such bodies are seen in the RBCs. They are eccentrically located in the RBC and less than 1 μm in diameter. Howell-Jolly bodies are remnants of the erythrocyte nucleus and thus are deoxyribonucleic acid (DNA). Under normal conditions, they are derived from nuclear fragmentation (karyorrhexis) or incomplete expulsion of the nucleus in the

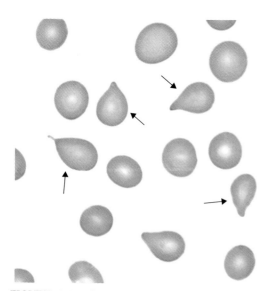

FIGURE 12-31 **Dacryocytes *(arrows)*.** (From Carr JH, Rodak BF: Clinical hematology atlas, ed 3, St Louis, 2009, Saunders.)

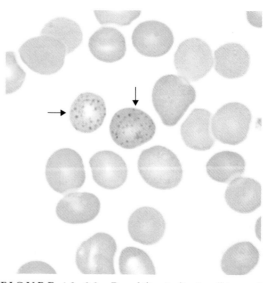

FIGURE 12-32 **Basophilic stippling in cell *(arrows)*.** (From Carr JH, Rodak BF: Clinical hematology atlas, ed 3, St Louis, 2009, Saunders.)

later stages of RBC maturation and are thought to be aberrant chromosomes in certain abnormal conditions. These nuclear remnants are normally removed from the reticulocytes in the peripheral blood by a pitting process as they pass through the spleen. Therefore, they are seen in peripheral blood after removal of the spleen, as well as in cases of abnormal erythrocyte formation, such as megaloblastic anemias and some hemolytic anemias.

Cabot's Rings

The threadlike red-violet strands known as *Cabot's rings* occur in ring, twisted, or figure-8 shapes in reticulocytes and are rare. Their origin is unknown, but they are thought to result from abnormal erythrocyte formation during mitosis and can be seen in megaloblastic anemias and lead poisoning.

Parasitized Red Cell (Malarial)

In patients with malaria, various stages of the malaria parasites may be seen in the erythrocytes (Fig. 12-35). Depending on the species of malaria organism present, the parasites may be confused with Cabot's rings, basophilic stippling, or platelets lying on top of RBCs.

ERYTHROCYTE ARTIFACTS AND ABNORMAL DISTRIBUTION PATTERNS

Platelet on Top of Erythrocyte

When a platelet rests on top of RBCs in the blood film, it may be confused with inclusions, especially the trophozoite stage of malaria organisms (Fig. 12-36). In such cases, the overlying platelets should be compared with those in the surrounding field. If the platelet is on top of the RBC, neither the platelet nor the RBC can be focused in the same plane, because the platelet is not in the RBC.

Crenation

Crenated cells on the blood film resemble echinocytes, with scalloped, spicular, or spiny projections regularly distributed around the cell surface. These crenated cells are an artifact resulting from incorrect preparation of the blood film, usually failure to dry it adequately.

Punched-Out Red Cells

Erythrocytes with a punched-out appearance rather than a normal area of central pallor are also drying artifacts (Fig. 12-37). They should not be confused with hypochromic RBCs. The remaining

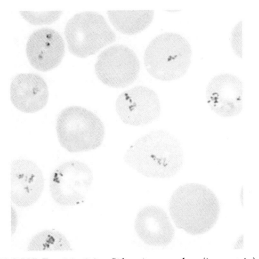

FIGURE 12-33 Siderotic granules (iron stain). (From Carr JH, Rodak BF: Clinical hematology atlas, ed 3, St Louis, 2009, Saunders.)

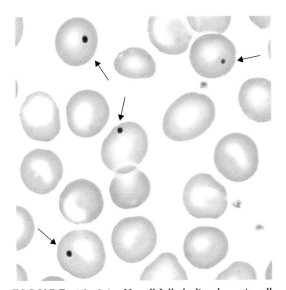

FIGURE 12-34 Howell-Jolly bodies shown in cells *(arrows)*. (From Carr JH, Rodak BF: Clinical hematology atlas, ed 3, St Louis, 2009, Saunders.)

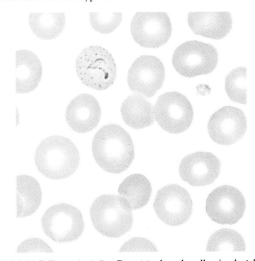

FIGURE 12-35 Parasitized red cells (malarial). (From Carr JH, Rodak BF: Clinical hematology atlas, ed 3, St Louis, 2009, Saunders.)

cell shows a normal staining reaction with this artifact.

Rouleaux Formation

Rouleaux represents an abnormal distribution pattern of RBCs, which stick together or become aligned in aggregates that look like stacks of coins (Fig. 12-38). This arrangement is a typical artifact in the thick area of blood films. It is clinically significant when found in the normal examination area and associated with elevated plasma fibrinogen or globulin, with a corresponding increase in the ESR (e.g., multiple myeloma).

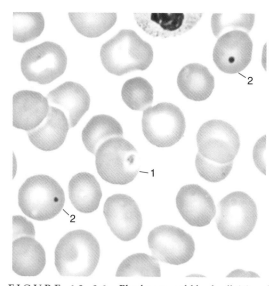

FIGURE 12-36 Platelets on red blood cell *(1)* and Howell-Jolly bodies *(2)*. (From Carr JH, Rodak BF: Clinical hematology atlas, ed 3, St Louis, 2009, Saunders.)

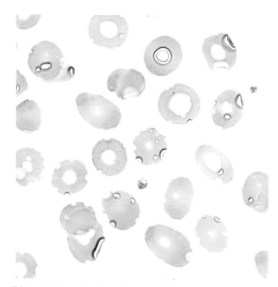

FIGURE 12-37 Drying artifact in red cells showing punched-out appearance. (From Carr JH, Rodak BF: Clinical hematology atlas, ed 3, St Louis, 2009, Saunders.)

Agglutination

Agglutination, irregular or amorphous clumping of RBCs in the blood film, represents another alteration in erythrocyte distribution. Clinically, this may be caused by the presence of a cold agglutinin (antibody) in the patient's serum and may indicate an autoimmune hemolytic state or anemia.

Nucleated Red Cells in Peripheral Blood

Normally, erythrocytes do not enter the blood until the reticulocyte stage of maturation, just after extrusion of the nucleus (Fig. 12-39). The presence of earlier nucleated forms of RBCs in the peripheral blood is abnormal. It indicates intense marrow stimulation, such as that seen in acute blood loss, megaloblastic anemias, or pathologic conditions associated with various malignancies.

Cells in the later stages of maturation are most often present, so the cytoplasm is orange-red because the cells contain hemoglobin. However, the nucleus is also present, although shrunken and dark blue in color. Earlier forms may occur and may be difficult to distinguish from small lymphocytes or plasma

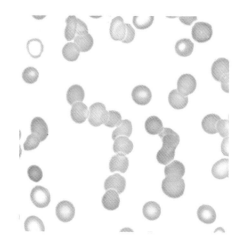

FIGURE 12-38 Rouleaux formation, an abnormal distribution pattern. (From Carr JH, Rodak BF: Clinical hematology atlas, ed 3, St Louis, 2009, Saunders.)

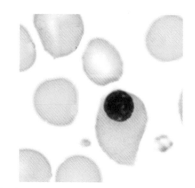

FIGURE 12-39 Nucleated red cell (orthochromic normoblast). (From Carr JH, Rodak BF: Clinical hematology atlas, ed 3, St Louis, 2009, Saunders.)

cells; the presence of pink in the RBC cytoplasm is helpful in such cases. The presence of nucleated RBC forms in the peripheral blood is characteristic of megaloblastic anemias. In these cases, the young erythrocytes are larger (macrocytic) and tend to have a more open chromatin pattern than corresponding stages of normocytic erythrocytes (dyssynchrony of nucleus and cytoplasm maturation).

It is important to remember that the WBC count must be corrected when nucleated RBCs are observed in the peripheral blood film, because these cells are counted as WBCs when present.

CLINICAL SIGNIFICANCE OF ERYTHROCYTE ALTERATIONS

Clinically, alterations in erythrocyte morphology are associated with many diseases and especially with anemia. Anemia is not a specific disease, but a condition in which there is a decrease in the oxygen-carrying capacity of the blood and therefore in the amount of oxygen reaching the tissues and organs. Its causes are many and varied, and the type of anemia present and its underlying cause must be determined before treatment can be effectively undertaken. It may or may not be the result of a disorder of the blood or blood-forming tissues.

TYPES OF ANEMIAS

Clinically, all patients with anemia have similar symptoms or complaints regardless of the cause of the anemia. The severity generally depends on the hemoglobin concentration of the blood, because most symptoms result from the decreased oxygen-carrying capacity. The primary complaints are fatigue and shortness of breath. Other common complaints are faintness, dizziness, heart palpitation, and headache.

Once the existence of anemia has been demonstrated, usually on the basis of the blood hemoglobin concentration, the underlying cause must be determined. In addition, the case history and physical examination, various laboratory procedures, including the appearance of the RBCs on the peripheral blood film, are helpful in establishing the diagnosis.

Anemias can be classified according to either the appearance of the RBCs (morphologic classification) or the physiologic cause of the anemia (etiologic or pathogenic classification) (Table 12-7). Morphologically, anemias are generally classified as:
1. Normochromic-normocytic
2. Macrocytic
3. Hypochromic-microcytic

Normochromic-Normocytic Anemias

Normochromic-normocytic anemias are characterized by normal-appearing RBCs on the peripheral blood film and RBC indices within the reference range. The cells produced by the marrow are normal, but the number of cells in circulation is reduced for a variety of reasons, including acute blood loss. Conditions resulting in increased plasma volume, such as overhydration, will also result in normochromic-normocytic anemia. If the bone marrow is suppressed (hypoplastic), as seen in cases of aplastic anemia, the RBCs that remain are normal, although the number is decreased. Suppressed marrow results in a deficiency of the myeloid series, which is seen as decreased leukocyte and platelet counts. If the marrow is infiltrated with a neoplasm or malignancy, such as leukemia or multiple myeloma, the remaining RBCs appear normal but are decreased in number. In certain hemolytic diseases and chronic kidney and liver diseases, the erythrocytes appear normal but also are reduced in number.

Macrocytic Anemias

Macrocytic anemias are primarily represented by the megaloblastic anemias resulting from vitamin B_{12} or folic acid deficiency, or a combination of both. The deficiency may be nutritional or may result from a malabsorption syndrome such as pernicious anemia, in which the patient is unable to absorb vitamin B_{12}. In either case, the deficiency leads to a nuclear maturation defect and megaloblastic anemia. The marrow shows certain changes in the myeloid series, including the erythrocytes, granulocytes, and megakaryocytes (platelets). Megaloblastic changes are characterized by larger cells having a more open chromatin pattern in the nucleus and by the presence of larger, hypersegmented mature neutrophils in the

TABLE 12-7

Etiologic Classification of Anemias	
Type	Example
Blood Loss	
Acute	Trauma
Chronic	Colon cancer
Impaired Production	
Aplastic anemia	Radiation exposure
Iron-deficiency anemia	Excessive menstrual bleeding
Sideroblastic anemia	Faulty iron utilization
Anemia of chronic diseases	Cancer
Megaloblastic anemia	Pernicious anemia
Hemolytic Anemia	
Inherited defects	Hereditary spherocytosis
Acquired disorders	Hemolytic disease of the newborn
Hemolytic-hemoglobin disorders	Sickle cell anemia, thalassemias

peripheral blood. The enlarged RBCs (macrocytes) have MCV values of 120 to 140 fL. Actual hyperchromasia is impossible, but the RBCs appear to contain more hemoglobin because of their increased size and therefore thickness. Although the anemia may be severe, the RBC count is decreased more than the hemoglobin concentration, since the cells that are present are large and almost completely filled with hemoglobin. Other changes seen in the blood film include anisocytosis (erythrocytes varying in size), poikilocytosis (erythrocytes varying in shape), and Howell-Jolly bodies.

Nutritional deficiency of vitamin B_{12} is relatively rare, but nutritional deficiency of folic acid is fairly common. It may be found in chronic alcoholism or other conditions in which the diet is not well balanced. Folate deficiency is also observed when the requirement is increased, as in pregnancy, infancy, certain hemolytic anemias, and hyperthyroidism. Celiac disease, tropical sprue, certain drugs, contraceptives, and liver disease may lead to malabsorption and megaloblastic anemia.

Megaloblastic erythrocytes have an abnormal developmental sequence. Although it is similar to the sequence of maturation of the normoblasts, megaloblasts are larger. As they develop, cells of the megaloblastic sequence have a more open or immature chromatin pattern in the nucleus, referred to as *asynchronous maturation* or *dyssynchronous development* of the nucleus and cytoplasm. In megaloblastic anemia, these changes are not limited to the erythrocyte series; all types of cells normally produced in the bone marrow are similarly affected, as evidenced by large, hypersegmented neutrophils. Lymphocytes are unaffected, and a small lymphocyte is a useful visual size marker.

Hypochromic-Microcytic Anemias

Hypochromic-microcytic anemias can be the most common types encountered, with iron-deficiency anemia being the type most frequently seen. Iron deficiency is not a simple classification, because there are several possible causes of this clinical condition. In simplified terms, iron-deficiency anemia may result from:

- Decreased iron intake (either from inadequate diet or impaired absorption)
- Increased iron loss (generally from chronic bleeding from a variety of causes)
- An error of iron metabolism (sideroblastic anemias)
- Increased iron requirements in infancy, pregnancy, and lactation

The cause of the anemia must be determined in order to treat it. If it results from a dietary deficiency of iron, a relatively simple and effective treatment is to administer iron, usually orally as ferrous sulfate tablets. However, if it is caused by another condition, the administration of iron will do no good, and it may do harm either in itself (e.g., in the thalassemias, in which iron overload is a possibility) or because it delays the use of appropriate therapy.

If the iron-deficiency anemia results from chronic bleeding, the cause of the bleeding must be determined. The bleeding is most often gastrointestinal, although women with excessive menstrual flow often develop iron-deficiency anemia. Gastrointestinal bleeding leading to iron-deficiency anemia may result from such causes as ulcer, carcinoma or other neoplasms, hemorrhoids, hookworm, or even the ingestion of salicylate (usually as aspirin). The treatment is different for each of these causes.

All iron-deficiency anemias produce similar changes in erythrocyte morphology. The RBCs are smaller than normal (microcytic), and the MCV is decreased. Unfortunately, the decreased size is not always as apparent on the blood film as it is in the MCV value. In iron-deficiency anemia, the amount of hemoglobin within each RBC is significantly decreased; such cells are hypochromic (deficient in color). This appears in the RBC volume, which is primarily a function of hemoglobin, but may not be evident on the slide because the hypochromic RBC spreads out or flattens and may appear to be of normal size or even larger than normal. The hypochromic cell is extremely pale, showing only a thin rim of color with a significantly increased area of central pallor, which occupies more than a third of the cell. The decreased hemoglobin per RBC is measured in the laboratory as decreased MCH and MCHC. Other changes characteristic of iron-deficiency anemia include anisocytosis and poikilocytosis, which vary in degree with the severity of the disease and are reflected by an increased RDW. Other tests that may be useful in the investigation of iron-deficiency anemias include examination of the stool for occult blood, determination of serum iron and total iron-binding capacity, radiographic study of the gastrointestinal tract, and rarely, bone marrow examination.

Another group of anemias that demonstrate mild to severe microcytosis and hypochromia are disorders in the synthesis of globin, a component of the hemoglobin molecule. These are the thalassemias, a group of inherited disorders of hemoglobin synthesis. Microcytosis, hypochromasia, and basophilic stippling are general observations. Anisocytosis, poikilocytosis, and target cells may be present, as well as decreased osmotic fragility. Actual differentiation of α and β forms of thalassemia require additional laboratory testing.

Hypochromic-microcytic anemias also include those resulting from disorders of porphyrin and heme synthesis. As a result, the hemoglobin molecule is malformed. The sideroblastic anemias are a heterogeneous group of disorders that have in common increased storage of iron, especially in the mononuclear phagocytic system. The bone marrow in these conditions shows sideroblasts, nucleated RBCs with granules of iron that can be demonstrated with Prussian blue stain. The granules occur characteristically in a full or partial ring around the nucleus. Besides microcytosis and hypochromasia, the peripheral blood from these patients shows siderocytes, nonnucleated RBCs with granules of iron (see Alterations in Erythrocyte Structure and Inclusions). Because the body is already overloaded with iron that is not being utilized appropriately, iron therapy in these anemias would be harmful to the patient.

A number of chemicals cause sideroblastic anemias by inhibiting heme synthesis. Lead poisoning produces an anemia that is characteristically mildly microcytic and hypochromic and is often characterized by basophilic stippling of the RBCs. It is most often seen in children who have ingested lead paint chips and may be seen in adults with industrial exposure to lead.

Hemolytic Anemias

One problem with a morphologic classification of anemias is that it does not deal conveniently with a broad etiologic class of anemias, the hemolytic anemias. These are sometimes classified as normochromic-normocytic based on calculated indices. However, the RDW is very increased in hemolytic anemia because of anisocytosis and poikilocytosis, unlike in the other normochromic-normocytic anemias. In addition, because of the increased number of young RBCs (reticulocytes), which are larger than mature cells, the MCV is increased in hemolytic anemia, although not as much as for the megaloblastic anemias.

The hemolytic anemias are generally classified as congenital or acquired. They are characterized by increased destruction or hemolysis of RBCs from a variety of causes, accompanied by increased erythrocyte production by the bone marrow. This is seen as polychromasia and even nucleated forms of RBCs on Wright-stained blood films and as increased reticulocyte counts. Anisocytosis and poikilocytosis with increased RDW are characteristic of hemolytic anemias in general. An inherited form of spherocytic anemia, hereditary spherocytosis, results from an inherited erythrocyte abnormality and is characterized by spherocytes in the peripheral blood. This condition is indistinguishable morphologically from certain acquired disorders that result in spherocytic anemia. In such cases a useful laboratory test is the *direct antiglobulin* test (DAT), formerly called the *Coombs test*.

The DAT is used to detect RBCs that have been coated with antibodies. This is one of the most useful procedures for distinguishing immune from nonimmune mechanisms that can underlie hemolytic anemias. When RBCs are precoated with an antibody, the DAT usually will be positive unless the amount of antibody on the cell membrane is too small. Erythrocytes can become sensitized when an autoimmune process is in effect. In this type of disorder, antibodies are produced by the patient's own immune system and react with specific antigens on the patient's own RBCs. These anemias can be temperature induced or drug induced.

Other changes of shape (poikilocytosis) are characteristic of certain hemolytic anemias. Elliptocytes are characteristic of hereditary elliptocytosis, an erythrocyte membrane disorder. Sickle cells are characteristic of sickle cell anemia, an inherited hemoglobin abnormality. Schistocytes, or fragmented cells, are characteristic of the microangiopathic hemolytic anemias and may be produced by mechanical fragmentation resulting from an intravascular pathologic condition or intravascular coagulation.

Leukocyte Alterations

Quantitative changes in leukocytes are measured by the white blood cell (WBC) count, the actual number of leukocytes in a certain volume of blood. Again, a WBC count above normal is *leukocytosis*; a count below normal is *leukopenia*. There can also be increases or decreases in number of any of the five WBC types enumerated collectively in the WBC count, and such changes are measured by the white cell differential. Quantitative changes in any of the cell types are described by the following terms: *neutrophilia* (increase), *neutropenia* (decrease); *eosinophilia, eosinopenia; basophilia, basopenia; lymphocytosis, lymphopenia;* and *monocytosis, monocytopenia.*

In addition, these increases or decreases may be relative or absolute. If the change is *absolute*, the particular cell type shows a numerical increase or decrease from its normal concentration in the blood. If it is *relative*, there is an alteration (either high or low) of the percentage of the particular cell type, as determined in the leukocyte differential, while the numerical concentration is within normal values. Finally, there may be both an absolute and a relative change when both the percentage and the numerical values are above or below normal.

As discussed earlier, qualitative or morphologic alterations in circulating leukocytes may be described in terms of a *shift to the left*, referring to the presence of younger or more immature cell forms than are normally found in the peripheral blood. Such changes may be found within any cell line, including erythrocytes.

As described and illustrated next, most alterations in leukocyte morphology can be classified as (1) toxic or reactive changes, (2) anomalous changes, or (3) leukemic or other malignant changes.

Reactive alterations are particularly characteristic of lymphocytes. **Reactive lymphocytes** can be seen in viral infections and are often associated with infectious mononucleosis, although many other conditions produce reactive cell forms. Changes generally include increased cytoplasmic basophilia with or without radial or peripheral localization, increased or decreased cytoplasmic volume, increased coarse azurophilic granulation, and alterations in the nuclear chromatin, which becomes either loose, delicate, and reticular or dark, heavy, and clumped. These changes are defined further later in this section.

TOXIC CHANGES AND GRANULOCYTE ALTERATIONS

Toxic changes are seen in neutrophils and are generally associated with a bacterial infection or a toxic reaction. Changes are seen on a blood film as toxic granulation, vacuolization, or the presence of Döhle bodies.

Toxic Granulation

Toxic granules are deeply staining basophilic or blue-black larger-than-normal granules found in the cytoplasm of neutrophils, bands, and metamyelocytes (Fig. 12-40). They resemble the primary granules seen in the promyelocyte, an early developmental stage of the neutrophil. Their presence is associated with acute bacterial infections, drug poisoning, and burns.

Döhle Bodies

Döhle bodies are round or oval, small, clear, light-blue–staining areas found in the neutrophil cytoplasm. They are remnants of cytoplasmic RNA from an earlier stage of neutrophil development and are often seen together with toxic granulation

in infections, in burns, after administration of toxic agents, and in pregnancy.

Toxic Vacuolization

Vacuoles are also signs of toxic change and imply the occurrence of phagocytosis. Sites of digestion of phagocytized material are seen as vacuoles in the cytoplasm of neutrophils and bands, and vacuoles are often found in association with toxic granulation.

Hypersegmentation of Nucleus

Neutrophils that are hypersegmented contain six or more lobes in their nuclei. They are characteristic of the megaloblastic anemias of vitamin B_{12} and folic acid deficiency and have been called *pernicious anemia* (PA) neutrophils. The megaloblastic neutrophil is larger than a normal-sized neutrophil.

Barr Bodies

A Barr body is a small knob attached to or projecting from a lobe of the neutrophil nucleus and consisting of the same nuclear chromatin or substance. It is often referred to as the *sex chromatin* or *sex chromosome* because it is seen in some neutrophils of normal females and is thought to be an inactivated X chromosome.

Auer Rods (Bodies)

Auer rods or bodies are slender, rod-shaped or needle-shaped bodies found in the cytoplasm; they stain reddish purple, similar to azurophilic granules (Fig. 12-41), and are composed of lysosomal material and fused primary granules. Auer rods can be observed in the cytoplasms of myeloblasts or monoblasts and are considered diagnostic in distinguishing myeloblastic from lymphoblastic leukemias.

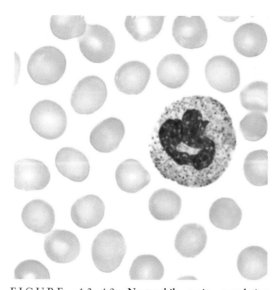

FIGURE 12-40 **Neutrophil: toxic granulation.** (From Carr JH, Rodak BF: Clinical hematology atlas, ed 3, St Louis, 2009, Saunders.)

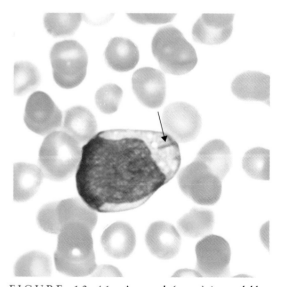

FIGURE 12-41 **Auer rod (*arrow*) in myeloblast.** (From Carr JH, Rodak BF: Clinical hematology atlas, ed 3, St Louis, 2009, Saunders.)

ANOMALOUS CHANGES

An *anomaly* is a "deviation from the rule" or an irregularity. Hematologic deviations from normal may be congenital or acquired.

Pelger-Huët Anomaly

Pelger-Huët anomaly is seen as a failure of the granulocyte nucleus to segment or form lobes normally. The neutrophil nuclei are band shaped or at most have two lobes. In addition, the chromatin is quite coarsely clumped. This is a benign anomaly that can be inherited or acquired. In its acquired form, it is known as pseudo–Pelger-Huët anomaly.

Chédiak-Higashi Anomaly

In Chédiak-Higashi anomaly, large amorphous granules are observed in the neutrophil cytoplasm; granules are also seen in the lymphocyte and monocyte cytoplasm. This syndrome is inherited and rare, and patients have been treated with bone marrow transplantation.

May-Hegglin Anomaly

May-Hegglin anomaly is inherited, and most patients have no clinical symptoms. Blue inclusion bodies similar to Döhle bodies are present in neutrophils but are usually larger and have more sharply defined borders. Platelets may be decreased in number, but some giant forms can be present.

Alder-Reilly Anomaly

Alder-Reilly anomaly is inherited and often associated with mucopolysaccharidoses. Heavy, dark, azurophilic granulation is observed in neutrophils, eosinophils, basophils, and sometimes lymphocytes and monocytes.

MALIGNANT OR LEUKEMIC CHANGES

The hematologic malignancies include a large and varied group of diseases that are beyond the scope of this book. However, this section provides some general comments and descriptions. The hematologic malignancies may be classified as:

1. *Acute myelocytic leukemia* (AML), also known as *acute nonlymphoblastic leukemia* (ANLL)
2. Chronic myeloproliferative disorders, including *chronic myelogenous leukemia* (CML)
3. *Acute lymphocytic leukemia* (ALL)
4. Chronic lymphoproliferative disorders, including *chronic lymphocytic leukemia* (CLL) and lymphomas

Leukemia is a disease of the blood-forming tissues that is an abnormal, uncontrolled proliferation of one or more of the various hematopoietic cells that progressively displaces normal cellular elements. There are usually, but not always, qualitative changes in the affected cells.

Classification

Leukemias are classified morphologically as *lymphocytic* (or lymphoid) and *myelogenous* (or myeloid). The youngest cell forms, or blasts, common to these leukemias are the *lymphoblast* and the *myeloblast*, respectively. It may be impossible to distinguish between the myeloblast and the lymphoblast morphologically, especially in the most serious or acute forms of the disease, when only blast forms are seen in the blood. The presence of *Auer rods* (rods or granules of lysosomal material, an azurophilic substance) in the cytoplasm is diagnostic of the myeloblast. Auer rods are not seen in all cases of myelogenous leukemia. Other considerations in the differentiation of myeloblasts and lymphoblasts are the N/C ratio, the number of nucleoli, and the nuclear chromatin pattern, but these differences are often inconclusive and may be misleading. If more mature cells are present, they may aid in the morphologic identification.

Leukemias can be classified as acute or chronic on the basis of clinical course (prognosis) and the number of blasts present. Acute leukemias usually occur with sudden onset. The patient usually has anemia, which is normocytic-normochromic and increases as the disease progresses. The platelet count is low to greatly decreased. The leukocyte count varies but is usually moderately to extremely elevated, with 50 to 100 × 10^9/L possible, although the count may be normal or even decreased. Blast cells are present in the peripheral blood film; generally, more than 60% blasts indicate an acute leukemic process. The bone marrow is hypercellular and consists predominantly of blast cells. Untreated acute leukemias can lead to death within 2 to 3 months. Death is often the result of *hemorrhage*, which increases in severity as the platelet count falls below 20 × 10^9/L, or *infection*, which results as the granulocyte count falls below 1.5 × 10^9/L. Treatment includes chemotherapy, transfusion therapy, and bone marrow transplantation.

Epidemiology

Leukemia can occur at any age, but certain forms appear to be age related. AML occurs at all ages but is primarily a disease of middle age. CML usually occurs between ages 20 and 50. CLL is generally a disease of later adult years, generally over 50. Treatment is usually only for complications of the disease. ALL is generally a disease of children under 10 years of age (seldom over 20 years) and peaks between the ages 3 and 7. ALL is the most prevalent form of malignancy in children.

Etiology

The exact cause of leukemia is unknown. Evidence suggests hereditary factors and genetic predisposition. Environmental causes have also been cited, especially exposure to gamma radiation, producing genetic mutations or chromosome damage, such as the Philadelphia chromosome seen in CML. Various chemicals and drugs have also been implicated, and viruses have been related to leukemia in mice and other animals. The *chronic myeloproliferative disorders* are a group of myeloid neoplasms in which there is malignant clonal proliferation of predominantly myeloid cells in the marrow and blood. These may be cells of the granulocytic, erythrocytic, or megakaryocytic cell lines. Diseases include CML (neutrophilic), polycythemia vera (erythrocytic), and essential thrombocythemia (megakaryocytic).

Signs and Symptoms

Chronic leukemias (myeloproliferative or lymphoproliferative disorders) begin slowly and insidiously and may exist for a long time without symptoms. Symptoms develop slowly and include fatigue, night sweats, weight loss, and fever. Anemia usually develops late in the disease, but hemolytic anemia may develop as the disease progresses. The platelet count is usually normal and may even increase in CML; in the later stages, however, both thrombocytopenia and anemia usually occur. The WBC count is usually greatly increased, often higher than $100 \times 10^9/L$, but it can be normal or even decreased. Morphologically, fewer than 10% myeloblasts will be seen in the peripheral blood in CML, and the blood tends to look like bone marrow because it contains all granulocyte developmental stages plus basophilia, an important finding. In CLL, very few to no lymphoblasts are seen in the peripheral blood. The blood characteristically shows a monotonous picture of lymphocytes that are all similar in size and morphology. In addition, many damaged or basket cells may be present because the lymphocytes tend to be fragile.

Laboratory Testing

Traditionally, morphologic criteria have been used to classify leukemias. The use of cytochemical and histochemical staining techniques and immunologic markers now makes it possible to identify abnormal hematopoietic precursors with more assurance. A testing battery of special studies using staining and immunologic methods is employed as part of the complete workup for a patient with leukemia. Special stains include myeloperoxidase, Sudan black stain, leukocyte alkaline phosphatase activity (LAP), TdT enzyme activity, nonspecific and specific esterase activity, and the periodic acid–Schiff (PAS) reaction. These tests are used to classify the acute leukemias in the French-American-British (FAB) system.

Prognosis

The average length of survival for patients with CML is relatively short, 3 to 4 years. CLL has an average survival of about 10 years, although prolonged survival for up to 35 years is possible, and about 30% of patients die of causes unrelated to the disease. Infection is the most common cause of death related to CLL. CML tends to proceed to an acute or accelerated stage called a *blast crisis*, and patients eventually die of hemorrhage or infection, as in acute leukemia.

OTHER MALIGNANT CHANGES

Malignant hematologic conditions other than leukemia include *plasma cell dyscrasias* (multiple myeloma, primary macroglobulinemia, Fc fragment or heavy-chain disease), *Hodgkin's disease* (or malignant lymphoma, Hodgkin's type), *non-Hodgkin malignant lymphomas*, and some unusual *tumors* closely resembling hematologic malignancies.

The laboratory has a significant role in the diagnosis and management or treatment of patients with these various hematologic diseases. Many laboratory procedures will be requested, such as cell and platelet counts, tests for the presence of anemia, coagulation studies, white cell differential count, blood film examination, cytochemical and histochemical stains, immunologic tests, and preparation and selection of appropriate blood products for transfusion therapy.

Again, the actual examination of the blood film in cases of such altered and complex morphology is left to the trained hematologist. Such changes should be recognized as abnormal during routine screening of blood films and referred to the pathologist or technologist with special training.

LYMPHOCYTE ALTERATIONS
Variant Lymphocytes (Reactive or Atypical Lymphocytes)

Reactive, atypical, or variant lymphocytes (also called *transformed lymphocytes* or *virocytes*) are particularly associated with infectious mononucleosis; however, many other viral infections also show such alterations (Fig. 12-42). Reactive lymphocytes generally show the different stages of immune responsiveness of B and T lymphocytes in the peripheral blood and immune system. In general, the cytoplasm increases in amount and appears to be reacting to a stimulus. Although the cells have been more specifically classified morphologically, they tend to have one or several of the characteristics described next.

The cytoplasm tends to become more intensely blue in color (cytoplasmic basophilia). The basophilia tends to be localized, either *peripherally*, with an increased blue color around the outer edge

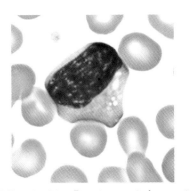

FIGURE 12-42 **Reactive, atypical, or variant lymphocyte.** (From Carr JH, Rodak BF: Clinical hematology atlas, ed 3, St Louis, 2009, Saunders.)

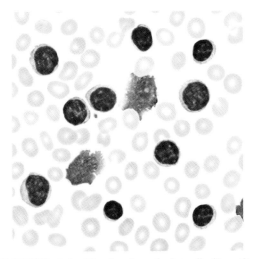

FIGURE 12-43 **Smudge or basket cells.** (From Carr JH, Rodak BF: Clinical hematology atlas, ed 3, St Louis, 2009, Saunders.)

of the cell, or *radially*, with areas of blueness radiating from the more central nucleus to the outer edges of the cell like spokes of a wheel. Radial and peripheral basophilia may be combined, in which case the cell is described as resembling a fried egg or a flared skirt. The reactive cell may also show increases or decreases in cytoplasmic volume. Cells with increased cytoplasmic volume, when observed on films prepared with Wright's stain, tend to show indentations by adjacent structures, especially RBCs. The cytoplasm appears to be flowing around and almost engulfing such structures. The cells also tend to have an increased number of nonspecific azurophilic granules in the cytoplasm.

Reactive or atypical lymphocytes also show nuclear changes. There is generally a sharper separation of chromatin and parachromatin. The nucleus may become loose and delicate, resembling an earlier developmental stage; this is referred to as a *reticular appearance*, thus the term *reticular lymphocyte*. In other cases, the nucleus becomes oval or kidney shaped with heavy clumps of deeply stained chromatin; these are called *plasmacytoid changes*, because the cells resemble plasma cells. The reactive lymphocyte may resemble the lymphoblast, and it may be necessary to rule out a leukemic process in such cases of reactive lymphocytosis.

Smudge or Basket Cells

Smudge or basket cells are damaged WBCs (Fig. 12-43). Smudge cells are cellular fragments consisting of battered or frayed nuclei with no cytoplasmic material. Basket cells are not counted as part of the white cell differential, and a few damaged cells are encountered in most peripheral blood films. They are not significant unless present in large numbers. They may be associated with CLL, and in some cases of CLL and acute leukemias, the number of basket cells may be greater than the usual lymphocyte count.

ADDITIONAL HEMATOLOGY PROCEDURES

The procedures and material discussed thus far are part of the testing often included in the so-called complete blood count (CBC). Two additional procedures, the reticulocyte count and erythrocyte sedimentation rate, are frequently performed in the clinical laboratory but are not part of the CBC.

Reticulocyte Counts

Reticulocytes are young erythrocytes that have matured enough to have lost their nuclei but not their cytoplasmic RNA. They do not have the full amount of hemoglobin. The number of reticulocytes is a measure of the regeneration or production of RBCs. Using the reticulocyte count and the immature RBC fraction is a means of establishing that a bone marrow/stem cell transplant is successful. Reticulocytes appear in a Wright-stained blood film as polychromatophilic RBCs because of the basophilic cytoplasmic remnant of the immature erythrocyte RNA.

Normal Erythropoiesis and Reticulocytes

In the circulating blood, 0.5% to 2.5% of the RBCs are usually reticulocytes. This is based on an average RBC lifespan of 120 days, with replacement of approximately 1% of the adult circulating erythrocytes each day. A reticulocyte count above this level, **reticulocytosis,** is a clinical indication that the body is attempting to meet an increased need for RBCs. An increase in reticulocytes is observed when RBCs are being hemolyzed in the body. Increased reticulocyte counts and polychromasia

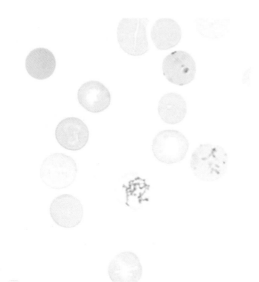

FIGURE 12-44 Reticulocytes stained with new methylene blue. (From Carr JH, Rodak BF: Clinical hematology atlas, ed 3, St Louis, 2009, Saunders.)

are characteristic of a hemolytic condition, subsequent to blood loss, treatment of anemia, or other causes. The demand for RBCs may be so great in some patients that nucleated erythrocytes are prematurely released from the bone marrow.

Specimen Requirements

Anticoagulated whole blood or capillary blood from the finger, toe, or heel may be used. Venous blood should be anticoagulated with EDTA. Heparinized blood should be avoided because the staining quality is poor. If anticoagulated whole blood is used, the test should be performed within 1 or 2 hours after the specimen is drawn because cells will continue to mature in the test tube, resulting in a decreased percent of reticulocytes seen.

Manual Methods for Counting Reticulocytes

RNA content can be detected in reticulocytes by exposing the living cells to a supravital stain. Manual methods for preparing reticulocyte slides for counts require supravital staining of the RBCs[7] (Fig. 12-44 and Procedure 12-5). In supravital staining, the living blood cells are mixed with the stain as opposed to making a film and staining it.

New methylene blue (NMB) or brilliant cresyl blue is used for the staining of reticulocytes. NMB dye is preferred; it provides consistent results and a sharp blue staining of the RNA reticulum. In addition to the dye, the stain should contain an ingredient to preserve the RBCs (provide an isotonic condition). The method described here requires that the stain prevent coagulation. Brilliant cresyl

blue contains sodium citrate, which prevents coagulation, and sodium chloride, which provides isotonicity. NMB contains sodium oxalate, which prevents coagulation, and sodium chloride. These supravital dyes precipitate the RNA in the reticulocytes, coloring it blue.

Reporting Reticulocyte Results

The classic reporting unit for the reticulocyte count is percent reticulocytes, based on counting 1000 erythrocytes, reticulocytes included. The reference values vary from 0.5% to 2.5% for adults, with a 2% to 10% accuracy for manually counted cells.

ABSOLUTE RETICULOCYTE COUNT

There is a relation between the percentage of reticulocytes calculated and the total erythrocyte count. A meaningful reticulocyte count should indicate the total production of erythrocytes, regardless of the concentration of erythrocytes in the blood. The reticulocyte count can also be reported as an absolute value by multiplying the reticulocyte count in percent by the total RBC count. This reporting method provides a comparable basis for following the progress or treatment of anemias and is the preferred way of reporting reticulocyte values.

RETICULOCYTE COUNT CORRECTED FOR A LOW HEMATOCRIT (ANEMIA)

Because a decreased hematocrit and an increased reticulocyte count ratio can exaggerate erythrocyte production response, the reticulocyte count can be corrected for the degree of anemia present by application of a factor involving hematocrit values. The patient's hematocrit is compared with a normal hematocrit (considered to be 42% for women and 45% for men) and then related to the patient's reticulocyte count, as follows:

$$\text{Corrected reticulocyte count}\,(\%)=\text{Patient's reticulocyte count}\,(\%)\times\frac{\text{Patient's hematocrit}}{\text{Normal hematocrit}}$$

RETICULOCYTE PRODUCTION INDEX

The use of this correction compensates for the amount of time it takes for reticulocytes to mature in the peripheral blood, especially when the anemia is severe and the subsequent erythropoietic response involves early release of RBCs from the bone marrow. A reticulocyte production index (RPI) factor can be applied to correct the reticulocyte count for abnormally early release of RBCs from the marrow into the peripheral blood. Premature release of cells from the marrow does not

Reticulocyte Count: New Methylene Blue Method

PRINCIPLE

Supravital stains (e.g., new methylene blue N or brilliant cresyl blue) bind, neutralize, and cross-link ribonucleic acid (RNA). These stains cause the ribosomal and residual RNA to co-precipitate with the few remaining mitochondria and ferritin masses in living young erythrocytes to form microscopically visible, dark-blue clusters and filaments (reticulum). An erythrocyte still possessing RNA is referred to as a *reticulocyte*. Counting of reticulocytes is important in assessing the status of production of erythrocytes in the bone marrow (erythropoiesis).

SPECIMEN

Whole blood that is anticoagulated with either EDTA or heparin is suitable. Capillary blood drawn into heparinized tubes or immediately mixed with stain may also be used. Mixing of the stain and blood should be performed promptly after blood collection. However, stained smears retain their color for a prolonged period.

REAGENTS, SUPPLIES, AND EQUIPMENT

Reagent

- New methylene blue solution (prepare according to manufacturer's instructions)
- Filter prepared solution daily or immediately before use to remove any precipitate

Supplies and Equipment

- Capillary tubes
- Slides
- Wright's or Wright-Giemsa stain
- Microscope, lens paper, and immersion oil
- Miller ocular disc (optional)

PROCEDURE

1. One-third of a capillary tube should be filled with well-mixed blood.
2. An equal amount of filtered stain is then drawn into the tube. The tube is rotated back and forth by hand.
3. An alternate method is to mix 2 drops of blood and 2 drops of filtered stain.
4. Allow this mixture to stand for at least 10 minutes.
5. Gently remix and expel small drops of the stain/blood mixture onto several microscope slides and prepare smears.
6. Air-dry.
7. Several slides may be counterstained with Wright's stain.
8. Using the 10× microscope objective, focus the smear. Add a drop of oil to the slide and move to the oil-immersion (100×) objective. The appropriate counting area is the portion of the smear where the erythrocytes are evenly distributed and not overlapping. Before beginning the count, scan the slide to check that reticulocytes can be located on that slide.
9. To count the reticulocytes, a minimum of 1000 (both reticulin-containing and nonreticulated) erythrocytes must be counted. Normally, 500 erythrocytes will be counted on each of two slides. If the number of reticulocytes on these two slides do not agree within 20%, a third slide of 500 erythrocytes must be counted. Be sure to count all cells that contain a blue-staining filament, fragment, or granule of reticulum in the erythrocyte. The counting field can be reduced by using paper hole reinforcers or small pieces of paper cut to fit the oculars with a small hole cut out in the middle of each. This makes counting easier than viewing the entire field.

   Note: A Miller ocular disc can be used to facilitate counting the number of reticulocytes and total RBCs.

Continued on following page

CALCULATIONS

If 57 reticulocytes are found when 1000 erythrocytes are examined (57 reticulocytes and 943 mature erythrocytes), the reticulocyte count is calculated as follows:

$$\frac{57}{1000} \times 100 = 5.7\% \text{ reticulocytes (uncorrected)}$$

REPORTING RESULTS

Reference values: 0.5% to 2.5%; neonates, 2.5% to 6.0% (corrected)

MILLER OCULAR DISC

Principle

A Miller ocular disc inserted into the eyepiece of the microscope permits a rapid survey of erythrocytes. This disc imposes two squares (one nine times the area of the other) onto the field of view.

Procedure

Reticulocytes are counted in the large square and erythrocytes in the small square in successive microscopic fields until at least 300 red blood cells (RBCs) are counted. This allows for an estimate of reticulocytes among a minimum population of 2700 erythrocytes. The absolute reticulocyte count can be determined by multiplying the reticulocyte percentage by the RBC count.

Calculations

$$\text{Reticulocytes (expressed in percentage)} = \frac{\text{No. of reticulocytes in large squares}}{\text{No. of RBCs in small squares} \times 9} \times 100$$

Example: Given that there are 40 reticulocytes in the large squares and 300 RBCs in the small squares:

$$\text{Reticulocytes (expressed in percentage)} = \frac{40}{300 \times 9} = 100 = 1.33$$

NOTE: Reticulocytes may also be counted by automated methods.

SOURCES OF ERROR

1. A refractile appearance of erythrocytes should not be confused with reticulocytes. Refractile bodies result from poor drying caused by moisture in the air.
2. Filtration of the stain is essential because precipitate can resemble a reticulocyte.
3. Erythrocyte inclusions should not be mistaken for reticulocytes. Howell-Jolly bodies appear as one or sometimes two deep-purple, dense structures.

   Heinz bodies stain a light blue-green and are usually present at the edge of the erythrocyte.

   Pappenheimer bodies are more often confused with reticulocytes and are the most difficult to distinguish. These purple-staining iron deposits generally appear as several granules in a small cluster. If Pappenheimer bodies are suspected, stain with Wright-Giemsa to verify their presence.
4. Falsely decreased reticulocyte counts can result from understaining the blood with new methylene blue.
5. High glucose levels can also cause reticulocytes to stain poorly.

CLINICAL APPLICATIONS

Certain disorders are associated with increased and decreased reticulocytes. Increased reticulocyte production can be observed following a significant blood loss, in a crisis associated with hemolytic anemia, and in pernicious anemia when treated. Decreased reticulocyte counts are associated with lack of erythrocyte production in the bone marrow. The lack of production is associated with aplastic anemia and other disorders.

PROCEDURE **12-5** (Continued)

NOTE: BD manufacturers Unopettes for reticulocyte counts. This system includes a capillary collection tube and fluid containing vessel. In addition, Bioanalytic GmgH manufactures a kit for reticulocyte counts.

REFERENCES

Brecher JW, Schneiderman M: A time-saving device for the counting of reticulocytes, Am J Clin Pathol 20:1–79, 1950.

Clinical and Laboratory Standards Institute: Method for reticulocyte counting (automated blood counters, flow cytometry, and supravital dyes): approved guideline, ed 2, Wayne, PA, 2004, CLSI Document H44-A2.

NCCLS: Method for reticulocyte counting: proposed standard, Villanova, PA, 1985, NCCLS Document H16-P.

Turgeon M: Clinical hematology, ed 4, Philadelphia, 2005, Lippincott Williams & Wilkins.

necessarily indicate increased marrow production. Abnormally early release of the RBCs from the marrow into the peripheral blood is indicated by the presence of nucleated RBCs or polychromatophilic macrocytes, also known as **shift cells,** on blood films prepared with Wright's stain. Reticulocytes normally spend approximately 2 to 3 days in the bone marrow before being released into the blood, and approximately 1% of the circulating RBCs are replaced each day. When the hematocrit and the rate of marrow release are normal, the apparent reticulocyte percentage may be considered an index of production, or maturation, and set equal to 1, as follows:

Normal reticulocyte production index (RPI) = 1

However, if reticulocytes are being released directly into the blood before maturation in the marrow, as evidenced by the presence of nucleated forms or shift cells on the blood film, the count is corrected by dividing the apparent reticulocyte count by 2 (the usual number of days of maturation).

If the presence of polychromatophilic RBCs is observed on a Wright-stained blood film, an RPI factor must be applied. The maturation time in days for the reticulocyte is[8]:

Maturation Factor (Days)	Hematocrit (% Units)
1	45
1.5	35
2	25
3	15

The corrected reticulocyte count is referred to as the *reticulocyte production index.* If no nucleated cells or shift cells are seen in the blood, the reticulocyte count is divided by 1 (i.e., left unchanged).

When both an abnormally low hematocrit and shift cells are present on the blood film, both corrections should be applied to the apparent reticulocyte count. The following general formula can be used:

$$RPI = \frac{1}{2}\left[\text{Patient's reticulocyte count (1\%)} \times \frac{\text{Patient's hematocrit}}{\text{Normal hematocrit}}\right]$$

The factor ½ represents division by a maturation factor of 2. The maturation factor can vary, depending on the severity of the anemia. Marrow can respond to anemia by a twofold to fivefold increase in erythrocyte production.

Precautions and Technical Factors With Manual Reticulocyte Counts

Careful focusing of the microscope is essential when reticulocytes are being counted. Stained platelet granules and leukocyte granules must not be mistaken for reticulocytes. Precipitated stain might also be mistaken for reticulum within the erythrocytes. To minimize this possibility, the dye must be filtered immediately before use. Immediate drying of the film will prevent the formation of the crystalline-like artifacts that sometimes appear in the RBC and resemble remnants of RNA.

The proportions of dye and blood must be altered if the patient is anemic. More blood must be used. If the procedure is followed carefully, the distribution of reticulocytes on the blood films will be good. With experience, the problem of agreement will be primarily a result of the distribution of reticulocytes on the films and not misidentification of reticulocytes. Reticulocytes have a lower specific gravity than mature RBCs and rise to the top of a blood/stain mixture. The specimen must be well mixed before the incubation period and immediately before the three slides are made. The slides must be made in a uniform manner to ensure random sampling.

Procedures employed for reticulocyte counts vary in different clinical laboratories, although the principles are the same. Variations include (1) the manner in which the stain and cells are mixed, (2) the total number of RBCs counted and the number of slides observed, (3) the use of a Miller disc in the eyepiece of the microscope to help define the field to be counted, (4) counterstaining of the reticulocyte film with Wright's stain, and (5) the use of corrections for the patient's hematocrit and the presence of shift cells.

Automated Reticulocyte Counts

With the use of an automated procedure (see Chapter 9), the process of counting reticulocytes is greatly enhanced. The flow cytometry principle is employed, cells are stained with a fluorochrome dye that preferentially stains RNA, and the cells are counted by a fluorescent technique. The RNA-containing reticulocytes will fluoresce when exposed to ultraviolet light. The instrument can count thousands of reticulocytes in just a few seconds with an accuracy of about 0.1%.

Clinical Uses for Reticulocyte Counts

The reticulocyte count is used to follow therapeutic measures for anemias in which the patient is deficient in, or lacking, one of the substances essential for manufacturing RBCs. When the deficiency has been diagnosed, therapy is begun. This consists of supplying the missing essential substances to the body and waiting for the body to react by increasing erythrocyte production. New RBCs will be released rapidly into the circulating blood, many before they are fully matured, in response to therapy. The corresponding increase in the reticulocyte count indicates a favorable response to therapy.

The response to therapy in iron-deficiency anemia (treated with iron) and pernicious anemia (treated with vitamin B_{12}) is followed by reticulocyte counts. As the total RBC count and the hemoglobin concentration reach normal levels, erythrocyte regeneration slows to the normal rate, allowing more time for maturation of the RBCs in the bone marrow. This is indicated by the presence of fewer reticulocytes in the circulating blood.

Reference Values[8]

Reticulocytes:
    Adults 0.5%-2.5%
    Newborn 2.5%-6.0%

Erythrocyte Sedimentation Rate

If blood is prevented from clotting (by using blood collected in citrate anticoagulant) and allowed to settle, sedimentation of the erythrocytes will occur. The rate at which the RBCs fall is known as the **erythrocyte sedimentation rate (ESR).** This rate depends on three main factors:
1. Number and size of erythrocyte particles
2. Plasma factors
3. Certain technical and mechanical factors

The most important factor determining the rate of fall of the RBCs is the size of the falling particle: the larger the particle, the faster it falls. The size of the falling particles depends on the formation of RBC *rouleaux,* which in turn depends on the presence of certain factors in the plasma. In normal blood the RBCs tend to remain separate from one another because they are negatively charged (zeta potential) and tend to repel each other. In many pathologic conditions, the phenomenon of rouleaux is caused by alteration of the erythrocyte surface charge by plasma proteins.

The protein that is most often involved is fibrinogen, although increases in gamma globulins or abnormal proteins also produce this effect. With increased concentrations of large molecules in the plasma, there is a greater tendency for erythrocytes to pile up in rouleaux formation.

Determination

The Westergren method is the preferred ESR method[9] (Procedure 12-6). The reference range is 0 to 20 mm in 1 hour for women and 0 to 15 mm in 1 hour for men. The reference range for ESR varies with age, gender, and the specific methodology used. The CLSI-approved method uses venous blood collected in sodium citrate anticoagulant.[10] Other anticoagulants are unsatisfactory.

Precautions and Technical Factors

The following precautions and technical factors are important in the performance of the ESR:
- An anticoagulant that not only prevents clotting but also preserves the shape and volume of the RBCs must be used. Anticoagulants that prevent erythrocyte sedimentation are unsuitable for this test.
- Because erythrocyte numbers influence the rate of fall in the ESR, the specimen must not be hemolyzed.
- Fibrin clots must not be present.
- The tube used for the test must be placed vertically in the rack; an angle different from this position can alter the rate of fall significantly. As the blood specimen stands after

Sedimentation Rate of Erythrocytes: Westergren Method

The Westergren method has been selected as the method of choice by the Clinical and Laboratory Standards Institute (CLSI).

PRINCIPLE

The erythrocyte sedimentation rate (ESR), also called the "sed rate," measures the rate of settling of erythrocytes in diluted human plasma. The rate of settling depends on variables such as the plasma protein composition, concentration of erythrocytes, and shape of the erythrocytes. The ESR value is determined by measuring the distance from the top of the erythrocyte sedimented in a special tube that is placed perpendicular in a rack for 1 hour. The clinical value of this procedure is in the diagnosis and monitoring of inflammatory or infectious states.

SPECIMEN

Fresh anticoagulated blood collected in sodium citrate is the preferred anticoagulant. The specimen must fill the entire evacuated collection tube in order to achieve the correct ratio of blood to anticoagulant. The ratio is 4 vol of blood to 1 vol of sodium citrate. Blood should be at room temperature for testing and should be no more than 2 hours old. If anticoagulated blood is refrigerated, the test must be set up within 6 hours. Hemolyzed specimens cannot be used.

REAGENT, SUPPLIES, AND EQUIPMENT

- Westergren pipettes
- Vertical rack—This special rack is equipped with a leveling bubble device to ensure that the tubes are held in a vertical position within 1 degree. The fittings on the rack should be clean and uncracked to prevent leakage of the diluted blood.

PROCEDURE

1. Mix the blood specimen thoroughly.
2. Wearing gloves, aspirate a bubble-free specimen into a clean and dry Westergren pipette. Fill to the 0 mark. Do not pipette by mouth.
3. Place the pipette into the vertical rack at 20°C to 25°C in an area free from vibrations, drafts, and direct sunlight.
4. After 60 minutes, read the distance in millimeters from the bottom of the plasma meniscus to the top of the sedimented erythrocytes.
5. Record the value as millimeters in 1 hour.

REPORTING RESULTS

The reference value of this test varies depending on age. In persons younger than 50 years of age, the average reference values are up to 10 mm/hr in males and 13 mm/hr in females. For persons older than 50 years of age, average reference values are up to 15 mm/hr in males and up to 20 mm/hr in females.

PROCEDURE NOTES

Sources of Error

Numerous sources of error have been cited for the ESR procedure. The age of the specimen is important, the test should be performed at 20°C to 25°C, and the blood should be at room temperature. Other sources of error include incorrect ratios of blood and anticoagulant, bubbles in the Westergren tube, and tilting of the ESR tube. Tilting of the tube accelerates the fall of erythrocytes, and an angle of even 3 degrees from the vertical can accelerate sedimentation by as much as 30%.

Clinical Applications

Clinical conditions associated with increased ESR values include anemia, infections, inflammation, tissue necrosis (e.g., myocardial infarction), pregnancy, and some types of hemolytic anemia.

REFERENCES

Clinical and Laboratory Standards Institute: Methods for the erythrocyte sedimentation rate (ESR) test: approved standard, ed 4, Wayne, PA, 2000, H2-A4.
Turgeon M: Clinical hematology, ed 5, Philadelphia, 2011, Lippincott Williams & Wilkins.

the venipuncture, the suspension stability of the erythrocytes increases.

- The test must be set up in the Westergren tube within 2 hours after the blood has been drawn to ensure a reliable ESR. Preferably the test should be set up within 1 hour. Specimens may be refrigerated for up to 6 hours but must be brought to room temperature before setting up the ESR.
- Temperature and vibrations can affect the ESR and should be taken into consideration.

Reporting of Test Results

The RBCs in the ESR tube are allowed to sediment for 1 hour. The results of the test are expressed in millimeters, the distance of fall for the top of the RBC column after 1 hour. Reporting an ESR result in this manner indicates that this test measures a distance of fall after a specified interval.

Clinical Significance

The ESR is a nonspecific screening test for inflammatory activity. It is a measure of the presence and severity of pathologic processes. In the vast majority of infections, there is at least some increase in the ESR; chorea and undulant fever are two exceptions. The ESR also increases in most cases of acute myocardial infarction and other inflammatory conditions. As patients recover, the ESR slowly returns to normal. The ESR may still be increased long after other clinical manifestations have disappeared, showing that the defense mechanisms of the body continue to be more active than normal.

Changes in the number and shape of erythrocytes also affect the ESR. In anemia the ESR is increased, more so in megaloblastic than iron-deficiency anemias. The rate of sedimentation is inhibited by variations in RBC shape, including spherocytes, acanthocytes, and sickle cell formation.

Increased numbers of erythrocytes, as seen in patients with polycythemia and failure of the right side of the heart, tend to cause a marked slowing of sedimentation (decreased ESR). When the hematocrit is greater than 48% to 50%, sedimentation is greatly slowed regardless of any factors present that might otherwise accelerate it.

A decrease in the ESR will result when the plasma fibrinogen level is decreased, as in patients with severe liver disease. The ESR is not increased in viral diseases, such as infectious mononucleosis and acute hepatitis, probably because fibrinogen production is not increased in these diseases despite a pronounced inflammatory reaction. The ESR is also not usually increased in chronic degenerative joint disease, but it is increased in inflammatory joint disease.

Reference Values*

Erythrocyte sedimentation rate:

50 Years and Over

Male	0 = 15 mm/hr
Female	0 = 20 mm/hr

CASE STUDIES

CASE STUDY 12-1

A 25-year-old woman has a 2-month history of difficulty in breathing and extreme fatigue. She has been on a "fad" diet for the past 6 months.

Physical examination revealed no enlargement of the spleen or liver. Laboratory data are:

Hemoglobin: 6.0 g/dL
Hematocrit: 18%
White cell count: 3.3×10^9/L
White cell differential:
   Neutrophils: 10%
   Lymphocytes: 80%
   Monocytes: 10%
   Eosinophils, basophils: 0%
Red cell count: 2.00×10^{12}/L
   RDW: 12
   Platelet count: 13.0×10^9/L
   Reticulocyte count: 0.6%

1. This patient's MCV is ___ fL.
   a. 90
   b. 85
   c. 80
   d. 75

2. This patient's MCH is ___ pg.
   a. 30
   b. 28
   c. 26
   d. 24

3. How would you classify this anemia morphologically?
   a. Hypochromic, microcytic
   b. Hypochromic, macrocytic
   c. Normochromic, normocytic
   d. Normochromic, microcytic

4. This patient's difficulty in breathing and extreme tiredness are most directly due to:
   a. low hemoglobin.
   b. low platelet count.
   c. low reticulocyte count.
   d. low white cell count.

5. The most probable type of anemia seen in this patient is:
   a. aplastic anemia from bone marrow depletion.
   b. folate-deficiency anemia.
   c. hemolytic anemia.
   d. iron-deficiency anemia.

CASE STUDY 12-2

An 80-year-old man is seen for an annual physical examination. He complains of shortness of breath on exertion and is often tired. His stool is black. Laboratory data are:

Hemoglobin: 8.2 g/dL
Hematocrit: 30%
White cell count: $4.2 \times 10^9/L$
White cell differential:
   Neutrophils: 60%
   Lymphocytes: 31%
   Monocytes: 7%
   Eosinophils: 2%
   Basophils: 0%
Red cell count: $4.0 \times 10^{12}/L$
   RDW: 20%
   Platelet count: $400 \times 10^9/L$
   Reticulocyte count: 1.2%
   Stool occult blood: Positive

1. This patient's MCV is ___ fL.
   a. 95
   b. 85
   c. 75
   d. 65

2. This patient's MCV is:
   a. within normal limits.
   b. below the reference range.
   c. above the reference range.
   d. unable to determine the reference range.

3. How would you classify this anemia morphologically?
   a. Hypochromic, microcytic
   b. Hypochromic, macrocytic
   c. Normochromic, normocytic
   d. Normochromic, microcytic

4. The most probable type of anemia seen in this patient is:
   a. aplastic anemia from bone marrow depletion.
   b. folate-deficiency anemia.
   c. hemolytic anemia.
   d. iron-deficiency anemia.

5. The anemia seen in this patient is most likely caused by which of the following?
   a. Bone marrow depletion of cells
   b. Blood loss from gastrointestinal bleeding
   c. Lack of adequate folic acid in the diet
   d. Lack of vitamin B12 the diet

CASE STUDY 12-3

A 65-year-old woman is seen in clinic. She complains of extreme fatigue, difficulty in breathing, and an extremely sore tongue. Laboratory data are:

Hemoglobin: 8.7 g/dL
Hematocrit: 25.5%
White cell count: $4.0 \times 10^9/L$
White cell differential:
   Neutrophils: 65%
   Lymphocytes: 31%
   Monocytes: 4%
Red cell count: $1.97 \times 10^{12}/L$
   RDW: 19%
   Platelet count: $134 \times 10^9/L$
   Reticulocyte count: 0.3%

1. What is this patient's MCV?
   a. 132
   b. 129
   c. 108
   d. 100

2. How would you classify this anemia morphologically?
   a. Microcytic
   b. Macrocytic
   c. Normochromic
   d. Unable to tell

3. The most probable type of anemia seen in this patient is:
   a. aplastic anemia from bone marrow depletion.
   b. megaloblastic anemia from folate or B_{12} deficiency.
   c. hemolytic anemia.
   d. iron-deficiency anemia.

4. From the hematologic results provided, which of the following erythrocyte changes would you *not* expect to find on a Wright-stained blood film from this patient?
   a. Anisocytosis
   b. Macrocytosis
   c. Poikilocytosis
   d. Polychromasia

5. This patient's total leukocyte count is:
   a. within normal limits.
   b. slightly decreased.
   c. decreased.
   d. slightly increased.

CASE STUDY 12-4

A 20-year-old female university student is seen in the student health clinic. She has a general feeling of sickness, an extremely sore throat, and swollen lymph nodes in her neck.

Blood is drawn for a CBC, and her throat is swabbed for a rapid strep test and culture. Laboratory data are:

Hemoglobin: 13.5 g/dL
Red blood cell: 3.9×10^{12}/L
Red cell indices: All within normal limits
White cell count: 14.5×10^9/L
White cell differential:
   Neutrophils: 7%
   Lymphocytes: 89%
   Monocytes: 3%
   Eosinophils: 1%
   Basophils: 0%
Platelet estimate: Normal, with normal morphology
Rapid throat culture: Negative; culture pending

1. Based on the laboratory results provided, which of the following applies?
   a. Absolute lymphocytosis
   b. Absolute neutropenia
   c. Absolute granulocytosis
   d. None of the above

2. Which of the following leukocyte changes would you expect to find on a Wright-stained blood film from this patient?
   a. Toxic granulation of neutrophils
   b. Hypersegmentation of neutrophils
   c. Variant lymphocytes
   d. Hypochromic red blood cells

3. This patient's quantitative platelet count is estimated at:
   a. 50 to 100×10^{12}/L.
   b. 100 to 150×10^{12}/L.
   c. 150 to 350×10^{12}/L.
   d. More than 450×10^{12}/L.

4. The estimated hematocrit for this patient would be ___ %.
   a. 20-24
   b. 25-29
   c. 26-35
   d. 36-39

5. The disease most likely exhibited by this patient is:
   a. infectious mononucleosis.
   b. leukemia.
   c. pneumonia.
   d. Group A β-hemolytic streptococci infection.

CASE STUDY 12-5

A 65-year old man has chills, high spiking fevers, cough, and signs of consolidation in the left lower lobe of his lung. Blood is drawn for a CBC, sputum is collected for Gram stain and culture, and a chest x-ray film is obtained. Laboratory data are:

Hemoglobin: 14.5 g/dL
HCT: 42%
Red cell indices: All within normal limits
White cell count: 24.0×10^9/L
White cell differential:
   Segmented neutrophils: 33%
   Band neutrophils: 61%
   Lymphocytes: 6%
Platelet estimate: Normal with normal morphology
Sputum Gram stain: Many gram-positive cocci in pairs; culture pending

1. From the laboratory results provided and your calculations, which of the following apply?
   a. Absolute lymphocytosis
   b. Absolute neutrophilia
   c. Neutropenia
   d. Reactive lymphocytosis

2. Which of the following leukocyte changes could you expect to find on a Wright-stained blood film from this patient?
   a. Hypersegmentation of neutrophils
   b. Variant lymphocytes
   c. Toxic granulation of neutrophils
   d. Hypochromia

3. This patient's red cell morphology on a peripheral blood smear will appear to be:
   a. microcytic, hypochromic.
   b. macrocytic, hypochromic.
   c. normocytic, normochromic.
   d. normocytic, hypochromic.

4. The patient appears to be suffering from a _____ infection.
   a. bacterial
   b. viral
   c. fungal
   d. parasitic

5. The patient's estimated red blood cell count would be:
   a. 2.4 to 3.0 × 10^{12} L.
   b. 3.1 to 4.0 × 10^{12} L.
   c. 4.1 to 4.6 × 10^{12} L.
   d. 4.7 to 5.2 × 10^{12} L.

6. The disease most likely exhibited by this patient is:
   a. infectious mononucleosis.
   b. leukemia.
   c. pneumonia.
   d. Group A β-hemolytic streptococci infection.

REFERENCES

1. Handin RI, Lux SE, Stossel TP: Blood, ed 2, Philadelphia, 2003, Lippincott, Williams & Wilkins.
2. Beutler E, Lichtman MA, Coller BS, Kipps TJ: Williams hematology, ed 5, New York, 1995, McGraw-Hill.
3. Clinical and Laboratory Standards Institute: Laboratory documents: development and control; approved guideline, ed 5, Wayne, PA, 2006, GP2-A5.
4. Clinical and Laboratory Standards Institute: Procedures and devices for the collection of diagnostic capillary blood specimens: approved standard, ed 5, Wayne, PA, 2004, H4-A5.
5. Clinical and Laboratory Standards Institute: Reference leukocyte differential count (proportional) and evaluation of instrumental methods: approved standard, Wayne, PA, 1992, H20-A.
6. Conn HJ, Darrow MS: Staining procedures used by the Biological Stain Commission, ed 2, Baltimore, 1960, Williams & Wilkins.
7. Clinical and Laboratory Standards Institute: Method for reticulocyte counting (automated blood counters, flow cytometry, and supravital dyes): approved guideline, ed 2, Wayne, PA, 2004, H44-A2.
8. Williams WJ, Beutler E, Erslev A, et al: Hematology, ed 4, New York, 1990, McGraw-Hill.
9. Westergren A: The techniques of the red cell sedimentation reaction, Am Rev Tuberc Pulmonary Dis 14:94, 1926.
10. Clinical and Laboratory Standards Institute: Methods for the erythrocyte sedimentation rate (ESR) test: approved standard, ed 4, Wayne, PA, 2000, CLSI Document H2-A4.
11. Henry JB, editor: Clinical diagnosis and management by laboratory methods, ed 19, Philadelphia, 1996, Saunders.

BIBLIOGRAPHY

Clinical and Laboratory Standards Institute: Procedure for determining packed cell volume by the microhematocrit method: approved standard, ed 3, Wayne, PA, 2000, CLSI document H7-A3.
Clinical and Laboratory Standards Institute: Reference procedures for the quantitative determination of hemoglobin in blood: approved standard, ed 3, Wayne, PA, 2000, H15-A3.
Jacobs DS, et al: Laboratory test handbook: concise with disease index, Hudson, Ohio, 1996, Lexi-Comp.
QBC Star Centrifugal Hematology System, QBC Diagnostics, 2005, www.qbcdiagnostics.com (retrieved May 8, 2006).
Turgeon M: Clinical hematology, ed 4, Philadelphia, 2005, Lippincott, Williams & Wilkins.

REVIEW QUESTIONS

1. The anticoagulant of choice for a complete blood count (CBC) is:
   a. EDTA.
   b. heparin.
   c. sodium citrate.
   d. oxalate.

Questions 2-4: Match each of the following cell types with its approximate life span in peripheral blood (a to e). An answer may be used more than once.

2. ___ Mature, inactivated B lymphocyte

3. ___ Neutrophil (PMN)

4. ___ Red blood cell
   a. Months to years
   b. 120 days
   c. 1 to 3 days
   d. About 10 hours
   e. Less than 8 hours

5. When seen on a Wright-stained peripheral blood film, a young red cell that has just extruded its nucleus is referred to as a:
   a. normoblast (metarubricyte).
   b. orthochromatic cell.
   c. polychromatophilic cell.
   d. reticulocyte.

6. Which of the following stains is classified as a Romanowsky stains?
   a. Brilliant cresyl blue
   b. New methylene blue
   c. Wright-Giemsa
   d. Prussian blue

Questions 7-11: Classify the following cells as myeloid (*a*) or lymphoid (*b*).

7. ___ B cells

8. ___ Basophils

9. ___ Eosinophils

10. ___ Neutrophils

11. ___ T cells

12. Which of the following is essential to the oxygen-carrying capacity of hemoglobin?
    a. Globin
    b. Heme
    c. Iron
    d. None of the above

Questions 13-16: *Match each of the following descriptions with the correct hemoglobin variant (a to d). Each answer will only be used once.*

13. ____ A hemoglobin variant associated with the presence of target cells on the blood film

14. ____ A hemoglobin variant resulting in sickle cell anemia in the homozygous state

15. ____ The principal form of hemoglobin found in the blood of normal adults

16. ____ The principal form of hemoglobin during intrauterine life and at birth
   a. Hemoglobin A
   b. Hemoglobin C
   c. Hemoglobin F
   d. Hemoglobin S

Questions 17-22: *Match each of the following descriptions with the correct hemoglobin derivative (a to f).*

17. ____ A stable derivative of hemoglobin bound to cyanide; used in the standard method of hemoglobin determination

18. ____ An irreversible combination of hemoglobin with a sulf group; incapable of transporting oxygen or reverting to functional hemoglobin

19. ____ Hemoglobin bound to carbon monoxide with an affinity 100 times that of oxygen

20. ____ Hemoglobin containing iron in a ferric, rather than a ferrous, state

21. ____ The form of hemoglobin that normally transports carbon dioxide from the tissues to the lungs

22. ____ The form of hemoglobin that normally transports oxygen from the lungs to the tissues
   a. Carboxyhemoglobin
   b. Hemiglobincyanide (cyanmethemoglobin)
   c. Methemoglobin
   d. Oxyhemoglobin
   e. Reduced hemoglobin
   f. Sulfhemoglobin

23. The use of daily hemoglobin control solution with automated equipment will detect which of the following? (More than one may apply.)
   a. Accuracy of the measuring device used
   b. Deterioration of the hemoglobin reagent
   c. Technical skill of the technologist
   d. Both a and b

Questions 24-29: *Match the following tests with their respective units of measurement (a to e).*

24. ____ Hematocrit (conventional)

25. ____ Hemoglobin

26. ____ Packed cell volume

27. ____ Platelet count

28. ____ Red cell count

29. ____ White cell count
   a. Cells $\times 10^9$ per liter
   b. Cells $\times 10^{12}$ per liter
   c. Grams per deciliter
   d. Liters per liter
   e. Percent

30. Assuming normochromic and normocytic red cells, a blood sample with a hemoglobin of 15 g/dL would be expected to show a hematocrit of ____ %.
   a. 25
   b. 35
   c. 45
   d. 55

Questions 31 and 32: *Match each of the following descriptions of methodology with the corresponding method for determining packed cell volume (hematocrit; a and b).*

31. ____ A centrifugation method that is rarely used; requires anticoagulated venipuncture blood and a relatively long centrifugation time

32. ____ A direct measurement of packed cell volume that may use capillary or venous blood
   a. Automated hematocrit by multiparameter instrument
   b. Spun microhematocrit

Questions 33-39: *Match the following situations regarding spun microhematocrit determinations with results (a, b, or c).*

33. ____ Capillary blood is drawn into a heparinized anticoagulated microhematocrit tube.

34. ____ Inadequate sealing of the microhematocrit tube

35. ____ Inclusion of the buffy coat in the measured packed cell volume

36. ____ Red blood cells show marked anisocytosis and poikilocytosis on the blood film.

37. ____ Use of a clotted blood sample

38. ____ Use of a hemolyzed blood sample

39. ___ Anticoagulated venous blood is drawn into an anticoagulated microhematocrit tube.
   a. Falsely high
   b. Falsely low
   c. Unaffected

Questions 40-43: Match each of the following definitions of red blood cell (RBC) indices with its common abbreviation (a to d).

40. ___ Hemoglobin concentration or color of the average RBC

41. ___ Measure of the degree of RBC size variability

42. ___ Volume or size of the average RBC

43. ___ Weight of hemoglobin in the average RBC
   a. MCH
   b. MCHC
   c. MCV
   d. RDW

Questions 44-46: Match the following blood cell indices with their respective (S.I.) units of measurement (a, b, or c).

44. ___ MCV

45. ___ MCH

46. ___ MCHC
   a. Femtoliters (fL)
   b. Picograms (pg)
   c. g/L

Questions 47 and 48: Match the following requirements for diluents with the appropriate manual cell count (a or b).

47. ___ Hemolysis of erythrocytes

48. ___ Provides isotonicity and prevents hemolysis
   a. Acetic acid
   b. Normal saline

Questions 49-54: Match the following situations regarding preparation of the peripheral blood film with the results seen in the blood film (a to g).

49. ___ Blood film covers half to three-quarters the length of slide

50. ___ Defined border at end of blood film (no feather edge)

51. ___ Dirty or chipped slides

52. ___ Dirty slides or excess fat in lipemic specimen or very high white cell count

53. ___ Large drop of blood, large angle, and slow stroke

54. ___ Small drop of blood, small angle, and fast stroke
   a. Good blood film
   b. Neutrophils accumulate in feather edge
   c. Unusually thick blood film
   d. Unusually thin blood film
   e. Vacuoles or bubbles in blood film

Questions 55-60: For blood films stained with a polychrome Romanovsky-type stain, match the cell components with the dye component (a, b, or c).

55. ___ Azurophilic granules

56. ___ Cytoplasmic RNA

57. ___ Eosinophilic granules

58. ___ Hemoglobin

59. ___ Neutrophilic granules

60. ___ Nuclear DNA
   a. Acidophilic (eosin)
   b. Basophilic (methylene blue)
   c. Acidophilic (eosin) and basophilic (methylene blue)
   d. Methylene azure (polychrome methylene blue)

Questions 61-64: Match each of the following alterations in staining with the most probable cause (a to d). Use only one alteration per cause.

61. ___ Faded or washed-out appearance of all cells

62. ___ Gross appearance of slide excessively blue, with blue-red erythrocytes and dark, granular leukocytes

63. ___ Gross appearance of slide excessively red with bright-red erythrocytes, pale-blue white cell, and brilliant-red eosinophilic granules

64. ___ Large amounts of precipitated stain
   a. Improper washing or old stain
   b. Overfixing, overstaining, underwashing; too-alkaline stain or buffer, or too-thick blood film
   c. Overwashing, understaining, underfixing
   d. Understaining, overwashing; too-acid stain, buffer, or water

65. A white blood cell (WBC) count and WBC differential are performed. WBC count: 7.0×10^9/L; of 100 WBCs classified: 70% neutrophils, 20% lymphocytes, 7% monocytes, 2% eosinophils, and 1% basophil. The absolute neutrophil cell count is ___ × 10^9/L.
   a. 2.10
   b. 3.55
   c. 3.99
   d. 5.10

Questions 66-71: Match each of the following causes or descriptions of anemia with the morphologic type (a, b, or c).

66. ___ Acute blood loss (trauma)

67. ___ Anemia associated with increased plasma volume (pregnancy and overhydration)

68. ___ Aplastic anemia from bone marrow suppression

69. ___ Iron deficiency due to diet or blood loss

70. ___ Thalassemia and other hemoglobinopathies

71. ___ Vitamin B_{12} or folate deficiency
   a. Hypochromic-microcytic
   b. Macrocytic
   c. Normochromic-normocytic

72. What is the term for erythrocytes that show normal color or staining reaction?
   a. Normochromic
   b. Normocytic
   c. Orthochromatic
   d. Polychromatophilic

73. What is an increased variation in size of erythrocytes on the blood film?
   a. Anisocytosis
   b. Microcytosis
   c. Macrocytosis
   d. Poikilocytosis

74. What is an increased variation in the shape of erythrocytes on the blood film?
   a. Anisocytosis
   b. Microcytosis
   c. Orthochromia
   d. Poikilocytosis

75. The presence of anisocytosis and poikilocytosis is reflected in which of the following red cell indices?
   a. MCV
   b. MCH
   c. MCHC
   d. RDW

76. A patient being treated for metastatic carcinoma was found to have a white cell count of 5×10^9/L with 5 metarubricytes (nucleated red cells) per 100 white WBCs. What is the corrected white cell count for this patient?
   a. 2.1×10^9/L
   b. 2.4×10^9/L
   c. 4.8×10^9/L
   d. 5.2×10^9/L

77. The presence of polychromasia on a Wright-stained peripheral blood film is associated with which of the following untreated anemias?
   a. Aplastic anemia
   b. Hemolytic anemia
   c. Iron-deficiency anemia
   d. Megaloblastic anemia

78. Which of the following leukemias is most frequently associated with the presence of the Philadelphia chromosome?
   a. Acute lymphocytic
   b. Acute myelogenous
   c. Chronic lymphocytic
   d. Chronic myelogenous

79. The presence of Auer rods in the peripheral blood is associated with which of the following cells?
   a. Lymphoblast
   b. Myeloblast
   c. Reactive lymphocyte
   d. Shift cell

80. Which of the following types of leukemia is most associated with children ages 2 to 10 years?
   a. Acute lymphoblastic
   b. Acute myelogenous
   c. Chronic lymphocytic
   d. Chronic myelogenous

81. Which of the following hematologic tests may not be part of the usual complete blood count?
   a. Hematocrit
   b. Hemoglobin
   c. Platelet estimate
   d. Reticulocyte count

82. Which of the following is a nonspecific screening test for inflammation?
   a. Erythrocyte morphology
   b. Erythrocyte sedimentation rate
   c. Leukocyte morphology and differential
   d. Platelet count

83. Which of the following tests is used to evaluate the response to therapy in the treatment of iron-deficiency anemia?
   a. Erythrocyte sedimentation rate
   b. Leukocyte morphology and differential
   c. Platelet count
   d. Reticulocyte count

CHAPTER 13

INTRODUCTION TO HEMOSTASIS

Learning Objectives

At the conclusion of this chapter, the student will be able to:

- Identify and describe the three components of the hemostatic system.
- Explain the role of platelets in hemostasis.
- Describe the three major steps of the mechanism of coagulation.
- Summarize the activity of the extrinsic pathway of coagulation.
- Summarize the activity of the intrinsic pathway of coagulation.
- List and describe the role of the various coagulation factors.
- Discuss the common laboratory tests used for coagulation and hemostasis.
- Describe the use of coagulation point-of-care tests.

Hemostasis is the cessation of blood flow from an injured blood vessel. The process of hemostasis balances numerous interdependent coagulation factors that prevent bleeding and involves a complex interaction among blood vessels, platelets, plasma coagulation factors, and inappropriate clotting. Thus, hemostasis is the process whereby the body retains the blood within the vascular system.

The result of activation of the hemostatic system is the formation of the **hemostatic plug** or **thrombus (clot)** at the site of injury to the blood vessel. Hemostasis also prevents pathologic or harmful **clotting** by controlling limitations on formation of the hemostatic plug.

Primary hemostasis results in the formation of a platelet plug. The most immediate response of the body to bleeding is **vasoconstriction;** the damaged blood vessel constricts, decreasing the blood flow through the injured area. **Platelet adhesion** is essential to the formation of a platelet plug. Platelets must be available in adequate numbers and must be functioning normally for this to occur.

Secondary hemostasis results in the formation of a blood clot because coagulation factors present in the blood interact, forming a fibrin network and a thrombus to stop the bleeding completely. Slow lysis of the thrombus begins, and final repair to the site of the injury takes place.

HEMOSTATIC MECHANISM

The hemostatic mechanism is the entire process by which bleeding from an injured blood vessel is controlled and finally stopped. It is a series of physical and biochemical changes normally initiated by an injury to the blood vessel and tissues and culminating in the transformation of fluid blood into a thrombus that effectively seals the injured vessel. The entire hemostatic mechanism can be divided into three components:

- Extravascular effects
- Vascular effects
- Intravascular effects

An unbalanced system or mechanism produces bleeding or thrombosis. These conditions can result from a defect in any of the phases of repair, as follows:

1. Vascular system itself may be prone to injury.
2. Platelets may be inadequate in number or function to form the temporary platelet plug.
3. Fibrin clotting mechanism may be inadequate.
4. Fibroblastic repair may be inadequate.

Excessive abnormal bleeding is usually the result of a combination of defects.

Extravascular Effects

The tissue surrounding the blood vessels constitutes the **extravascular component.** Extravascular effects consist of (1) the physical effects of the surrounding tissues (e.g., muscle, skin, elastic tissue), which tend to close and seal the tear in the injured vessel, and (2) the biochemical effects of certain *tissue factors* that are released from the injured tissue and react with plasma and platelet factors. These latter *coagulation factors* are found in the **extrinsic system of coagulation.**

Vascular Effects

The blood vessels themselves constitute the **vascular component.** The inner monolayer of cells of the blood vessel, the vascular endothelium, is important to hemostasis. This layer of cells provides an inert surface protecting the circulating procoagulants from inappropriate activation until coming in contact with subendothelial collagen. Trauma or injury can disrupt the endothelium and expose the underlying basement membrane of the vessel that contains collagenous material. When circulating platelets make contact with this collagenous material, biochemical and structural changes occur and result in the formation of platelet aggregates and fibrin clots. Platelet aggregates (platelet plug) can plug gaps in the endothelial lining and prevent more stimulation by the collagen layer.

Vascular effects also involve the blood vessels themselves, which constrict almost instantaneously when injured (vasoconstriction). This phenomenon tends to last a relatively short time, but it may be enhanced and prolonged by local release of a vasoconstricting substance, **serotonin.** Serotonin is released from the platelets as they adhere to the margins of the injury in the wall of the blood vessel. It promotes local, direct, biochemically stimulated narrowing of the torn blood vessel and of locally intact blood vessels in the same vicinity as the injury.

Intravascular Effects

The **intravascular component** of the hemostatic mechanism includes the platelets and plasma coagulation proteins that circulate in the blood vessels. The intravascular coagulation factors participate in an extremely complicated sequence of physiochemical reactions that transform the liquid blood into a firm **fibrin clot.** This process requires the initiation of a platelet plug, which is followed by reinforcement with fibrin derived from the activation of the **intrinsic system of coagulation.** All the coagulation factors necessary for the intrinsic system are contained within the blood. Many natural inhibitors and accelerators are brought into action during this time.

Functions of Platelets

Platelets have three important functions:

1. To react to injury of vessels by forming an aggregate plug of platelets that can physically slow down or stop blood loss
2. To help activate and participate in plasma coagulation to serve more effectively as a barrier to extensive blood loss
3. To maintain the endothelial lining of the blood vessels

To provide normal primary hemostasis, there must be an adequate number of normally functioning platelets. In the past, the bleeding time (BT) test was used as a general screening test for platelet function but now has largely been replaced by more specific platelet function tests.

Formation of Platelet Plug

When endothelial cells are damaged or displaced or become degenerate, the platelets in the bloodstream are exposed to the underlying collagen. The contact with collagen results in activation or changes in platelet function, which in turn result in **platelet adherence** to the damaged area of the blood vessel. **Fibronectin** is secreted by endothelial cells and platelets and assists in bonding platelets to the collagen substrate. An additional protein factor, **von Willebrand factor** (VIII:vWF), acts as the glue necessary for optimal platelet-collagen binding to occur. Adherence to the collagen initiates platelet activation. On activation, platelets take on a different shape, becoming more spherical with long, irregular arms. This greatly increases the surface area of the platelet and facilitates interaction with other platelets and proteins in the coagulation cascade process. Platelets also aggregate with one another because of changes that occur on their outer coats, a phenomenon known as **platelet aggregation.** The mass of platelets grows and forms the primary hemostatic plug in vivo. This plug must be stabilized by the fibrin strands produced during plasma protein coagulation for more lasting rather than temporary effects.

Platelets in Coagulation

The role of platelets in the coagulation process is varied. Platelets secrete substances that serve to promote vasoconstriction, platelet aggregation, and vessel repair. During platelet activation, alterations result in the formation of receptors capable of binding several plasma proteins, most importantly fibrinogen.

Platelet factor 3 (PF3) is a phospholipoprotein (phospholipid) that resides on or within the plasma membrane of the platelets. PF3 is required in the activation of certain coagulation factors. One important function of this activation process is facilitating the formation of thrombin.

The endothelium of blood vessels is repaired and maintained with help from products that are secreted by the platelets, such as platelet-derived growth factor (PDGF).

QUANTITATIVE PLATELET DISORDERS

The normal range of circulating platelets is $150 \times 10^9/L$ to $450 \times 10^9/L$. When the quantity of platelets decreases to levels below this range, a condition of thrombocytopenia exists. If the quantity of platelets increases, thrombocytosis is the result. Disorders of platelets can be classified as quantitative (thrombocytopenia or thrombocytosis) or qualitative (thrombocytopathy).

Thrombocytopenia

A correlation exists between severe thrombocytopenia and spontaneous clinical bleeding. If platelets are absent or severely decreased below $100 \times 10^9/L$, clinical symptoms usually include the presence of **petechiae** or **purpura.** Petechiae appear as small, purplish hemorrhagic spots on the skin or mucous membranes; purpura is characterized by extensive areas of red or dark-purple discoloration.

Thrombocytopenia can result from a wide variety of conditions, such as after the use of extracorporeal circulation in cardiac bypass surgery or in alcoholic liver disease. Heparin-induced thrombocytopenia (HIT) and associated thrombotic events, relatively common side effects of heparin therapy, can cause substantial morbidity and mortality. Thrombocytopenia in itself rarely poses a threat to affected patients, but disorders associated with it—which include deep venous thrombosis, **disseminated intravascular coagulation (DIC),** pulmonary embolism, cerebral thrombosis, myocardial infarction, and ischemic injury to the legs or arms—can produce severe morbidity and mortality.

Serum from patients with heparin-induced thrombocytopenia (HIT) contains immunoglobulin G (IgG) that, in the presence of small amounts of heparin, activates normal platelets and causes them to aggregate and release the contents of their granules, including serotonin.

Most thrombocytopenic conditions can be classified into major categories. These categories are:

1. Disorders of production
2. Disorders of destruction and disorders of utilization
3. Disorders of platelet distribution and dilution

Thrombocytosis

Thrombocytosis is generally defined as a substantial increase in circulating platelets over the normal upper limit of $450 \times 10^9/L$.

COAGULATION

When a blood vessel is injured, coagulation is the mechanism that allows plasma proteins, coagulation factors, tissue factors, and calcium to work together on the surface of the platelets to form a fibrin clot. Most clinical conditions requiring coagulation studies involve the intrinsic system of coagulation. This section discusses the coagulation factors and their nomenclature.

The blood coagulation mechanism involves many coagulation factors; knowing which factor is not performing its proper function is critical. The proper formation of a blood clot after a scratch or cut depends on healthy functioning of all the coagulation factors. In an individual with a weakness or deficiency in one or several coagulation factors, severe trauma from serious injury or surgical treatment can result in collapse of the clotting mechanism. This will result in a most drastic manifestation, severe hemorrhage. Persons whose clotting mechanism is adequate for everyday living but who, during such common surgical procedures as dental extraction or tonsillectomy, experience severe bleeding.

It is generally agreed that all the elements necessary for clot formation are normally present in the circulating blood, and that the fluidity of blood depends on a balance between the coagulant and anticoagulant.

The mechanism of coagulation takes place in the following three major steps, with the formation of a fibrin thrombus being the major goal:
1. Formation of thromboplastin
2. Formation of thrombin
3. Formation of fibrin

Coagulation Factors

The coagulation factors are fundamentally protein, with the exception of calcium and the phospholipid of the platelets.

The coagulation factors are divided into three categories: substrate, cofactors, and enzymes. Fibrinogen (factor I) is considered the substrate because the formation of a fibrin clot from fibrinogen is seen as the major goal of the coagulation process. **Cofactors** are proteins that accelerate the reactions of the enzymes involved in the process. Cofactors include coagulation factors III (tissue factor), V (labile factor), and VIII (antihemophilic factor, AHF) and high-molecular-weight kininogen (HMWK, Fitzgerald factor). Most of the remaining coagulation factors are enzyme precursors, or **zymogens,** which become active enzymes after proteolytic or structural change. Except for coagulation factor XIII (fibrin-stabilizing factor, fibrinase), which is a transamidase, the enzyme factors functioning in coagulation are serine proteases, which require vitamin K for proper formation. This becomes important when discussing anticoagulation with warfarin. Except possibly for coagulation factor VIII, coagulation proteins usually are produced in the liver. Other factors are produced in endothelial cells and the megakaryocytes.

The process of coagulation is a series of biochemical reactions in which inactive zymogens are converted to active enzyme forms, which then activate other zymogens. The coagulation process is a true coagulation cascade of factor activities, all interrelated to other factors. It is a carefully controlled process that responds to injury while continuing the maintenance of blood circulation.

Nomenclature

To standardize the complex nomenclature used by researchers involved in coagulation studies, the Scientific and Standardization Committee of the International Society on Thrombosis and Haemostasis (ISTH) has established an ongoing updating process.[1] Twelve coagulation factors are described and designated by Roman numerals; other coagulation factors are known by name only (Table 13-1).

Roman numerals have been assigned to the various coagulation factors in the order of their discovery and do not indicate anything about the sequence of the reactions. No coagulation factor has been assigned Roman numeral VI. The numerals are used to denote the coagulation factors as they exist in the plasma, except for coagulation factor III, tissue thromboplastin, which is not normally present in plasma but is found in tissue. Factor III is not a single substance but a variety of substances, which is why the ISTH committee has made "tissue thromboplastin" the standard designation and relegated factor III to an historical reference.

The lowercase *a* denotes activated forms and cofactors for the coagulation factors. All coagulation factors except tissue thromboplastin (factor III) circulate in an inactive, or precursor, form.

In addition to the coagulation factors denoted by Roman numerals, other essential coagulation reactants include phospholipid (or phospholipoprotein), the phospholipoprotein of platelets (PF3); prokallikrein (commonly called *prekallikrein* [PK]), the active form of kallikrein; kininogen; and protein C, a vitamin K–dependent factor that is an inactivator of thrombin-activated factors V and VIII.

Prekallikrein is the zymogen to plasma kallikrein, which activates factor XI. Prokallikrein is

TABLE 13-1

	Coagulation Factors	
Factor*	Name	Synonym(s)
I	Fibrinogen	
II	Prothrombin	
III	Tissue thromboplastin	Tissue factor
IV	Ionized calcium	
V	Labile factor	Proaccelerin, accelerator globulin (AcG)
VI	Stable factor	Proconvertin, serum prothrombin conversion accelerator (SPCA)
VII	(Not assigned)	
VIII:C	Antihemophilic factor (AHF)	Antihemophilic globulin (AHG), antihemophilic factor A, subunit VIII:C
VIII:vWF	von Willebrand factor (vWF)	Subunit VIII:vWF
IX	Plasma thromboplastin component (PTC)	Antihemophilic factor B (AHB), Christmas factor
X	Stuart-Prower factor	Stuart factor
XI	Plasma thromboplastin antecedent (PTA)	Antihemophilic factor C
XII	Hageman factor	Glass factor, contact factor
XIII	Fibrin-stabilizing factor (FSF)	Fibrinase
Others	Prekallikrein (PK) High-molecular-weight kininogen (HMWK) Fibronectin Antithrombin III Protein C Protein S	Fletcher factor HMW kininogen, Fitzgerald factor

*When factors have been activated, they have the designation *a* after the Roman numeral.

the proenzyme to tissue kallikrein, the activation pathway of which is not clearly understood.

Fibrinogen (Factor I)

Fibrinogen is the soluble precursor of the clot-forming protein, fibrin, and is involved in the common pathway of both the extrinsic and intrinsic clotting pathways. Fibrinogen is a globulin with a molecular weight of 340,000 daltons. It is present in the plasma of normal persons at a concentration of 200 to 400 mg/dL. A minimum of 50 to 100 mg/dL is required for normal coagulation.

Fibrinogen is synthesized by the liver but does not require vitamin K for its production. In severe liver disease, a moderate lowering of the plasma fibrinogen level may occur, although rarely to the degree that hemorrhage results.

By the action of thrombin, two peptides are split from the fibrinogen molecule, leaving a fibrin monomer. Fibrin monomers aggregate to form the final polymerized fibrin clot.

Fibrinogen is relatively unaffected by heat and storage (is stable) but may be irreversibly precipitated at 56°C. It has a half-life of 120 hours.

Prothrombin (Factor II)

Thrombin is generated from a precursor, **prothrombin,** and is involved in the common pathway of both the extrinsic and the intrinsic clotting pathway. Prothrombin is synthesized by the liver through the action of vitamin K. It is a protein (globulin) with a molecular weight of about 70,000 daltons and is normally present in the plasma in a concentration of approximately 8 to 15 mg/dL. Prothrombin is utilized in the clotting mechanism to such a degree that little remains in the serum. In normal plasma, there is an excess of prothrombin relative to the amount of thrombin needed to clot fibrinogen. A wide margin of safety has been provided for this important substance. About 20% to 40% of the normal concentration must be present to ensure hemostasis. Prothrombin is heat stable and has a half-life of 70 to 110 hours.

Tissue Thromboplastin (Factor III)

Thromboplastin, or *tissue factor* (TF), is the name given to any substance capable of converting prothrombin to thrombin. In coagulation, two separate mechanisms utilize thromboplastin: as intrinsic or blood thromboplastin and as extrinsic or tissue thromboplastin. All injured tissues yield a complex mixture of as-yet unclassified substances that possess potential thromboplastic activity. During clotting of whole blood, platelets appear to be the source of thromboplastin.

Tissue thromboplastin is a high-molecular-weight lipoprotein that is found in almost all body tissues. The molecular weight depends on the type of tissue from which the particular thromboplastin is derived; it can range from 45,000 to more than 1 million daltons. Tissue thromboplastin is found in brain, lung, vascular endothelium, liver, placenta, or kidneys.

Ionized Calcium (Factor IV)

Calcium in the ionized state is essential for coagulation. The term **ionized calcium** is now used for calcium when it participates in this process (this was formerly called "factor IV"). Ionized calcium is necessary to activate thromboplastin and to convert prothrombin to thrombin; the exact mechanism by which calcium acts is not completely understood. Only a small amount of ionized calcium is required for blood coagulation. Ionized calcium is essential for clotting, which makes possible the use of anticoagulants that bind calcium; by binding of calcium, fibrin formation cannot take place, and clotting does not occur.

Calcium appears to function mainly as a bridge between the phospholipid surface of platelets and several clotting factors. Binding sites on several factors allow bridging with the calcium-phospholipid complex.

Factor V (Proaccelerin or Labile Factor)

Factor V is essential for the prompt conversion of prothrombin to thrombin in the clotting of whole blood and is involved in the common pathway of both the extrinsic and intrinsic clotting pathways. It is synthesized in the liver; acquired deficiencies have been observed in liver disease. When factor V levels decrease to 5% to 25% of normal, bleeding occurs. Factor V is a globulin with a molecular weight of about 330,000 daltons. It is labile, its activity being destroyed in the clotting process. The activity of factor V in plasma deteriorates even when the plasma is frozen; it is the most unstable of the coagulation factors and is also known as **labile coagulation factor.** Its activity decreases within a few hours when human blood or plasma is stored at or above room temperature. It has a half-life of about 25 hours in the plasma.

Factor VII (Proconvertin, Stable Factor, Serum Prothrombin Conversion Accelerator)

Factor VII is not destroyed or consumed in the clotting process and is known as **stable factor.** It is present in both plasma and serum and is essential only for the extrinsic clotting pathway. It is a beta globulin with a molecular weight of 60,000 daltons. It is synthesized in the liver and requires vitamin K for its production. For normal coagulation, minimum levels are 5% to 10% of the normal amount. An acquired deficiency of factor VII results from any disorder that decreases its synthesis in the liver. It has a very short biological half-life, 4 to 6 hours, which results in a rapid disappearance from the blood when factor VII production is halted. This may occur during drug therapy with coumarin or in a congenitally deficient patient. Factor VII remains at a high level in stored blood as well as in serum. Factor VII activates tissue thromboplastin and accelerates the production of thrombin from prothrombin. Its presence can be monitored by the prothrombin test.

Factor VIII (Antihemophilic Factor [AHF], VIII:C, VIII:vWF, Factor VIII Clotting Activity)

Factor VIII is actually a combination of two functional subunits circulating as a complex: coagulation factors VIII:C and VIII:vWF (von Willebrand factor). The entire circulating molecule can be designated VIII/vWF.

FACTOR VIII:C

Factor VIII:C represents the ability of the factor VIII molecule to correct coagulation abnormalities associated with classic hemophilia A. A hereditary deficiency of VIII:C corresponds with classic hemophilia A; deficiencies can be acquired as well. The subunit designated coagulation factor VIII:C acts in the intrinsic clotting pathway as a cofactor to factor IXa in the conversion of X to Xa. This unit is measured by the factor VIII assay and the activated partial thromboplastin time (APTT) test.

FACTOR VIII:VWF

The other factor VIII subunit, called *factor VIII:vWF* or **von Willebrand factor,** facilitates platelet adherence to subendothelial surfaces. Factor VIII:vWF is necessary for normal platelet adhesion. It is the portion of the molecule responsible for binding platelets to endothelium and supports normal platelet adhesion and function. This subunit is not involved in the coagulation pathway. It is present in plasma, platelets, megakaryocytes, and endothelial cells.

The larger part of the factor VIII complex is made up of the VIII:vWF subunit. It is strongly antigenic, and a portion of the molecule participates in platelet aggregation induced by the antibiotic ristocetin. Laboratory tests using immunoassay are used to measure antigenic activity, while the basis of another test is the portion of the molecule that makes possible platelet aggregation in the presence of ristocetin.

The production site of factor VIII is not certain; possible sites are endothelial cells and megakaryocytes for the VIII:vWF subunit. Factor VIII is a beta globulin with a high molecular weight of more than 1 million daltons. It is lost rapidly from the bloodstream; the VIII:C subunit has a half-life of 6 to 10 hours. This rapid clearance occurs in normal persons as well as in those with a congenital deficiency of the factor (classic hemophilia A).

HEMOPHILIA A

Hemophilia refers to a sex-linked recessive coagulation disorder. The terms *antihemophilic factor* (AHF) and *antihemophilic globulin* (AHG) have been used to designate the procoagulant present in normal plasma but deficient in the plasma of patients with hemophilia. It has been demonstrated that the coagulation defect can be corrected by the use of normal plasma-mixing study. Mixing normal plasma with plasma from a patient with hemophilia A will correct the deficiency of AHF present in this patient's plasma. Further, mixing normal plasma with patient plasma is a convenient way to differentiate factor deficiency from an acquired deficiency caused by antibody deactivation or specific pathologic factor inhibitors.

The term **hemophilia A,** the classic "bleeder's disease," is adopted to designate the hereditary disease caused by a deficiency in the factor VIII:C subunit. Patients with severe hemophilia A have a history of bleeding into joints and intramuscular hemorrhage. These patients usually have normal levels of the VIII:vWF subunit and a normal BT.

Von Willebrand disease (vWD) is hereditary and is found in several different subtypes; the clinical manifestations will vary with the severity of the disease. Symptoms can include abnormal bleeding in childhood, easy bruising, bleeding gums, gastrointestinal bleeding, and abnormal bleeding after dental procedures. Patients with vWD have a deficiency of von Willebrand factor (VIII:vWF subunit of coagulation factor VIII); this factor is required for normal platelet adhesion to endothelium in the hemostatic process.

Factor IX (Plasma Thromboplastin Component)

Factor IX is a stable protein factor, an alpha or beta globulin, with a molecular weight of 55,000 to 62,000 daltons. It has a half-life of about 20 hours, is not consumed during clotting, and is not destroyed by aging. It is present in both serum and plasma, and there is probably no significant loss of the factor in blood or plasma stored at 4°C for 2 weeks. Factor IX is an essential component of the intrinsic thromboplastin-generating system. It is synthesized in the liver and requires vitamin K for its production.

HEMOPHILIA B

The disease resulting from a deficiency of factor IX is known as **hemophilia B.** It is inherited as a sex-linked recessive disorder, and its clinical symptoms are similar to those of hemophilia A. Hemophilia B can be classified as mild, moderate, or severe, paralleling the level of coagulation factor IX present.

Factor X (Stuart-Prower Factor)

This relatively stable factor is not consumed during the clotting process and therefore is found in both serum and plasma. It is an alpha globulin weighing 59,000 daltons that requires vitamin K for its synthesis in the liver. Factor X is essential to the intrinsic pathway, working with other substances to generate thromboplastin that converts prothrombin to thrombin. It helps to form the final common pathway through which products of both the intrinsic and the extrinsic thromboplastin-generating system act. Factor X is stable for several weeks to 2 months when stored at 4°C. It has a half-life of 24 to 65 hours.

Factor XI (Plasma Thromboplastin Antecedent)

Factor XI is a beta globulin weighing 160,000 to 200,000 daltons. Its synthesis takes place in the liver, and vitamin K is not required for its production. It circulates as a complex with another protein, high-molecular-weight kininogen (HMWK). Only part of factor XI is consumed during the clotting process, so it is present in the serum as well as the plasma. It is essential for the intrinsic thromboplastin-generating mechanism.

Factor XII (Hageman Factor)

Factor XII is a stable gamma globulin weighing 80,000 daltons. It is not consumed during the clotting process and is found in both serum and plasma. It is synthesized in the liver and does not depend on vitamin K for its synthesis. Factor XII is converted to an active form when it comes in contact with glass and is therefore also known as the *contact factor* or *glass factor*. The natural counterpart of glass is not known, but platelets or damaged endothelium may be involved in this primary activation process. Factor XII is involved in the initial phase of the intrinsic coagulation pathway. Deficiency of this factor does not place a patient at risk for abnormal bleeding.

Factor XIII (Fibrin-Stabilizing Factor, Fibrinase)

Factor XIII is an alpha globulin with a high molecular weight. Its site of production is not fully known but is believed to be in the liver for the plasma factor. Platelet factor XIII is synthesized by megakaryocytes. Evidence indicates that factor XIII is an enzyme (fibrinase) that catalyzes the polymerization of fibrin; polymerizing the fine fibrin clots produces a stable fibrin clot. This factor is inhibited by ethylenediaminetetraacetic acid (EDTA).

Factor XIII is used up in the polymerization of fibrin. It acts to stabilize the fibrin clot and further acts to assist in linking the endothelial cell protein fibronectin to collagen and fibrin residues; this is extremely important in tissue growth and repair. Deficiencies cannot be detected by routine testing methods.

Prokallikrein (Prekallikrein, Fletcher Factor)

Prokallikrein is a precursor for a serine protease, kallikrein, which also activates plasminogen. It is involved in the intrinsic coagulation pathway. Kallikrein is a chemotactic coagulation factor used to recruit phagocytes, and it can stimulate the complement cascade. PK is found in the plasma in association with HMWK. It is produced in the liver but is not dependent on vitamin K for its synthesis. PK is the precursor for the plasma zymogen that converts to active kallikrein.

High-Molecular-Weight Kininogen (HMWK, Fitzgerald Factor)

HMWK can be acted on to yield kinin. It serves as a cofactor for reactions involving coagulation factor XII and activation of coagulation factor VII. HMWK is involved in the intrinsic coagulation pathway. It is the precursor molecule of **bradykinin,** an important inflammatory mediator involving vascular permeability and dilation, pain production at sites of inflammation, and synthesis of prostaglandin. HMWK is produced in the liver and is not dependent on vitamin K for its synthesis.

Properties of Coagulation Factors

Coagulation factors can be divided into three groups based on their properties:

FIBRINOGEN GROUP

The fibrinogen group (thrombin sensitive) consists of coagulation factors I, V, VIII, and XIII. Thrombin acts on all these factors. Thrombin enhances factors V and VIII by converting them to active cofactors. It also activates factor XIII and converts fibrinogen (factor I) to fibrin. All these factors are consumed in the coagulation process. Coagulation factors V and VIII are relatively labile and are not present in stored plasma. In addition to their presence in plasma, fibrinogen factors are also found within platelets.

PROTHROMBIN GROUP

The prothrombin group (vitamin K dependent) consists of coagulation factors II, VII, IX, and X. Vitamin K is essential for synthesis of all these factors. Coumarin-type drugs, which inhibit vitamin K, cause a decrease in these factors. Factors VII, IX, and X are not consumed in the coagulation process and are present in serum as well in plasma. These factors are stable and are well preserved in stored plasma.

CONTACT GROUP

The contact group consists of coagulation factors XI and XII, prokallikrein (Fletcher factor), and HMWK (Fitzgerald factor). These factors are not consumed in the coagulation process, are not dependent on vitamin K for their synthesis, and are relatively stable.

Mechanism of Coagulation

The complex mechanism of coagulation takes place in three major stages.

Stage 1: Generation of Thromboplastic Activity

The thromboplastic activity necessary to convert prothrombin to thrombin is produced in stage 1 through the interaction of platelets with coagulation factors XII, XI, IX, and VIII (intrinsic pathway) or through the release of tissue thromboplastin from the injured tissues (extrinsic pathway). Plasma coagulation factor VII is activated by the tissue thromboplastic substances released by the injured tissue and initiates the extrinsic pathway. Various tests will detect stage 1 deficiencies, but the test of choice for screening and identification is the APTT test.

Stage 2: Generation of Thrombin

The plasma or tissue thromboplastin, plus factor VII produced in stage 1, in the presence of factors V and X, converts prothrombin to the active enzyme thrombin. Laboratory tests are available to detect deficiencies in stage 2. The one-stage prothrombin time (PT) test detects deficiencies best in stages 2 and 3. Abnormal formation of a clot results from a deficiency of any of the coagulation factors or the presence of an inhibitor or anticoagulant. The anticoagulants EDTA, oxalate, and citrate remove calcium to prevent clotting in vitro. Heparin and warfarin (Coumadin) drugs prevent the conversion of prothrombin to thrombin, also preventing the clotting mechanism from functioning in vivo.

Stage 3: Conversion of Fibrinogen to Fibrin

Thrombin converts fibrinogen to fibrin, and a fibrin clot is formed that is stabilized by the presence of factor XIII. The thrombin time (TT) test measures the concentration and activity of fibrinogen in stage 3. The presence of calcium ions is necessary in all three stages of the clotting mechanism.

PATHWAYS FOR COAGULATION CASCADE

The final product in the clotting process is the production of a stable fibrin clot. A series of events must take place involving many reactions and feedback mechanisms before the clot is formed. By means of the intrinsic or extrinsic pathway, or both, leading to a common pathway, the various precursors, factors, and other reactants respond normally in an orderly, controlled process—the coagulation cascade.

Intrinsic versus Extrinsic Coagulation Pathway

All factors required for the intrinsic pathway are contained within the blood. The extrinsic pathway is activated by tissue thromboplastin (factor III), which is released from the damaged cells and tissues outside the circulating blood.

Intrinsic Pathway (Activation of Factor X)

In the intrinsic pathway, the circulating blood contains all the necessary components that lead to the activation of factor X. It is thought that tissue injury, after exposure to foreign substances such as collagen, activates the intrinsic pathway. Injury to endothelial cells can begin this process. In this pathway a complex involving factors VIII and IX, in association with calcium and phospholipid on the platelets, ultimately activates factor X. To accomplish this, factor IX is first activated by the action of factor XIa (in the presence of calcium ions), which has previously been activated by factor XII (Fig. 13-1). Factors XI and XII are known as "contact" factors because their activation is ini-

tiated by contact with subendothelial basement membrane that is exposed at the time of a tissue or blood vessel injury.

Although the complex reactions that occur in the intrinsic pathway take place relatively slowly, they account for the majority of the coagulation activities in the body. A laboratory test that monitors the intrinsic pathway leading to fibrin clot formation is the APTT. The APTT measures factors XII, XI, X, IX, VIII, V, II, and fibrinogen.

Extrinsic Pathway (Activation of Factor X)

The term *extrinsic* is used to indicate the pathway taken when tissue thromboplastin, a substance not found in the blood, enters the vascular system and, in the presence of calcium and factor VII, activates factor X. Factor VII is activated to its VIIa form in the presence of ionized calcium (factor IV) and tissue thromboplastin (factor III). Factor VIIa activates coagulation factor IX to IXa, which in turn activates factor X to Xa. Thromboplastin is released from the injured wall of the blood vessel. Only activated factor VII is needed in the extrinsic pathway, bypassing factors XII, XI, IX, and VIII (used in the intrinsic pathway to activate factor X to its activated form, Xa [Fig. 13-2]). In addition to quickly providing small amounts of thrombin, which leads to fibrin formation, the thrombin generated in the extrinsic pathway can enhance the activity of factors V and VIII in the intrinsic pathway. To monitor the extrinsic pathway leading to fibrin clot formation in the laboratory, the PT test is performed. The PT measures factors VII, X, V, II, and I.

Common Pathway (Formation of Fibrin Clot from Factor X)

By means of either the extrinsic or the intrinsic pathway, or a combination of both pathways, the common pathway, the activation of factor X to Xa occurs. The activation of factor X is the point where the two pathways converge to form the common pathway. Once Xa is formed, another cofactor, V, in the presence of calcium and PF3, converts prothrombin (factor II) to the active enzyme, thrombin. The activation of thrombin is slow, but once generated, it further amplifies the coagulation process. Thrombin acts to convert fibrinogen to fibrin (Fig. 13-3). Activation of factor XIII during this process results in the formation of a stronger, more durable clot.

Fibrin Clot and Clot Retraction

The result of converting fibrinogen to fibrin is a visible fibrin clot. The fibrin clot is formed loosely over the site of injury, reinforcing the platelet

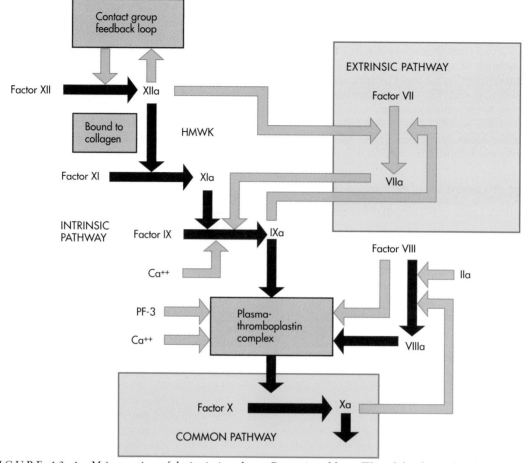

FIGURE 13-1 Major reactions of the intrinsic pathway. Generation of factor IXa and the plasma-thromboplastin complex (a, activated). *HMWK,* High-molecular-weight kininogen; *Ca++,* ionized calcium; *PF-3,* platelet factor 3. (Redrawn from Powers LW: *Diagnostic hematology,* St Louis, 1989, Mosby.)

plug and closing off the wound. After a time, the clot begins to retract and becomes smaller—**clot retraction.** This retraction is attributed to the action of the platelets and other cells that have been trapped in the clot. The fibers of fibrin are pulled closer together by cytoplasmic processes initiated by the platelets. Clot retraction can also be observed in a test tube (in vitro). The liquid remaining after the clot has retracted is serum. Normal clot retraction in vitro should be complete by 4 hours at 37°C.

FIBRINOLYSIS

Besides having a system for clot formation, the body also has a means by which the fibrin clot may be removed and the flow of blood reestablished. The mechanism for clot removal is not completely understood.

As soon as the clotting process has begun, **fibrinolysis** is initiated to break down the fibrin clot that is formed. Normally, the fibrinolytic system

functions to keep the vascular system free of fibrin clots or deposited fibrin. Evidence indicates that the **fibrinolytic system** and the coagulation system are in equilibrium in normal persons. As a general rule, fibrinolysis is increased whenever coagulation is increased.

The active enzyme that is responsible for digesting fibrin or fibrinogen is **plasmin.** Plasmin is not normally found in the circulating blood but is present in an inactive form, **plasminogen.** Plasminogen is converted to plasmin by certain proteolytic enzymes. These plasminogen activators are found in small amounts in most body tissues, in very low amounts in most body fluids, and in urine. The decomposition products of fibrin and fibrinogen, called *fibrin degradation products* (FDPs) or *fibrin split products* (FSPs), are formed during fibrinolysis and are removed from the blood by the mononuclear phagocytic system. As breakdown products of fibrin, D-dimers result only when fibrin that has been stabilized by factor XIII crosslinking has been digested.

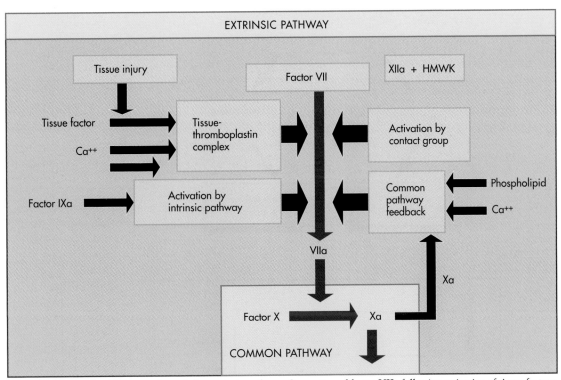

FIGURE 13-2 Major reactions of the extrinsic pathway. Generation of factor VIIa following activation of tissue factors. (Redrawn from Powers LW: Diagnostic hematology, St Louis, 1989, Mosby.)

NORMAL PROTECTIVE MECHANISMS AGAINST THROMBOSIS

To maintain a balance, the body has a number of proteins that inhibit coagulation and help prevent unwanted thrombus formation. In the blood circulation, the predisposition to thrombosis depends on the balance between procoagulant and anticoagulant factors. Several important biological activities normally protect the body against thrombosis, as follows:
1. Normal flow of blood
2. Removal of activated clotting factors and particulate material
3. Natural in vivo anticoagulant systems: antithrombin III (AT-III), heparin cofactor II (HC-II), and protein C and its cofactor, protein S
4. Cellular regulators

Normal Blood Flow

Normal flow of blood prevents the accumulation of procoagulant material, which reduces the possibility of local fibrin formation.

Removal of Materials

Activated clotting factors are removed by hepatocytes. This process and naturally occurring inhibitors limit intravascular clotting and fibrinolysis by inactivation of such factors as XIa, IXa, Xa, and IIa. Removal of particulate material is also important in preventing the initiation of coagulation.

Natural Anticoagulant Systems

The in vivo existence of natural anticoagulant systems is essential to prevent thrombosis. These natural anticoagulants include AT-III, HC-II, and protein C/protein S.

Deficiencies of AT-III, protein C, or protein S, as well as their inhibitors (antibodies), will contribute to a hypercoagulable state. Enzyme-linked immunosorbent assay (ELISA) tests will reveal deficiencies of these proteins.

Antithrombin III

AT-III is considered the major inhibitor of thrombin. It inhibits thrombin formation by forming a stable, one-to-one complex with thrombin. AT-III is the principal physiologic inhibitor of thrombin and factor Xa. It is also known to inhibit factors IXa, XIa, and XIIa.

The AT-III laboratory assay relies on the principle that in the presence of heparin, thrombin is neutralized at a rate that is proportional to the antithrombin (AT-III) concentration. After defibrination, plasma is assayed in a two-stage procedure that uses standardized amounts of heparin,

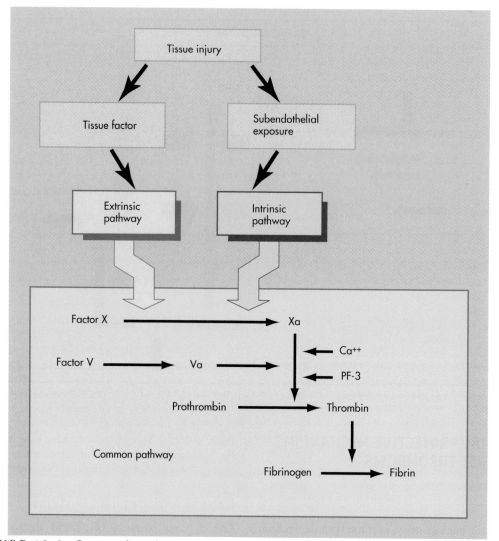

FIGURE 13-3 Overview of coagulation. Relationships among the three pathways—common, extrinsic, and intrinsic—emphasizing the major events of the common pathway. *PF-3,* Platelet factor 3. (Redrawn from Powers LW: Diagnostic hematology, St Louis, 1989, Mosby.)

fibrinogen, and thrombin. The resulting clotting time is interpreted using a calibration curve.

Heparin Cofactor

AT-III heparin cofactor and HC-II are two heparin-dependent thrombin inhibitors present in human plasma. Heparin is produced endogenously by mast cells, and heparin-like molecules are found in the endothelium.

Protein C and Protein S

Protein C is synthesized in the liver and circulates as an inactive zymogen. Protein C is converted to an active form, *activated protein* C (APC), by thrombin in the presence of **thrombomodulin,** which is found on the endothelial cells. APC in the presence of

the cofactor protein S cleaves factor Va and factor VIIIa into their inactive Vi and VIIIi forms (*i* indicating inactive). Its interaction with protein C and protein S shows that thrombin acts not only as a **procoagulant,** but also as an anticoagulant.

APC resistance, also known as *factor V Leiden,* is a genetic variation of the factor V protein that alters the binding site for APC and prevents APC from inactivating factor Va. The heterozygous form of this genetic variation occurs in up to 20% of people tested. It accounts for 20% to 50% of cases of inherited thrombophilia.

Cellular Regulators

Cellular regulators include enzymes, which are cellular proteases that block the activation or action of plasmin. In addition, cells that regulate coagulation include not only hepatic cells but also monocytes, macrophages, and platelets. The production of protein S cofactor by endothelial cells is believed to play a significant regulatory role in the initiation, propagation, and suppression of hemostasis and thrombosis.

TESTS FOR HEMOSTASIS AND COAGULATION

Screening Tests for Disorders of Hemostatic System

Diagnosis of disorders of the hemostatic system should begin with a physical examination and clinical history of the patient and family members. It is also important to include a complete drug history, which will often provide information about the type of disorder that may be affecting the patient. Hemostatic disorders can be secondary to several primary diseases, such as liver disorders, renal failure, and certain carcinomas. Screening tests for hemostasis and coagulation include tests for the condition of the blood vessels (vascular coagulation factors), for platelets, and for the coagulation and fibrinolytic systems—divided according to the main lines of defense against hemorrhage (see Hemostatic Mechanism). A comprehensive and carefully obtained clinical history is considered the most valuable screening test.

Tests for the vascular factors include the capillary fragility test (also known as the *cuff test*, *tourniquet test*, or *capillary resistance test*) and BT tests. Current tests for platelets include the platelet count, platelet aggregation assays, and platelet adhesiveness studies. There are various tests for the plasma coagulation factors and whole blood coagulation factors involved in coagulation: the venous clotting time, PT, and APPT (Table 13-2).

Tests for Vascular Coagulation Factors

Bleeding Time Tests

Bleeding time (BT) tests measure the time required for cessation of bleeding after a standardized capillary puncture to a capillary bed. The time required will depend on capillary integrity, the number of platelets, and the platelet function. There must be an adequate number of circulating platelets for a normal BT. If a platelet count is less than 50×10^9/L, the BT is almost always prolonged. Platelet dysfunction is better assayed by more specific tests such as platelet aggregation, and the use of the BT test for platelet function is not considered as useful as in the past.

The BT test is positive (prolonged BT) in von Willebrand disease (vWD), thrombocytopenic purpura, and constitutional capillary inferiority. Normal BTs are found in hemophilia and other defects of the clotting mechanism. BT tests especially focus on the number of platelets present and their ability to form a plug. Besides low platelet count, prolonged BTs are also generally found with platelet dysfunction or when the patient has recently ingested aspirin-containing compounds, and it is recommended that BTs not be done in these patients. In any patient a BT test should not be done unless a platelet count has been done shortly before the BT.

TEMPLATE BLEEDING TIME TEST (MIELKE MODIFICATION)

A number of different BT tests have been devised. The test now in use is a modification by Mielke and colleagues of the original Ivy bleeding time test; two incisions of a standardized depth are made, and the average of the two bleeding times is reported.[2,3] A blood pressure cuff is used to maintain the blood pressure at 40 mm Hg during the test. The chief difficulty in performing BT tests in general is the production of adequate and standardized skin punctures; a valid test result depends greatly on the way the skin wound is made. Capillary bleeding is tested, and wounds more than 3 mm deep are likely to involve vessels of greater than capillary size, whereas wounds that are shallow are not likely to adequately test the capillaries and the hemostatic coagulation factors involved. A standardized, disposable BT test system (e.g., Simplate) is preferred, whereby compliance with infection control measures is also achieved. A CLSI guideline document provides information about performing template BT tests.[4]

Tests for Platelet Function

Platelet dysfunction may be acquired, inherited, or induced by platelet-inhibiting agents. It is clinically important to assess platelet function as a potential cause of a bleeding diathesis, especially in critically ill patients who may develop life-threatening hemorrhages. The most common causes of platelet dysfunction are related to uremia, liver disease, vWD, and exposure to agents such as acetylsalicylic acid (ASA, aspirin). Current methods to assess platelet function include platelet aggregation studies and whole-blood in vitro test systems such as the closure time.

Platelet Closure Times

Closure time (CT) is a test system to assess platelet-related primary hemostasis with greater accuracy and reliability than BT. The CT assay is an important aid in the assessment of platelet dysfunction

TABLE 13-2

Laboratory Tests for Hemostasis and Coagulation	
Test	Purpose/Factor Assessment
Bleeding time (BT)	Platelet factors: function and number
	Vascular factors: capillary integrity
Capillary fragility (cuff test, tourniquet test)	Vascular factors (condition of blood vessels)
Platelet count	Platelet factors: platelet numbers
Platelet aggregation	Platelet factors: platelet function
Platelet adhesion (platelet retention)	Platelet factors: platelet function
Clot retraction	Platelet factors: platelet function
Activated partial thromboplastin time (APTT)	Plasma factors: deficiencies in intrinsic and common pathways; identifies stage I deficiencies (factors XII, XI, IX, VIII, V, II, I); monitors heparin therapy
Prothrombin time (PT)	Plasma factors: deficiencies in extrinsic and common pathways; identifies stage II and III deficiencies (factors VII, X, V, II, I); monitors coumarin therapy
Thrombin time (TT)	Plasma factors: measures concentration and activity of fibrinogen in stage III; monitors coumarin therapy
Fibrinogen	Plasma factors: deficiencies of fibrinogen, alteration in conversion of fibrinogen to fibrin
Specific Factor Assays	Plasma Factors
Factor VIII:C	Deficiency: hemophilia A
Factor VIII:vWF	Deficiency: von Willebrand disease
Factor IX	Deficiency: hemophilia B

and bleeding risk caused by uremia, vWD, congenital platelet disorders, and exposure to agents such as aspirin. CTs are indicated when a disorder of platelet function is suspected by a personal or family history of easy bruising, nosebleeds (epistaxis), menorrhagia, or postoperative bleeding, especially after dental extraction or tonsillectomy. CT is not recommended as a screen for potential bleeding risk. CTs may be prolonged when the platelet count is less than 100,000/mm^3 even if platelet function is normal. In addition, CT will be prolonged when hematocrit levels are less than 35%, because of the contributory effect of red blood cells on platelet behavior. These restrictions should be considered before performing CT testing.

Suspected vWD, inherited platelet disorders, and evaluation of acquired disorders of platelet function (hepatic disease, renal disease, drug effects) are appropriate clinical reasons for CT screening. It may also be useful to monitor the response of therapeutics, such as desmopressin (DDAVP) infusions, renal dialysis, and platelet/antiplatelet drug therapy. Abnormal CTs, indicating possible defective platelet function, should be further investigated with standard platelet aggregation tests.

Closure times are performed on a PFA-100, an instrument and test cartridge system in which the process of platelet adhesion and aggregation after vascular injury is simulated in vitro. This system allows for rapid evaluation of platelet function on samples of anticoagulated whole blood. Membranes consisting of collagen/epinephrine (CEPI) and collagen/adenosine-5′-diphosphate (CADP) and the high shear rates generated under standardized flow conditions result in platelet attachment, activation, and aggregation, building a stable platelet plug at the aperture. The time required to obtain full occlusion of the aperture is reported as the CT in seconds.[5]

Platelet Aggregation Studies

The response of platelets during the hemostatic process includes a change in shape, an increase in surface adhesiveness, and the tendency to aggregate with other platelets to form a plug. Measurement of platelet aggregation is an essential part of the investigation of any patient with suspected platelet dysfunction. An aggregating agent is added to a suspension of platelets in **platelet-rich plasma (PRP),** and the response is measured turbidometrically as a change in the transmission of light. The various commercially available instruments devised to conduct this test are called *aggregometers* or *platelet function analyzers.* The platelet function CT automates the measurement of aggregation in the presence of various aggregating reagents.

When an aggregating reagent (e.g., thrombin, adenosine diphosphate [ADP], epinephrine, serotonin, arachidonic acid, ristocetin, snake venoms, collagen) is added to PRP being stirred in a cuvette at a constant temperature, platelets start to aggregate, and the transmission of light increases. The PRP appears turbid at the beginning of the test. With the addition of the aggregating reagent, larger platelet aggregates begin to form, and thus the PRP begins to clear, with a corresponding increase in the light being transmitted. The increased change in optical density or transmission of light is recorded as a function of time on a moving strip recording. The platelet response curve consists of distinct phases that vary with the concentration and type of aggregating reagent used. The response curve can indicate whether an observed clinical picture is caused by a platelet dysfunction or vWD.

Automated Platelet Function Analysis

Conventional platelet aggregometry and platelet adhesiveness testing is too time consuming and labor intensive for many applications where point-of-care tests or rapid turnaround times are indicated. Several automated platelet function analyzers have been developed.

Impedance platelet counting uses two separate anticoagulated samples, one of which contains ADP and collagen. The platelet count is measured in an impedance hematology analyzer and the percent aggregation calculated.[6]

Platelet aggregation under flow conditions can measure quantitative, qualitative, and vWF defects. Citrated whole blood is aspirated under constant vacuum through apertures coated with platelet agonists. These agonists include epinephrine/collagen and collagen/ADP. The platelets undergo adherence, activation, and aggregation, ultimately plugging the aperture. The time required for closure is measured and the results evaluated to identify inherited dysfunction such as Glanzmann's thrombasthenia and Bernard-Soulier syndrome. vWD can be detected and DDAVP monitored in patients who are responsive to desmopressin therapy (stimulates release of vWF). This test system is insensitive to defects or deficiencies in the classic coagulation factors or fibrinogen. In a similar process, nonanticoagulated whole blood is passed through small holes in a blood conduit. In one hole, a collagen fiber is present to activate the platelets, and CT is measured. This system simulates in vivo clotting and platelet function under physiologic conditions.[7]

Tests for Plasma Coagulation Factors

To assess potential defects in the coagulation cascade, screening tests are first performed. Common screening tests of the plasma coagulation system are the one-stage **prothrombin time (PT),** or prothrombin assay; the **activated partial thromboplastin time (APTT);** and the **thrombin time (TT).** Other related tests for coagulation are bleeding time, platelet counts, and the older clot retraction test (see Table 13-2). Once it has been determined by the screening tests that the patient has a coagulation disorder, the exact coagulation factor deficiency or abnormality should be identified.

In the monitoring of anticoagulant therapy, measurement of prothrombin is most often done when the patient is receiving coumarin drugs. Heparin therapy is usually followed by determining the APTT and TT, although the whole-blood coagulation time is occasionally used.

The manual methods for coagulation tests have been replaced by automated and semiautomated equipment. Automated methodology is based on manual methods. Several instruments are available that can do coagulation tests for PT and APTT. Two nonautomated techniques for performing plasma-clotting tests are discussed in this section: the assay for prothrombin and the APTT.

Specimens for Coagulation Tests

In the coagulation laboratory, the ultimate goal is to reflect the patient's actual state of hemostatic function in vivo. Any factor that causes the test to misrepresent the actual state of coagulation function in the patient can lead to adverse outcomes for the patient.

According to CLSI, "Coagulation tests are exquisitely susceptible to error introduced by suboptimal specimen quality. This is due to the fact that the very act of obtaining a blood sample initiates the hemostatic response, the physiologic system that the testing is designed to assess."[8]

Specimens for coagulation tests must be collected in the least traumatic manner; the premature activation of the clotting process must be avoided to ensure valid test results. The blood must be drawn carefully to avoid:

1. Contamination of the specimen with tissue thromboplastin
2. Contact with the surface of an inappropriate specimen container
3. Use of an inappropriate anticoagulant
4. Improper temperature conditions
5. Any technique that would produce hemolysis of the specimen

CLSI guidelines cover the essentials for the proper collection, transport, and processing of blood specimens for coagulation testing.[9] Coagulation assays are highly vulnerable to preanalytical variability because of:

1. Complexity of the biochemical and cellular reactions measured in assays such as the PT and APTT
2. Lability of several coagulation proteins
3. Calcium dependence of many of these reactions
4. Highly excitable nature of blood platelets[8]

ANTICOAGULANTS

The majority of coagulation laboratory errors arise in the preanalytical (preevaluation) phase. Ensuring the quality of citrated blood samples is critical for accurate test results.[10] Screening coagulation assays are performed on plasma that has been processed from blood anticoagulated with a 3.2% sodium citrate solution. The citrate reversibly binds calcium ions and prevents the various steps in the coagulation process, beginning with the activation of factors IX and VII. Binding the calcium does not inhibit the contact phase of coagulation, so it is critical that no activation of this process be made while the blood is being collected or processed. An example of contact-phase effects is premature activation of factors XI and XII if blood comes in contact with glass. For this reason, only nonreactive materials can be used for collection tubes or testing steps when performing coagulation tests.

The ratio of blood to anticoagulant is critical for clotting tests, necessitating only the use of evacuated-tube systems with the proper vacuum; expiration dates must be observed, and outdated tubes must not be used. By a long-established convention for coagulation tests, nine volumes of carefully drawn blood are mixed with one volume of citrate anticoagulant (1:10 ratio). The standard ratio of anticoagulant to sample is 1:10 for persons with hematocrit between 20% and 60%. Ratios must be changed for persons who are extremely polycythemic. For specimens from patients with extremely high hematocrit, when there is a reduced plasma volume, the use of a reduced anticoagulant volume is needed. CLSI recommends that "the final concentration in the blood should be adjusted in patients who have hematocrits above 0.55 L/L (55%)."[10] Clots are unacceptable in a specimen because clots change the activity of clotting factors.

COLLECTION TECHNIQUE

The screening coagulation tests are performed on plasma. A clean, rapid venipuncture is necessary to prevent tissue thromboplastin from contaminating the blood sample. Tissue thromboplastin (in the tissue juices) can be found in blood samples when the vessel has been cut or traumatized, and even a slight amount can alter coagulation test results for both normal and abnormal

samples. Hemolyzed red blood cells act similar to tissue thromboplastin in activating plasma coagulation factors, and thus hemolysis of the sample must be avoided. Glass surfaces affect hemostasis; certain coagulation factors will be prematurely activated by contact with glass. Nonreactive materials and nonwettable surfaces, which will not interact or activate the coagulation mechanism, should be used; silicone-coated glass or plastic containers are recommended for collecting specimens for coagulation tests. Temperature also affects hemostasis; for example, factors V and VIII are very labile if left at room temperature for any length of time, and factors VII and XI are activated prematurely by cold temperatures. For most coagulation testing, a room-temperature specimen is recommended.[10]

Either a syringe or an evacuated-tube system can be used to collect the specimen. A clean entry into the vein must be made. The blood should flow quickly and smoothly into the container.

Evacuated-Tube System

A common collection system uses evacuated collection tubes, which are available with 3.2% buffered citrate anticoagulant. There is less direct contact with the actual blood specimen when these tubes are used, an important safety issue. In the evacuated-tube system, blood should be collected into the citrated tubes for coagulation studies before blood has been drawn for other tests. BD and CLSI has recommended the proper order of draw[9] (see Chapter 2).

It is important to maintain the correct blood/anticoagulant ratio. Therefore the vacuum citrate tube must be allowed to fill completely, and only tubes within their expiration dates should be used.

SPECIMEN PROCESSING

Once the sample is drawn, some changes can begin quickly in vitro. Transportation to the laboratory for testing should be done as quickly and carefully as possible. CLSI allows PT specimens to remain uncentrifuged for up to 24 hours (as long as the tube stays capped). Specimens to be tested for APTT should be centrifuged and the plasma tested or separated from the cells within 60 minutes of being drawn if the patient is receiving heparin. Otherwise, CLSI states that the APTT specimens do not need to be centrifuged for up to 4 hours. The tubes should be kept stoppered during centrifuging and until the plasma is removed for testing. The platelet-poor ($<10 \times 10^9$/L) plasma-anticoagulant mixture should be separated from the cellular elements unless testing is done immediately; when immediate testing is done, the plasma may remain on the packed cells.

It is important to check the sample for micro-clot formation. If present, specimens are unacceptable for testing because clotting has been initiated. Specimens that have visible hemolysis are also unacceptable for testing because of possible coagulation factor activation and interference in endpoints for many of the analytical testing instruments being used. Most instruments using an optical detector may also have problems with endpoint determinations using samples that are extremely icteric or lipemic. The plasma to be tested should be kept refrigerated in a tightly covered clean tube until it is tested.

Performance of Coagulation Assays

General guidelines apply to most coagulation tests. CLSI guidelines outline recommendations for determination of coagulant activities, specifically assays for measurement of PT and APTT.[10,11] Specific manufacturer's instructions for each instrument must be followed explicitly. For coagulation assays, an ongoing program of quality control should be in place and carefully followed to comply with Clinical Laboratory Improvement Amendments of 1988 (CLIA '88) regulations. Records must be maintained for documentation purposes.

Quality Control

Normal and abnormal controls should be run when testing is begun each day and at the beginning of each new work shift or with each test run of assays. Control specimens are reconstituted daily from a lyophilized aliquot, or frozen controls are used. Controls must be used within their established viability periods (usually 8 to 16 hours). Once a control is thawed or reconstituted, it should not be refrozen or reused. Control samples should be handled and tested under conditions similar or identical to those for the patient samples being tested. Patient values are not reported unless the control values are within the established reference range. CLSI guidelines cover the essentials in regard to issues of quality control for coagulation testing.[12]

Laboratories must develop their own reference ranges representing a normal population for the particular facility. Reference ranges should be reestablished when a new lot of reagents is implemented, with major changes in collection techniques, or when new instruments are introduced into the laboratory.

Prothrombin Assay

The original assay for PT was devised on the assumption that when an optimal amount of calcium and an excess of thromboplastin are added to decalcified plasma, the rate of coagulation depends on the concentration of prothrombin in the plasma.[12]

Prothrombin time is the time required for the plasma to clot after an excess of thromboplastin and an optimal concentration of calcium have been added. The assay measures the functional activity of the extrinsic (and common) coagulation pathway. PT tests generation of thrombin (stage 2) and conversion of fibrinogen to fibrin (stage 3) of the clotting mechanism and screens for deficiencies of factors I, II, V, VII, and X. A normal PT assay shows that the factors of stages 2 and 3 of the coagulation mechanism are probably not disturbed.

The measurement of PT is the method of choice for monitoring anticoagulant therapy with vitamin K antagonists (warfarin-type oral anticoagulant drugs, e.g., Coumadin), especially for preventing postoperative thrombosis and pulmonary embolism, and to screen for coagulation factor deficiencies in hemorrhagic diseases. If the degree of anticoagulation is insufficient, rethrombosis or embolism can occur, but an excess of anticoagulation can produce a fatal hemorrhage.

The reagents necessary for the prothrombin assay are primarily calcium chloride and thromboplastin. Thromboplastin reagents with an assigned ISI (international sensitivity index) are used. Each prothrombin control must be prepared before use according to the manufacturer's directions. Control values and limits will vary with the brand of control used. The laboratory will establish its own range for the control specimens. Proper use of the control can detect (1) deterioration of the thromboplastin and (2) use of an improper incubation temperature.

PRECAUTIONS AND TECHNICAL FACTORS

Prothrombin assays should be done within 24 hours of blood collection, if the specimen remains capped. After that time, plasma must be frozen. Freezing should occur at −20°C for up to 2 weeks and −70°C for up to 6 months.

When the thromboplastin-calcium reagent is used, it is important to mix the suspension very well. The blood for this test must be free of clots; if any clots are present, a new specimen must be drawn. The ratio of anticoagulant to blood specimen should be 1:10.

AUTOMATED PROTHROMBIN ASSAYS

Automated or semiautomated assays are employed for conducting coagulation testing. The endpoint of the reaction is the formation of a fibrin clot. The older Fibrometer (BBL Microbiology Systems, BD), which is used as a backup instrument in many laboratories, is a semiautomated, electromechanical instrument for coagulation assays. It consists of a Fibrometer coagulation timer, a thermal preparation block or incubator, and an automatic pipetting system. The Fibrometer consists of a timer, several warming wells, and a clot detector (probe arm with electrodes).

Automated or semiautomated coagulation systems are available. Clot formation is timed automatically and is detected by a photocell that reads the optical density change when the clot is formed. The unit contains a heating block that brings the reagents and plasma samples to 37°C during the testing process. These analyzers automatically pipette the necessary reagents and samples or require manual pipetting before analysis. All routine coagulation assays may be performed with these instruments, including PT, APTT, specific coagulation factor assays, TT, and fibrinogen tests. Reagents are stored at room or refrigerator temperature. Refrigeration helps to maintain reagent integrity.

REPORTING PROTHROMBIN RESULTS: INTERNATIONAL NORMALIZED RATIO

For many years, the results of assays to measure prothrombin were reported in seconds, using prothrombin time tests, or PTs. The prothrombin time is not actually a quantitative assay for prothrombin. The **international normalized ratio (INR)** was first used instead of seconds to report results for prothrombin assays when the test was being used to monitor patients receiving oral anticoagulant therapy. The reference values for PT in seconds range from 10 to 13 seconds. Therapeutic range is considered to be longer than 25 seconds. Experience has shown that the INR is used by physicians more often than the PT in seconds for any purpose, not only for patients receiving oral anticoagulant therapy. Therefore, in most clinical settings, the PT is no longer reported in seconds only.

The World Health Organization (WHO) originally helped devise use of the INR for patients receiving long-term anticoagulant therapy to ensure that tests done in different laboratories would yield comparable results. Even though different thromboplastins and different instrumentation are used in various laboratories, the INR makes standardization of oral anticoagulant therapy possible. The use of the INR effectively calibrates the results of a particular PT reagent or instrument system to results of an international reference reagent.[12]

Manufacturers of thromboplastin reagents provide the **international sensitivity index (ISI)** for each lot of reagents. The ISI is a mathematical indicator of the responsiveness of the PT testing system to deficiencies of the vitamin K coagulation factors. The WHO reference thromboplastin is highly responsive and has an assigned ISI of 1.0. The ISI is obtained by comparing the manufacturer's thromboplastin reagent with the WHO international reference thromboplastin. The ISI for a specific test system is used to convert the observed PT ratio to its INR equivalent. The INR is the ratio between the sample PT over the mean normal PT (MNPT) raised to the power of a calculated ISI of the standardized thromboplastin reagent (TP): INR = (patient PT/MNPT) ISI.

The INR reference range is 0.9 to 1.13 in persons age 1 year or older, and increasing INR values correspond to increased anticoagulation. Most patients receiving warfarin are required to maintain INR values between 2 and 3, or 2.5 and 3.5 for oral anticoagulant therapy because of a mechanical value. The INR becomes elevated with deficiencies in coagulation factors in the extrinsic pathway. These deficiencies most often result from the use of oral anticoagulant therapy, which depletes the vitamin K–dependent coagulation factors (II, VII, IX, X) or from liver disease.

Activated Partial Thromboplastin Time

The APTT, like the prothrombin time assay, is automated using the same instrumentation as the PT. But in the APTT assay an activator, calcium chloride, is mixed with a phospholipid component of thromboplastin (a platelet substitute) before addition to the plasma being tested. Only a partial component of thromboplastin is used, thus giving the test its name. The activator used depends on the manufacturer of the reagents; one activator is a *kaolin* suspension[13] (a finely divided silicate clay). The APTT test is the most useful routine screening procedure for factor deficiencies of the intrinsic and common pathways. The APTT adds the kaolin, an activator of factor XII, which allows more complete activation, shortens the clotting times, and improves reproducibility over the formerly used "partial thromboplastin time" (PTT) test.

The APTT measures deficiencies mainly in factors VIII, IX, XI, and XII but can detect deficiencies of all factors except VII and XIII. The tests are based on the observation that when whole thromboplastin is used, as for prothrombin assays, the times obtained for hemophilic plasma are about the same as those for normal plasma. With a partial thromboplastin solution or platelet substitute, the times obtained for hemophilic plasma are much longer than those for normal plasma.

The principal use of the APTT test is in the management of patients receiving heparin therapy. The sensitivity of the thromboplastin reagent must be evaluated before this test is used as a heparin control. Most thromboplastin reagents are insensitive to low-molecular-weight (LMW) heparins. Anti-Xa assays should be used to monitor LMW heparin. LMW heparin generally does not require monitoring, except in extremes of patient weight, pregnancy, renal disease, and children.

A phospholipid substitute for platelets acts as a partial thromboplastin. It is more sensitive to the absence of coagulation factors involved in intrinsic thromboplastin formation than are the more complete tissue thromboplastins used in prothrombin assays.

Activation in the procedure is obtained by separate addition of a kaolin suspension.[14] Kaolin ensures maximal activation of the coagulation factors. Addition of kaolin speeds up the slow contact phase of the coagulation cascade. Activators used can vary with the manufacturer of the reagents being used. By activation of the contact coagulation factors, more consistent and reproducible results are achieved.

The APTT test result will be prolonged in contact and intrinsic coagulation factor deficiencies. The presence of an inhibitor, such as the lupus anticoagulant, in the patient's plasma may also be the cause of a prolonged APTT. The APTT is used to monitor heparin concentration during intravenous administration. The APTT is not sensitive to minor abnormalities in some common-pathway coagulation factors but is useful to screen mild to moderate deficiencies of factors VIII and IX and the contact coagulation factors. Deficiencies of these coagulation factors represent the most common and potentially serious disorders. If an abnormal APTT is determined, differential studies should be done for specific coagulation factor deficiencies.

The principle of the APTT test is the assumption that during anticoagulation, the calcium present in the blood is bound to the anticoagulant. After centrifugation, the plasma contains all the intrinsic coagulation factors except calcium (removed during anticoagulation) and platelets (removed during centrifugation). Under carefully controlled conditions and with properly prepared reagents, calcium, a phospholipid platelet substitute (the partial thromboplastin), and an activator (kaolin) are added to the plasma to be tested. The time required for the plasma to clot is the APTT. The normal times proposed by the reagent manufacturer should be followed.

Normal control results must always fall within the acceptable control range; if they do not, a problem exists with the reagents, the equipment, or the technique being used. When the control is out of range, the entire test must be repeated. Most laboratories also include controls in the "high" and "low" ranges at least once a day. The ranges for

controls are established by the laboratory before each new lot is placed into service.

PRECAUTIONS AND TECHNICAL FACTORS

Use of kaolin provides maximal activation of the coagulation factors and therefore more consistent and reproducible results. Kaolin in suspension settles out very quickly; when kaolin is used, it is necessary to mix the solutions vigorously before any pipetting is done. Many automated instruments provide continual mixing. Citrated blood should be centrifuged within 1 hour of collection. Plasma allowed to sit longer than the recommended time can lead to abnormal results.

REPORTING RESULTS

APTT tests are reported in seconds to the nearest tenth of a second, along with the control specimen reference values established for the laboratory. Results must be clearly marked for "patient" or "control." Generally, a normal APTT is less than 35 seconds, with a range from 25 to 40 seconds. Control plasmas must be run every 8 hours and their values must fall within the laboratory's reference range. Deviations in control results can be due to deterioration over time, temperature changes, different reagent lots, the technique being used, or instrument malfunction, if automation or semiautomation is being employed.

D-Dimer Assay

The D-dimer assay is actually two different tests, with each having a specific application and each being completely misleading when used for the wrong application. D-Dimer is the cross-linked breakdown product of fibrin. There are two analytical avenues for testing for D-dimer: ELISA and particle agglutination. Particle agglutination is used for detecting D-dimers associated with disseminated intravascular coagulation (DIC) and does not require a high degree of sensitivity because they are being generated systemically. The particle agglutination tests generally detect D-dimers at about 500 ng/mL. The ELISA testing for D-dimer is a more sensitive order of magnitude, detecting below 10 ng/mL. This level of sensitivity is necessary to rule out venous thromboembolism (VTE). Using a particle agglutination test to rule out VTEs will result in many false-negative results, and using ELISA D-dimer testing for diagnosing DIC will result in false-positive results.[14]

Other Tests for Coagulation

Other tests for specific coagulation factors include:
- Prothrombin consumption test
- Thromboplastin generation test

- Plasma recalcification time (plasma clotting time)
- Thrombin time (TT)
- Fibrinogen titer
- Quantitative tests for fibrinogen
- Russell viper venom time
- Reptilase time
- von Willebrand factor and other coagulation factor assays
- Assays for the hypercoagulable state, antithrombin III, protein C and activated protein C, protein S, and circulating lupus anticoagulant

Point-of-Care Tests for Coagulation Assays

Because turnaround time is of great importance in certain clinical situations, **point-of-care testing (POCT)** for some coagulation assays is used. During surgical procedures for patients receiving heparin anticoagulant therapy, POCT tests for activated clotting time (ACT) can be performed. Several studies have shown that frequent home monitoring of oral anticoagulant therapy time reduces the number of major bleeds or thrombotic events.

Coagulation Analyzers

Some POCT analyzers use only capillary blood, and others use capillary blood, whole blood, plasma, or all three. Coagulation analyzers can be used in surgical suites, intensive care units, dialysis units, or other patient care units. Fresh whole blood is added to a sample well on a test cartridge, which is inserted into the instrument after a prompt signal appears. The blood sample is drawn by capillary action into the test channel, where it mixes with the reagents. An electro-optical system detects the point at which blood flow ceases and the clot forms; this is the endpoint of the assay. The result appears in a display window. Results with whole blood are higher than for the typical laboratory analyzers, which use plasma. Results are converted to equivalent plasma values, and INRs are given for prothrombin assays. Coagulation POCT results should be included in the patient's chart in the same manner as for traditional coagulation test results.

Quality Control

Quality control programs must be used with any POCT coagulation analyzer. CLIA '88 regulations mandate that two levels of control, normal and abnormal, be assayed during each 8-hour shift for automated coagulation systems, traditional methods, and POCT. The manufacturers of these coagulation POCT analyzers are working to improve their electronic quality control, but at present, conventional liquid coagulation controls remain the CLIA '88–acceptable type. Use of liquid controls is expensive for POCT coagulation assays because the control specimen is viable for only a specific time (usually 8 to 16 hours). Also, often only a few patients are tested by POCT during this time, unlike traditional in-laboratory coagulation testing, in which many tests are performed during an 8-hour shift. Each time a control specimen or patient specimen is tested, a test cartridge is used, increasing the cost for the testing.

Problems and Drawbacks

Reagents for coagulation POCT are considerably more expensive than reagents for conventional coagulation assays. Another potential drawback of coagulation POCT is that with the ease of using these analyzers and with the availability of almost instantaneous data, the advantages of their use may be negated if data are lost or never transferred to the patient's permanent record. Validation of coagulation POC analyzers can be daunting. Calibration to dissimilar laboratory-based methods requires comparison of laboratory wet reagents to POCT dry reagents with different reaction kinetics. The coefficient of variation (CV) of the INRs generated on a POCT instrument may range from 9% to 13%, whereas plasma-based assays typically do not exceed 5%. For this reason, clinicians require that the POCT be done on one instrument consistently, and that if the INR must be generated on an alternate system, its respective interval must be consulted.[15]

Training of Users

It is important that any person who is to use the coagulation POCT analyzers be adequately trained in their use and that the training be documented. Ideally, the users should be trained under the auspices of the laboratory, and the quality control measures should be monitored by laboratory staff. Some manufacturers of coagulation POCT analyzers provide users, including physicians, patients (in their homes), and other health care workers, with a system of quality management. This includes in-depth training in the use of the analyzer and technical support, if needed, in the future. Training must include information about the importance of good specimen collection techniques and the use of quality control measures.

CASE STUDIES

CASE STUDY 13-1

A 23-year-old man has a long history of abnormal bleeding into his joints.

Laboratory Data

Prothrombin assay: Normal

APTT: Greatly prolonged

Factor VIII assay: Greatly decreased

Factor IX assay: Normal

Platelet count: Normal

Template bleeding time: Normal

Which of the following disorders is the most likely for this patient?

a. Classic hemophilia A

b. Classic hemophilia B

c. von Willebrand disease

d. Severe liver disease

CASE STUDY 13-2

A 45-year-old female patient has severe liver disease with jaundice, purpura (bleeding into the tissues), and a platelet count of 120×10^9/L.

Which one of the following prothrombin time (PT) and bleeding time (BT) profiles is most likely for this patient?

a. Prolonged PT, prolonged BT

b. Normal PT, prolonged BT

c. Normal PT, normal BT

d. Prolonged PT, normal BT

CASE STUDY 13-3

A 25-year-old man was admitted to the hospital for surgical repair of an abdominal hernia. He was in good physical condition, but his family history included minor bleeding problems among some of his relatives.

Laboratory Data

Prothrombin time: Normal

APTT: Prolonged

Factors VIII assay: Normal

Factors VIII:C: Normal

Factors VIII:vWF: Normal

Factor IX assay: Decreased

Platelet count: Normal

Platelet aggregation test: Normal

Template bleeding time: Normal

Based on the history and laboratory results, this patient most likely has which of the following disorders?

a. Classic hemophilia A

b. Classic hemophilia B

c. von Willebrand disease

d. Severe liver disease

REFERENCES

1. International Society on Thrombosis and Haemostasis (ISTH): Scientific and Standardization Committee; International Union of Pure and Applied Chemistry–International Federation of Clinical Chemistry (IUPAC-IFCC), Commission/Committee on Quantities and Units (in Clinical Chemistry): Nomenclature of quantities and units in thrombosis and haemostasis, Thromb Haemost 71:375, 1994.
2. Ivy AC, Shapiro PF, Melnick P: The bleeding tendency in jaundice, Surg Gynecol Obstet 60:781, 1935.
3. Mielke CH, Kaneshiro IA, Maher JM, et al: The standardized normal Ivy bleeding time and its prolongation by aspirin, Blood 34:204, 1969.
4. Clinical and Laboratory Standards Institute: Performance of the bleeding time test: approved guideline, ed 2, Wayne, Pa, 2005, H45-A2.
5. Hassett AC, Bontempo FA: Closure time platelet function screening, transfusion medicine update, Institute for Transfusion Medicine, www.itxm.org (retrieved November 2005).
6. Lennon MJ, Gibbs NM, Weightman WM, et al: A comparison of plateletworks and platelet aggregometry for the assessment of aspirin-related platelet dysfunction in cardiac surgical patients, J Cardiothorac Vasc Anesth 18:136, 2004.
7. Mammen EF, Comp PC, Gosselin R, et al: PFA-100 system: a new method for assessment of platelet dysfunction, Semin Thromb Hemost 24:195, 1998.
8. Lawrence JB: CE Update, Laboratory Medicine Vol. 34, No 1:49–57, Jan. 2003.
9. Clinical and Laboratory Standards Institute: Collection, transport, and processing of blood specimens for coagulation testing and performance of coagulation assays: approved guideline, ed 4, Wayne, Pa, 2003, H21-A4.
10. NCCLS: Determination of coagulation factors coagulant activities: approved guideline, Wayne, Pa, 1997, NCCLS Document H48-A.
11. Clinical and Laboratory Standards Institute: One-stage prothrombin time (PT) test and activated partial thromboplastin time test (APTT): approved guideline, Wayne, Pa, 1996, H47-A.
12. International Committee for Standardization in Haematology: International Committee on Thrombosis and Haemostasis: ICSH/ICTH recommendations for reporting prothrombin time in oral anticoagulant control, Thromb Haemost 53:155, 1985.
13. Proctor RR, Rapaport SL: The partial thromboplastin time with kaolin, Am J Clin Pathol 36:212, 1961.
14. Houdiijk WP: Efficacy of d-dimer, Adv Admin Lab 13:72, 2004.
15. Fritsma GA, Marques MB: Top ten problems in coagulation (2004), *Advance* 16:22, 2004.

BIBLIOGRAPHY

Accumetrics: Verify Now Aspirin, San Diego, 2005.

Cheng X et al: Prevalence, profile, predictors, and natural history of aspirin resistance measured by the Ultegra rapid platelet function assay-ASA in patients with coronary heart disease: clinical studies/outcomes, presentation number C-25, International Federation of Clinical Chemistry (IFCC)/American Association for Clinical Chemistry (AACC) meeting, Orlando, Fla, July 2005.

Clinical and Laboratory Standards Institute: Assays of von Willebrand factor antigen and ristocetin cofactor activity: approved guideline, Wayne, Pa, 2002, H51-A.

Clinical and Laboratory Standards Institute: Point-of care monitoring of anticoagulation therapy: approved guideline, Wayne, Pa, 2004, H49-A.

Clinical and Laboratory Standards Institute: Procedures for validation of INR and local calibration of PT/INR systems: approved guideline, Wayne, Pa, 2004, H54-A.

Ford A: Immunoassay market overflowing with change, CAP Today 19(6):18, 2005.

Helena Laboratories Point of Care: Plateletworks Point of Care, Beaumont, 2004, Texas.

Katz B, Marques MB: Point-of-care testing in oral anticoagulation: what is the point? MLO, March 2004, pp 30-35, www.mlo-online.com (retrieved August 2005).

Margolius HS: Kallikreins and kinins: some unanswered questions about system characteristics and roles in human disease, Hypertension 26:221, 1995.

Schmaier AH: The kallikrein-kinin and the renin-angiotensin systems have a multilayered interaction, Am J Physiol Regul Integr Comp Physiol 285:R1, 2003.

Turgeon ML: Clinical hematology: theory and procedures, ed 4, Philadelphia, 2005, Lippincott, Williams & Wilkins.

REVIEW QUESTIONS

1. Which of the following is the anticoagulant of choice for routine coagulation assays?
   a. Heparin
   b. Sodium oxalate
   c. Sodium citrate
   d. Sodium fluoride

2. The prothrombin assay requires that the patient's citrated plasma be combined with which one of the following?
   a. Thromboplastin
   b. Calcium chloride and thromboplastin
   c. Calcium chloride
   d. Kaolin

3. What does the silicate (kaolin) do in the test system for APTT?
   a. Binds calcium so that clotting does not occur
   b. Activates tissue thromboplastin
   c. Facilitates platelet adherence to endothelial surfaces
   d. Allows more complete activation of coagulation factor XII, thus shortening the clotting times

4. Which of the following peripheral blood cells is involved in hemostasis?
   a. Thrombocytes
   b. Lymphocytes
   c. Erythrocytes
   d. Granulocytes

Questions 5-8: Filling in the blank with the factor number, is the following statement correct? A = True, B = False.

Factor ___ is used only in the extrinsic coagulation pathway.

5. ___ III

6. ___ V

7. ___ VII

8. ___ VIII

Questions 9-12: Filling in the blank with the factor number, is the following statement correct? A = True, B = False.

Factor ___ is part of the common coagulation pathway.

9. ___ V

10. ___ X

11. ___ XI

12. ___ XII

13. The bleeding time test is almost always prolonged when the platelet count is:
    a. $<10 \times 10^9$/L.
    b. $<50 \times 10^9$/L.
    c. $<100 \times 10^9$/L.
    d. $>100 \times 10^9$/L.

Questions 14-17: Filling in the blank with the factor number, is the following statement correct? A = True, B = False.

Factor ___ will be inhibited by coumarin-type drugs.

14. ___ II

15. ___ VII

16. ___ VIII

17. ___ X

18. Fibrinogen is synthesized in the:
    a. liver.
    b. endothelium.
    c. platelets.
    d. plasma.

19. Primary hemostasis results in:
    a. formation of a thrombus.
    b. retraction of the clot.
    c. formulation of a platelet plug.
    d. presence of vitamin K.

Questions 20-23: Which of the following completed statements about platelets is (are) correct, and which is (are) incorrect? A = True, B = False.

For control of most bleeding:

20. ___ PF3 is important in activation of some coagulation factors.

21. ___ Platelet adhesion is essential.

22. ___ VIII: vWF acts as a glue for platelet-collagen binding to occur.

23. ___Aggregate with one another because of interchemical changes in each platelet.

24. Clot removal is accomplished by which of the following systems?
    a. Fibrinolysis
    b. Hemostasis
    c. Thrombosis
    d. Anticoagulation

Questions 25-28: A = True, B = False.

This test can assess potential defects in the coagulation cascade.

25. ___ Platelet count

26. ___ Bleeding time

27. ___ Prothrombin assay

28. ___ Activated partial thromboplastin time

29. Hemostasis is defined as a process to:
    a. localize an injury.
    b. restore normal anatomy.
    c. stop bleeding from an injured blood vessel.
    d. facilitate the removal of a clot.

30. Hemophilia A is a disorder associated with a deficiency of:
    a. factor VIII.
    b. factor IX.

    c. circulating platelets.
    d. vitamin K–dependent coagulation factors.

Questions 31-34: Fill in the blank with the factor number, is the following statement correct? A = True, B = False.

Factor ___ is measured by the prothrombin assay.

31. ___ V

32. ___ VII

33. ___ VIII

34. ___ IX

35. Which of the following is the most accurate POCT coagulation test used to monitor heparin?
    a. Prothrombin
    b. Activated partial thromboplastin time
    c. Bleeding time
    d. Platelet count

RENAL PHYSIOLOGY AND URINALYSIS

Learning Objectives

At the conclusion of this chapter, the student will be able to:

- Compare the characteristics of historic and modern urinalysis.
- Define routine urinalysis and describe its three main components.

- Explain the clinical usefulness of urinalysis and classify tests pertaining to diseases or conditions affecting the kidney or urinary tract and metabolic disease.

Continued

Learning Objectives—cont'd

- Describe the basic anatomic components of the urinary system and the function of each.
- Discuss the chemical composition of normal urine.
- Identify and compare various urine specimen requirements for a routine urinalysis, including preservation and storage requirements.
- Discuss the differences between various types of urine collection, including mid-stream clean-catch, quantitative, and timed specimens.
- Identify and describe normal and abnormal physical properties (especially color and transparency) that might be encountered in urine specimens, and correlate physical findings with chemical and microscopic findings.
- Discuss the relationship between urine volume and specific gravity.
- Define the term *specific gravity*.
- Test a urine specimen for chemical constituents by using a multiple-reagent strip, and demonstrate correct technique.
- For each of the analytes discussed in this chapter, describe the following: clinical importance, principle of the test, specificity and sensitivity, interferences, and additional considerations.
- Discuss the pathophysiology and significance of proteinuria due to glomerular damage, tubular damage, prerenal disorders, lower urinary tract disorders, asymptomatic proteinuria, and consistent microalbuminuria.
- Compare the pathophysiology of hematuria, hemoglobinuria, and myoglobinuria, and explain how to differentiate among the respective analytes when a positive reagent strip test for blood is seen.

- Discuss the pathophysiology and clinical importance of tests for nitrite and leukocyte esterase and how they relate to each other.
- Discuss the pathophysiology and clinical importance of bilirubin and urobilinogen, and identify the laboratory findings in various types of jaundice.
- Describe conditions when urine should be examined microscopically.
- Perform a microscopic examination of the urine sediment.
- Identify and discuss the various urine sediment constituents that might be encountered, including pathophysiology and clinical importance.
- Describe the formation and significance of casts and how they are classified and reported.
- List the normal crystals encountered in acid and alkaline urine, and describe the most frequently encountered forms of each.
- List the abnormal crystals of metabolic and iatrogenic origin, and describe the most frequently encountered forms of each.
- Discuss the relationships among sediment, chemical, and physical findings in the urine.
- Discuss the components of a quality assessment system for urinalysis.
- Recognize discrepant results when reviewing urinalysis findings (physical, chemical, and sediment), before results are reported.
- Analyze a case study in terms of the relevance of the laboratory findings to the clinical condition.

OVERVIEW OF URINALYSIS

History of Urinalysis

Hippocrates, Aristotle, and the ancient Egyptians inferred diagnoses from urine evaluation, but it was not until the Middle Ages that uroscopy reached diagnostic dominance. A major reason for its rise to prominence was the publication of Johannes de Ketham's *Fasciculus Medicinae* in 1491. This was the first illustrated medical book printed. It depicts a urine wheel: a large circle surrounded by thin-necked, urine-filled flasks. This wheel shows how the color and consistency of urine could be matched to a diagnosis. Disease was thought to result from the imbalance of humours, reflected by one of the urine colors. In the corners of the urine wheel, four small circles contain descriptions of the four temperaments/humors[1]:

1. Sanguineous (blood)
2. Choleric (yellow bile)
3. Phlegmatic (phlegm)
4. Melancholic (black bile)

Modern Urinalysis

Urine yields a great amount of valuable information quickly and economically. **Urinalysis** remains one of the three major in vitro diagnostic screening tests, after serum chemistry profiles and complete blood counts. The physical, chemical, and microscopic analysis of the urine is known as *urinalysis*. In general, a urinalysis will provide information that reflects a patient's general health, as well as a clinical picture of the patient and potential disease (Box 14-1).

Urine samples are readily available, and many of the routine tests are relatively simple to perform using chemically impregnated strips. When manually performed, a test strip is immersed into a urine specimen, and a color reaction is observed by visual comparison with a color chart at an appropriate time. Semiautomated or fully automated systems are used in laboratories with a high volume of tests.

Quality Assessment and Quality Control

The urinalysis laboratory, as with all departments of the clinical laboratory, requires a quality assessment program to ensure that results of testing are meaningful. For many years, preanalytical improvements have centered on blood specimens. Urine collection and processing often have lagged behind and represent areas with opportunity for improvement.[2]

Preanalytical phases of urine testing consists of six phases:

1. Test ordering
2. Sample collection
3. Specimen transport to the laboratory
4. Specimen receipt in the laboratory
5. Preparation of samples for testing
6. Transportation of samples to the section of the laboratory where testing occurs

Each of these subphases contains between two and five steps, so the average preanalytical urine testing workflow consist of at least 22 steps. Common areas of preanalytical variability in urine testing include patient-related factors, specimen collection, specimen identification and labeling, specimen transfer and transport, and specimen processing.[2] Their effect on the outcomes of urine testing is described in more detail in this chapter.

The specifics of a given quality assurance program must meet Clinical Laboratory Improvement Amendments of 1988 (CLIA '88) regulations (see Chapter 8). Quality assessment elements include record keeping, the procedure manual, materials and equipment, proficiency testing, and continuing education and training.

The use of multiple-reagent strips generally ensures rapid and reliable screening of all specimens, providing a greater range of abnormal constituents than was possible before these strips came into routine use. Tests must be performed in a technically correct manner, and the reagent strips and tablets must be stored properly so that they react as they were designed to react; this is ensured by the use of control specimens.

Control solutions must be used each day by each shift of workers. Several quality control products are commercially available and suitable for use in the laboratory. Most are obtained in lyophilized form (freeze-dried human urine) and require reconstitution before use. Positive and negative controls are available, and both should be used in the routine testing program. The products are assayed for expected results with common reagent strips and methods. The assayed values available for a product will be a factor in determining which product a laboratory uses.

Urinalysis control solutions may be used both as a check on the urinalysis reagents and procedures and as a means of evaluating the ability of the laboratory personnel to perform and interpret the tests correctly. New bottles of reagent strips and tablets should be tested when first opened. All previously opened bottles of reagent strips and tablets should be tested at the beginning of each shift. Controls should be included whenever new reagents are used. Control solutions should be employed that check for both false-negative and false-positive results, the relative sensitivity at different concentrations, and the stability of the reagents.

Results should be recorded or documented in such a way as to ensure that the laboratory remains in control and that problems are corrected when detected. The notation system used will vary from laboratory to laboratory; control results may be tabulated on daily and weekly graphs similar to those used for clinical chemistry analyses. Control specimens should be tested as follows:

1. Test all opened bottles of reagent strips or tablets each morning.
2. Test each new bottle on opening.
3. Record data on the record sheet daily.

All bottles should be covered tightly when not in use. The manufacturer's directions for storage should be carefully followed. If any discoloration appears on the reagent strips or tablets, discard the bottle immediately. Record the date when a bottle is first opened. Note the expiration date, and do not use any product after that date.

Although infrequently used, refractometers should be checked when used for accuracy, and the data should be recorded in an acceptable manner. The method of checking refractometers is described later (see Specific Gravity).

Probably the oldest and still the most useful tool in quality control of urinalysis is a final inspection of all the results that make up the urinalysis before they are reported on the patient's laboratory record. Correlation of expected findings is discussed in this chapter whenever applicable. To correctly inspect the testing output for correlated results, laboratory staff must know the limitations of the tests and the reasons for their use. Physical properties, chemical test results, and constituents seen in the urinary sediment should be correlated, and if discrepancies are seen, they should be corrected or explained before results are reported.

RENAL ANATOMY AND PHYSIOLOGY[3]

Renal Anatomy

In general, urine can be considered a fluid composed of the waste materials of the blood. It is formed in the kidney and excreted from the body by way of the urinary system.

Anatomy of the Kidney

The urinary system consists of two kidneys, located in the retroperitoneal space on either side of the vertebral column (between T11-12 and L3); two ureters; the bladder; and the urethra (Fig. 14-1). Blood enters the kidney through the renal artery. This artery branches into smaller and smaller units, finally becoming the afferent arterioles entering the glomerular tuft. Blood leaves the glomerulus through the efferent arterioles. These arterioles run close to the corresponding renal tubules of the nephron so that reabsorption and secretion between the blood and glomerular filtrate can occur. The kidney is a highly vascular organ. Normally, one-fourth of the cardiac output is contained within the kidneys at a given time.

Gross examination of the kidneys reveals two bean-shaped, reddish brown organs. Each kidney weighs about 150 g. Much of the medial border is occupied by an indentation, the **hilum,** through which the renal vessels, nerves, lymphatics, and the renal pelvis enter or leave the **renal sinus,** the space enclosed by the renal parenchyma. The

bisected kidney through the hilum shows that the parenchyma consists of an outer **cortex,** which forms a continuous subcapsular band of tissue, and an inner **medulla,** which is discontinuous, interrupted by projections of the cortex toward the renal sinus, the renal **columns** (columns of Bertin). The medulla consists of several triangular structures, the **pyramids,** with their bases toward the cortex and their tips, called **papillae,** projecting into minor calyces.

Renal Physiology

The functional unit of the kidney is the nephron (Fig. 14-2), where urine is formed. The formed urine flows from the kidney into the ureter and is passed to the bladder for temporary storage. It is eliminated from the body through the urethra.

The kidney may be described as having the following main functions:

1. Removal of waste products, primarily nitrogenous wastes from protein metabolism, and acids
2. Retention of nutrients such as electrolytes, protein, water, and glucose
3. Acid-base balance
4. Water and electrolyte balance
5. Hormone synthesis, such as erythropoietin, renin, and vitamin D

These functions are carried out by means of filtration, reabsorption, and secretion.

Glomerulus

Each nephron consists of a tuft of anastomosing capillaries called the **glomerulus.** Blood enters the glomerulus from the renal circulation through the afferent arteriole and leaves through the efferent arteriole. Urine formation begins with the glomerulus, the structure that delivers the blood to the nephron; it is the "working portion" of the kidney.

Glomerular (Bowman's) Capsule

As blood circulates through the glomerulus, it is filtered into Bowman's capsule. The glomerular capillaries are covered by the inner layer of Bowman's capsule, forming a semipermeable membrane that allows passage of all substances with molecular weights less than about 70,000 daltons. The fluid that passes through this membrane is basically blood plasma without proteins and fats. It is an *ultrafiltrate* of blood and is called the **glomerular filtrate.** Because it has most of the solutes of plasma, the glomerular filtrate is **iso-osmolar** with plasma. That is, it has about the same osmolality as plasma, 232 to 300 mOsm/L, with a specific gravity of about 1.008. The formation of the glomerular

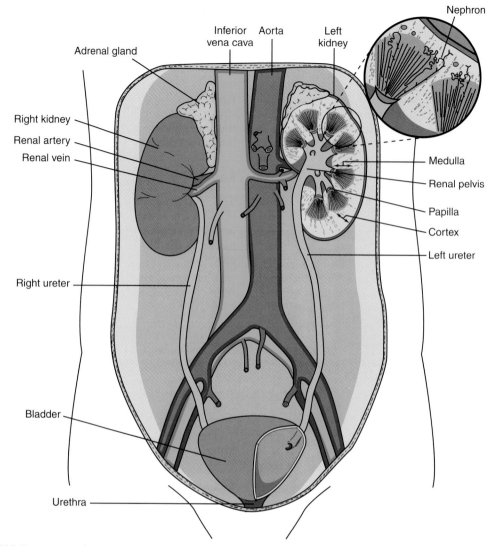

FIGURE 14-1 **The urinary system.** (From Brunzel NA: Fundamentals of urine and body fluid analysis, ed 2, Philadelphia, 2004, Saunders.)

filtrate is the first step in urine formation. About 180 L of glomerular filtrate are produced daily, but only 1 or 2 L of urine are eliminated from the body. Therefore, most of the glomerular filtrate is reabsorbed back into the blood.

Proximal Convoluted Tubule

Reabsorption from the renal tubules back into the blood begins at the proximal convoluted tubule, where about 80% of the fluid and electrolytes filtered by the glomerulus is reabsorbed.

Reabsorption may be **active reabsorption,** with an expenditure of energy required for the analyte to be reabsorbed, usually against a concentration gradient, from a region of lower to a region of higher concentration. Alternately, the reabsorption may be **passive reabsorption,** in which case an analyte

moves passively down a concentration gradient, from a region of higher to a region of lower concentration. In addition, an analyte can move passively along with another analyte that may be actively reabsorbed.

Most of the water in the glomerular filtrate is passively reabsorbed along with sodium ions, which are actively reabsorbed by the sodium pump mechanism. Chloride, bicarbonate, and potassium ions, together with 40% to 50% of the urea present in the filtrate, are passively reabsorbed with water at the proximal tubules. Other analytes that are actively reabsorbed in the proximal convoluted tubules include glucose, protein as albumin (a small amount of albumin is filtered into Bowman's capsule and subsequently reabsorbed), amino acids, uric acid, calcium, potassium, magnesium, and phosphate.

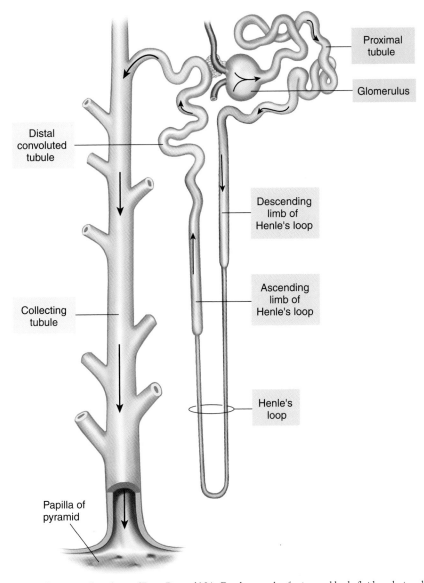

FIGURE 14-2 **Diagram of nephron.** (From Brunzel NA: Fundamentals of urine and body fluid analysis, ed 2, Philadelphia, 2004, Saunders.)

The proximal tubule has a limit to the amount of an analyte that will be completely reabsorbed from the glomerular filtrate. This is referred to as the **renal plasma threshold.** This differs with each analyte. When the plasma concentration of an analyte is greater than its renal plasma threshold, it will remain in the glomerular filtrate and be excreted in the urine. For example, the renal plasma threshold for glucose is about 180 mg/dL. When a patient with diabetes mellitus has a blood glucose concentration greater than 180 g/dL, excess glucose will be eliminated in the urine.

The proximal convoluted tubules are also a site of active secretion of body wastes. The secretion includes hydrogen ions, phosphate, organic acids, and certain drugs such as penicillin. Hydrogen ions

are secreted in exchange for sodium ions, which are reabsorbed with bicarbonate into the plasma. This exchange depends on the presence of the enzyme carbonic anhydrase, which is present in proximal and distal renal tubular cells and red blood cells.

Solutes and water are reabsorbed in equal proportions at the proximal tubules, so the tubular fluid is still iso-osmolar with plasma when it leaves the proximal tubules.

Loop of Henle

The descending and ascending loops of Henle function to reduce the volume of the urine while reabsorbing or recovering sodium and chloride. The descending portion of the loop is the concentrating portion. The interstitial fluid outside the tubules in the medulla of the kidney becomes hypertonic as a result of increased concentrations of sodium, chloride, and urea in the tubules. This occurs because the descending portion is freely permeable to water but not to solutes. As the loop passes farther into the medulla, water moves from the loop into the interstitium. This further concentrates the urine in the tubule. The water released into the interstitium is then reabsorbed back into the blood vessels that accompany the tubules. In other words, as the fluid (to be urine) moves down the descending loop, water moves out and into the bloodstream in a **countercurrent mechanism.**

The ascending loop of Henle serves as the diluting segment because of the ability to actively secrete sodium and chloride but prevent water loss. Therefore the fluid within the tubule loses sodium and chloride and eventually is either hypertonic or isotonic compared with plasma when it reaches the distal convoluted tubule.

Distal Convoluted Tubule

There are two main functions of the nephron at the distal tubule. The final reabsorption of sodium occurs at this point (maintaining water and electrolyte balance), and excess acid is removed from the body (acid-base balance).

Sodium is actively reabsorbed with some bicarbonate at this point. The primary mechanism for sodium reabsorption is by the sodium-potassium pump under the control of the hormone **aldosterone.** Aldosterone is released from the adrenal medulla in response to angiotensin II, which is a product of the renin response to either hypotension or low plasma sodium. Aldosterone stimulates active absorption of sodium ion in exchange for potassium that is excreted by tubular cells (the sodium-potassium pump). Overall, there is an increase in plasma sodium and water, with a decrease in body potassium levels.

When it is necessary to retain more sodium ions, ammonia is formed from glutamine and combines with hydrogen ions to form ammonium ions. This allows for a greater exchange of hydrogen ions for sodium ions. The pH of the final urine is affected by the distal tubules, especially by an excretion of hydrogen and ammonium ions in exchange for sodium. In general, the blood pH is maintained within very narrow limits at about 7.4, whereas urine generally has a pH of 5 or 6. Water is also reabsorbed under the influence of **antidiuretic hormone (ADH).**

Collecting Tubules

The collecting tubules are the site for the final concentration of urine. The fluid that will eventually be urine is still isotonic when it leaves the distal tubule and enters the collecting ducts. Although the collecting ducts are permeable to water, reabsorption is under the control of ADH, or vasopressin, a hormone produced by the pituitary gland. ADH is produced in response to increased plasma osmolality and has the effect of preventing excess excretion of water (antidiuresis). A lack of ADH results in production of more dilute urine (diuresis).

Ureters, Bladder, and Urethra

The fluid that leaves the collecting ducts and enters the ureters is now urine. There are two ureters, narrow tubes that carry urine from the kidneys to the bladder. Muscles in the ureter walls continually tighten and relax, forcing urine downward, away from the kidneys. If urine backs up or is allowed to stand still, a kidney infection can develop. About every 10 to 15 seconds, small amounts of urine are emptied into the bladder from the ureters.

The **bladder** is a triangle-shaped, hollow organ located in the lower abdomen. It is held in place by ligaments that are attached to other organs and the pelvic bones. The bladder's walls relax and expand to store urine and contract and flatten to empty urine through the urethra. Two circular **sphincter muscles** keep urine from leaking by closing tightly like a rubber band around the opening of the bladder. **Innervation of the bladder** alerts a person when it is time to urinate, or empty the bladder.

The **urethra** is a hollow tube that allows urine to pass outside the body. The brain signals the bladder muscles to tighten, which squeezes urine out of the bladder. At the same time, the brain signals the sphincter muscles to relax to let urine exit the bladder through the urethra. When all the signals occur in the correct order, normal urination occurs.

Histology

All the structures that make up the urinary system, from the glomerular capsule to the terminal portion of the urethra, are lined with epithelial cells. Each portion of the urinary system is characterized by a specific type of epithelial cell. These cells generally are classified as either *renal* (meaning from the kidney or nephron itself), *transitional,* or *squamous* epithelial cells (see Microscopic Analysis of Urinary Sediment). A few of these cells are constantly sloughed off into the urine, but increased numbers or cytologic changes of any of these cells may have clinical significance and be important in determining the cause of renal dysfunction.

COMPOSITION OF URINE

The composition of urine varies greatly, depending on such factors as diet, nutritional status, metabolic rate, general state of the body, and state of the kidney or its ability to function normally.

Urine is a complex aqueous mixture consisting of 96% water and 4% dissolved substances, most derived from the food eaten or waste products of metabolism. The dissolved substances consist primarily of salt (sodium and some potassium chloride) and urea (the principal end product of protein metabolism).

In addition to urea, the principal organic substances found in urine are uric acid and creatinine. Urea, uric acid, and creatinine are nitrogenous waste products of protein metabolism that must be eliminated from the body because increased levels are toxic. Urea makes up about half of the dissolved substances in urine; it is the end product of amino acid and protein breakdown. The amount of creatinine excretion is related to the muscle mass of the body, not diet. Each individual excretes a constant amount of creatinine daily; therefore, urine creatinine measurements are used to assess the completeness of timed urine collections. Blood (plasma) creatinine levels are used to indicate renal function because creatinine is normally filtered through the glomerulus, and none is reabsorbed back into the blood. An increase in the plasma creatinine indicates impaired glomerular filtration and thus impaired renal function. The glomerular filtration rate is calculated from the urine and plasma creatinine levels, together with 24-hour urine volume and patient's height and weight.

In addition to sodium and chloride, the main inorganic substances present in urine include potassium, calcium, magnesium, and ammonia, plus phosphates and sulfates.

Normal Urine

Normal urine contains a few cells from the blood and lining of the urinary tract but little or no protein and no casts (although a few hyaline casts may be present). The reference values shown in Table 14-1 are typical of what may be "normally" encountered when the urine is examined for physical and chemical properties. Any of the substances tested for in routine urinalysis may be present in various disease states (Box 14-2).

Normal but concentrated urine typically crystallizes certain chemicals out of solution at room or refrigerator temperature. A routine urinalysis usually shows crystals of uric acid or its salts, the urates, at an acid pH, whereas phosphates typically crystallize out of solution in concentrated urine of an alkaline pH. Such crystallization appears grossly

TABLE 14-1

Urine Reference Values (Physical and Chemical)	
Property	Reference Value
Color	Yellow
Transparency	Clear
pH	5-7
Specific gravity	1.003-1.035 (adult random urine)
Protein, albumin	Negative Trace (in a concentrated specimen)
Blood (hemoglobin)	Negative
Nitrite	Negative
Leukocyte esterase	Negative
Glucose	Negative
Ketones	Negative
Bilirubin (conjugated)	Negative
Urobilinogen	<1 mg/dL

BOX 14-2

Clinical Usefulness of the Routine Urinalysis

Indicators of the State of the Kidney or Urinary Tract

Appearance (color, transparency, odor, and foam)
Specific gravity
Chemical tests (protein, blood, nitrite)
Leukocyte esterase
Urinary sediment (cells, casts, certain crystals)

Indicators of Metabolic and Other Conditions or Disease

pH (crystal identification; occasionally for acid-base status)
Appearance (pigments, concentration/dilution)
Glucose and ketones (diabetes mellitus)
Bilirubin (jaundice, liver disease)
Urobilinogen (hemolytic anemias, some liver diseases)

Indicators of Other Systemic (Nonrenal) Conditions or Disease

Hemoglobin (intravascular hemolysis)
Myoglobin (rhabdomyolysis)
Light-chain proteins (multiple myeloma, other gammaglobulinopathies)
Porphobilinogen (some porphyrias)

as cloudiness or turbidity of the urine, and the crystals are identified morphologically by microscopic examination. Although they are the primary constituents of urine, urea and sodium chloride do not crystallize out of urine specimens.

Identification of a Fluid as Urine

It is sometimes necessary to determine whether a specimen is urine or a body fluid such as amniotic fluid. This is done by measuring urea, creatinine, sodium, and chloride levels, which are all significantly higher in urine than in other body fluids.

COLLECTION AND PRESERVATION OF URINE SPECIMENS

Important considerations in the proper collection and handling of urine for routine examination include the container used, the collection procedure, and the conditions of storage and preservation from the time of collection until the specimen is tested. For routine urinalysis, the urine specimen must be collected in a suitable, clean, dry container. In most cases, the first specimen freely voided in the morning is preferred, although a specimen collected 2 to 3 hours after eating is preferable for testing of glucose. The specimen must be examined when fresh, ideally within 30 minutes, or suitably preserved, such as by refrigeration for up to 6 to 8 hours. Changes in urine left at room temperature more than 2 hours are shown in Table 14-2.

Types of Urine Specimens

Clinical information obtained from a urine specimen is influenced by the collection method, timing, and handling. Various types of collection and transport containers for urine specimens are available. A specimen must be carefully collected, preserved, and processed before analysis in order for the reported results to be reliable. If urine testing cannot be performed within 2 hours of collection, the specimen should be stored at 4°C as soon as possible after collection. Specimens can be stored under refrigeration for 6 to 8 hours, with no gross alterations in constituents.

Random Specimen

A random urine specimen is the most common type for analysis.[4] Random specimens, or specimens collected at any time, can give an inaccurate view of a patient's health because the specimen is too diluted and analyte values are artificially lowered. Although there are no specific guidelines on how the collection should be conducted, avoiding the introduction of contaminants into the specimen is

recommended. This requires explicit instructions to patients about not touching the inside of the cup or cup lid with their body.

First Morning Specimen

The first urine voided in the morning is the specimen of choice for urinalysis and microscopic examination. This urine is generally more concentrated because of the length of time the urine is allowed to remain in the bladder overnight. The specimen contains relatively high levels of cellular elements and analytes (e.g., glucose, protein). Any urine that is voided from the bladder during the 8-hour (typically overnight) collection period should be pooled and refrigerated so that a true 8-hour sample is obtained. To test for the presence of urine sugar, the best specimen to use is one voided 2 to 3 hours after a meal. This is the one exception to the recommended use of the first morning specimen.

Midstream Clean-Catch Specimen

Midstream clean-catch urine is the preferred type of specimen for culture and sensitivity testing because of the reduced incidence of cellular and microbial contamination. Patients are required first to cleanse the urethral area and then to void

TABLE 14-2

Changes in Urine Left at Room Temperature		
Constituent	Observed Change	Mechanism of Change
pH	Increased (alkaline)	Breakdown of urea to ammonia
Cells	Decreased number	Lysis
Casts	Decreased number	Lysis-dissolution
Glucose	Decreased	Glycolysis (by bacterial action)
Ketones	Decreased	Conversion of diacetic acid to acetone and evaporation of acetone from specimen
Bilirubin	Decreased (color change from yellow to green)	Oxidation to biliverdin
Urobilinogen	Decreased (color change from colorless to orange-red)	Oxidation to urobilin

Modified from Ringsrud KM, Linné JJ: Urinalysis and body fluids: a color text and atlas, St Louis, 1995, Mosby.

the first portion of the urine stream into the toilet. These first steps significantly reduce the incidence of contamination of the urine specimen. A midstream sample of urine is then collected into a clean container. This method of collection can be conducted at any time of day or night.

24-Hour or Timed Specimen

The most common tests requiring the 24-hour urine specimen include those measuring creatinine, urine urea nitrogen, glucose, sodium, potassium, and substances (e.g., catecholamines, 17-hydroxy-steroids) that are affected by diurnal variations. The bladder is emptied before beginning the timed collection. Then, for the duration of the designated 24-hour period, all urine is collected and pooled into a collection container, with the final collection at the end of the period. Usually the specimen is refrigerated. Accurate timing is critical to determining the concentration of various analytes and calculated ratios.

Catheter Collection Specimen

This assisted procedure is conducted when a patient is confined to bed or cannot urinate independently. A healthcare provider can use an existing catheter or can insert a Foley catheter into the bladder through the urethra to collect the urine specimen.

Suprapubic Aspiration Specimen

This method is used when a bedridden patient cannot be catheterized or a sterile specimen is required. The urine specimen is collected by needle aspiration through the abdominal wall into the bladder.

Pediatric Specimen

For infants and small children, a special urine collection bag is adhered to the skin surrounding the urethral area. Once the collection is completed, the urine is poured into a collection cup or transferred directly into an evacuated tube with a transfer straw. Urine collected from a diaper is not recommended for laboratory testing, because contamination from the diaper material may affect test results. If a 24-hour pediatric specimen is required, a special tube can be attached to the bag, which in turn is connected to a collection bottle.

Containers for Urine Collection

It is essential that the containers[5] used to collect the urine specimen be clean, dry, and free of particles or interfering substances. Containers should not be reused. Several types of containers are suitable for this purpose. Disposable inert plastic containers with leak-resistant lids, plastic bags, or jars are most often used.

Any bedpans that are used to collect voided urine must be scrupulously clean and free of cleaning agents or bleach. Labels must remain fixed to the urine specimen container at all times and must be on the container, not on the lid.

Urine Collection Cups

Urine collection container cups come in a variety of shapes and sizes, with either snap-on or screw-on lids. CLSI guidelines for urine (GP-16A2) recommend the use of a primary collection container that holds at least 50 mL, has a wide base, and has an opening of at least 4 cm. The wide base prevents spillage, and a 4-cm opening is an adequate target for urine collection.

Leak-resistant cups should be used to protect healthcare personnel from exposure to the specimen and protect the specimen from exposure to contaminants. Some urine transport cup closures have special access ports that allow closed-system transfer of urine directly from the collection device to the tube.

Urinalysis Tubes

Evacuated tubes, similar to those used in blood collection, are filled through a straw device from cups with integrated transfer devices built into their lid, or from direct sampling devices, and are used to access catheter sampling ports.

For testing purposes, conical-bottom test tubes provide the best sediment collection for microscopic analysis. Some tubes are specially designed to be used with a pipettor that allows for standardized sampling. Fill volumes of urinalysis tubes usually range from 8 to 15 mL.

BD manufactures a plastic urine preservative tube. This tube contains chlorhexidine, ethylparaben, and sodium propionate and maintains sample integrity for up to 72 hours without refrigeration.

24-Hour Collection Containers

Urine collection containers for 24-hour specimens should hold up to 3 L and may be colored to protect light-sensitive analytes (e.g., porphyrins, urobilinogen) from degradation.

If a preservative is required, the least hazardous type should be selected and added to the collection container before the urine collection begins. Common 24-hour preservatives are hydrochloric acid, boric acid, acetic acid, and toluene. Warning labels should be placed on the container. A corresponding material safety data sheet (MSDS) should be given to the patient, and the healthcare provider should explain any potential hazards.

Urine Culture Containers

CLSI guidelines recommend sterile collection containers for microbiology specimens. These containers should have secure closures to prevent specimen loss and to protect the specimen from contamination.

Urine Transport Tubes

Transport tubes should be compatible with automated systems and instruments used by the laboratory. Collection containers and transport tubes should be compatible with the pneumatic tube system if one is used for urine specimen transport in the facility. A leakproof device in this situation is critical.

Urine Volume for Routine Urinalysis

The minimum volume for routine urinalysis is usually 12 mL, but 50 mL is preferable. The minimum amount necessary for the usual processing procedure is 12 mL; the urine is placed in a disposable centrifuge tube, centrifuged, and concentrated 12:1 so that 1 mL of sediment is retained for the microscopic analysis of the sediment. This volume also allows for a convenient, standardized volume of urine for assessment of physical properties, such as color and transparency, which are often observed in the centrifuge tube.

Smaller volumes may be accepted for chemical analysis from oliguric patients or from infants. If only 3 mL of urine is collected, a 12:1 concentration of sediment may still be made. In some situations, a drop of unconcentrated urine placed on the desired portion of a reagent strip or observed microscopically may be the only option available.

Collection of Urine Specimens

ROUTINE SPECIMENS

A specimen for urinalysis should be collected in a clean, dry container, and the specimen should be fresh. For routine screening, a freshly voided, random, preferably midstream (freely flowing) urine specimen is usually suitable. For most routine urinalysis, including protein content and urinary sediment constituents, the concentrated first morning specimen is the most satisfactory one to use.

Occasionally a catheterized specimen may be needed. This type of specimen is obtained by a physician or designee and is obtained by introducing a catheter into the bladder, through the urethra, for the withdrawal of urine. Catheterization may be required under special circumstances or for obtaining a sterile urine specimen for bacteriologic examination. The risk of introducing infection is always present when an invasive procedure such as catheterization is performed. Under most conditions, a free-flowing (midstream) voided specimen is satisfactory for bacteriologic cultures.

When both a bacteriologic culture and a routine urinalysis are needed on the same specimen, the culture should always be done first, then the routine tests, to avoid contamination of the specimen before culturing on bacteriologic media. Procedure 14-1 describes the collection of urine specimens suitable for culture.

COLLECTION OF TIMED URINE SPECIMENS

The patient is carefully instructed about details of the urine collection process[6] if the collection will be done on an outpatient basis. The bladder is emptied at the starting time (e.g., 8 AM), and this time is noted on the collection container. The first urine voided at the beginning of the collection is always discarded. All subsequent voidings are collected and put into the container, up to and including the urine voided at 8 AM the following day. This last urine specimen will complete the 24-hour collection.

For timed collections of other than 24 hours, the sample collection principle applies. These timed collection specimens are preserved by refrigeration between collections, with the appropriate chemical preservative added to the container before the beginning of the collection process.

The total volume of the timed collection sample is measured and recorded, and the sample well mixed, before a measured aliquot is withdrawn for analysis.

COLLECTION OF URINE FOR CULTURE

A clean-catch, midstream urine specimen is desirable for culture (see Procedure 14-1). It is important that the glans penis in the male and the urethral orifice in the female be thoroughly cleaned with a mild antiseptic solution by means of sterile gauze or cotton balls. The patient should be instructed to urinate forcibly and allow the initial stream of urine to pass into the toilet or bedpan. Throughout the urination process for the female, the labia should be separated so that no contamination results. The midstream specimen should be collected in a sterile container, and no portion of the perineum (female) should come in contact with the collection container. After the specimen has been collected, the remaining urine is discarded.

Patient Collection Instructions for Midstream, Clean-Catch Urine Specimen for Culture

1. Wash your hands thoroughly with soap and water.
2. Open the lid of the urine container provided. Be careful to not touch the inside.
3. Cleanse your genital area using the following procedure:

MAN
   a. If you are uncircumcised, draw back the foreskin before cleansing.
   b. Clean the tip of your penis using a sterile cleansing towelette, beginning at the tip and moving toward the base. Repeat the cleansing process using a second towelette.

WOMAN
   a. Squat over the toilet, and use the fingers of one hand to separate and hold open the folds of the skin in your genital area.
   b. Clean the urinary opening and surrounding area with a sterile cleansing towelette, moving from front to back. Repeat the cleansing process using a second towelette.
4. Discard the towelettes in a trash receptacle (not in the toilet).
5. Begin urinating into the toilet bowl. After the urine has flowed for several seconds into the toilet, catch the midportion of the urine flow in the collection container. When sufficient urine has been collected (approximately half full), continue urinating into the toilet.
6. Tightly screw the cap on the specimen container.
7. Wash your hands thoroughly with soap and water.
8. Promptly give the specimen container to the nurse or laboratory personnel, or leave in the place specified.
9. Ensure that the specimen label contains your proper identification.

Preservation of Urine Specimens

If a fresh specimen of urine is left at room temperature for a period, the urine rapidly undergoes changes. Decomposition of urine begins within 30 minutes after collection. Specimens left at room temperature will soon begin to decompose, primarily because of the action of urea-splitting bacteria, which produces ammonia on combining with hydrogen ions, ammonia forms ammonium ions, causing an increase in urine pH, which will contribute to the decomposition of casts and certain cells, if present in the urine. The various laboratory tests planned for a urine specimen should be performed promptly after collection. No longer than 1 or 2 hours should elapse before the tests are done, unless the urine is preserved in some way.

The best method of preservation is immediate refrigeration during and after collection. The specimen may be kept 6 to 8 hours under refrigeration with no chemical preservative added, with no gross alterations. Specimens can be frozen (at 24°C to 16°C) after collection. Several chemical preservatives are available as additives for routine urine specimens.[6] Preservatives have different roles but usually are added to reduce bacterial action or chemical decomposition or to solubilize constituents that might otherwise precipitate from the solution. Specimens for some types of analysis should not have preservatives added because of the possibility of interference with analytical methods. Generally, the length of preservation capacity ranges from 24 to 72 hours.

In addition to refrigeration or freezing, common chemical preservatives are hydrochloric acid, boric acid, and acetic acid. Boric acid allows urine to be kept at room temperature while still providing results comparable to those of refrigerated urine. Other preservatives include the following[7]:

- Toluene, a solution lighter than urine or water, prevents the growth of bacteria by excluding contact of urine with air. A thin layer of toluene is added, just enough to cover the surface of the urine. The toluene should be skimmed off or the urine pipetted from beneath it when the urine is examined. Toluene (toluol) is the best all-around preservative because it does not interfere with the various tests done in the routine urinalysis.

- Formaldehyde (formalin), a liquid preservative, acts by fixing the formed elements in the urinary sediment, including bacteria. it may interfere with the reduction tests for urine sugar, however, and may form a precipitate with urea that interferes with the microscopic examination of the sediment. Preservative tablets that produce formaldehyde are commercially available. The tablets are more convenient to use than the liquid formalin and do not interfere with the usual chemical and microscopic examination.
- Thymol, a crystalline substance, works to prevent the growth of bacteria. Thymol may interfere with tests for urine protein and bilirubin.
- The BD Vacutainer Plus Plastic UA Preservative Tube contains a proprietary additive (chlorhexidine, ethylparaben, sodium propionate) that maintains sample integrity of up to 72 hours without refrigeration. When a specimen is directly transferred from a collection cup into a preservative tube, it provides a stable environment for the specimen until testing can be conducted and reduces the risk of bacterial overgrowth or specimen decomposition.

Specialized additives include nitric acid for mercury analysis, sodium bicarbonate and EDTA for porphyrins, and sodium bicarbonate for urobilinogen analysis.[4]

The most common preservative of urine for culture and sensitivity (C&S) testing is boric acid, which comes in tablet, powder, or lyophilized form. Clinical evidence suggests that nonbuffered boric acid may be harmful to certain organisms and that buffered boric acid preservatives can reduce the harmful effects of the preservative on the organisms.[4] C&S preservatives are designed to maintain the specimen in a state equivalent to refrigeration by deterring the proliferation of organisms that could result in a false-positive culture or bacterial overgrowth.

Preserved urine specimens can be stored at room temperature until time of testing. Product claims regarding duration of preservative potency should be obtained from the particular manufacturer.

Specimen Preservation Guidelines[4]

1. CLSI guidelines for microbiological urine testing recommend refrigeration of specimens at 2°C to 8°C or the use of chemical preservatives if the specimen cannot be processed within 2 hours of collection.
2. Chemical preservatives should be nonmercuric and environmentally friendly. The American Hospital Association and the Environmental Protection Agency issued a Memorandum of Understanding for the "virtual elimination of mercury containing waste from the healthcare industry waste stream" by 2005 (http://www.epa.gov/mercury).
3. To ensure accurate test results, the proper specimen-to-additive ratio must be maintained when using a chemical preservative. Maintaining the correct ratio is especially important when transferring samples into a preservative tube. The indicated fill lines on the tube are used to ensure proper fill.
4. An evacuated tube system is designed to achieve proper fill volume to ensure the proper specimen-to-additive ratio and proper preservative function. Evacuated systems also reduce the potential exposure of the healthcare worker to the specimen.

Labeling and Processing of Urine Specimens

As with any type of laboratory specimen, certain criteria must be met for proper collection and transportation of urine specimens.

Labels

Include the patient name and identification information on labels. Make sure that the information on the container label and the requisition match. If the collection container is used for transport, the label should be placed on the container, not on the lid, because the lid can be mistakenly placed on a different container. Ensure that the labels used on the containers are adherent under refrigerated conditions.

Collection Date and Time

Include the date and time of the urine collection on the specimen label. This will confirm that the collection was done correctly. For timed specimens, verify start and stop times of collection. Document the time at which the specimen was received in the laboratory for verification of proper handling and transport after collection.

Collection Method

The method of collection should be checked when the specimen is received in the laboratory to ensure the type of specimen submitted meets the needs of the test ordered.

Proper Preservation

Check whether there is a chemical preservative present or whether the specimen has not been refrigerated for longer than 2 hours after collection. Verify that the method of preservation used is appropriate for the selected test.

Light Protection

Verify that specimens submitted for testing of light-sensitive analytes are collected in containers that protect the specimen from light.

PHYSICAL PROPERTIES OF URINE

The first part of a routine urinalysis usually involves an assessment of physical properties including volume, color, transparency, and odor (Table 14-3). Another physical property, specific gravity, is discussed later in this section. Simple observations are extremely useful both for the eventual diagnosis of the patient and for the laboratory personnel who perform the complete urinalysis. Such tests often give clues leading to findings in subsequent portions of the urinalysis. For example, if a urine specimen is cloudy and red, the presence of red blood cells (RBCs) will probably be revealed by microscopic analysis of the urinary sediment. If RBCs are not found, all parts of the urinalysis must be carefully rechecked for accuracy. Chemical tests for blood (hemoglobin) might be falsely negative when ascorbic acid is present in urine; however, the presence of blood might be indicated by an abnormal red color and confirmed by the presence of RBCs in the urinary sediment. If hemoglobin is present without RBCs, the only indication of ascorbic acid interference might be the abnormal color of the urine.

Certain tests are performed when abnormal physical properties are observed. For example, a chemical test for the pigment bilirubin is necessary

TABLE 14-3

Physical Properties of Urine		
Physical Property	**Description**	**Possible Cause**
Normal color	Yellow	Urochrome, uroerythrin, urobilin
Abnormal color	Pale	Dilute urine
	Amber (dark yellow or orange-red)	Concentrated urine or bilirubin
	Brown (yellow-brown or green-brown)	Bilirubin or biliverdin
	Orange (orange-red or orange-brown)	Urobilin (excreted colorless as urobilinogen)
	Bright orange	Azo-containing dyes or compounds
	Red	Blood or heme-derived pigment, urates or uric acid, drugs, foodstuffs
	Clear red	Hemoglobin
	Cloudy red	Red blood cells
	Dark red-brown	Myoglobin
	Dark red or red-purple	Porphyrins
	Black (dark brown and black)	Melanin, homogentisic acid, phenol poisoning
	Green, blue, or orange	Drugs, medications, foodstuffs
Normal transparency	Clear	Normal or dilute urine
Abnormal transparency	Hazy, cloudy, turbid	Mucus, phosphates, urates, crystals, bacteria, pus, fat, casts
Normal odor	Aromatic	Normal
Abnormal odor	Ammoniacal, putrid or foul	Breakdown of urea by bacteria (old urine)
		Urinary tract infection
	Sweet or "fruity"	Ketone bodies
	Sweaty feet, maple syrup, cabbage or hops, mousy, rotting fish, rancid	Specific amino acid disorder for each
Normal foam	White, small amount	Normal
Abnormal foam	White, large amount	Protein
	Yellow, large amount	Bilirubin

when it is suspected on the basis of abnormal color of the urine. In several situations the laboratory evaluates the complete urinalysis for reliability before reporting results to the physician, or abnormal constituents are found in subsequent tests because abnormal physical properties were noted.

Volume

Normal Volume

Although it is a physical property, the volume of the urine is not measured as part of a routine urinalysis. In certain conditions, the volume of urine excreted in 24 hours is a valuable aid to clinical diagnosis. In normal adults with normal fluid intake, the average 24-hour urine volume is 1200 to 1500 mL. It can, however, normally range from 600 to 1600 mL. The total volume of urine excreted in 24 hours must be measured when quantitative tests are performed, because it enters into the calculation of results in these tests.

Under normal conditions, a direct relationship exists between urine volume and water intake. That is, if water intake is increased, the kidney will protect the body from excessive retention of water by eliminating a larger volume of urine than normal. Conversely, if water intake is decreased, the kidney will protect the body against dehydration by eliminating a smaller amount of urine.

Abnormal Volume

Patient conditions that can result in abnormal urine volumes include:
- **Polyuria:** consistent elimination of an abnormally large volume of urine, more than 2000 mL/24 hours
- **Diuresis:** any increase in urine volume, even if the increase is only temporary
- **Oliguria:** excretion of an abnormally small amount of urine, less than 500 mL/24 hours
- **Anuria:** complete absence of urine formation
- **Nocturia:** excretion of more than 400 mL urine at night

Color

The color of normal urine seems to result from the presence of three pigments: urochrome, uroerythrin, and urobilin. **Urochrome** is a yellow pigment and is present in larger concentrations than the other two pigments. **Uroerythrin** is a red pigment, and **urobilin** is an orange-yellow pigment. The color of normal urine varies considerably, even in one person in a single day. Numerous words have been used to describe the range of normal color.

In general, normal urine is some shade of yellow. The terms *yellow, straw,* and *amber* may be used. *Straw* is generally used to describe a lighter-colored urine with normal yellow pigment. *Amber* refers to a darker color, with red or orange pigments in addition to yellow. Abnormalities in color (see Table 14-3) may have various possible causes.

Pale urine suggests that the urine is dilute; urine that is more highly colored has a greater concentration of normal waste products because its volume is diminished.

Transparency

When voided, urine is normally clear; most urines will become cloudy when allowed to stand. Cloudiness of a specimen when voided is usually of clinical significance and should not be disregarded. Numerous words have been used in attempts to describe the degree of transparency of a urine specimen. According to the Clinical and Laboratory Standards Institute (CLSI), standardized terms such as *clear, hazy, cloudy,* and *turbid* should be used to reduce ambiguity and subjectivity. Schweitzer and colleagues[8] advocate the use of a limited number of descriptors:
- Clear: no visible particulate matter present
- Hazy: some visible particulate matter present; newsprint is not distorted or obscured when viewed through the urine
- Cloudy: newsprint can be seen through the urine, but letters are distorted or blurry
- Turbid: newsprint cannot be seen through the urine

Common constituents that cause cloudiness in urine, either normal or possibly significant or pathologic, are summarized in Table 14-4.

Odor

Normal urine has a characteristic, faintly aromatic odor because of the presence of certain volatile acids (see Table 14-3). If urine is allowed to stand, it acquires a strong ammoniacal odor. This is caused by the breakdown of urea by bacteria to form ammonia. This odor is important as an indication that the urine specimen is probably too old for the urinalysis to have clinical significance. Urine heavily contaminated with bacteria may have a particularly unpleasant odor, which may be described as foul or putrid. Foul-smelling urine will indicate urinary infection only if the specimen is known to be fresh.

Another characteristic odor that is significant clinically is a so-called fruity, or sweet, odor. This results from the presence of acetone and acetoacetic acid, an important finding in the urine of diabetic patients at risk of diabetic coma.

TABLE 14-4

Common Constituents Causing Cloudiness in Urine	
Generally Normal	Possibly Pathologic
Amorphous phosphates and urates	Amorphous urates
Normal crystals	Abnormal crystals
	Red blood cells
	White blood cells
	Casts
	Fat (lipids)
Epithelial cells (squamous, transitional)	Epithelial cells (renal, transitional, malignant)
Bacteria (old urine)	Bacteria (fresh urine)
	Other microorganisms (yeast, fungi, parasites)
Mucus	
Sperm, prostatic fluid	Chyluria (lymph, rare)
Powders, antiseptics	Fecal matter (from fistula)

Specific Gravity

Urine is a mixture of substances dissolved and suspended in water. In normal urine, these dissolved substances are primarily urea and sodium chloride. **Specific gravity** is a measure of the amount of dissolved substances in a solution. The specific gravity of urine is used as a measure of the ability of the kidney to regulate the composition and osmotic pressure of the extracellular fluid by concentrating or diluting the urine.

Specific gravity is defined as the weight of a solution compared with the weight of an equal volume of water. More specifically, it is the ratio of the density (weight per unit volume) of a solution to the density (weight per unit volume) of an equal volume of water at a constant temperature. From this definition, it is clear that the specific gravity of water is always 1.000. Because it is a ratio, specific gravity has no units. It is always reported to the third decimal place.

Clinical Aspects

Clinically, the specific gravity of urine may be used to obtain information about two general functions: the state of the kidney and the patient's state of hydration.

If the kidney is performing adequately, it is capable of producing urine with a specific gravity ranging from about 1.003 to 1.035. If the renal epithelium is not functioning adequately, it will gradually lose the ability to concentrate and dilute the urine. The ability to concentrate urine is one of the first functions lost when the kidney is impaired. Deficiency or failure to respond to ADH will also result in failure to concentrate urine. The specific gravity of the protein-free glomerular filtrate is about 1.008. Without any active work on the part of the kidney, this will increase to 1.010 as a result of simple diffusion as the filtrate passes through the kidney tubules. Thus, if the kidney has completely lost its ability to concentrate and dilute the urine, the specific gravity will remain at 1.010. If it is known that the kidney is functioning adequately, the state of hydration may be reflected by the specific gravity. For example, if the urine is consistently very concentrated, dehydration is implied.

Although normal specific gravity may range from 1.003 to 1.035, the specific gravity of a 24-hour collection is usually between 1.016 and 1.022 with normal diet and fluid intake. Because the specific gravity reflects the amount of dissolved substances present in solution, it varies inversely with the volume of urine (this is because a fairly constant amount of waste is produced each day). If the urinary volume increases because of increased water intake, and the amount of waste produced remains constant, the specific gravity of the urine decreases. In other words, if the urinary volume is high, the specific gravity is low, and vice versa, assuming the kidney is functioning normally. With an individual on a restricted fluid diet for 12 hours, the normal kidney is capable of concentrating urine to a specific gravity of about 1.022 or more. A person without fluids for 24 hours should produce urine with a specific gravity of 1.026 or more. If the individual is placed on a very high-fluid diet, the normal kidney is capable of diluting the urine to a specific gravity of about 1.003. The concentrated first urine specimen passed in the morning should have a specific gravity greater than 1.020 if the kidney is functioning normally.

Two frequently observed cases in which specific gravity does not vary inversely with urinary volume are diabetes mellitus and certain types of renal disease. With diabetes mellitus, an abnormally large urinary volume associated with an abnormally high specific gravity is observed. This is caused by the presence of large amounts of dissolved glucose, which raises the specific gravity of the urine. In certain types of renal disease, such as glomerulonephritis, pyelonephritis, and various anomalies, there is a combination of low specific gravity and low urinary volume. This results from the inability of the renal tubular epithelium either to excrete normal amounts of water or to concentrate the waste products. The specific gravity in these cases may eventually be fixed at about 1.010.

The loss of concentrating ability is seen in diabetes insipidus, an impairment of ADH. This rare condition results in extremely large volumes of urine with very low specific gravity, ranging from 1.001 to 1.003.

Abnormally high specific gravity values, usually greater than 1.035 and up to 1.050 or more, may also be encountered after certain diagnostic x-ray procedures in which a radiographic dye is injected intravenously to obtain a pyelogram of the kidney. Such high specific gravity readings will be accompanied by delayed false-positive reactions for protein with the sulfosalicylic acid procedure, and the dye may crystallize out of the urine as an abnormal, colorless crystal resembling plates of cholesterol.

Measures of Urine Solute Concentration (Specific Gravity and Osmolality)

Although specific gravity is a convenient measure of the urine solute concentration, it is not the only one available. Other measures are osmolality, refractive index, and ionic concentration. All the methods of measuring solute concentration are influenced by the number of molecules present in solution, in addition to the size and ionic charge.

OSMOLALITY BY OSMOMETER

This is another method of determining solute concentration. **Osmolality** is a measure of the number of solute particles per unit amount of solvent; thus it depends only on the number of particles in solution. It is determined with an osmometer by measuring the freezing point of a solution, because the freezing point is depressed in proportion to the amount of dissolved substances present. In normal persons with a normal diet and fluid intake, the urine will contain about 500 to 850 mOsm/kg of water. Osmolality is preferred to specific gravity as a measurement of urine concentration. Urine and plasma osmolality as a ratio is used to evaluate renal tubular concentration, which depends on the patient's state of hydration.

SPECIFIC GRAVITY AS REFRACTIVE INDEX BY REFRACTOMETER

A previously popular method for measurement of solute concentration, reported in the urinalysis laboratory as specific gravity, is refractive index. The **refractive index** of a solution is the ratio of the velocity of light in air to the velocity of light in solution. This ratio varies directly with the number of dissolved particles in solution. Although not identical to specific gravity, refractive index varies and corresponds with specific gravity. Measurement is made with a refractometer that is calibrated to give results in terms of specific gravity (Fig. 14-3). The

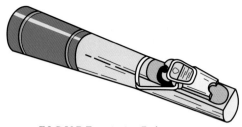

FIGURE 14-3   Refractometer.

specific gravity scale by refractometer is valid only for urine. It cannot be used to determine the specific gravity of salt or glucose solutions.

The refractometer has the advantage of requiring only a drop of urine. Automated instruments are available that use pass-through models of refractometers. These use a larger volume of urine (about 2 mL). Refractometer results are valid up to 1.035; specimen with greater than 1.035 should be diluted and remeasured.

Although the refractometer actually measures the refractive index, the scales of the instrument are calibrated in terms of total solids (g/100 mL) for plasma or serum, or in terms of specific gravity for urine. Up to a value of 1.035, the urinary refractive index and specific gravity agree. Few normal urines have values greater than 1.035; higher values suggest the presence of unusual solutes in the specimen, such as glucose, protein, or radiopaque compounds. Beyond a value of 1.035, the refractive index is poorly correlated with the specific gravity.

The refractive index changes with temperature, but the Goldberg refractometer compensates for temperature changes in the solution being measured. It is not necessary to correct for changes in temperature of the urine.

QUALITY CONTROL

The refractometer should be checked daily or at time of use with deionized or distilled water and with a solution of known specific gravity. The distilled water should read 1.000 ± 0.001. The instrument contains a zero set screw to adjust the reading to water. Follow the manufacturer's directions. The known solution may be a commercial control solution or one of the following (SG, specific gravity):

NaCl	0.513 mol/L	3% w/v	SG = 1.015
NaCl	0.856 mol/L	5% w/v	SG = 1.022
Sucrose	0.263 mol/L	9% w/v	SG = 1.034

CORRECTIONS FOR ABNORMAL DISSOLVED SUBSTANCES

Because refractive index is a measure of dissolved particles in solution, the presence of substances such as glucose, protein, or radiopaque dyes will act to raise the specific gravity when measured with the refractometer as compared with reagent strips. It is sometimes desirable to correct refractometer readings for dissolved substances to access the concentrating ability of the kidneys.

Correction for Glucose

Subtract 0.004 from the refractometer value for each gram of glucose per deciliter of urine. Urine specimens from diabetic patients often contain 3 or 4 g glucose/dL urine, resulting in a specific gravity value by refractometer 0.012 to 0.016 higher than by reagent strip, on the same specimen.

Correction for Protein

Subtract 0.003 from the refractometer value for each gram of protein per deciliter of urine. Urine specimens rarely contain 1 g or more of protein/dL urine; therefore, correction for protein is rarely necessary.

Radiopaque Media

With values greater than 1.035, unusual substances such as radiopaque media or certain antibiotics should be suspected when not explained by other findings such as high glucose concentration. The presence of unusual crystals of these substances in the microscopic analysis of the urine sediment is often associated with very high specific gravity readings with the refractometer. Alternatively, their presence may be indicated by a delayed false-positive sulfosalicylic acid test for urine protein. These substances will not be measured by the reagent strip method.

Use of Reagent Strips for Specific Gravity

Reagent strips have replaced the refractometer in many laboratories. These strips actually measure **ionic concentration,** which relates to specific gravity. Values are reported as specific gravity. However, substances that are dissolved in urine must ionize to be measured by this method. The waste products that constitute normal urinary constituents and that indicate the concentration and dilution ability of the kidney do ionize. Certain substances that may be present in urine (e.g., glucose, certain radiopaque dyes) do not ionize; therefore, specific gravity results obtained with a refractometer will be significantly higher than with the reagent strip if the urine contains significant quantities of a nonionizable, dissolved substance.

PRINCIPLE

The reagent strips for specific gravity actually measure ionic concentration. Reagent strip tests for specific gravity are based on a pK_a change of

certain pretreated polyelectrolytes in relation to the ionic concentration of urine. The polyelectrolytes in the reagent strip contain acid groups that dissociate in proportion to the number of ions in solution. This produces hydrogen ions, which reduce the pH (hydrogen ion concentration). The pH change is indicated by the color change of an acid-base indicator. The system is buffered so that any change in color is related to pK_a change, and not pH of the urine itself. Therefore, reagent strips measure only ionizable substances. (The pK_a is the negative logarithm of the ionization constant of an acid.)

Readings are made at 0.005 intervals from 1.000 to 1.030 by comparison with a color chart. Therefore, precision is significantly less than by refractometer, which is read at 0.001 intervals. Reagent strip tests generally correlate to within 0.005 of the refractometer. Urines with specific gravity greater than 1.025 are not reliably measured with ionic concentration methodology and should be tested with the refractometer. The procedure for measuring urine specific gravity with reagent strips is the same as that used for all reagent strips (Procedure 14-2).

CORRECTIONS AND LIMITATIONS

Dissolved substances must ionize to be detected by the reagent strips for specific gravity. Substances that do not ionize (e.g., glucose, radiopaque dyes) will not affect the reagent strips, giving different values from those obtained with a refractometer. Although this may give a better picture of the concentrating ability of the kidney, to interpret specific gravity results properly, it is important that the clinician understand which methodology is used by the laboratory and whether the results are "corrected" or not.

Highly buffered alkaline urine may cause low readings, and 0.005 may be added to readings from urines with pH of 6.5 or greater. Automated instruments apply this correction. Unlike readings with the refractometer, elevated specific gravity readings may be obtained in the presence of only moderate (100 to 750 mg/dL) amounts of protein. Urine specimens containing urea at concentrations greater than 1 g/dL will cause low readings relative to more traditional methods.

CHEMICAL TESTS IN ROUTINE URINALYSIS

Reagent Strip Tests

These tests are generally done by using multiple-reagent strips. Tests for protein and glucose are basic to any urinalysis. Other chemical tests have become routine as they have been added to the

General Procedure for Urine Reagent Strips

1. Test fresh, well-mixed, uncentrifuged urine at room temperature.
2. Completely immerse all chemical areas of the reagent strip briefly, not more than 1 second.
3. Remove excess urine from the reagent strip. Draw the strip along the lip or rim of the urine container as it is removed, then touch the edge of the strip to absorbent paper or gauze.
4. Avoid possible mixing of chemicals from adjacent reagent areas; hold the strip horizontally while waiting and reading results.
5. Read each chemical reaction at the time stated by the manufacturer.
6. Use adequate light. Hold the strip close to the color block on the chart supplied by the manufacturer, and match carefully for each chemical test. Be sure the strip is properly oriented to the color chart. Multistix are held perpendicular to the bottle, whereas Chemstrips are held parallel to the bottle.
7. Read the results in consistent units as established for your laboratory.

readily available multiple-reagent strips. Different combinations are available for use in different clinical situations. For example, in an obstetric clinic, tests for glucose, protein, blood, and leukocyte esterase are especially desirable. In certain cases, positive findings in the chemical screen may require confirmation with other chemical tests or may indicate the likelihood of certain findings in the microscopic examination of the urine sediment.

Most of the chemical tests done as part of the routine urinalysis use dry reagent strips. Reagent strips are available both as single tests for a specific chemical substance and as combinations of single tests, referred to as **multiple-reagent strips.**

Reagent strips are plastic strips that contain one or more chemically impregnated test sites on an absorbent pad. When the chemicals on the test site come into contact with urine or a control solution, a chemical reaction occurs. The reaction is indicated by a color change, which is compared with a special color chart that is provided with the reagent strip, usually printed on the bottle. Results can be read visually or in special instruments that automatically read specific reagent strips (see Chapter 10).

The intensity of the color formed is generally proportional to the amount of substance present in the specimen or control when observed at a specific time. Some areas are used as screening tests; others are used to estimate (semiquantitate) the amount of substance present and are reported in a plus system or in numerical values (e.g., mg/dL, g/dL). The method of reporting results will vary from laboratory to laboratory.

Advantages to dry reagent strip tests over the more traditional chemical tests on which they are based include:

1. Convenience: rapid results with a minimum of time and personnel
2. Cost-effectiveness
3. Stability
4. Relative ease in learning to use
5. Disposability
6. Smaller sample volumes required
7. Space savings: storage, use, and cleanup

Because they are so apparently easy to use, reagent strip tests are candidates for abuse. Reliable, reproducible results depend on correct technique. Manufacturers' directions must be followed exactly. Any person using reagent strips should understand the principle and specificity of each chemical test area, be aware of precautions or limitations and interferences that occur, and know the sensitivity and significance of positive or negative results.

In certain cases, additional confirmatory tests may be used when positive results are obtained with the reagent strip tests. These are usually in the form of tablet tests.

Manufacturer's Directions

General directions that apply to all reagent strip tests are included in this section (Fig. 14-4). It is imperative that the specific directions of the manufacturer be followed for all reagent strip tests. Tests are continually changed and reformulated in this highly competitive market. Each container of reagent strips is supplied with a product insert. This contains the most up-to-date information for

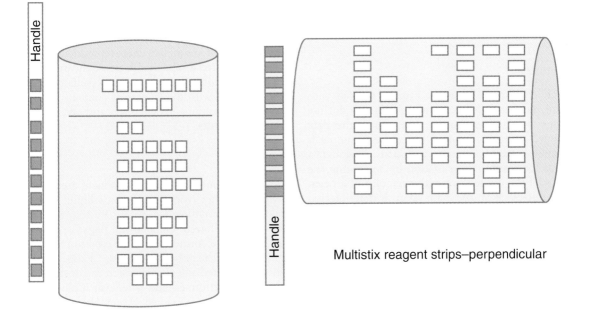

Chemstrip reagent strips–parallel

Multistix reagent strips–perpendicular

FIGURE 14-4 **Reading reagent strips (orientation to bottle).**

the successful performance of the test in question. Inserts include directions for use, warnings, procedure limitations, specimen-handling information, storage, and expected values. Information on interfering substances that may produce false-negative or false-positive reactions is also included. For each new lot number of reagent strips, the laboratorian should study the product insert, compare it to the previous insert, noting any changes, and file it with the laboratory procedure manual.

In this discussion, tests are arranged in order of clinical utility or physiologic significance, not in the order in which they are placed on a reagent strip. Chemical tests indicating disease of the kidney or urinary tract—pH, specific gravity, protein, blood, nitrite, and leukocyte esterase—are described first. Chemical tests indicating metabolic and other disease are then described: glucose, ketones, bilirubin, and urobilinogen. Many reagent strips include a test for specific gravity, as described previously. Each parameter is described in terms of clinical importance, principle of the test, specificity (what is being tested), sensitivity (minimum detectable level), and interferences (false-positive and false-negative reactions).

Sampling or Wetting

The specimen to be tested must be fresh or adequately preserved, well mixed (not centrifuged), and at room temperature. The first step in using the reagent strip is adequately sampling the specimen or wetting the reagent strip. Although this sounds easy, it is a common source of error. The strip must be adequately moistened so that all test areas of the strip are brought into contact with the sample. Care must be taken not to leave the strip in contact with the sample too long, or chemicals will be leached out of the strip and unavailable for the chemical reaction to occur. Therefore the strip is inserted into the specimen only briefly, for 1 second or less. Another problem is runover between chemicals on adjacent pads. This is avoided by drawing the edge of the strip along the edge of the urine container as it is removed, touching the edge of the strip to absorbent paper, and holding the strip horizontally while waiting for and reading results.

Storage and General Precautions

Reagent strips must be kept in tightly capped containers. They will deteriorate[8] rapidly when exposed to moisture, direct sunlight, heat, or volatile substances. Each container contains a desiccant, or drying agent, within the product to protect it from moisture; the desiccant should not be removed. Store containers at recommended temperatures, generally at room temperature, under 30°C, but not refrigerated or frozen. Keep strips in their original containers. Do not mix strips from different containers. Remove only the number of strips needed at a time, and close the container tightly. Do not touch the test areas. Keep the test areas away from detergents, bleach, or other contaminating substances.

Stability

Each container of reagent strips is marked with a lot number and an expiration date. Do not use strips after the expiration date. Write the date opened on each container. Once the container is opened, use strips within 6 months. Watch test areas for possible deterioration by comparing the color of the dry reagent with the color of a negative test block on the color chart. If deterioration is suspected, test the strip with a known control solution. Discard the entire bottle of strips if any reagent pads are discolored or when quality control is consistently out of range.

Timing

Read the results at the time stated by the manufacturer for each chemical test. This is absolutely necessary if results are to be semiquantitated. Different results will be seen for the same specimen at different times. An advantage of using an automated or semiautomated instrument to read reagent strips is that it controls the exact time at which all the chemical reactions are read.

Reading Results

Whenever results depend on color comparison, individual interpretation is a possible source of error. Adequate light is essential in visual interpretation. Hold the strip next to the most closely matched color block for each chemical test (see Fig. 14-3). Be sure to follow the manufacturer's instructions to orient the reagent strip correctly to the color chart when reading results. The use of automated or semiautomated instruments will eliminate individual differences in color interpretation and improve the reproducibility of results. Report results in a consistent manner as established for your institution.

Although multiple-reagent strips were developed to be read visually, several instruments have been developed to electronically measure the intensity of the color reactions produced on the reagent strips (see Chapter 10). These reflectance photometers measure the intensity of light produced by the chemical reaction between the analyte in question and the chemicals impregnated on each test portion of the reagent strip. The intensity of light produced is proportional to the amount of analyte in the specimen being tested. Actual instruments vary in the way the strips are inserted into the instrument, the degree of

automation, and the manner in which patient specimens are identified and results are displayed or printed. The advantages of semiautomated and automated systems include more reproducible readings and printed results that decrease the incidence of transcription (clerical) errors. Results can also be interfaced with the laboratory computer system to further minimize clerical errors and save time in reporting results.

Controls

Several commercial control products are readily available either lyophilized or as a liquid. Manufacturers' directions for reconstitution and use should be followed. Generally, a negative control and a positive control should be used to test every parameter of the reagent strip in use. Reagent strips should be tested at least once each day or shift that the test is performed and whenever a new bottle of reagent strips is opened. Acceptable results are generally within one color block of the assigned target, as stated by manufacturer. The only acceptable result for a negative control solution is negative. According to CLSI, quality control should "adhere to all local, state and federal regulations, as well as manufacturers' instructions."[9]

pH

One function of the kidney is to regulate the acidity of the extracellular fluid. Some information about this function, as well as other information, may be obtained by testing the urinary pH.

The pH is the unit that describes the acidity or alkalinity of a solution. In ordinary terms, acidity refers to the "sourness" of a solution, whereas alkalinity refers to its "bitterness." Lemon juice is an example of a sour, or acidic, solution; baking soda (sodium bicarbonate) is a bitter, or alkaline, substance in solution. In chemical terms, acidity refers to the hydronium ion (H_3O^+) concentration of a solution, and alkalinity refers to its hydroxyl ion (OH^-) concentration. These concentrations are usually expressed in terms of pH.

All solutions can be placed somewhere on a scale of pH values from 0 to 14. Some solutions, however, are neither acidic nor basic. These solutions are neutral and are placed at 7 on the pH scale. Water is an example of a neutral solution; its pH is 7. Water is neutral because the concentration of hydronium ions is equal to the concentration of hydroxyl ions.

A solution with more hydronium ions than hydroxyl ions is an acidic solution. On the pH scale, an acidic solution has a value ranging from 0 to 7. The farther it is from 7, the greater the acidity. For example, solutions of pH 2 and pH 5 are both acidic, but a solution of pH 2 is more acidic than a solution of pH 5. In simpler terms, a solution of pH 2 is more "sour" than a solution with a higher pH value. For example, lemon juice has a pH of about 2.3, whereas orange juice has a pH of about 3.5.

An alkaline solution has a pH value greater than 7. It can be any value from 7 to 14; the farther it is from 7, the greater the alkalinity, or the more "bitter" the solution.

Clinical Importance

Regulation of the pH of the extracellular fluid is an extremely important function of the kidney. Normally, the pH of blood is about 7.4 and varies no more than 0.05 pH unit. If the blood pH is 6.8 to 7.3, marked **acidosis** will be seen clinically; if it is 7.5 to 7.8, marked **alkalosis** will be observed. A pH less than 6.8 or greater than 7.8 will result in death. The carbon dioxide produced in normal metabolism results in a tremendous amount of acid, which must be eliminated from the blood and extracellular fluid, or death will result. This acid is normally eliminated from the body by the lungs and the kidneys.

Because the kidney is generally working to eliminate excess acid, the pH of urine is normally between 5 and 7, with a mean of 6. The kidney is capable of producing urine ranging in pH from 4.6 to 8. The urine is normally acidified through an exchange of hydrogen ions for sodium ions in the distal convoluted tubules. In renal tubular acidosis, this exchange and the ability to form ammonia are impaired, resulting in a relatively alkaline urine. Certain metabolic acid-base disturbances may also be reflected in measurements of urinary pH as the kidney attempts to compensate for changes in blood pH. Such acid-base disturbances are classified as *metabolic* or *respiratory* acidosis and alkalosis, and measurements of titratable acidity, ammonium ion, and bicarbonate concentration are used in these distinctions.

Although the kidney is essential in controlling the pH of blood and extracellular fluid, measurements of urinary pH are not necessarily used to obtain information about this role. The routine urinalysis includes a measurement of urinary pH for the following reasons:

1. Freshly voided urine usually has a pH of 5 or 6. However, on standing at room temperature, urea is converted to ammonia by bacterial action. The production of ammonia raises the hydroxyl ion concentration, resulting in an alkaline urine specimen. Therefore, unless it is known that a urine specimen is fresh, an alkaline pH probably indicates an old urine specimen.
2. Alkalinity of freshly voided urine, especially if persistent throughout the day, may indicate a urinary tract infection. Other urinalysis findings in infection include positive reagent strip tests for nitrite and leukocyte esterase and large numbers of bacteria and possibly white cells (neutrophils) in the urine sediment.
3. The urinary pH helps in the identification of crystals of certain chemical compounds that are often seen in the urine sediment. Certain crystals are associated with acid urine, pH less than 7, and others with alkaline urine, pH 7 and greater. Knowledge of the urine pH is important in the identification of crystals and may be the major reason for testing the pH of a urine specimen.
4. If the urine specimen is dilute and alkaline, various formed elements, such as casts and RBCs, will rapidly dissolve.
5. Persistently acidic urine may be seen in a variety of metabolic disorders, especially diabetic acidosis resulting from an accumulation of ketone bodies in the blood.
6. Persistently alkaline urine may be seen in some infections, in metabolic disorders, and with the administration of certain drugs.
7. It is sometimes necessary to control the urinary pH in the management of kidney infections, in patients with renal calculi (stones), and during the administration of certain drugs. This is done by regulating the diet; meat diets generally result in acidic urine and vegetable diets in alkaline urine.

Reagent Strip Tests for pH

PRINCIPLE

Reagent strip tests use a methyl red and bromthymol blue double-indicator system that measures urine pH in a range from 5 to 9. They are available as multiple-reagent strips in combination with other tests for urinary constituents. The methyl red is used to indicate a pH change from 4.4 to 6.2, with a color change from red to yellow. Bromthymol blue indicates a pH change from 6 to 7.6, as seen by a color change from yellow to blue.

INTERFERENCES

No interferences are known. The pH value is not affected by the buffer concentration of the urine.

ADDITIONAL COMMENTS

The specimen must be tested when fresh because bacterial growth may result in a significant shift to an alkaline pH, giving falsely alkaline values. Be careful not to wet the reagent strip excessively so that the acid buffer from the protein area runs into the pH area, causing an orange discoloration.

Protein

Clinical Importance

In the detection and diagnosis of renal disease, probably the most significant finding involves urinary protein. The presence of protein, when correlated with certain chemical tests, especially tests for blood, nitrite, and leukocyte esterase, and findings in the microscopic analysis of the urine sediment, is part of the eventual diagnosis.

The occurrence of protein in the urine is termed **proteinuria.** Proteinuria is an abnormal condition, probably the most important pathologic condition found in a routine urinalysis. In general, proteinuria may be the result of:

1. Glomerular damage
2. Tubular damage
3. Prerenal disorders or overflow from the excessive production of low-molecular-weight proteins such as hemoglobin, myoglobin, or immunoglobulins
4. Lower urinary tract disorders
5. Asymptomatic disorders

Proteinuria may be classified as to the amount (quantity) or degree of protein excreted per day (24 hours) as follows:

Amount of Proteinuria	Grams Excreted per Day
Mild (minimal)	<1 g/day
Moderate	1 to 3 or 4 g/day
Large (heavy)	>3 or 4 g/day

Note that the amount of protein per 100 mL in a random urine specimen is related to 24-hour urine volume. Thus, heavy proteinuria, with 3 g of protein eliminated per day and a 24-hour urine volume of 1500 mL, would correspond to 200 mg protein/dL in a random urine specimen. If the 24-hour urine volume were 500 mL, there might be 600 mg protein/dL.

Normally, the glomerular filtrate, the initial stage in the formation of urine, is an ultrafiltrate of blood plasma without cells, larger protein molecules, or certain fatty substances. Normal urine contains less than 10 mg/dL of protein as albumin. This is not detectable by normal tests for urinary protein. The normal glomerular membrane allows the passage of proteins with molecular weights of 50,000 to 60,000 daltons or less. Albumin has a molecular weight of about 67,000 daltons. This is a fairly small molecule, and some albumin is normally filtered through the glomerulus. However, this is normally reabsorbed in the convoluted tubules. Therefore, proteinuria (measurable amounts of protein in urine) may be the result of increased permeability of the glomerulus or decreased reabsorption by the renal tubules.

Tamm-Horsfall protein is a high-molecular-weight glycoprotein (mucoprotein) that is normally secreted by renal tubular epithelial cells. It is a product of the kidney and is not present in the blood plasma. This is the protein that forms the basic matrix of most urinary casts. Casts are an important pathologic urinary finding and are associated with proteinuria. The occurrence of casts with proteinuria distinguishes an upper urinary tract (kidney) disorder from a disorder of the lower urinary tract (bladder).

The implications of protein in the urine in association with renal disease are extremely serious, and prompt diagnosis and treatment are vitally important. In addition, the loss of protein from the blood plasma will result in severe water balance problems, because the osmotic pressure of the blood is largely dependent on the concentration of plasma proteins. This is readily seen in the edema often associated with kidney disorders.

Although proteinuria is indicative of renal disease, additional tests are needed for the final diagnosis. These include observations of the urine sediment (especially for the presence and types of casts), a determination of the amount of protein excreted per day by quantitative tests, the type of protein by electrophoresis, and the patient's clinical history.

Glomerular Damage

Proteinuria (generally albuminuria) is a consistent finding in glomerular disease. If the glomerular membrane is damaged, larger protein molecules find their way into the glomerular filtrate and are detected in the urine. This increased glomerular permeability usually begins with the passage of the smaller albumin molecules, and the larger globulin molecules remain in the blood plasma.

A variety of causes, including toxins, infections, vascular disorders, and immunologic reactions, may result in glomerular damage and increased filtration with proteinuria. Poststreptococcal **acute glomerulonephritis (AGN)** is an example of glomerular proteinuria. This is an immunologic sequela of a bacterial infection, usually a throat infection caused by group A β-hemolytic streptococcus. Urinalysis findings include proteinuria, hematuria (RBCs), and casts (RBC, blood, or granular).

Early in cases of glomerular damage, only the small protein molecules (albumin) are filtered through the glomerulus. As the glomerular damage progresses, virtually all proteins present in the plasma find their way into the urine. Albumin is responsible for the osmotic pressure. Decreased amounts result in generalized swelling or edema throughout the body. In the **nephrotic syndrome,** heavy (massive) proteinuria (3 or 4 g/day) is seen. So much protein is lost from the body through the urine that the ability of the liver to synthesize sufficient albumin to maintain the normal blood albumin is lost, and **hypoalbuminemia** results. In addition to massive proteinuria, the nephrotic syndrome is associated with the presence of free fat, tubular epithelial cells containing fat (oval fat bodies), and fatty casts in the urine sediment.

Tubular Damage

A very small amount of protein (albumin) does find its way into the glomerular filtrate. In normal situations, all this protein is reabsorbed back into the blood through the renal convoluted tubules. Although the concentration of protein that normally filters into the glomerular filtrate is extremely small, and only 1 in 180 parts of the glomerular filtrate is eliminated from the body as urine (the rest is reabsorbed), failure to reabsorb any protein from this large volume of glomerular filtrate will result in fairly large amounts of protein in the urine. In other words, another cause of proteinuria is decreased reabsorption of protein by the renal tubular cells. The amount of proteinuria in tubular damage is generally mild to moderate. Examples of tubular proteinuria include pyelonephritis, acute tubular necrosis, polycystic kidney disease, heavy metal and vitamin D intoxication, phenacetin damage, hypokalemia, Wilson's disease, galactosemia, Fanconi's syndrome, and posttransplantation syndrome.

Acute pyelonephritis is an infection of the pelvis and parenchyma of the kidney. It is usually the result of infection ascending from the lower urinary tract into the kidney. In addition to moderate proteinuria, urinalysis findings may include nitrite, leukocyte esterase, white blood cells (WBCs, neutrophils), and casts (WBC, cellular, granular, or bacterial). The presence of casts in the urine locates the infection in the kidney.

Drug-induced **acute interstitial nephritis** (an allergic response) is also associated with moderate proteinuria. The presence of eosinophils is especially characteristic, together with neutrophils, RBCs, and cellular or granular casts.

Only mild proteinuria may be seen with acute renal failure or acute tubular necrosis. However, the sediment may contain renal tubular epithelial cells and casts (epithelial, granular, or waxy).

Prerenal Disorders

Prerenal or overflow disorders may result in proteinuria from disorders in body sites other than the kidney. Overflow from excessive production of low-molecular-weight proteins such as hemoglobin, myoglobin, or immunoglobulins may result in such proteinuria. The presence of light-chain immunoglobulins (Bence Jones protein) associated with multiple myeloma is an example.

Prerenal proteinuria may also be the result of a change in hydrostatic pressure in the kidney glomerulus. Increased blood pressure may force more proteins than normal through the glomerulus, resulting in the mild proteinuria seen with hypertension, congestive heart failure, and dehydration.

Lower Urinary Tract Disorders

Infections of the lower urinary tract may result in a mild proteinuria. The proteinuria may result from infection of the ureters or bladder with exudation through the mucosa (lining). Other urinalysis findings include positive chemical tests for nitrite (depending on the infecting organism) and leukocyte esterase, and the presence of WBCs and bacteria in the sediment. Casts are not present in lower urinary tract infection; they originate in the kidney.

Asymptomatic Proteinuria

In certain situations, small amounts of urinary protein may occur transiently in normal persons. In particular, urinary protein may be found in young adults after excessive exercise or exposure to cold or in **orthostatic proteinuria,** which occurs in persons engaged in normal activity but disappears when they lie down.

In general, the proteinuria associated with renal disease is consistent, whereas that found in normal persons is transient. The long-term significance of asymptomatic proteinuria is unclear. To determine the cause of the proteinuria, it is often necessary to determine quantitatively the amount of protein in a 24-hour urine collection. Tests for orthostatic proteinuria are made on urine collections obtained both when the patient is at rest (first morning, collected immediately after rising) and after the patient has been walking and standing, but not sitting, for about 2 hours.

Consistent Microalbuminuria

Although screening tests for proteinuria should not be so sensitive that they detect the very small amount of protein that may be normally present in urine, it is sometimes desirable to detect the consistent passage of very small amounts of protein (microproteinuria). This is especially true of patients with diabetes mellitus. In these patients, it is thought that the early development of renal complications can be predicted by the early detection of consistent microalbuminuria. This early detection is desirable because better control of blood glucose levels may delay the progression of renal disease. The methodology for the detection of microalbuminuria includes nephelometry, radial immunodiffusion, and radioimmunoassay. With Chemstrip Micral Urine Test Strips (Roche Diagnostics) for microalbumin, albumin present in the patient's urine binds specifically with a soluble antibody-gold conjugate present on a zone of the test strip. This test strip is useful in monitoring the progression of nephropathy in diabetic patients once it has been diagnosed, but it is not suitable as a diagnostic test.

Reagent Strip Tests for Protein

PRINCIPLE

Reagent strip tests for urinary protein involve the use of *pH indicators*, substances that have characteristic colors at specific pH values. At a fixed pH, certain pH indicators will show one color in the presence of protein and another color in its absence. This phenomenon is referred to as the "protein error of indicators." The pH of the urine is held constant by means of a buffer, so any change of color of the indicator will indicate the presence of protein.

SPECIFICITY

The reagent strip tests for urinary protein are more sensitive to albumin than to other proteins such as globulin, hemoglobin, Bence Jones protein, and mucoprotein. If these proteins are present in the urine without albumin, false-negative results may be obtained. In other words, a negative reagent strip does not rule out the presence of protein. Therefore, depending on the patient population, it may be necessary for a given laboratory to test all urine specimens with both a reagent strip and a precipitation method for urinary protein so as not to miss certain abnormal proteins, such as those seen in new, undiagnosed cases of multiple myeloma.

SENSITIVITY (MINIMUM DETECTABLE LEVEL): MANUFACTURER'S VALUES

Multistix/Albustix	15 to 30 mg/dL albumin
Micro-Bumintest	4 to 8 mg/dL albumin
Chemstrip	6 mg/dL albumin (in 90% tested)

INTERFERENCES

If the urine is strongly pigmented, there may be interference with the color reaction. Bilirubin or drugs that give a vivid orange color, such as phenazopyridine (Pyridium) and other azo-containing compounds, may result in this interference.

False-Positive Results

If the urine is exposed to the reagent strip for too long, the buffer may be washed out of the strip, resulting in the formation of a blue color whether protein is present or not.

If a urine specimen is exceptionally alkaline or highly buffered, the reagent strip tests may give a positive result in the absence of protein.

Contamination of the urine container with residues of disinfectants containing quaternary ammonium compounds or chlorhexidine may show a positive result because of increased alkalinity.

Chemstrip products may give false-positive results during therapy with phenazopyridine and when infusions of polyvinylpyrrolidone (blood substitutes) are administered.

False-Negative Results

When proteins other than albumin are present, the reagent strip will give a negative result in the presence of protein.

ADDITIONAL COMMENTS

The reagent strip tests for protein are not affected by turbidity, radiographic contrast media, most drugs and their metabolites, or urine preservatives, which occasionally affect other protein tests.

The color must be matched closely with the color chart when results are being read. The protein portion of the reagent strip is difficult to interpret, especially at the trace level. When results are in doubt, the slightly more sensitive sulfosalicylic acid (SSA) protein test or a test for microalbuminuria such as Micro-Bumintest (Bayer) might be helpful.

Blood (Hemoglobin and Myoglobin)

Clinical Significance

Together with tests for protein and the microscopic analysis of the urine sediment, tests for blood in urine are used as indicators of the state of the kidney and urinary tract. Chemical tests for blood in urine react with RBCs, hemoglobin, and myoglobin (which is muscle hemoglobin). Although the chemical tests are more sensitive to the presence of hemoglobin and myoglobin than to intact RBCs, most positive reactions are actually caused by the presence of red cells (erythrocytes). Blood may represent bleeding at any point from the glomerulus to the urethra, and the actual location is important to the diagnosis and treatment of the patient. Although the chemical detection of blood in urine is a serious finding, the presence of a few RBCs in urine is normal, and hematuria may be associated with benign conditions.

It is clinically significant to differentiate between RBCs and hemoglobin in the urine. Because tests for hemoglobin are positive in the presence of both free hemoglobin and erythrocytes, it would seem that this differentiation is made mainly by the finding of RBCs in the microscopic analysis of the urine sediment. The presence of hemoglobin and the absence of RBCs in the urine does not necessarily mean that the hemoglobin was originally free urinary hemoglobin. Red cells rapidly lyse in urine, especially when the specific gravity is low (<1.010) or the pH is alkaline. For this reason, urine should be absolutely fresh when examined for the presence of RBCs.

Hematuria

Hematuria is the presence of RBCs in the urine. It results from many of conditions, including lesions of the kidney and bleeding at any other point in the urinary tract. It may be an early sign of kidney or bladder tumor (benign or malignant) or may result from stone formation in the kidney or bladder. Hematuria may be a sign of glomerular damage or interstitial nephritis (infection of the kidney) or may be seen with a lower urinary tract infection such as cystitis (bladder infection). Generalized bleeding disorders or anticoagulant therapy may also result in hematuria.

Hematuria is a sensitive early indicator of renal disease and should not be missed. Although blood will not be present in every voided specimen in every patient with renal disease, occult blood (blood that is not grossly visible but is found by laboratory tests) may be present in almost every renal disorder. There may be little correlation between the amount of blood and the severity of the disorder, but its presence may be the only indication of renal disease. Hematuria is associated with glomerular damage and is typically seen in glomerulonephritis. Other laboratory findings besides hematuria indicate the presence of renal disease. Protein is usually present along with blood, and the presence of casts (especially RBC casts) and dysmorphic RBCs in the urine sediment are particularly useful.

Hemoglobinuria

Hemoglobinuria, or the presence of free hemoglobin in the urine, results from a variety of conditions and disease states. It may be the result of hemolysis in the bloodstream **(intravascular hemolysis),** in the kidney or lower urinary tract, or in the urine sample itself. The detection of intravascular hemolysis is important because the passage of free hemoglobin through the glomerulus and subsequent uptake by renal proximal convoluted epithelial cells are damaging to the nephron. Hemoglobin is carried in the bloodstream bound to a protein, **haptoglobin.** This hemoglobin-haptoglobin complex is a large molecule that is not filtered through the glomerulus. However, there is a limited amount of haptoglobin in the blood, and once it is saturated, the excess hemoglobin is filtered through the glomerulus into the renal tubules. Some of the excreted hemoglobin is absorbed into the renal tubular cells, converted to ferritin and **hemosiderin,** and subsequently excreted several days after an acute hemolytic episode. These hemosiderin-containing cells and granules may be observed in the urine sediment, especially when stained with Prussian blue.

Hematologic disease states resulting in hemoglobinuria include hemolytic anemias, hemolytic transfusion reactions, paroxysmal nocturnal hemoglobinuria, paroxysmal cold hemoglobinuria, and favism. Severe infectious diseases such as yellow fever, *Bartonella* infection, and malaria also result in hemoglobinuria, as do poisonings with strong acids or mushrooms, severe burns, and renal infarction. Finally, significant amounts of free hemoglobin occur whenever excessive numbers of RBCs are present as a result of various renal disorders, infectious or neoplastic diseases, or trauma in any part of the urinary tract.

Myoglobinuria

Myoglobinuria is the presence of myoglobin in the urine; it is a rare finding. Chemical tests for occult blood are equally sensitive to the presence of hemoglobin and myoglobin. Myoglobin is released after **rhabdomyolysis,** acute destruction of muscle fibers. Myoglobinuria may result from traumatic muscle injury (e.g., from traffic accidents), excessive unaccustomed exercise, and beating or other crush injury. It is also seen in certain infections, after exposure to toxic substances and drugs, and in rare hereditary disorders.

The detection of myoglobinuria is important because myoglobin is rapidly cleared from the blood and excreted into the urine as a red-brown pigment. Large amounts of myoglobin are damaging to the kidney and may result in anuria. It seems that myoglobin is more damaging than hemoglobin to the kidney.

Differentiation of Hematuria, Hemoglobinuria, and Myoglobinuria

The differentiation of these conditions may be difficult. It is done with a combination of gross observations of urine and serum (or plasma) and certain chemical tests (Table 14-5). The occurrence of blood in urine will result in coloration ranging

TABLE 14-5

Differentiation of Red Blood Cells, Hemoglobin, and Myoglobin in Urine			
Finding	Red Cells	Hemoglobin	Myoglobin
Reagent strip for blood	Positive	Positive	Positive
Urine sediment for red cells	Present	Absent (few)	Absent (few)
Urine appearance	Cloudy red	Clear red	Clear red-brown
Plasma appearance	Normal	Pink to red (hemolysis)	Normal
Total serum creatine kinase (CK)	Normal	Slight elevation (10 times normal upper limit)	Marked elevation (40 times normal upper limit)
Total serum lactate dehydrogenase (LDH)	Normal	Elevated	Elevated
LDH_1 and LDH_2	Normal	Elevated	Normal
LDH_4 and LDH_5	Normal	Normal	Elevated

Modified from Ringsrud KM, Linné JJ: Urinalysis and body fluids: a color text and atlas, St Louis, 1995, Mosby.

from normal to smoky, pink, amber, red to red-brown, brown, or frankly bloody. In general, with hemoglobin and myoglobin, the urine specimen is brown or red-brown. Although the presence of RBCs would result in cloudiness, and hemoglobin or myoglobin by itself would leave a clear specimen, other constituents often accompany all three entities, leading to cloudiness of the specimen. A gross observation of the serum or plasma accompanying these specimens is useful. If the urine contains only RBCs, the serum would have a normal color. If intravascular hemolysis has occurred, the serum would appear to be hemolyzed (red). If rhabdomyolysis occurs, the myoglobin released into the blood is rapidly cleared into the urine, and the serum appears normal in color.

In all three cases, the reagent strip test for blood is positive. If present, RBCs should be detectable in the microscopic examination of the urine sediment. With both hemoglobin and myoglobin, RBCs would be absent, or very few would be present. In the case of rhabdomyolysis resulting in myoglobinemia and myoglobinuria, greatly elevated serum creatine kinase (CK) is typical because of the destruction of muscle. CK levels are not affected as greatly by hemolysis. Unfortunately, myoglobin-induced renal failure may not be seen clinically until a week or more after the clinical event, and by then myoglobin is no longer present in the urine.

Reagents Strip Tests for Blood

PRINCIPLE AND SPECIFICITY

Reagent strip tests for blood (hemoglobin, myoglobin) in urine make use of the peroxidase activity of the heme portion of the hemoglobin molecule. The reagent strips are impregnated with an organic peroxide, together with the reduced form of a chromogen. A positive reaction is seen when the peroxidase activity of the heme portion of the hemoglobin or myoglobin molecule catalyzes the release of oxygen from peroxide on the reagent strip. The released oxygen reacts with the reduced form of a chromogen, forming an oxidized chromogen, which is indicated by a color change. This reaction is summarized as follows:

$$
\begin{array}{ccc}
\text{Peroxide} & \text{Heme} & \text{Water} \\
+ & \rightarrow & + \\
\text{Reduced} & \text{(Peroxide} & \text{Oxidized} \\
\text{chromogen} & \text{activity)} & \text{chromogen}
\end{array}
$$

The reagent strips are equally sensitive to hemoglobin and myoglobin. Intact RBCs are hemolyzed when they come into contact with the reagent strip, and the released hemoglobin reacts as described. It is essential that well-mixed urine be tested for the presence of blood. This is especially important when only a few intact RBCs are present in the urine specimen. If intact RBCs are allowed to settle and the supernatant urine is tested, false-negative results will be obtained.

SENSITIVITY (MINIMUM DETECTABLE LEVEL): MANUFACTURER'S VALUES

Multistix/Hemastix 0.015 to 0.062 mg/dL hemoglobin (equivalent to 5-20 intact RBCs/μL)

Chemstrip 5 RBCs/μL, or hemoglobin corresponding to 10 RBCs/μL in 90% of urine specimens tested

INTERFERENCES
False-Positive Results

- Strong oxidizing cleaning agents, such as hypochlorite bleach, because of oxidation of the chromogen in the absence of peroxidase

- Microbial peroxidase activity associated with urinary tract infection
- The presence of blood as a contaminant from menstruation (no clinical significance)

False-Negative or Delayed Results

- Ascorbic acid in urine specimens containing more than 25 mg/dL. This is seen after ingestion of large doses of vitamin C or when ascorbic acid is included as a reducing agent in certain parenteral antibiotics, such as tetracycline. Both Multistix and Chemstrip reagent strips claim no interference at reasonable or normally encountered levels. Chemstrip products include a blood-iodate scavenger to reduce false-negative results. Multistix products containing diisopropylbenzene dihydroperoxide as the organic peroxide are less subject to interference with ascorbic acid.
- Testing the supernatant urine from centrifugation or settling when only a few intact RBCs are present. Urine must be well mixed when tested.
- Elevated specific gravity (high salt concentration) or elevated protein may reduce the lysis or RBCs necessary for a reaction to occur.
- When formalin is used as a urinary preservative
- Treatment with captopril (an antihypertensive)
- Extremely high nitrite levels (>10 mg/dL), seen (rarely) in severe urinary tract infections

ADDITIONAL COMMENTS

The presence of ascorbic acid in urine is a potential problem in the reagent strip tests for blood, as in any reagent strip test that depends on the release of oxygen and subsequent oxidation of a chromogen. When present in sufficient quantity, the ascorbic acid (a strong reducing agent) reacts with the released hydrogen peroxide (rather than the chromogen), causing inhibited (negative) results or a delayed color reaction.

When the reagent strip test for blood is negative but RBCs are observed in the urine sediment, the presence of ascorbic acid should be suspected. This may be confirmed by testing the urine with a reagent strip for ascorbic acid or by the patient's clinical history.

CONFIRMATORY TESTS

- Microscopic examination of the urinary sediment
- Reagent strip test for ascorbic acid if the test for blood is negative and RBCs are seen in the urine sediment, or if blood is suspected on the basis of the appearance of the urine specimen

Nitrite

Clinical Importance

Tests for the presence of **nitrite** in the urine have been included in the routine urinalysis as a rapid method of detecting urinary tract infection (UTI). Screening tests for nitrite are most useful when combined with tests for leukocyte esterase, another indicator of UTI. The presence of urinary nitrite indicates the existence of a UTI. It is especially useful in detecting asymptomatic infections. When certain bacteria are present in the urinary tract, they will convert nitrate, a normal constituent of urine, to nitrite, an abnormal constituent. Nitrate converters are generally gram-negative bacteria, such as the common Enterobacteriaceae. Gram-positive organisms such as enterococci and yeast do not generally convert nitrate to nitrite. However, there must also be sufficient nitrate (primarily derived from vegetables in the diet) in the urine for conversion to nitrite to take place.

Urine must be retained (incubated) in the bladder for a sufficient period (generally 4 hours) for this reaction to take place. Thus, a first morning urine collection is the specimen of choice in testing for nitrite. A specimen collected at least 4 hours after previous voiding is also acceptable. Unfortunately, a common complaint with UTI is frequent urination, making collection of an adequate specimen difficult.

The early detection of UTI is important for the prevention of kidney damage. It is believed that most UTIs begin in the lower urinary tract, as a result of fecal contamination. Most infections are caused by organisms that are normally present in the feces, such as *Escherichia coli*. The infection is introduced into the normally sterile urinary tract via the urethra and ascends to the bladder, ureters, and finally the kidney. The early detection and subsequent treatment of UTI are important in preventing infection of the kidney and subsequent renal failure. From this discussion, it should be apparent that because of anatomic differences, UTI is much more common in women than men. In fact, other than just after birth or with incontinence (often associated with aging or disability), UTI is typically a disease of women.

Traditionally, UTIs are diagnosed through quantitative urine culture, in which the organism that causes the infection is cultured and identified (see Chapter 16). Nitrite tests are screening tests that aid quantitative urine cultures. The existence of UTIs is also suggested by other findings in the routine urinalysis. Microscopic findings include the presence of WBCs and bacteria in lower UTIs; this plus the presence of casts, especially WBC or pus casts, indicates upper UTI (pyelonephritis). Chemical test results suggestive of UTI include the presence of leukocyte esterase and protein and a more alkaline urinary pH.

Reagent Strip Tests for Nitrite

PRINCIPLE

Reagent strip tests for nitrite are based on the **Griess test.** This involves a **diazo reaction.** Nitrite will react with an aromatic amine (*p*-arsanilic or sulfanilic acid) in an acid medium to produce a diazonium salt. The diazonium salt is then coupled with another aromatic ring (quinoline) to give an azo dye, which is seen as a pink or red color.

SPECIFICITY

The Griess test is specific for nitrite.

RESULTS

Results are reported as positive or negative. Any overall pink coloration is a positive reaction. Pink spots or pink edges are a negative reaction. The intensity of color formation does not necessarily indicate the degree of bacterial infection. Any pink coloration suggests a significant infection.

SENSITIVITY (MINIMUM DETECTABLE LEVEL)

Multistix	0.06 to 0.1 mg/dL nitrite ion
Chemstrip	As low as 0.05 mg/dL nitrite

INTERFERENCES

False-Positive Results

- Medications such as phenazopyridine or other azo-containing compounds or dyes that color urine red or that turn red in an acidic medium
- In vitro conversion of nitrate to nitrite as a result of bacterial contamination of the specimen; prevented by testing fresh urine specimens

False-Negative or Delayed Results

- Insufficient time in the bladder for the conversion of nitrate to nitrite, even with significant bacterial infection
- Insufficient dietary nitrate present for bacteria to reduce nitrate to nitrite, such as with starvation, fasting, or intravenous feeding
- Presence of bacteria that further reduce nitrite to nitrogen
- Sensitivity may be reduced in concentrated urine with low pH (<6). This is not typically seen with bacterial infection.

- Ascorbic acid in concentration of 25 mg/dL or greater in specimens with small amounts of nitrite, resulting from the reduction of the diazonium salt by ascorbic acid

ADDITIONAL COMMENTS

The nitrite test is primarily useful if positive. If the nitrite test area shows a negative reaction, UTI cannot be ruled out. Organisms must contain the reductase enzyme necessary to reduce nitrate to nitrite. This is true of most of the gram-negative enteric pathogens that cause UTIs. The gram-positive enterococci and yeast, however, do not contain this enzyme. The urine must be retained in the bladder for 4 hours or more for adequate conversion of nitrate to detectable nitrite. Obtaining such specimens may be difficult because urgency and frequent urination are common in patients with UTIs. Thus, lack of sufficient incubation time is a major obstacle to positive reagent strip results with significant infection.

CONFIRMATORY TESTS

Microscopic examination of the urine sediment, Gram stain, and quantitative urine culture can be used to confirm the nitrite test.

Leukocyte Esterase

Clinical Importance

Chemical tests for leukocyte esterase have been included on the urine reagent strip tests as another means of detecting UTI. These tests are based on the measurement of leukocyte esterase, which is present in azurophilic or primary granules of granulocytic leukocytes. These granulocytes include polymorphonuclear neutrophil leukocytes (PMNs or neutrophils), monocytes (histiocytes), eosinophils, and basophils. In practice, positive reactions occur with increased neutrophils. Conditions associated with sufficient quantities of other granulocytes to give positive reactions are extremely rare, if they ever occur. Lymphocytes and the various epithelial cells that make up the kidney and urinary tract do not contain leukocyte esterase and are not measured in this test.

The detection of leukocyte esterase as an indicator of infection is useful because neutrophils are generally increased in response to bacterial infection. When bacteria infect the urinary tract, at any point from the urethra to the kidney, the presence of increased numbers of WBCs, particularly neutrophils, is typical. Neutrophils are also seen in the urine sediment. However, a frequent problem is the rapid lysis of neutrophils in urine, a result of their phagocytic activity. Once lysed, they are not detectable in the microscopic analysis of the sediment. However, the test for leukocyte esterase depends on its release from the azurophilic or primary granules of granulocytes. Thus the leukocyte esterase test is positive whether lysed or intact cells are present in the urine.

Urine normally contains a few (up to 5) WBCs per high-power field (hpf) in the microscopic analysis of the urinary sediment. This normal occurrence of WBCs is not sufficient to cause a positive reaction with the leukocyte esterase test. The reaction requires 5 to 15 leukocytes/hpf to give a positive reaction. Therefore the absence of leukocyte esterase does not rule out a UTI. However, the presence of leukocyte esterase is helpful, especially with an elevated (alkaline) urine pH and the chemical detection of nitrite in the urine, together with the presence of bacteria and WBCs in the urine sediment.

Increased leukocyte esterase may be seen in conditions in which bacteria are not seen in the urine sediment or cultured. These include inflammatory conditions that may occur without bacterial infection, bacterial infection after treatment with antibiotics, and infections by organisms such as trichomonads and chlamydia, which are not seen on standard culture media.

Negative or low results for leukocyte esterase may be seen in the urine of immunosuppressed patients who have significant bacterial infection, because of the inability to produce adequate granulocytes.

Reagent Strip Tests for Leukocyte Esterase

PRINCIPLE

Reagent strip tests for leukocyte esterase use a diazo reaction, similar to the reagent strip tests for nitrite. The test area contains an ester that is hydrolyzed by leukocyte esterase to form its alcohol (which contains an aromatic ring) and acid. The aromatic ring is then coupled with a diazonium salt, present in the test area, to form an azo dye, which is seen as the formation of a purple color. Chemstrips use an indoxyl ester, and Multistix use a pyrrole amino acid ester.

SPECIFICITY

The reaction is specific for esterase that is present in granulocytic leukocytes, primarily neutrophils in urine.

SENSITIVITY (MINIMUM DETECTABLE LEVEL): MANUFACTURER'S VALUES

Multistix   5 to 15 cells/hpf in clinical urine
Chemstrip   10 to 25 cells/μL

INTERFERENCES

The presence of substances that color urine, such as azo-containing compounds, nitrofurantoin, riboflavin, and bilirubin, may make color interpretation difficult.

False-Positive Results

Strong oxidizing agents such as chlorine bleach and urinary preservatives such as formalin (formaldehyde); preservatives should not be used.

False-Negative or Reduced Results

- Drugs (antibiotics) such as cephalexin, cephalothin, tetracycline, and gentamicin
- Elevated glucose (>3 g/dL)
- High specific gravity
- Oxalic acid (metabolite of ascorbic acid)
- High levels of albumin (>500 mg/dL)

ADDITIONAL COMMENTS

The presence of repeated trace and positive values are clinically significant and indicate the need for further testing to determine the cause of the presence of neutrophils (granulocytes) in the urine (pyuria). Tests may include microscopic analysis of the urine sediment, Gram stain, and quantitative urine culture. The test is not affected by the presence of blood, bacteria, or epithelial cells. Results of leukocyte esterase testing are especially useful when combined with reagent strip tests for nitrite.

Glucose (Sugar)

Clinical Importance

Chemical screening tests for glucose (**dextrose**) are generally included in every routine urinalysis. Unlike the parameters previously discussed, these tests are used to diagnose and monitor a metabolic condition, rather than a renal or urinary tract condition. The occurrence of glucose in the urine indicates that the metabolic disorder diabetes mellitus should be suspected, although several other conditions result in glucosuria.

Any condition in which glucose is found in the urine is termed **glycosuria** (or **glucosuria**). Tests for glucosuria were among the earliest laboratory tests. The "taste test" was used by the Babylonians and the Egyptians to detect diabetes by tasting for the presence of sugar (sweet) in what would normally be a salty solution, and Hindu physicians noticed that "honey urine" attracted ants.

The occurrence of measurable glucose in the urine is not normal. The blood glucose concentration normally varies between 60 and 110 mg/dL, depending on the method of analysis. After a meal it may increase to 120 to 160 mg/dL. Normally, all the glucose in the blood is filtered by the glomerulus and reabsorbed into the blood. However, if the blood glucose concentration becomes too high (usually >180 to 200 mg/dL), the excess glucose will not be reabsorbed into the blood and will be eliminated from the body in the urine. Other factors that might result in glucosuria are reduced glomerular blood flow, reduced tubular reabsorption, and reduced urine flow.

The lowest blood glucose concentration that will result in glycosuria is termed the **renal threshold,** and it varies somewhat from person to person. The most common condition in which the renal threshold for glucose is exceeded is diabetes mellitus. In simplified terms, diabetes mellitus is a deficiency in the production of, or an inhibition in the action of, the hormone insulin. Insulin has the effect of lowering the blood glucose concentration. As a result of the deficiency of insulin, the blood glucose concentration exceeds the renal threshold, and glucose is spilled over into the urine.

Diabetic patients have used tests for urine glucose to self-monitor the adequacy of insulin control. Although these urine tests have been replaced by home blood glucose testing for unstable diabetic patients, urine glucose testing is less expensive, is noninvasive, and remains useful for patients who do not have to make frequent insulin dose adjustments. Tests for diabetes mellitus include tests for blood glucose as well as for urinary glucose. Additional tests, such as those for glycated hemoglobin, may also be used to monitor diabetes mellitus.

Although diabetes mellitus is suspected in patients with glycosuria, the occurrence of glycosuria is not diagnostic; glycosuria has many other causes. For example, glycosuria may be observed after large amounts of sugar or foods containing sugar are eaten, during acute emotional strain when the liver liberates glucose for energy, and after exercise. Glycosuria may also be associated with pregnancy, certain types of meningitis, hypothyroidism, certain tumors of the adrenal medulla, and some brain injuries.

In addition, certain abnormal conditions are characterized by the presence in the urine of sugars other than glucose. These are generally **reducing sugars,** which require detection by methods other than those employed in the reagent strip tests that are specific for glucose. **Galactosuria** is the presence of the sugar galactose in the urine. It results from a metabolic error whereby the enzyme galactose-1-phosphate uridyltransferase is lacking, so galactose is not metabolized, resulting in increased galactose in the blood (galactosemia) and urine. This condition results in permanent physical and mental deterioration, which may be controlled by early detection and dietary restriction of galactose. Therefore, urine from young pediatric patients should be screened with a nonspecific copper reduction test for reducing substances that will detect galactose and other reducing sugars in addition to glucose. State-required newborn metabolic

screening tests for inherited disease often include a test for galactosemia.

Other reducing sugars, such as lactose, may be seen in the urine late in pregnancy or early lactation. Lactose intolerance in infancy and failure to gain weight may occur because of intestinal lactase deficiency, and lactosuria may be seen.

Reagent Strip Tests for Glucose Oxidase

PRINCIPLE AND SPECIFICITY

The reagent strip tests for urinary sugar are specific for glucose because they are based on the use of the enzyme **glucose oxidase.** An *enzyme* may be described as a *biological catalyst,* a substance that must be present before a chemical reaction will occur. As with most enzymes, glucose oxidase is absolutely specific. It will react only in the presence of glucose, and it will not react with any other substance.

Reagent strip tests for urine glucose are double-sequential enzyme reactions. Glucose oxidase will oxidize glucose to gluconic acid and at the same time reduce atmospheric oxygen to hydrogen peroxide. In the presence of the enzyme peroxidase, the hydrogen peroxide formed will oxidize the reduced form of a dye to the oxidized form, which is indicated by the color change of an oxidation-reduction indicator. This reaction is diagrammed as follows:

Step 1:

$$\text{Glucose (in urine)} + O_2 \text{ (from air)} \xrightarrow{\text{Glucose oxidase}} \text{Gluconic acid} + H_2O_2$$

Step 2:

$$H_2O_2 + \text{Reduced form of dye} \xrightarrow{\text{Peroxidase}} \text{Oxidized form of dye} + H_2O$$

The glucose oxidase, the peroxidase, and the reduced form of the oxidation-reduction indicator are all impregnated onto a dry reagent strip. Reagent strips differ in the chromogen used as the oxidation-reduction indicator. They all contain glucose oxidase and peroxidase.

Laboratory personnel must remember that nonglucose reducing substances (NGRSs) will not be detected by tests that are specific for glucose. Therefore, specimens from infants and young pediatric patients and specimens in which NGRSs are suspected should be subjected to non-specific (usually copper reduction) tests for reducing substances in addition to the specific tests for glucose.

SENSITIVITY (MINIMUM DETECTABLE LEVEL): MANUFACTURER'S VALUES

Multistix/Diastix 75-125 mg/dL glucose (as low as 40 mg/dL in dilute urine containing less than 5 mg/dL ascorbic acid)

Chemstrip 40 mg/dL in 90% of urine specimens tested

INTERFERENCES

Because reagent strip tests are all specific for glucose, most interferences lead to reduced or false-negative results.

False-Positive Results

- Contamination by bleach or other strong oxidizing agents may oxidize the reduced form of the dye present on the reagent strip, causing a color change in the absence of glucose. This shows the importance of using contamination-free urine containers and work surfaces.
- Trace values may be seen in very dilute urine specimens because of increased sensitivity at low specific gravity.
- Reagent strips exposed to air by improper storage have been shown to give false-positive results.[4]

False-Negative or Delayed Results

- Large urinary concentrations of ascorbic acid from therapeutic doses of vitamin C or from drugs such as tetracyclines, in which ascorbic acid is used as a reducing agent. Ascorbic acid blocks or delays the reaction by acting as a reducing agent reacting with the released hydrogen peroxide (rather than the chromogen in the reagent strip). Multistix products are inhibited by ascorbic acid concentrations of 50 mg/dL (500 mg/L) or greater in specimens containing small amounts (75 to 125 mg/dL) of glucose. Chemstrip is unaffected by ascorbic acid concentration less than 100 mg/dL (1000 mg/L). With questionable ascorbic acid interference, repeat tests on urine voided at least 10 hours after the last administration of vitamin C, or test for ascorbic acid.
- Ketone bodies at moderate levels (>40 mg/dL) in specimens containing small amounts (75 to 12 mg/dL) of glucose. This combination of high ketone and low glucose is unlikely in a diabetic patient.
- Sodium fluoride is an enzyme inhibitor. Do not use as a preservative.
- Refrigerated specimens, because of decreased enzyme activity. Urine must be at room temperature when tested.

When the presence of a reducing sugar other than glucose (e.g., galactose) is suspected in the

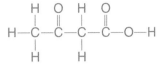

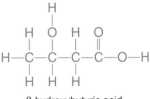

Acetoacetic acid

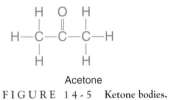

β-hydroxybutyric acid

Acetone

FIGURE 14-5   Ketone bodies.

urine, a nonspecific test, Clinitest, should be performed. The Clinitest method is an older procedure of the detection of reducing carbohydrates. The method detects the presence of any reducing substance to reduce copper II (cupric) ions to copper I (cuprous) ions in the presence of heat and alkali. A positive reaction is semiquantitated as a change in color ranging from blue to green, yellow, and orange, depending on the amount of sugar in the urine. This reagent tablet test will detect as low as 250 mg/dL of sugar.

Ketone Bodies

Clinical Importance

Ketone bodies are a group of three related substances: acetone, acetoacetic (or diacetic) acid, and β-hydroxybutyric acid. Their structural similarity is illustrated in Fig. 14-5. They are normal products of fat metabolism and not normally detectable in the blood or urine.

In fat **catabolism** (the phase of metabolism in which fats are broken down for energy), aceto-acetic acid is produced first. It is converted either reversibly to β-hydroxybutyric acid or irreversibly to acetone. All three types of ketone bodies are utilized as a source of energy and are eventually converted to carbon dioxide and water. When the body uses normal amounts of fat, the tissues are able to use the entire ketone production as an energy source. If more fat than normal is metabolized, however, the body is unable to use all the ketone bodies. The clinical result is an increased concentration of ketones in the blood (**ketonemia**) and urine (**ketonuria**). **Ketosis** is the combination of increased ketones in both the blood and the urine.

Whenever fat (rather than carbohydrate) is used as the major source of energy, ketosis and ketonuria may result. The two outstanding causes of ketone accumulation are diabetes mellitus and starvation. In diabetes mellitus the body is unable to use carbohydrate as an energy source and attempts to compensate by resorting to fat catabolism, which results in accumulation of the ketones. In starvation the body is depleted of stored carbohydrate and must resort to fat as an energy source. Similarly, ketosis is seen in patients with dehydration and conditions associated with fever, vomiting, and diarrhea. The same situation may occur in patients with severe liver damage. Most carbohydrate is stored as liver glycogen. In liver damage, there is no stored glycogen; thus the body must again resort to fat for energy. Also, a **ketogenic diet** will result in ketone accumulation. A ketogenic diet is high in fat and low in carbohydrates—specifically, a diet containing more than 1.5 g of fat per 1 g of carbohydrate. Low-carbohydrate diets used for weight reduction may be ketogenic diets.

Because the presence of ketone bodies in urine is an early indication of a lack of adequate insulin control, diabetic patients often use reagent strips that combine tests for glucose and ketones for home monitoring of their disease. The physiologic effect of ketone accumulation in the blood and urine (ketosis) is serious. Acetoacetic acid and β-hydroxybutyric acid contribute excess hydrogen ions to the blood, resulting in acidosis. Acidosis is an extremely serious condition and results in death if allowed to continue. Therefore the body attempts to compensate for excess acid in the blood by eliminating acid through the urine. The kidney is capable of producing urine with a pH as low as 4.5. Thus the occurrence of ketones in the urine is associated with a low urinary pH. Before insulin was used in the treatment of diabetes mellitus, acidosis was the cause of death in two-thirds of all patients. In the treatment of diabetes mellitus, it is important to control the amount of insulin so that ketosis and acidosis do not occur. A typical urine specimen from an uncontrolled diabetic is pale and greenish, contains a large amount of sugar, has a high specific gravity by refractometer, has a low pH, and contains ketone bodies.

When ketones accumulate in the blood and urine, they do not occur in equal concentrations.

Of the ketones, 78% are present as β-hydroxybutyric acid, 20% as acetoacetic acid, and only 2% as acetone. However, the reagent strip tests for ketones are most sensitive to the presence of acetoacetic acid. No simple laboratory tests exist for β-hydroxybutyric acid.

Reagent Strip Tests for Ketone Bodies

PRINCIPLE

The reagent strip tests for ketone bodies are based on Legal's (Rothera's) test, a color reaction with sodium nitroprusside (nitroferricyanide). Acetoacetic acid will react with sodium nitroprusside in an alkaline medium to form a purple color. If glycine is added, the test is slightly sensitive to acetone. Multistix and Ketostix have been formulated to react only with acetoacetic acid. They do not react with acetone. The Chemstrip products include glycine and detect both acetoacetic acid and larger amounts of acetone. None of the reagent strips detect β-hydroxybutyric acid.

ACETEST TABLET TEST

The Acetest (Bayer Diagnostics) is a tablet test for acetone and acetoacetic acid, based on a color reaction with sodium nitroprusside. The principle is virtually identical to that of the reagent strip tests. In addition to urine, Acetest tablets can be used to test whole blood, plasma, or serum. This test may be useful in testing urines containing interfering colors.

INTERFERENCES

The presence of various pigments, drugs, or substances causing abnormal, highly colored urine specimens presents problems in the reading of ketone results. False-positive reactions may result from the formation of a color that may be interpreted as positive, or true positive reactions may be masked in these urine specimens.

False-Positive Results

- Specimens containing phthaleins (bromsulphalein, phenolsulfonphthalein), very large amounts of phenylketones, or the preservative 8-hydroxyquinoline
- Highly concentrated urine specimens (high specific gravity) or specimens containing large amounts of levodopa metabolites may give weak positive reactions.
- 2-Mercaptoethanesulfonic acid (mesna) or other compounds containing sulfhydryl groups. A positive reaction is seen initially, but the color fades to normal by the time specified for reading the color reaction. This interference is especially problematic when automatic

reagent strip readers are employed, because these instruments are programmed to read the various chemical reactions more quickly than with visual readings. If such interference is suspected, reagent strips should be checked visually and the visual result reported. If the color persists and interference is still suspected, a drop of glacial acetic acid may be added to the test area on the reagent strip or the Acetest tablet. If the color is caused by a sulfhydryl group, it will fade, whereas color caused by diacetic acid will remain.

False-Negative or Reduced Results

Conversion of acetoacetic acid to acetone, with subsequent evaporation from the specimen, in improperly stored specimens; urine specimens must be tested when freshly voided or immediately refrigerated.

ADDITIONAL COMMENTS

When a patient is monitored with repeated determinations of acetone and acetoacetic acid in plasma or urine, the concentrations of these compounds may start at very high levels and fall but may still give results that correspond to "large" on the color chart. Repeated reports of "large" do not reflect the changes as they occur. In some cases it is desirable to dilute subsequent specimens to monitor and observe a decrease in ketone excretion. The urine specimen is diluted 1:2, 1:4, and so on, until a "large" value is no longer seen. The report in such cases should state at what dilution a "large" value is no longer obtained (e.g., large, 1:4 dilution moderate).

Bilirubin and Urobilinogen

As mentioned earlier, the routine urinalysis provides information on the function and disorders of the kidney and urinary tract, as well as other metabolic or systemic disorders. Tests for urine bilirubin and urobilinogen are used as indicators of liver function.

Normal Liver Function

The liver is a large and complex organ necessary for numerous body functions; it is responsible for many metabolic, storage, excretory, and detoxifying processes. More specifically, the liver is a major factor in the metabolism of carbohydrates, lipids, and proteins, in terms of both intermediary metabolism and the synthesis of many essential compounds. Many enzymes and coenzymes needed for carbohydrate, lipid, and protein metabolism are present only in liver cells. Glycogen is formed, stored, and converted back to glucose in the liver.

Energy derived from food is made available to the cells of the body through glycolysis of the high-energy bonds in adenosine triphosphate (ATP), which are formed by oxidative phosphorylation in the liver cells.

The liver is the site of detoxification of various substances. These toxic substances may be formed in normal body metabolism and converted or detoxified by the liver; an example is the formation of urea from the ammonia produced in protein metabolism. Toxic substances introduced into the blood from the intestine (e.g., dyes, heavy metals, drugs) are excreted by the liver. The liver is essential in the formation and secretion of bile, bile pigments, and bile salts, which are necessary for digestion. These substances are derived from bilirubin, a major byproduct of the destruction of RBCs. In addition, the liver is the site of formation and synthesis of many of the factors involved in the clotting of blood.

These important functions of the liver may be altered when the liver is diseased or damaged. Numerous laboratory tests are available to determine both the existence of liver disease and the extent, location, and type of damage so that appropriate treatment can be initiated. No one test will give a complete clinical view of liver function; instead, a carefully selected group of tests may be necessary, depending on the process in question. These include tests for the presence and concentration of bilirubin in the blood and the urine.

Normal Formation and Excretion of Bilirubin and Urobilinogen

Bilirubin is a normal product resulting from the breakdown of RBCs. Individual RBCs do not exist indefinitely in the body; they are degraded after approximately 120 days. As part of erythrocyte degradation, the heme portion of the hemoglobin molecule is converted to the bile pigment bilirubin by the mononuclear phagocytic system (MPS), primarily by MPS cells in the liver, spleen, and bone marrow. A total of approximately 6 g of hemoglobin is released each day as RBCs are eliminated from the body. The cells of the MPS initially phagocytose the RBCs, then convert the released hemoglobin through a complex series of reactions in which the heme portion of the molecule is finally converted to bilirubin.

Bilirubin is a vivid yellow pigment. An increase in the concentration of bilirubin in the blood indicates the presence of jaundice. Although it is useful in the bile, bilirubin is a waste product that must eventually be eliminated from the body. When formed by the MPS cells, bilirubin is not soluble in water. Therefore it is transported from the MPS cells through the blood to the liver cells linked to albumin as a bilirubin-albumin complex. This insoluble form of bilirubin is referred to as **free bilirubin** or **unconjugated bilirubin.**

Bilirubin is normally excreted from the body by the liver by way of the intestine. It is excreted by the liver rather than the kidney because the bilirubin-albumin complex cannot pass through the glomerular capsule of the kidney. When free bilirubin reaches the liver, it is made water soluble by conjugation with glucuronic acid and other hydrophilic substances to form **bilirubin glucuronide.**

The water-soluble bilirubin glucuronide, referred to as **conjugated bilirubin,** can be eliminated from the body by way of the kidney or the intestine. Normally, conjugated bilirubin is excreted by the liver into the bile and transported to the common bile duct and then to the gallbladder, where it is concentrated and emptied into the small intestine.

In the intestine, bilirubin is converted to **urobilinogen** by the action of certain bacteria that make up the intestinal flora. Urobilinogen is actually a group of colorless chromogens, all of which are referred to as *urobilinogen.* Part of the urobilinogen formed in the intestine is absorbed into the portal blood circulation and returned to the liver, where it is re-excreted into the bile and returned to the intestine. A very small amount of urobilinogen escapes this liver clearance and is therefore excreted from the body by way of the urine. This represents only about 1% of the urobilinogen produced in 1 day.

Part of the urobilinogen in the intestine is converted to **stercobilinogen** (colorless), which is oxidized to the colored **stercobilin;** this latter substance gives feces its normal color. The net effect is that, in normal circumstances, 99% of the urobilinogen formed from bilirubin is eliminated by way of the feces.

Urobilin (formerly known as *urochrome*) is a breakdown product of heme. Urobilin is produced when urobilinogen is oxidized by intestinal bacteria. Once urobilinogen is exposed to the environment upon urination, it is oxidized to urobilin, which makes the urine appear dark in instances of common bile duct obstruction. It is a sensitive marker for biliary obstruction, and early acute hepatitis as well.

Urine normally contains only a very small amount of urobilinogen and no bilirubin. Unconjugated (albumin-bound) bilirubin cannot be excreted by the kidney and is absent in urine. However, conjugated bilirubin can pass through the renal glomerulus, and if it is present in abnormal concentration in the blood, it will be excreted by the kidney.

Clinical Importance

Tests for urinary bilirubin and urobilinogen should be performed when indicated by abnormal color of the urine or when liver disease or a hemolytic condition is suspected from the patient's history. Because these tests are part of most multiple-reagent strips, they are included in the routine urinalysis. The presence of bilirubin in the urine is an early sign of liver cell disease (hepatocellular disease) and of obstruction to the bile flow from the liver. It is especially useful in the early detection and monitoring of hepatitis, a highly infectious disease of particular importance to laboratory workers. The presence of urobilinogen in the urine is increased in any condition that causes an increase in the production of bilirubin glucuronide and any disease that prevents the liver from performing its normal function of returning urobilinogen to the intestine through the bile. Information about urinary bilirubin and urobilinogen, in addition to serum bilirubin levels, is useful in determining the cause of jaundice. (See also Chapter 11.)

Bilirubin

CLINICAL SIGNIFICANCE

Tests for urinary bilirubin (along with urobilinogen) are important in the detection of liver disease and the determination of the cause of jaundice. Normally there is no detectable bilirubin in the urine, even with the most sensitive methods. However, finding even very small amounts of bilirubin in urine is important because it may be present in the earliest phases of liver disease.

Jaundice is a condition that occurs when the serum bilirubin concentration becomes greater than normal and there is an abnormal accumulation of bilirubin in the body tissues. Bilirubin is a vivid yellow pigment, so its accumulation in the tissues results in yellow pigmentation of the skin, the sclera or white of the eyes, and the mucous membranes. The causes of jaundice are numerious and must be discovered as soon as possible so that treatment may be started. There are several classifications of the various types of jaundice; one describes three types: hemolytic (prehepatic), hepatic (hepatocellular), and obstructive (posthepatic). Laboratory findings in various types of jaundice are summarized in Table 14-6.

Hemolytic (Prehepatic) Jaundice

Hemolytic jaundice, also known as **prehepatic jaundice,** occurs in conditions in which there is increased destruction of RBCs, such as hemolytic anemias and hemolytic disease of the newborn. The liver is basically normal, so there is an

TABLE 14-6

		Laboratory Findings in Various Types of Jaundice			
Type of Jaundice	Clinical Example	Blood Bilirubin (Unconjugated)	Urine Bilirubin (Conjugated)	Urine Urobilinogen	Color of Feces
Normal		0-1.3 mg/dL	Negative	<1 mg/dL	Normal, brown
Hemolytic (prehepatic)	Hemolytic anemia	Increased	Negative	Increased	Increased (dark brown)
	Hemolytic disease of newborn				
Hepatic (hepato-cellular)	Neonatal physiologic Hepatitis (viral, toxic) Cirrhosis	Increased (varies)	Increased (varies)	Increased or absent	Normal or pale
Obstructive (posthepatic)	Gallstones Tumor	Normal	Increased	None (decreased)	Pale chalky-white ("acholic")

Modified from Ringsrud KM, Linné JJ: Urinalysis and body fluids: a color text and atlas, St Louis, 1995, Mosby.

increased formation of conjugated bilirubin and subsequently of urobilinogen. Increased formation of urobilinogen from bilirubin results in increased levels of urobilinogen in the blood. The liver is overwhelmed by the increased production of bilirubin and urobilinogen and unable to excrete the urobilinogen back into the intestine. Therefore, more urobilinogen is eliminated in the urine. However, all the bilirubin that is conjugated by the liver goes into the intestine, where it is converted to urobilinogen, and no bilirubin is found in the urine.

Hepatic (Hepatocellular) Jaundice

Hepatic jaundice, also called **hepatocellular jaundice,** results from conditions that involve the liver cells directly and prevent normal excretion of bilirubin. This type is probably the most varied and difficult jaundice to understand. Findings differ, depending on the disease or condition and the stage of disease, and include:

1. Failure to conjugate bilirubin, with increased concentration of free (albumin-bound) bilirubin in blood
2. Failure to transport conjugated bilirubin into the bile canaliculi, with increased conjugated bilirubin backing up (regurgitating) into the blood and urine
3. Failure of the liver to re-excrete the recirculated urobilinogen, with increased concentration of urobilinogen in the blood and the urine

Neonatal physiologic jaundice results when there is an enzyme deficiency in the immature liver and thus failure to conjugate bilirubin, resulting in increased unconjugated (free) bilirubin in the blood with no bilirubin in the urine.

Disturbances of the transport mechanisms by which conjugated bilirubin is passed into the

bile canaliculi are characteristic of hepatocellular jaundice. In conditions such as viral hepatitis, toxic hepatitis (caused by heavy metal or drug poisoning), and cirrhosis, there is a diffuse overall hepatic cell involvement. In these cases, the bilirubin conjugated by the liver is not excreted into the bile; instead, conjugated bilirubin backs up into the blood and then can be eliminated by the kidney. Of the conjugated bilirubin that reaches the gut, urobilinogen is formed, part of which is absorbed into the portal circulation and returned to the liver for excretion. However, the diseased liver cells may be unable to remove the urobilinogen from the blood, resulting in excretion of urobilinogen into the urine. As the disease progresses to later stages, the liver is unable to form and pass conjugated bilirubin into the bile, so conjugated bilirubin regurgitates (backs up) into the blood and is eliminated from the body by way of the urine. Such patients would have little or no urobilinogen in the urine.

Obstructive (Posthepatic) Jaundice

Posthepatic jaundice, also known as **obstructive jaundice,** occurs when the common bile duct is obstructed by stones, tumors, spasms, or stricture. As a result, the conjugated bilirubin is regurgitated back into the liver sinusoids and the blood. If the blockage is sufficiently extensive, liver cell function may be impaired, and both free and conjugated bilirubin may be found in the blood. The conjugated bilirubin will be excreted by the kidney and therefore will be found in the urine. Conjugated bilirubin is unable to reach the intestine, so no urobilinogen is formed, and it is absent in the blood and urine. Because urobilinogen is not formed, urobilin is absent, and the stools have a characteristic chalky-white to light-brown color, also referred to as **acholic.**

REAGENT STRIP TESTS FOR BILIRUBIN

Principle

The reagent strip tests for bilirubin are based on a diazo reaction. Bilirubin is coupled with a diazonium salt in an acid medium to form azobilirubin. A positive reaction is seen as the formation of a colored compound. Tests differ in the diazonium salt used and thus the color produced.

Specificity

Tests are specific for bilirubin. However, the presence of other highly colored pigments in the urine causes problems in interpreting results. This is especially true when metabolites of drugs such as phenazopyridine are present. These metabolites give the gross urine specimen a characteristic vivid red-orange color that may be mistaken for bilirubin and may mask or give atypical color reactions on the reagent strip.

Sensitivity (Minimum Detectable Level): Manufacturer's Values

Multistix	0.4 to 0.8 mg/dL
Chemstrip	0.5 mg/dL in 90% of urine specimens tested

Interferences

The reagent strip tests for bilirubin are difficult to read, and the color formed after reaction with urine must be carefully compared with the color chart supplied by the manufacturer. Proficiency in reading these results comes with experience and is essential for reliable results.

Atypical colors, which are unlike any of the color blocks, may indicate that other bile pigments derived from bilirubin are present in the urine and may be masking the bilirubin reaction. Testing the urine with a more sensitive test, such as the Ictotest tablet test, may be indicated. Large amounts of urobilinogen may affect the color reaction but not enough to give a positive result.

False-Positive or Atypical Results

- Substances that color the urine red or that turn red in an acid medium, such as phenothiazine, chlorpromazine, and metabolites of phenazopyridine (Pyridium) or ethoxazene (Serenium)
- Metabolites of etodolac (Lodine)
- A yellow-orange to red color with indican (indoxyl sulfate). Indoles are formed from bacterial overgrowth in the gut or in surgically constructed urinary bladders made from intestine

False-Negative or Decreased Results

- Oxidation of bilirubin to biliverdin, especially when exposed to ultraviolet light

- In vitro hydrolyzation of bilirubin diglucuronide to free bilirubin; tests are most sensitive to the conjugated form of bilirubin.
- Ascorbic acid in concentration of 25 mg/dL or more
- Elevated nitrite concentration, as seen in UTI, may decrease sensitivity.

Additional Comments

The presence of highly pigmented compounds may be mistaken for bilirubin in the gross urine specimen and may mask the reaction of small amounts of bilirubin. The Icotest can be done when interpretation of the bilirubin pad on the chemical analysis strip is difficult or questionable to read.

Urine specimens must be tested when fresh, or bilirubin will oxidize to biliverdin. The test is specific for bilirubin; it will not react with biliverdin.

Urobilinogen and Porphobilinogen

CLINICAL IMPORTANCE OF UROBILINOGEN

Urobilinogens are normal byproducts of erythrocyte degradation; they are formed from bilirubin by bacterial action in the intestine and are excreted in the feces as stercobilin. Increased destruction of RBCs may be accompanied by large amounts of urobilinogen in the urine. Urobilinogen is seen in the various hemolytic anemias, in pernicious anemia, and in the hemolytic phase of malaria. In the absence of increased erythrocyte destruction, the tests may be considered liver function tests. One of the first effects of liver damage is impairment of the mechanism for removing urobilinogen from the blood circulation and re-excreting it through the intestine. This results in removal of urobilinogen by the kidney and its presence in the urine. Tests for urinary urobilinogen are thus useful for the early detection of liver damage. Urobilinogen is found in the urine in conditions such as infectious hepatitis, toxic hepatitis, portal cirrhosis, congestive heart failure, and infectious mononucleosis.

Normally, 1% of all the urobilinogen produced is excreted in the urine, and 99% is excreted in the feces. Under certain conditions, however, urobilinogen is completely absent from the urine and the feces. When the normal intestinal bacterial flora is destroyed, as by antibiotic therapy, urobilinogen cannot be produced. Urobilinogen is also absent if the liver does not conjugate bilirubin, or if there is biliary tract obstruction, such as from gallstones, resulting in failure of conjugated bilirubin to reach the intestinal tract.

CLINICAL IMPORTANCE OF PORPHOBILINOGEN

Another substance that is related to urobilinogen is porphobilinogen. **Porphobilinogen** is a normal, colorless precursor of the porphyrins. The porphyrins are a group of compounds utilized in the synthesis of hemoglobin. The heme portion of hemoglobin is a type of porphyrin, namely, ferroprotoporphyrin-9. In normal persons, porphyrins are eliminated from the body in the urine and feces, mainly as coproporphyrin I, with a small amount of coproporphyrin III. However, certain errors of porphyrin metabolism lead to increased excretion of other porphyrins in the urine. These conditions are collectively called **porphyrias,** and in some porphyrias, porphobilinogen is present in the urine. *Porphobilinogenuria* is seen in acute attacks of acute intermittent porphyria, variegate porphyria, and hereditary coproporphyria. An acute attack may be precipitated by drugs affecting the liver (e.g., barbiturates, sulfa drugs, heavy metals, hydantoins, hormones), by infection, and by diet. The discovery of porphobilinogen in urine is a critical value that can eliminate or reduce adverse effects from drugs or anesthetics.

Tests for urobilinogen that use the Ehrlich aldehyde reaction will detect urobilinogen and porphobilinogen, in addition to other Ehrlich-reactive compounds.

REAGENT STRIP TESTS FOR UROBILINOGEN

Principle

The reagent strip tests for urobilinogen (unlike other reagent strip tests) differ in basic principle and specificity.

Multistix tests for urobilinogen are based on a modified **Ehrlich aldehyde reaction.** In this reaction, urobilinogen (also porphobilinogen and other Ehrlich-reactive compounds) reacts with *p*-dimethylaminobenzaldehyde in concentrated hydrochloric acid to form a colored (cherry-red) aldehyde. This is also the basis of the **Watson-Schwartz test.** An inverse Ehrlich's aldehyde reaction is the basis of the **Hoesch test,** which is used for the detection of porphobilinogen in urine.

Chemstrip reagent strips employ a diazo reaction in which a diazonium salt reacts with urobilinogen in an acid medium to form a red azo dye.

Specificity

The Multistix reagent strips react with substances known to react with Ehrlich reagent. These substances include porphobilinogen and various intermediate Ehrlich-reactive substances, such as sulfonamides, *p*-aminosalicylic acid (PAS), procaine, and 5-hydroxyindoleacetic acid (HIAA). Therefore, urine specimens that give a positive reaction with these reagent strips should be confirmed by using another method, such as Chemstrip, which is specific for urobilinogen; the Hoesch test for porphobilinogen; or the Watson-Schwartz test for urobilinogen, porphobilinogen, and intermediate Ehrlich-reactive compounds.

The Chemstrip reagent strips react with urobilinogen and stercobilinogen. Differentiation between these two substances is not diagnostically important because stercobilinogen is found in feces, not urine. Porphobilinogen and other Ehrlich-reactive substances are not detected with some reagent strips. This is helpful because many interfering Ehrlich-reactive substances are often encountered in routine urinalysis. The existence of unsuspected or undiagnosed porphyria would be missed completely with this test.

Sensitivity (Minimum Detectable Level): Manufacturer's Values

Multistix   As low as 0.2 mg/dL
Chemstrip   Approximately 0.4 mg/dL

The absence of urobilinogen cannot be determined. Results of 1 mg/dL or less should be reported as normal, rather than negative. Normally, up to 1 mg/dL urobilinogen is present in urine.

Interferences

The presence of intermediate Ehrlich-reacting substances other than urobilinogen is a problem in any test based on the Ehrlich aldehyde reaction, such as Multistix. All strips are affected by highly colored pigments or their metabolites in the urine specimen. Strips based on the diazo reaction (Chemstrip) show interferences similar to reagent strip tests for bilirubin.

False-Positive Results

- Intermediate Ehrlich-reacting substances, such as sulfonamides, PAS metabolites, procaine, and HIAA, will react in tests based on the Ehrlich aldehyde reaction (Multistix).
- Methyldopa (Aldomet) will give a strong color reaction with Ehrlich's reagent.
- Highly colored pigments and their metabolites, including ethoxazene (Serenium), drugs containing azo dyes (e.g., phenazopyridine), nitrofurantoin, riboflavin, and *p*-aminobenzoic acid, may cause atypical or positive reactions with all reagent strips.
- Reactivity with Multistix increases with temperature and may give a false-positive reaction if the urine is tested at body temperature, because of a "warm aldehyde reaction." Test urine at room temperature (22°C to 26°C).

False-Negative or Decreased Results

- Oxidation of urobilinogen (colorless) to urobilin, an orange-red pigment. The urine specimen should be tested as soon as possible after collection.
- Formalin as a preservative with all reagent strips
- Greater than 5 mg/dL nitrite with Chemstrip

- Although porphobilinogen may be detected with tests based on the Ehrlich aldehyde reaction, Multistix is not a reliable test for the detection of porphobilinogen.
- Tests based on a diazo reaction (Chemstrip) will not detect porphobilinogen in the urine.

Additional Comments

The absence of urobilinogen is not detectable with any reagent strip.

It is extremely important that fresh urine specimens be tested, because urobilinogen is very unstable when exposed to room temperature or daylight. Urobilinogen, a colorless compound, is rapidly oxidized to urobilin, an orange-red pigment, which is not detected with either reagent strip test. This oxidation takes place so readily that most urine specimens that contain urobilinogen will show an abnormal color caused by partial oxidation to urobilin. The presence of urobilinogen and that of urobilin have the same clinical significance.

It is also extremely important that urine specimens be fresh and properly stored for testing for porphobilinogen. Porphobilinogen is a colorless compound that polymerizes (oxidizes) to a colored compound, porphobilin. Porphobilin gives a characteristic dark red or red-purple color, referred to as *port-wine red*. Fresh urine containing porphobilinogen is not usually colored, but some patients may have a dark red urine, or it may darken on standing as porphobilinogen polymerizes. To extend reactivity, the pH may be adjusted to 7 with sodium bicarbonate.

Summary

Table 14-7 summarizes the information in this section on chemical tests in routine urinalysis and provides additional testing data.

MICROSCOPIC ANALYSIS OF URINE SEDIMENT

Urine sediment refers to all solid materials suspended in the urine specimen. Microscopic examination of urine sediment is especially helpful in assessing the presence of kidney and urinary tract disease. The presence of certain findings in the microscopic examination will help explain abnormal physical and chemical tests.

The need for cost containment in health care has prompted some laboratories to omit the microscopic analysis of the urine sediment as part of every routine urinalysis. Various protocols now call for the microscopic analysis only when abnormal findings are seen in the physical and chemical analysis of the urine, or when determined by laboratory protocol (including the patient's condition

or clinical history) or requested by the physician. The CLSI states, "The decision to perform microscopic examinations should be made by each individual laboratory based on its specific patient population."[1]

Specimen Requirements

Type of Specimen

Although any freely voided collection is acceptable, the ideal specimen for microscopic analysis of the urine sediment is a fresh, voided, first morning specimen. A first morning specimen (an 8-hour concentration) is preferable because it is the most concentrated. This provides a greater chance of detecting abnormal constituents. In addition, the formed elements (cells and casts) are less likely to disintegrate in more concentrated urine.

Preservation

A fresh urine specimen is particularly important for reliable results. If the urine cannot be examined within 2 hours, it should be refrigerated as soon as possible after collection. Specimens left at room temperature for more than 2 hours are not acceptable. However, an "unacceptable" specimen should not be discarded until clinical personnel have been consulted and a mutually agreeable decision has been reached.

Although refrigeration prevents decomposition of urine sediment constituents, amorphous deposits of urates and phosphates tend to precipitate out of solution as the urine cools. These findings are important in that they may obscure the presence of pathologic constituents that are present.

If the specimen must be kept in the refrigerator for more than a few hours, a chemical preservative might be considered. Formalin may be used as a preservative to fix the various cellular elements and casts, but it interferes with many chemical tests. Other preservatives, such as toluene or thymol, may be used to prevent bacterial contamination. None of the preservatives is completely satisfactory; fresh collections are preferred. If preservatives that may interfere with various chemical tests are added, it is advisable to split the well-mixed specimen so that the sediment constituents are preserved, yet the chemical constituents are not affected.

Protection from Contamination

In addition to being a fresh first morning collection, the urine specimen should be clean and free of external contamination. This is sometimes a problem, especially with female patients, because

TABLE 14-7

Confirmatory Urinalysis Tests*		
Substance	Test	Comments
Protein	Sulfosalicylic acid (SSA) test	Based on acid precipitation of protein with strong acid (SSA).
		Reagent strip test is most sensitive to albumin.
		SSA reacts with any protein; in addition to albumin: globulins, glucoproteins, and immunoglobulins.
		Delayed false-positive results with diagnostic radiographic media.
Micro-albuminuria	Micro-Bumintest (Bayer)	Tablet test for very small amounts of albumin; may be used to test for early presymptomatic diabetic nephropathy; principle as for reagent strip test but will detect as low as 4-8 mg albumin/dL.
Blood	Microscopic examination	If microscopic analysis shows more than two red blood cells per high-power field and reagent strip is negative, test for presence of ascorbic acid or otherwise account for discrepancy.
Hemoglobin, myoglobin	Centrifugation; then test supernatant with reagent strip test for blood	Separate hemoglobin from myoglobin by urine and plasma appearance, total serum creatine kinase (CK), total serum lactate dehydrogenase (LDH), and LDH isoenzymes.
Hemosiderin	Rous test	Based on positive Prussian blue reaction of hemosiderin with potassium ferrocyanide.
Glucose and other reducing substances	Clinitest (Bayer)	Tests for reducing substances in addition to glucose, based on reduction of copper II to copper I in presence of heat and alkali.
		Detects glucose, galactose, lactose, fructose, and pentose (L-xylulose) but not sucrose.
		False-positive results may be seen with large quantities of ascorbic acid, salicylates, and large quantities of some penicillins.
		Used routinely for pediatric specimens (<1 year old) to detect nonglucose reducing sugars.
Carbohydrates	Thin-layer chromatography	Common tests are for fructose, sucrose, dextrose, lactose, xylose, galactose, and arabinose, because these are sugars most often found in urine.
Salicylates	Ferric chloride test	Rapid (spot) test for salicylate poisoning; also detects very large amounts of acetoacetic acid.
Bilirubin	Ictotest (Bayer)	Used when very small amounts of bilirubin are suspected, because test more sensitive than reagent strip test; based on diazo reaction.
Urobilinogen, porphobilinogen	Watson-Schwartz test	This is Ehrlich aldehyde reaction.
		Will differentiate urobilinogen, porphobilinogen, and intermediate Ehrlich-reacting substances if Bayer reagent strip shows more than 1 Ehrlich unit.
Porphobilinogen	Hoesch test	Specific for porphobilinogen; based on inverse Ehrlich reaction.
Ascorbic acid	EM Quant (Merckoquant)	Use when interference is suspected from any of reagent strip tests that depend on presence of hydrogen peroxide; reagent strip tests for blood are especially susceptible.

NOTE: Some of the listed procedures are no longer performed in the United States.

vaginal contamination will result in the presence of epithelial cells, red cells, and white cells. In such cases it may be necessary to use a clean-voided midstream specimen, which is also required for quantitative urine culture. It may also be necessary to pack the vagina or use a tampon in some cases to avoid vaginal and menstrual contamination.

Normal Sediment

Normally, urine contains little or no sediment, reflecting that normal urine is clear. However, a few constituents may be seen in any urine specimen. These generally consist of a very few RBCs, WBCs, hyaline casts, epithelial cells, and crystals.

TABLE 14-8

Reference Values for Urine Sediment	
Constituent	Reference Value
Red blood cells	0-2/hpf
White blood cells	0-5/hpf (female > male)
Casts	0-2 hyaline/lpf identify with hpf
Squamous epithelial cells	Few/lpf
Transitional epithelial cells	Few/hpf
Renal tubular epithelial cells	Few/hpf
Bacteria	Negative
Yeast	Negative
Abnormal crystals	Negative
Sperm (males only)	Present

hpf, High-power field; *lpf,* low-power field.

Each laboratory must establish its own reference values for normal urine on the basis of methodology and patient population. The reference values in Table 14-8 are typical of what might be encountered in "normal" urine.

Techniques for Examination of Urine Sediment

The urine sediment consists of a great variety of material. Some constituents are normal, whereas others are abnormal and represent serious conditions. It is important to learn to identify both the normal and abnormal constituents. In general, normal constituents are more easily seen under the microscope and must be recognized so they do not obscure the presence of the less obvious but more serious abnormal constituents. Recognition of abnormal constituents is extremely important in the diagnosis and treatment of various renal diseases. They often provide information about the state of the kidney and urinary tract. In addition, microscopic analysis of the sediment will help confirm and account for findings in the chemical examination of urine. For example, protein in the urine is often associated with the presence of casts and cellular elements in the sediment.

Traditionally, the urine sediment has been examined microscopically by placing a drop of urine on a microscope slide, applying a coverglass, and observing the preparation under the low-power (10×) and high-power (40×) objectives of a brightfield microscope. The CLSI recommends using a standardized method (see Procedure 14-3).

Because the preparation is a wet mount, oil immersion cannot be used in this examination.

The brightfield examination of unstained sediment is difficult, and various microscopic techniques, such as phase-contrast and polarizing microscopy, have been developed to aid in the identification of the various entities that might be present in the urine sediment. Other useful techniques in the examination of the urine sediment may include the use of stains and cytocentrifugation.

Microscopic Techniques

BRIGHTFIELD MICROSCOPY

Using the brightfield microscope is the traditional method of observation of the urine sediment and the most difficult. When the sediment is examined with brightfield illumination, correct light adjustment is essential. To give contrast between the unstained structures and the background liquid, the light must be sufficiently reduced by correct positioning of the condenser and use of the iris diaphragm. As described in Chapter 5, the condenser should be left in a generally uppermost position (at most only 1 or 2 mm below the specimen) and the desired contrast achieved by opening or closing the iris diaphragm. The condenser should not be "racked down." The correct light adjustment requires care and experience. Correct light adjustment is essential, and various translucent elements that may occur in the urine sediment are easily overlooked with this technique. Of particular difficulty are hyaline casts, mucous threads, and various cells (e.g., red cells) that have lost their hemoglobin content.

If only a brightfield microscope is available, the use of a suitable stain is encouraged. Phase-contrast microscopy is helpful, and a combination of phase-contrast and brightfield microscopy is recommended. The hemoglobin pigment present in blood casts and RBC casts is more apparent with brightfield illumination, as are certain cellular details and the presence of highly refractile fat (free and in cells or casts). Most crystals are more easily visualized with brightfield or brightfield and polarizing microscopy.

PHASE-CONTRAST MICROSCOPY

Phase-contrast microscopy is useful in the examination of unstained urine sediment, particularly for delineating translucent elements such as hyaline casts and mucous threads, which have a refractive index similar to that of the urine in which they are suspended. Some laboratories use a phase-contrast microscope for the routine examination of the urine sediment. However, some elements are better visualized with brightfield, and the microscopist must be able to change from phase to brightfield with ease.

PLANE-POLARIZING MICROSCOPY

Polarized light microscopy provides information on absorption color and differing refractive indices obtainable in brightfield microscopy, as well as optical properties of substances such as crystals. Crystal identification is of value in the examination of urine sediment as well as body fluids, including joint fluids.

Laboratory Procedure

Procedure 14-3 uses a 12:1 concentration of the urine specimen and employs parts of the KOVA system. Well-mixed urine is measured and centrifuged in a special graduated centrifuge (KOVA) tube. The urine is decanted, and exactly 1 mL is retained for microscopic examination by using a special disposable pipette with a built-in plastic disk (KOVA Petter). Results are reported according to the system in Table 14-9. Directions are included for both standardized slides and traditional glass microscope slides with coverglasses, using both unstained and stained sediment. If a phase-contrast microscope is used, staining is generally unnecessary, but if only a brightfield microscope is used, staining is recommended.

Specimen Preparation (Concentration)

When the urine sediment is to be examined, a concentrated portion of the urine is used. The sediment is concentrated before examination to ensure detection of less abundant constituents. To concentrate the sediment, a well-mixed measured portion of urine is centrifuged. The clear supernatant is decanted, and the solid material, which settles to the bottom during centrifugation, is examined under the microscope. (The supernatant may be further tested for chemical constituents, such as urine protein.) The various parts of the sediment are identified and enumerated to give semiquantitative results. For these results to have any meaning, a constant amount of urine must be centrifuged and a constant volume of supernatant removed.

Standardization

Various aids to standardization of the preparation and examination of the urine sediment are available. Complete systems or portions of systems may be used by a given a laboratory. Complete systems include specially designed, graduated centrifuge tubes with devices or pipettes that allow for the easy decanting of the supernatant urine and retention of an exact volume of undisturbed concentrated urine sediment. Systems differ in the final volume of urine sediment, although they generally begin by centrifuging 12 mL of well-mixed urine.

Traditionally, sediment was examined by placing a drop of concentrated sediment on a glass microscope slide and applying a coverglass. However, the size of the drop varied (it was generally not a measured drop), and results varied depending on the size of the coverglass used. Standardized systems employ specially designed slides of acrylic plastics with wells or applied coverglasses. They differ in the number of tests per slide, slide chamber volume (depth and surface area), availability of graded slides, and type of coverglass material (plastic or glass).

CLSI recommends the use of commercial standardized systems to ensure comparison between laboratories and consistency within laboratories.[1] According to CLSI guidelines, the following factors must be standardized, regardless of whether a standardized system is used:

1. *Urine volume.* Standardized systems use 12 mL. Volumes of 10 and 15 mL are also used. The final concentration of sediment should be reported with results.

2. *Time of centrifugation.* Five minutes is recommended.

3. *Speed of centrifugation.* CLSI recommends a relative centrifugal force (RCF) of 400 g. Others recommend 450 g or 400 to 450 g. Normograms can be used to relate the revolutions per minute (rpm) to RCF by measuring the radius of the centrifuge head in centimeters from the center pin to the bottom of a horizontal cup, using the following formula:

$$RCF\,(g) = 11.8 \times 10^{-6} \times Radius\,(cm) \times rpm^2$$

4. *Concentration factor of the sediment.* This is based on the volume of urine centrifuged and the final volume of sediment remaining after the supernatant urine is removed. Standardized systems facilitate retention of a specific volume of urine sediment.

5. *Volume of sediment examined.* Standardized slides contain chambers that hold a specific volume of concentrated sediment. With a traditional slide and coverglass, the volume of concentrated sediment placed on the glass slide should be measured; 20 μL is typically used. The volume examined may be calculated based on the volume of sediment placed on the slide, size (area) of the coverglass, diameter of the microscope objective, and concentration of urine sediment used.

6. *Reporting format.* Every person in an institution who performs a microscopic examination of the urine sediment should use the same terminology, reporting format, and reference ranges.

Microscopic Examination of the Urine Sediment

GENERAL PROCEDURE

1. Pour exactly 12 mL of well-mixed urine into a labeled, graduated centrifuge (KOVA) tube.
   a. If less than 12 mL is available, use 3 mL.
   b. If less than 3 mL is available, examine the sediment without concentration. State this information on the report.
2. Centrifuge at a relative centrifugal force of 450 for 5 minutes. Let the centrifuge come to a stop without using the brake. Use of the brake will cause resuspension of the sediment and falsely low results.
3. Decant 11 mL of clear supernatant urine into a test tube, leaving 1 mL of sediment in the KOVA tube.
   a. Insert the KOVA Petter into the centrifuge tube. Push it to the bottom of the tube until it is firmly seated. Holding the Petter in place, decant the supernatant urine. This will leave exactly 1 mL of sediment in the bottom of the tube.
   b. If a 3-mL specimen is used, do not use a KOVA Petter. Decant all liquid quickly, retaining a small drop in which to resuspend the sediment. This is approximately equivalent to a 12:1 concentration.
   c. If a KOVA Petter is not available, pour off 11 mL of supernatant urine in one even motion so as not to resuspend the sediment. Use a disposable pipette to bring the volume of sediment to exactly 1 mL with the clear supernatant urine. Removal of more than 11 mL and readjustment to 1 mL are preferable to removal of less than 11 mL.
4. If using a brightfield microscope, use supravital staining. Add 1 or 2 drops of stain to the sediment and mix thoroughly. If the amount of original specimen is limited, or if the urine is very alkaline, split the concentrated sediment and stain only one portion.
5. Thoroughly resuspend the sediment by gently squeezing the KOVA Petter.
6. Add the resuspended sediment to a standardized microscope slide, following the manufacturer's directions.
   - If traditional glass slides and coverglasses are used, place 20 mL (measured volume) of resuspended sediment on a glass microscope slide and cover with a 22 × 22 mm coverglass. The size of the drop and the size of the coverglass are important. The fluid should completely fill the area under the coverglass without overflowing the area or causing the coverglass to float. Take care that no bubbles appear when placing the coverglass over the sediment. If bubbles appear, a new preparation must be made on a clean slide. Bubbles are confusing and make enumeration impossible because they prevent random distribution of the substances to be counted.
7. Place the preparation on the microscope stage, and focus. Adjust the light, using the low-power objective, by carefully positioning the condenser and iris diaphragm. The tendency is to have too much light, but the light must not be overly reduced. Be sure that the sediment itself is brought into focus, rather than the coverglass. It is easier to achieve focus with specimens that are stained. Finally, vary the fine adjustment continuously to maintain focus.
8. Be systematic in the examination. With standardized slides, scan the entire preparation. With traditional microscope slides and coverglasses, begin by looking around the four sides of the coverglass, then the center. First, look for the substances that are identified and graded under low power. Change to high power, refocus and readjust the light, and search for the substances that are identified and graded under high power. All gradings are based on the average number of structures seen in a minimum of 10 microscope fields. Describe separately the structures searched for under low power and high power. Casts and cells are most important; look for these most carefully, observing the less important crystals and miscellaneous structures almost in retrospect.

Low-Power Examination

With the low-power (×10) objective, search for the following:
   a. Casts. With standardized slides, scan the entire area for the presence of casts. With traditional slides, look for casts around all four edges of the preparation, then in the center, because casts tend to roll to the edges of the coverglass.

Continued on following page

PROCEDURE **14-3** (Continued)

- When a cast is discovered, change to high power to identify it.
- Grade and report casts on the basis of the average number seen per low-power field, as shown in Table 14-9. If more than one type of cast is found in a single specimen, identify and grade each type separately.
  b. Crystals and amorphous material. Look for these structures in the same way as for casts.
  - Normal crystals are reported as few, moderate, or many per high-power field, if present. However, crystals may be more apparent under low power.
  - Abnormal crystals are graded as the average number seen per low-power field, when present (see Table 14-9). Abnormal crystals must be confirmed by chemical test or clinical history before they are reported.
  - Crystals are generally identified by shape rather than size. Therefore a combination of low-power and high-power observation is necessary in the detection and identification.
  c. Squamous epithelial cells. When these are present, report as few, moderate, or many per low-power field.
  d. Mucus (mucous threads). These are reported as present when easily seen or prominent under low power. They are more apparent with phase-contrast microscopy.

High-Power Examination

With high-power (×40) objective, search for the following:
  a. Red blood cells. Grade and report based on the average number seen per high-power field (see Table 14-9). Report the presence of unusual forms, such as dysmorphic red cells, if encountered.
  b. White blood cells. Grade and report based on the average number seen per high-power field (see Table 14-9). These are usually neutrophils (PMNs). If unusual cell types, such as lymphocytes or eosinophils, are morphologically identifiable, report this finding.
  c. Normal crystals. Identify and report as few, moderate, or many per high-power field for each type of crystal encountered.
  d. Casts. Identify with high power, but grade under low power.
  e. Epithelial cells: renal tubular, oval fat bodies (renal tubular cells with fat), and transitional. When these are present, estimate and report as few, moderate, or many per high-power field.
  f. Miscellaneous. This category includes various cell forms and other structures that may be encountered in the urine sediment, such as yeast, bacteria, trichomonads, and fat globules. When these are present, identify the cell or structure and report as few, moderate, or many per high-power field. Report sperm as present in males only. It is considered a contaminant in routine urinalysis specimens from females and is not reported.

Representative Grading Scale for Microscopic Structures	
Structure	Quantitation Representative Numerical Range
RBCs/hpf	0-5, 5-10, 10-25, 25-50, 50-100, >100 (too numerous to count), with or without clumps
WBCs/hpf	0-5, 5-10, 10-25, 25-50, 50-100, >100 (too numerous to count), with or without clumps
Epithelial cells/lpf	Specify type 0-5 (rare), 5-20 = few, 25-100 = moderate, >100 = many
Casts/lpf	Specify type (hyaline, granular, etc.) 0-5, 5-10, >10
Crystals/hpf	Specify type 0-5 (rare), 5-10 (moderate), >20 (many)
Bacteria/lpf	Rare, few, many

NOTE: Quantitate an average of 10 representative fields. Do not quantitate trichomonads, sperm, budding yeast, or mucus, but note their presence on the report. *hpf,* High-power field; *lpf,* low-power field.

CONSTITUENTS OF URINE SEDIMENT

In general, the constituents of the urine sediment are either biological or chemical. The biological part, also called the **organized sediment,** includes RBCs (erythrocytes), WBCs (leukocytes), epithelial cells, fat of biological origin, casts, bacteria, yeast, fungi, parasites, and spermatozoa. (Casts are long cylindrical structures that result from the solidification of material within the lumen of the kidney tubules.) The biological portion is the more

TABLE 14-9

Reporting System for Normal Urine Sediment	
Average Number per Low-Power Field	
Casts (identify with high power)	Negative
Abnormal crystals	Negative
Squamous epithelial cells	
Mucus (if prominent)	
Average Number per High-Power Field	
Red blood cells	0-2
White blood cells	0-2
Normal crystals	Few
Epithelial cells (renal, oval fat bodies, transitional)	Few
Miscellaneous (bacteria, yeast, *Trichomonas*, free fat)	Few
Sperm (males only)	Present

Few, Some cells are present; *Moderate*, easily seen; *Many*, prominent.
Magnification low-power objective (10×) × 10× ocular = 100×.
Magnification high-power (40×) objective × 10× ocular = 400×.

important part of the sediment; the cells and casts are of primary importance but are also the most difficult to detect.

The chemical portion, also called **unorganized sediment,** consists of crystals of chemicals and amorphous material. In general, it is less important than the biological portion. However, some abnormal crystals have pathologic significance. In addition, the constituents of the crystalline or chemical portion are sometimes so numerous that they tend to obscure the more important parts, which must be searched for with great care.

Cellular Constituents

Red Blood Cells (Erythrocytes)

CLINICAL IMPORTANCE

A few RBCs are present in the urine of normal persons. The number varies, but generally five or fewer per high-power field (≤5/hpf) in the concentrated sediment is considered "normal."[2] As discussed earlier, the condition in which RBCs are found in the urine is termed *hematuria*. The degree of hematuria may vary from a frankly bloody specimen on gross examination to a specimen that shows no change in color. Hematuria may be the result of bleeding at any point along the urogenital tract and may be seen with almost any disease of the urinary tract, including

renal disease or dysfunction, infection, tumor or lesions, stone formation, and generalized bleeding disorders, or it may result from anticoagulant usage. Hematuria is a sensitive early indicator of renal disease.

To determine the cause of hematuria, it is necessary to determine the site of bleeding. This involves various types of information, both laboratory and clinical. Part of this information will depend on other findings in the microscopic examination and other portions of the routine urinalysis. For example, bleeding through the glomerulus will often be accompanied by RBC casts, as seen in acute glomerulonephritis or disease of the glomerulus. This is an extremely serious situation, and RBC casts must be looked for carefully when erythrocytes are found. There may be little correlation between the amount of blood and the severity of the disorder, but the hematuria may be the only indication of renal disease. The occurrence of hematuria without accompanying protein and casts usually indicates that the bleeding is in the lower urogenital tract.

MICROSCOPIC APPEARANCE

Red cells are not easy to find under the microscope. Their detection requires careful examination. The high-power objective is used, and the light must be reduced by proper adjustment of the condenser and iris diaphragm, or the RBCs will be missed. Their detection also requires continual refocusing with the fine adjustment of the microscope. The phase-contrast microscope is very useful in detecting RBCs. Even after hemolysis has occurred, the erythrocyte membrane is clearly visible with this technique.

In absolutely fresh urine, RBCs will be unaltered or intact and appear much as they do in diluted whole blood. They are seen as pale, yellowish orange, intact biconcave disks that are especially apparent as they roll over. Red cells have a generally smooth appearance, as opposed to the granular appearance of white cells, and are about 7 μm in diameter (Fig. 14-6, *A*). However, RBCs rapidly undergo morphologic changes in urine specimens and are rarely observed as described. This is because urine is rarely an isotonic solution with RBCs (the solute concentration within the red cell is rarely the same as the solute concentration of urine). The urine may be more or less concentrated than the blood, and the changes described next will result.

When the urine is hypotonic or dilute, as evidenced by low specific gravity, the RBCs appear swollen and rounded because of diffusion of fluid into them. If the urine is hypertonic or concentrated (high specific gravity), the RBCs appear **crenated** (see Fig. 14-6, *B*) and shrunken because

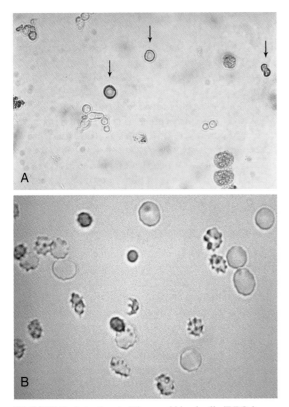

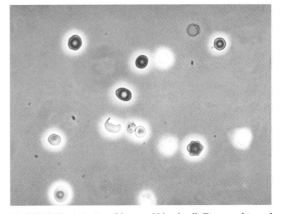

FIGURE 14-7   Ghost red blood cell. Dysmorphic and crenated RBCs. A single ghost RBC is located at top of view. (Phase contrast, ×400.) (From Brunzel NA: Fundamentals of urine and body fluid analysis, ed 2, Philadelphia, 2004, Saunders.)

FIGURE 14-6   A, Three red blood cells (RBCs): two viewed from above appear as biconcave disks, and one viewed from the side appears hourglass shaped *(arrows)*. Also present are budding yeast and several white blood cells. (Brightfield, sedistain, ×400.) B, Crenated RBCs. RBCs in hypertonic urine (concentrated, high specific gravity). Many cells in this field of view have lost their typical biconcave shape and are crenated. (From Brunzel NA: Fundamentals of urine and body fluid analysis, ed 2, Philadelphia, 2004, Saunders.)

they lose fluid to the urine. When crenated, the RBCs have little spicules, or projections, that cause them to be confused with WBCs. However, a crenated RBC is significantly smaller than a WBC and has a generally smooth, rather than granular, appearance. Also, when the urine is dilute and alkaline, the RBCs will often appear as shadow cells or ghost cells. In this situation the RBCs have burst and released their hemoglobin; all that remains is the faint colorless cell membrane, a "ghost" or "shadow" of the original cell. This membrane is clearly visible with phase-contrast illumination. Ghost cells are often seen in old urine specimens. Eventually, even the ghosts will disappear as the cell completely disintegrates (Fig. 14-7).

Dysmorphic RBCs may also be seen. These distorted or misshapen RBCs may indicate the presence of glomerular disease. The distortion is best seen with phase-contrast illumination. It is also possible to see nucleated RBCs or sickle

cells (in sickle cell disease) in urine, but this is extremely rare.

STRUCTURES CONFUSED WITH RED CELLS

Red cells not only are difficult to detect in a urine specimen but also are often confused with other structures found in urinary sediment.

Red cells are often confused with white cells (leukocytes), but the leukocyte is larger and has a generally granular appearance plus a nucleus. If morphologic differentiation is impossible, a drop of 2% acetic acid may be added to a new preparation or introduced under the coverglass. Acetic acid will lyse the RBCs and at the same time stain (or accentuate) the nuclei of leukocytes. With a Sternheimer-Malbin stain, RBCs in acidic urine may stain slightly purple or not at all. If the urine is alkaline, the alkaline hematin that is formed stains dark purple. The reagent strip tests for blood and leukocyte esterase are also helpful.

Yeast may also be confused with RBCs in urine, but yeast cells are generally smaller than RBCs, are spherical rather than flattened, and vary considerably in size within one specimen. In addition, because yeast reproduces by budding, the occurrence of buds or little outgrowths should identify yeast.

A very rare ovoid form of *calcium oxalate* may also be confused with RBCs, especially when viewed with brightfield illumination. However, calcium oxalate crystals are more refractile and, unlike red cells, polarize light. Thus they are easily differentiated with polarizing microscopy.

Bubbles or *oil droplets* are also confused with RBCs, especially by the inexperienced viewer. These vary considerably in size, are extremely refractive or reflective, and are obvious under the microscope.

OTHER CONSIDERATIONS

The presence of RBCs may be indicated by a tiny red button in the bottom of the centrifuge tube after centrifuging.

Red cells in the sediment should correlate with a positive reagent strip test for blood. Because chemical tests are more sensitive to hemoglobin than to intact RBCs, however, it is possible to have a negative reagent strip test when only a few intact red cells are present and no hemolysis has occurred. This is rare. Reagent strip sensitivity is reduced in urine with high specific gravity; the RBC must lyse in order to react. In this situation, RBCs may be demonstrated by adding water to the sediment to lyse cells, then retesting with the reagent test for blood.

When large amounts of vitamin C are present, reagent strip results may be negative or delayed even though RBCs are seen in the sediment. In such cases the sediment result can be confirmed by the use of a reagent strip test for ascorbic acid. Another clue would be the gross appearance of the urine sediment or a red button of cells in the bottom of the centrifuge tube.

If the reagent strip test for blood is positive and RBCs are absent in the urine sediment, the presence of hemoglobin or myoglobin in the urine should be considered.

White Blood Cells (Leukocytes)

CLINICAL IMPORTANCE

The presence of a few WBCs or leukocytes in the concentrated urine sediment is normal. Again, reference values vary, but more than a few (as many as five per high-power field) is considered abnormal. The term *white blood cell* or *leukocyte* in urine usually refers to the presence of a neutrophil (polymorphonuclear neutrophil, or PMN); unless otherwise specified, it is assumed that this is what is meant. However, any WBC type present in blood can also be found in the urine sediment. The presence of lymphocytes and eosinophils is of particular diagnostic significance, as described later.

The presence of large numbers of WBCs in the sediment indicates inflammation at some point along the urogenital tract. The inflammation may result from a bacterial infection or other causes. The presence of WBCs is often associated with bacteria, but both bacteria and white cells can be present alone, without the other. In bacterial infections, ingested bacteria may be seen within the cell. These cells are extremely labile and rapidly disappear from the specimen. If the leukocytes originate in the kidney, rather than lower in the urinary tract (e.g., in the bladder),

they may form cellular casts. Therefore, the presence of casts (usually cellular or granular) along with WBCs and bacteria would help distinguish an upper (kidney) from a lower (bladder) UTI. Protein is usually present along with casts, and it may or may not be present in a lower UTI. The condition in which increased numbers of leukocytes are found in urine is termed **pyuria.** Pyuria may cause clouding of the urine, and when this is severe enough, the urine will have a characteristic milk-white appearance. Under the microscope, the WBCs may appear singly or in clumps. The presence of clumps is associated with acute infection.

MICROSCOPIC APPEARANCE

Leukocytes must be searched for with the high-power objective, reduced light, and continual refocusing with fine adjustment. Typically, WBCs are about 10 to 14 µm in diameter, about twice the size of RBCs; however, this size difference may not be obvious, and WBCs often appear about the same size as RBCs. Leukocytes have thin cytoplasmic granulation and a nucleus. Even if the nucleus is not distinct, the center of the cell appears granular (Fig. 14-8). White cells are fragile and will disintegrate in old alkaline urine specimens. Various stages of disintegration may be observed in a single urine specimen. Neutrophil leukocytes are especially vulnerable in dilute alkaline urine specimens, and about 50% can be lost within 2 to 3 hours if the urine is kept at room temperature. In addition, the lobed nucleus tends to consolidate, and the neutrophil appears as a mononuclear cell as the cell begins to degenerate. If the urine is dilute, the cell cytoplasm may expand out in petals, without granules, before the neutrophil disintegrates.

Phase-contrast microscopy is especially useful in the detection and identification of WBCs in the urine sediment (Fig. 14-9), as is the use of a stain such as the Sternheimer-Malbin stain (Fig. 14-10). However, precipitation of the stain in the highly alkaline urines associated with WBCs and bacteria may pose a problem. When stained, neutrophilic leukocytes show a red-purple nucleus and violet or blue cytoplasm, although the same urine specimen may have a variety of staining reactions, and extremely fresh cells may fail to stain.

STRUCTURES CONFUSED WITH WHITE CELLS

Other structures may be mistaken for leukocytes. Most often this occurs with RBCs and epithelial cells. White cells are generally larger than red cells, appear granular, and have a nucleus. A 2% acetic acid solution may aid in the identification of WBCs

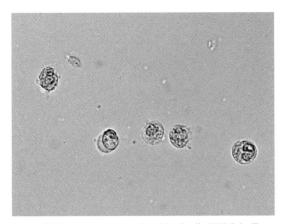

FIGURE 14-8 **Five white blood cells (WBCs).** (From Brunzel NA: Fundamentals of urine and body fluid analysis, ed 2, Philadelphia, 2004, Saunders.)

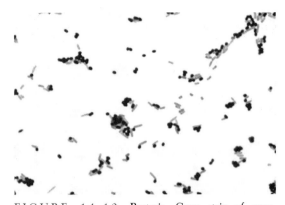

FIGURE 14-10 **Bacteria. Gram stain of gram-negative rods and gram-positive cocci. (Brightfield, ×1000.)** (From Brunzel NA: Fundamentals of urine and body fluid analysis, ed 2, Philadelphia, 2004, Saunders.)

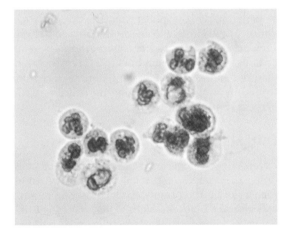

FIGURE 14-9 **Leukocytes (WBCs) stained with 0.5% toluidine blue. (Brightfield, ×400.)** (From Brunzel NA: Fundamentals of urine and body fluid analysis, ed 2, Philadelphia, 2004, Saunders.)

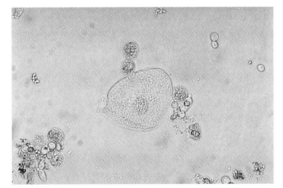

FIGURE 14-11 **Several WBCs with characteristic cytoplasmic granules and lobed nuclei surrounding a squamous epithelial cell. Budding yeast cells are also present. (Brightfield, sedistain, ×400.)** (From Brunzel NA: Fundamentals of urine and body fluid analysis, ed 2, Philadelphia, 2004, Saunders.)

(Figs. 14-11 and 14-12). There are several different morphologic types of epithelial cells, but in general they are larger than WBCs and have smaller nuclei. Renal epithelial cells are most like white cells; however, the nucleus is generally round, more distinct, and surrounded by more cytoplasm (Fig. 14-13).

OTHER LEUKOCYTES IN SEDIMENT

Other WBC cell types that may be seen in the urine sediment include the following.

Glitter Cells

Glitter cells are larger, swollen neutrophilic leukocytes that appear in hypotonic urine with a specific gravity of about 1.010 or less. Their cytoplasmic granules are in constant random (brownian) movement, giving a glittering appearance.

These cells are especially striking under phase-contrast illumination. When stained, glitter cells have a light-blue or almost colorless cytoplasm, and the brownian motion of the granules may or may not be observed. Once thought to indicate chronic pyelonephritis, glitter cells are also seen in dilute urine specimens from patients with lower UTIs.

Eosinophils

Eosinophils may be present in the urine sediment. They are morphologically similar to neutrophils and difficult to distinguish, especially with a wet preparation, under both brightfield and phase-contrast illumination. Eosinophils are typically larger than neutrophils and oval or elongated. The cytoplasmic granules may not be prominent, but the presence of two or three distinct lobes of the nucleus with fresh specimens is

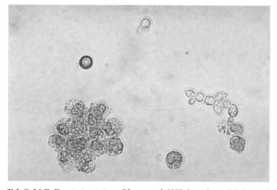

FIGURE 14-12 Clump of WBCs. One RBC and budding yeast are also present. (Brightfield, sedistain, ×400.) (From Brunzel NA: Fundamentals of urine and body fluid analysis, ed 2, Philadelphia, 2004, Saunders.)

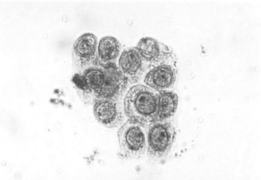

FIGURE 14-13 Fragment of renal collecting duct epithelial cells stained with 0.5% toluidine blue. (Brightfield, ×400.) (From Brunzel NA: Fundamentals of urine and body fluid analysis, ed 2, Philadelphia, 2004, Saunders.)

helpful. Cytocentrifugation is useful in confirming the presence of eosinophils. However, they do not stain as well with Wright stain as they do in blood smears. Use of special eosinophil stains, such as **Hansel stain,** is helpful. Increased eosinophils are associated with drug-induced interstitial nephritis, as seen with treatment with penicillins. Detection is important because the treatment is fast and effective (i.e., discontinuation of the drug).

Lymphocytes and Other Mononuclear Cells

A few small lymphocytes are normally present in urine, even though they are rarely recognized. They are difficult to distinguish from RBCs, especially with the normal wet preparation of the urine sediment, under both brightfield and phase-contrast illumination. These lymphocytes are only slightly larger than RBCs, with a single round nucleus and scant cytoplasm. The presence of many small lymphocytes is seen in the first few weeks after renal transplant rejection and is a useful early indicator of this rejection process. If their presence is suspected, identification of lymphocytes is most easily confirmed by cytocentrifugation and staining with Wright stain. Because they are not granulocytes, lymphocytes will not react with the reagent strips for leukocyte esterase.

Monocytes, histiocytes, and macrophages may also be present in the urine sediment. They are difficult to recognize on the standard wet preparation but are generally larger than, and resemble, aging neutrophils. Their cytoplasm is usually abundant, vacuolated, and granulated. These cells are granulocytes and are capable of reacting with the reagent strips for leukocyte esterase. However, the sensitivity of the strips may not be sufficient to detect these cells, which, even when present, are seen in relatively small numbers. Monocytes and histiocytes are

associated with chronic inflammation and radiation therapy. Macrophages may be present with various inclusions within the cytoplasm. These include ingested fat, hemosiderin, RBCs, and crystals. As with lymphocytes, identification of other mononuclear cells is most easily confirmed by cytocentrifugation and staining with Wright stain.

Epithelial Cells

Except for the single layer of renal epithelial cells lining the tubules of the nephron, the structures that make up the urinary system are lined by several layers of epithelial cells. The layer of epithelial cells closest to the lumen of organs such as the urethra and bladder (besides contaminating cells of the male and female genital tracts) is continually sloughed off **(exfoliated)** into the urine and replaced by cells originating from deeper layers. Therefore a few squamous epithelial cells are seen in most urine specimens. The single-layered renal epithelial cells are also sloughed into the urine. The identification of the various epithelial cell types may be difficult yet clinically significant. They include squamous, transitional (urothelial), and renal epithelial cells.

Squamous Epithelial Cells

Squamous epithelial cells line the urethra and bladder trigone in the female and the distal portion of the male urethra. They also line the vagina, and many of the squamous epithelial cells found in urine are the result of perineal or vaginal contamination in females or foreskin contamination in males. They are the most frequently encountered and the least significant type of epithelial cell in urine specimens. Squamous epithelial cells can be divided into intermediate and superficial squamous

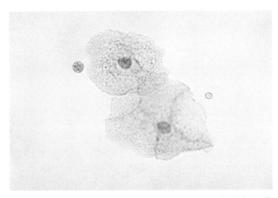

FIGURE 14-14 Two squamous epithelial cells stained using Sternheimer-Malbin stain. (Brightfield, ×100.) (From Brunzel NA: Fundamentals of urine and body fluid analysis, ed 2, Philadelphia, 2004, Saunders.)

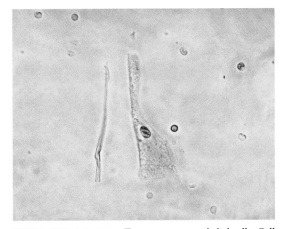

FIGURE 14-16 Two squamous epithelial cells. Cell on the left is presenting a side view, demonstrating flatness of these cells. (Brightfield, sedistain, ×200.) (From Brunzel NA: Fundamentals of urine and body fluid analysis, ed 2, Philadelphia, 2004, Saunders.)

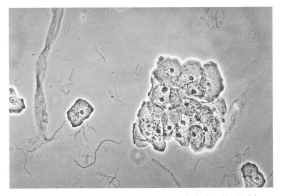

FIGURE 14-15 Squamous epithelial cells. Ribbon-like mucous threads are also present. (Phase contrast, ×100.) (From Brunzel NA: Fundamentals of urine and body fluid analysis, ed 2, Philadelphia, 2004, Saunders.)

cells. They form the most superficial layer of cells that line the mucosa and are continually sloughed off and replaced by newer, deeper cells.

Squamous epithelial cells are very large, flat cells that consist of a thin layer of cytoplasm and a single distinct nucleus (Figs. 14-14, 14-15, and 14-16). The nucleus is about the size of an RBC or lymphocyte, and the cell is about five to seven times the size of an RBC, about 30 to 50 μm. A thin flat cell, the squamous epithelial cell may be rectangular or round. Epithelial cells are large enough to be seen easily under low power and sometimes roll into cigar shapes, which are mistaken for casts. When stained, these cells show a purple nucleus and an abundant pink or violet cytoplasm. They are easily recognized until they begin to degenerate, when they may eventually appear as an amorphous mass.

The presence of squamous epithelial cells is of little clinical significance unless they are in large numbers. When the urine is contaminated by vaginal secretions or exudates, sheets of squamous epithelial cells accompanied by many rod-shaped bacteria or yeasts, or both, may be seen.

CLUE CELLS

Another type of squamous epithelial cell that might be encountered in the urine is of vaginal origin and is referred to as a clue cell. **Clue cells** are vaginal squamous epithelial cells that are covered or encrusted with a bacterium, *Gardnerella vaginalis*. They are usually searched for in wet mounts of vaginal swabs, and their presence indicates bacterial vaginitis caused by *Gardnerella*. Clue cells are coccobacilli and give the cytoplasm a characteristic refractile, stippled, or granular appearance with shaggy or bearded cell borders. Most of the cell surface should be covered with bacteria, and the bacteria should extend beyond the cytoplasmic margins, in order for the cell to be called a clue cell. The occasional keratohyaline granules in the cytoplasm of squamous epithelial cells should not be mistaken for clue cells.

Transitional Epithelial (Urothelial) Cells

Transitional epithelial cells occur in multiple layers. They line the urinary tract, from the kidney pelvis in both females and males to the base of the bladder in the female and the proximal part of the urethra in the male. As the cell layers become deeper, the cells become thicker and rounded, increasingly resembling renal epithelial cells or WBCs. Their size varies with the depth and place of origin in the transitional epithelium. In general, however, transitional epithelial cells are about four to six times the size of an RBC (20 to 30 μm) and appear smaller and plumper than squamous epithelial cells. They are spherical or polyhedral in shape. Because they readily take on water, urothelial cells are often spherical from swelling, similar to a balloon of water. They are generally larger than renal

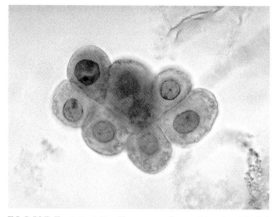

FIGURE 14-17 Fragment of transitional epithelial cells. (From Brunzel NA: Fundamentals of urine and body fluid analysis, ed 2, Philadelphia, 2004, Saunders.)

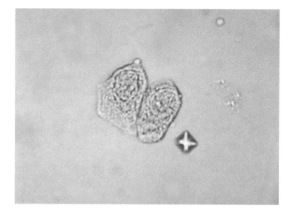

FIGURE 14-18 Two renal collecting duct cells stained with 0.5% toluidine blue. The polygonal shape and nuclear detail distinguish these cells from leukocytes. (Brightfield, ×400.) (From Brunzel NA: Fundamentals of urine and body fluid analysis, ed 2, Philadelphia, 2004, Saunders.)

tubular cells and have a round nucleus (sometimes two nuclei) similar in size and appearance to the nucleus seen in a squamous epithelial cell. The more superficial bladder epithelial cells are large, flat cells of a squamous nature. Transitional epithelial cells stain with a dark blue nucleus and varying amounts of pale blue cytoplasm, which may have occasional inclusions. Some of these cells have tails and are indistinguishable from the caudate cells of the renal pelvis.

A few transitional epithelial cells are present in the urine of normal persons. Increased numbers are seen in the presence of infection. Clusters or sheets of these cells are seen after urethral or ureteral catheterization and with urinary tract lesions. Urothelial cells may show malignant changes, and such cells should be referred for cytologic examination. Radiation therapy may result in large cells with multiple nuclei and vacuoles (Fig. 14-17).

Renal Epithelial Cells

Renal epithelial cells are the single layer of cells that line the nephron from the proximal to the distal convoluted tubules, plus the cells lining the collecting ducts to the pelvis of the kidney. Their occurrence in urine is important because it implies a serious pathologic condition and destruction of renal tubules, as does the presence of epithelial casts. Identification of renal epithelial cells is difficult in wet preparations with either brightfield or phase contrast. Morphology varies, depending on the site of origin within the nephron. Intact renal epithelial cells are from three to five times the size of RBCs—that is, slightly larger to twice as large as a neutrophil. Cells from the proximal convoluted tubules are relatively large and elongated or oval, with a granular cytoplasm. The granularity makes the proximal tubular cells, in particular, appear as

small or fragmented granular casts. The nucleus is extremely difficult to see in these renal epithelial cells in wet preparations. The use of cytocentrifugation and staining with Wright stain will help visualize the nucleus and show these structures to be cells rather than casts, but the traditional cytologic examination with the Papanicolaou (Pap) stain is recommended.

Renal epithelial cells resemble both WBCs and smaller transitional epithelial cells. Morphologically, they closely resemble leukocytes, especially degenerating WBCs, but they are typically larger and have a distinct single round nucleus (Fig. 14-18). Renal cells of the collecting tubules tend to be polyhedral or cuboid; one side tends to be flat, unlike the rounded cell more typical of transitional epithelial cells. (Unlike transitional epithelial cells, renal cells do not absorb water and swell; therefore they tend to retain their polyhedral shape.) When these cells are stained, the nucleus stains a dark shade of blue-purple and the cytoplasm a lighter shade of blue-purple. Cytocentrifugation and a Pap stain are helpful.

As with all epithelial cells, renal epithelial cells will not react with the leukocyte esterase reagent strips; this may be helpful in distinguishing them from neutrophils. Renal epithelial cells are associated with the presence of protein in the urine and are often found in association with casts. The presence of epithelial or granular casts will help confirm their identification, and when renal cells are suspected, casts should be sought with great care. The phase-contrast microscope is particularly useful in such situations.

RENAL EPITHELIAL FRAGMENTS

These fragments or groups of three or more renal epithelial cells originate from the collecting ducts. Their presence is more serious than the

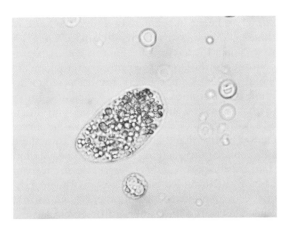

FIGURE 14-19 Oval fat body. A cell with numerous highly refractile fat globules and other inclusions. (Brightfield, ×400.) (From Brunzel NA: Fundamentals of urine and body fluid analysis, ed 2, Philadelphia, 2004, Saunders.)

presence of individual renal epithelial cells because they indicate renal tubular injury with disruption of the basement membrane.

OVAL FAT BODIES

A special type of renal epithelial cell is filled with fat (lipid) droplets. **Oval fat bodies (OFBs)** are sometimes referred to as **renal tubular fat (RTF)** or renal tubular fat bodies. They indicate serious pathology and must not be overlooked when present in the urine sediment. The fat droplets are generally contained within degenerating or necrotic renal epithelial cells, although some OFBs may be macrophages that have filled with fat. The fat droplets contained within these cells are highly refractive, coarse droplets that vary greatly in size (Fig. 14-19). OFBs are more easily visualized with brightfield than phase-contrast microscopy. Although they are cells filled with fat, the cell nucleus is usually invisible.

Certain aids to the identification of OFBs are available. When stained with Sternheimer-Malbin stain, fat globules do not become colored but appear highly refractive in a blue-purple background. When stained with fat stains such as Sudan III or oil red O, globules of triglyceride or neutral fat appear orange or red. Polarized light is useful for indicating the presence of cholesterol esters in the fat. Cholesterol esters show a typical Maltese cross pattern when viewed with polarizing filters. Triglycerides or neutral fat do not show this pattern with polarized light. The appearance of a Maltese cross pattern is also seen with starch, a common urine contaminant. Fat should be confirmed by careful microscopic examination or specific staining. OFBs are often seen along with fat droplets and fatty casts in the urine sediment, and the other two components should be searched for carefully when one is present.

OFBs resulting from tubular epithelial degeneration of the nephron are associated with large amounts of protein in the urine, as in the nephrotic syndrome. The fatty material in the tubular cells may be the lipoprotein that passes through the damaged glomerulus in this syndrome. The lipoprotein may be ingested by the renal tubular cell, which metabolizes it into cholesterol. Clinically, the presence of neutral fat (triglyceride) and the presence of cholesterol are equal.

FAT GLOBULES

Although not a cellular constituent, fat globules are discussed here because of their relationship to OFBs. Fat globules may be found in the urine sediment as highly refractive droplets of various sizes. When their source is biological (rather than contamination), a serious pathologic condition implying severe renal dysfunction exists. Such lipiduria is also associated with the nephrotic syndrome and its various causes, with diabetes mellitus, and with conditions that result in severe damage to renal tubular epithelial cells, such as ethylene glycol or mercury poisoning. Fat globules are found in association with OFBs and fatty casts. Fat stains orange or red with Sudan stains or oil red O. The identification may be aided by the use of polarized light; cholesterol will show a Maltese cross pattern. Fat in urine may also come from extraneous sources, such as unclean collection utensils or oiled catheters. This occurs less often with the use of disposable urine collection containers.

HEMOSIDERIN

Occasionally, renal epithelial cells with granules of hemosiderin in the cytoplasm are seen in the urine sediment. This occurs several days after a hemolytic episode, when free hemoglobin has passed through the glomerulus into the nephron. The hemosiderin granules appear as yellow or colorless granules that are morphologically similar to amorphous urates. Unlike urates, they will stain blue with a Prussian blue stain for iron (Rous test). Besides their presence in desquamated renal epithelial cells, granules of hemosiderin may be seen as free granules in the sediment, in macrophages, and in casts.

VIRAL INCLUSION BODIES

Renal tubular epithelial cells may also be seen with viral inclusion bodies. This is especially characteristic of infection with cytomegalovirus. Viral inclusion bodies are difficult to recognize on wet preparations. Cytocentrifugation and staining with Pap stain are helpful in recognizing this condition.

Casts

Formation and Significance

Casts are both the most difficult and the most important constituent of the urine sediment to discover. Their importance and their name derive from the manner in which they are produced. Casts are formed in the lumen of the tubules of the nephrons (working units of kidney) by solidification of material in the tubules. They are important because anything contained within the tubule is flushed out in the cast. Thus a cast represents a biopsy of an individual tubule and is a means of examining the contents of the nephron. It is believed that casts may be formed at any point along the nephron, either by precipitation of protein or by grouping together (conglutination) of material within the tubular lumen. In either case, the basic structure of the cast is a protein matrix. All casts have a matrix of Tamm-Horsfall mucoprotein; in addition, plasma proteins may be present.

Before casts can form within the renal tubules, certain conditions must exist. Because the cast is made of protein, there must be a sufficient concentration of protein within the tubule. In addition, the pH must be low enough to favor precipitation, and there must be a sufficient concentration of solutes. For the same reasons, casts are not likely to be found in dilute alkaline urine because such conditions do not favor cast formation. This also means that the urine must be examined when fresh; as urine becomes alkaline with aging, the casts will disintegrate.

Because casts represent a biopsy of the kidney, they are extremely important clinically. They often contain RBCs, WBCs, epithelial cells, fat globules, and bacteria. These inclusions are not normally present within the renal tubule; they represent an abnormal situation. The formation of casts implies that there was at least a temporary blocking of the renal tubules. Although a few hyaline casts consisting only of precipitated Tamm-Horsfall mucoprotein may be seen in "normal" urine, increased numbers of casts indicate renal disease rather than lower urinary tract disease. The number of hyaline casts may increase in mild irritations of the kidney associated with dehydration or physical exercise. The presence of other types of casts represents a serious (pathologic) situation.

Identification and Morphology

Casts are extremely difficult to see and must be searched for carefully with reduced light and the low-power objective. Casts are found and enumerated under low power but must be identified as to type by means of the high-power objective. The refractive index of the cast is almost the same as that of glass, which means that the image is difficult to see under the microscope. For this reason, phase-contrast and interference-contrast microscopy are useful in the examination of the urine sediment. Phase-contrast microscopy gives sufficient contrast so that structures are not overlooked, and differential interference microscopy provides an appreciation of the shape and inclusions within these structures. Stains such as the Sternheimer-Malbin stain are also particularly useful for the discovery of casts in the urine sediment. Casts that might otherwise be overlooked in brightfield examination, especially by the inexperienced observer, become obvious when so stained, although the presence of mucous strands in the sediment might be confusing, especially in searching for hyaline casts.

As might be imagined from the shape of the tubular lumen, casts are cylindrical bodies and have rounded ends. To be identified as a cast, a structure should have an even and definite outline, parallel sides, and two rounded ends. Although they vary somewhat in size, casts should have a uniform diameter (about seven or eight times the diameter of a red cell) and be several times longer than wide.

Although casts should have parallel sides and two rounded ends, this is not always the case. Casts take on the shape of the tubule in which they are formed. They may be serpentine or convoluted and are often folded. One end may taper off to a tail or point. Such structures have been referred to as **cylindroids,** but they should be considered to be, and enumerated along with, hyaline casts. Cylindroids are often confused with strands of mucus, and care must be taken to avoid this mistake. In addition, casts may be fragmented or broken, and waxy casts typically show blunt rather than rounded ends. Judgment is necessary in the enumeration of such structures. The whole urine sediment picture must be considered so that important pathologic findings are reported. Conversely, the occurrence of only one questionable cast, with no other pathologic indicators, should not be reported.

Classification of Casts

Classification of casts is not always simple. In the laboratory, classification is done mainly on the basis of morphologic groupings: hyaline, cellular, granular, waxy, fatty, pigmented, or inclusion. A urine specimen may contain more than one morphologic type, and a particular cast may be of mixed morphology; for example, one end may be hyaline and the other cellular.

Casts are believed to arise either by precipitation of protein within the renal tubule or by conglutination (clumping) of material within the tubular lumen. Both types of casts may contain inclusions.

Casts formed by protein precipitation may trap any other substance that may be present, including leukocytes, fat, bacteria, RBCs, desquamated renal tubular epithelium, and crystals. Casts formed by either mechanism may appear coarsely or finely granular or waxy as cells disintegrate when the cast is retained in the tubule before being flushed out of the kidney. Structures will also disintegrate if the urine specimen stands.

Again, casts have a protein matrix, and the presence of casts in the urine is almost always accompanied by proteinuria. Tamm-Horsfall protein, the specific mucoprotein secreted by the renal tubular cells, has been identified immunologically and found to be present in all casts. Other immunoproteins have been identified in certain casts, although they are not found exclusively in any particular type of cast or disease state.

The following morphologic classification is based on appearance, physical properties, and existence of cellular components. The appearance of a cast when seen in the urine may not be the same as when it was originally formed in the renal tubule. If the cast is retained in the kidney (as in oliguric patients), its cells change in appearance. As the cells degenerate in the cast, their cytoplasm becomes granular. This is followed by loss of cell membranes, resulting in large or coarse granules. As these granules degenerate further, the cast shows smaller or fine granules. The final step in this degeneration is complete lack of structure, with the protein changed or coagulated into a thick, very refractive, opaque substance with a waxlike appearance, referred to as a **waxy cast.** These are the most serious casts pathologically because the formation of the waxy material implies a greatly lengthened transit time or a shutdown of the portion of the kidney where the structure evolved. Such casts are sometimes referred to as *renal failure casts.*

The width or diameter of a cast is important clinically. Most casts have a fairly constant diameter, as do the tubules in which they are formed, although casts from small children are narrower than those from adults. Narrow casts probably result from swelling of the tubular epithelium, as in an inflammatory process, with narrowing of the tubular lumen. They are not particularly important and tend to be of a hyaline type. Broad casts are a much more serious finding. Their diameter is several times greater than normal, believed to result from their formation in dilated renal tubules or in collecting tubules. (Several nephrons empty into a common collecting tubule, which has a greater diameter than the renal tubule.) Severe chronic renal disease or obstruction (stasis) will often result in dilation and destruction of renal tubules. Cast formation in the collecting tubules must result from urinary stasis in the group of nephrons feeding

---

> **BOX 14-3**
> ## Morphologic Classification of Casts
>
> - Hyaline cast
> - Cellular cast
>   White blood cell (leukocyte, neutrophil, pus) cast
>   Red blood cell (blood, hemoglobin, hemoglobin pigment) cast
>   Epithelial cell cast
>   Bacterial cast
> - Granular cast
> - Waxy cast
> - Fatty cast
>   Oval fat body cast
> - Pigmented casts
>   Hemoglobin (blood) cast
>   Myoglobin cast
>   Bilirubin cast
>   Drug pigment cast
> - Inclusion casts
>   (Granular cast)
>   (Fatty cast)
>   Hemosiderin cast
>   Crystal cast

---

a single collecting tubule. If not, the fluid pressure would be much too great for cast formation to occur. This cast formation represents serious stasis, and the presence of a significant number of broad casts in the urine sediment is considered a poor prognostic sign. Broad casts can be of almost any type, but because of the degree of stasis necessary for their formation, most tend to be waxy.

The types of casts encountered in the microscopic analysis of the urine sediment are described next in a morphologic classification (Box 14-3).

Hyaline Casts

Hyaline casts are colorless, homogeneous, nonrefractive, semitransparent structures (Fig. 14-20). They are the most difficult casts to discover under the microscope and the least important clinically. They require careful adjustment of light with the brightfield microscope; the light is adjusted to give contrast by lowering the condenser slightly and closing the iris diaphragm. Phase-contrast and interference microscopy are especially valuable tools in the search for hyaline casts. Stain is also useful; hyaline casts stain a uniform pale pink or pale blue. However, they may take up a minimum of stain and remain difficult to visualize. Hyaline casts also may be difficult to distinguish from mucous threads when they are present in the urine, both when stained and when observed by phase-contrast microscopy.

Hyaline casts result from solidification of Tamm-Horsfall protein, which is secreted by the renal

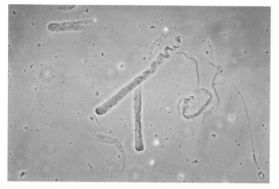

FIGURE 14-20 **Three hyaline casts. The cast with the tapered end is frequently called a *cylindroid*. (Phase contrast, ×100.)** (From Brunzel NA: Fundamentals of urine and body fluid analysis, ed 2, Philadelphia, 2004, Saunders.)

tubular cells and may be seen without significant proteinuria. They will include any material that may be present in the tubular lumen at the time of formation, such as cells or cellular debris.

Although hyaline casts are generally of the classic shape for identification as a cast (i.e., parallel sides, uniform diameter, definite borders, and rounded ends), interesting modifications, representing molds of the tubular lumen where they are formed, may be observed. Some hyaline casts are broad, whereas others are thin and elongated; serpentine and folded forms are not unusual. Cylindroids are hyaline casts with one end that has not rounded off; they have the same significance and should be enumerated and reported as hyaline casts.

Hyaline casts are soluble in water and even more soluble in slightly alkaline solution. They are therefore more likely to be found in concentrated, acidic urine and may not form in advanced renal failure because of the inability to concentrate the urine or maintain the normal acid pH. In addition, hyaline casts dissolve if the urine stands and becomes alkaline. Hyaline casts may be further classified, according to their inclusions, as hyaline cellular (red, white, or epithelial), hyaline granular, and hyaline fatty casts.

Simple hyaline casts are the least important clinically, and a few (less than two per low-power field) may be seen in urine from normal persons. They may be seen in increased numbers after strenuous exercise; however, the sediment returns to normal in 24 to 48 hours. Simple hyaline casts may be seen in large numbers (20 or 30 per low-power field) in moderate or severe renal disease.

Cellular Casts

Cellular casts contain intact WBCs, RBCs, or epithelial cells. They are called *white cell* (or *pus*) casts, *red cell* (or *blood*) casts, and *epithelial* casts. *Bacterial* casts have also been described. A truly cellular cast

appears to result from clumping, or conglutination, of cells rather than simply precipitation of protein and entrapment of cells, although they are still incorporated in a protein matrix. Alternatively, smaller numbers of the same cell types may be embedded in a hyaline cast.

Cellular casts indicate the presence of cells in the renal tubules. When this occurs, although there are a variety of causes and different degrees of severity, a serious situation exists.

It may be difficult if not impossible to distinguish the type of cell in a cast, especially when cells begin to deteriorate. In these situations the best indicator is probably the nature of other constituents in the urine sediment. Leukocytes and bacteria in the sediment would be associated with leukocyte (white cell) casts, whereas epithelial casts are more likely to be accompanied by cells appearing to be renal epithelium. Glitter cells are often seen when phagocytic neutrophils are present. When a morphologic distinction is impossible, the cast should be reported merely as a "cellular cast" rather than possibly misidentifying it. The clinician will use other findings in the urine specimen, both chemical and microscopic, to infer the cell type or source.

Cellular casts are more easily detected under the microscope than hyaline casts because the cells give them a definite structure compared with the homogeneous solidified protein of the hyaline cast. Cellular casts must still be sought with care, however, and proper illumination of the brightfield microscope is essential. Phase-contrast or interference microscopy and stains and cytocentrifugation are useful tools in the examination of the urine sediment for cellular casts.

WHITE BLOOD CELL CASTS

WBC casts are also referred to as *leukocyte casts*, or *pus casts*, when neutrophilic leukocytes are present. When leukocytes are present in a cast, it is obvious that the cells originated in the kidney. The leukocytes may enter the nephron from the blood by passing through the glomerulus into the glomerular capsule in glomerular diseases. More often, they probably enter the nephron from the blood by squeezing through the cells making up the renal tubules, often in response to a bacterial infection within the tubular interstitium. Such phagocytic neutrophils are typically seen in *pyelonephritis*, a renal infection of the interstitium. In such cases, leukocytes and bacteria are also present in the urine sediment. The presence of casts (particularly WBC casts), along with white cells and bacteria, is used to distinguish an upper from a lower UTI.

WBC casts are seen fairly easily in the urine sediment with the brightfield microscope (Fig. 14-21). The cells are fairly prominent, and the

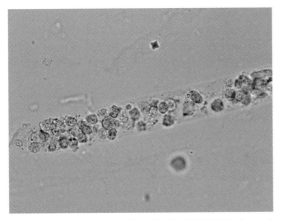

FIGURE 14-21 **White blood cell (WBC, leukocyte) cast. (Brightfield, ×400.)** (From Brunzel NA: Fundamentals of urine and body fluid analysis, ed 2, Philadelphia, 2004, Saunders.)

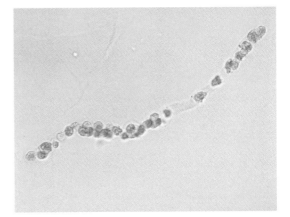

FIGURE 14-22 **Renal tubular epithelial cell cast. (Brightfield, ×400.)** (From Brunzel NA: Fundamentals of urine and body fluid analysis, ed 2, Philadelphia, 2004, Saunders.)

characteristic multilobular nucleus can usually be seen. Small leukocytes stain purple to violet, whereas large cells may be pale blue, in a pink matrix. As the cells disintegrate within the cast, their cytoplasm becomes granular, cell borders merge, and nuclei become indistinct, resulting in a granular cast when the cells are no longer distinguishable. The number of cells in a cast varies; some casts are packed with cells, and others show only a few cells in a hyaline matrix. WBC casts packed with cells still have a protein matrix and should have parallel sides and rounded ends. It is sometimes difficult to distinguish such a white cell cast from a clump of leukocytes **(pseudoleukocyte cast),** which may originate lower in the urinary tract. The presence of strands of mucus to which the WBCs adhere is another complication. However, it is still important not to report such pseudocasts as casts, which imply renal involvement or disease.

EPITHELIAL CELL CASTS

As indicated earlier, to be called an epithelial cell cast, the epithelial cell must be renal tubular in origin. Epithelial casts represent a most serious situation, although they are infrequently seen in the urine. They may be seen in cases of exposure to nephrotoxic substances, such as mercury or ethylene glycol (antifreeze), or in infections with viruses, such as cytomegalovirus or hepatitis virus. Epithelial casts result from destruction or desquamation of the cells that line the renal tubules. These cells are responsible for the work done by the kidney. The damage may be irreversible, depending on the severity of the disease process. The time needed to replace renal epithelial cells, if the basement membrane is left intact, is unknown; however, cells do not show maximum concentrating ability for several months after severe loss of tubular epithelium.

The epithelial cast often appears to consist of two rows of renal epithelial cells, implying tubular desquamation (Fig. 14-22). However, the cells may also vary in size, shape, and distribution, showing a varying amount of protein matrix. A haphazard arrangement of cells in the cast in varying stages of degeneration implies cellular damage and desquamation from different portions of the renal tubule. The epithelial cast does not remain constant once formed, but rather undergoes a series of changes. These changes result from cellular disintegration as the cast remains within the kidney, because of decreased urine flow (stasis). Therefore a range of epithelial casts, from cellular to coarsely granular, finely granular, and finally waxy, may be seen. The waxy type represents the most serious situation, since prolonged blockage of renal flow is required for them to form. All these types of casts are often seen in the same specimen; such specimens are referred to as "telescoped" urine sediments. Epithelial casts may be difficult to distinguish from white cell casts, as previously discussed. When stained, the cells have a blue-purple nucleus and lighter blue-purple cytoplasm in a pink matrix. Phase-contrast and interference microscopy are also helpful in this examination, as is cytocentrifugation.

RED BLOOD CELL (BLOOD AND HEMOGLOBIN) CASTS

The observation of RBC casts in the urine sediment is a significant diagnostic finding and indicates a serious renal condition. Their presence must not be missed. The RBCs enter the nephron by leakage through the glomerular capsule. It is possible that RBCs bleed into the renal tubules at a point beyond the glomerular capsule; however, this would be a much less common path because RBC casts are almost always associated with diseases that affect the glomerulus, such as acute

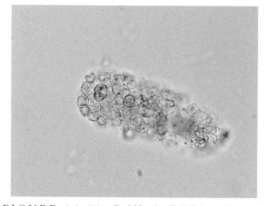

FIGURE 14-23 Red blood cell (RBC, erythrocyte) cast, unstained. (From Brunzel NA: Fundamentals of urine and body fluid analysis, ed 2, Philadelphia, 2004, Saunders.)

glomerulonephritis and lupus nephritis. Once RBCs are present in the lumen of the nephron, they clump together to form red cell casts. RBC casts are probably the most fragile casts in the urine sediment, which may explain why they are rarely observed and why fragments are more often found. When physical conditions indicate that RBC casts may be present, it is imperative that the urine specimen be absolutely fresh and gently treated. The casts may be so fragile that they disintegrate under the microscope as the observer watches.

Blood (RBC) casts have a characteristic orange-yellow color caused by hemoglobin, which makes them unlike anything else seen in the urine sediment (Fig. 14-23). Stain may or may not be useful in the identification of blood casts; however, the casts may have intact RBCs, which stain colorless or lavender in a pink matrix. Both phase-contrast and interference microscopy are useful in detecting RBC casts. The characteristic color is best seen with brightfield observation of the unstained sediment.

The number of cells present in the blood cast is variable. Often, only a few intact cells are seen in a hyaline matrix; this may be referred to as a *hyaline RBC cast*. If many cells are clumped together to form the cast, the matrix is often not visible. These casts are more fragile and, unfortunately, more serious clinically.

Red cell casts or casts derived from RBCs are often divided into red blood cell casts, blood casts, and hemoglobin casts. It is also possible to see **mixed-cell casts,** which are a combination of all types. The **red blood cell cast** contains at least some recognizable RBCs. They may be present in a generally hyaline matrix or may appear as a solid mass of conglutinated RBCs with little or no matrix between the packed cells. When the RBCs degenerate, no longer showing a cell margin but remaining recognizable as probably being derived

from blood, they are called a **blood cast.** (This is analogous to the cellular or coarsely granular cast derived from white cells or epithelial cells.) The **hemoglobin (pigment) cast** shows a homogeneous matrix with no cell margins or recognizable RBCs. Both blood and hemoglobin casts have a characteristic orange-yellow color. The hemoglobin pigment cast is then analogous to the waxy cast, representative of urinary stasis, and a more chronic than acute condition.

The occurrence of RBCs within a cast, regardless of the number of cells, represents a serious situation. The finding of RBCs in the urine sediment, in conjunction with red cell casts of any type, indicates renal (usually glomerular) involvement.

BACTERIAL CASTS

Casts made up of bacteria in a protein matrix have been described. Bacterial casts are an important finding and are diagnostic of acute pyelonephritis or intrinsic renal infections. They are probably mistaken for granular casts, which they resemble. The use of phase-contrast or interference-contrast microscopy and supravital stain is helpful. However, bacterial casts are most easily recognized if a dry or cytocentrifuged preparation is stained with Gram stain. The bacteria in the cast may be packed closely together, sparsely distributed throughout, or concentrated in an area of a cast matrix. In addition to the bacteria, WBCs may be present within the cast.

Granular Casts

The granules seen in granular casts may result from the breakdown of cells within the cast or the renal tubule, or they may be aggregates of plasma proteins, including fibrinogen, immune complexes, and globulins in a Tamm-Horsfall matrix. Once all the cells have become granules, it is impossible to determine what type of cell was originally present in the renal tubule. Such a distinction is useful, because red cell casts indicate glomerular injury, epithelial cell casts indicate renal tubular damage, and white cell casts indicate interstitial inflammation or infection. Often, casts are seen that are basically granular but show some cells in transition to granules. When cells are present, they should be identified if possible. Once again, phase-contrast and interference microscopy are helpful in this distinction, as is cytocentrifugation. The end product of this disintegration is the waxy cast.

The size of the granules within the granular cast varies; they become progressively smaller as the cells disintegrate. The number of granules also varies, and casts range from those that are completely filled with granules to those that are basically hyaline and contain only a few granules.

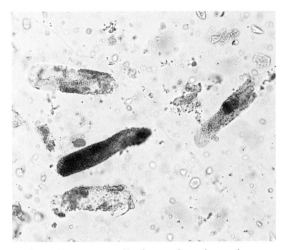

FIGURE 14-24   Finely granular and coarsely granular casts. (From Brunzel NA: Fundamentals of urine and body fluid analysis, ed 2, Philadelphia, 2004, Saunders.)

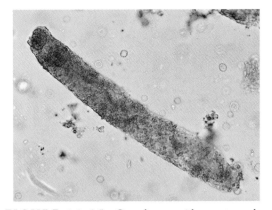

FIGURE 14-25   Granular cast with coarse granules. (From Brunzel NA: Fundamentals of urine and body fluid analysis, ed 2, Philadelphia, 2004, Saunders.)

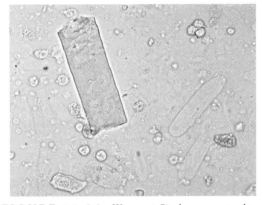

FIGURE 14-26   Waxy cast. Single waxy cast and two hyaline casts. Note the difference in refractility between these two types of casts. (From Brunzel NA: Fundamentals of urine and body fluid analysis, ed 2, Philadelphia, 2004, Saunders.)

Such granules may have been present in the renal tubule and trapped in a protein matrix as the cast was formed. Although granular casts are sometimes reported as coarsely or finely granular, the term *granular* is sufficient (Fig. 14-24). The distinction between coarsely and finely granular is subjective but relatively easily made. If the cast has a definite hyaline matrix with only a few granules, it is reported as hyaline. When large numbers of granules are present, it is described as granular. When many somewhat shortened granular casts are seen, the possibility that they are actually proximal renal tubular epithelial cells should be considered (see earlier discussion). They are more easily visualized with stained brightfield preparations, and cytocentrifugation and staining with Wright and Pap stains are especially helpful.

Coarsely Granular Casts

Coarsely granular casts contain large granules that appear to be degenerated cells (Fig. 14-25). They tend to be darker, shorter, and more irregular in outline than finely granular casts. They show a darker color and large granules that make them easier to find than either hyaline or finely granular casts. Coarsely granular casts stain with dark purple granules in a purple matrix.

FINELY GRANULAR CASTS

Finely granular casts look much like hyaline casts; however, the presence of fine granules makes them more distinctive and easier to find. When viewed with phase-contrast or interference microscopy, hyaline casts generally show a fine granulation. They are usually grayish or pale yellow in the unstained sediment and stain with fine, dark purple granules in a pale pink or pale purple matrix.

Waxy Casts

Waxy casts resemble hyaline casts, and they may be mistaken as such but are much more significant clinically. The waxy cast is homogeneous, as is the hyaline cast, but it is yellowish and more refractive, with sharper outlines. It appears hard, whereas the hyaline cast has a delicate appearance. Waxy casts tend to be wider than hyaline casts (they are described as "broad casts" or "broad waxy casts") and usually have irregular broken ends and fissures or cracks in their sides (Fig. 14-26). Fairly long forms are also seen. Phase-contrast and interference microscopy and staining are useful in the examination of waxy casts. They generally stain with greater intensity than hyaline casts, making them easier to visualize (Fig. 14-27).

Waxy casts are thought to be the final step in the disintegration of cellular casts and are especially serious because they imply renal stasis. They are associated with severe, chronic renal disease and renal amyloidosis. Waxy casts are seen only rarely and in small numbers in acute renal diseases.

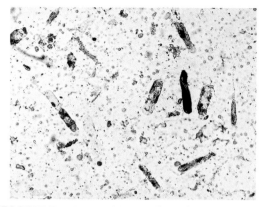

FIGURE 14-27 **Mixture of casts from "telescoped" urine specimen.** (From Brunzel NA: Fundamentals of urine and body fluid analysis, ed 2, Philadelphia, 2004, Saunders.)

Fatty Casts

The importance and probable mechanism of formation of fatty casts are discussed with oval fat bodies and fat globules (see previous sections). These three structures are often seen together in the same urine specimen, along with extremely large amounts of protein (>2000 mg/dL) and the pale, foamy appearance of the specimen associated with the nephrotic syndrome. They are also seen in diabetes mellitus with renal degeneration and in toxic renal poisoning, as from ethylene glycol or mercury.

Fatty casts contain droplets of fat, which are highly refractile under the microscope (Fig. 14-28). Although phase-contrast and interference microscopy are useful, the characteristic refractile appearance of fat droplets might be better appreciated with the brightfield microscope. If the droplets are neutral fat or triglyceride, they will stain bright orange or red with Sudan III or oil red O stains. If cholesterol is present, the fat droplets will show a Maltese cross pattern with polarized light. With Sternheimer-Malbin the cast matrix will stain, but the refractile fat globules will not stain.

Fatty casts may be seen as a protein matrix almost completely filled with fat globules or as fat globules contained within a basically hyaline, cellular, or granular cast. In addition to free fat globules, intact oval fat bodies may be seen within the cast matrix; these are sometimes referred to as *oval fat body casts.*

Other Casts

Various other structures found in the urine sediment may rarely be incorporated into the protein matrix of a cast. Pigmented casts may be seen, including hemoglobin (already described), myoglobin, bilirubin, and drugs such as phenazopyridine. Hemosiderin casts contain granules of hemosiderin. Crystal casts, which contain urates, calcium

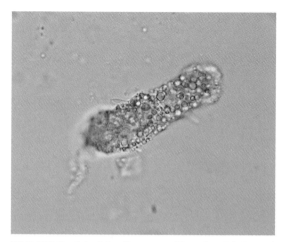

FIGURE 14-28 **Fatty cast. Note the globules and their characteristic refractility. (Brightfield, ×400.)** (From Brunzel NA: Fundamentals of urine and body fluid analysis, ed 2, Philadelphia, 2004, Saunders.)

oxalate, or sulfonamides, have also been seen. However, these must not be mistaken for crystals adhering to strands of mucus; rather, the protein matrix must be visualized in a true crystal cast.

Structures Confused with Casts

MUCOUS THREADS

The refractive index of mucous threads is similar to that of hyaline casts; however, mucous threads are long, ribbonlike strands with undefined edges and pointed or split ends. They also appear to have longitudinal striations. Mucous threads are most apparent, and cause the most confusion, with phase-contrast or interference microscopy. They are often seen together with hyaline casts. Although difficult to distinguish, hyaline casts are generally more formed or structured than mucous threads.

ROLLED SQUAMOUS EPITHELIAL CELLS

Squamous epithelial cells may be mistaken for casts when they have rolled into a cigar shape. However, they have pointed ends rather than rounded ones and are shorter than casts, and a single round nucleus may be discovered with careful focusing.

DISPOSABLE DIAPER FIBERS

Diaper fibers are easily confused with waxy casts, appearing almost identically as highly refractile with blunt ends. They may be seen in urine specimens from infants or from geriatric patients or other adults who must use diapers. Unlike waxy casts, diaper fibers are rarely accompanied by other pathologic findings, especially proteinuria. The use of polarizing microscopy may be useful; waxy casts do not polarize light; diaper fibers do (Fig. 14-29).

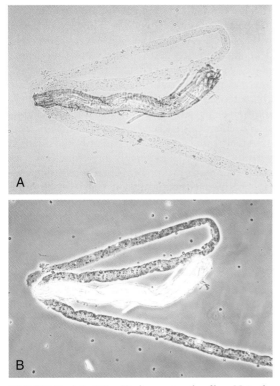

FIGURE 14-29 Hyaline cast and a fiber. Note the difference in form and refractility. A, Brightfield, × 100. B, Phase contrast, ×100. (From Brunzel NA: Fundamentals of urine and body fluid analysis, ed 2, Philadelphia, 2004, Saunders.)

OTHER STRUCTURES

Bits of hair or threads of material fibers are also mistaken for casts by the beginner. However, these are extremely refractive structures that have nothing in common with the appearance of protein microscopically. Likewise, scratches on the glass slide or coverglass may be mistaken for casts at first. Again, they are much too definite and obvious to be important. Finally, hyphae of molds are sometimes mistaken for hyaline casts; this is similar to mistaking yeast for RBCs. Hyphae are much more refractive than hyaline casts and are jointed and branching, as may be observed on closer examination.

Crystals and Amorphous Material

Clinical Significance

Crystals and amorphous precipitates of certain chemicals make up what has been called the *unorganized urine sediment*. These materials are generally obvious under the microscope. Because they are so striking, there is a natural tendency to pay considerable attention to them, but they are the most insignificant part of the urine sediment and deserve little attention. In the past, great emphasis was placed on the identification of these materials.

However, it is generally preferable to search carefully for more pathologic constituents and note only briefly the occurrence of crystals.

The presence of crystals in the urine specimen is called **crystalluria.** As urine specimens stand, especially when refrigerated, many lose clarity and become cloudy because of the precipitation of amorphous material and crystals. However, crystalluria generally is important only when present in urine when voided (at body temperature). It is necessary to identify crystals and amorphous materials that may be present, both normal and so-called abnormal forms, for various reasons.

If crystals are abundant, they will obscure such important structures as RBCs, WBCs, and casts. The more important structures must be sought with extreme care when crystals and amorphous materials are present. The use of a stain (e.g., Sternheimer-Malbin) may be especially useful in these situations.

The precipitation of certain crystals may accompany kidney stone formation **(lithiasis).** When crystals are seen in the urine of patients with lithiasis, the chemical composition of the **calculi** (stones) may be implied. This is one reason for the attention formerly given to urinary crystals. However, stone formation may exist without the presence of crystals in the urine, and crystals are often present without stone formation.

Amino acids such as cystine, leucine, and tyrosine may crystallize in urine and indicate serious metabolic or inherited disorders. Administration of sulfonamide drugs may cause the formation of sulfonamide crystals, especially in acidic urine. The formation of sulfonamide crystals within the kidney may result in blockage of renal output and severe renal damage. This problem was greater when sulfonamide drugs were first introduced. Currently used drugs are more soluble and thus less likely to precipitate. However, crystals are occasionally seen when high doses are given. More recently, crystals of the protease inhibitor indinavir sulfate have been associated with renal blockage and stone formation in human immunodeficiency virus (HIV)–positive individuals.

When the concentration of a salt in solution is greater than the solubility threshold for that salt, crystals will precipitate out of solution. Therefore, crystals are more likely to be seen in concentrated urine specimens with high specific gravity. This is often observed in the urine of persons with dehydration and fever.

Classification of Urine Crystals

The various crystals that are encountered in urine specimens are usually classified as *normal* or *abnormal*. These are further subclassified as normal *acid*

Crystals Found in Urine Sediment

Normal Acid Crystals

Amorphous urates
Uric acid
Acid urates
Monosodium or sodium urates
Calcium oxalate (also seen in neutral and alkaline
  urine)

Normal Alkaline Crystals

Amorphous phosphates
(Calcium oxalate)
Triple phosphates
Calcium carbonate

Abnormal Crystals of Metabolic Origin

Cystine
Tyrosine
Leucine
Cholesterol
Bilirubin
Hemosiderin

Abnormal Crystals of Iatrogenic Origin
(Drugs)

Sulfonamides
Ampicillin
Radiographic contrast media
Acyclovir
Indinavir sulfate

---

crystals (crystals seen in normal urine of an acidic pH), normal *alkaline* crystals (crystals seen in normal urine of an alkaline pH), abnormal crystals of metabolic origin, and abnormal crystals of iatrogenic origin. **Iatrogenic** refers to crystals that result from medication or treatment, that is, inadvertently caused by the physician. The various crystals found in the urine sediment are categorized in Box 14-4. The crystals in each category are arranged in approximately the order of importance or frequency in which they are encountered.

Identification and Reporting of Urine Crystals

Identification of crystals is usually done on the basis of shape or morphology. This is aided by knowledge of the urine pH. Certain forms are seen in urine of an acid pH (generally ≤6.5), whereas others are associated with urine of an alkaline pH (generally ≥7.0). Although pH 7 is neutral, crystals present in urine of pH 7 are generally forms seen in a more alkaline pH.

The normal crystals are usually reported on the basis of morphology alone. They are observed with both low-power and high-power objectives, depending on size, and reported as few, moderate, or many per high-power field. Unlike the urine sediment constituents already described, crystals are characterized by *shape* rather than size. Although some crystals are typically large or small, crystals of chemicals such as uric acid may vary from extremely small crystals that can only be visualized with high power to extremely large forms that are easily seen with low power. The *color* of the crystals, both macroscopically on the basis of urine appearance and microscopically, is also helpful. In some cases, *solubility* with heat, acids, or alkalis is useful in the final identification.

The abnormal crystals generally require confirmation before they are reported to the clinician. They are observed under low and high power, depending on size, and reported on the basis of the average number per low-power field, as shown in Table 14-9. Confirmation may consist of a chemical test, such as a diazo reaction for sulfonamides or a cyanide nitroprusside reaction for cystine. When chemical confirmatory tests are unavailable, confirmation may consist of the patient's drug history or history of various imaging procedures, such as intravenous pyelography or computed tomography (CT).

Most crystals are birefringent when viewed with polarized light. The strength of birefringence depends both on the chemical composition of the crystal in question and on the thickness of the crystal. Thick crystals will show stronger birefringence than thin ones. As with synovial fluid crystals, phosphates or phosphate-containing crystals generally show weaker birefringence than urates or uric acid. The ability to polarize light is very helpful in the identification of crystalline structures versus structures of biological origin, such as cells, microorganisms, and casts, which do not polarize light.

Normal Crystals

NORMAL ACID CRYSTALS

These crystals are seen in normal urine of an acidic pH (≤pH 6.5). In most cases, crystals seen at this pH are some form of uric acid or calcium oxalate. Uric acid is especially pleomorphic; when an unusual crystal is first encountered, it is often found to consist of uric acid or a salt of this acid. However, most of the abnormal crystals that have been encountered in urine are also associated with an acidic pH. Therefore, care must be taken to rule out the presence of pathologic crystals, before unusual forms are assumed to be a form of uric acid.

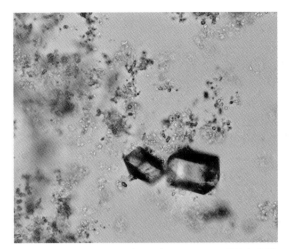

FIGURE 14-30 Amorphous urates. (Brightfield, × 400.)

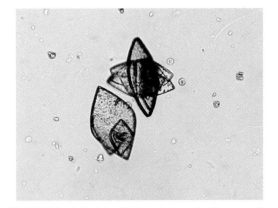

FIGURE 14-31 Uric acid crystals. Common diamond shape. (From Brunzel NA: Fundamentals of urine and body fluid analysis, ed 2, Philadelphia, 2004, Saunders.)

Amorphous Urates

Urates represent the amorphous material found in urine of an acid pH. Chemically, amorphous urates are a sodium salt of uric acid (sodium, potassium, magnesium, or calcium). *Amorphous* means without shape or form. The urates show a characteristic yellowish red, shapeless granulation (Fig. 14-30). They are strongly birefringent when viewed with polarized light. When present in sufficient numbers, they form a characteristic fluffy pink or orange precipitate referred to as "brick dust."

Amorphous urates tend to precipitate out of urine that is highly concentrated, as in dehydration and fever. Such urine specimens are typically highly colored (dark amber) and show large amounts of brick dust. Although of an alarming appearance to the patient, such specimens are of minimal concern clinically.

Amorphous urates will change to uric acid when acidified with glacial uric acid. They will dissolve when warmed to 60°C and when treated with 10% sodium hydroxide (NaOH). Their solubility when heated is useful in differentiating them from amorphous phosphates, which are insoluble when heated. However, this differentiation is usually made on the basis of urine pH; urates are seen in acidic urine and phosphates in alkaline urine. When treated with ammonium hydroxide, urates will change to ammonium biurate, the ammonium salt of uric acid.

Uric Acid

Uric acid crystals have a variety of shapes and colors. Typically, they are yellow or reddish brown, similar to the chemically related amorphous urates. The typical shape is the *whetstone*. Other shapes include rhombic plates or prisms, somewhat oval forms with pointed ends ("lemon shaped"), and barrel-shaped forms. Wedges, rosettes, irregular plates, and laminated forms are also seen. Uric acid crystals are usually recognized by color, but some, especially the rhombic plates, may appear colorless. Unusual crystals of an acid pH are generally forms of uric acid. A hexagonal form of uric acid may be mistaken for cystine crystals, which are abnormal and important to detect. Several of the sulfonamides may mimic uric acid. When this situation is suspected, a drug history should be obtained and confirmatory test for sulfonamides performed.

Uric acid crystals are often seen in urine specimens, especially after the specimen has been standing. However, they are pathologic only when seen in fresh urine immediately after it is voided. Amorphous urates and uric acid, together with elevated serum uric acid, may be associated with gout or stone formation. The uric acid concentration in urine depends on dietary intake of purines and breakdown of nucleic acid. Therefore, large amounts of urates or uric acid are often seen in the urine of patients with leukemia or lymphoma who are receiving chemotherapy.

Uric acid is strongly birefringent and gives a beautiful play of colors when viewed with polarized light (Fig. 14-31). As with amorphous urates, uric acid is soluble when heated to 60°C and when treated with 10% NaOH. However, uric acid crystals remain (are insoluble) when treated with glacial acetic acid.

Acid Urates

These rare forms of uric acid are seen in urine of acidic or neutral pH. Acid urates may be sodium, potassium, or ammonium urates and are observed as brown spheres or clusters that resemble ammonium biurate. They are often seen in urine together with amorphous urates. They have the same significance as amorphous urates or uric acid. Acid urates

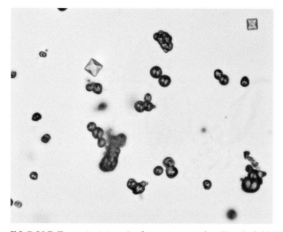

FIGURE 14-32 Acid urate crystals. (Brightfield, ×200.) (From Brunzel NA: Fundamentals of urine and body fluid analysis, ed 2, Philadelphia, 2004, Saunders.)

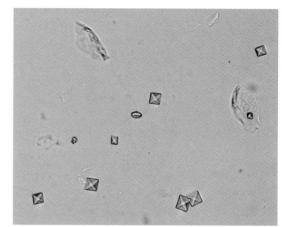

FIGURE 14-34 Calcium oxalate crystals. Octahedral (envelope) form of dehydrate crystals. (Brightfield, ×200.) (From Brunzel NA: Fundamentals of urine and body fluid analysis, ed 2, Philadelphia, 2004, Saunders.)

FIGURE 14-33 Monosodium urate. (Brightfield, ×200.) (From Brunzel NA: Fundamentals of urine and body fluid analysis, ed 2, Philadelphia, 2004, Saunders.)

resemble the alkaline counterpoint of uric acid, namely, ammonium biurate. They also resemble sulfamethoxazole, an abnormal crystal of pathologic significance, and are important to recognize for this reason (Fig. 14-32).

As with amorphous urates and uric acid, the acid urates are soluble at 60°C and in 10% NaOH and are changed to uric acid when treated with glacial acetic acid.

Monosodium or Sodium Urates

The sodium urates are another rare form of uric acid that might be seen in urine. Monosodium urate is the form of uric acid seen in the synovial fluid of patients with gout. If present in urine, it appears as tiny, slender, colorless needles (Fig. 14-33).

Calcium Oxalate

Calcium oxalate crystals have a characteristic shape referred to as an "envelope." These are octahedrons that vary somewhat in size but are typically

small, colorless, and glistening. Occasionally, they are seen as rectangular forms with pyramidal ends. Less frequently, they may appear in a dumbbell or an ovoid shape that may resemble that of RBCs. Unlike red cells, however, calcium oxalate will polarize light (Fig. 14-34).

Although most common in acidic urine, calcium oxalate crystals may also be seen in neutral or alkaline urine specimens. They are of little clinical significance, although they may be present in association with stone formation; calcium oxalate is the most common constituent found in kidney stones. A correlation exists between calcium stones and excess oxalate and uric acid in the urine. (Uric acid may be the nidus for stone formation.) Excess oxalate may result from ingestion of foodstuffs containing oxalic acid, such as spinach and rhubarb, and from ingestion of vitamin C, because oxalic acid is a breakdown product of ascorbic acid. Calcium oxalate crystals may also be seen in cases of ethylene glycol or methoxyflurane poisoning.

NORMAL ALKALINE CRYSTALS

These forms are the "normal" crystals seen in urine of an alkaline pH (generally ≥ pH 7.0). They are usually phosphate- or calcium-containing crystals. However, the alkaline counterpoint of uric acid, ammonium biurate, is also seen. Phosphates have little clinical significance, although they are associated with an alkaline pH and infection.

Amorphous Phosphates

The amorphous material found in alkaline urine is amorphous phosphate. Generally, the phosphates give a finer or more "lacy" precipitate than the amorphous urates and are colorless (Fig. 14-35). Phosphates are the most common cause of turbidity in alkaline urine and are seen as a fine, white

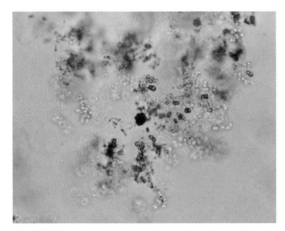

FIGURE 14-35 **Amorphous phosphates. (Bright-field, ×400.)** (From Brunzel NA: Fundamentals of urine and body fluid analysis, ed 2, Philadelphia, 2004, Saunders.)

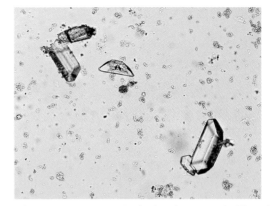

FIGURE 14-36 **Triple phosphate crystals. Typical "coffin-lid" form. (Brightfield, ×100.)** (From Brunzel NA: Fundamentals of urine and body fluid analysis, ed 2, Philadelphia, 2004, Saunders.)

precipitate microscopically. They do not dissolve when heated but are soluble in acetic acid and dilute hydrochloric acid. Phosphates resemble, and are often seen with, bacteria; care must be taken not to overlook bacteria when phosphates are present. Use of phase-contrast microscopy is helpful.

TRIPLE PHOSPHATE

Triple (ammonium magnesium) phosphates (also referred to as *struvite*) are colorless crystals and typically show great variation in size, from tiny to relatively huge crystals. They have a characteristic "coffin-lid" shape that is impossible to miss (Fig. 14-36). They may also be seen as large, long prisms that are difficult to distinguish from calcium phosphate. Both triple and calcium phosphates have similar clinical significance, and either may be reported as phosphates. Less often, triple phosphates occur in a fernlike form as they dissolve into solution. They are soluble in dilute acetic acid.

Ammonium Biurate

This ammonium salt is the alkaline counterpart of uric acid and amorphous urates in urine. The crystals are spherical with radial or concentric striations and long prismatic spicules, resembling thorn apples (Fig. 14-37). They are yellow and may be mistaken for some forms of the sulfonamide drugs that may precipitate out of urine. Sulfa crystals, however, are usually seen in acidic urine. Ammonium biurates are often present in old alkaline urine specimens, especially those that contain unusual sediment constituents and have been retained for teaching purposes. They are much less frequently seen in fresh urine collections. They are soluble at 60°C with acetic acid and in strong alkali. Ammonium biurates will convert to uric acid with concentrated hydrochloric acid or acetic acid.

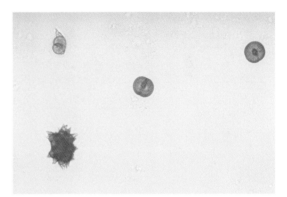

FIGURE 14-37 **Ammonium biurate crystals. Spheres and "thorn-apple" form. (Brightfield, ×200.)** (From Brunzel NA: Fundamentals of urine and body fluid analysis, ed 2, Philadelphia, 2004, Saunders.)

Calcium Phosphate

Calcium phosphates are colorless crystals occasionally seen in normal alkaline urine. Typically, they appear as slender prisms with a wedgelike end, occurring singly or arranged in rosettes (Fig. 14-38). They may resemble, and appear with, triple phosphate crystals as long prisms of calcium monohydrogen phosphate, also known as *brushite*. Calcium phosphate may also appear as flat plates, which might be mistaken for large, degenerating squamous epithelial cells (Fig. 14-39).

Calcium phosphate is insoluble when heated to 60°C, slightly soluble in dilute acetic acid, and soluble in dilute hydrochloric acid.

Calcium Carbonate

Calcium carbonate crystals are tiny, colorless granules that typically occur in pairs ("dumbbells") but also may occur singly (Fig. 14-40). Because they are so small, calcium carbonate crystals

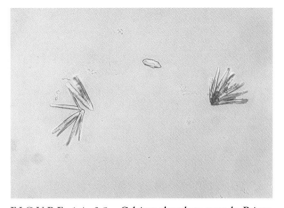

FIGURE 14-38 Calcium phosphate crystals. Prisms are arranged singly and in rosette forms. (Brightfield, ×100.) (From Brunzel NA: Fundamentals of urine and body fluid analysis, ed 2, Philadelphia, 2004, Saunders.)

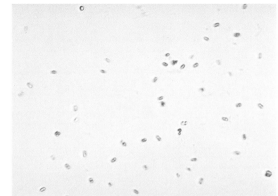

FIGURE 14-40 Calcium carbonate crystals. Numerous single crystals (dumbbell shape). (From Brunzel NA: Fundamentals of urine and body fluid analysis, ed 2, Philadelphia, 2004, Saunders.)

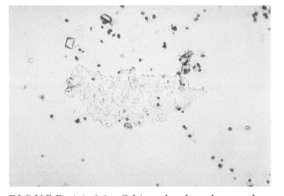

FIGURE 14-39 Calcium phosphate sheet or plate. (Brightfield, ×100.) (From Brunzel NA: Fundamentals of urine and body fluid analysis, ed 2, Philadelphia, 2004, Saunders.)

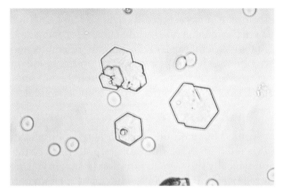

FIGURE 14-41 Cystine crystals. Thin, colorless, laminated hexagons. (Brightfield, ×400.) (From Brunzel NA: Fundamentals of urine and body fluid analysis, ed 2, Philadelphia, 2004, Saunders.)

represent part of the amorphous material seen in normal alkaline urine specimens. They are soluble in acetic acid with effervescence.

Abnormal Crystals

With only a few, very rare exceptions, the abnormal urinary crystals are seen in urine specimens of an acid pH, 6.5 or less. Normal crystals of urine may be reported on the basis of microscopic examination (morphology) and pH. However, the abnormal crystals require further confirmation. Whenever possible, this should be a chemical confirmation, although a history of medications or treatment procedures may be the only possible confirmation. Unlike the normal crystals, which are reported as few, moderate, or many, the abnormal crystals are reported as the number seen per average low-power field.

Abnormal crystals may be further classified as metabolic (physiologic) or iatrogenic (see Table 14-9). The abnormal crystals of metabolic origin

are the result of certain disease states or inherited conditions. These include cystine, tyrosine, leucine, cholesterol, bilirubin, and hemosiderin. Iatrogenic crystals are the result of medication or treatment and thus are inadvertently caused by the physician. Examples of iatrogenic crystals include the various sulfonamides, ampicillin, radiographic contrast media, acyclovir, and indinavir sulfate.

ABNORMAL CRYSTALS OF METABOLIC ORIGIN

Cystine

Cystine crystals are colorless, refractile, hexagonal plates that are often laminated (Fig. 14-41). They may be seen in the urine of patients with the hereditary condition cystinuria. This is an amino acid transport disorder affecting cystine, ornithine, lysine, and arginine (COLA). Of these amino acids, only cystine crystallizes out in the urine. This crystallization of cystine is serious because these patients tend to form cystine stones, which

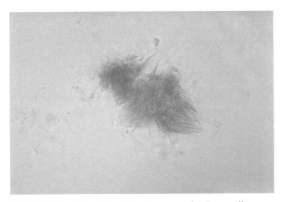

FIGURE 14-42 **Tyrosine crystals. Fine, silky needles.** (From Brunzel NA: Fundamentals of urine and body fluid analysis, ed 2, Philadelphia, 2004, Saunders.)

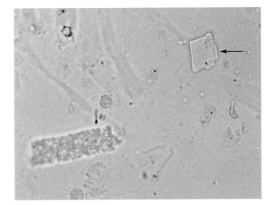

FIGURE 14-43 **Cholesterol crystal (arrow).** (From Brunzel NA: Fundamentals of urine and body fluid analysis, ed 2, Philadelphia, 2004, Saunders.)

may lead to kidney damage. Patients with cystinuria must always be well hydrated to prevent such stone formation. The crystals may be mistaken for a form of uric acid that is also hexagonal.

The presence of cystine should be confirmed with the cyanide-nitroprusside reaction. Cystine is reduced to cysteine by sodium cyanide. The free sulfhydryl groups that result react with nitroprusside to give a red-purple color. Cystine crystals are most insoluble in urine of an acid pH. However, they remain insoluble up to pH 7.4. They are soluble in alkali (especially ammonia) and dilute hydrochloric acid. They are destroyed by the presence of bacteria, because of the formation of ammonia. Cystine crystals are insoluble in boiling water, acetic acid, alcohol, and ether.

Tyrosine

Tyrosine crystals are rare but may be present as the result of inherited amino acid disorders (hereditary tyrosinosis, oasthouse urine disease) and, together with leucine, in patients with massive liver failure.

Tyrosine crystals are colorless, fine, silky needles arranged in sheaves or clumps and appear black as the microscope is focused (Fig. 14-42). They occur in urine of an acid pH. Tyrosine is soluble in alkali and dilute mineral acid. Tyrosine crystals are relatively soluble when heated but are insoluble in alcohol and ether. They are confirmed with a nitrosonaphthol test or by amino acid analysis using high-performance liquid chromatography (HPLC).

Leucine

Leucine crystals are yellow, oily-looking spheres with radial and concentric striations. They are of metabolic origin and extremely rare. Leucine and tyrosine crystals usually appear together and are associated with severe liver disease. Leucine is found in urine of an acid pH.

Cholesterol

Droplets of cholesterol that polarize as a Maltese cross are seen in the urine sediment as free fat, in oval fat bodies, and in fatty casts. However, cholesterol crystals or plates are extremely rare in freshly voided urine sediment; they have been seen rarely after the specimen has been refrigerated. When seen, they have the same clinical significance as the more common globules or droplets.

As with most abnormal crystals, cholesterol crystals are associated with urine of an acidic or neutral pH. Cholesterol crystals are large, flat, hexagonal plates with one or more notched corners (Fig. 14-43).

When apparent cholesterol crystals are seen in large numbers, the presence of another drug or its crystals should be suspected. Crystals of radiographic media (e.g., meglumine diatrizoate) are found in urine collected immediately after intravenous radiographic studies. They are morphologically similar to cholesterol but are associated with a very high specific gravity (>1.035 by refractometer) and a false-positive, delayed sulfosalicylic acid test for protein. Radiographic media crystals should not be mistaken for cholesterol.

If present, crystals of cholesterol should be associated with other findings, such as free fat, oval fat bodies, or fatty casts. They are more likely to be seen in urine specimens that have been retained and refrigerated.

Absolute, chemical confirmation of cholesterol may be difficult. However, cholesterol crystals are very soluble in chloroform, ether, and hot alcohol.

Bilirubin

The presence of crystals of precipitated bilirubin is occasionally seen in the urine sediment of patients with bilirubinuria. This finding has about the same clinical significance as the chemical detection of bilirubin in urine, and these crystals

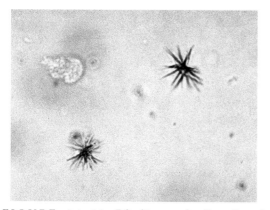

FIGURE 14-44 Bilirubin crystals. (From Brunzel NA: Fundamentals of urine and body fluid analysis, ed 2, Philadelphia, 2004, Saunders.)

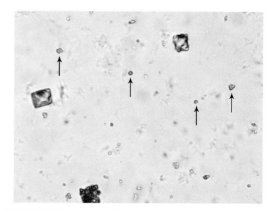

FIGURE 14-45 Hemosiderin granules in urine sediment appear yellow-brown. Numerous granules and a clump are present in this field of view. Arrows identify four granules. (From Brunzel NA: Fundamentals of urine and body fluid analysis, ed 2, Philadelphia, 2004, Saunders.)

should not be reported in the absence of bilirubin. Bilirubin crystals are seen as reddish brown needles that cluster in clumps or as spheres (Fig. 14-44).

Hemosiderin

The pathophysiology of hemosiderin is discussed in the section on renal epithelial cells. However, this abnormal crystal might be mistaken for amorphous urates, a common urine sediment finding.

Hemosiderin may be seen in acid or neutral urine a few days after a severe intravascular hemolytic episode. In unstained urine sediment, hemosiderin appears as coarse, yellow-brown granules. These may be seen as free granules, or they may be contained within renal epithelial cells, macrophages, or casts. Hemosiderin may be confirmed with the **Rous test,** a wet Prussian blue stain for iron (Fig. 14-45). Cytocentrifuged preparations of the urine sediment may also be stained with Prussian blue, as in hematologic stains for iron content.

ABNORMAL CRYSTALS OF IATROGENIC ORIGIN

Sulfonamides

The presence of these iatrogenic crystals in the urine sediment is an important pathologic finding. Sulfonamides are likely to cause renal damage because the crystals precipitate in the nephron, causing bleeding (hematuria) and oliguria as a result of mechanical blockage of the renal tubules, which may lead to renal failure or shutdown. Precipitation or crystallization of the sulfonamides is prevented by adequate hydration of the patient and possibly alkalization of the urine with diet or medication.

In the past, as previously noted, much attention was given to the various forms of sulfonamides that might be encountered in the urine. However,

current pharmacology uses more soluble forms of these drugs, and sulfonamide crystals are now an uncommon finding.

The sulfonamides are most likely to precipitate in urine with a low acid pH. The crystals are generally yellow to brown but may be colorless. Shape varies with the actual drug, and the various sulfonamides mimic various forms of uric aid, urates, and biurates. They have been described as colorless needles in sheaves or rosettes, arrowheads, or whetstones; as brownish shocks of wheat with central binding; as colorless to greenish brown fan-shaped needles; and as dense brown or irregularly divided spheres.

All forms of sulfonamides may be confirmed by hydrolysis with heat and acid and application of a diazo reaction. Further confirmation may be made by requesting a list of medications administered to the patient. The more frequently encountered sulfonamide forms that crystallize in the urine are described next.

Sulfamethoxazole

Sulfamethoxazole is the sulfonamide crystal found most often in the urine sediment. It is supplied as acetylsulfamethoxazole together with trimethoprim under the trade names Bactrim and Septra. Although this is a common drug, occasionally it has been seen to crystallize in urine after unusually high dosage. When present, it is seen as a dense brown or an irregularly divided sphere (Fig. 14-46).

Acetylsulfadiazine

Acetylsulfadiazine is a dangerous form of sulfonamide because of its relative insolubility. It is now rarely used. It is seen as yellow-brown sheaves of wheat with eccentric binding.

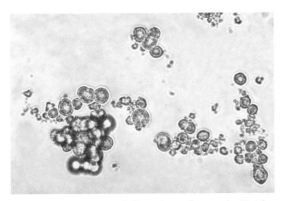

FIGURE 14-46 **Sulfamethoxazole crystals. (Bright-field, ×400.)** (From Brunzel NA: Fundamentals of urine and body fluid analysis, ed 2, Philadelphia, 2004, Saunders.)

Sulfadiazine

Sulfadiazine is another form of sulfonamide that is used only rarely. It appears as dense brown globules. These crystals are morphologically similar to ammonium biurates and acid urates.

Ampicillin

Ampicillin crystals appear as long, thin, colorless needles in acidic urine. They are seen only rarely, as the result of large doses of the drug, which may be necessary for treatment of bacterial meningitis.

Radiographic Contrast Media

Crystals of compounds used for diagnostic radiographic procedures, such as meglumine diatrizoate (Renografin, Hypaque), may be precipitated in the urine for a brief period after injection. They are primarily important because they might be misidentified as cholesterol crystals. Occasionally their presence is of clinical importance, such as in dehydrated elderly patients, who may experience renal blockage from crystalline precipitation.

Crystals of meglumine diatrizoate may be seen in the urine sediment as flat, four-sided plates, often with a notched corner. They closely resemble cholesterol plates and should not be mistaken for them. They may also occur as long, thin prisms or rectangles.

The presence of radiographic media should be suspected when many crystals resembling cholesterol plates are seen and the specific gravity by refractometer is extremely high (>1.035). Because radiographic media do not ionize, however, the specific gravity by reagent strip is unaffected by their presence. When they are present, the urine may show a delayed false-positive sulfosalicylic acid precipitation test for protein. This should not be mistaken for true protein precipitation. The presence of radiographic media may be confirmed by a clinical history of recent imaging procedures.

Acyclovir

Acyclovir is another drug form that may be seen in the urine sediment in rare cases of patients treated with high doses. Unlike most abnormal crystals, which are seen in acidic urine, acyclovir crystals have been seen in urine of pH 7.5. They appear as colorless slender needles that are strongly birefringent with polarized light. They may be confirmed by obtaining a drug history.

Indinavir Sulfate

With the use of protease inhibitors in the treatment of HIV infection, the presence of crystals of indinavir sulfate (Crixivan) has been observed. According to product literature, 4% of patients treated with indinavir sulfate have renal stone formation.[5] As with other drugs that might precipitate in the urine, it is important that patients be well hydrated to avoid crystallization of the drug. The presence of these crystals in the urine might be an early sign of stone formation, especially when the patient has clinical evidence of stones, such as pain and hematuria.

Crystals of indinavir sulfate are slender colorless needles or slender rectangular plates that tend to be arranged in fan-shaped or starburst forms, bundles, or sheaves. They resemble some forms of sulfonamides. Unlike most abnormal crystals, indinavir sulfate is most insoluble at an alkaline pH. The crystals are strongly birefringent with polarized light. Confirmation may depend primarily on the patient's drug history of indinavir use. Confirmation is possible by mass spectrometry or HPLC, but this is beyond the scope of the routine laboratory.

Other Cellular Constituents

Spermatozoa

Spermatozoa may be present in the urine of both men and women. Laboratory protocol should be established and followed as to when the presence of sperm is to be reported. In fertility studies and cases of possible sexual abuse, the presence of spermatozoa may be an important finding.

Spermatozoa are easily recognized by their oval body (head) and long delicate tail. The head is about 4 to 6 μm long (smaller and narrower than RBC), and the tail is about 40 to 60 μm long. Spermatozoa may be motile in wet preparation (an aid to identification), or they may be stationary. Phase-contrast microscopy is especially helpful in identification (Fig. 14-47).

Bacteria

Under normal conditions, the urinary tract is free of bacteria, but most urine specimens contain at least a few bacteria because of contamination when

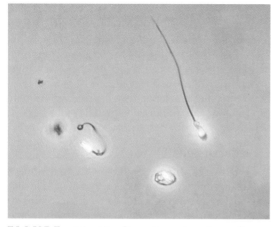

FIGURE 14-47 Spermatozoa in urine sediment. One typical and two atypical forms. (Phase contrast, ×400.) (From Brunzel NA: Fundamentals of urine and body fluid analysis, ed 2, Philadelphia, 2004, Saunders.)

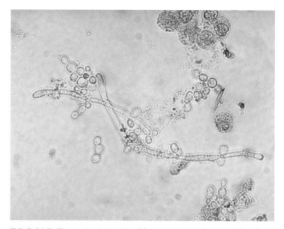

FIGURE 14-48 Budding yeast and pseudohyphae. Leukocytes also present singly and as a clump. (Brightfield, sedistain, ×400.) (From Brunzel NA: Fundamentals of urine and body fluid analysis, ed 2, Philadelphia, 2004, Saunders.)

the urine is voided. Bacteria multiply rapidly when urine stands at room temperature. In specimens that are obtained in a manner suitable for urine culture and kept under sterile conditions, the presence of bacteria may indicate a UTI. In this case the bacteria are likely to be associated with the presence of WBCs, although this is not always true. Bacterial infection should be confirmed by quantitative urine culture.

Bacteria are recognizable morphologically in wet preparation under high power. They are extremely small, only a few micrometers long. They may be either rods or cocci and may occur singly, in pairs, in chains, or in tetrads. Rods are more easily recognized than cocci because of their larger size, although some rods are extremely short and difficult to distinguish from cocci. Bacteria are often motile, which helps in their identification. Occasionally, unusually long rod-shaped forms with central swelling are seen. These **protoplasts** are the result of damage to the cell wall by antibiotics (especially penicillins) used in therapy.

Bacteria are most often seen in alkaline urine and may be confused with amorphous material at first, but this will not be a problem as the microscopist gains experience in observation. Phase-contrast microscopy is very useful in the visualization of bacteria, which are difficult to see with brightfield illumination. Although not normally part of urinalysis, Gram staining a drop of concentrated sediment is helpful in recognition of bacteria in difficult specimens. On Wright-stained cytocentrifuged preparations, all bacteria will stain deep blue-purple (basophilic).

In lower urinary tract (bladder) infections, bacteria are generally but not always associated with the presence of WBCs (leukocytes, PMNs). Mild proteinuria and a positive reagent strip test

for nitrites or leukocyte esterase may also be seen. With upper urinary tract (kidney) infections, bacteria may be seen along with WBCs and casts (leukocyte, cellular, granular). The patient may have moderate proteinuria and a positive reagent strip test for nitrites or leukocyte esterase.

Yeast

Yeast cells are occasionally seen in urine, especially from female and diabetic patients. They are often present as the result of contamination of the urine from a vaginal yeast infection. Yeast cells are associated with the presence of sugar in the urine. Sugar is the energy source for yeast cells, which grow and multiply rapidly when it is present. For this reason, yeast cells are often discovered in the urine of diabetic patients, along with a high sugar content, low pH, and ketones. Yeast cells are also common contaminants from skin and air, and infections are seen in debilitated and immunosuppressed or immunocompromised patients.

Yeast cells are often mistaken for RBCs. They are generally smaller than erythrocytes and show considerable size variation, even within a specimen. Yeast cells have a typically ovoid shape, lack color, and have a smooth and refractive appearance. The most distinguishing characteristic is the presence of little buds, or projections, because of their manner of reproduction. Pseudomycelial forms of *Candida* species (type of yeast usually present) may also be seen. These are elongated cells that may be up to 50 μm long and resemble mycelia of true fungi. These **pseudohyphae** may be branched and have terminal buds (Fig. 14-48). They are clinically significant in the urine of debilitated patients with severe *Candida* infection, as seen in immunosuppressed patients.

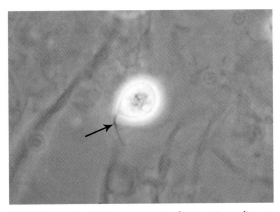

FIGURE 14-49 *Trichomonas vaginalis* in urine sediment. Arrow points to the protruding posterior axostyle. (**Phase contrast, ×400.**) (From Brunzel NA: Fundamentals of urine and body fluid analysis, ed 2, Philadelphia, 2004, Saunders.)

Other mycelial forms of yeast have been observed; these should not be mistaken for casts.

Parasites

TRICHOMONAS VAGINALIS

Trichomonas vaginalis is the parasite most frequently seen in urine specimens. This protozoan is primarily responsible for vaginal infections, but it can also infect the urethra, periurethral glands, bladder, and prostate. It generally resides in the vagina in women and prostate in men, where it feeds on the mucosal surface and ingests bacteria and leukocytes that may be present. The organism is motile, which is an aid to its identification. When an infection is suspected, direct swabs of the vagina or urethra are examined, although the organisms may be seen contaminating the urine sediment.

T. vaginalis is a unicellular flagellated organism, a protozoan. It has a characteristic pear-shaped appearance, with a single nucleus, four anterior flagella, and an undulating membrane, as well as a sharp, protruding posterior axostyle (Fig. 14-49). The most distinguishing feature of this trichomonad is its motility: a rapid, jerky, rotating, nondirectional motion that is easily recognized in wet preparations. The organisms are larger than typical leukocytes (up to 30 μm long) and may resemble transitional epithelial cells, especially when no longer motile. Phase-contrast microscopy is particularly useful in visualization, especially of the flagella. When stained, the cells lose their characteristic motility as they round up and die, appearing very similar to degenerating transitional epithelial cell forms (see Chapter 16).

OTHER PARASITES

Various other parasites may be seen in urine, mostly as the result of fecal or vaginal contamination. Some may be common to particular geographic areas and patient populations. All of these require special knowledge for identification, but they may be noticed initially during urinalysis and then referred to a microbiologist for identification.

Enterobius vermicularis, or pinworm, is a fairly common helminth infecting the intestinal tract that may occasionally be found in the urine in larval or egg (ova) form (see Chapter 16). Other parasites occasionally seen in urine include *Trichuris* (whipworm), *Schistosoma haematobium*, *Strongyloides*, and *Giardia*, as well as various amoebae. *S. haematobium* ova can be introduced directly into the urine from the bladder wall mucosa.

Various insects or "bugs" possibly seen in urine specimens include lice, fleas, bedbugs, mites, and ticks.

Tumor Cells

Tumor cells related to malignant conditions (e.g., transitional cell carcinoma) and other cell forms with altered cytologic features may be found in the urine sediment. These cell forms cannot be diagnosed from the usual sediment preparation but require special collection, cytocentrifugation, and stains and examination by qualified personnel in cytology. If tumor cells are suspected from the examination of the sediment, the specimen should be referred accordingly. The presence of RBCs in the chemical examination of the urine is an early diagnostic clue.

Contaminants and Artifacts

Many objects and structures in the urine sediment are contaminants or artifacts that distract the observer's attention from the important urinary constituents. These are the objects that beginning microscopists tend to see first when attempting a microscopic examination of the urine sediment. It seems to be a general rule that if an object is easy to see, it is unimportant.

Starch

Granules of starch are common contaminants in the urine sediment. They are the result of the use of barrier-protective gloves in all areas of the laboratory and medical care. *Starch* refers to cornstarch, a carbohydrate often used to line surgical or barrier-protective gloves. It is different from talc, or talcum, which is hydrated magnesium silicate, a chunky, irregular crystal.

Starch is a ubiquitous structure that is easily recognized, but it must not be confused with globules or droplets of cholesterol. Both starch and cholesterol globules are birefringent and polarize as a

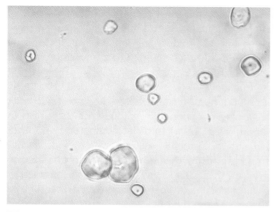

FIGURE 14-50 Starch granules. (Brightfield, × 400.) (From Brunzel NA: Fundamentals of urine and body fluid analysis, ed 2, Philadelphia, 2004, Saunders.)

Maltese cross (white cross on a black background) when viewed with polarized light. Starch is most easily recognized with brightfield microscopy (Fig. 14-50). It is seen as an irregular, generally round granule with a central dimple or slit. Even when viewed with polarized light, the Maltese cross formation produced by starch is more irregular than the very round, regular formation produced by droplets of cholesterol.

Fibers (Including Disposable Diaper Fibers)

Disposable diaper fibers are particularly troublesome in their resemblance to waxy casts. They may be seen in the urine of both infants and incontinent adults. They should be suspected when other findings associated with waxy casts, such as protein, are absent. As described earlier, diaper fibers will polarize light, but waxy casts will not.

Other contaminants may be introduced into the urine specimen on collection or by laboratory personnel during specimen processing or examination. These include cotton threads, wood fibers, synthetic fibers, and hair. They are all highly refractile structures that should not be mistaken for casts.

Air Bubbles

Air bubbles are highly refractile and structureless and easily recognized. They may be introduced as the coverglass is applied to the urine sediment or as the sediment is introduced into the standardized slide.

Oil Droplets

Oil droplets may be the result of contamination from such lubricants as vaginal cream, catheter lubricant, and mineral oil. They may be confused with RBCs or fat globules of physiologic origin. Oil droplets are highly refractile and structureless.

Contaminating oil should be distinguished from fat of physiologic origin. True lipiduria is usually associated with other findings, such as proteinuria, fatty casts, and oval fat bodies, as described previously.

Glass Fragments

Colorless, highly refractile, pleomorphic fragments of glass (probably from very small pieces of coverglass) might appear similar to crystals.

Stains

The various supravital stains used in the examination of the urine sediment may precipitate, especially when added to urine of an alkaline pH. This may be seen as an amorphous purple granulation or as brown-to-purple needle-shaped crystals in clusters. Sudan III fat stain may also precipitate as clusters of needle-shaped crystals that are bright red or red-orange. When such precipitation occurs, identification of pathologic structures that might be present is difficult.

Pollen Grains

Pollen grains may be seen as a urine contaminant, especially on a seasonal basis. They are fairly large and regularly shaped, with a thick cell wall. Pollen grains may resemble the eggs of some parasitic worms.

Fecal Contamination

The presence of fecal elements in urine is usually the result of contamination during collection. If there is a **fistula** (an abnormal connection) between the colon and the urinary tract, fecal constituents may be seen in the urine. This is a serious pathologic condition that leads to recurrent infection of the urinary tract.

The presence of feces in the urine is usually observed as an overall yellow-brown color of the gross urine specimen. Microscopic findings include plant fibers, skeletal muscle fibers, and microorganisms. Rarely, columnar epithelial cells from the gut mucosa or squamous epithelial cells from the anal mucosa are seen.

When detection of a fistula is clinically indicated, patients may be fed activated charcoal, which is carefully searched for in the urine. The presence of charcoal in the urine demonstrates an abnormal connection between the gut and the urinary tract.

Specimen Changes on Standing

Changes (see Table 14-2) that may occur as the urine stands include the following. RBCs become distorted because of the lack of an isotonic solution. Erythrocytes either swell or become crenated, which makes them difficult to recognize, and they finally disintegrate. WBCs rapidly disintegrate in hypotonic solutions. Casts disintegrate, especially as the urine becomes alkaline, because they must have sufficient acidity and solute concentration to exist. Other components that are found only in acidic urine will disappear as the urine becomes alkaline. The increase in alkalinity results from the growth of bacteria and production of ammonia. Finally, bacteria multiply rapidly, obscuring various components.

CASE STUDIES

CASE STUDY 14-1

A 20-year-old female college student with a sore throat is seen in the student health service. A throat swab is cultured and reported positive for group A β-hemolytic streptococci. She is treated with an intramuscular injection of penicillin. Two weeks later, she wakes up in the morning and finds that she has decreased urine volume, and her urine is dark red. She also has a fever and swelling in her feet. She returns to the student health service, where urine is collected for urinalysis. The following urinalysis results were obtained (SSA, Sulfosalicylic acid; hpf, high-power field; lpf, low-power field):

Physical Appearance
Color: Red
Transparency: Cloudy

Chemical Screening
pH: 6
Specific gravity: 1.025
Protein (reagent strip): 100 mg/dL
Protein (SSA): 2+
Blood: Large
Nitrite: Negative
Leukocyte esterase: Negative
Glucose: Negative
Ketones: Trace
Bilirubin: Negative
Urobilinogen: Normal

Microscopic Examination
Red blood cells: 10-25 per hpf; dysmorphic forms present
White blood cells: 0-2 per hpf
Casts: 2-5 red blood cell casts per lpf
Crystals: Moderate amorphous urates

1. This patient's proteinuria is probably caused by which of the following?
   a. Glomerular damage
   b. Lower urinary tract disorders
   c. Prerenal disorders
   d. Tubular (or interstitial) damage

2. The presence of dysmorphic red blood cells (RBCs) and RBC casts indicates which of the following?
   a. Bleeding from kidney stone formation
   b. Kidney disease located in the glomerulus
   c. Kidney infection
   d. Probable menstrual contamination

3. The trace reagent strip reaction for ketone and the presence of amorphous urates in the urine sediment of this patient are probably the result of which of the following?
   a. A false-positive ketone reaction caused by sensitivity of the test
   b. Dehydration caused by fever, with concentration of urine
   c. The presence of dysmorphic RBCs and RBC casts
   d. The presence of protein

4. Which of the following conditions is exhibited by this patient?
   a. Acute cystitis
   b. Acute drug-induced interstitial nephritis
   c. Acute glomerulonephritis
   d. Acute pyelonephritis

CASE STUDY 14-2

An 8-year-old girl complains of feeling like she needs to urinate all the time. Her urine burns when she does void, and it is cloudy. She is seen at her pediatrician's office, where urine is collected for routine urinalysis and culture. The following urinalysis results were obtained:

Physical Appearance
Color: Pale
Transparency: Cloudy

Chemical Screening
pH: 7.5
Specific gravity: 1.010
Protein (reagent strip): Trace
Protein (SSA): Trace
Blood: Negative
Nitrite: Positive
Leukocyte esterase: Positive
Glucose: Negative
Ketones: Negative
Bilirubin: Negative
Urobilinogen: Normal

Microscopic Examination
Red blood cells: 0-2 per hpf

White blood cells: 50-100 per hpf; clumps of white cells seen

Casts: None seen

Crystals: Moderate amorphous phosphates

Bacteria: Many rods

1. The positive reagent strip test for nitrite in this patient is probably caused by which of the following?
   a. An infection from gram-negative bacteria
   b. An infection from gram-positive bacteria
   c. A yeast infection
   d. An old urine specimen, unsuitable for examination

2. The positive reagent strip test for leukocyte esterase in this patient is caused by the presence of which of the following?
   a. Bacteria
   b. Protein
   c. Red blood cells
   d. White blood cells

3. This patient's alkaline pH is caused by the presence of which of the following?
   a. Bacteria
   b. Leukocyte esterase
   c. Nitrite
   d. Protein

4. This patient's proteinuria is probably caused by which of the following?
   a. Glomerular damage
   b. Lower urinary tract infection
   c. Prerenal disorders
   d. Upper urinary tract infection

5. Which of the following conditions is exhibited by this patient?
   a. Acute cystitis
   b. Acute drug-induced interstitial nephritis
   c. Acute glomerulonephritis
   d. Acute pyelonephritis

CASE STUDY 14-3

A 45-year-old man has been a paraplegic since being involved in a motorcycle accident 20 years ago. He has a history of recurrent urinary tract infections (UTIs) as a result of infection from an indwelling catheter. He now has severe back pain, with fever, chills, and vomiting. He has been exposed to "the flu" and seeks medical attention. A midstream urine specimen is collected for examination and culture. The following routine urinalysis results were obtained:

Physical Appearance

Color: Yellow

Transparency: Cloudy

Chemical Screening

pH: 6.5

Specific gravity: 1.010

Protein (reagent strip): 100 mg/dL

Protein (SSA): 2+

Blood: Moderate

Nitrite: Negative

Leukocyte esterase: Positive

Glucose: Negative

Ketones: Negative

Bilirubin: Negative

Urobilinogen: Normal

Microscopic Examination

Red blood cells: 2-5 per hpf

White blood cells: 10-25 per hpf

Casts: 5-10 WBC casts per lpf

Bacteria: Moderate rods

1. This patient's proteinuria is probably caused by which of the following?
   a. Glomerular damage
   b. Lower urinary tract disorders
   c. Prerenal disorders
   d. Tubular (or interstitial) damage

2. Concerning the positive leukocyte esterase and the negative nitrite in this patient, which of the following statements is correct?
   a. The leukocyte esterase test is probably a false-positive reaction.
   b. The negative nitrite reaction is probably caused by insensitivity of the test or lack of sufficient incubation of urine in the bladder.
   c. The positive leukocyte esterase reaction indicates that an upper UTI is present.
   d. The presence of a bacterial infection is ruled out because of the negative nitrite reaction.

3. Concerning the positive reagent strip test for blood and the relatively low level of RBCs seen in the urine sediment of this patient, which of the following statements is correct?
   a. The presence of hematuria is not consistent with the disease exhibited by this patient.
   b. The presence of protein is probably interfering with the chemical test for blood.
   c. The reagent strip test is extremely sensitive and consistent with the microscopic findings.
   d. The reagent strip test is probably falsely positive because of the presence of ascorbic acid.

4. The presence of white blood cells, bacteria, and cellular casts in this urine specimen indicate which of the following?
   a. UTI located in the kidney
   b. UTI located in the bladder
   c. An inflammatory condition of the urinary tract
   d. The presence of a kidney stone

5. In this patient, the cells present in the casts were probably derived from which of the following?
   a. Epithelial cells
   b. Lymphocytes
   c. Neutrophils
   d. Red blood cells

Continued

6. Which of the following conditions is exhibited by this patient?
   a. Acute cystitis
   b. Acute drug-induced interstitial nephritis
   c. Acute glomerulonephritis
   d. Acute pyelonephritis

CASE STUDY 14-4

A 12-year-old boy has a history of several infections in the past few months. He is now very lethargic and swollen, with generalized edema. He tells his mother that his urine is very foamy when he urinates and that he feels "awful." He is seen by his pediatrician, and urinalysis is performed with the following results:

Physical Appearance
Color: Pale
Transparency: Cloudy
Foam: Abundant white foam

Chemical Screening
pH: 6.0
Specific gravity: 1.010
Protein (reagent strip): >2000 mg/dL
Protein (SSA): 4+
Blood: Trace
Nitrite: Negative
Leukocyte esterase: Negative
Glucose: Negative
Ketones: Negative
Bilirubin: Negative
Urobilinogen: Negative

Microscopic Examination
Red blood cells: 0-2 per hpf
White blood cells: 0-2 per hpf
Casts: 5-10 fatty casts per lpf; 2-5 hyaline casts per lpf
Epithelial cells: Few renal epithelial cells; many oval fat bodies present
Other: Moderate free fat globules seen

1. The abundant white foam in this urine specimen is caused by the presence of which of the following?
   a. Blood
   b. Casts
   c. Fat
   d. Protein

2. The edema seen in this patient is caused by the presence of which of the following?
   a. Blood
   b. Casts
   c. Oval fat bodies
   d. Protein

3. The presence of fatty casts, oval fat bodies, renal epithelial cells, and free fat in this case indicates which of the following?
   a. A lower UTI
   b. An allergic reaction
   c. An upper UTI
   d. Severe renal dysfunction, probably glomerular

4. Which of the following conditions is exhibited by this patient?
   a. Acute drug-induced interstitial nephritis
   b. Acute glomerulonephritis
   c. Acute pyelonephritis
   d. Nephrotic syndrome

CASE STUDY 14-5

A 9-year-old boy has a history of a recent viral infection. He now feels faint and is feverish, and he is generally not well. He has to urinate frequently and is very thirsty. His breath smells fruity. He is seen in an urgent care clinic, where blood is drawn and urine collected for routine urinalysis. The following urinalysis results were obtained:

Physical Appearance
Color: Pale
Transparency: Clear

Chemical Screening
pH: 5.0
Specific gravity (refractometer): 1.029
Specific gravity (reagent strip): 1.005
Protein (reagent strip): Negative
Blood: Negative
Nitrite: Negative
Leukocyte esterase: Negative
Glucose: >2000 mg/dL
Ketones: Large
Bilirubin: Negative
Urobilinogen: Negative

Microscopic Examination
Red blood cells: 0-2 per hpf
White blood cells: 0-2 per hpf

1. The difference in the specific gravity values in this specimen is probably caused by which of the following?
   a. Ability of the refractometer to measure only nonionizing substances
   b. Difference in the principles of the methods
   c. Failure to use proper quality control
   d. Instrument error

2. This patient is at risk of losing consciousness as a result of which of the following?
   a. Diabetic coma
   b. Diabetic shock
   c. Infection
   d. Kidney failure

3. Which of the following conditions is exhibited by this patient?
   a. Anorexia nervosa
   b. Diabetes insipidus
   c. Diabetes mellitus
   d. Galactosemia

CASE STUDY 14-6

A 60-year-old man with a history of alcoholism is seen in an urgent care clinic; he complains of extreme pain in his upper abdomen. He has been experiencing pain on and off for the past 10 days. Now he is yellow (jaundiced) and feels extremely ill. He also mentions that his stool specimens have lost their normal color and look like clay. Blood is drawn for testing and urine collected for urinalysis. The following urinalysis results were obtained:

Physical Appearance
Color: Brown (yellow-brown)
Transparency: Clear
Foam: Abundant yellow foam

Chemical Screening
pH: 6.5
Specific gravity: 1.020
Protein (reagent strip): Negative
Blood: Negative
Nitrite: Negative
Leukocyte esterase: Negative
Glucose: Negative
Ketones: Negative
Bilirubin: Large
Urobilinogen: Normal

Microscopic Examination
Red blood cells: 0-2 per hpf
White blood cells: 0-2 per hpf

1. The abnormal urine color is caused by which of the following?
   a. Bilirubin
   b. Free bilirubin
   c. Unconjugated bilirubin
   d. Urobilinogen
   e. More than one of the above

2. The lack of color in the feces is caused by an absence of which of the following?
   a. Bilirubin glucuronide
   b. Free bilirubin
   c. Unconjugated bilirubin
   d. Urobilinogen

3. This patient's jaundice is the result of the presence of which of the following?
   a. Bilirubin glucuronide
   b. Unconjugated bilirubin
   c. Urobilinogen
   d. More than one of the above

4. From the patient history and the urinalysis, this patient's jaundice is probably the result of which of the following?
   a. Acute alcoholism leading to a cirrhotic liver
   b. Hemolytic jaundice
   c. Infectious hepatitis
   d. Obstructive jaundice associated with gallstones

REFERENCES

1. Angeletti LR, Gazzaniga V: Theophilus' Auctoritas: the role of De urinis in the medical curriculum of the 12th-13th centuries, Am J Nephrol 19:165–171, 1999.
2. Stankovic AK, DiLauri E: Quality improvements in the Pre-analytical phase: focus on urine specimen workflow, Clin Lab Med (vol. 28), no. 2, 339–350, 2008.
3. Ringsrud KM, Linné JJ: Urinalysis and body fluids: a color text and atlas, St Louis, 1995, Mosby, pp 25-27. This section is reprinted with permission.
4. Clinical and Laboratory Standards Institute: Routine urinalysis and collection, transportation, and preservation of urine specimens: approved guideline, ed 2, Wayne, PA, 2001, GP16-A2.
5. Clinical and Laboratory Standards Institute: Urinalysis and collection, transportation, and preservation of urine specimens: approved guideline, ed 2, Wayne, PA, 2001, CLSI Document GP16-A2, pp 4, 7, 10–12.
6. Skobe C: The basics of specimen collection and handling of urine testing, Lab Notes 14(2), 2004 (http://www.bd.com/vacutainer/labnotes/Volume14Number2/ Retrieved May 2005).
7. Cohen HT, Spiegel DM: Air-exposed urine dipsticks give false-positive results for glucose and false-negative results for blood, Am J Clin Pathol 96:398, 1991.
8. Schweitzer SS, Schumann JL, Schumann GB: Quality assurance guideline of the urinalysis laboratory, J Med Technol 3(11):569, 1986.
9. Drug package insert, West Point, PA, 1996, Merck & Co.

BIBLIOGRAPHY

Bayer Health Care Diagnostics Division: Modern urine chemistry, Tarrytown, NY, 2004, Bayer HealthCare.
Brunzel NA: Fundamentals of urine and body fluid analysis, ed 2, Philadelphia, 2004, Saunders.
Busby DE, Atkins RC: The detection and measurement of microalbuminuria: a challenge for clinical chemistry, Med Lab Obs 37(2):8, 2005.
College of American Pathologists: Clinical microscopy (glossary of terms). In 1996 Proficiency Testing Program, Northfield, IL, 1996, The College, p 12.
Haber MH: A primer of microscopic urinalysis, ed 2, Garden Grove, Calif, 1991, Hycor Biomedical.
Haber MH: Urine casts: their microscopy and clinical significance, ed 2, Chicago, 1976, American Society of Clinical Pathologists.
Haber MH: Urinary sediment: a textbook atlas, Chicago, 1981, American Society of Clinical Pathologists.
Henry JB, Lauzon RL, Schumann GB: Basic examination of urine. In Henry JB, editor: Clinical diagnosis and management by laboratory methods, ed 21, Philadelphia, 2008, Saunders.
Kaplan LA, Pesce AJ: Clinical chemistry: theory, analysis, and correlation, ed 5, St Louis, 2010, Mosby.
Mahon CR, Smith LA: Standardization of the urine microscopic examination, Clin Lab Sci 3:328, 1990.
Nikon Microscopy: http://www.microscopyu.com/articles/polarized/polarizedintro.html (retrieved August 2005).

Pietrach CA, et al: Comparison of the Hoesch and Watson-Schwartz tests for urinary porphobilinogen, Clin Chem 23:166, 1977.

Schneider's Children's Hospital at North Shore, Department of Urology: http://www.schneiderchildrenshospital.org/peds_html_fixed/peds/urology/urinaryant.htm. Retrieved August 2005.

Schumann GB: Urine sediment examination, Baltimore, 1980, Williams & Wilkins.

Schumann GB, Schumann JL, Marcussen N: Cytodiagnostic urinalysis of renal and lower urinary tract disorders, New York, 1995, Igaku-Shoin Medical Publishers.

REVIEW QUESTIONS

1. **The parts or a part of a routine urinalysis are (is):**
   a. physical.
   b. chemical.
   c. microscopic.
   d. all of the above.

2. **The formation of urine begins in the:**
   a. nephron.
   b. glomerulus.
   c. ureter.
   d. bladder.

3. **The principal end product of protein metabolism in the urine is:**
   a. uric acid.
   b. creatinine.
   c. glucose.
   d. urea.

Questions 4-8: Match the following descriptions of urine volume with their appropriate definitions (a to e).

4. ___ **Anuria**

5. ___ **Diuresis**

6. ___ **Nocturia**

7. ___ **Oliguria**

8. ___ **Polyuria**
   a. Any increase in urine volume, even temporary
   b. Complete absence of urine formation
   c. Consistent elimination of 2000 mL urine per 24 hours
   d. Excretion of 500 mL urine per 24 hours
   e. Excretion of 400 mL urine at night

Questions 9-18: Match the following abnormal urine colors with their causes (a to j).

9. ___ **Amber**

10. ___ **Black (or brown) on standing**

11. ___ **Bright orange**

12. ___ **Brown (yellow-brown or green-brown)**

13. ___ **Clear red**

14. ___ **Cloudy red**

15. ___ **Dark red or red-purple**

16. ___ **Dark red-brown**

17. ___ **Orange (orange-red or orange-brown)**

18. ___ **Pale**
    a. Bilirubin
    b. Concentrated urine
    c. Dilute urine
    d. Hemoglobin
    e. Melanin or homogentisic
    f. Myoglobin
    g. AZO-containing dye
    h. Porphyrins
    i. Red blood cells (hematuria)
    j. Urobilin

19. **A urine specimen with a strong ammonia odor is most often the result of:**
    a. diabetes mellitus.
    b. improper handling and storage.
    c. ingestion of certain foodstuffs.
    d. urinary tract infection.

Questions 20-23: Indicate whether the following statements concerning specific gravity are A = True or B = False.

20. ___ If the kidney is unable to concentrate or dilute urine, the specific gravity will be fixed at about 1.010.

21. ___ Reagent strips for specific gravity and the refractometer measure different things.

22. ___ Reagent strips measure any substance that is dissolved in the urine.

23. ___ Specific gravity is a measure of the amount of dissolved substances in solution.

Questions 24-28: Indicate whether the following statements concerning the measurement of urine pH are A = True or B = False.

Urine pH:

24. ___ Is an indicator of proteinuria

25. ___ Is helpful in the identification of crystals in the urine

26. ___ Is unaffected by diet

27. ___ Is useful in the assessment of specimen acceptability for examination

28. ___ May be used as an indication of urinary tract infection

29. Detection of which of the following urine constituents is most helpful in the detection and diagnosis of renal disease?
    a. Blood
    b. Leukocyte esterase
    c. Nitrite
    d. Protein

Questions 30-33: Match the following protein types with the following statements (a to e).

30. ___ Albumin

31. ___ Globulin

32. ___ Hemoglobin

33. ___ Light-chain immunoglobulins (Bence Jones protein)
    a. Associated with gammaglobulinopathies such as multiple myeloma
    b. May be seen in urine as the result of intravascular hemolysis
    c. Molecule is generally too large to be filtered through the glomerulus
    d. The protein most often associated with glomerular damage

34. The reagent strip test for protein is most likely to show a positive reaction with which of the following?
    a. Albumin
    b. Hemoglobin
    c. Light-chain immunoglobulins
    d. Both a and b

35. Which of the following is not detected by the reagent strip test for blood?
    a. Hemoglobin
    b. Hemosiderin
    c. Myoglobin
    d. Red blood cells

36. Reagent strip tests that depend on the release of oxygen and subsequent oxidation of a chromogen, resulting in a color change, are subject to false-negative reactions because of the presence of:
    a. ascorbic acid.
    b. azo-containing drugs or compounds.
    c. chlorine bleach.
    d. low specific gravity.

Questions 37-41: Indicate whether the following statements concerning the reagent strip test for nitrite in the urine are A = True or B = False.

37. ___ Tests for nitrite tend to be positive when large numbers of gram-positive bacteria are present.

38. ___ Tests for nitrite tend to be positive when large numbers of gram-negative bacteria are present.

39. ___ Negative reactions for nitrite rule out the presence of urinary tract infection.

40. ___ Results are most useful if positive, as an indicator of urinary tract infection.

41. ___ Results may be falsely negative in the presence of severe urinary tract infection by gram-negative organisms in starving, fasting, or hospitalized patients being fed intravenously.

42. Reagent strip tests for urinary leukocyte esterase are most useful in the detection of:
    a. immunosuppression.
    b. malignancy.
    c. renal transplant rejection.
    d. urinary tract infection.

43. Reagent strip tests for urinary leukocyte esterase are most useful when results are evaluated together with the results for the reagent strip test for:
    a. blood.
    b. nitrite.
    c. protein.
    d. specific gravity.

44. A positive reagent strip test for glucose is most often associated with which of the following conditions?
    a. Anorexia nervosa
    b. Diabetes insipidus
    c. Diabetes mellitus
    d. Starvation

Questions 45-47: Indicate whether the following statements concerning bilirubin and urobilinogen are A = True or B = False.

45. ___ In cases of obstructive jaundice, urine bilirubin and urobilinogen are both increased.

46. ___ Increased urine urobilinogen is associated with hemolytic jaundice and liver disease.

47. ___ Jaundice results from the presence of an increased concentration of any form of bilirubin in the blood.

Questions 48-57: Match the following urine constituents with the classic test principles (a to i). Test principles may have more than one constituent.

48. ___ Bilirubin

49. ___ Blood

50. ___ Glucose

51. ___ Ketones

52. ___ Leukocyte

53. ___ Nitrite

54. ___ pH

55. ___ Protein

56. ___ Reducing sugars

57. ___ Specific gravity
   a. Copper reduction test
   b. Diazo reaction
   c. Double-pH indicator system
   d. Enzyme reaction based on glucose oxidase
   e. Measures esterase
   f. Peroxidase activity of heme
   g. pK$_a$ change of polyelectrolytes (ionic concentration)
   h. Protein error of indicators
   i. Reaction with sodium nitroprusside

Question 58-60: *Match the following microscopic findings with the statements concerning red blood cells (a to c).*

58. ___ Dysmorphic red cells

59. ___ Hematuria

60. ___ Shadow or swollen red cells
   a. A sensitive early indicator of renal disease
   b. Distorted or misshapen red cells that may indicate glomerular damage
   c. Presence associated with dilute or hypotonic urine

Questions 61-68: *Match the leukocytes or epithelial cells with the following statements (a to i).*

61. ___ Eosinophils

62. ___ Glitter cells

63. ___ Lymphocytes

64. ___ Neutrophils (PMNs)

65. ___ Oval fat bodies

66. ___ Renal epithelial cells

67. ___ Squamous epithelial cells

68. ___ Transitional epithelial cells
   a. Indicate active kidney disease or tubular injury
   b. May be seen with infection and after urethral catheterization
   c. Presence an early indicator of renal transplant rejection

   d. Presence associated with drug-induced interstitial nephritis
   e. Presence associated with the nephrotic syndrome
   f. Presence usually indicates vaginal contamination
   g. Swollen neutrophils exhibiting brownian motion; associated with hypotonic urine; specific gravity 1.010
   h. Type of leukocyte most often seen in urine; indicates inflammation somewhere in the urogenital tract

69. **The presence of which of the following types of casts has the least clinical significance?**
   a. Fatty
   b. Granular
   c. Hyaline
   d. Red or white blood cell
   e. Waxy

Questions 70-75: *Match the following type of casts with the disease states or conditions (a to h).*

70. ___ Epithelial cell cast

71. ___ Fatty cast

72. ___ Hyaline or granular cast

73. ___ Red blood cell cast

74. ___ Waxy cast

75. ___ White blood cell cast
   a. Acute glomerulonephritis
   b. Acute pyelonephritis
   c. Chronic renal disease or renal failure
   d. Nephrotoxic poisoning
   e. Diabetic nephropathy
   f. CMV infection
   g. Strenuous exercise

Questions 76-90: *Indicate whether the following statements concerning crystals found in the urine sediment are A = True or B = False.*

76. ___ Ammonium biurate crystals are a common finding in freshly voided alkaline urine.

77. ___ Cystine is an abnormal crystal that can be associated with stone formation.

78. ___ Hemosiderin may be seen as free granules in cells or casts several days after an acute hemolytic episode.

79. ___ Most abnormal crystals are seen in urine of an alkaline pH.

80. ___ Most crystals seen in urine exhibit birefringence.

81. ___ Most kidney or bladder stones are made up of calcium oxalate or a calcium-containing compound.

82. ___ The amorphous material seen in alkaline urine is amorphous urate.

83. ___ The crystalline form of cholesterol (large, flat, hexagonal plate) is a common finding seen in most cases of the nephrotic syndrome.

84. ___ The identification of normal crystals is based primarily on the urine pH and the morphology of the crystal.

85. ___ The presence of abnormal crystals requires confirmation before they are reported.

86. ___ The presence of crystals is most significant when they are seen in an absolutely fresh urine specimen.

87. ___ The presence of crystals of the sulfonamides is a common finding in the urine and is of no clinical significance.

88. ___ The use of phase-contrast microscopy is especially helpful in the identification of urine crystals.

89. ___ The use of polarizing microscopy is not particularly helpful in the identification of urine crystals.

90. ___ Uric acid crystals in the urine sediment indicate that the patient probably has gout.

Questions 91-94: Match the type of urine specimen with the appropriate statement or application.

91. ___ Random

92. ___ First morning

93. ___ Midstream

94. ___ 24-hour specimen
   a. Contains high level of analytes and cellular elements
   b. Preferred for culture and sensitivity testing
   c. Used for substances affected by diurnal variation
   d. Most common type of specimen collected

95. When urine decomposes, the pH:
   a. becomes more alkaline.
   b. becomes more acidic.
   c. does not change.

96. Urine can be refrigerated for __ hours after collection with no gross alterations.
   a. 2
   b. 4
   c. 6
   d. 8

97. The preservative that allows urine to be kept at room temperature with results comparable to refrigeration is:
   a. hydrochloric acid.
   b. boric acid.
   c. toluene.
   d. all of the above.

CHAPTER 15

EXAMINATION OF BODY FLUIDS AND MISCELLANEOUS SPECIMENS

Learning Objectives

At the conclusion of this chapter, the student will be able to:

- Define *cerebrospinal fluid*, and describe the components of routine examination, including gross examination, cell counts, morphologic examination, and common chemical tests.

- Differentiate a traumatic tap from a hemorrhage on the basis of gross appearance of the spinal fluid.

- Identify the serous fluids, and describe the components of their routine examination.

- Define the term *effusion*, and differentiate a transudate from an exudate.

- Define *synovial fluid*, and describe the components of its routine examination.

- Describe and perform the microscopic examination of synovial fluid for gout and pseudogout, using compensated polarizing microscopy for the identification of crystals.

- Describe the components of a semen analysis.

- Describe the function and properties of amniotic fluid.

- Name three types of studies of saliva.

OVERVIEW OF BODY FLUIDS

Sterile body fluid can be found in various body cavities under normal conditions. In various disorders and diseases, the quantity of these fluids can increase significantly. Fluid specimens aspirated from different anatomic sites (Table 15-1) can be analyzed for the total number of red and white blood cells, differentiation of white blood cell types, chemical composition, and microorganisms. Standard Precautions must be practiced when handling all types of body fluids.

The type of examination performed on the body fluid depends on the source of the specimen. The specimen must be fresh. Cell counts cannot be done on a clotted specimen; anticoagulants must be used to prevent coagulation of the specimen when a cell count is needed. Aliquots of many types of specimens, such as cerebrospinal fluid, are sent to a particular division of the clinical laboratory: hematology, chemistry, microbiology, immunology, or cytology.

CEREBROSPINAL FLUID

Cerebrospinal fluid (CSF) acts as a shock absorber for the brain and spinal cord, circulates nutrients, lubricates the central nervous system (CNS), and may contribute to the nourishment of brain tissue. CSF is found inside all the ventricles, in the central canal of the spinal cord, and in the subarachnoid space around both the brain and the spinal cord (Fig. 15-1).

CSF specimens must be immediately delivered to the laboratory for examination. The four or five collection tubes must be handled using Standard Precautions. Tubes are designated for routine testing in hematology, microbiology, clinical chemistry, and immunology/serology.

CSF is normally clear, colorless, and sterile. The average, healthy adult has 90 to 150 mL of CSF, and the newborn infant, 10 to 60 mL. CSF has four main functions:

1. Serves as a mechanical buffer that prevents trauma
2. Regulates the volume of the intracranial contents
3. Provides nutrient medium for the central nervous system (CNS)
4. Acts as an excretory channel for metabolic products of the CNS

A physician performs a spinal tap, or lumbar puncture (LP), only if serious diagnostic concerns exist, because LP involves potential harm to the patient. Indications for LP are:

- Diagnosis of meningitis (bacterial, fungal, mycobacterial, amebic)
- Diagnosis of hemorrhage (subarachnoid, intracerebral, cerebral infarct)
- Diagnosis of neurologic disease (e.g., multiple sclerosis, demyelinating disorders, Guillain-Barré syndrome)
- Diagnosis and evaluation of suspected malignancy (e.g., leukemia, lymphoma, metastatic carcinoma)
- Introduction of drugs, radiographic contrast media, and anesthetics

The greatest risk of LP involves paralysis or death resulting from tonsillar herniation in patients with increased intracranial pressure. LP also carries a risk of infection.

CSF differs from serous and synovial fluids because of the selective permeability of the membranes and adjacent tissues containing CSF. This is referred to as the *blood-brain barrier*. As a result, CSF is not an ultrafiltrate of plasma. Rather, active transport occurs among the blood, CSF, and brain in both directions, giving differing concentrations of substances in each direction.

Many drugs do not enter CSF from the blood. Electrolytes such as sodium, magnesium, and chloride are more concentrated in spinal fluid than in plasma or plasma ultrafiltrates, whereas bicarbonate, glucose, and urea are less concentrated in CSF. Protein enters CSF in very small amounts. Very few cells are found in normal spinal fluid.

Collection of Cerebrospinal Fluid

A certain degree of risk to the patient is inherent in the procedure for obtaining a specimen of spinal fluid. These specimens must be handled with the utmost care. In general practice, three or four

T A B L E 1 5 - 1

Body Fluids	
Fluid	Synonyms
Bronchoalveolar lavage	Bronchial washings
Cerebrospinal fluid	Spinal fluid Lumbar puncture fluid Ventricular fluid Meningeal fluid
Peritoneal fluid	Dialysate fluid Paracentesis fluid Ascitic fluid
Pericardial fluid	Fluid from around the heart Pericardiocentesis fluid
Pleural fluid	Chest fluid Thoracic fluid Thoracentesis fluid
Seminal fluid	Semen
Synovial fluid	Joint fluid

sterile tubes containing about 5 mL each are collected during the spinal tap. These tubes are numbered in sequence of collection and immediately brought to the laboratory. In some cases, four tubes may not be collected, as with neonates or babies or a problematic tap.

The opening pressure is measured as the LP is done. It is important that any cell count or glucose determinations be done as soon as possible after collection to prevent deterioration of cells and potentially decreased glucose concentrations. As with other body fluids, CSF is potentially infectious, and it must always be collected and handled using Standard Precautions. CSF specimens may be highly infectious and should be treated with extreme care.

The tubes that are sequentially collected and labeled in order of collection are generally dispersed. The order for analysis (after gross examination of all tubes) may differ from one institution to another. Each laboratory has a protocol for the processing of spinal fluid. Students and new staff members need to familiarize themselves with the established protocol for that laboratory.

An example of a sequence is :

Tube 1: Chemical tests

Tube 2: Microbiology studies

Tube 3: Total cell counts and differential cell count

Tube 4: Immunology/serology studies and repeat RBC

Routine Examination of Cerebrospinal Fluid

Gross Appearance

All tubes collected by LP are evaluated as to gross appearance. Normal CSF is crystal clear and looks similar to distilled water. Color and clarity are noted by holding the sample beside a tube of water against a clean white paper or a printed page.

TURBIDITY

Slight haziness in the specimen or turbidity may indicate an increased white blood cell (WBC) count.

Turbidity in spinal fluid may result from the presence of large numbers of leukocytes (WBCs) or from bacteria, increased protein, or lipid. If radiographic contrast media have been injected, the CSF will appear oily, and when mixed, turbid. This artifactual turbidity is not reported.

CLOTS

In addition to the gross observations of turbidity and color, CSF should be examined for clotting. Clotting can result from increased protein. Gel formation on standing is caused by an increased fibrinogen content resulting from a "traumatic tap." Rarely, clotting may be associated with subarachnoid block or meningitis.

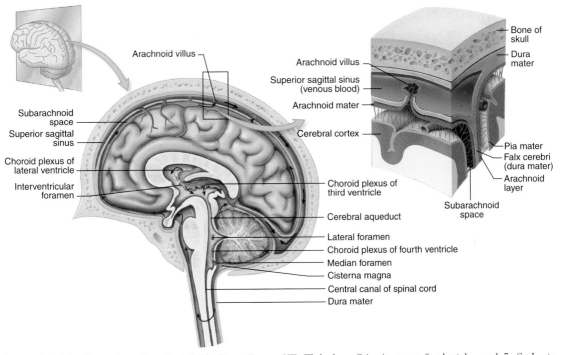

FIGURE 15-1 **Flow of cerebrospinal fluid.** (From Patton KT, Thibodeau GA: Anatomy & physiology, ed 7, St Louis, 2010, Mosby.)

COLOR

Bloody fluid can result from a traumatic tap or from subarachnoid hemorrhage. Any presence of color should be noted. If blood in a CSF specimen results from a traumatic tap (inclusion of blood in the specimen from LP itself), the successive collection tubes will show less bloody fluid, eventually becoming clear. If blood in a specimen is caused by a subarachnoid hemorrhage, the color of the fluid will look the same in all the collection tubes. In addition, subarachnoid bleeding may be indicated by the presence of xanthochromia.

Xanthochromia

The presence of a pale pink to pale orange or yellow color in the supernatant CSF is called **xanthochromia.** It is the result of the release of hemoglobin from hemolyzed red blood cells (RBCs), which begins 1 to 4 hours after hemorrhage. Pale pink or pale orange xanthochromia caused by oxyhemoglobin peaks in 24 to 36 hours and gradually disappears in 4 to 8 days. Because hemolysis of RBCs will occur in vitro as well as in vivo, the examination for xanthochromia must be done within 1 hour of collection, or false-positive results will be obtained.

When the hemorrhage is old, the supernatant fluid will show **yellow xanthochromia.** The yellow color is caused by bilirubin, formed from hemoglobin from the lysed RBCs. This appears about 12 hours after a bleeding episode, peaks in 2 to 4 days, and gradually disappears in 2 to 4 weeks. When the CSF protein level is more than 150 mg/dL because of damage to the blood-brain barrier, a yellow color may be seen, similar to the color of normal serum or plasma.

Also, subarachnoid bleeding is associated with the microscopic observation of erythrophagia, which is the ingestion of RBCs by macrophages in the CSF.

Red and White Blood Cell Counts

Cell counts on CSF are usually performed using automated equipment. However, manual methods may be used under some circumstances (see Procedures in Chapter 12).

The viscosity of some body fluids (especially joint fluids), variations in cell size (especially when tumor cells are present), and background debris, which is generally higher than cell counts, can create problems when using automated equipment. Fluids can be contaminated with pathogenic microorganisms, and special disinfecting procedures and disposable equipment are employed to prevent contamination. Semiautomatic micropipettes may be used to prepare dilutions, and disposable counting chambers may be used. Traditional hemocytometers must be thoroughly disinfected after use.

Cell counts should be done as soon as possible after the specimen is obtained; cells lyse on prolonged standing, and the counts become invalid. If the cell count cannot be done immediately, the tubes should be refrigerated. At room temperature, 40% of WBCs will lyse in 2 hours. With refrigeration, WBC lysis is not prevented but reduced to 15%. With refrigeration, RBCs are relatively stable.[1]

Normally, there are no RBCs in CSF. The normal WBC count in CSF is 0 to 8 cells/µL. More than 10 cells/µL is considered abnormal. Increased WBC counts can be observed in infectious diseases (e.g., meningitis) and noninfectious conditions (e.g., trauma, multiple sclerosis).

Red Blood Cell Counts in Subarachnoid Hemorrhage

Most cases of subarachnoid hemorrhage are diagnosed by computed tomographic (CT) scanning of the brain. If the CT result is negative, a lumbar puncture for the analysis cerebrospinal fluid is frequently performed. The diagnosis of subarachnoid hemorrhage includes:

- Elevated opening pressure
- Presence of red blood cells
- Presence of xanthochromia

A CSF from a traumatic tap can complicate the diagnosis of subarachnoid hemorrhage. A current trend is to perform an RBC count on both the first and last CSF tubes collected (tube #1 and tube #4). When an abnormal number of RBCs is demonstrated in tube #1 but tube #4 exhibits a decreased RBC count, this is strong evidence for a traumatic tap. If a specimen shows incomplete clearing, this probably represents a likely traumatic tap that may or may not be superimposed on a subarachnoid hemorrhage.[1]

CYTOCENTRIFUGATION

Cytocentrifugation requires the use of a special cytocentrifuge such as the Cytospin (Shandon, Pittsburgh, Pa). It is a slow centrifugation method that provides better cell yield and morphologic preservation than ordinary centrifugation. The technique is relatively easy to learn and perform and gives an excellent yield with a small amount of sample. The sample is slowly centrifuged from 200 to 1000 rpm for 5 to 10 minutes. During centrifugation, the fluid portion of the specimen is absorbed into a filter paper, and the cellular portion is concentrated in a circle 6 mm in diameter on a microscope slide. The cytocentrifuged preparation is stained with Wright stain or with a variety of stains for hematologic or cytologic studies.

SMEARS FROM CENTRIFUGED SPINAL FLUID SEDIMENT

If a cytocentrifuge is not available, the CSF is centrifuged for 5 minutes at 3000 rpm. The supernatant is removed, and the sediment is used to prepare smears on glass slides. The smears are dried rapidly and stained with Wright stain. Recovery of cells is not as good as with other techniques, and the cells tend to be distorted or damaged.

OTHER CONCENTRATION TECHNIQUES

Special sedimentation methods and membrane filter techniques are also used. These are more time consuming and expensive than cytocentrifugation and require more technical expertise. These methodologies are typically unavailable in small hospital laboratories.

Morphologic Examination

The protocol for performing a differential cell count on CSF varies among laboratories. Some laboratories do differential counts on all specimens; others use a minimum total cell count benchmark before performing a cell differential. Counts may be done on a smear made from the centrifuged CSF sediment, using recovery with a filtration or sedimentation method, or preferably on a cytocentrifuged preparation.

DIFFERENTIAL CELL COUNT

Exactly 100 WBCs are counted and classified, and the percentage of each cell type is reported. Depending on the method of preparation, morphologic identification may be difficult. In some cases, cells can be identified only as "polynuclear" or "mononuclear." With other preparation techniques, identification is more specific. Any of the cells found in blood may be seen in CSF, including neutrophils, lymphocytes, monocytes, eosinophils, and basophils. A predominance of polynuclear cells usually indicates a bacterial infection (Fig. 15-2), whereas the presence of many mononuclear cells indicates a viral infection (Fig. 15-3).

In addition, cells that originate in the CNS may be seen. These include ependymal (Fig. 15-4), choroidal, and pia-arachnoid mesothelial (PAM) cells. If any tumor cells or unusual cells are encountered, the CSF specimen should be referred for cytologic examination.

Chemistry Tests

Several chemical determinations can be done on spinal fluid. The same chemical constituents are generally found in CSF and plasma, but because of the blood-brain barrier and selective filtration, normal CSF values are different from plasma values. Abnormal CSF values may result from alterations in the permeability of the blood-brain barrier or from production or metabolism by neural cells in various pathologic conditions. There are relatively few important CSF chemical findings. Some of the more routine analyses are described here.

PROTEIN

Protein tests and protein electrophoresis are common analyses and of diagnostic significance for a variety of conditions and disease states. Protein fractions in CSF are generally the same as in plasma, but the ratios vary. The normal CSF protein varies with methodology and site of collection, with a reference range of 12 to 60 mg/dL. Increased CSF protein levels are the most common pathologic finding and are seen with meningitis, hemorrhage, and multiple sclerosis. Low values are associated with leakage of fluid from the CNS

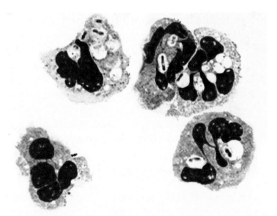

FIGURE 15-2 **CSF cells.** (From Carr JH, Rodak BF: Clinical hematology atlas, ed 3, St Louis, 2009, Saunders.)

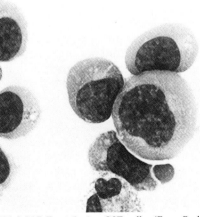

FIGURE 15-3 **CSF cells.** (From Rodak BF, Fritsma GA, Doig K: Hematology: clinical principles and applications, ed 3, St Louis, 2007, Saunders.)

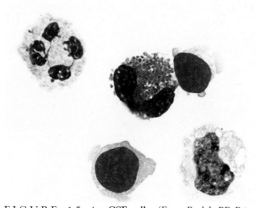

FIGURE 15-4 **CSF cells.** (From Rodak BF, Fritsma GA, Doig K: Hematology: clinical principles and applications, ed 3, St Louis, 2007, Saunders.)

because of damage to the blood-brain barrier. Electrophoresis may be done when evaluation of CSF protein fractions is needed.

GLUCOSE

The glucose level in spinal fluid should be measured immediately. It is about two-thirds of that in blood, but the amounts may vary. Both levels should be measured simultaneously because the difference between these values is clinically significant. Bacteria and cells utilize glucose. The glucose level in CSF is especially reduced in bacterial meningitis but not in viral meningitis, primary brain tumor, or vascular accidents. Glucose is decreased in metastatic tumor and insulin shock and elevated in diabetic coma.

LACTATE

Determination of lactate levels in CSF can be used in the diagnosis and management of meningitis, although its usefulness is controversial and method dependent. A lactate level greater than 25 mg/dL is seen in bacterial, fungal, and tubercular meningitis and is more consistent than a decrease in glucose level. The elevated serum lactate levels remain during initial treatment, but a fall indicates successful treatment. Increased lactate levels occur in oxygen deprivation and are seen in any condition involving decreased oxygen flow to the brain.

Microbiological Examination

Gram stain and culture are done. CSF specimens are normally sterile. Gram stain is most useful in the diagnosis of acute bacterial meningitis because the organisms can actually be seen in the Gram-stained specimen. Tuberculosis (acid-fast stain) and *Cryptococcus* infections (India ink preparations) may also be detected with microscopic

examination of the spinal fluid. CSF cultures, both bacterial and viral, may be part of the routine protocol.

Serology Tests

The Venereal Disease Research Laboratories (VDRL) test is a well-known serologic test for syphilis that is done on spinal fluid. The fluorescent treponemal antibody absorption (FTA-ABS) test is more sensitive but less specific.

SEROUS FLUIDS (PERICARDIAL, PLEURAL, AND PERITONEAL)

The fluids of the pericardial, pleural, and peritoneal cavities are called **serous fluids.** They normally are formed continuously in the body cavities and are reabsorbed, leaving only very small volumes. The normal appearance of these fluids is pale and yellow colored. The fluid becomes more turbid as the total cell count rises, an indication of inflammation. Increases in the amounts of these body cavity fluids formed are seen in inflammation and when the serum protein level falls.

Serous fluids are aspirated by a physician if they are mechanically inhibiting the function of the associated organs, as well as for diagnostic purposes. The specimen is collected into various containers, depending on the laboratory testing to be done. An EDTA tube is used for cell counts and smear evaluation, sterile tubes are used for cultures, and oxalate or fluoride tubes for protein, glucose, or other chemistry tests. If a large volume of fluid is aspirated, it is collected in a container with an appropriate additive to prevent clotting. If the fluid clots, it is useless for many analyses.

Serous fluids have a composition similar to serum and are the fluids contained within the closed cavities of the body. These cavities are lined by a contiguous membrane that forms a double layer of mesothelial cells called the *serous membrane.* The cavities are the pleural, pericardial, and peritoneal cavities. A small amount of serous fluid fills the space between the two layers and serves to lubricate the surfaces of these membranes as they move against each other. The fluids are ultrafiltrates of plasma that are continuously formed and reabsorbed, leaving only a very small volume within the cavities. An increased volume of any of these fluids is referred to as an **effusion.**

Transudates and Exudates

Normal serous fluids are formed as an ultrafiltrate of plasma as it filters through the capillary endothelium and are called **transudates.** Normally, serum protein exerts colloidal osmotic pressure

TABLE 15-2

Differentiation of Serous Effusions: Transudate from Exudate*		
Observation or Test	Transudate	Exudate
Appearance	Watery, clear, pale yellow Does not clot	Cloudy, turbid, purulent, or bloody May clot (fibrinogen)
White cell count	Low, <1000/μL, with more than 50% mononuclear cells (lymphocytes, monocytes)	500-1000/μL or more, with increased polymorpho- nuclear neutrophil leukocytes (PMNs) Increased lymphocytes with tuberculosis or rheumatoid arthritis
Red cell count	Low, unless from a traumatic tap	>100,000/μL, especially with a malignancy
Total protein	<3 g/dL	>3 g/dL (or greater than half the serum level)
Lactate dehydrogenase	Low	Increased (>60% of the serum level because of cellular debris)
Glucose	Varies with serum level	Lower than serum level with some infections and high cell counts

Modified from Ringsrud KM, Linné JJ: Urinalysis and body fluids: a color text and atlas, St Louis, 1995, Mosby.
*Note that some values are variable between the two effusions. Clinical considerations must always be used in combination
with the laboratory findings.

and helps impair movement of fluid into the serous cavity. If plasma protein levels decrease, the colloidal osmotic pressure falls and effusion results as movement of the transudate into the serous cavity increases. Serous fluid formation is also affected by capillary pressure and permeability.

An increase in serous fluid volume (effusion) occurs in many conditions. In determining the cause of an effusion, it is helpful to determine whether the effusion is a transudate or an exudate. In general, the effusion is a transudate (ultrafiltrate of plasma) as the result of a systemic disease. An example of a transudate is ascites, an effusion into the peritoneal cavity, which might be caused by liver cirrhosis or congestive heart failure. Transudates may be the result of a mechanical disorder affecting movement of fluid across a membrane.

Exudates are usually effusions that result from an inflammatory response to conditions that directly affect the serous cavity. These inflammatory conditions include infections and malignancies.

Although it may be difficult to determine whether an effusion is a transudate or an exudate, the distinction is important from a practical standpoint. If the effusion is a transudate, further testing is generally unnecessary. If it is an exudate, however, further testing is required for diagnosis and treatment. If infection is suspected, Gram stain and culture are indicated; suspected malignancies might require cytologic tests and biopsy.

Serous effusions have been classified as transudates or exudates on the basis of the amount of protein. Generally, effusions with a total protein content less than 3 g/dL are considered transudates,

and those with a total protein more than 3 g/dL are exudates. Unfortunately, there is considerable overlap in separating the effusions. A more reliable method of separating transudates and exudates is the simultaneous measurement of the fluid and serum for protein and lactate dehydrogenase. Appearance of the fluid, cell counts, and spontaneous clotting are also useful in the differentiation. These findings are summarized in Table 15-2.

Description of Individual Serous Fluids

Pleural Fluid

Normally, about 1 to 10 mL of **pleural fluid** is moistening the pleural surfaces. It surrounds the lungs and lines the walls of the thoracic cavity. If inflammation occurs, plasma protein level falls, congestive heart failure is present, or lymphatic drainage decreases, there can be an abnormal accumulation of pleural fluid.

Pericardial Fluid

The pericardial space enclosing the heart normally contains about 25 to 50 mL of a clear, straw-colored ultrafiltrate of plasma called **pericardial fluid.** This fluid forms continually and is reabsorbed by the nearby lymph vessels (lymphatics), leaving a small but constant volume. When an abnormal accumulation of pericardial fluid occurs, it fills up the space around the heart and can mechanically inhibit the normal action of the heart (cardiac tamponade). In these patients, immediate aspiration of the excess fluid is indicated.

Peritoneal Fluid

Normally, less than 100 mL of clear, straw-colored **peritoneal fluid** is present in the peritoneal cavity (abdominal and pelvic cavities). An abnormal accumulation of peritoneal fluid is indicated by severe abdominal pain and may be caused by a ruptured abdominal organ, hemorrhage resulting from trauma, postoperative complications, or an unknown condition. The excess fluid is aspirated. Such an accumulation must always be considered in the light of other findings.

Collection of Serous Fluids

Serous fluids are collected under strictly antiseptic conditions. The aspiration may be for diagnostic purposes or for mechanical reasons to prevent an excess accumulation of fluid from inhibiting the actions of the lungs or heart. A pleural effusion may compress the lungs, a pericardial effusion may cause cardiac tamponade, and ascites (peritoneal effusion) may elevate the diaphragm, compressing the lungs. At least three anticoagulated tubes of fluid are generally collected and used as follows:

1. Ethylenediaminetetraacetic acid (EDTA) tube for gross appearance, cell counts, morphology, and differential
2. Suitably anticoagulated tube (e.g., heparin) for chemical analysis
3. Sterile heparinized tube for Gram's stain and culture

Additional tubes, or the entire collection with a suitable preservative, are collected for cytologic examination for tumor cells. Sequentially collected tubes are observed for a possible traumatic tap.

In some extreme cases, fluid may be collected into a sterile bag containing anticoagulant or a suitable preservative and transported to the laboratory for examination.

Routine Examination of Serous Fluids

The routine examination of serous fluids generally includes an observation of gross appearance; cell counts, morphology, and differential; and Gram stain and culture. Certain chemical analyses and cytologic examination for tumor cells and tumor markers are performed when indicated.

Gross Appearance

Normal serous fluid is pale and straw colored; this is the color seen in a transudate. Turbidity increases as the number of cells and the amount of debris increase. An abnormally colored fluid may appear milky (chylous or pseudochylous), cloudy, or bloody on gross observation. A cloudy serous fluid is often associated with an inflammatory reaction, either bacterial or viral. Blood-tinged fluid may result from a traumatic tap, and grossly bloody fluid may be seen when an organ (e.g., spleen, liver) or a blood vessel has ruptured. Bloody fluids are also seen after myocardial infarction and in malignant disease states, tuberculosis, rheumatoid arthritis, and systemic lupus erythematosus.

Clotting

To observe the ability of the serous fluid to clot, the specimen must be collected in a plain tube with no anticoagulant. Ability of the fluid to clot indicates a substantial inflammatory reaction.

Red and White Blood Cell Counts

Cell counts are done on well-mixed anticoagulated serous fluid in a hemocytometer. The fluid may be undiluted or diluted, as indicated by the cell count. The procedure is essentially the same as that described for CSF red and white cell counts. If significant protein is present, acetic acid cannot be used as a diluent for WBC counts because of the precipitation of protein. In this case, saline may be used as a diluent, and the RBC and WBC counts are done simultaneously. The use of phase microscopy is helpful in performing these counts.

Leukocyte (WBC) counts greater than 500 cells/μL are usually clinically significant. If there is a predominance of neutrophils (polynuclear cells), bacterial inflammation is suspected. A predominance of lymphocytes suggests viral infection, tuberculosis, lymphoma, or malignancy. WBC counts greater than 1000/μL are associated with exudates.

Erythrocyte (RBC) counts greater than 10,000 cells/μL in pleural fluids may be seen in an effusion associated with malignancies, infarcts, and trauma.

Morphologic Examination and White Cell Differential

Morphologic examination and WBC differential for serous fluid are essentially the same as described for CSF. Again, slides prepared by cytocentrifugation are preferred to smears prepared after normal centrifugation. Slides are generally stained with Wright stain, and a differential cell count is done. The WBCs generally resemble those seen in peripheral blood, with the addition of mesothelial lining cells. Generally, 300 cells are counted and differentiated as to percentage of each cell type seen. If any malignant tumor cells are seen or appear to be present, the slide must be referred to a pathologist or qualified cytotechnologist.

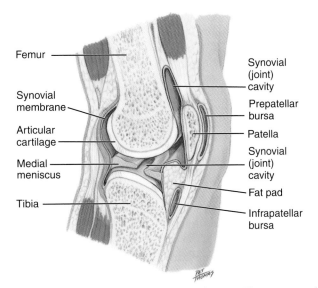

FIGURE 15-5 **Schematic representation of the knee.** (From Applegate E: The anatomy and physiology learning system, ed 2, Philadelphia, 2000, Saunders.)

Microbiological Examination

Microbiological examination will include Gram stain and culture on all body effusions of unknown etiology (see Chapter 16).

Chemical Analysis

PROTEIN

Total protein is measured in the fluid and the plasma. The level and ratio are helpful in distinguishing an exudate from a transudate. Protein electrophoresis is used in some cases.

LACTATE DEHYDROGENASE

Lactate dehydrogenase is also measured in the fluid and the plasma. The level and ratio, together with the total protein levels and ratios, are used to distinguish an exudate from a transudate. Increased levels are seen as a result of cellular debris from infection or malignancy.

GLUCOSE

In bacterial infections, serous fluids have a lower concentration of glucose than blood. Glucose level is decreased because bacteria use glucose as a metabolic substrate. Glucose determinations on serous fluids should be accompanied by a simultaneous blood glucose collection.

OTHER TESTS

Determinations of amylase, lipase, other enzymes, ammonia, and lipids, among others, are also done in various conditions.

SYNOVIAL FLUID

Synovial fluid is the fluid contained in joints (Fig. 15-5). Arthrocentesis constitutes a liquid biopsy of the joint. Normal joints have very little synovial fluid. Aspiration of this fluid from the joints by arthrocentesis provides information about joint diseases. A variety of disorders (e.g., rheumatoid arthritis, gout) produce changes in the number and types of cells, the chemical composition, and crystals in the fluid. In addition, arthrocentesis may alleviate elevated intraarticular pressure.

Synovial membranes line the joints, bursae, and tendon sheaths. Normal synovial fluid is an ultrafiltrate of plasma with the addition of a high-molecular-weight mucopolysaccharide called **hyaluronate** or **hyaluronic acid.** The presence of hyaluronate differentiates synovial fluid from other serous fluids and spinal fluid. Hyaluronic acid is responsible for the normal viscosity of synovial fluid, which serves to lubricate the joints so that they move freely. Hyaluronate is secreted by the synovial fluid cells (synoviocytes) that line the joint cavity. This normal viscosity is responsible for some difficulties in the examination of synovial fluid, especially in performing cell counts.

Normal Synovial Fluid

Normal synovial fluid is straw colored and viscous, resembling uncooked egg white. The word *synovial* comes from *syn,* "with," and *ovi,* "egg." About 1 mL of synovial fluid is present in each large joint such as the knee, ankle, hip, elbow, wrist, and shoulder.

In normal synovial fluid, the WBC count is low, less than 200 cells/µL, and the majority of the WBCs are mononuclear, with less than 25% neutrophils. RBCs and crystals are normally absent, and the fluid is sterile. Because the fluid is an **ultrafiltrate of plasma,** normal synovial fluid has essentially the same chemical composition as plasma without the larger protein molecules. A small amount of protein is secreted by the synovial cells, resulting in less than 3 g/dL of total protein.

Aspiration and Analysis

Synovial fluid differs from other body cavity fluids because of the importance of finding crystals in the specimen and because it is normally very viscous.

The aspiration and analysis of synovial fluid may be done to determine the cause of joint disease, especially when accompanied by an abnormal accumulation of fluid in the joint (effusion). The joint disease might be crystal induced, degenerative, inflammatory, or infectious. Morphologic analysis for cells and crystals, together with Gram stain and culture, will help in the differentiation. Aspiration is also done for effusions of unknown etiology and for pain or decreased joint mobility. Effusion of synovial fluid is usually present clinically before aspiration, and therefore it is often possible to aspirate 10 to 20 mL of the fluid for laboratory examination. The volume (normally about 1 mL) may be extremely small, however, so the laboratory receives only a drop of fluid in the aspiration syringe.

In the management of joint disorders, the differential diagnosis is essential so the correct treatment can be instituted. Analysis of synovial fluid can be invaluable in this diagnosis. It can give an immediate diagnosis in some disorders and provide valuable information on other joint diseases. If fluid volume or resources are limited, the most important aspects of analysis are microbiological study and an examination for crystals with compensated polarized light microscopy.

Classification of Synovial Fluid in Joint Disease

The differential diagnosis of diseased synovial fluid usually classifies the fluid as noninflammatory, inflammatory, infectious, crystal-induced, or hemorrhagic. Although the disease states in this grouping overlap, it is helpful.

Noninflammatory Fluid

Noninflammatory synovial fluid is seen in degenerative joint disease such as osteoarthritis, traumatic arthritis, and degenerative joint disease. The fluid is usually clear and viscous; WBC count is less than 2000 cells/µL, with less than 25% neutrophils. The glucose and protein contents are approximately the same as in normal synovial fluid. Collagen fibrils or cartilage fragments may be seen, especially with phase microscopy.

Inflammatory Fluid

Inflammatory effusions are associated with immunologic disease such as rheumatoid and lupus arthritis. The fluid is cloudy and yellow, has low viscosity, and has a moderately high WBC count—2000 to 20,000 cells/µL, with more than 50% neutrophils. The glucose content is normal, and the protein content is high. The fluid may form spontaneous fibrin clots.

Infectious Fluid

Infectious infusions suggest a bacterial infection. The fluid is generally cloudy and has low viscosity. The fluid may be yellow, green, or milky. WBC count is very high: 500 to 200,000 cells/µL, with more than 90% neutrophils. The glucose content is characteristically very low. The protein content is high, and fibrin clot formation is common. Most infections are bacterial. *Staphylococcus aureus* and *Neisseria gonorrhoeae* are the most common infecting agents, although streptococci, *Haemophilus*, tuberculosis, fungi, or anaerobic bacteria are also seen. The most common type of organism found varies with the age of the patient.

Crystal-Induced Fluid

Crystal-induced effusions are seen in gout and pseudogout. The fluid is yellow or turbid and has a fairly high but variable white cell count (500 to 200,000 cells/µL), with an increased percentage of neutrophils (up to 90%). Crystals of monosodium urate (MSU) are seen with gout, and calcium pyrophosphate dihydrate (CPPD) crystals with pseudogout. Crystals are recognized by morphology and appearance when examined by polarized microscopy, with the addition of a full-wave compensator.

Hemorrhagic Fluid

Hemorrhagic effusions are characterized by the presence of RBCs from bleeding or hemorrhage in the joint. This may be the result of traumatic injury (e.g., fracture) or tumor. Coagulation deficiencies (e.g., hemophilia) and treatment with anticoagulants may also result in hemorrhagic effusions.

Collection of Synovial Fluid

Synovial fluid is collected by needle aspiration, which is called **arthrocentesis.** It is done by experienced persons under strictly sterile conditions. The fluid is collected with a disposable needle and plastic syringe to avoid contamination with confusing birefringent material.

The fluid should be collected both anticoagulated and unanticoagulated. Ideally the fluid should be divided into the following three parts:

1. Sterile tube for microbiological examination
2. Tube with liquid EDTA (preferred) or sodium heparin for microscopic examination
3. Plain tube (without anticoagulant) for clot formation, gross appearance, and chemical and immunologic procedures; this should be a plain tube without a serum separator

Normal synovial fluid does not clot. To test for clot formation, the fluid must be collected in a plain tube without anticoagulant. However, infectious and crystal-induced fluids tend to form fibrin clots, making an anticoagulant necessary for adequate cell counts and an even distribution of cells and crystals for morphologic analysis. If an anticoagulant is used, sodium heparin or liquid EDTA is the additive of choice. There is some disagreement as to whether anticoagulated or plain tubes should be used for analysis of crystals; the decision may need to be individualized. Ideally, both tubes would be made available so that if artifactual anticoagulant crystals are suspected, the plain clot tube could be examined.

Although an anticoagulant will prevent the formation of fibrin clots, it will not affect viscosity. Therefore, if the fluid is highly viscous, it can be incubated for several hours with a 0.5% solution of hyaluronidase in phosphate buffer to break down the hyaluronate. This reduces the viscosity, making the fluid easier to pipette and count.

Routine Examination of Synovial Fluid

The routine examination of synovial fluid should include: (1) gross appearance (color, clarity, and viscosity); (2) microbiological studies; (3) WBC and differential cell counts; (4) polarizing microscopy for crystals; and (5) other tests as necessary. The most important tests are the microbiological studies, especially Gram stain, and crystal analysis. If the quantity of aspirated fluid is limited, these should be done first.

Gross Appearance

The first step in the analysis of synovial fluid is to observe the specimen for color and clarity. Noninflammatory fluid is usually clear. To test for clarity, read newspaper print through a test tube containing the specimen. As the cell and protein contents increase or crystals precipitate, the turbidity increases, and the print becomes more difficult to read. In a traumatic tap of the joint, blood will be seen in the collection tubes in an uneven distribution, which diminishes as the aspiration continues. It may also be seen as an uneven distribution with streaks of blood in the aspiration syringe. A truly bloody fluid is uniform in color and does not clot. Xanthochromia in the supernatant fluid indicates bleeding in the joint, but this is difficult to evaluate because the fluid is normally yellow. A dark red or dark brown supernatant is evidence of joint bleeding rather than a traumatic tap.

Viscosity

Viscosity is most easily evaluated at the time of arthrocentesis by allowing the synovial fluid to drop from the end of the needle. Normally, synovial fluid will form a string 4 to 6 cm in length. If it breaks before it reaches 3 cm in length, the viscosity is lower than normal. Inflammatory fluids contain enzymes that break down hyaluronic acid. Anything that decreases the hyaluronic acid content of synovial fluid lowers its viscosity.

Viscosity has been evaluated in the laboratory by means of the mucin clot test. However, this test is of questionable value, because results rarely change the diagnosis and are essentially the same as with the string test for viscosity.

Red and White Blood Cell Counts

The appearance of a drop of synovial fluid under an ordinary light microscope can be helpful in estimating the cell counts initially and in demonstrating the presence of crystals. The presence of only a few WBCs per high-power (×40) field suggests a noninflammatory disorder. A large number of WBCs would indicate inflammatory or infected synovial fluid.

The total WBC count and differential count are very important in diagnosis. When cells are counted in other fluids, such as blood, the usual diluting fluid is dilute acetic acid. This cannot be used with synovial fluid because it may cause mucin clotting. Instead, a solution of saline containing methylene blue is used. If it is necessary to lyse RBCs, either hypotonic saline or saponinized saline can be used as a diluent. The undiluted synovial fluid, or if necessary, suitably diluted fluid, is mounted in a hemocytometer and counted as described for CSF counts. Because acetic acid cannot be used as a diluent, both red and white cells are enumerated at the same time. This is most easily accomplished by using a phase-contrast rather than a brightfield microscope.

WBC counts less than 200 cells/µL, with less than 25% polymorphonuclear cells (neutrophils) and no RBCs, are normally observed in synovial fluid. Monocytes, lymphocytes, and macrophages are seen. A low WBC count (200 to 2000/µL) with predominantly mononuclear cells suggests a noninflammatory joint fluid, whereas a high WBC count suggests inflammation, and an extremely high count with a high proportion of polymorphonuclear cells strongly suggests infection.

Morphologic Examination

As with CSF, cytocentrifuged preparations of synovial fluid are preferred for the morphologic examination and WBC differential. These preparations may also be used for crystal identification. The procedure is generally the same as that described for CSF. Slides should be prepared as soon as possible after collection to prevent distortion and degeneration of cells. Digestion with hyaluronidase may be necessary with highly viscous fluids. If neutrophils are increased, they are especially prone to disintegration, making them difficult to recognize.

If a cytocentrifuge is not available, smears are made, as for CSF, from normally centrifuged sediment. Smears should be thin because hyaluronic acid will distort the cells. Smears are sometimes prepared from the fluid at the time of aspiration. The smears are air dried and stained with Wright stain.

Lupus erythematosus (LE) cells may be found in stained slides from patients with systemic lupus erythematosus and occasionally in fluid from patients with rheumatoid arthritis. The in vivo formation of LE cells in synovial fluid probably results from trauma to the WBCs.

Eosinophilia may be seen in metastatic carcinoma to the synovium, acute rheumatic fever, and rheumatoid arthritis. It is also associated with parasitic infections and Lyme disease and has also occurred after arthrography and radiation therapy.

Microscopic Examination for Crystals

A drop of synovial fluid is placed on a slide and a coverglass applied, as for the examination of urine sediment (see Chapter 14). To avoid confusion from extraneous particles that might polarize, it is recommended that slides and coverglasses be cleaned with alcohol and carefully dried with gauze or lens paper just before examination. It is also recommended that the coverglass be immediately sealed with clear fingernail polish to reduce drying from evaporation. If nail polish is used, the slide should be allowed to dry for 15 minutes before microscopic examination to prevent damage to the objective. An unsealed preparation can be examined during this waiting period if desired. Any crystals at the junction of the nail polish and synovial fluid should be ignored.

The unclotted synovial fluid is first examined with an ordinary brightfield or, preferably, phase-contrast microscope. Crystals are reported as being present or absent and, if they are present, as intracellular, extracellular, or both. The initial examination is followed by compensated polarized light microscopy. After examination of the wet preparation, a cytocentrifuged preparation may also be examined for the presence and identity of crystals.

BRIGHTFIELD OR PHASE-CONTRAST MICROSCOPIC EXAMINATION

Needle-shaped, intracellular MSU crystals seen in a simple wet preparation of synovial fluid are characteristic of gouty arthritis. Pseudogout, a crystal-deposition disease distinct from gout, is demonstrated by the presence of rhomboid CPPD crystals.

Cholesterol crystals are a rare finding in synovial fluid from persons with rheumatoid arthritis and are not seen in normal synovial fluid. Lipid crystals showing a Maltese cross formation with polarized light have also been reported as causing acute arthritis. These should not be confused with starch (a common contaminant) or with a rare form of MSU seen as a spherulite or "beachball."

Crystals of hydroxyapatite (HA) have been reported as causing apatite gout. They are too small to be seen with ordinary microscopy. Clumps of these crystals, however, may be seen as spherical microaggregates.

Crystals of calcium oxalate may occur in oxalate gout, in patients receiving chronic renal dialysis, or in the rare primary oxalosis.

Polyester fibers have been seen in the synovial fluid of patients who have had joint replacement, indicating deterioration of the artificial joint. These birefringent fibers are difficult to evaluate in the synovial fluid, especially on cytocentrifuged preparations that contain fibers derived from the filter paper.

Iatrogenic or extraneous crystals may be present in the synovial fluid. Starch might be introduced from gloves. These crystals show a Maltese cross pattern that might be confused with lipid droplets of cholesterol or spherulites of urates. Other substances lining gloves appear as tiny rectangles that might be mistaken for CPPD.

If the joint has been treated with corticosteroids, crystals may be seen that resemble both MSU and CPPD. The crystals are generally extracellular and show numbers significantly greater than is typical of MSU or CPPD, but identification without the clinical history is very difficult. Other substances that might be present and confusing are collagen fibrils, fibrin strands, and fragments of cartilage.

The crystals seen in synovial fluid are summarized in Tables 15-3 and 15-4.

POLARIZED LIGHT MICROSCOPY

More definitive microscopic identification of crystals in synovial fluid can be made with the use of polarized light (see Chapter 5). Both wet and cytocentrifuged preparations may be examined for the presence and identity of crystals. A polarizing microscope with a first-order red compensator (quartz compensator) is used. To set up the microscope, a polarizing filter (called a *polarizer*) is placed between the light source (bulb) and the specimen. A second polarizing filter (called an *analyzer*) is placed above the specimen, between the objective and the eyepiece. One of the polarizing filters (usually the polarizer) is rotated until the two are at right angles to each other. This is seen as the extinction of light through the microscope (one sees a black field because all light waves are canceled when the filters are at right angles to each other). This is diagrammed in Chapter 5, Fig. 5-11.

Certain objects or crystals have the ability to rotate or polarize light so they are visible when viewed through crossed polarizing filters. This property is called **birefringence,** and objects are termed *weakly birefringent* or *strongly birefringent* depending on how completely they polarize light. Strongly birefringent crystals appear bright (white) against a dark background; weakly birefringent crystals appear less bright.

Monosodium Urate

In synovial fluid, MSU crystals appear as strongly birefringent, needle-shaped or rod-shaped crystals from 1 to 30 μm in length (Fig. 15-6). They may be intracellular or extracellular, and this distinction is recorded. The presence of intracellular crystals is characteristic of acute gout; extracellular crystals imply a more chronic condition. Crystals from a tophus may be quite large. MSU crystals are found in almost 100% of patients with acute gouty arthritis and in 75% of those with chronic gout.

TABLE 15-3

Clinically Significant Crystals in Synovial Fluid					
Crystal	Morphology	Strength of Birefringence	Crystal Color When Parallel to Slow Wave	Crystal Size (μm)	Comments
MSU	Long, slender needles	Strong	Yellow	1-30	Seen in gout
CPPD	Short, chunky rectangles or rhomboids	Weak	Blue	1-20	Seen in pseudogout (or more)
Hydroxyapatite	Shiny clumps	Difficult to detect	N/A	0.5-1	Need electron microscope to visualize
Cholesterol plates	Large, flat, notched plates	Variable	Variable	10-100	Extremely rare, chronic effusion
Fat droplets (cholesterol)	Round spheres	Strong	Blue-yellow Maltese cross	2-15	Maltese cross appearance similar to starch
Cartilage fragments	Irregular	Strong	Variable	10-50	No definite crystal morphology
Polyethylene "wear" fragments	Long threads	Strong	Variable	Variable	Appearance similar to Cytospin filter paper fibers
Calcium oxalate	Bipyramidal (octahedrons)	Strong/variable	N/A	2-10	Seen in oxalate gout, especially with renal dialysis
Hematin	Vivid yellow-brown diamond shape	Weak	Might confuse with CPPD; use bright-field to avoid confusion	—	Seen 2-4 weeks after hemorrhage

CPPD, Calcium pyrophosphate dihydrate; *MSU,* monosodium urate; *N/A,* not applicable.

TABLE 15-4

			Crystal Color		
		Strength of	When Parallel		
Crystal	Morphology	Birefringence	to Slow Wave	Crystal Size (µm)	Comments
Corticosteroids	Variable Similar to MSU with blunt, jagged edges	Strong	Yellow	2-15 or more; variable	Common artifact from injection Solution in alcohol Polarize like MSU Appear similar to MSU or CPPD
Starch	Variable Globule with irregular edges and central dimple Similar to tiny CPPD	Strong	Blue-yellow Maltese cross Yellow	2-15	Common contaminant Maltese cross similar to cholesterol Use brightfield to identify Similar to hydroxyapatite or CPPD
Filter paper fibers		Strong	Variable	10-50 or more	Similar to polyester fragments
Lipids from cells		Strong	Blue-yellow Maltese cross	≈1-2	Indicate degeneration of cells
Nail polish					Causes confusion; avoid edges of coverslip

CPPD, Calcium pyrophosphate dihydrate; *MSU*, Monosodium urate.

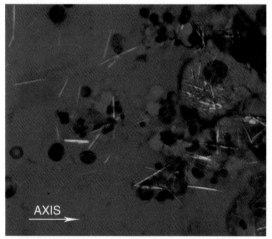

FIGURE 15-6 Monosodium urate crystals (fine, needlelike) appear yellow, and calcium pyrophosphate crystals (rodlike) appear blue in synovial fluid viewed using polarizing microscopy, with the longitudinal axis parallel to the axis of the red compensator. (From Brunzel NA: Fundamentals of urine and body fluid analysis, ed 2, Philadelphia, 2004, Saunders.)

Calcium Pyrophosphate Dihydrate

CPPD crystals are also found in synovial fluid. These crystals are weakly birefringent, rod shaped, rectangular, or rhomboid. Occasionally they are needle shaped. They may be very short and chunky, varying from 1 to 20 µm in length and up to about 4 µm in width. These crystals are characteristic of pseudogout (also referred to as *pyrophosphate gout* or *calcium pyrophosphate dihydrate crystal deposition disease*). Pseudogout is seen in patients with degenerative arthritis and in arthritides associated with hypothyroidism, hyperparathyroidism, hemochromatosis, and other conditions. Symptoms of pseudogout resemble those of gout, rheumatoid arthritis, and osteoarthritis.

COMPENSATED POLARIZED LIGHT

MSU and CPPD crystals that have been identified by polarized light are further identified by adding a full-wave compensator. This is also referred to as a *first-order red plate* (filter) or a *full-wave retardation plate*. Morphology and intensity of birefringence, although helpful, are not sufficient in separating these crystals.

Birefringent crystals have different properties when viewed with polarized light with the addition of a compensator. When the compensator is in place, the background appears magenta rather than black. The compensator may be inserted above the analyzer or the polarizer. It is inserted in such a manner that the axis of slow vibration of the compensator (called the *slow wave*) is at an angle of 45 degrees to the crossed polarizers. In determining the type of crystal in question, the direction of the slow wave must be known. Crystals are identified by observation of the color of the long axis of the crystal in its relationship or orientation to the direction of the slow wave.

Crystals of MSU and CPPD have opposite characteristics when viewed with compensated polarized light. Crystals of MSU appear yellow when the long axis of the crystal lies parallel to the slow wave of the red compensator. These crystals appear blue when the long axis of the crystal lies perpendicular to the slow wave. This may be demonstrated by looking for crystals in the fluid that are so oriented, or by observing a crystal in a parallel orientation and then repositioning the slow wave at right angles to its original position. Alternatively, if the microscope has a rotating stage, the stage may be moved so that the crystal is rotated 90 degrees. In the case of MSU, the crystal will change from a yellow to a blue color. Crystals that appear yellow when parallel and blue when perpendicular to the slow wave exhibit **negative birefringence.** That is, the sign of birefringence is negative. The term *negative* should be avoided in reporting findings in synovial fluid so that it is not taken to mean the crystal in question is absent. Crystals are reported as being "present" or "absent" and are identified as to crystal type.

In the case of CPPD, the crystal appears blue when the long axis of the crystal is parallel to the direction of the slow wave. The same crystal will appear yellow when it lies perpendicular to the slow wave, which can be demonstrated as previously described. The sign of birefringence in this case is positive **(positive birefringence),** which by definition is blue when the long axis is parallel to the slow wave. A determination of the type of birefringence with CPPD crystals may be troublesome because it may be very difficult to determine their long axis, which may be very short and almost square.

Microbiological Examination

Pathogenic organisms can be identified by use of Gram stain and by culturing the synovial fluid. Cultures for suspected bacteria or mycobacterial or fungal infections are an essential part of the synovial fluid analysis. Gonococcal arthritis is a joint disease that is sometimes difficult to diagnose unless special techniques and care are used.

Chemistry Tests

GLUCOSE

The determination of glucose in the synovial fluid is valuable when infectious diseases are suspected. For example, a significantly lower glucose level in synovial fluid than in serum or plasma suggests infection of the joint. Samples of the patient's synovial fluid and blood must be obtained at the same time for a comparison of the two values to be valid.

PROTEIN

Total synovial protein level is increased in several conditions. With inflammatory joint disease, such as rheumatoid arthritis, the total protein level approaches that of plasma. Normally it is about a third of the plasma value. Values are also increased in gout and infectious arthritis.

OTHER TESTS

These include lactate dehydrogenase, uric acid, and lactate determinations.

Immunologic Tests

The synovial fluid normally contains a lower immunoglobulin concentration than plasma. This is not the case in rheumatoid arthritis, in which the level of immunoglobulin is about equal to that in plasma, which suggests production of immunoglobulins in the affected joint.

Rheumatoid factor has been reported in the synovial fluid as well as in the serum of patients with rheumatoid arthritis. The presence of rheumatoid factor in the synovial fluid but not in the serum can be helpful in the diagnosis of this disease. Other immunologic tests include antinuclear antibodies, which are associated with systemic lupus erythematosus (SLE), and the demonstration of decreased complement levels.

SEMINAL FLUID

The main function of seminal fluid is to transport sperm to female cervical mucus. After deposition in the female reproductive tract, sperm remain in seminal plasma for a short time while attempting to enter the mucus.

Semen Analysis

A fresh specimen is needed. The specimen may be collected in a clean, sterile, glass or plastic container. Ideally, seminal fluid should be analyzed within 30 minutes of collection. It is mandatory that the specimen be kept at 37°C and examined within 1 to 2 hours of collection. After 60 minutes of storage in a plastic container, sperm motility is significantly reduced. Most laboratories examine two specimens collected a few days apart. Collection, proper transport, and prompt examination are critical factors in the analysis of seminal fluid. Again, Standard Precautions should be adhered to when handling semen, blood, and other body fluids.

It is recommended that a 3- to 5-day period of sexual abstinence be observed before specimen

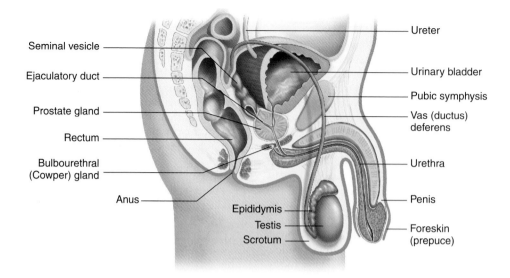

FIGURE 15-7 **Male reproductive system.** (From Patton KT, Thibodeau GA: Anatomy & physiology, ed 7, St Louis, 2010, Mosby.)

TABLE 15-5

Seminal Fluid—Structures and Secretions	
Structure	% Contribution to Total Volume of Semen
Testes & epididymis	<5
Seminal vesicles	60
Prostate gland	30
Bulbourethral glands	<5

From Patton KT, Thibodeau GA: Anatomy & physiology, ed 7, St Louis, 2010, Mosby.

collection; 2 days may be sufficient, but the period should not exceed 5 days. Condoms treated with spermicide or lubricants with spermicidal properties must be avoided during specimen collection. In addition, patients must be advised to keep the specimen warm if collected at home and to deliver it promptly to the laboratory.

Semen analysis is typically done for assessment of fertility or infertility, forensic purposes, determination of the effectiveness of vasectomy, and determination of the suitability of semen for artificial insemination procedures.

Semen (seminal fluid) consists of a combination of products of various male reproductive organs (Fig. 15-7). The total volume of semen is formed by secretions from various structures (Table 15-5).

During ejaculation the products are mixed, producing the normal viscous semen specimen, or ejaculate. This ejaculated human semen is a viscous, yellow-gray fluid that forms a fairly firm gel-like clot immediately after ejaculation. At room temperature, this clot liquefies spontaneously and completely within 5 to 60 minutes. If the liquefaction process requires more than 1 hour, the specimen is considered abnormal. Liquefaction must be complete before any laboratory analysis can be done.

Macroscopic Examination

Macroscopic examination of seminal fluid includes time for complete liquefaction, appearance, volume, viscosity (consistency), and pH.

Wet Mount Analysis

Wet mount analysis is used to determine the approximate sperm count and motility. A drop of the thoroughly mixed, liquefied semen specimen is placed on a clean glass slide under a coverslip. The volume of semen delivered onto the slide and the dimensions of the coverslip must be standardized. A standardized volume of 10 μL covered with a 22 × 22 mm coverglass will result in a fixed depth of about 20 μm and allow for an estimate of sperm number, morphology, motility, and velocity. The freshly made preparation is allowed to stabilize for 1 to 3 minutes before microscopic analysis. This is done by observing 10 to 20 microscope fields, using a ×40 or ×60 (high-power) objective.

Normally, mature sperm cells make up the majority of cells seen (Fig. 15-8). Other cells typically seen are epithelial cells from the male genital tract, immature germ cells, and WBCs. Percentages of the various types of cells are determined and reported. The approximate sperm count is reported

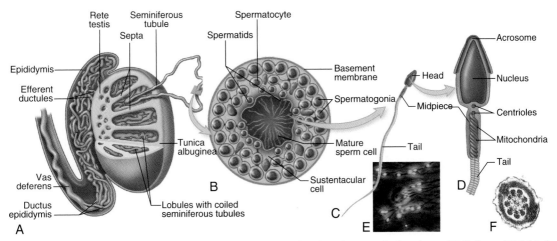

FIGURE 15-8 **Sperm formation.** (From Patton KT, Thibodeau GA: Anatomy & physiology, ed 7, St Louis, 2010, Mosby. E, Courtesy Lennart Nilsson. F, From Stevens A, Lowe J: Human histology, ed 3, Philadelphia, 2005, Mosby.)

as few, several, many, or numerous. Although subjective, this estimate should correlate with the actual chamber sperm count. The relative percentage of motile sperm is determined while the sperm count is estimated. Because mobility and velocity are temperature dependent, a microscope with a warm stage should be used. At least 200 motile and nonmotile sperm are counted in at least five different microscope fields, and the percentage of motile sperm is calculated as follows:

$$\% \text{ Motility} = \frac{\text{Total sperm} - \text{Nonmotile sperm}}{\text{Total sperm}} \times 100$$

Normally, 50% or more sperm are motile.

Other Tests

Qualitative semen analysis is subjective and generally requires further testing, including tests or observations of agglutination, viability, counting chamber sperm counts, and sperm antibody assays. In addition, sperm morphology can be evaluated by performing a differential count of morphologically normal and abnormal sperm types on a hematoxylin-eosin stained smear.

AMNIOTIC FLUID

Amniotic fluid is the nourishing and protecting liquid contained by the amnion (Fig. 15-9) of a pregnant woman. It consists of mostly water but also contains *proteins, carbohydrates, lipids* and *phospholipids, urea,* and *electrolytes,* all of which aid in the growth of the fetus. In the late stages of gestation, most of the amniotic fluid consists of fetal urine.

The volume of amniotic fluid increases until about 34 weeks' gestation, at which time the

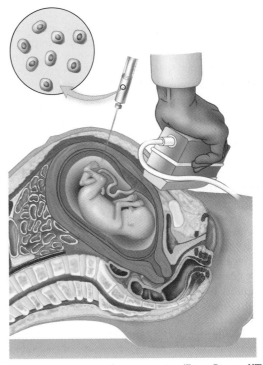

FIGURE 15-9 **Amniocentesis.** (From Patton KT, Thibodeau GA: Anatomy & physiology, ed 7, St Louis, 2010, Mosby.)

amount of amniotic fluid is about 800 mL. This amount reduces to about 600 mL at the time of birth (about 40 weeks).

Amniotic fluid is continually being swallowed and "inhaled" and replaced through being "exhaled." It is essential that the amniotic fluid be breathed into the lungs by the fetus in order for the lungs to develop normally.

TABLE 15-6

Assays for Fetal Lung Maturity	
Test Name	Recommended Use
Fluorescence polarization (Fetal lung maturity)	Assess fetal lung maturity (FLM) to time delivery of fetus for optimal outcome Assess need for intratracheal administration of exogenous surfactant in premature births Test of choice for urgent clinical situations
Lamellar body counts	Use in obstetric situations involving premature labor, premature rupture of membranes, management of eclampsia, fetal distress, and elective delivery at term Test requires less than 10 minutes to determine FLM
Phosphatidylglycerol	Often ordered for assessment of FLM when mother has diabetes Positive result indicates maturity Negative result unhelpful
Lecithin-sphingomyelin ratio	Traditional test for predicting fetal lung maturity Requires a minimum of 4 hours for results Test of choice for rapid screening is fluorescence polarization

Modified from ARUP Laboratories, Inc: Fetal lung maturity: neonatal respiratory distress syndrome www.aruplab.com. Accessed March 3, 2010.

The analysis of amniotic fluid, tapped from the mother's abdomen, is called *amniocentesis*. The fluid contains fetal cells that can be examined for genetic defects, and chemical analysis (e.g., fibronectin and other assays; Table 15-6) can determine fetal lung maturity.

Fetal fibronectin (fFN) is a protein produced during pregnancy and functions as a biological glue, attaching the fetal sac to the uterine lining. Fetal fibronectin (fFN) is performed if a woman is 26 to 34 weeks pregnant and having symptoms of premature labor. The goal then is to intervene to prevent the potentially serious health complications of a preterm baby.

A cervical or vaginal fluid sample is collected and analyzed for fFN. During the first trimester and for about half of the second trimester (up to 22 weeks of gestation), fFN is normally present in the cervicovaginal secretions of pregnant women. In most pregnancies, after 22 weeks, this protein is no longer detected until the end of the last trimester (1 to 3 weeks before labor). The presence of fFN during weeks 24 to 34 of a high-risk pregnancy, along with symptoms of labor, suggests that the "glue" may be disintegrating ahead of schedule and alerts doctors to a possibility of preterm delivery.

A negative fFN result is highly predictive that preterm delivery will not occur within the next 7 to 14 days. A negative fFN can reduce unnecessary hospitalizations and drug therapies. High levels can be due to causes other than risk of preterm delivery. The American College of Obstetrics and Gynecology currently does not recommend routine fFN screening of pregnant women, as its use has not been shown to be clinically effective in predicting preterm labor in low-risk, asymptomatic pregnancies.

SALIVA

Saliva, a clear, alkaline, and viscous fluid secreted by mucous glands of the mouth, can be used for various analyses. Microbial studies of viruses and bacteria and chemical testing of hormones, therapeutic drugs, and drugs of abuse can be performed on saliva. Saliva may be tested in the blood bank to detect secretors of certain antigens. The most common way of collecting a specimen is to have a patient chew on wax or absorbent dental cotton for several minutes and then collect the saliva.

CASE STUDIES

CASE STUDY 15-1

A 15-year-old high school student with fever, chills, and severe headache is seen in an urgent care clinic. He felt nauseated and vomited before reporting to the clinic. At the clinic his temperature is 104°F; he has neck rigidity and complains of back pain. Some small petechial spots are noted on his chest and back and in the mouth. Blood is drawn for a complete blood count (CBC) and blood glucose, and a lumbar puncture (LP) is performed. Cerebrospinal fluid (CSF) is collected sequentially in three sterile tubes and examined.

Blood Results

White cell count: 25×10^9/L

Differential: 80% neutrophils, 10% lymphocytes, 10% monocytes

Glucose: 95 mg/dL

Cerebrospinal Fluid Results

CSF pressure: Increased

Gross appearance: All tubes equally cloudy, not bloody

Glucose: 15 mg/dL

CSF white cell count: 12,000/μL; 90% neutrophils

Gram stain: Many gram-negative cocci in pairs, some intracellular

1. What type of infection is suggested by this patient's white cell count and differential on venous blood?
   a. Bacterial
   b. Viral
   c. Parasitic
   d. Cannot differentiate

2. What is the significance of the gross appearance of the spinal fluid in this patient?
   a. Indicates possible bleeding
   b. Indicates possible infection
   c. Is insignificant
   d. Either a or b

3. What is the significance of the CSF glucose in this patient?
   a. Possible viral infection
   b. Possible bacterial infection
   c. Possible hemorrhage
   d. All of the above

4. Based on the Gram stain, what is the likely diagnosis for this patient?
   a. Bacterial meningitis
   b. Viral meningitis
   c. Fungal meningitis
   d. Stroke

CASE STUDY 15-2

A 75-year-old woman has had a long history of joint pain in the large joints. She now has shoulder pain and a swollen, red knee joint. She has a slight fever and bilateral muscle weakness in the lower limbs. Blood is drawn for hematology, radiographs of her knee are taken, and arthrocentesis is performed on her knee.

Hematology Results

Hemoglobin: 11.9 g/dL

White cell count: 12×10^9/L

Radiographic Findings

Calcification in the cartilage and meniscus (chondrocalcinosis)

Synovial Fluid Findings

Appearance: Cloudy and watery

Microscopic exam: Many neutrophils. Intracellular and extracellular crystals present, appearing as small, chunky rectangles that show weak birefringence and appear blue when parallel and yellow when perpendicular to the slow wave of vibration of compensated polarized light.

1. The pattern of birefringence in this patient is consistent with:
   a. calcium pyrophosphate dihydrate (CPPD).
   b. cholesterol.
   c. hydroxyapatite (HA).
   d. monosodium urate (MSU).

2. The disease exhibited by this patient is referred to as:
   a. gout.
   b. osteoarthritis.
   c. pseudogout.
   d. rheumatoid arthritis.

REFERENCE

1. MacDonnell K, Fan G: CSF cell count on clear fluid, Med Lab Obs (MLO), vol. 42(5):50–51, 2010.

BIBLIOGRAPHY

Brunzel NA: Body fluid: clinical importance and utility of cell counts, American Association for Clinical Chemistry Annual Meeting, Orlando, July 2005, Fla.

Butch AW: Performance of the Iris iQ200 for body fluid cell counting, American Association for Clinical Chemistry Annual Meeting, Orlando, July 2005, Fla.

College of American Pathologists: Hematology; Clinical microscopy; Body fluids (glossaries). In 1996 Proficiency Testing Program, Northfield, Ill, 1996.

Huicho L, Sanchez D, Contreras M, et al: Occult blood and fecal leukocytes as screening tests in childhood infection diarrhea, Pediatr Infect Dis J 12:474, 1993.

Kjeldsberg CR, Knight JA: Body fluids: laboratory examination of amniotic, cerebrospinal, seminal, serous and synovial fluids, ed 3, Chicago, 1993, American Society of Clinical Pathologists Press.

McCarty DJ, editor: Arthritis and allied conditions: a textbook of rheumatology, ed 12, Baltimore, 1992, Lippincott Williams & Wilkins.

Ringsrud KM, Linné JJ: Urinalysis and body fluids: a color text and atlas, St Louis, 1995, Mosby.

Schumacher RH Jr, Reginato AJ: Atlas of synovial fluid analysis and crystal identification, Philadelphia, 1991, Lea & Febiger.

Smith GP, Kjeldsberg CR: Cerebrospinal, synovial, and serous body fluids. In Henry JB, editor: Clinical diagnosis and management by laboratory methods, ed 19, Philadelphia, 1996, Saunders, pp 457–506.

Turgeon ML: Immunology and serology in laboratory medicine, ed 4, St Louis, 2009, Mosby.

Turgeon ML: Clinical hematology, ed 4, Philadelphia, 2005, Lippincott Williams & Wilkins.

REVIEW QUESTIONS

1. **Which of the following fluids is not an ultrafiltrate of plasma?**
   a. Cerebrospinal fluid (CSF)
   b. Peritoneal fluid
   c. Pleural fluid
   d. Synovial fluid

2. Regarding gross appearance, normal spinal fluid is:
   a. crystal clear.
   b. pale yellow.
   c. slightly cloudy.
   d. xanthochromatic.

Questions 3-8: Match the following causes with the gross appearances of cerebrospinal fluid (a to f).

3. ___ Bilirubin from past hemorrhage

4. ___ Infection

5. ___ Normal appearance

6. ___ Recent hemorrhage

7. ___ Subarachnoid hemorrhage

8. ___ Traumatic tap
   a. Cloudy fluid in all tubes
   b. Crystal clear fluid in all tubes
   c. Pale pink or pale orange xanthochromasia in supernatant
   d. Three sequentially collected tubes are equally bloody.
   e. Three sequentially collected tubes are progressively less bloody; the third is clear or almost clear.
   f. Yellow xanthochromasia in supernatant fluid

9. An increased CSF white cell count with a preponderance of neutrophils is most characteristic of which of the following?
   a. Bacterial meningitis
   b. Tuberculosis
   c. Viral meningitis
   d. Yeast infection

10. A lower-than-normal CSF glucose level in relation to blood glucose is most characteristic of which of the following?
    a. Bacterial meningitis
    b. Brain tumor
    c. Diabetic coma
    d. Viral meningitis

Questions 11-19: Match the following fluids with the definitions.

11. ___ Cerebrospinal fluid

12. ___ Effusion

13. ___ Exudate

14. ___ Pericardial fluid

15. ___ Peritoneal fluid

16. ___ Pleural fluid

17. ___ Serous fluids

18. ___ Synovial fluid

19. ___ Transudate
    a. Normal serous fluids
    b. An effusion that is usually the result of an inflammatory process
    c. An increase in serous fluid volume
    d. Around the abdominal and pelvic organs
    e. Around the brain and spinal cord
    f. Around the heart
    g. Around the joints
    h. Around the lungs
    i. Normal fluids contained within the closed cavities of the body

20. The presence of which of the following distinguishes synovial fluid from other extravascular fluids?
    a. Glucose
    b. Hyaluronic acid
    c. Lactate dehydrogenase
    d. Protein

Questions 21-30: Match the following joint diseases with the type of fluid (you may use an answer more than once).

21. ___ Degenerative joint disease

22. ___ Fracture

23. ___ Gonorrhea

24. ___ Gout

25. ___ Hemophilia

26. ___ Immunologic disease

27. ___ Lupus arthritis

28. ___ Osteoarthritis

29. ___ Pseudogout

30. ___ Staphylococcal infection
    a. Crystal-induced fluid
    b. Hemorrhagic fluid
    c. Infectious fluid
    d. Inflammatory fluid
    e. Noninflammatory fluid

31. Which of the following anticoagulants is preferred for microscopic examination of the synovial fluid?
    a. Liquid EDTA
    b. Lithium heparin
    c. Oxalate
    d. Plain serum separator tube

32. The viscosity of synovial fluid may be assessed by which of the following?
    a. Mucin clot test
    b. String test
    c. Specific gravity
    d. More than one of the above

33. The presence of monosodium urate (MSU) crystals in the synovial fluid is characteristic of which of the following?
    a. Gout
    b. Osteoarthritis
    c. Pseudogout
    d. Rheumatoid arthritis

34. The presence of calcium pyrophosphate dihydrate (CPPD) crystals in the synovial fluid is characteristic of which of the following?
    a. Gout
    b. Osteoarthritis
    c. Pseudogout
    d. Rheumatoid arthritis

35. The final identification of crystals in crystal-induced arthritis is best accomplished with which of the following?
    a. Brightfield microscopy
    b. Compensated polarized light microscopy
    c. Phase-contrast microscopy
    d. Polarized light microscopy

Questions 36-41: Match each statement with the crystals seen in crystal-induced arthritis.
A = Calcium pyrophosphate (CPPD) crystals;
B = Monosodium urate (MSU) crystals.

36. ___ Appear blue when parallel and yellow when perpendicular to the slow wave of vibration of compensated polarized light

37. ___ Appear yellow when parallel and blue when perpendicular to the slow wave of vibration of compensated polarized light

38. ___ Exhibit weak birefringence

39. ___ Exhibit strong birefringence

40. ___ Typically seen as chunky rectangles

41. ___ Typically seen as long, slender needles

Questions 42-44: Indicate whether the following statements concerning sperm are A = True or B = False.

42. ___ In normal semen, spermatozoa are the minority of cells seen.

43. ___ Qualitative semen analysis is subjective, and further testing is generally required.

44. ___ Qualitative semen analysis must take place before liquefaction of the specimen.

CHAPTER 16

INTRODUCTION TO MICROBIOLOGY

Learning Objectives

At the conclusion of this chapter, the student will be able to:

- Learn the importance of collection requirements for the various specimens used in microbiological studies.
- Describe the various Gram stain reactions for common bacteria.
- Prepare and examine a Gram-stained smear for common bacteria.
- Select and inoculate the appropriate media for frequently collected specimens: urine, throat swabs, genitourinary exudates, and blood.
- Collect an appropriate specimen for a urine culture, quantitatively plate it, and interpret results.
- Collect a throat swab for a throat culture on sheep blood agar, plate it, and interpret results.

- Collect blood for culture, and describe how to process and interpret the result of the culturing.
- Explain the major sexually transmitted diseases and the laboratory tests used in their diagnosis.
- Collect genitourinary specimens for culture.
- Explain the purpose and process of antimicrobial susceptibility testing.
- Explain the factors to consider in the selection of an antimicrobial agent.
- Explain the characteristics of fungi and the common methods used to detect fungi in the laboratory.
- Explain the specimen collection and identification process for common intestinal parasites.

INTRODUCTION TO MICROORGANISMS

The field of medical or clinical microbiology involves the isolation and identification of organisms so small they cannot be seen with the naked eye. They can be observed only with a microscope and are therefore known as **microorganisms** or **microbes.** Some microorganisms inhabit the human body normally and do not cause disease; these are called **normal flora** or **normal microbiota.** Other microorganisms can cause disease; these are called **pathogens.**

Several different groups of microorganisms are studied in the microbiology laboratory, including bacteria, viruses, rickettsiae, fungi, protozoa and other parasites, and algae. Organisms in each of these groups can cause disease. Medical microbiology is concerned with identifying pathogens and developing effective ways to eliminate or control them.

The field of medical microbiology is generally divided into areas of specialization according to the type of microorganism being studied. For example, the study of bacteria is **bacteriology,** the study of viruses is **virology,** the study of fungi is **mycology,** the study of rickettsiae is **rickettsiology,** and the study of parasites is **parasitology.** This chapter focuses more on bacteriology than other areas of microbiology, although the general skills discussed can be applied to specialties other than bacteriology. As with other divisions of the clinical laboratory, if the basic skills are understood and learned

well, other specific tests and procedures can be performed more easily.

The routine procedures such as specimen collection, initial media inoculation, handling of media, staining of slides, and microscopic examination of the slides are extremely important for the final identification process. This chapter discusses techniques involved in these routine procedures, including the growth (culture) and identification of various common pathogenic microorganisms. Monoclonal antibodies (single antibody molecule type) have been employed in many tests involving antigen-antibody reactions, which are described in this chapter and in other chapters where applicable.

Direct molecular diagnostic techniques have added a new dimension to the microbiology laboratory. Genetic probes are also being applied; these known, labeled sequences of deoxyribonucleic acid (DNA) or ribonucleic acid (RNA) are used to detect complementary sequences in target specimens. Currently in the microbiology laboratory, application of DNA probes includes the detection of bacterial, fungal, mycobacterial, and parasitic pathogens.

Normal Flora (Biota)

Microorganisms are present under normal conditions in certain sites of the body. Examples of normal flora (biota) are the normal constituents of the human intestinal tract, especially the large intestine and colon. These microorganisms benefit from this association because they derive essential food materials from the host. The host also benefits because the microorganisms synthesize and aid in the digestion of vitamins that are essential for human life. Usual inhabitants also may be found in the mouth and oral cavity, in the nose, and on the surface of the skin. Normal bacteria in the oral cavity can prevent pathogenic bacteria from colonizing (temporary or permanent presence) this cavity, preventing possible "strep throat." Examples of body sites that normally are **sterile,** or that contain no normal flora, are the blood, cerebrospinal fluid, and urinary bladder.

Pathogenic Microorganisms

Although microorganisms are generally beneficial and essential for life, some are harmful to their hosts. These are the disease-producing, or pathogenic, microorganisms. It is important to be able to distinguish normal flora from pathogens in the specimens being cultured from specific sites. The discussion in this chapter is primarily concerned with pathogenic microorganisms.

An **opportunistic pathogen** is an organism that does not usually cause disease in a person with an intact immune system but can cause disease when the host's immune system has been compromised by disease or another condition that has damaged or changed the immune status. Infectious microorganisms can be present in the hospital or health care facility and become a major problem if they infect patients. **Healthcare–associated infections (HAIs)** or **nosocomial infections** are infections that patients acquire during a course of treatment in a health care facility; the organism is neither present nor incubating in the patient before he or she is admitted to the hospital or health care facility.

Onset of symptoms 48 hours after admission is considered the time frame for acquisition of an HAI infection.[1] Infection control is critical to prevent this from occurring, and health care facilities of all types have active infection control departments for this purpose. In contrast, a **community-associated infection** is acquired by persons not hospitalized within the last year or persons who have not had a medical procedure such as dialysis or catheterization. The bacterium *Staphylococcus aureus* has become resistant to many antimicrobial agents and is the cause of many infections acquired in health care facilities. This resistant strain is called *methicillin-resistant Staphylococcus aureus* (MRSA) and can also be acquired in the community. These community-associated infections are usually skin infections such as boils or abscesses.[2]

Pathogenic microorganisms in medical microbiology include bacteria, fungi, parasites, viruses, and rarely algae. There are many bacterial pathogens; this chapter discusses only the more frequently encountered members. The fungi consist of molds and yeast, and as with bacteria, fungi can also be beneficial. However, many serious infections are caused by pathogenic and opportunistic fungi. The parasites are divided into protozoa (e.g., *Giardia lamblia*), nematodes or roundworms (e.g., *Enterobius vermicularis*), trematodes or flukes (e.g., *Fasciolopsis buski*), and cestodes or tapeworms (*Taenia solium*). Viruses infect animals, plants, and bacteria in a different manner than bacteria. They also differ in their structure and viral cycle from the previous groups.

Also studied in microbiology are invertebrate animals called *arthropods*. Arthropods themselves rarely cause disease but frequently serve as vectors in certain microbial infections. Malaria is an example of a parasitic disease transmitted by the *Anopheles* mosquito. A representative tickborne disease is Lyme disease, the causative or etiologic agent being the spirochete, *Borrelia burgdorferi*, a helical and motile bacterium. A bite from a tick of the genus *Ixodes* is the transmission route for this spirochete, and diagnosis of Lyme disease depends on finding antibodies in the serum or spinal fluid.

Prokaryotic and Eukaryotic Cell Differences

Cells are defined as prokaryotic or eukaryotic depending on their structure (Fig. 16-1). Bacterial cells are prokaryotes and are less complex in structure than eukaryotic cells. **Prokaryotes** (Greek for "before nucleus") do not have a nucleus or any membrane-bound organelles such as mitochondria, and their **ribosomes** (site of protein synthesis) are a smaller size than eukaryotic ribosomes. Their DNA is in a single circular chromosome located in a **nucleoid** region within the bacterial cell. They have a **cell wall** made of **peptidoglycan** that aids bacterial cells in maintaining their shape and helps in preventing lysis caused by increased osmotic pressure. Features of the cell wall contribute to the staining properties of bacterial cells. The Gram stain is the most widely used stain in microbiology, and the reactions, gram-positive or gram-negative, correlate to the cell wall structure of bacteria. Inside the cell wall is a **cell membrane** (lipid bilayer that surrounds the cytoplasm), and many bacteria are enclosed within a polysaccharide or protein **capsule,** also called the *slime layer*.

An important structure formed by gram-positive bacteria is the **spore** or **endospore.** Bacteria form spores by a process called *sporulation* when the environment becomes hostile (e.g., nutrient depletion). Spores are resistant to heat, cold, drying conditions, and chemicals and therefore are able to survive under extremely unfavorable conditions. Spore-forming bacteria can revert to the

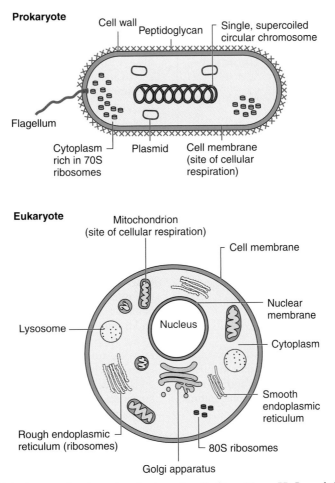

FIGURE 16-1 **Major features of prokaryotic and eukaryotic cells.** (From Murray PR, Rosenthal KS, Pfaller MA: Medical microbiology, ed 5, Philadelphia, 2005, Mosby.)

vegetative or active state when the conditions become favorable again. This process is referred to as *germination*.

Bacteria have external structures such as fimbriae or pili and flagella. **Flagella** are threadlike structures anchored within the cell membrane. The rotational motion (described as "runs" and "tumbles") of the flagella enables the bacterial cell to move. Flagella vary in their number and position on the bacteria, and this pattern is helpful in identifying the species. **Pili** are hairlike structures on the exterior of bacterial cells that promote adherence to surfaces. For many bacteria, adherence to tissue begins the infection process, and therefore pili are termed a *virulence factor* (factor that contributes to the disease process).

Eukaryotes (Greek for "true nucleus") are animal, plant, and fungal cells. They have a membrane-bound **nucleus, organelles** (e.g., mitochondria, lysosomes), **cytoskeleton,** cell membrane, and larger **ribosomes.** Also, because eukaryotic cells have mitochondria, they possess smaller ribosomes that are present in these organelles. Their DNA is

enclosed within a nucleus and is complexed with histone proteins. Eukaryotic cells are more complex than prokaryotic cells, and the ultrastructure of both cell types is observed using electron microscopy. In medical microbiology, the eukaryotes are the parasites and the fungi.

CLASSIFICATION OF MICROORGANISMS: TAXONOMY

In discussing microorganisms, it is necessary to refer to the method by which living things are classified or named. By using biological classification methods, it is possible for the laboratory microbiologist to identify microbes systematically. The scientific study of the classification process is known as **taxonomy.** One aspect of taxonomy is the traditional classification system, which provides an orderly method for placing microbes into categories. This was previously done by morphologic and biochemical testing; advanced genetic testing is now used and has resulted in a number of name changes. A second aspect is nomenclature, the method used

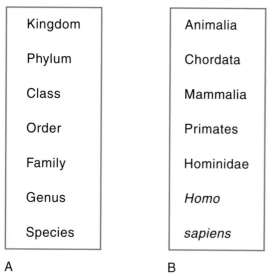

Kingdom	Animalia
Phylum	Chordata
Class	Mammalia
Order	Primates
Family	Hominidae
Genus	*Homo*
Species	*sapiens*

A   B

FIGURE 16-2 Taxonomic hierarchy. A, Categories of biological classification. B, Biological classification of humans.

to name the microorganisms. Lastly, taxonomy involves identification of the microorganisms, which is the process of determining whether or not a microorganism belongs to a particular defined taxonomic group.

Classification and Nomenclature

All living things are classified by the same scheme, and a hierarchy is followed. The top of the scheme has members with the broadest relationship and progresses to members with the closest relationship. The following is the breakdown of the classification scheme beginning at the top: kingdom, phylum, class, order, family, genus, and species (Fig. 16-2, A).

There are five kingdoms at the top of the scheme: Animalia, Plantae, Protista, Fungi, and Monera (also referred to as *Prokaryotae*). Bacteria belong to the kingdom Monera, parasites to the kingdom Protista, and the yeasts and molds to the kingdom Fungi.

The classification scheme is divided so that systematic designations are given to all living things (see Fig. 16-2, B). Conventionally, the microbes studied in the medical microbiology laboratory will have two names, the genus name and the species name. The **species** category represents microorganisms with the closest physiologic and genetic relationship and is the basic unit of the biological world. The **genus** is the next larger classification. Members of the same genus share common features, but they differ from one another sufficiently to remain in a separate species classification; a genus can include several species, all of which

differ somewhat from one another. These Latin or Greek names are printed in italics. The genus name is always capitalized, and the species name is always lowercase. For example, the genus *Streptococcus* includes several species. Depending on the species, the organisms can cause different diseases in humans. *Streptococcus pyogenes* is a pathogen that causes pharyngitis, scarlet fever, and other infections, whereas *Streptococcus pneumoniae* can cause pneumonia and meningitis. Other species of the genus *Streptococcus* are members of the normal flora. It is common to see the genus name abbreviated, especially after first use, followed by the species designation, such as *S. pyogenes*. Another convention frequently used when discussing a genus without reference to a particular species is to abbreviate species to sp. (singular) and spp. (plural). An example would be *Staphylococcus* spp. At other times, when there is a nonspecific or informal reference to all members of a group, no capital or italics is used; examples include staphylococci and β-hemolytic streptococci.

At times in medical microbiology, groups of microorganisms are large, and the family division is used to include all these members. The family division is above the genus designation, and similar genera are grouped into families. An example is the family *Enterobacteriaceae*, which has more than 30 genera. These members are categorized by their key features, which include biochemical reactions. This large family includes the member *Escherichia coli*, a common cause of urinary tract infections.

Classification by Morphology and Biochemical Properties

Organisms have traditionally been classified in medical microbiology by placing them into groups based on the similarity of their phenotypical or observable characteristics for all members of a particular group. This includes observation of their morphology on culture and Gram stain, and on their biochemical reactions when they are tested for metabolic characteristics.

PROTECTION OF LABORATORY PERSONNEL, DECONTAMINATION, DISINFECTION, AND STERILIZATION

All clinical laboratories have procedures in place that must be followed for the general safety and protection of the workers (see Chapter 2). Because the material to be examined in the microbiology laboratory is likely to contain infectious pathogens, it is necessary to protect the microbiologist from any potentially infectious specimens.

Microbiology laboratories pose a hazard in addition to the hazards of blood and body fluid specimens (involving Standard Precautions). Potentially hazardous infectious cultures of pathogenic agents are present in these laboratories and require extra precautionary measures, such as working under a biological safety hood. It is also important to have safety and precautionary measures in place (e.g., biological safety cabinet) if bacterial identification is suspected to involve one of those included in the Centers for Disease Control and Prevention (CDC) list of bioterrorism agents[3] (see Chapter 2, Table 2-2 and Box 2-3). Workers in a microbiology laboratory must pay special attention to all measures employed by the laboratory for their protection and safety. Protection from infection from pathogenic microbiological agents requires specific additional safety practices when working in a microbiology laboratory setting.

Classification of Biological Agents Based on Hazard to Personnel

The CDC has published a list that classifies biological or etiologic agents based on the assessment of the relative risk of working with them.[4] The following discussion provides examples of the more common agents encountered. Personnel must adhere to Standard Precautions (safe laboratory practice to prevent infection) when processing patient specimens because the nature of the etiologic agent in these specimens is usually not known.

Biosafety Level 1

Biosafety Level 1 agents are well known, do not usually cause disease in healthy adult people, and are of minimal hazard to laboratory personnel. The level 1 agents are used for laboratory instruction for introductory microbiology laboratory courses. Good standard working practices should be used in handling these agents. An example of a Biosafety Level 1 agent is *Bacillus subtilis*.

Biosafety Level 2

Biosafety Level 2 agents are those most often identified in patient specimens in the routine microbiology laboratory. They include all the common agents of infectious diseases. The general principles of safety and infection control discussed must be used for handling these agents. These include (1) the use of specific training in handling pathogenic agents, (2) limited access to the laboratory, (3) precautions with contaminated sharps, and (4) use of a biological safety cabinet as necessary when aerosolization of the agent is possible. Biosafety Level 2 agents include such organisms as human

immunodeficiency virus (HIV), *Salmonella* spp., and *Shigella* spp.

Biosafety Level 3

Agents in this category are not usually encountered in the routine microbiology laboratory. Agents in Biosafety Level 3 include certain arboviruses, arenaviruses, and cultures of *Mycobacterium tuberculosis* (specimen handling can be done at a Biosafety Level 2) and certain mold stages of systemic fungi. Laboratories where these agents are in use must have laboratory personnel with specific training in handling pathogenic and potentially lethal agents. All procedures manipulating infectious materials must be done in a biological safety cabinet with special engineering features for careful control of air movement. Personnel are required to wear protective clothing and other special barrier devices when working at this level.

Biosafety Level 4

Biosafety Level 4 agents are not found in routine microbiology laboratories. Access to these laboratories is highly controlled. All work is confined to a biological safety cabinet that has special engineering features for control of air movement. The Biosafety Level 4 laboratory has special features to prevent dissemination of these exotic agents into the environment. A Biosafety Level 4 agent includes the filoviruses, of which Ebola (hemorrhagic fever) is a member, and other arboviruses and arenaviruses not included in Biosafety Level 3. In the United States, the CDC is an example of a facility with a Biosafety Level 4 laboratory.

General Safety Practices in the Microbiology Laboratory

Access to the microbiology laboratory should be limited to those persons who understand the potential risk involved in simply being in this area. Specific high-risk work can be done in an area separate from the main microbiology laboratory, where access is strictly limited.

The air-handling system of the microbiology laboratory should operate to move air from low-risk areas to high-risk areas and not the reverse. Ideally, air should not be recirculated after it has been in this area. If special procedures are done that generate aerosols that are infectious, a biological safety cabinet should be in place. Several diseases may be contracted by inhalation of the infectious particles, including tularemia, tuberculosis, brucellosis, histoplasmosis, and legionnaires' disease. These infectious particles are known as **aerosols;** several processes carried out in microbiological studies can create aerosols. Techniques such as mincing, vortexing, and preparation of direct smears have been known to produce aerosol droplets. These selected procedures should be carried out in a biological safety cabinet (see Protection from Aerosols, Chapter 2).

It is essential that strict adherence to the policies of Standard Precautions be maintained. One important aspect of this is the conscientious use of barrier precautions, the most common barrier being the use of gloves for handling patient specimens. Protective laboratory clothing, such as laboratory coats, should always be worn in the laboratory. These coats should be removed before leaving the laboratory (see Personal Protective Equipment, Chapter 2).

Another important consideration is the transportation and handling of laboratory specimens. Specimen containers must always be transported to the laboratory in plastic, leakproof, sealed bags, and the outside surface of the container should not be contaminated with any of the specimen contents.

Hands should be washed thoroughly before leaving the microbiology laboratory, according to the laboratory's established protocol; hands must also be washed in case of contamination. The microbiologist should not work with uncovered open cuts or broken skin; these should be covered with a bandage or some suitable material before putting on gloves.

Each health care facility will have its own policies for safety protocol specifically pertaining to the microbiology laboratory, and these must be followed when working in that area.

Waste Disposal and Disinfection Process

Any material that has become contaminated with an infectious agent must be decontaminated before final disposal. All such materials must first be placed into clearly marked biohazard containers. These materials include media that have been inoculated, along with any remaining patient specimens. The biohazard bags or containers are then disposed of according to procedures established by the health care facility. Any sharp objects (needles, blades) must be placed in special puncture-resistant sharps containers for disposal before decontamination. The actual decontamination can be done by steam sterilization (e.g., autoclave), incineration, or burning.

The work area should be disinfected before and after use each day. Disinfectants such as phenol or a diluted solution of bleach are typically used for cleaning. Diluted bleach is a very effective disinfectant against viral agents. The longer the surface is allowed to remain wet with the cleaning agent, the more effective the disinfection will be. Disinfection is an ongoing process in the microbiology laboratory.

Incinerators and Flame Burners

Many microbiology laboratories now use incinerators to sterilize inoculating loops and needles. These units are electrical as opposed to flame burners that operate on gas. Therefore the hazard of gas in a laboratory can be avoided by using this type of sterilization method, but cautions regarding electrical hazards must be followed. If open-flame burners are used in the laboratory to sterilize the inoculating loops and needles, special care must be taken. Turning off burners may minimize fire hazards whenever they are not in use. In addition, burners should be kept away from material that is flammable. When inoculating loops or needles are sterilized, care must be taken to prevent splattering of material during the process.

Disinfection and Sterilization Techniques

It is essential to use sterile media for growing pure cultures of bacteria and to avoid contamination by any of the microorganisms widely distributed in nature (organisms in the air, on the hands, and on laboratory equipment and supplies). In general, all equipment, glassware, and media used in the microbiology laboratory must be sterile to ensure the preparation of pure cultures of microorganisms. Contaminated media must also be placed in special biohazard bags before being discarded to prevent infection of those responsible for its removal.

Sterilization refers to the killing or destruction of all microorganisms, including bacterial spores. Sterilization may be achieved in various ways, generally involving physical means such as heat or filtration and chemical means such as oxidation.

Disinfection is the process of destroying pathogenic organisms, but not necessarily all microorganisms or bacterial spores (endospores). Physical (moist or dry heat) or chemical (e.g., bleach, phenol, alcohols, aldehydes) means may be used.

Antisepsis is the process used to decrease the number of microorganisms that are present on the skin. Typical antiseptic agents are iodine, alcohols, and chlorhexidine products. Alcohol is often used to disinfect the skin before venipuncture.

Use of Chemical Disinfectants

In microbiology laboratories, disinfection is done daily and when any spill occurs that may have infectious microorganisms present. Chemical disinfectants such as a 1:10 dilution of bleach or a 2% to 5% phenol solution are two types of disinfectants used to clean benchtops and other surfaces.

Use of Heat or Burning

The effect of heat on organisms is generally known, and heat is a widely used and efficient physical means of sterilization. Heat may be employed in the form of dry heat or moist heat. Dry heat destroys bacteria by oxidation, whereas moist heat works by denaturing proteins. The type of sterilization method that is used will depend on the nature of the material being treated.

STERILIZATION BY DRY HEAT

Dry-heat sterilization is carried out in a hot-air chamber similar to an oven. The temperature must be kept at 171°C for at least 1 hour. If the temperature is decreased, the time must be increased. Glassware can be sterilized in this manner.

STERILIZATION BY MOIST HEAT

One method of employing moist heat is by boiling water. Boiling in water is sufficient to kill vegetative forms of bacteria, but the spores remain. Certain species of bacteria, including the genus *Bacillus*, have the ability to form spores under unfavorable conditions but return to the vegetative or active state when favorable conditions return. Spores are highly resistant forms of bacteria and thus pose a problem in sterilization.

The most effective means of sterilization with moist heat involves steam under pressure, using a special device called an **autoclave.** It is the method of choice for any material that is not injured by moisture, high temperature, or high pressure. Most types of media used in microbiology are sterilized in the autoclave. Some equipment also is sterilized in this manner, as are some infected materials that will be discarded. Basically, the autoclave is a heavy metal chamber with a door or lid that can be fastened to withstand the internal steam pressure, a pressure gauge, a safety valve, and a temperature gauge. The material is exposed to pure steam in the autoclave at 121°C for 15 minutes. This temperature is achieved by applying pressure. Generally, 15 lb above atmospheric pressure is required to reach 121°C. This time and temperature will kill all forms of bacterial life, including spores. Temperature chart recorders must be used for documentation of autoclave maintenance, and quality assurance programs require that the maintenance of the autoclave be checked and documented regularly. This may be done by one of several methods, using biological or chemical indicators.

Use of Filtration

In the preparation of certain media that are used in microbiology, none of the preceding methods of sterilization is applicable because they result in deterioration of the media. In these cases, some other means may be used, such as filtration through thin membrane filters composed of plastic polymers or cellulose esters. Heat-sensitive solutions such as vaccines or antibiotic solutions can be sterilized by filtration.

High-efficiency particulate air (HEPA) filters are used to filter the air in biological safety cabinets. Isolation and operating rooms also use HEPA filters. These filters are capable of filtering 99.97% of microorganism larger than 0.3 μm.[5]

SPECIMENS FOR MICROBIOLOGICAL EXAMINATION

When a patient has particular disease symptoms and a microbiological infection is suspect, the causative agent must often be identified. Positive identification of the causative agent is essential in selecting the best treatment for the patient. Therefore it is important that only appropriate specimens be sent to the laboratory. Information accompanying the specimen (other than patient information) must include its source (e.g., wound culture, sputum), date and time of collection, person collecting the specimen, physician, and any antibiotics the patient may be taking.

In the patient with a possible kidney or urinary tract infection, a urine specimen will be collected for bacterial analysis. If the patient has a sore throat, the throat will be swabbed, and this specimen will be submitted for testing. Gastroenteritis will require the examination of stool specimens. Examination of infected wounds will require swabs, aspirates, or appropriate material from the area of infection. Other sources from which material or swabs are submitted to the laboratory for culture and identification include blood and body fluids (e.g., pleural, peritoneal, cerebrospinal), genital area, ears, eyes, respiratory tract (upper and lower), and various tissues.

Specimen Collection Requirements for Culture

The microbiologist must be aware of the types of infective agents that may be responsible for a disease and test for these accordingly. Likewise, for each source of infected material, the personnel collecting the specimen must have appropriate procedures to follow to ensure that the specimen will be optimal.

The treatment of a disease or infection often involves the use of antimicrobial agents that destroy various pathogens. Antibiotics are often administered before the causative agent is identified in bacterial culture; such identification takes 1 day or longer, and the patient requires immediate treatment. If antibiotics are given before specimen collection, often it will be impossible to recover the pathogenic bacteria, so the appropriate specimen should be obtained before antibiotics are administered.

It is important to remember that material should be collected for culture from the location where the suspected organism is most likely to be found. An example is the culture of specimens from draining lesions containing *Staphylococcus aureus*. This type of specimen should be collected with as little external contamination as possible from areas around the lesion. If the surrounding area is cultured along with the lesion, normal skin flora may grow in the culture. Another example is the collection of sputum to assist in the diagnosis of a lower respiratory tract infection. Sputum is needed for this culture, not saliva from the oral cavity, which may yield only normal mouth flora.

Pertinent information that accompanies the specimen (e.g., source) will help ensure that the correct medium is inoculated, aiding in the correct identification of the pathogen. Also, a quality specimen will yield a report physicians will be able to interpret for the best treatment of their patients.

Specimen Containers

Correct identification of a causative agent requires isolation and growth of a pure culture of that organism in the laboratory. To do this, the original specimen must be collected in a sterile container and must not be contaminated at any stage in its subsequent transfer to or isolation in the laboratory. It is also important, for the protection of laboratory personnel and others handling the specimen, that the specimen be placed entirely within the appropriate container and not allowed to contaminate the outside. Proper transport procedures must be followed to minimize any risks to hospital personnel.

A variety of disposable containers have been manufactured for collecting microbiology specimens. One of the most useful pieces of collecting equipment is a swab system that has a plastic shaft and calcium alginate, Dacron, or rayon polyester tips. When choosing a particular type of swab, it is necessary to consider the source and what type of organisms may be recovered from that source. Two considerations are in culturing the genital area for sexually transmitted organisms. Wooden shafts should not be used to culture *Chlamydia trachomatis*, and cotton and calcium alginate can inhibit or be toxic to *Neisseria gonorrhoeae*. Genital swabs can be transported with charcoal, which acts as a detoxifying agent. These swab systems, tipped with the appropriate fiber and packaged in a capped sterile container, are available commercially and may be used for the collection of material from the throat,

nose, eyes, or ears; from wounds and surgical sites; from urogenital orifices; and from the rectum.

Many innovations have been made in sterile, disposable culture units of various types. To prolong the survival of microorganisms that have been collected, transport media can be used. This is especially desirable when a significant delay occurs between collection and culturing. Swabs of infectious material can be prevented from drying out by immersion in a transport or holding medium until culture is done. Transport media are designed to sustain bacteria without allowing appreciable growth. The whole culture unit must be properly labeled and promptly sent to the laboratory.

If the suspected organism is an anaerobe, conventional transport tubes should not be used. The crucial factor in the successful final culturing of anaerobic (oxygen-sensitive) organisms is the transport of a tissue biopsy or needle aspirate. Some anaerobic transport systems are designed for liquid specimens and will support the viability of anaerobes (Fig. 16-3). The specimen is injected through the rubber stopper, avoiding the introduction of air. Atmospheric oxygen, which kills such organisms, must be kept out until the specimen has been processed anaerobically by the laboratory. If only a swab must be used, special double-stoppered collection tubes containing an oxygen-free inner tube are available (Fig. 16-4; see Requirements for Bacterial Cultivation).

Transport to the Laboratory

Once the specimen has been placed in the appropriate container, it should be delivered to the laboratory in a timely manner and not allowed to

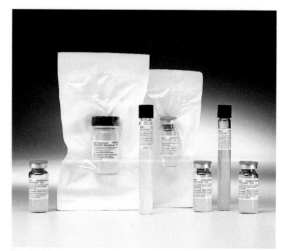

FIGURE 16-3 **Anaerobic transport system designed to support the viability of anaerobes present in liquid specimens.** (Courtesy and copyright Becton, Dickinson and Company Sparks, Md. Port-A-Cul is a trademark of Becton, Dickinson and Company.)

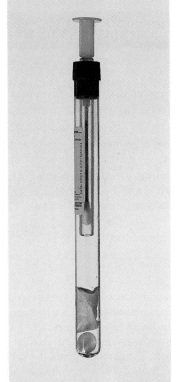

FIGURE 16-4 **Anaerobic transport system designed to support the viability of anaerobes present in swab specimens (Vacutainer Anaerobic Specimen Collector [BD Diagnostics Systems, Sparks, Md.]).** (From Forbes BA, Sahm DF, Weissfeld AS: Bailey and Scott's diagnostic microbiology, ed 12, St Louis, 2007, Mosby.)

stand at the patient care unit or clinic. Although many organisms remain alive for long periods after collection, some are **fastidious,** requiring special conditions for culture, including rapid inoculation into a suitable culture medium, in order to be detected. In fact, some organisms are so fragile that arrangements must be made to take a special culture medium to the patient so that the material can be placed directly on it. *N. gonorrhoeae* is best recovered by immediately placing the specimen on media when performing cultures for detection of this organism. Newer DNA/RNA methods approved by the Food and Drug Administration (FDA) for testing of *N. gonorrhoeae* and *C. trachomatis* make collection easier (see Gonorrheal Infections and Chlamydial Infections).

Handling and Storing Specimens in the Laboratory

Immediate culture of freshly collected specimens is always best but not always practical. If culture must be delayed, refrigeration at 4°C to 6°C provides a safe method for temporary storage of most pathogenic organisms or specimens until they can be tested. Exceptions are those samples that must be immediately cultured (specimens that may contain gonococcal organisms) or certain meningitis-causing bacteria in cerebrospinal fluid, such as meningococci *(Neisseria meningitidis),* that are susceptible to low temperatures and also require immediate culturing. Most pathogenic organisms are not greatly affected by small changes in temperature, but they are generally susceptible to drying out. Laboratory personnel are responsible for knowing which organisms require immediate inoculation and which can be safely stored until culturing can be done.

Refrigeration will prevent overgrowth of other organisms (normal flora) that are present. This will make the isolation of the significant microbe easier. Refrigeration is particularly effective for specimens of urine, feces, sputum, and material on swabs from a variety of sources. It is not effective for anaerobic organisms, cerebrospinal fluid, or genital cultures for *N. gonorrhoeae;* these specimens should be kept at room temperature until cultured. Specimen collection and handling requirements should be checked when testing for specific microorganisms or using unique biological samples. Only when the specimens are properly collected and handled by the laboratory will the final results of the culturing be valid. Serum samples for serology testing can be stored in the freezer for 1 week before testing.

Types of Microbiology Specimens Collected

Blood

A blood sample for culture is a very important specimen cultured in microbiology, because of the critical nature of an infection of this type. Special blood-collecting equipment is used. Sterile collecting bottles containing the proper nutrient broth media, blood-collecting sets with needles and tubing that allow the blood to flow into the collecting bottle, and the proper skin-cleaning supplies are necessary to ensure a properly collected blood specimen for culture.

Special care must be taken to clean the venipuncture site carefully before puncture to avoid possible contamination of the blood sample with skin contaminants. One method uses an initial cleaning with a 70% solution of alcohol to remove dirt and lipids. A circular motion moving from the venipuncture site out is used. A 1% to 10% povidone-iodine solution is used, followed by an alcohol rinse[6] (see Venous Blood Collection in Chapter 3 and Blood Cultures in this chapter). The protocol is determined by the facility.

Collecting and Processing Laboratory Specimens for Throat Culture

1. Ask the patient to open his or her mouth.
2. Using a sterile tongue blade to hold the tongue down and a sterile swab to collect the specimen, take the specimen directly from the back of the throat, being careful not to touch the teeth, cheeks, gums, or tongue when inserting or removing the swab (see Chapter 3, Fig. 3-7).
3. The tonsillar fauces and rear pharyngeal wall should be swabbed, not just gently touched, in order to remove organisms adhering to the membranes. White patches of exudate in the tonsillar area are especially productive for isolating the streptococcal organisms.
4. The swab containing the specimen can be placed in a special container with transport media. Commercial collection sets containing both swabs and transport media are available. Streptococci survive on dry swabs for up to 2 to 3 hours and on swabs in transport (holding) media at 4°C for 24 to 48 hours.
5. The specimen container must be labeled with the necessary patient identification.

Cerebrospinal Fluid

A physician collects cerebrospinal fluid (CSF) through a lumbar puncture. Rapid handling of CSF samples in the laboratory is extremely important because of the serious nature of meningitis, and organisms recovered in meningitis are sensitive to temperature change, so refrigeration is not done. CSF is typically placed in sterile tubes. The tubes are sent to the laboratory immediately for testing, including culture and Gram stain. The CSF specimen should be centrifuged if the specimen in the tube is greater than 1 mL, and 5 to 10 mL is recommended for detection (see Chapter 15).

Stool

Stool specimens contain large numbers of bacteria (normal flora), and a stool specimen is usually cultured only to isolate certain types of pathogenic enteric organisms. Stool specimens should be cultured within 2 hours. If this cannot be done, transport media special for stool samples can be used. Swabs of the rectal area can be used for infants, but this is not the preferred method of collection for other age groups. Stool specimens are also collected for identification of parasites (see later discussion).

Respiratory

When a specimen of sputum is collected, the patient must cooperate fully to ensure that a proper specimen is obtained. Sputum is usually collected in the morning, and it should be sent to the laboratory and processed immediately. Deep coughing will usually bring up a good sputum specimen. It is necessary to avoid collecting saliva. A wide-mouthed sterile container is best used for collecting this type of specimen.

An acceptable or suitable sputum specimen that is free from contamination with saliva can be Gram-stained and checked microscopically for the presence of squamous epithelial cells. Finding an average of more than 10 squamous epithelial cells per low-power field indicates the specimen is saliva and is therefore not an acceptable specimen to culture.[7]

Other respiratory specimens sent to the microbiology laboratory include bronchial washings, lavages, and brushings, which are collected by a physician in a procedure called *bronchoscopy*. These specimens are excellent for recovery of many agents of pneumonia and should be processed promptly (smear and culture). Induced sputums are collected by respiratory therapy technicians by stimulating the patient to produce sputum. Bronchoscopy can be used when a patient cannot produce a sputum sample. Also, aspiration or suctioning can be done when patients have tracheostomies.

A common upper respiratory specimen obtained by way of a swab is the throat culture for detection of group A beta-hemolytic streptococci causing pharyngitis (Procedure 16-1 and Fig. 16-5). The specimen can be used for the classic culture on sheep blood media or for one of the rapid direct tests utilizing extraction of the cell wall polysaccharide antigen and its recognition by antibody. These rapid tests have gained popularity, especially in physicians' offices, because results are available within minutes instead of hours (see Rapid Detection Methods).

Swabs of Various Fluids

Swabs are used to collect cultures from various openings of the body, such as the nose, throat (see Respiratory), mouth, vagina, anus, and wounds.

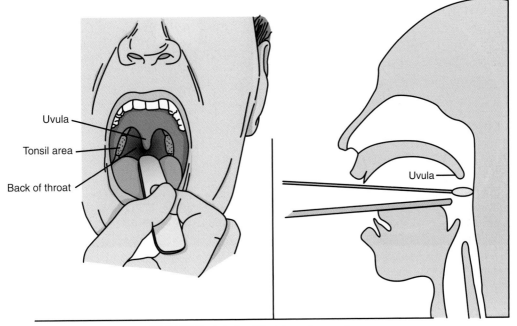

FIGURE 16-5   Obtaining a throat culture.

These swabs must be collected carefully and placed in the proper transport media before they are taken to the laboratory for processing. If swabs are not properly handled, the microorganisms may dry out, or their numbers may be insufficient for culture.

Urine

The collection of urine for microbiological studies also requires the cooperation of the patient. A clean-catch midstream sample, usually the first morning specimen, is suitable for culture, provided care has been taken to clean the urethral area before the collection (see Chapter 14). Urine in the bladder is normally sterile. A sterile container must be used for the collection of urine for culture. When a patient is too ill or cannot void properly, a specimen is obtained by catheterization. After collection, specimens should be sent to the laboratory for immediate processing or refrigeration, or a preservative can be used to maintain bacterial counts.

BASIC EQUIPMENT AND TECHNIQUES USED IN MICROBIOLOGY

Microbiologists use special equipment and techniques to grow and isolate pure cultures of microorganisms. Most work in the microbiology laboratory involves efforts to culture, characterize, and identify the various microbes being studied. The

information gained through these studies provides knowledge in three important areas: (1) culture of organisms present in the patient specimens, (2) classification and identification of the organisms when isolated, and (3) interpretation for the use of an appropriate antimicrobial agent. Such efforts require the use of specific techniques and equipment for culturing specimens, and stained slides for microscopic examination (see also Smear Preparation and Stains Used in Microbiology).

Inoculating Needle or Loop

A common tool of the microbiologist is the **inoculating transfer needle** or **loop.** Disposable and reusable types are used. Disposable inoculating loops are made of plastic and can be discarded after use. The classic reusable type may be either a straight wire or a wire with a loop at one end inserted into a suitable holder. The wire is usually platinum or an alloy such as Nichrome that can be sterilized by being heated to glowing without being affected and return to room temperature fairly rapidly. An object that can be safely heated until it is red is sterilized almost instantaneously. The needle or loop is used to culture specimens and transfer microorganisms from one medium to another or from a culture to a microscope slide. Because it can be sterilized quickly, the loop can be used repeatedly for this purpose. When a transfer is to be made, the needle or loop is sterilized in an incinerator or flame, then used to perform the transfer, and resterilized before it is set aside.

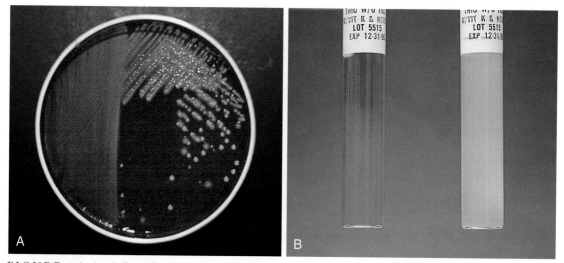

FIGURE 16-6 A, Example of bacterial growth on a solid medium. B, Liquid or broth media. Clear broth *(left)* indicates no growth, and turbid broth *(right)* indicates bacterial growth. (From Forbes BA, Sahm DF, Weissfeld AS: *Bailey and Scott's diagnostic microbiology,* ed 12, St Louis, 2007, Mosby.)

Incinerators

The **incinerator burner** is also a common piece of equipment in the microbiology laboratory. Many laboratories use this sterilization method for inoculating loops and needles because no gas is necessary to operate the burner. Sterilization is simply done by inserting the loop or needle into the central part of the burner, which is at a high temperature. **Bunsen burners** are used in the open-flame method, where the inoculating loop is sterilized by insertion into the flame.

Solid and Liquid Media

Solid media are prepared by adding agar to the nutrients of the particular medium being made. The melted agar (heated to about 100°C) is poured into a Petri dish or agar plate and left to solidify in an inverted position to prevent condensation on its surface. An agar plate is a shallow plastic or glass plate with a loose-fitting cover of the same material, shape, and depth as the dish but slightly larger in diameter. The plates are also stored in an inverted position after inoculation; they are labeled on the back of the portion of the plate where the medium is contained (Fig. 16-6, A). Slant cultures are solid media in tube form and can be used for storage, transportation, or biochemical testing. When preparing slants, the medium is dispensed into tubes and then autoclaved. The melted agar medium is allowed to harden while set at an angle.

Liquid media or **broth media** are prepared by placing the broth media in test tubes (Fig. 16-6, B). Wound and anaerobic cultures are processed using solid and liquid media. Broth media can be used to recover organisms of insufficient number

that were not represented on the agar plates; therefore a broth culture can back up the solid culture plates. When bacteria grow in a broth medium, the appearance of the medium will change from clear to turbid. Blood cultures are another example of using liquid media. Blood is collected, placed into a broth medium (in bottles), incubated, and if positive, can be Gram stained and subcultured for identification.

Culturing Techniques

Dilution streak technique is a method used in microbiology to obtain isolated colonies and semi-quantitation of bacterial colonies. A *colony* is a growth of bacteria that began as one bacterium and divided multiple times to produce a visible growth. When plating a specimen on solid agar, the aim is to inoculate successively smaller quantities over four areas of the plate (quadrants) of the original material so that by the fourth area, growth of isolated colonies can be seen. Some laboratories use a three-quadrant streak method to achieve isolation of colonies.

In general, a small amount of material (inoculum) is streaked onto the periphery of the plate, or the specimen can be dropped onto the periphery of the plate by a sterile pipette (Fig. 16-7). Streaking is achieved by drawing the sterilized inoculating loop back and forth across the surface of the medium. The first streak is continued across approximately one quarter of the plate (first quadrant). The inoculating loop is sterilized and allowed to cool between all quadrants and at the end. The plate is then turned and streaked again, beginning at the periphery, overlapping the previously inoculated

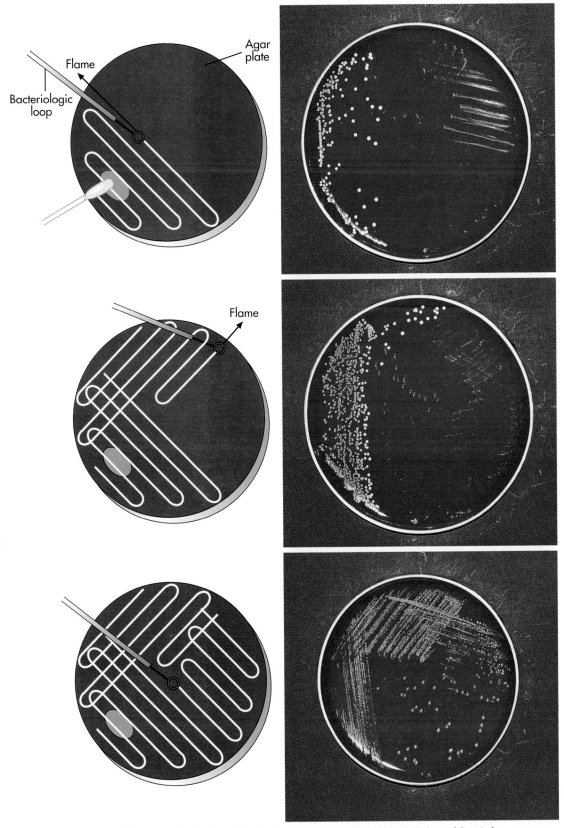

FIGURE 16-7 **Dilution streak technique.** (From Forbes BA, Sahm DF, Weissfeld AS: Bailey and Scott's diagnostic microbiology, ed 12, St Louis, 2007, Mosby.)

area a few times, and continuing across the second quadrant. The plate is turned once again and streaked a third time, beginning at the periphery, drawing the loop through the second streak a few times, and continuing across the third quadrant. Finally, the fourth quadrant is streaked by beginning at the periphery, drawing the loop through the third streak a few times and continuing across the fourth quadrant. In a specimen that has many bacteria present, isolated colonies will generally be found in the fourth quadrant.

Incubators

Temperature is an important factor in recovering bacteria, and most human pathogens multiply best at 35°C (host temperature). Incubators are chambers that have controlled environments. In the microbiology laboratory, routine incubators are set at 35°C ±2°C, have 3% to 5% carbon dioxide (CO_2), and are humidified. Most bacteria are enhanced by CO_2; certain bacteria do not grow when CO_2 is absent. Some microbiology laboratories use a candle jar for a CO_2 atmosphere (use only white, unscented candles). In most microbiology laboratories, two other incubators are set at 30°C, primarily for cultivation of fungi, and 42°C, for recovery of *Campylobacter* spp., which are intestinal pathogens.

IDENTIFICATION OF BACTERIA

To identify the etiologic or causative agent of an infection correctly, the microbiologist must carry out several steps involving a general knowledge of microorganisms and their modes of action. This section and those following discuss basic aspects of diagnostic microbiology, including routine specimen collection and identification processes for common bacteria, fungi, and parasites found in clinical specimens.

One of the principal roles of working in a microbiology laboratory is to isolate, identify, and present interpretive information about bacteria that cause disease in humans. The identification of most bacteria involves microscopic observations (smear preparation and staining), bacterial cultivation, and biochemical tests. Table 16-1 contains microscopic and macroscopic (colony) morphology of gram-positive organisms that are routinely recovered in clinical microbiology. Table 16-2 contains biochemical testing for identification of these gram-positive organisms. Fig. 16-8 shows an algorithm of gram-positive cocci. Table 16-3 contains biochemical testing of selected gram-negative organisms that are routinely recovered in clinical microbiology. Fig. 16-9 shows an algorithm of gram-negative enteric bacilli.

TABLE 16-1

Microscopic and Macroscopic (Colony) Morphology of Selected Gram-Positive Cocci		
Organism	Microscopic Morphology	Macroscopic (Colony) Morphology
Staphylococcus aureus	Pairs and clusters	Medium to large; most creamy yellow; translucent; smooth; slightly raised; most beta-hemolytic but some are gamma-hemolytic
Coagulase-negative staphylococci	Pairs and clusters	Small to medium; unpigmented; opaque; smooth; slightly raised or some convex; gamma-hemolytic
Group A beta-hemolytic streptococci	Pairs and chains	Small; gray-white; transparent to translucent; matte or glossy; large zone of beta-hemolysis
Group B beta-hemolytic streptococci	Pairs and chains	Small; gray-white; translucent to opaque; glossy; flat; narrow zone of beta-hemolysis
Group C beta-hemolytic streptococci	Pairs and chains	Two colony sizes (pinpoint and small); gray-white; transparent to translucent; glistening; large zone of beta-hemolysis
Group F beta-hemolytic streptococci	Pairs and chains	Pinpoint to small; gray-white; transparent to translucent; matte; small to large zone of beta-hemolysis
Group G beta hemolytic streptococci	Pairs and chains	Two colony sizes (pinpoint and small); gray-white; matte; large zone of beta-hemolysis
Streptococcus pneumoniae	Lancet shaped pairs, short chains, possible halo around pairs (due to capsule)	Small; gray; transparent to translucent; glistening; some mucoid; convex then umbilicated; alpha-hemolytic
Viridans streptococci	Pairs and chains	Pinpoint to small; gray; translucent; smooth to matte; domed; alpha-hemolytic
Enterococcus spp.	Pairs and chains	Small; cream to white; smooth; can exhibit alpha-, beta-, or gamma-hemolysis

TABLE 16-2

Testing for the Identification of Selected Gram-Positive Cocci									
Organism	Hemolysis on BAP	Catalase	Coagulase	PYR	Bacitracin	Lancefield typing	Optochin	Bile Solubility	Bile Esculin	Salt Tolerance (6.5% NaCl broth)
S. aureus	β, δ	+	+*							
Coagulase-negative staphylococci	δ	+	−							
Group A beta-hemolytic streptococci	β	−		+	+†	A				
Group B beta-hemolytic streptococci	β	−		−	−‡	B				
Group C beta-hemolytic streptococci	β	−		−	−	C				
Group F beta-hemolytic streptococci	β	−		−	−	F				
Group G beta-hemolytic streptococci	β	−		−	−	G				
S. pneumoniae	α	−					+§	+		
Viridans streptococci	α	−		−			−‖	−	−	−
Enterococcus spp.	α, β, δ	−¶		+					+	+

*There are some animal isolates of the staphylococci that are coagulase-positive. S. lugdunensis and S. schleiferi may be positive with the slide coagulase test.
†Positive: any zone of inhibition around the disc (0.4U).
‡Negative: no zone of inhibition.
§Positive: zone of inhibition >14mm.
‖Negative: no zone of inhibition.
¶Some enterococci demonstrate pseudocatalase (weak release of bubbles).

Smear Preparation and Stains Used in Microbiology

Identification of a particular species of bacteria involves morphologic examination under the microscope. The shapes and staining reactions of bacteria are observed in this way. If unstained bacteria are placed on a glass slide and observed under the microscope, they appear as transparent, colorless structures and may be homogeneous or granular. To make the bacteria stand out from the background, staining techniques are used. If they are unstained, the use of phase-contrast microscopy is helpful in visualization. Various staining procedures may be used, depending on the information desired (see Staining Techniques).

Smear Preparation

To stain bacteria, the material to be examined is spread thinly on a glass microscope slide and allowed to dry. The film should be thin enough that individual bacterial cells can be seen. If the material to be examined is a liquid, such as a broth culture, it may be transferred by means of a sterile swab, pipette, or inoculating loop and spread directly on the dry slide. If it is taken from an isolated colony from an agar plate, a drop of sterile water in which to suspend the bacteria must be placed on the slide first.

Many specimens are sent to microbiology in a two-swab system: one for culture and the other for Gram stain. If the specimen is submitted to microbiology on a single swab, however, culture media must be inoculated first and then the swab rolled onto the surface of the dry, clean glass slide. Slides are not sterile and thus are prepared last after all other culture media are inoculated.

The material is spread thinly but evenly over the appropriate area of the slide. This material may be from a patient specimen, a suspension of bacteria in a liquid medium, or a colony from a solid medium. All slides prepared must be labeled with sufficient patient identification information. It is sometimes helpful to draw a circle, using a wax pencil, on the underside of the slide directly under the area where

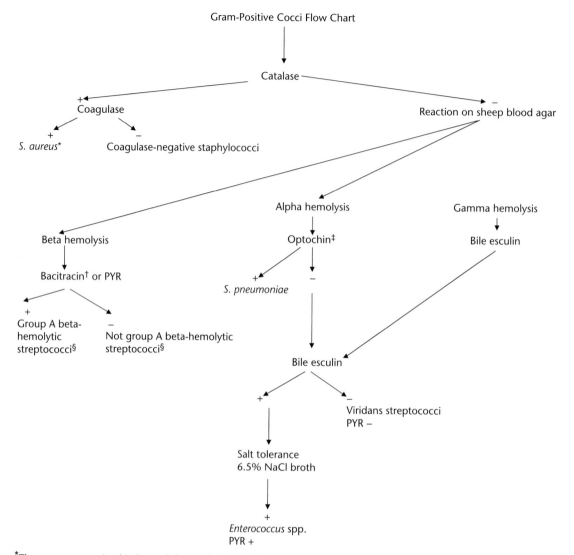

Gram-Positive Cocci Flow Chart

Catalase

+ Coagulase

+ S. aureus*

− Coagulase-negative staphylococci

Reaction on sheep blood agar

Alpha hemolysis

Gamma hemolysis

Beta hemolysis

Optochin‡

Bile esculin

Bacitracin† or PYR

+ S. pneumoniae

−

+ Group A beta-hemolytic streptococci§

− Not group A beta-hemolytic streptococci§

Bile esculin

+

− Viridans streptococci PYR −

Salt tolerance 6.5% NaCl broth

+ Enterococcus spp. PYR +

*There are some animal isolates of the staphylococci that are coagulase-positive. *S. lugdunensis* and *S. schleiferi* may be positive with the slide coagulase test.
†Positive: any zone of inhibition around the disc (0.04 U).
‡Positive: zone of inhibition >14 mm; zone of inhibition between 6 and 14 mm, perform bile solubility.
§Lancefield typing is performed to differentiate between beta-hemolytic streptococci.

FIGURE 16-8 Algorithm for identification of selected gram-positive cocci.

the specimen has been placed so the examination area may be found more easily under the microscope.

After the material has air-dried completely, it must be fixed to the slide. The fixing process prevents many of the bacterial cells from washing off the slide in subsequent staining operations. Fixation is achieved by heat or by placing the slide in 95% methanol for 1 minute.

Several staining procedures are used in the microbiology laboratory, but the Gram stain is used routinely and yields valuable information. Gram stains are also used for the examination of cultures to determine purity and for preliminary identification of bacterial microorganisms. Properly prepared and stained preparations of specimens may give

clues to the media for inoculation or further tests to be done. Gram stain results on specimens such as CSF, sputum, and wound cultures can be of great value regarding early treatment of the patient.

Types of Stains

To observe gross morphologic features, a **simple stain** such as methylene blue can be used. However, the most widely used staining method in microbiology is a **differential stain.** The Gram stain is an example of a differential stain; it separates bacteria into two groups based on their reaction, gram-positive and gram-negative. In addition to these two divisions, observation of morphologic features is noted. Another

TABLE 16-3

Key Biochemical Reactions of Selected Enterobacteriaceae										
Organism	IND	CIT	H₂S	LDC	LDA	UREA	ODC	MOT	TSI	GAS
Escherichia coli	+	–	–	+	–	–	+	+	A/A	+
Shigella spp.	V	–	–	–	–	–	V	–	K/A	–
Edwardsiella tarda	+	–	+	+	–	–	+	+	K/A	+
Salmonella spp. (most)	–	+	+	+	–	–	+	+	K/A	V
Citrobacter spp.	V	+	V	–	–	V	V	+	V/A	+
Klebsiella pneumoniae	–	+	–	+	–	+	–	–	A/A	+
Enterobacter spp.	–	+	–	+	–	V	+	+	A/A	+
Serratia marcescens*	–	+	–	+	–	–	+	+	A/A	V
Proteus mirabilis	–	V	+	–	+	+	+	+	K/A	+
Proteus vulgaris	+	– (V)	+	–	+	+	–	+	K/A	V
Morganella morganii	+	–	–	–	+	+	+	+	K/A	+
Providencia rettgeri	+	+	–	–	+	+	–	+	K/A	V
Providencia spp.	+	+	–	–	+	–†	–	+	K/A	V

IND, Indole; *CIT*, citrate utilization; *H₂S*, hydrogen sulfide; *LDC*, lysine decarboxylase; *LDA*, lysine deaminase; *UREA*, urease; *MOT*, motility; *TSI*, triple sugar iron agar.

*Enterobacter spp. and *Serratia marcescens* cannot be differentiated by the above tests, an additional gelatinase test can be performed, *S.marcescens* is positive and *Enterobacter* is negative.

†*Providencia stuartii* is urease variable.

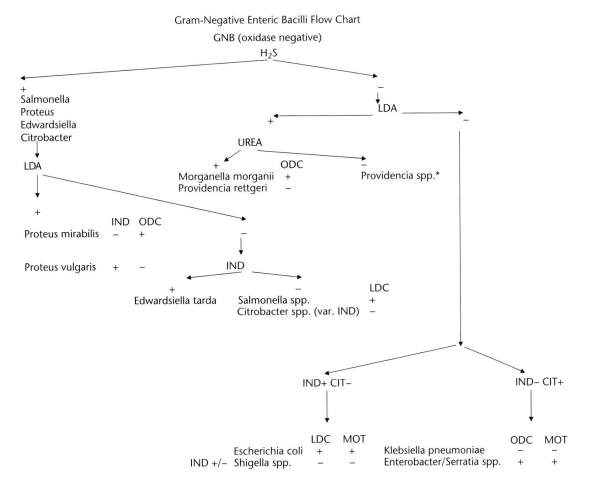

* *Providencia stuartii* is urea variable.

FIGURE 16-9 Gram-negative bacilli algorithm for identification of selected Enterobacteriaceae.

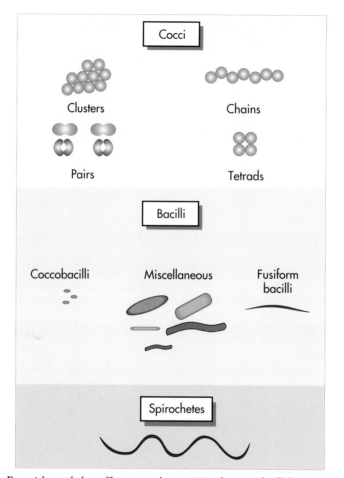

FIGURE 16-10 Bacterial morphology. Shown are characteristic shapes and cellular arrangements of bacteria. (From Forbes BA, Sahm DF, Weissfeld AS: Bailey and Scott's diagnostic microbiology, ed 12, St Louis, 2007, Mosby.)

differential stain is the acid-fast stain used to diagnose tuberculosis. Other stains include capsule stains, flagella stains, stains for metachromatic granules, spore stains, and stains for fungi (see Staining Techniques).

Morphology of Bacteria

Each species of bacteria has a characteristic shape (Fig. 16-10). Spherical or round bacteria are **cocci** (singular *coccus*), rod-shaped bacteria are **bacilli** (singular *bacillus*), and spiral-shaped bacteria are **spirochetes** and **spirilla** (singular *spirochete* and *spirillum*). Within the bacilli there can be curved rods called *vibrios*, small round rods called *coccobacilli*, and long, thin, or fat bacilli. The particular species may be further classified according to whether the cells normally occur singly, in pairs, in chains, or in clusters. The prefix *diplo-* describes bacteria that occur in pairs, *strepto-* describes bacteria occurring in chains, and *staphylo-* refers to irregular clumps or clusters of bacterial cells. At times, certain bacteria will exhibit **pleomorphism,** or variations in form. In this case the bacteria will have a varied

appearance on the same smear, such as long bacilli and coccobacilli in the same viewing field.

Although bacteria can be seen under the ordinary brightfield microscope, they are extremely small structures. They are normally observed under oil immersion with a 100× objective, giving a total magnification of 1000 times when the 10× ocular is used. Bacteria are measured in micrometers (1 μm = 1/1000 millimeter) and vary in size. *Staphylococcus* ranges from 0.5 to 1.5 μm in diameter; this is near the limit of resolution of the common light microscope, 0.2 μm. The bacilli show an even greater size variation. *Haemophilus influenzae* is a very small rod, about 0.2 μm wide by 0.5 μm long. *Bacillus anthracis* is a relatively large rod, 1 to 3 μm wide by 8 μm long. For comparison, a red blood cell is approximately 7 μm in diameter.

Morphology and staining characteristics of bacteria can lead the microbiologist to the initial identification of the bacterium. For the final identification, it is necessary to know the cultural characteristics of the bacterium and to perform biochemical testing, as discussed later.

PROCEDURE 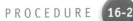 16-2

Staining With Methylene Blue

1. Spread a thin film of material on a clean microscope slide, air-dry, and fix. Place the slide on the staining rack.
2. Flood the surface of the slide with methylene blue staining solution. Allow the stain to remain on the slide for 2 minutes.
3. Wash the slide gently with running water to remove excess stain, and air-dry.
4. Examine the smear with the oil-immersion lens, noting the size, shape, and uniformity of staining of the microorganisms present.

Staining Techniques

The use of staining techniques is a common tool used by microbiologists to begin the identification process. Stains are chemical substances that contain dyes. Certain bacterial structures have affinities for particular dyes. Most microbiology laboratories purchase stains from commercial companies that are ready to use. Special stains are useful for showing the morphology of bacteria and specific structures such as capsules, flagella, spores, and granules. Simple stains (e.g., methylene blue) or more complex differential stains are used to show special cellular details. The way bacteria react to differential stains (e.g., Gram stain) depends on the chemical composition of the cell wall.

SIMPLE STAINS

Simple staining procedures employing crystal violet, fuchsin, methylene blue, or safranin have only limited use in the microbiology laboratory. These are termed *simple stains* because only one stain is used, and all structures present are stained the same color. When a simple stain is used, organisms should be observed for size, shape, and uniformity of staining.

Methylene Blue Stain

Procedure 16-2 outlines the technique for using one simple stain in microbiology, the methylene blue stain.

DIFFERENTIAL STAINS

Differential stains are used to distinguish between groups of bacteria. The most frequently used differential stain is the Gram stain.

Gram Stain

The **Gram stain** is used to differentiate various types of bacteria that have similar morphologic features (Procedure 16-3). The cell wall of

PROCEDURE 16-3

Staining With Conventional Gram Stain

1. Flood the fixed slide with crystal violet stain and wait 10 seconds.*
2. Rinse with water.
3. Flood with Gram's iodine solution and wait for 10 seconds.*
4. Rinse with water.
5. Decolorize quickly with the alcohol-acetone solution, or with 95% alcohol if the alcohol-acetone decolorization proves to be too rapid. Continue until no more color is extracted by the solvent. This usually takes 10 to 20 seconds,* but be careful not to overdecolorize.
6. Rinse with water.
7. Flood with safranin for 10 seconds.*
8. Rinse with water, air-dry, and examine using the oil-immersion lens.

*Times may vary depending on the laboratory's procedure; either 30 or 60 seconds.

the particular bacterium contributes to the Gram-staining reaction of the organism. The Gram stain method uses four different reagents: (1) the primary stain crystal violet; (2) the addition of Gram's iodine, which serves as a mordant; (3) decolorization with an alcohol-acetone solution; and (4) counterstaining with safranin. (A mordant is a substance that combines with a particular dye, forms an insoluble complex, and fixes the color in the substance dyed.)

The Gram stain method divides bacteria into two broad groups (Fig. 16-11). Bacteria that stain purple/blue as a result of retention of the crystal violet–iodine complex are termed **gram-positive.** Bacteria that stain red/pink from the counterstain safranin are termed **gram-negative.** The mechanism involved in retention of the crystal violet–iodine complex in gram-positive organisms but not in gram-negative organisms results from the difference in cell wall structure between the two groups. Gram-positive cells have a thick peptidoglycan layer with many teichoic acid cross-linkages. Gram-negative cells have a thinner peptidoglycan layer with an additional outer membrane similar to the cell membrane.

In the first step of the procedure for Gram staining, all organisms present are stained violet by the primary stain, crystal violet. The Gram's iodine added forms a crystal violet–iodine complex,

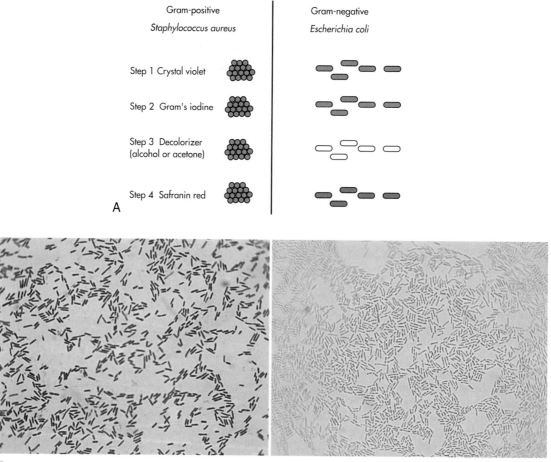

A

B

FIGURE 16-11 Gram stain method. **A,** In gram-positive bacteria such as *Staphylococcus aureus,* the crystal violet is retained in the thick peptidoglycan layer. These bacteria will appear purple/blue. In gram-negative bacteria such as *Escherichia coli,* the crystal violet–iodine complex is washed out during the decolorizing step, and then bacteria are counterstained with safranin. These bacteria will appear red/pink. **B,** Gram stains of gram-positive *(left)* and gram-negative *(right)* bacteria observed under oil immersion. (**A** from Murray PR, Rosenthal KS, Pfaller MA: Medical microbiology, ed 5, St Louis, 2005, Mosby; **B** modified from Atlas RM: Principles of microbiology, St Louis, 1995, Mosby.)

which is fixed or retained in gram-positive but not in gram-negative organisms.

Decolorization is done with a mixture of acetone and 95% alcohol; this removes all color from gram-negative organisms but does not affect gram-positive bacteria, which remain purple/blue. When a slower decolorization is warranted, 95% alcohol can be used alone. Because the gram-negative organisms are colorless after this step, they are counterstained with the red stain safranin so they can be visualized under the microscope.

Differentiation of bacteria is particularly helpful in determining the subsequent tests and means of culture for eventual identification of the bacteria. It is also a guide to treatment for patients because certain antibiotics are generally effective against gram-positive bacteria, whereas gram-negative bacteria are not as susceptible to their action, and vice versa.

Acid-Fast Stain

The acid-fast stain is used mainly to detect organisms that cause tuberculosis. Because of the possible aerosolization of these organisms, it is important to handle the specimens carefully, using a biological safety cabinet. These organisms would partially stain gram -positive if a Gram stain were used and would appear beaded. A differential stain for this group is the **acid-fast stain,** and mycobacteria will appear different from other groups of bacteria. Once stained, they retain the primary dye color, and decolorization is difficult, even with an acid-alcohol solution, and thus the term **acid-fast bacteria (AFB).** The acid-alcohol reagent decolorizes bacteria that do not have cell walls containing mycolic acid; these bacteria will be counterstained and all appear the same. The acid-fast bacteria (containing mycolic acid) will not decolorize and appear the color of the primary stain.

Staining for Acid-Fast Organisms Using Kinyoun Carbolfuchsin Method

1. Heat-fix the smears for 2 hours at 65°C to 70°C or for 15 minutes at 80°C.
2. Flood the smears with Kinyoun's carbolfuchsin stain for 5 minutes at room temperature.
3. Rinse with water.
4. Decolorize by adding acid-alcohol reagent. This requires approximately 2 minutes for smears of average thickness.
5. Rinse with water.
6. Counterstain with methylene blue or malachite green for 1 to 3 minutes.
7. Rinse with water, air-dry, and examine using the oil-immersion lens.

Staining for Acid-Fast Organisms Using Auramine-Rhodamine Method

1. Heat-fix the smears for 2 hours at 65°C to 70°C or for 15 minutes at 80°C.
2. Flood the slide with auramine-rhodamine for 15 minutes at room temperature.
3. Rinse with water.
4. Decolorize with acid-alcohol for 2 to 3 minutes.
5. Rinse with water.
6. Flood the slide with potassium permanganate for 2 to 4 minutes.
7. Rinse with water, and examine slides using a fluorescence microscope.

The *Ziehl-Neelsen* acid-fast method uses carbolfuchsin as the primary stain, heat to facilitate penetration of the stain, a mixture of 3% hydrochloric acid and 95% ethanol as the decolorizer, and methylene blue as the counterstain. The *Kinyoun* acid-fast modification uses a slightly different carbolfuchsin preparation, phenol to facilitate penetration of the stain, and either methylene blue or malachite green as a counterstain (Procedure 16-4). The Kinyoun method is referred to as the "cold" method because heat is not necessary as a result of the phenol. After the first step of the acid-fast staining procedure, all bacteria present on the slide appear red. Following decolorization with acid-alcohol reagent, the acid-fast bacteria appear red, and all other bacteria are colorless. After counterstaining with methylene blue, the acid-fast bacteria appear red, and all other cells appear blue (if malachite green is used, all other cells appear green).

A third method of staining acid-fast bacteria is by using fluorochrome stains. **Fluorochromes** are dyes that absorb ultraviolet light and emit light of higher wavelengths. Fluorescent microscopes have filters that excite fluorochromes and detect the emitted light (see Chapter 5). This method is more sensitive than the Ziehl-Neelsen and Kinyoun methods because the acid-fast bacteria will fluoresce and stand out as bright yellow-orange against a dark background. The slides can also be rapidly screened under a lower magnification, which decreases the reading time per slide. The

fluorochrome method uses auramine and rhodamine as the primary stains (Procedure 16-5). The decolorizer is acid-alcohol reagent, and the counterstain is potassium permanganate.

Microscopy Techniques Used

Although brightfield microscopy is used for most routine microscopic examinations in the microbiology laboratory, the use of varying microscopy techniques is important in some microbiological assays.

BRIGHTFIELD MICROSCOPY

For most routine microscopy needs, the brightfield microscope is used. With this type of illumination, the organism appears dark against a bright background. Gram stains are usually examined with an ordinary brightfield microscope using the oil-immersion objective (100×).

FLUORESCENT MICROSCOPY

In fluorescent microscopy, the specimen is self-illuminating and a light image is observed against a dark background. A special darkfield fluorescent microscope is used (see Chapter 5). The acid-fast staining method using the fluorochromes, auramine and rhodamine, is a rapid screening method for detection of *Mycobacterium* spp., including *M. tuberculosis*, the causative agent of tuberculosis.

Immunofluorescent techniques are used in many laboratories for identification of certain microorganisms. In this technique it is possible to pretreat certain antibodies with fluorescent dye

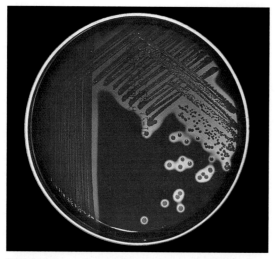

FIGURE 16-12 Pure culture of *Staphylococcus aureus* on a sheep blood agar plate. Each colony began as an individual parent bacterial cell that multiplied many times to become visible. (From Forbes BA, Sahm DF, Weissfeld AS: Bailey and Scott's diagnostic microbiology, ed 12, St Louis, 2007, Mosby.)

and then to react them with microorganisms. If the microorganism is specific for the complementary antigen, they will complex. The antibody-antigen complex is fluorescent and can be observed using the fluorescent microscope. This technique can be used to identify the bacterial pathogen *Legionella pneumophila* (legionnaires' disease) and certain viral infections.

Bacterial Cultivation

To begin the process of identification of microorganisms, a culture must be grown, and the organisms that are biochemically tested must be in a pure culture. This is necessary for accuracy and also because the pure culture is used to test for susceptibility and resistance to antimicrobial agents.

Primary Culture, Subculture, and Pure Culture

When culturing specimens from patients, the **primary culture** plates are streaked in the dilution streak technique to obtain isolated colonies. Many cultures are mixtures of more than one species of bacteria, so a **subculture** must be performed to separate the different types of bacteria present. To separate the bacteria, a single isolated colony is taken and then subcultured onto additional media so that several colonies will appear, all arising from single bacteria. The growth of several colonies originating from a single colony, and thus a single cell, is known as a **pure culture** (Fig. 16-12). It is assumed that a colony is begun by one parent bacterial cell

that multiplies many times, until a visible aggregate or colony forms.

Types of Culture Media

Many (but not all) microorganisms may be grown in the laboratory away from their natural habitat. To grow microorganisms artificially, it is necessary to provide the proper nutrients and growth conditions. The growth of microorganisms on artificial material is referred to as **culture** of the microorganism, and the mixture of nutrients on which the microorganism is grown is the **culture medium.**

Bacteria are grown on specially prepared culture media. The isolation and identification of viable pathogenic organisms on culture media are still the standard for diagnosis of infectious disease processes. Specimens are plated and inoculated on several different growth media, depending on the suspected etiologic agent. Choosing appropriate culture media is essential for the isolation, growth, and final identification of pathogenic organisms. By studying the cultural characteristics of a particular bacterium, certain growth patterns may be seen, and the presumptive species identification may be made.

The media used in microbiology are generally prepared from measured quantities of known substances that are formulated to give highly repeatable culture results. Media of this type are produced synthetically and consist of the specific amino acids, sugars, salts, vitamins, and minerals needed to ensure the proper growth of certain bacterial species. They are usually produced commercially and are used for diagnostic purposes. Commercially prepared media in disposable culture plates or tubes have generally replaced on-site preparation. The Clinical and Laboratory Standards Institute (CLSI), formerly the National Committee for Clinical Laboratory Standards (NCCLS), has published recommendations for manufacturers of commercial media[8] (see Quality Control of Media).

Agar is used extensively in the preparation of solid media; it is a seaweed extract that is liquid when heated and solid when cooled. It does not affect bacterial growth and is an excellent base for nutrient media. Agar can be melted and poured into tubes or plates, where it will solidify when cooled. The more agar used, the more solid the final medium will become. Plates and agar slants are prepared with agar as the base.

In addition to agar plates or Petri dishes to observe growth characteristics of the microorganisms, culture studies include the use of agar slants for maintenance of cultures, certain biochemical studies, or semisolid media for motility. Broths or liquid media are also sometimes used as culture media. Broths are meat extracts of protein materials, either peptone, an intermediate product of protein digestion, or digested protein. Broths are used for all wound and anaerobic cultures. They can serve as a backup medium to the agar plates, and if the organism is low in numbers, the broth will support the growth. The broth can be subcultured to agar plates for identification.

Colony Characteristics (Appearance) of Bacterial Cultures

When inoculated onto suitable semisolid or solid nutrient media with the proper temperature and moisture, bacteria rapidly multiply and form macroscopic colonies. Under ideal conditions, the growth of a microbial cell is a geometric progression over time. For example, a single bacterium such as *Escherichia coli*, with a generation time of 20 minutes, would produce 1,073,741,824 (1×2^{30}) cells in 10 hours. Certain limiting factors, however, ultimately terminate growth. A culture that is a closed system will eventually stop growing as a result of exhaustion of essential nutrients, accumulation of toxic products, or development of an unfavorable pH.

The type of culture medium used (liquid or solid) can affect the appearance or growth of the colonies. In liquid media, bacterial growth does not have a characteristic appearance, and organisms cannot be separated from "mixed cultures." By contrast, on solid media the appearance of a culture is extremely useful in initially differentiating the colony type, and pure cultures can be isolated.

Bacteria multiply by binary fission, where the bacterial cell will divide and produce two daughter cells. Macroscopic bacterial colonies form in 24 to 48 hours. The colonies originate from individual cells, although each colony is a mass of individual cells, each of which functions independently. Different species of bacteria form colonies that differ in appearance; therefore, colony appearance is useful in identifying the species of bacteria. Colony characteristics that are observed for the purpose of identification include:

1. Bacteria without slime capsules produce colonies that appear dry and rough.
2. Bacteria with slime capsules produce colonies that appear shiny and wet (mucoid).
3. Bacteria may possess a pigment that gives a characteristic color (e.g., white, red, yellow, orange) to the colony.
4. Bacteria may spread or swarm across the media, which indicates that they are motile.

Bacterial colonies should be observed for their relative size, shape or form, elevation, texture, marginal appearance, and color. This information, in addition to morphologic appearance under the microscope, various staining reactions (e.g., Gram

stain), and results of biochemical tests performed, helps in the eventual identification of a particular species of bacteria (see Tables 16-1 to 16-3 and Figs. 16-8 and 16-9).

Requirements for Bacterial Cultivation

Bacteria, as with all living things, have specific requirements to sustain life and reproduce. The culture requirements for bacteria include a source of nutrients, the proper temperature, an adequate supply of oxygen (or in some cases the absence of oxygen), and the correct pH.

OXYGEN REQUIREMENTS: AEROBES AND ANAEROBES

An important factor that must be considered in culturing microorganisms is the presence or absence of oxygen. Pathogenic organisms are either obligate **aerobes,** utilizing oxygen for their growth; obligate **anaerobes,** intolerant to oxygen; or microaerophiles, growing best in an atmosphere of reduced oxygen tension. Aerobes can be incubated in room air. Most clinically significant aerobes are really **facultative anaerobes,** which can grow under either aerobic or anaerobic conditions. Most of the common pathogenic bacteria grow well in the presence of oxygen.

Some pathogenic organisms are incapable of growth in oxygen and are classified as *obligate anaerobic organisms*. All specimens for anaerobic studies must be cultured as soon as possible after collection to avoid loss of viability. Special methods are required for the isolation and study of anaerobic bacteria. Anaerobes are able to derive energy from their food sources and are actually inhibited by atmospheric oxygen; to culture these anaerobes or anaerobic organisms, atmospheric oxygen must be excluded.

Specimens originating from sites where an anaerobic agent is suspected are cultured on both aerobic and anaerobic media. Enriched media as well as differential and selective media are inoculated (see Classification of Media). The enriched and selective media are needed because anaerobes are fastidious and most anaerobic infections are polymicrobic, or polymicrobial (i.e., mixed with aerobic and other anaerobic organisms). Inoculated plates are immediately placed in an anaerobic environment for incubation. Jars, chambers, or commercially produced pouches and bags can be used (Fig. 16-13). Cultures are incubated for 48 hours at 35°C. Usually these cultures should not be exposed to any oxygen until after 48 hours of incubation. If plates are in a chamber or an anaerobic bag, they can be observed after 24 hours without oxygen exposure. Anaerobic conditions can be attained by commercial hydrogen or CO_2 generator systems for use with jars and pouches. In anaerobic

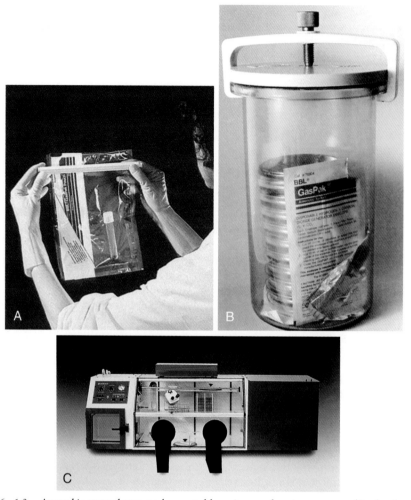

FIGURE 16-13 **Anaerobic atmospheres can be created by using pouches, jars, or anaerobic chambers. A, Anaerobic pouch. B, Anaerobic jar. C, Anaerobic chamber.** (**A** courtesy and copyright Becton Dickinson and Company; **B** from Forbes BA, Sahm DF, Weissfeld AS: *Bailey and Scott's diagnostic microbiology,* ed 12, St Louis, 2007, Mosby; **C** courtesy Anaerobe Systems, Morgan Hill, Calif.)

chambers, a gas mixture is used to keep an oxygen-free environment. Specimens and media are placed in the chamber by an air lock, therefore maintaining the anaerobic environment.

Thioglycolate broth is used to grow anaerobic and aerobic organisms. It contains thioglycolate and 0.075% agar; both serve to create an anaerobic environment in the bottom of the tube (see Common Types of Media). Strict aerobes will grow at the top of the media, where oxygen is available. Prereduced media are commercially available for the isolation of anaerobic bacteria, and each facility has recommended enriched and selective media for primary plating of anaerobic specimens.

NUTRIENTS

The proper nutrient elements must be available because microorganisms differ in their food requirements. Some grow on media containing simple mixtures of inorganic salts, since they are able to synthesize their own organic compounds. Others, especially many pathogens, require complex mixtures of nutrients, including many of the B vitamins and certain amino acids. In general, the culture medium must be able to supply carbon and energy sources, usually in the form of carbohydrates. Peptone is used in a variety of culture media because it contains nitrogen in a form (amino acids and simple nitrogen compounds) that can be used by most microorganisms. Certain bacteria require media to which serum, blood, or ascitic fluid has been added.

TEMPERATURE

All organisms have a minimum temperature below which development ceases, an optimum temperature at which growth is best or luxuriant, and a maximum temperature above which death occurs. Bacteria can grow at a wide range of temperatures. Some grow at cold temperatures (10°C), and others grow in hot springs (50°C). However, the pathogens generally have a narrow temperature range, with optimum growth at 35°C; therefore, most cultures are incubated at 35°C. Because the heat of an incubator promotes drying, the incubator should always be equipped with containers of water or some other suitable source of humidity.

HYDROGEN ION CONCENTRATION (pH)

Another factor affecting the growth or culture of microorganisms is the pH of the medium. A culture medium not only must contain the proper nutrients in the correct concentrations, but also must have the correct degree of acidity or alkalinity. Most clinical pathogens prefer media that are approximately neutral: pH range of 6.5 to 7.5.

The pH of media is controlled by use of **buffers,** or substances that resist changes in hydrogen ion concentration. Buffers are especially useful for microorganisms that produce acid as part of their metabolism. These microorganisms would kill themselves by their own acid production if a suitable buffer were not present. Conversely, some bacteria produce alkaline products such as ammonia; these also must be buffered, or the culture would destroy itself.

STERILE CONDITIONS

To obtain a pure culture of a microorganism, the culture medium must be sterile. Not only is sterilization necessary for separation of the inoculated organism, but contamination by other microbes may influence or prevent the growth of the desired microorganism. Commercially prepared media are sterilized and packaged and are used by most laboratories. If a laboratory makes media, sterilization is performed by use of the autoclave.

MOISTURE

Water is necessary for metabolic reactions to take place in the bacterial cell and must be present in the medium for growth to occur. Also, if the medium dries out, the concentration of the solutes in the medium increases, which could affect the bacteria negatively. Incubator chambers are humidified to prevent drying of media.

Incubation Time and Temperature for Routine Cultures

A certain amount of time is needed for any final identification of cultures. Most cultures require 2 days, although anaerobic cultures require longer incubation times, usually 3 to 5 days for final identification if there is growth in the cultures. Genital cultures are routinely kept 3 days before

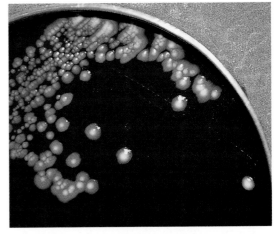

FIGURE 16-14 Buffered charcoal–yeast extract (BCYE) is an enrichment medium formulated specifically to grow the pathogen *Legionella pneumophila*. (From Forbes BA, Sahm DF, Weissfeld AS: Bailey and Scott's diagnostic microbiology, ed 12, St Louis, 2007, Mosby.)

a final report is documented. Although 2 days is generally required for identification, most bacteria can be seen growing on media within 24 hours. Routine cultures are incubated at 35°C ±2°C, with an atmosphere of 3% to 5% CO_2 and a source of humidity (see Incubators).

Storage of Media

Media are generally stored under refrigeration (4°C) to prevent deterioration and dehydration. Certain media require special storage; such information will be provided with the media. In general, a medium should be allowed to warm up to room temperature before it is inoculated, or microorganisms may be destroyed.

Classification of Media

Different types of media are used in diagnostic microbiology to aid not only in supporting growth but also in identification. Therefore, media are placed in categories by their function: enrichment, supportive, selective, and differential.

ENRICHMENT MEDIA

Enrichment media permit one bacterial pathogen to grow by using specific nutrients for the growth of that pathogen. An example of enrichment media is buffered charcoal–yeast extract agar that supports the growth of *Legionella pneumophila*, the causative agent of legionnaires' disease (Fig. 16-14).

SUPPORTIVE MEDIA

Supportive media contain nutrients that allow most nonfastidious organisms to grow at their normal rate. These media do not give one organism

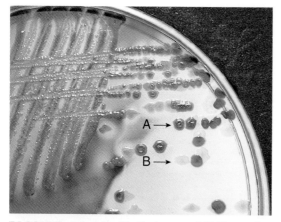

FIGURE 16-15 MacConkey agar (MAC) is a selective and differential medium used frequently for primary plating of specimens to isolate and differentiate gram-negative bacilli. Gram-negative bacilli that ferment lactose will appear pink/red *(A)*. Gram-negative bacilli that do not ferment lactose will appear clear or slightly pink *(B)*. (From Forbes BA, Sahm DF, Weissfeld AS: Bailey and Scott's diagnostic microbiology, ed 12, St Louis, 2007, Mosby.)

any growth advantage over another. The organism's own metabolism affects the progress of its growth.

SELECTIVE MEDIA

Selective media are prepared by adding dyes, antibiotics, or other chemical compounds that inhibit certain bacteria while allowing others to grow. MacConkey agar is a selective medium that contains crystal violet and bile salts to inhibit the growth of gram-positive bacteria (Fig. 16-15). In primary cultures, MacConkey agar is the most frequently used selective agar for recovery of gram-negative bacteria.

DIFFERENTIAL MEDIA

Differential media contain factors that give colonies of particular organisms distinctive and easily recognizable characteristics. MacConkey agar is a differential medium that contains lactose and neutral red as the factors for differentiation (see Fig. 16-15). Certain organisms ferment lactose to an acid product that changes the pH of the media. The indicator present, neutral red, will give the bacterial colonies a deep pink/purple color at an acid pH. Non–lactose-fermenting bacteria are colorless or pale pink. Therefore, microbiologists can differentiate between lactose-fermenting bacteria and non–lactose-fermenting bacteria based on their appearance on MacConkey agar. This is an important distinction because stool pathogens such as *Salmonella* and *Shigella* spp. are non–lactose-fermenting gram-negative organisms. As previously noted, MacConkey agar is a selective medium as well as a differential medium.

Common Types of Media

The eventual identification of a particular microorganism requires its culture on various media (selective, enrichment, or differential). No one system is universally employed in the identification of pathogens (see Biochemical and Enzymatic Tests). Many types of media are available for culture purposes. Some are used for primary plating of routine cultures, and others are used only rarely. Descriptions and intended uses of available media can be found in either the Difco Manual[9] or the REMEL Technical Manual.[10]

CHOCOLATE AGAR (CHOC)

Chocolate agar is an enrichment medium that promotes the growth of fastidious bacteria. Chocolate agar is prepared by adding blood to a nutrient base medium, then gently heating the preparation. The heat lyses the red blood cells, causing the medium to turn brown, thus the name "chocolate." This gives a richer medium than ordinary blood agar, providing hemin (X factor) and nicotinamide adenine dinucleotide (NAD, or V factor) for growth. The X and V growth factors are required by some fastidious organisms, such as *Haemophilus* spp. Choc is also used in the cultivation of the pathogenic *Neisseria* spp. These organisms cause gonorrhea and meningitis and can be difficult to grow. They require an atmosphere of 3% to 7% CO_2 in addition to selective media for growth.

COLUMBIA COLISTIN–NALIDIXIC ACID AGAR WITH BLOOD

Columbia colistin-nalidixic acid (CNA) agar is a selective and differential medium used to recover gram-positive bacteria. The antibiotics colistin and nalidixic acid inhibit most gram-negative organisms. The 5% sheep blood aids in differentiation of hemolytic organisms (see sheep blood agar).

EOSIN–METHYLENE BLUE AGAR

Eosin–methylene blue (EMB) agar is both a selective and a differential medium used in the primary plating of routine cultures. It inhibits the growth of gram-positive organisms, selecting for gram-negative growth; many gram-negative organisms have a characteristic appearance on EMB. Laboratories use EMB for urine cultures in conjunction with sheep blood agar. Many urinary tract infections can be caused by gram-negative bacilli that will grow differentially on EMB because of the addition of lactose. This aids the microbiologist in identification. Different gram-negative bacilli ferment lactose to an acid product, and with the dyes eosin and methylene blue, these bacilli appear purple or blue-black. *Escherichia coli* has a characteristic metallic sheen when grown on EMB.

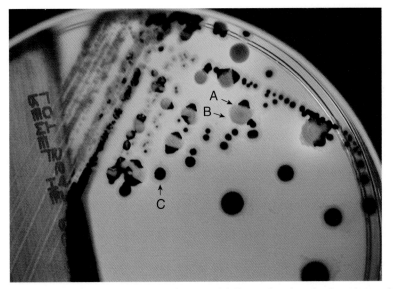

FIGURE 16-16 Hektoen enteric agar (HE) is a selective and differential medium for the isolation of enteric pathogens. *Escherichia coli* is a lactose-fermenting gram-negative bacillus and appears yellow on HE *(A)*. *Shigella* spp. do not ferment lactose and will appear green or transparent *(B)*. *Salmonella* spp. are also non–lactose-fermenters but produce hydrogen sulfide (H_2S); therefore the colonies will appear green or transparent with black centers *(C)*. (From Forbes BA, Sahm DF, Weissfeld AS: Bailey and Scott's diagnostic microbiology, ed 12, St Louis, 2007, Mosby.)

MacConkey agar, also selective and differential, can be used instead of EMB in urine cultures.

HEKTOEN ENTERIC AGAR

Hektoen enteric (HE) agar is a selective and differential media for the isolation of enteric pathogens such as *Salmonella* and *Shigella* spp. HE contains bile salts and two indicators, bromthymol blue and acid fuchsin, for the inhibition of gram-positive organisms. This medium also slows the growth of most nonpathogenic enteric gram-negative bacilli and contains lactose for additional aid in differentiating pathogenic from nonpathogenic enteric bacteria (Fig. 16-16). Most nonpathogens will ferment lactose to an acid pH and appear yellow because of the indicator bromthymol blue. *Salmonella* and *Shigella* spp. do not ferment lactose, so no color change will occur. There are additional components, sodium thiosulfate and ferric ammonium citrate, for the detection of hydrogen sulfide (H_2S) production. Organisms that produce H_2S will form a black precipitate. Colonies of *Salmonella*, an H_2S producer, will appear green or transparent with black centers, and *Shigella*, a non-H_2S producer, will appear green or transparent.

LÖWENSTEIN-JENSEN MEDIUM

Löwenstein-Jensen (LJ) medium is used to cultivate and isolate *Mycobacterium* species. It is an egg-based medium containing whole eggs, potato flour, and glycerol to support the growth of mycobacteria. It is the best medium for recovery of *M. tuberculosis*, the genus responsible for tuberculosis. The presence of malachite green in the medium inhibits the growth of other bacteria that may be present in the specimen. Specimens are inoculated onto LJ medium and incubated at 35°C with 5% to 10% CO_2 and high humidity, then observed weekly for 8 weeks. Alternate media used to cultivate *Mycobacterium* spp. are Middlebrook 7H10 and 7H11. Strains resistant to isoniazid (antimycobacterial agent) grow better on these media than on egg-based media.

LYSINE IRON AGAR

Lysine iron agar (LIA) slants (see Fig. 16-19) contain lysine, peptones (nutrient source), glucose (small amount), ferric ammonium citrate (indicator), and sodium thiosulfate (sulfur source). Bacteria can be identified by which enzyme they possess. This medium is used to determine whether an organism can decarboxylate lysine or deaminate lysine by the action of the enzymes lysine decarboxylase or lysine deaminase, respectively. If the organism possesses lysine decarboxylase, the medium in the butt will appear purple (original color of medium). If the organism is lysine decarboxylase negative, the butt will appear yellow (see Biochemical or Enzymatic Tests).

An organism that is lysine deaminase positive will have a burgundy slant, and if negative, the slant will remain purple. An organism cannot be positive for both enzymes. Ferric ammonium citrate and sodium thiosulfate are present for detection of H_2S, as noted by a black color.

LIA slants are inoculated by first stabbing the butt through the center, then streaking the slant surface. LIA aids in the differentiation of enteric pathogens from nonpathogens. Some nonpathogens that may be confused with *Salmonella* spp. are lysine deaminase positive (burgundy slant), such as *Proteus*. Both *Salmonella* and *Shigella* are lysine deaminase negative (purple slant), and *Salmonella* is lysine decarboxylase positive (purple butt), further aiding in identification.

MACCONKEY AGAR (MAC)

MacConkey is both a selective and a differential medium for gram-negative bacilli and can be used in the primary plating of routine cultures (see Fig. 16-15). It differentiates between lactose-fermenting and non–lactose-fermenting gram-negative bacilli. Crystal violet and bile salts are present to inhibit gram-positive organisms. The medium is also used in the diagnosis of gastroenteritis, and the organisms that cause these infections do not ferment lactose. Organisms that ferment lactose to an acid pH will appear pink-red because of the addition of the pH indicator neutral red. Lactose fermenters will appear as pink-red, and non–lactose fermenters will appear clear or slightly pink.

MacConkey is the most frequently used selective and differential medium for isolation of gram-negative bacilli. It is used preferentially over EMB because MAC inhibits swarming by *Proteus* spp.

PHENYLETHYL ALCOHOL AGAR

Phenylethyl alcohol (PEA) agar is essentially sheep blood agar with phenylethyl alcohol added. The medium inhibits the growth of gram-negative organisms, except *Pseudomonas aeruginosa*, and permits growth of gram-positive cocci. PEA is also used to isolate anaerobic organisms, particularly when mixed with other flora. Therefore, PEA is enriched and selective. Hemolysis cannot be observed on the PEA plate.

SABOURAUD DEXTROSE AGAR WITH ANTIBIOTICS

Sabouraud dextrose agar with antibiotics (SAB) is a selective medium that promotes the growth of fungi while inhibiting bacterial growth. To inhibit bacteria, SAB has a low pH. It should be incubated at 30°C. Chloramphenicol is included to inhibit bacterial growth, and cycloheximide may be included to inhibit nonpathogenic or saprophytic fungi.

SELENITE BROTH

Selenite broth is an enrichment medium used for stool cultures (L-cystine for recovery of *Salmonella*). The selenite acts selectively to inhibit the growth of gram-positive organisms and coliform bacilli while favoring *Shigella* and *Salmonella*, two causative agents of gastroenteritis. The medium suppresses growth of organisms other than *Shigella* and *Salmonella* for 12 to 18 hours. After this time, coliform bacilli and enterococci grow rapidly, causing overgrowth. Therefore, after 18 hours of incubation, cultures grown in selenite broth must be subcultured to a suitable differential medium (e.g., HE, xylose-lysine-desoxycholate [XLD]).

SHEEP BLOOD AGAR

Sheep blood agar (SBA or BA) is an all-purpose medium that supports the growth of most bacteria. SBA is therefore used for primary plating and for subculturing. It is a good general medium for the growth of pathogens because the blood adds many of the substances pathogens require. SBA is also useful in distinguishing different types of organisms, such as streptococci, by their ability to hemolyze the red blood cells (erythrocytes) present in the medium; therefore it is a differential medium. The three designations for differentiation of organisms are alpha (α) hemolysis—green (or partial) hemolysis; beta (β) hemolysis—clear (or complete) hemolysis; and gamma (γ) hemolysis—no hemolysis (see Fig. 16-23).

THAYER-MARTIN AGAR (MODIFIED THAYER-MARTIN AGAR)

Thayer-Martin agar is a selective and enriched medium for *Neisseria gonorrhoeae* and *N. meningitidis*. It is a modification of chocolate agar, containing hemoglobin and a supplement that includes NAD and vitamins. Several antimicrobial agents are present in the medium to inhibit the growth of normal flora and fungi (e.g., *Candida albicans*).

THIOGLYCOLATE BROTH (THIO BROTH)

Thioglycolate broth (see Fig. 16-6, *B*) is a liquid medium that can be used to isolate a wide range of bacteria, but it is used particularly for the cultivation of anaerobic organisms when additional supplements are added, such as vitamin K and hemin. It contains thioglycolate and agar to encourage anaerobic growth by decreasing oxygen tension in the bottom of the tube. The medium is in a reduced state and contains the indicator resazurin, which turns pink if the medium is oxidized. All cultures in which an anaerobic organism is suspected are inoculated into thioglycolate broth.

TRIPLE SUGAR IRON AGAR SLANTS

Triple sugar iron (TSI) slants (see Fig. 16-20) contain glucose, sucrose, and lactose (fermentable sugars), phenol red pH indicator, peptone (nutrient source), sodium thiosulfate (sulfur source), and ferric ammonium citrate (indicator). It is essential that the slants be inoculated with a pure culture, so a single, well-isolated colony should be used for the inoculum. The medium is inoculated by stabbing (use a straight inoculating needle) the butt through the center to the bottom, then streaking the slant.

TSI medium is especially useful as a first step in the identification of gram-negative bacilli. It is used to test the ability of gram-negative bacilli to ferment glucose, sucrose, or lactose and produce H_2S. Fermentation of sugars is accompanied by acid production, which is indicated by a change in the color of the phenol red indicator from red to yellow (yellow in acid pH and red in alkaline pH). Ferric ammonium citrate and sodium thiosulfate are present for detection of H_2S, as noted by a black color. Bubbles or splitting of the agar indicates gas production (see Biochemical or Enzymatic Tests).

Other media similar to TSI include Kligler's iron agar (KIA). This medium differs in that it tests fermentation of only glucose and lactose; sucrose is not included.

UREA AGAR

Urea agar is used to test the ability of a microorganism to utilize urea by action of the enzyme urease. Breakdown of urea by the action of urease results in the production of ammonia, which raises the pH of the medium, as indicated by a color change of the phenol red indicator to a bright pink-red or magenta color. The organism is streaked onto the slant only. The butt is not stabbed. Some organisms give a pink color only in the slant; in others, both the butt and the slant will be pink.

XYLOSE-LYSINE-DESOXYCHOLATE AGAR

Xylose-lysine-desoxycholate (XLD) agar is a selective and differential agar for the recovery of *Salmonella* and *Shigella* spp. The medium contains a phenol red indicator, desoxycholate, ferric ammonium sulfate, sodium thiosulfate, lysine, xylose, lactose, and sucrose. Desoxycholate inhibits gram-positive organisms and many nonenteric gram-negative bacilli, and therefore they do not grow. *Shigella* spp. are differentiated from other gram-negative enteric bacilli by not fermenting xylose, lactose, or sucrose. Because *Shigella* spp. do not ferment these carbohydrates, the colonies appear transparent or red (color of medium). *Salmonella* spp. possess the enzyme decarboxylase, which can act on the amino acid lysine. This reaction is called *decarboxylation* and can aid in differentiating *Salmonella* from other enteric organisms. The reaction yields colonies that are transparent or red. *Salmonella* spp. produce H_2S using sodium thiosulfate with the indicator ferric ammonium sulfate. This causes the transparent or red colonies to develop black centers. To differentiate enteric nonpathogens from the enteric pathogens, lactose and sucrose are included to make the colonies of the nonpathogenic organisms appear yellow.

Quality Control of Media

CLSI has developed recommendations for use of abbreviated quality control (QC) testing for commercially prepared media.[8] If a manufacturer has followed the CLSI recommendations, the performance of its media is consistent and adequate, and these media do not require further QC testing in the local laboratory.

Some commercially prepared media, however, require QC testing at the diagnostic laboratory, and CLSI has identified these media. For this testing, QC organisms can be purchased along with their expected results; the relevant CLSI publication should be consulted for this information.[8] All media prepared in the laboratory must be tested before being used for routine culture. The laboratory must maintain a stock of organisms for QC testing of the media for CLIA-mandated participation in quality assurance programs.

Biochemical or Enzymatic Tests

Many bacteria cannot be identified based on microscopic or cultural characteristics alone. The biochemical properties and reactions of bacteria form the basis for an important series of identification procedures. Biochemical identification is an important function of the microbiology laboratory. Biochemical tests rely on bacterial physiology and the end products produced in reactions of bacterial cells. Important biochemical reactions involve oxidation, fermentation, hydrogen sulfide production, urea hydrolysis, and indole production from the breakdown of tryptophan.

In each biochemical procedure, the unknown bacterium causes a change of some type in the medium, to which a specific test substance has been added. The change may be indicated by the formation of gas or by the formation of color. In some media a pH indicator is used to show, for example, when an acid is produced during fermentation. Enzymatic breakdown of the amino acid tryptophan produces indole, which can be detected by a color change in an indicator. Biochemical tests may be done individually or may be incorporated into culture media.

Colonies on primary cultures or colonies from subcultures can be used to perform biochemical tests. Some of these are rapid tests and take only minutes; others require hours of incubation for results to be seen. Together with macroscopic morphology (colony characteristics) and microscopic morphology, biochemical testing gives the clues for identification of the organism in question.

Modifications of the traditional biochemical tests have been made to facilitate inoculation of media, shorten the incubation time, automate

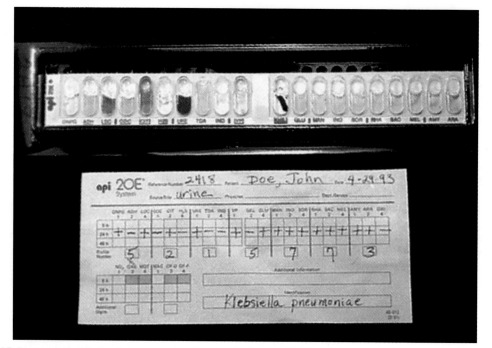

FIGURE 16-17 Biochemical test panel used to identify bacteria (API [bioMerieux, Hazelwood, Mo]). Each cupule is a separate test that is scored positive or negative. These scores are added to generate a biocode that can be matched to a database of biocodes to give the identity of the organism tested. (From Forbes BA, Sahm DF, Weissfeld AS: *Bailey and Scott's diagnostic microbiology,* ed 12, St Louis, 2007, Mosby.)

procedures, or in some way facilitate the identification of species based on reaction patterns.

In multitest systems, conventional biochemicals are arranged in a series. A biocode is generated and a database accessed for identification of the organism (Fig. 16-17). Automated systems are now used most frequently and can be in a microtiter tray format or in a multiple-well system. The substrates are rehydrated on inoculation with a suspension of the organism. In diagnostic microbiology laboratories, automated systems have made it easier to accommodate a large volume of work. These systems also perform antimicrobial susceptibility testing with the identification and can be interfaced with the laboratory computer information system.

This section describes some of the more traditional biochemical tests that can aid in preliminary, presumptive, or final identification of organisms. These tests are reliable and inexpensive to perform, two reasons why these traditional tests are still used for the identification of microorganisms.

Bile Esculin Agar

Bile esculin agar is used to aid in the identification of enterococci. Included in this media is 40% bile that inhibits the growth of most gram-positive organisms other than enterococci and some streptococci. The organisms such as enterococci that can hydrolyze the esculin in the media will turn

the indicator, ferric ammonium citrate, a black color.

Bile Solubility Test

Some organisms contain an active autocatalytic enzyme that will lyse the organism. With the addition of a bile salt, sodium desoxycholate, the lytic process is accelerated. When a drop of bile salt reagent is added to isolated colonies of *Streptococcus pneumoniae* on a blood agar, there will be visible autolysis of the colony within 30 minutes. *S. pneumoniae* gives a positive reaction, which is the disappearance of the suspected colony, leaving a flat area. Other streptococcal species will not be affected by the addition of the bile salt reagent.

Catalase Test

In this test the enzyme catalase breaks down hydrogen peroxide into oxygen and water. The catalase test is usually performed on a glass slide. A small amount of organism is placed on the slide, and a drop of 3% hydrogen peroxide is added to the organism. If bubbles of oxygen are immediately seen, the organism is positive for the enzyme catalase. The bubbles represent the release of oxygen in the enzymatic reaction. This test is often used to differentiate staphylococci from streptococci. All staphylococci are catalase positive and will produce bubbling. The genus *Streptococcus* does not produce catalase and consequently is catalase negative, producing no visible bubbling.

Citrate Utilization

Citrate agar is used to detect utilization of sodium citrate as a sole source of carbon, and ammonium phosphate as a sole source of nitrogen. This test is useful in determining the identification of members of the Enterobacteriaceae. Most organisms that can grow on this medium (slant) will turn the indicator, bromthymol blue, from green to blue. Some organisms can grow on this medium without turning the indicator blue (alkaline reaction), and evidence of growth is a positive reaction in this case (usually further incubation allows time for blue color development).

Coagulase Test

There are two types of coagulase. The first type, bound coagulase, or the clumping factor, can be detected by a rapid slide test. Clumping factor is bound to the cell wall and reacts with fibrinogen, causing visible clumping of bacterial cells. A positive reaction is visible clumping, and a negative test is a homogeneous suspension of the bacteria and the reagent. Commercial kits are available to test for clumping factor, and generally it takes only a few minutes to obtain the result. If the test is weak or delayed, a tube test for unbound coagulase should be performed (Fig. 16-18, A).

The second type of coagulase is the free, or unbound, coagulase. This test is carried out in a test tube and performed in rabbit plasma. The action of unbound coagulase causes a fibrin clot to form, and a positive test can be observed in 4 hours of incubation at 35°C. If the test appears negative, the time is extended to 24 hours. The test should initially be read at 4 hours because a positive test can revert to negative after 24 hours (see Fig. 16-18, B).

The coagulase test is done to differentiate *Staphylococcus aureus* from other members of the genus *Staphylococcus*. *S. aureus* is a common cause of many serious infections, and rapid identification aids in treatment of patients. Most other *Staphylococcus* species are coagulase negative, and because these staphylococci are usually members of the normal flora, they are together referred to as *coagulase-negative staphylococci*. If one of these members is isolated from a sterile source, the identification to species level can be performed if indicated.

Lysine Iron Agar

The lysine iron agar (LIA) test, in conjunction with the TSI, is helpful in screening stool specimens for enteric pathogens. The LIA tests for

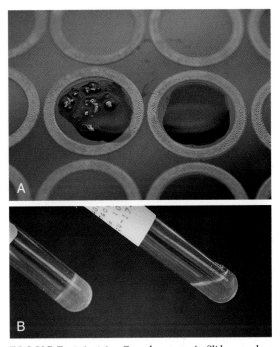

FIGURE 16-18 Coagulase test. **A,** Slide coagulase test for bound coagulase or clumping factor. *Left,* Positive test showing visible clumps. *Right,* Negative test with no clumps. **B,** Tube coagulase test for unbound or free coagulase. *Left,* Tube is positive, showing a fibrin clot. *Right,* Tube is negative with no clot. (From Forbes BA, Sahm DF, Weissfeld AS: Bailey and Scott's diagnostic microbiology, ed 12, St Louis, 2007, Mosby.)

the enzymes lysine deaminase and lysine decarboxylase (Fig. 16-19). H_2S can also be determined, but TSI may be a more reliable medium for this test. The medium is inoculated with an inoculating needle, using a small amount of growth from a pure colony of the organism being tested, by stabbing the butt of the medium through the center to the bottom of the tube and then streaking the slant (see Common Types of Media).

After incubation at 35°C for 18 to 24 hours in ambient air, reactions are noted. Reactions in the slant and butt are recorded as acid (A), alkaline (K), red (R), and the presence of H_2S (blackening of the agar). An acid reaction is indicated by a yellow color and an alkaline reaction by a purple color. A *K/K reaction* (purple/purple) refers to a negative test for lysine deaminase (slant) and a positive test for lysine decarboxylase (butt). An *R/A reaction* (red/yellow) refers to a positive test for lysine deaminase (slant) and a negative test for lysine decarboxylase (butt). A *K/A reaction* (purple/yellow) refers to glucose fermentation only and negative tests for the two enzymes. H_2S is recorded as positive if a black precipitate is seen. Table 16-4 shows the various reactions and interpretations.

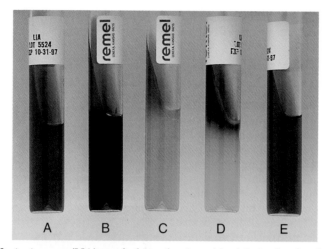

FIGURE 16-19 Lysine iron agar (LIA) tests for lysine deaminase (slant), lysine decarboxylase (butt), and H_2S production. **A,** Alkaline slant/alkaline butt (K/K or purple/purple) is negative for lysine deaminase but positive for lysine decarboxylase. **B,** Alkaline slant/alkaline butt, black precipitate (K/K H_2S+) is negative for lysine deaminase, positive for lysine decarboxylase, and positive for H_2S production. **C,** Alkaline slant/acid butt (K/A or purple/yellow) is negative for both enzymes. **D,** Red slant/acid butt (R/A) is positive for lysine deaminase and negative for lysine decarboxylase. **E,** Uninoculated tube. (From Forbes BA, Sahm DF, Weissfeld AS: *Bailey and Scott's diagnostic microbiology,* ed 12, St Louis, 2007, Mosby.)

PYR Test

PYR is a substrate, L-pyrrolidonyl-β-naphthylamide, that is acted on by the enzyme pyrrolidonyl arylamidase. It is a rapid test to identify *Enterococcus* spp. and group A β-hemolytic streptococci. Commercially prepared filter paper impregnated with PYR is available or can be prepared. The filter paper is inoculated with the organism in question, and a color developing reagent, *N,N*-dimethylaminocinnamaldehyde, is added. A positive test is the development of a bright red color within 5 minutes. A negative test would be no color change or a yellow-orange color. This is a rapid test for group A β-hemolytic streptococci (causative agent of strep throat), because they are the only β-hemolytic streptococci that have a positive reaction in the PYR test.

Rapid Urease Test

Organisms that produce the enzyme urease are able to hydrolyze urea-releasing ammonia as an end product. The production of ammonia changes the alkalinity, thus causing the pH indicator phenol red to change from yellow to magenta. This test can be used to screen lactose-negative colonies on differential media that have been plated with a stool specimen, thereby assisting in the differentiation of the pathogenic *Salmonella* and *Shigella* species, which are urease negative, from the urease-positive nonpathogens such as *Proteus* spp. Many diagnostic microbiology laboratories use this rapid test for detection of the yeast *Cryptococcus neoformans* (causative agent of pneumonia and meningitis) in sputum samples. It is a rapid method to screen

TABLE 16-4

Observations of Lysine Iron Agar (LIA)		
Notation	Color Change	Metabolic Change
K/K	Purple slant, purple butt	Lysine decarboxylation
K/A	Purple slant, yellow butt	No enzymatic reactions, only glucose fermentation
R/A	Red slant, yellow butt	Lysine deamination
H_2S	Black in butt	H_2S production

A, Acid; H_2S, hydrogen sulfide; *K,* alkaline; *R,* red.

sputum, and *C. neoformans* is positive, with other yeasts usually negative.

Salt Tolerance Test

The salt tolerance test is utilized to determine whether an organism can grow in the presence of sodium chloride (NaCl). A heart infusion broth containing 6.5% NaCl is inoculated with an organism, and if the organism is inhibited by the salt, the broth will be clear. If an organism can grow in 6.5% NaCl, the broth will be cloudy. This test helps identify enterococci, which grow well in 6.5% NaCl.

Spot Indole Test

Organisms that produce the enzyme tryptophanase can break down the amino acid tryptophan to yield indole. Indole can be detected by its ability to combine with certain aldehydes to form a colored compound. Indole reagent is added to (and should saturate) filter paper, then a portion of the isolated colony to be tested is rubbed onto the filter paper. Indole-positive organisms will result in the rapid development of a blue color on the filter paper if the indicator aldehyde is 1% paradimethylaminocinnamaldehyde. This test can be used to differentiate swarming *Proteus* species from one another and as a presumptive identification of *E. coli*. Positive organisms such as *E. coli* will give a blue-green color on the filter paper, and negative organisms remain colorless.

Spot Oxidase Test

Organisms that produce the enzyme cytochrome oxidase are able to oxidize the test reagent tetramethyl-*p*-phenylenediamine dihydrochloride (Kovac's oxidase reagent), forming a colored end product. A dark purple end product will be visible when an organism producing the enzyme is added to filter paper that has been impregnated with the reagent. The test is primarily done for presumptive identification of *Neisseria* spp. and *Pseudomonas aeruginosa*, both of which are oxidase positive. Oxidase-positive organisms will turn the filter paper a dark purple within 10 seconds. Oxidase-negative organisms will remain colorless or keep the color of the original colony.

Triple Sugar Iron Agar and Kligler's Iron Agar

Triple sugar iron agar (TSI) or Kligler's iron agar (KIA) can provide initial presumptive identification of gram-negative bacilli, especially members of the Enterobacteriaceae family, the usual enteric intestinal pathogens screened. Use of these media can determine primary characteristics of these organisms: ability to ferment the sugars glucose, lactose, and sucrose (KIA only glucose and lactose); production of H_2S (visualized by black, iron-containing precipitate); and gas production (visualized by bubbles or splitting of medium). The medium is inoculated with a needle using a small amount of growth from a pure colony of the organism being tested, stabbing the butt of the medium through the center to the bottom of the tube, then streaking the slant (Fig. 16-20). (See also Common Types of Media.)

After incubation at 35°C for 18 to 24 hours in ambient air, reactions are noted and the organism presumptively identified based on fermentation reactions, H_2S production, and gas formation. Because such a variety of reactions occur in the TSI slants, there must be a scheme for observing and recording these reactions. Reactions in the slant and butt are recorded as acid (A) or alkaline (K), and the production of H_2S and gas (G) is noted. An acid reaction is indicated by a yellow color and an alkaline reaction by a red color. Table 16-5 lists various observations and interpretations.

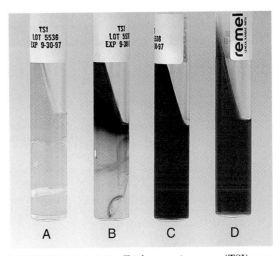

F I G U R E   1 6 - 2 0   Triple sugar iron agar (TSI) tests for fermentation of glucose (butt), lactose and/or sucrose (slant), H_2S production, and gas production. A, Acid slant/acid butt with gas (A/A or yellow/yellow gas+) is fermentation of glucose, lactose and/or sucrose, and gas production. B, Alkaline slant/acid butt with black precipitate (K/A or red/yellow H_2S+) is glucose fermentation and H_2S production. C, Alkaline slant/alkaline butt (K/K or red/red) is no fermentation of the three sugars. D, Uninoculated tube. (From Forbes BA, Sahm DF, Weissfeld AS: Bailey and Scott's diagnostic microbiology, ed 12, St Louis, 2007, Mosby.)

T A B L E   1 6 - 5

Observations of Triple Sugar Iron Agar (TSI)		
Notation	Color Change	Metabolic Change
A/A	Yellow slant, yellow butt	Glucose fermented, lactose or sucrose or both fermented
K/A	Red slant, yellow butt	Glucose fermented, lactose and sucrose not fermented
K/K	Red slant, red butt	None of the three sugars fermented, or no reaction
H_2S	Black in butt	H_2S production
G	Bubbles or splitting of agar in butt	Gas production

A, Acid; *G*, gas; *H_2S*, hydrogen sulfide; *K*, alkaline.

Failure of the organism to ferment any of the three sugars results in a K/K reaction (or no reaction), indicated by a red slant and butt. A K/A reaction (red slant and yellow butt) results when only glucose is fermented. Organisms fermenting only glucose will initially give an A/A reaction or yellow slant and butt; the small amount of glucose present is used up as the incubation continues. The slant is under aerobic conditions and reverts to alkaline (or red) in 18 to 24 hours. In the butt, however, anaerobic conditions exist; there is no

TABLE 16-6

General Interpretive Guidelines for Urine Cultures		
Result	Specific Specimen Type/Associated Clinical Condition, If Known	Workup
>10^4 CFU/mL of a single potential pathogen or for each of two potential pathogens	CCMS urine/pyelonephritis, acute cystitis, asymptomatic bacteriuria, or catheterized urines	Complete*
>10^3 CFU/mL of a single potential pathogen	CCMS urine/symptomatic males or catheterized urines or acute urethral syndrome	Complete
Three or more organism types with no predominating organism	CCMS urine or catheterized urines	None. Because of possible contamination, ask for another specimen.
Either two or three organism types with predominant growth of one organism type and 10^4 CFU/mL of the other organism type(s)	CCMS urine	Complete workup for the predominating organism(s);† description of the other organism(s)
>10^2 CFU/mL of any number of organism types (set up with a 0.001- and 0.01-mL calibrated loop)	Suprapubic aspirates, any other surgically obtained urines (including ileal conduits, cystoscopy specimens)	Complete

From Forbes BA, Sahm DF, Weissfeld AS: Bailey and Scott's diagnostic microbiology, ed 12, St Louis, 2007, Mosby.
CCMS, Clean-catch midstream; CFU/mL, colony-forming units per milliliter.
*A complete workup includes identification of the organism and appropriate susceptibility testing.
†Predominant growth = 10^4 to >10^5 CFU/mL.

reversion to alkaline pH, and the acid (or yellow) reaction remains.

An A/A reaction (yellow slant and butt) results when glucose and lactose and/or sucrose are fermented. The medium contains 10 times more lactose and sucrose than glucose. Therefore, organisms fermenting lactose and/or sucrose do not use up the sugars except after prolonged incubation. Fermentation of sucrose and/or lactose is indicated by acid (yellow) conditions in the slant. With prolonged incubation (48 to 72 hours), however, lactose and sucrose may also be used up, and formerly acid reactions may revert to alkaline. Therefore the time of incubation is critical; the time recommended to obtain typical reactions is 18 to 24 hours.

URINE CULTURES

Cultures are done on urine to diagnose bacterial infections of the urinary tract (bladder, ureter, kidney, and urethra). Urinary tract infections (UTIs) are of two main types: (1) lower UTIs of the bladder or urethra, such as cystitis, an infection of the bladder; and (2) upper UTIs of the ureters and kidneys, such as pyelonephritis, an infection of the renal parenchyma (kidney). Routine urine cultures are usually done by using one selective culture medium and one nonselective or supportive medium.

Collecting the Specimen

The urine specimen for culture must be collected in a clinically reliable manner; proper cleaning of the collection site, especially for females, is very important. Collecting a clean-catch, midstream urine sample uses the least invasive technique and consequently is most often performed (see Specimens for Microbiological Examination). If a patient cannot urinate, a catheterized specimen can be obtained. Using straight catheters (in-and-out type) is more invasive than collecting clean-catch urine but eliminates contamination. If the catheterized specimen is from a patient with an indwelling Foley catheter, the urine from the tubing (not the bag) is sent to the laboratory (never the actual catheter). Urine is collected during cystoscopy as well and is sent to microbiology for culture (see Chapter 14).

The specimen must be collected into a sterile container and, if not cultured immediately in the laboratory, must be refrigerated to prevent bacterial growth. Urine is normally sterile within the bladder but is easily contaminated during the collection process if caution is not used in cleaning the collection site.

Quantitative urine culture methods are required to differentiate true infections from contamination. The presence of bacteria in clean-catch urine does not necessarily indicate a UTI unless the number of organisms is significant. Urine cultures are reported in **colony-forming units per milliliter of urine (CFU/mL).** An increased number of white blood cells (leukocytes) present (polymorphonuclear neutrophils, PMNs) in the urine specimen, in conjunction with the results of the urine culture, increases the diagnostic value of both tests. Table 16-6 provides interpretive guidelines for urine cultures and is used to assess the validity of the specimen when many clean-catch specimens are contaminated.

Methods for Detection of Urinary Tract Infections

Rapid-Screening Test Strips

Rapid-screening test strips have been developed to test for UTIs. Nitrite tests have been incorporated into reagent strips used in many laboratories for routine urine analysis. Common organisms that cause UTIs, such as species of *Escherichia*, *Proteus*, *Klebsiella*, *Enterobacter*, and *Pseudomonas*, contain enzymes that reduce nitrate in the urine to nitrite (see Chapter 14). Organisms must possess the nitrate reductase enzyme necessary to carry out this process.

The rapid-screening test strips for UTIs are most useful when the test for nitrite is combined with that for leukocyte esterase. Chemical test strips are available that combine nitrite and leukocyte esterase tests. Multiple-reagent test strips contain test pads for these constituents. Leukocyte esterase is an enzyme present in the granules of neutrophils. Neutrophils are generally increased in UTIs, so the presence of leukocyte esterase in the urine is an indicator of infection (see Chapter 14). The absence of leukocyte esterase, however, does not rule out UTI. The finding of nitrite-positive and leukocyte esterase–positive urine using chemical screening tests is helpful in detecting UTIs, especially in combination with the presence of bacteria and leukocytes in the urine sediment. To identify the organism causing the infection, a quantitative urine culture is done.

Quantitative Culture Methods

To determine a true UTI, quantitative methods are used to determine the number of CFUs/mL of urine specimen, and cultures are done to identify the organism(s) causing the infection.

STREAK PLATE METHOD

A streak plate method for quantitating the growth of microorganisms in the urine is the classic culture method typically used in many clinical laboratories (Procedure 16-6). A calibrated standardized inoculating loop containing 0.001 or 0.01 mL of urine is used to transfer the well-mixed specimen to the culture plates and streak the plates (Fig. 16-21). The larger volume (0.01 mL) gives a greater amount of inoculum and can be used to gain more accurate quantitation, particularly in cytoscopy specimens where bacteria may be low in numbers.

In common practice, a supportive medium (e.g., SBA) and a selective and differential medium

---

PROCEDURE **16-6**

Quantitative Urine Streak Plate

1. Ensure that the urine specimen is well mixed.
2. Sterilize the calibrated inoculating loop and allow it to cool, or use a disposable calibrated loop, and insert it into the bubble-free surface of the specimen (see Figure 16-18).
3. Touch the loop to the center of the sheep blood agar and spread in a line across the diameter of the plate. Without resterilizing, spread the urine by zigzagging across the inoculum. Repeat the process and streak the MacConkey or EMB plate (see Figure 16-19).
4. Incubate the culture plates at 35°C in an inverted position for 18 to 24 hours.
5. Interpret the results.

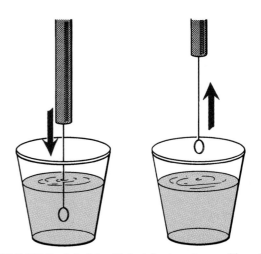

FIGURE 16-21 Method for inserting a calibrated loop into urine to ensure that the proper amount of specimen will adhere to the loop. (From Forbes BA, Sahm DF, Weissfeld AS: Bailey and Scott's diagnostic microbiology, ed 12, St Louis, 2007, Mosby.)

(e.g., MAC, EMB) are streaked with the urine specimen. This is done in such a way that the drop of urine is spread as uniformly as possible on the plate (Fig. 16-22). After streaking and incubation, the number of colonies seen is multiplied by 1000 (for the 0.001-mL loop) or 100 (for the 0.01-mL loop) to give CFU/mL of urine. SBA gives a total colony count because most common organisms grow on it. The selective medium indicates whether gram-negative bacilli are present. The

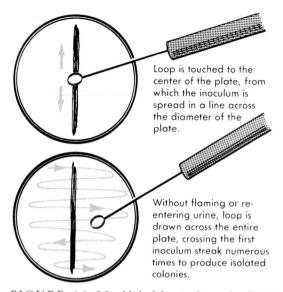

Loop is touched to the center of the plate, from which the inoculum is spread in a line across the diameter of the plate.

Without flaming or re-entering urine, loop is drawn across the entire plate, crossing the first inoculum streak numerous times to produce isolated colonies.

FIGURE 16-22 Method for streaking a loopful of urine with a calibrated loop to produce isolated colonies and countable colony-forming units of organisms. (From Forbes BA, Sahm DF, Weissfeld AS: Bailey and Scott's diagnostic microbiology, ed 12, St Louis, 2007, Mosby.)

EMB and MacConkey media also indicate whether the organisms are lactose positive or lactose negative. The most common cause of UTIs is *E. coli*, which is associated with a large percentage of UTIs in ambulatory and hospitalized patients. *E. coli*, *Klebsiella* spp., and *Enterobacter* spp. are lactose fermenters that show pink colonies on MacConkey (lactose positive), whereas *Proteus* spp. and *Pseudomonas aeruginosa* are lactose negative (do not ferment lactose) and show clear or slightly pink colonies. *Proteus* spp. may be recognized on SBA by their spreading growth. Gram-positive organisms such as staphylococci and enterococci grow well on SBA but are inhibited on EMB or Mac-Conkey agars.

INTERPRETING RESULTS OF QUANTITATIVE URINE CULTURES

Normal urine is sterile. Plates that show no growth may be discarded and reported as no growth after 48 hours of incubation. In many UTIs, the laboratory findings show the presence of 100,000 (10^5) or more bacteria colonies per milliliter of urine specimen. After the incubation period, the number of colonies growing on the plates is counted and multiplied by 1000 (if 0.001-mL urine has been plated) to determine the number of microorganisms per milliliter of original urine specimen. A count of 100,000 CFU/mL urine indicates a UTI in asymptomatic patients. A count of 1000 CFU/mL urine may be significant for a UTI in a symptomatic male patient. Therefore, it is always important to combine the results

of colony counts with the clinical information available. (See Table 16-6 for the interpretative guidelines for urine cultures.)

The growth characteristics of the colonies on the plates are also observed. As discussed previously, the EMB or MacConkey plates are observed for presumptive identification of gram-negative organisms, and growth on the blood agar plates is noted. Any cultural observations should agree with the results of the Gram stain if one was performed. Further biochemical tests can be done to identify the suspected organism.

Gram Stain of Urine Specimens

Gram stains are not done routinely on urine specimens, but if requested, the smear can be made directly from a well-mixed specimen. Using a sterile pipette, place 1 drop of uncentrifuged urine on the slide and let air-dry. Fix the slide, perform the Gram stain, and observe using the 100× oil-immersion objective. If at least one organism per field (after examining at least 20 fields) is seen, this correlates with a significant **bacteriuria** (presence of bacteria in urine) of greater than 100,000 CFU/mL urine.[11]

In patients with a severe UTI, progression to a **bacteremia** (presence of bacteria in blood) is possible. If this is suspected, a Gram stain result could aid in a rapid diagnosis and direct treatment with the appropriate antimicrobial agent. In other patients, three or more morphologic types of bacteria may be detected, indicating a contaminated specimen from the perianal, vaginal, or urethral areas.

THROAT CULTURES

Throat cultures are done primarily to differentiate the Lancefield group A β-hemolytic streptococcal (*Streptococcus pyogenes*) sore throat (pharyngitis) from a viral throat infection. Sore throats caused by the group A streptococcal organism must be identified and treated because, if untreated, sequelae can occur in some patients, leading to scarlet fever or acute rheumatic fever, followed by chronic rheumatic heart disease. Acute glomerulonephritis can also follow an untreated group A streptococcal throat infection in some patients.

Collecting the Specimen

The proper collection of the sample is important. Two sterile swabs are used to collect the specimen. Throat cultures are done by swabbing the rear pharyngeal wall and the tonsillar area (see Fig. 16-5 and Procedure 16-1). Before culturing the specimen, one swab will be used for rapid testing for group A β-hemolytic streptococci. If the rapid test is positive, a culture is not necessary. If the rapid test is negative, a confirmatory culture is done to confirm the rapid test with the second swab to account for possible false-negative results. If only one swab is sent, a sheep blood agar plate is cultured first, then the rapid test performed. Transport to the laboratory should be within 2 hours in transport media, and specimens can be stored for 24 hours at room temperature.

Methods for Detection of Group A Beta-Hemolytic Streptococci

Rapid testing is done routinely in many microbiology laboratories. The rapid diagnosis of pharyngitis caused by group A β-hemolytic streptococci (*S. pyogenes*) can prevent complications such as scarlet fever. All negative rapid tests are confirmed by culture. Some laboratories perform culture only for group A β-hemolytic streptococci, in which case only one swab is necessary.

Rapid Detection Methods: Nonculture Techniques

Numerous commercial products are available for the rapid detection of group A β-hemolytic streptococcal pathogens. Instead of waiting for an overnight incubation period for culture plate methods, these results are available within a much shorter time, 15 to 30 minutes, and antibiotic therapy can be started immediately. Rapid streptococcal antigen detection systems include enzyme immunoassays, latex agglutination, and optical immunoassays. The optical immunoassay uses antigen-antibody interactions on an inert surface that can be detected by changes in light reflectance because of an alteration in the thickness of the reactants on the surface. This technology is used in the Strep A OIA (BioStar, Boulder, CO) optical immunoassay for group A streptococcus, using a reflective surface for enhanced detection of antigen-antibody reactions. With this technology, antigen can be detected (or the presence of an antigen-antibody complex) by allowing the sample containing antigen to react with an appropriate reflective surface to which a specific antibody is attached. Light reflecting off the surface film containing bound antibody is viewed as one color, and group A–specific antigen binding increases the thickness of the film, causing the surface to appear a different color.

Most rapid tests for group A β-hemolytic streptococci usually first require extraction of any group A–specific antigen from the specimen on the throat swab. The group A–specific carbohydrate antigen is present in the cell wall of the

Plating Throat Cultures

1. Using the throat swab obtained from the patient, roll the swab onto one edge of a sheep blood agar plate, being certain to transfer as much of the specimen onto the plate as possible.
2. Sterilize the inoculating loop, and use it to streak the plate out from the inoculated area. The streaking is done to isolate the bacterial colonies as much as possible. Make three or four cuts into the agar to observe hemolysis more readily after incubation.
3. Incubate for 18 to 24 hours at 35°C, then examine the culture plates for pathogens. If pathogens are present, do appropriate testing for final identification, or perform subculture if there is an inadequate number of isolated colonies for testing.

streptococcal organisms. The swab is incubated with an enzyme or acid solution to extract the group A–specific carbohydrate antigen. Specific procedures will vary with the product, and the manufacturer's directions must always be followed carefully for optimal results. Controls should be used with all methods.

Most laboratory comparisons of conventional culture methods and rapid testing methods have shown excellent specificity. If results are positive using these methods, it is sufficient reason to begin antibiotic therapy because the rapid test is very specific for the group A β-hemolytic streptococcal antigen.

Many laboratories perform additional rapid antigen methods for detection of other pathogens, such as respiratory syncytial virus (RSV, bronchiolitis in infants) and influenza A and B (flu, respiratory illness) viruses. With increased surveillance for possible epidemic or pandemic (worldwide epidemic) influenza, the rapid detection of influenza A has become an important rapid test in the clinical microbiology laboratory.

Culture on Sheep Blood Agar

Culture on SBA will isolate bacterial pathogens from the pharyngeal area, if present (Procedure 16-7). For recovery of other pathogens, such as *Corynebacterium diphtheriae* or *Neisseria gonorrhoeae*, special media specific for their growth must be added.

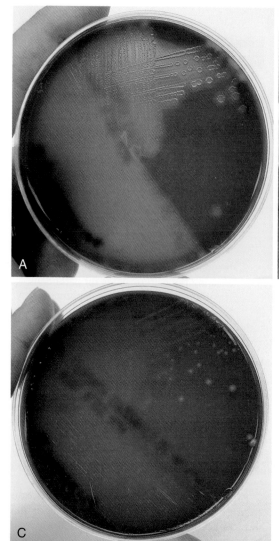

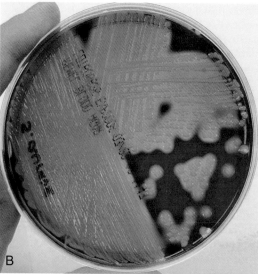

FIGURE 16-23 Three characteristic types of hemolysis on sheep blood agar. A, Alpha hemolysis of *Streptococcus pneumoniae.* B, Beta hemolysis of *Staphylococcus aureus.* C, Gamma hemolysis of *Enterococcus faecalis.* (From Forbes BA, Sahm DF, Weissfeld AS: Bailey and Scott's diagnostic microbiology, ed 12, St Louis, 2007, Mosby.)

INTERPRETING RESULTS OF THROAT CULTURE PLATES

After suitable incubation has taken place, the colony morphology and the appearance of hemolysis on SBA are used in the identification of streptococci.

APPEARANCE OF HEMOLYSIS

After incubation, hemolysis on SBA can be observed. Hemolysis is best determined by holding the culture plate directly in front of a light source. This phenomenon is useful in distinguishing different types of streptococci by their ability to hemolyze the red blood cells (RBCs) present in the medium. As previously noted, hemolysis is of three types, depending on the type of streptococci:

1. **Alpha hemolysis** is incomplete or partial hemolysis of the RBCs in the medium. *Viridans streptococci* (part of the normal flora of the throat) and *Streptococcus pneumoniae* (which can also be a cause of meningitis and pneumonia) exhibit this characteristic type of hemolysis, which is seen macroscopically as a green discoloration of the medium surrounding the colony (Fig. 16-23, A).

2. **Beta hemolysis** is complete hemolysis of the RBCs in the medium. *Streptococcus pyogenes* (common throat pathogen) is β-hemolytic, and the hemolysis appears macroscopically as a clear zone surrounding the surface colonies or in the stabs in the blood agar; this represents complete hemolysis of RBCs in the media (see Fig. 16-23, B).

3. **Gamma hemolysis** is no hemolysis of the RBCs in the medium. Macroscopically there is no change in the color of the medium. Some *Enterococcus* spp. characteristically show this type of hemolysis (see Fig. 16-23, C).

Throat cultures are done primarily to detect the presence of the Lancefield group A β-hemolytic streptococci, so plates are read with this organism in mind. β-Hemolytic streptococci typically appear as gray/white, round, small colonies, with a large zone of β hemolysis. Other pathogens may sometimes be clinically significant. Normal throat cultures show a predominance of α-hemolytic streptococci (viridans streptococci) and commensal *Neisseria* spp. Other organisms can also constitute normal flora.

IDENTIFICATION OF GROUP A BETA-HEMOLYTIC STREPTOCOCCI

One test used to identify group A β-hemolytic streptococci from other beta streptococci is the PYR test (see Biochemical or Enzymatic Tests). Group A β-hemolytic streptococci are the only β-hemolytic streptococci with a positive reaction in this test. A pure culture must be used to avoid false-positive results caused by other organisms that may be in the normal flora. Other β-hemolytic streptococci, such as groups C and G, can cause pharyngitis (without the severe sequelae), but they are PYR negative. Another organism that can be confused with group A β-hemolytic streptococci is *Arcanobacterium haemolyticum*; Gram stain results will rapidly differentiate the two because *A. haemolyticum* is a gram-positive bacillus.

Another test to identify group A β-hemolytic streptococci is by using bacitracin susceptibility. This traditional test has been performed for β-hemolytic streptococci by subculturing the β streptococci onto SBA, then adding the disk to the subculture. The bacitracin disk (with 0.04 unit) is placed in the center of the inoculated area aseptically, and the plate is incubated at 35°C. Any zone of inhibition of growth around the disk is indicative of bacitracin susceptibility and a positive test for group A β-hemolytic streptococci.

SEROLOGY TESTS

Many rapid products are available for testing cultures of β-hemolytic streptococci. These kits test for groups A, B, C, F, and G β-hemolytic streptococci by latex slide agglutination. Direct detection of the group A (or B, C, F, G) streptococcal antigen is done by extracting the antigens. For the latex agglutination tests, any extracted group A–specific antigen is mixed on a slide with specific latex-coated antibody, resulting in a visible agglutination, which occurs within a minute. This method gives a definitive identification for the particular Lancefield group that agglutinates, but it does not give a species designation.

BILE SOLUBILITY OR OPTOCHIN SUSCEPTIBILITY TESTS

Throat cultures are primarily done to diagnose pharyngitis caused by group A β-hemolytic *Streptococcus pyogenes*, but occasionally the question may arise of whether *Streptococcus pneumoniae* is present in large numbers. More often, this organism is identified in sputum specimens rather than throat cultures, because it is a common cause of pneumonia. If the culture is suspect, the bile solubility (see Biochemical and Enzymatic Tests) and optochin test can be performed. *S. pneumoniae* is an α-hemolytic streptococcus and can be differentiated from viridans streptococci (normal flora) by the addition of desoxycholate (*S. pneumoniae* will be lysed by the bile salt; other α-streptococci will not). The optochin (ethylhydrocupreine hydrochloride) disk is applied to a pure subculture of the organism on SBA and incubated at 35°C with 3% to 5% CO_2 overnight. *S. pneumoniae* will be inhibited (zone of inhibition >14 mm) by optochin impregnated onto the disk.

If the bile salt detergent reagent is used, a drop of the reagent is added to isolated colonies on a SBA plate, and visible dissolution of the *S. pneumoniae* colonies is noted within 30 minutes if they are present. The optochin disk, when used, is placed on a subculture of the suspected colonies on a blood agar plate, and the plate is incubated overnight. Zones of inhibition of ≥14 mm are seen around the optochin disk as presumptive identification for *S. pneumoniae*.

GENITOURINARY CULTURES

Microbiological examination of genitourinary tract specimens is done primarily to determine the cause of urethritis, vaginitis, and cervicitis. Organisms recovered from these sources are often sexually transmitted; *Neisseria gonorrhoeae* and *Chlamydia trachomatis* are two examples. These infections can cause pelvic inflammatory disease (PID), leading to infertility. Chlamydial infections have surpassed gonorrheal infections as the most prevalent sexually transmitted bacterial disease in the United States.

Other microorganisms that can cause vaginitis in females include *Gardnerella vaginalis* and *Trichomonas vaginalis*. A parasite and commonly recognized sexually transmitted organism, *T. vaginalis* can be identified in a wet mount of vaginal secretions (see Tests for Parasites). *G. vaginalis* is one cause of bacterial vaginosis (BV), a polymicrobial condition resulting from the disruption of the normal flora in the vagina (see later discussion). *G. vaginalis* organisms are short, gram-negative bacilli or coccobacilli. When the exfoliated vaginal epithelial cells are covered with tiny gram-variable bacilli and coccobacilli, they are known as "clue cells" (see Chapter 14). The smear also can show mixed flora because BV is a polymicrobic infection, with anaerobic bacteria (small gram-negative bacilli), *Mobiluncus* spp. (curved gram-variable or gram-negative bacilli), and *G. vaginalis*. Smears, not culture, are diagnostic for BV.

Genitourinary fungal infections are also common and often the cause of vaginitis in women, especially those receiving antibiotic therapy that inhibits the growth of normal vaginal bacterial flora. A common fungal infection is caused by *Candida albicans* (see Tests for Fungi). Herpes simplex virus is another frequent cause of genitourinary infections.

Collecting the Specimen

It is essential that genitourinary tract specimens, usually from the vaginal cervix or inflamed perineal areas in women and the urethra in men, be appropriately collected so the organisms may be detected. Specimens must be handled carefully to avoid any contamination with other viable infectious material.

Culture

For detecting chlamydial organisms from the endocervix, first a swab is used to remove purulent discharge present. Then a second swab is collected by vigorously swabbing to recover epithelial cells. Generally, swabs for cell culture should have a plastic shaft, and the tip can be Dacron or rayon. Chlamydiae are obligate intracellular pathogens and do not grow in artificial media. Cell culture techniques are used to grow chlamydiae, with the McCoy line being the most popular. Once collected, the specimen should be placed in a transport medium, such as 0.2 M sucrose-phosphate (2SP) or other suitable transport medium, and sent to the laboratory.

A separate sample must be taken for detection of gonococcal organisms (see Gonorrheal Infections), in which case the specimen is preferably inoculated immediately onto the appropriate culture medium and a smear made for Gram stain. JEMBEC systems are used to culture *N. gonorrhoeae* directly (Fig. 16-24). The system includes a medium (modified Thayer-Martin) in a snap-top box and a CO_2-generating sodium bicarbonate pellet. The medium is inoculated with the swab in a W or Z pattern and placed in the bag provided, which should be sealed and sent to the laboratory. If not immediately plated, genitourinary specimens should be transported to the laboratory within 24 hours at room temperature. Commercially available systems for

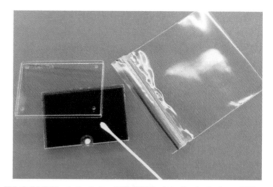

FIGURE 16-24 JEMBEC plate for isolation of *Neisseria gonorrhoeae.* The system includes modified Thayer-Martin medium in a snap-top box and a CO_2-generating sodium bicarbonate pellet. After inoculation, the medium is placed in a zip-locking plastic envelope. (From Forbes BA, Sahm DF, Weissfeld AS: Bailey and Scott's diagnostic microbiology, ed 12, St Louis, 2007, Mosby.)

transport and storage of genitourinary tract specimens enhance the survival of the organisms, if present. Kits include collection swabs (preferably Dacron or rayon) and transport tubes containing specially formulated media.

Nucleic Acid Testing

Hybridization and amplification methods have been licensed for testing *C. trachomatis* and *N. gonorrhoeae*. PACE 2 (Gen-Probe) is a hybridization method that allows detection of both pathogens from the same specimen. Viable organisms are not needed for this procedure, so transport is not an issue, which has facilitated specimen transport from distances. Disadvantages of this method are that no antimicrobial susceptibility testing is performed, and data for resistance surveillance are not available.

PACE 2 collection kits are available commercially and include two swabs, one to remove excess mucus and the second for collection. It is recommended the swab be rotated for 10 to 30 seconds in the endocervical canal to obtain sufficient sampling and placed into the transport tube. Males should not urinate for 1 hour before collection. The swab should be inserted into the urethra 2 to 4 cm using a rotating motion, then placed into the transport tube. Transport is at 2°C to 25°C, as is storage, and testing should be done within 7 days.

A nucleic acid amplified method is APTIMA Combo 2 (Gen-Probe) for detection of *C. trachomatis* and *N. gonorrhoeae*. The amplified methods have been shown to be more sensitive than culture and have become the test of choice for diagnosis of genital *C. trachomatis*.[7] In cases where the treatment has failed, culturing *C. trachomatis* is recommended. Disadvantages with this method include no antimicrobial susceptibility testing, and amplified methods cannot be used in legal cases. Urine can also be used as a source in the amplified method.

Endocervical swab collection follows the PACE 2 protocol. If urine will be collected, the patient should not urinate for at least 1 hour before collection. A first-catch urine sample is collected (20 to 30 mL), and 2 mL of the specimen is transferred to a transport tube. Transport and storage are at 2°C to 30°C, and testing should be performed within 60 days of collection for swabs and 30 days for urine.

Methods for Detection of Common Genitourinary Tract Infections

The physician must alert the laboratory to the probable organisms causing the genitourinary infection so that the identification process can be initiated using the appropriate culture medium and assay protocol.

Gram Stain

Gram-stained smears from urethral discharge are examined for the presence of polymorphonuclear neutrophils (PMNs) and gram-negative intracellular diplococci (within PMNs) indicative of gonococci in men only. Vaginal flora contaminates smears in women, and if done, the positive smear is only presumptive evidence of gonorrhea.

Gonorrheal Infections

When N. gonorrhoeae is suspected, a special agar medium and CO_2 atmosphere for incubation are required for optimal recovery from the clinical specimen being tested. Various supplemental media can also be inoculated. Modified Thayer-Martin agar is a selective medium for N. gonorrhoeae and contains various antimicrobials to inhibit the growth of other types of bacteria and fungi. Chocolate agar is also a supportive medium for N. gonorrhoeae, but it does not inhibit the growth of normal flora because it does not contain antibiotics.

After 24 to 48 hours of incubation on modified Thayer-Martin and chocolate agar, colonies of N. gonorrhoeae appear small, gray, translucent, and shiny. Gram staining should be done of one of these colonies, and if the organism is N. gonorrhoeae, the characteristic gram-negative diplococci ("coffee-bean" appearance) will be observed. In addition, the biochemical oxidase test (N. gonorrhoeae is positive) should be performed for presumptive identification purposes. Further testing may be required depending on the nature of the specimen and can be done using biochemical testing, serology, or nonamplified DNA methods. Several manufacturers have developed kits for this purpose.

Nucleic acid methods are widely used for gonorrheal infections (see previous discussion).

Chlamydial Infections

Infection with Chlamydia trachomatis is a prevalent sexually transmitted disease in the United States. It is important that the specimen be collected properly from the appropriate site by using a technique that dislodges the necessary epithelial cells where the chlamydial organism resides, and not to collect only an exudate. As with gonorrheal infections, nucleic acid methods are also widely used for chlamydial infections (see Nucleic Acid Testing).

If a culture is requested the specimen must be transported to the laboratory immediately. C. trachomatis is a fastidious organism, requiring complex or extensive nutritional requirements. Nonculture methods other than nucleic acid testing include direct immunofluorescent antibody studies using monoclonal antisera and enzyme-linked immunosorbent assay (ELISA).

Trichomonal and Yeast Infections

Trichomonas vaginalis can be observed on a direct wet mount of the vaginal fluid. This is the simplest and most rapid means of detection of this parasitic organism (see Tests for Parasites). Fungal elements can also be visualized at the same time. By addition of a 10% potassium hydroxide (KOH) reagent to the preparation, host cell protein is dissolved, allowing any fungal elements to be seen more easily (see Tests for Fungi). KOH also makes the discharge alkaline, causing it to emit a fishy, aminelike odor that is characteristically associated with BV. This can be done at the bedside.

Bacterial Vaginosis

BV is produced by a mixed infection with anaerobic and facultative organisms. These organisms live on or in a host but may also survive independently. BV is characterized by a foul-smelling vaginal discharge, and Gram stain will show a mixed flora and decreased amount of Lactobacillus spp. (normal flora). The vaginal discharge can be observed microscopically for diagnosis of BV; in a wet preparation, sloughed epithelial cells, many of which are covered with tiny gram-variable bacilli and coccobacilli, will be seen (clue cells).

BLOOD CULTURES

Blood is normally sterile, and no microorganisms should be present. Infections involving bacteria in the bloodstream are serious, reflecting the importance of blood cultures in the microbiology laboratory.

Bacteremia (bacteria in the blood) can have serious consequences for the patient. Blood cultures can provide a clinical diagnosis when a patient presents with a bacteremia. Bacteria can be detected in the blood in the absence of disease, especially after dental extractions or any incident involving a loss of integrity of the capillary endothelial cells; this is called a *transient bacteremia*. **Septicemia** or **sepsis** indicates a situation in which the bacteria in the blood or a toxin produced by the bacteria is causing harm to the host (patient). **Fungemia,** the presence of fungi in the blood, can be found in immunosuppressed hosts.

When a patient is septic, the bacteria can release **exotoxins** (toxins released to the surrounding environment) or **endotoxins** (part of the cell wall of gram-negative bacteria). Particularly in the case of endotoxins, a progressive syndrome can occur called **septic shock.** Symptoms of septic shock are fever, chills, lowered blood pressure (hypotension), respiratory distress, and disseminated intravascular coagulation (DIC). Endotoxins can activate complement and the clotting factors, leading to DIC. This is a serious complication of septic shock in which the clotting factors are used at a high rate. Once they are depleted, excessive bleeding occurs.

Organisms Commonly Isolated from Blood

Portals of entry for organisms that can cause bacteremia are the genitourinary tract (25%), respiratory tract (20%), abscesses (10%), surgical wound infections (5%), biliary tract (5%), miscellaneous sites (10%), and uncertain sites (25%).[12] Organisms commonly cultured from blood are gram-positive cocci such as *Staphylococcus aureus,* coagulase-negative staphylococci, the viridans streptococci, *Streptococcus pneumoniae,* and *Enterococcus* spp. Common gram-negative organisms found in blood are *Escherichia coli, Klebsiella pneumoniae, Pseudomonas aeruginosa, Enterobacter* spp., and *Proteus* spp. Two anaerobic groups also frequently recovered are *Bacteroides* and *Clostridium* spp.[12] Many of these organisms are likely to be found in the health care facility's environment and as normal flora; they may colonize the skin, oropharyngeal area, and gastrointestinal tract of hospitalized patients.

The incidence of bacteremia or septicemia has increased, most likely as a result of several factors: (1) the decreased immunocompetency status of several patient populations (patients live longer with proper therapy), (2) the increased use of invasive procedures such as intravenous catheters and vascular prostheses, (3) the prolonged survival of debilitated and seriously ill patients, (4) the increase in the aging population in general, and (5) the increased use of therapeutic drugs, such as broad-spectrum antibiotics, suppressing normal flora and allowing emergence of resistant strains of bacteria. These factors have made the interpretation of significant growth of microorganisms in the blood more difficult.

Candida albicans is the most common cause of fungemia. The incidence of fungemia is increased in immunocompromised patients. Standard blood culture systems are usually sufficient to isolate most fungi.

Collecting the Specimen

Collection of blood for culture requires a more exacting protocol than blood for most other laboratory tests. It is critical that additional care be taken to clean the skin at the venipuncture site in a special way to prevent any contamination from normal skin organisms present. CLSI has published recommendations for the collection of blood for culture, along with its information on venipuncture for routine laboratory testing.[13] Timing of the collection is also critical. Transient bacteremia can occur incidentally after dental, colonoscopic, or cystoscopic procedures. In this case, bacteria may be present in the blood only for a brief period after the procedure. **Intermittent bacteremia** can result from wound abscesses or other infections, and in this case, bacteria are present in the blood for a time, followed by a period with no bacteria. For **continuous bacteremia,** in which the organisms are from an intravascular source and are present in the blood consistently, the timing is not as critical. Ideally, blood should be collected before any antimicrobial agents are administered, because previous antimicrobial therapy may delay the growth of some organisms. A single culture is usually not sufficient to diagnose bacteremia.

Generally, two or three culture sets are drawn within 24 hours. The blood specimens can be drawn from separate sites or at timed intervals, depending on the patient's symptoms. Collecting more than three sets in a single day is discouraged; additional cultures do not add to the recovery of significant organisms. Typically, if subacute bacterial endocarditis is suspected, three sets are drawn within 24 hours, and if they do not grow, two or three additional sets are drawn in the next 24-hour period.[7]

The volume of blood being tested is a major factor in detecting bacteria in blood cultures; for adults, 10 to 20 mL of blood should be collected for each of the culture bottles. Smaller amounts are collected from children. Protocol for specific blood culture collection is established by each health care facility.

Cleansing the Collection Site

Because it is necessary to avoid any normal skin flora contaminating the collection, it is critical that extra precautions be taken to cleanse the venipuncture site when blood is collected for culture. Proper disinfection of the skin is essential. The skin is cleansed by using 70% alcohol and a povidone-iodine solution in a concentric, outward-moving circle beginning with the chosen venipuncture site. Allow the iodine to dry for one minute. If the phlebotomist must palpate the vein after disinfection, the gloved finger must be disinfected in the same manner as the skin. An alternative disinfectant scrub is chlorhexidine gluconate, which can be used if a patient is allergic to the povidone-iodine solution. The blood is collected directly into the blood culture bottles that contain broth. In this way the bacteria are in a nutrient broth immediately for growth.

Culture Media for Blood

The medium into which the blood is drawn is of an enrichment type, which encourages the growth and multiplication of all organisms present, even stray bacterial contaminants found as part of the normal skin flora.

The basic culture medium for blood is a liquid that contains both a nutrient broth and an anticoagulant. Most commercially available blood culture media contain trypticase soy broth, brain-heart infusion agar, peptone supplement, or thioglycolate broth. In addition, an anticoagulant, 0.025% to 0.05% sodium polyanethol sulfonate (SPS), is used in blood culture bottles because it does not harm the bacteria.[12] A blood/medium ratio of 1:5 or 1:10 is adequate for most laboratories. Blood cultures are generally drawn in sets. Each set contains an aerobic and an anaerobic bottle.

If the blood to be cultured is not drawn directly into the culture medium, it must be collected into a collection tube with an anticoagulant; the best anticoagulant is SPS. It is preferable to draw directly into the blood culture bottles with culture medium, avoiding additional SPS added to the transport tubes. These tubes are then sent to the laboratory for inoculation into the culture media.

Methods for Examination of Blood Cultures

Incubating the Blood Cultures: Traditional Method

After 6 to 18 hours of incubation at 35°C, most bacteria will be present in large enough numbers to detect. Detection includes doing blind subcultures on the aerobic bottle and direct smears on both anaerobic and aerobic bottles. The blind subcultures are made after the first 6 to 18 hours of incubation, and the bottles are reincubated for 5 to 7 days. A "blind" subculture means that culture bottles are subcultured to an appropriate medium (e.g., CHOC, SBA, MAC) even if visible growth of organisms is not noted. In addition to the blind subculture, a routine direct smear is made, Gram stained, and examined for all culture bottles. This is done because some organisms do not produce turbidity, hemolysis, or gas in the growth medium—evidence of "growth." When there is macroscopic evidence of growth, Gram staining of the medium is a rapid identification procedure. A number of rapid tests can be done using the broth blood culture.

The blood culture bottles are examined visually at least once a day for 7 days. Growth of organisms is indicated by hemolysis of RBCs, gas bubbles in the medium, turbidity, or the appearance of small colonies in the broth, on the surface of the RBC layer, or sometimes along the walls of the bottle. After 7 days, if no evidence of growth is noted, a report is made: "no aerobic and/or anaerobic growth after 7 days of incubation." If specific infections are suspected (e.g., bacterial endocarditis, fungemia, brucellosis, anaerobic bacteremia), the bottles should be held for extended incubation.

Subcultures of positive blood cultures are done to a variety of media types so that the growth of most organisms, anaerobes included, can be supported. All isolates from blood cultures should be stored on an agar slant in case additional testing is required.

Any presumptive positive finding must be reported to the physician as soon as possible. The presumptive result must be verified by using conventional procedures and a pure culture of the organism isolated. The physician will use the report on any isolated organism to determine its significance for the patient.

Automated Blood Culture Systems

Most laboratories now use an automated system to culture blood. The advantages of an automated system are (1) a more rapid detection time for many pathogens, (2) monitoring of growth without visual inspection or subculture of the culture bottles, and (3) the ability to use the report in conjunction with a computerized laboratory management information system.

One automated system, Bactec (BD Diagnostic Systems), allows a faster detection time for many pathogens, continuously monitors growth without visual inspection or subcultures, and can automatically handle large numbers of blood culture bottles. Bottles are incubated in the incubator chamber, where constant rocking occurs to enhance growth. Also in the chamber is a detector that measures CO_2 produced by bacterial metabolism. Gas-permeable sensors use fluorescence to detect the CO_2. The fluorescence is measured without entering the bottle. The system is alarmed to make personnel aware of positive samples. These systems improve the time to detection and show a reduced frequency of false-positive results.

The blood culture bottles in the automated systems are subcultured and Gram stained once they are flagged as "positive." Identification proceeds as in any blood culture system (see previous discussion). The traditional method is time-consuming and cumbersome; therefore, most laboratories use an automated system for detecting growth in blood cultures.

ANTIMICROBIAL SUSCEPTIBILITY TESTS

An important function of the medical microbiology laboratory is to test the isolated organisms for susceptibility to antimicrobial agents. The laboratory report showing susceptibility or resistance to a particular antibiotic largely determines whether the agent is used or withdrawn. In choosing an appropriate antimicrobial agent, the one with the most activity against the pathogen, the least toxicity to the host, the least impact on the normal flora, and the appropriate pharmacologic considerations—in addition to being the least expensive—should be selected to attain a more certain outcome for the treatment of the patient's infectious process.

In doing tests for antimicrobial susceptibility, the laboratory must maintain a high level of accuracy in the testing procedures, results must have a high degree of reproducibility, and good correlation must exist between the results and the patient's clinical response.

Susceptibility and Resistance

Antimicrobial susceptibility testing is performed on isolates from patients when clinically appropriate. A result of **susceptible** indicates that the patient most likely will respond to treatment with the antimicrobial agent. A result of **resistant** indicates that

treatment with the agent will most likely fail. Each isolate is tested against a battery of antimicrobial agents when appropriate. An **intermediate** result can mean that a high dose (if possible with the agent) may be necessary for a successful treatment outcome.

Patterns of susceptibility and resistance are constantly changing. Many microorganisms, including bacteria and fungi, have developed resistance even to the newest antimicrobial agents.

Minimum Inhibitory Concentration and Minimum Bactericidal Concentration

The lowest concentration of an antimicrobial agent that will visibly inhibit the growth of the organism being tested is known as the **minimal inhibitory concentration (MIC).** This is detected by the lack of visual turbidity, matching that of a negative control included with the test. Many factors must be considered in choosing the specific antimicrobial agent; the MIC is one important consideration. MIC is determined by dilution antimicrobial susceptibility testing methods.

The ability of an antimicrobial agent to inhibit the multiplication of an organism is measured by the MIC. Because MIC is a measure of an organism's inhibitory status, when the antimicrobial agent is removed, the organism could begin to grow again. In this case, the antimicrobial agent is called **bacteriostatic.** For certain infections, it may be necessary to determine the ability of the agent to kill the organism, or whether it is **bactericidal.** To determine this ability, a bactericidal activity test can be performed using a modification of the broth dilution susceptibility testing method; a **minimal bactericidal concentration (MBC)** is thus determined. The MBC results in a 99.9% reduction in the bacterial population.

Methods for Determination of Antimicrobial Susceptibility

Susceptibility and resistance are functions of the site of the infection, the microorganism itself, and the antimicrobial agent being considered. In other words, if the antimicrobial treatment is to be successful, the agent must be at the correct concentration at the infection site, and the organism must be susceptible to the agent. By using a standard method, the microbiology laboratory can produce consistent results to aid the physician in the therapeutic choice.

Two principal methods are employed to determine antimicrobial susceptibility: **agar disk diffusion,** or **Kirby-Bauer method,** employing antibiotic-impregnated disks; and **dilution testing.**

Most microbiology laboratories use automated instrument methods and perform the disk diffusion when questions arise about automated-format results. The disk diffusion method is also used for some organisms that have fastidious requirements, with media modifications to accommodate their fastidious nature. An example is *Streptococcus pneumoniae*, which has become increasingly resistant. *S. pneumoniae* must be tested by disk diffusion with Mueller-Hinton agar plus 5% sheep blood and incubated with CO_2 in order for this organism to grow.

Each hospital laboratory, with the infectious disease department and pharmacy, must determine which of the many antimicrobial agents are appropriate for testing against the various organisms in its particular setting. The number of antimicrobials being tested against a single isolated organism usually is limited by the particular method being used. Disk diffusion plates (with 150 mm of agar) can usually accommodate 12 disks, whereas some of the commercially available panels can test more drugs on the same panel.

It is important to remember that any in vitro test for antimicrobial susceptibility is an artificial measurement and will give only an estimate of the effectiveness of an agent against a microorganism in vivo. The only absolute test of antimicrobial susceptibility is the patient's clinical response to the dosage of the antibiotic.

The classic method for testing the susceptibility of microorganisms is the broth dilution method, yielding a quantitative result for the amount of antimicrobial agent needed to inhibit the growth of a specific microorganism, or the MIC. CLSI has published the complete protocol for this method.[14,15] Laboratories have now adapted the broth dilution methods to a microbroth method, either automated or done manually, because it saves time, is cost-effective, and promotes efficiency from replicate inoculation of the prepared systems being used.

The isolated organism being tested is first inoculated into a broth medium, whether a diffusion method or a macrodilution or microdilution method is used.

Preparation of Inoculum

The number of organisms in an inoculum can be determined in different ways. One practical method is to compare the turbidity of the test liquid medium with that of a standard that represents a known number of bacteria in suspension. Chemical solutions of standard turbidity have been prepared using barium sulfate. Tubes with varying concentrations of this chemical were developed by McFarland to approximate numbers of bacteria in solutions of equal turbidity, as determined by doing colony counts in a counting chamber[12] (see Disk Diffusion).

MCFARLAND STANDARDS

The standard used most frequently is the McFarland 0.5 standard, which contains 99.5 mL of 1% v/v sulfuric acid and 0.5 mL of 1.175% barium chloride to obtain a barium sulfate solution with a very specific optical density. This provides a turbidity comparable to that of a bacterial suspension containing approximately 1.5×10^8 CFU/mL.

Microdilution Method

The microdilution method utilizes plastic microdilution trays or panels and is used in many laboratories to give MIC results as part of the routine protocol for microbiology laboratory tests. This method permits a quantitative result to be reported (the MIC), indicating the amount of a drug needed to inhibit the microorganism being tested. Most laboratories purchase the microdilution panels commercially; the prepared wells each hold a microamount of the various concentrations of the antimicrobial agents being tested, with the necessary controls supplied for growth and sterility tests. These panels have been prepared under strict quality control standards, which assure the laboratory of consistent performance when they are used according to the manufacturer's directions. Usually a variety of panels containing different drug combinations are available for testing groups of organisms.

One completely automated system is the Vitek System (bioMerieux Vitek), in which the antimicrobial agents are contained in wells in a plastic card. The system includes a filler/sealer module, a reader incubator, a computer module, a data terminal, and a printer. The cards are incubated, and the wells are monitored for optical density. Results can be obtained in 6 to 8 hours for antimicrobial susceptibility testing. The Vitek System can be combined with identification testing, further simplifying the amount of work in a busy laboratory. Another automated system is the MicroScan Walkaway System (Siemens). This system uses a broth microdilution format. The inoculation is manual; a multipronged device delivers diluted organism to each well of a microdilution tray. This tray is incubated, and susceptibility results are available in 3.5 to 5.5 hours. As with the Vitek System, Microscan also offers identification testing in conjunction with susceptibility testing.

Disk Diffusion (Kirby-Bauer Method)

Methods utilizing disks impregnated with various antimicrobial agents and placed on an agar culture plate inoculated with the organism to be tested were used extensively before the advent of microdilution methodology.

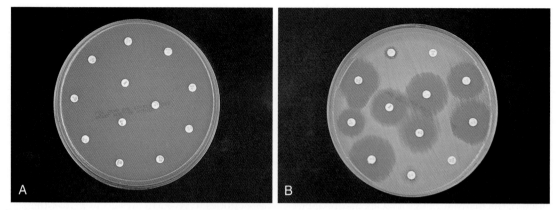

FIGURE 16-25 Agar disk diffusion. **A,** Mueller-Hinton agar has been inoculated with the test organism, and the antibiotic disks have been added to the media. No incubation has yet occurred. **B,** After 16 to 18 hours incubation, the zones of inhibition are apparent. The zones of inhibition are measured and compared to a table of values for each antibiotic. (From Forbes BA, Sahm DF, Weissfeld AS: Bailey and Scott's diagnostic microbiology, ed 12, St Louis, 2007, Mosby.)

For this test, the standardized inoculum is prepared as described and is swabbed over the surface of the agar plate. Paper disks containing a single concentration of the chosen antimicrobial agent are placed onto the inoculated surface, and the plate is incubated for 16 to 18 hours. The antimicrobial agent on the disk diffuses into the medium in a gradient extending from the disk in a circle, inhibiting the growth of the organism wherever the concentration of the agent is sufficient. Large zones of inhibition are an indication of more antimicrobial activity (Fig. 16-25). An area in which there is no zone indicates complete resistance to the drug. This test is also known as the *Kirby-Bauer method.*

With the disk diffusion method, several drugs can be tested against one organism isolate at the same time. Bondi and colleagues[16] first described this method in 1947. In 1966, Bauer and associates[17] standardized the method and correlated it with MICs. They introduced standardized filter paper disks and enabled this method to yield qualitative results that correlated well with results obtained by MIC tests. The results can be correlated directly with MIC values, but clinical interpretation of this method depends on performing the test with the established protocol.

Disks are commercially available for this method, and a special disk dispenser is used to distribute the appropriate disks on the inoculated plate. If there is a zone of inhibition around the disk containing the agent, the zone is measured with calipers and compared to the established breakpoints for susceptible, intermediate, or resistant. Much work has been done to standardize the disk procedure, and many laboratories use the Bauer modification.[17]

The disk diffusion test is more flexible than the commercially prepared microdilution panels, which are available only in standard panels of antimicrobials. The disk diffusion method allows a laboratory to choose any number of appropriate antimicrobial agents on the agar plate used for the test (usually 12 will fit on one plate). Because of this flexibility, it is also a cost-effective test.

The disk diffusion method is subject to CLSI requirements that cover disk concentrations, standardization of media, formula, pH, agar depth, inoculum density, temperature, zone sizes, interpretive tables, and reference strains of bacteria for controls.

SELECTION OF MEDIA FOR PLATING

For antimicrobial susceptibility testing, Mueller-Hinton (MH) agar plates are used. The plates should be stored in the refrigerator until used and should be checked periodically.

HANDLING AND STORAGE OF ANTIBIOTIC DISKS

Disks for antimicrobial susceptibility testing are usually supplied in separate containers with a suitable desiccant to prevent deterioration. Most antimicrobial disks should be refrigerated until used, but some require freezing to maintain their potency. The manufacturer's instructions for storage and handling should be followed.

PREPARATION OF INOCULUM

A tube of trypticase soy broth (5 mL) is inoculated with a pure culture of the organism to be tested, using four or five isolated colonies of similar morphology, and is incubated at 35°C for 4 hours or until the culture is visibly cloudy. Most microbiologists use a second method in which colonies are picked from those grown overnight on nonselective media, suspended in broth or saline, and matched to the 0.5 McFarland standard.

The turbidity of the test organism is compared with that of a McFarland barium sulfate standard. The standard must be vigorously mixed before use. The turbidity of the broth culture may be adjusted by diluting with uninoculated broth. If the 4-hour broth tube does not have sufficient growth, it can be reincubated until adequate growth is observed.

MH plates should be inoculated within 15 minutes of preparation of the inoculum.

INOCULATION OF MUELLER-HINTON AGAR PLATE

A sterile swab is dipped into the standardized, well-mixed broth culture inoculum, and any excess fluid is removed from the swab by squeezing it on the side of the tube. The swab is streaked across the plate in three directions to ensure that the plate surface is covered with the inoculum. The disks should be applied within 15 minutes of inoculating the MH plate.

APPLICATION OF DISKS

The appropriate disks are applied to all the plates, using a disk dispenser if one is available. Special disk dispensers are available with different combinations of antimicrobial-impregnated disks. Each disk should be firmly pressed down onto the surface of the agar with flamed and cooled forceps to ensure complete contact with the agar. The disks should be distributed so that no two disks are closer than 24 mm from center to center. Once a disk has been placed, it should not be moved, because some diffusion of the antibiotic occurs almost immediately. The plates are incubated at 35°C for 16 to 18 hours in ambient air.

READING OF RESULTS

After incubation, the diameters of the zones of inhibition are measured with calipers or a zone reader and recorded to the nearest whole millimeter (see Fig. 16-25). Reading zone sizes is done using a dark background and reflected light. At times there may be a haze of growth produced by some bacteria, and transmitted light is better to read the zones of inhibition. Within the limitations of the test, the diameter of the inhibition zone is a measure of the relative susceptibility to a particular agent. The diameters are compared with a table of breakpoint values for each antimicrobial to see whether the organism is susceptible, intermediate, or resistant to that particular agent. These results are reported to the physician. The term *susceptible* implies that an infection caused by the strain tested may be expected to respond favorably to the particular antimicrobial agent. Resistant strains, on the other hand, are not inhibited by the usual therapeutic concentration of the antimicrobial agent.

QUALITY CONTROL IN THE MICROBIOLOGY LABORATORY

Quality control is necessary in microbiology as in the other areas of the laboratory. Established QC procedures must be performed and results recorded.

Control of Equipment

Equipment used in the microbiology laboratory can be easily controlled; for example, the temperatures of incubators, refrigerators, water baths, and freezers can be monitored daily. All monitoring data must be recorded as part of the laboratory's ongoing quality assurance program. Every laboratory handling biological material must have a biological safety cabinet for handling hazardous specimens and organisms.

Control of Media

Most media are purchased already prepared from companies. These media are generally of high quality and provide good batch-to-batch consistency of results. Commercially prepared media must be stored and used in accordance with manufacturers' directions and must be used within the specified expiration dates. The QC measures used during manufacture of commercial media should follow CLSI recommendations[8] (see Quality Control of Media). If the laboratory prepares the media, strict controls must be used in the preparation. The best way to control the quality of media is by performance testing: checking the media with cultures of known stock microorganisms. Control strains of bacteria are available commercially.

Control of Reagents and Antisera

Reagents should be tested daily (some tests not performed frequently can have controls at the time of testing), using both positive and negative controls. New batches of reagents must also be tested in the same manner. Reagents should be dated when they are prepared, as with reagents in other areas of the laboratory. New reagents should be tested with known control cultures. Gram-staining reagents are best checked by staining and examining slides prepared with known suspensions of gram-negative and gram-positive organisms. In the same manner, acid-fast testing controls are prepared from acid-fast–positive and acid-fast–negative organisms.

Control of Antimicrobial Tests

Laboratories must periodically monitor their performance of methods used for antimicrobial testing, following CLSI recommendations.[15] Control organisms are specific strains of common organisms available for this purpose. These are maintained by subculturing weekly. Typically, weekly quality control is done for disk diffusion and automated systems with known organisms that should give a certain range of zones of inhibition or MICs, respectively.

Control of Specimens, Specimen Collection, and Specimen Rejection

If proper protocols and procedures are not in place regarding the collection of patient specimens and the procedures for handling these specimens in the laboratory, the identification of pathogens is not very meaningful, and quality assurance is not being practiced. Strict adherence to proper procedures for sample collection must be enforced and repeat collections made if the circumstances demand it.

If specimens are not collected appropriately (according to the protocol of the facility), they should be rejected as unacceptable. If a new specimen cannot be collected, the person may request to process the original specimen. In this case, a statement should be included with the result about the inappropriate condition of the specimen. Specimens are rejected because of improper labeling or improper transport, transport medium, or transport temperature, as well as leaking containers. Sputum specimens are assessed for quality by Gram staining, and viewing under low power for squamous epithelial cells. The presence of more than 10 cells per low-power field is evidence of contamination with saliva.[7]

TESTS FOR FUNGI (MYCOLOGY)

The study of fungi (yeasts and molds) is called **mycology** and is carried out in the medical microbiology laboratory. If a laboratory only processes mycology specimens and does not perform identification testing of fungi, the cultures can be referred to a reference laboratory.

Many patients with immunosuppression, such as those with HIV/AIDS or cancer, live longer lives with appropriate treatment. Also, transplantation (solid organ or bone marrow) requires immunosuppression, and great strides have been made in these areas for successful outcomes. Opportunistic infections can occur in patients with diabetes mellitus or other chronic, debilitating diseases and in those with impaired immunologic function resulting from drug therapy with corticosteroids. Therefore, an increase in opportunistic infections is evident.

In recent years, more fungal infections have occurred in immunocompromised patients. When an organism is isolated in an immunocompromised patient, it must be considered a significant finding

and used in the course of treatment. Many fungi are considered opportunistic, causing disease under immune suppression. These infections can be difficult to treat because fungi are eukaryotic cells, having the same type of cell structure as mammalian cells.

Genus- and species-level identification of molds can be a very difficult procedure and is beyond the scope of this text. Included in this section will be introductory topics such as collection of specimens, staining, media, general macroscopic and microscopic morphology, and common tests for yeast identification.

Characteristics of Fungi

Fungi include both yeasts and molds and differ significantly from bacteria. Fungi are eukaryotes, possessing a true nucleus with a nuclear membrane and mitochondria, whereas bacteria are prokaryotes, lacking these structures. The fungi that are seen in the clinical laboratory, yeasts and molds, can be separated into the two groups based on the macroscopic appearance of the colonies formed.

Yeasts are one-celled organisms that reproduce by budding. Yeasts produce moist, opaque, creamy, or pasty colonies on Sabouraud media, whereas molds produce fluffy, cottony, woolly, or powdery colonies. All yeasts look similar microscopically and therefore need to be differentiated based on biochemical test results.

Molds have a basic structure that is made up of tubelike projections called **hyphae.** Hyphae continue to grow, forming an intertwined mass collectively known as **mycelia** (singular mycelium). **Vegetative** hyphae make up the main body of the mold and are the actively growing part of the mold. **Aerial** hyphae are extensions that rise above the main body and can have reproductive structures (asexual spores) attached. These spores are not the same type of structure as bacterial endospores, which are not reproductive structures.

Some yeasts produce **pseudohyphae,** which are elongated buds that do not separate, similar to mycelia (Fig. 16-26). Pseudohyphae are constricted, unlike true hyphae, which have parallel walls and do not have constrictions. Types of mycelium can be recognized microscopically, which can assist in the early identification of certain molds. Molds have their characteristic "fuzzy" or woolly appearance because of their mycelia.

Fungi as a Source of Infection

Fungi normally live a nonpathogenic existence in nature, enriched by decaying nitrogenous material. Humans become infected with fungi through accidental exposure by inhalation of spores or by

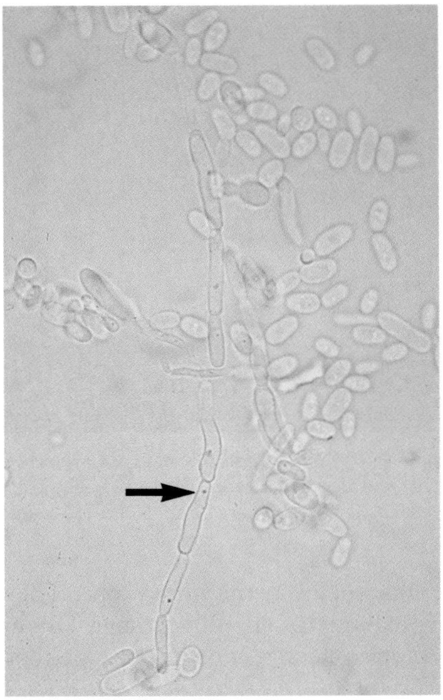

FIGURE 16-26 Pseudohyphae consisting of elongated cells *(arrow)* with constrictions at attachment sites (430×). (From Forbes BA, Sahm DF, Weissfeld AS: Bailey and Scott's diagnostic microbiology, ed 12, St Louis, 2007, Mosby.)

their introduction into tissue through trauma. Any alteration in the immunologic status of the host can result in infection by fungi that are normally nonpathogenic; most yeast infections are opportunistic. The most frequently isolated yeast is *Candida albicans*, which can be part of the normal flora of the gastrointestinal tract in healthy persons.

Fungal infections (or **mycoses**) can be superficial, cutaneous, subcutaneous, or systemic. A *superficial mycosis* is one confined to the outermost skin and hair layer, with symptoms of discoloration, scaling, or abnormal skin pigmentation. *Cutaneous infections* affect the keratinized layer of the skin, hair, or nails. Symptoms of these infections include itching, scaling, or ringlike patches (ringworm) of the skin; brittle or broken hairs; and thick, discolored nails. *Subcutaneous infections* affect the deeper layers of the skin, including muscle and connective tissue; these infections do not usually disseminate through the blood to other organs. Symptoms include ulcers that progress and do not heal and the presence of draining sinus tracts. *Systemic mycoses* affect the lungs and can disseminate to internal organs or the deep tissues of the body. The original site of these systemic infections is the lung, from which the organisms can disseminate via the bloodstream (hematogenous spread) to other sites in the body. Infiltrates may be seen in the pulmonary system on x-ray films. Symptoms can be very general, such as fever and fatigue; other symptoms include a chronic cough and chest pain.

Collection of Specimens for Fungal Studies

Any tissue or body fluid can be cultured for fungi, and swabs are the least desirable specimen in mycology. Other specimens cultured for fungi include hair, skin, nails and nail scrapings, urine, blood or bone marrow, tissue, other ordinarily sterile body fluids, and cerebrospinal fluid. **Fungemia,** or fungi in the bloodstream, is most often caused by C. *albicans.* Many specimens collected for fungal identification will be contaminated with bacteria or rapidly growing fungi. Therefore the media used should contain antibiotics to inhibit these organisms and allow the pathogens to grow. The selection of the type of specimen to be tested, along with collection techniques for specimens used in fungal studies, is directly related to the diagnosis of fungal infections. It is extremely important that specimens be appropriately collected from the proper site so that the fungi are recovered.

It is also important that a specimen for fungal studies be transported to the laboratory as quickly as possible. Because many pathogenic fungi grow slowly, any delay in transporting or processing a specimen can compromise the quality of the specimen and the eventual prospects of isolating the causative organism.

Methods for Detection of Fungi

Because of the increase in the number of fungal infections, primarily in immunocompromised patients, there is an increased need for the detection of these infecting organisms so that treatment may be started.

To begin the identification process in the laboratory, specimens for fungal studies should be directly examined microscopically and cultured immediately to ensure the recovery of the suspected fungal organism from the specimen.

Direct Microscopic Examination of Fungi

Examination of the specimen microscopically is an important part of the microbiology laboratory's fungal identification process. It provides a rapid method, which in some cases leads to an immediate tentative diagnosis; this in turn may result in the early initiation of treatment. Direct microscopic examination can often provide the first microbiological evidence of fungal etiology in patients with suspected fungal infections; several stains can be used for this purpose. Direct examination can also show specific morphologic characteristics and present a rationale for choice of special media to be inoculated immediately. The initial stain used is generally a Gram stain, but other direct stains

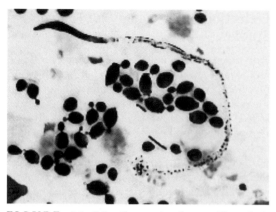

FIGURE 16-27 **Gram stain of yeast.** (From de la Maza LM, Pezzlo MT, Baron EJ: Color atlas of diagnostic microbiology, St Louis, 1997, Mosby.)

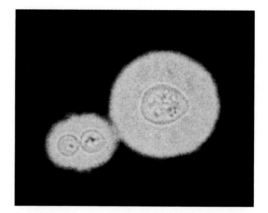

FIGURE 16-28 **India ink stain of *Cryptococcus neoformans*.** (From de la Maza LM, Pezzlo MT, Baron EJ: Color atlas of diagnostic microbiology, St Louis, 1997, Mosby.)

or procedures can give more specific information regarding the identity of the infecting organism.

GRAM STAIN

This is the stain typically used for most clinical microbiological specimens. The Gram stain will detect most fungi, if present in the specimen (see Smear Preparation and Stains Used in Microbiology). Yeast will appear gram positive (purple, blue/black) and will often show its budding tendencies when examined microscopically using the oil-immersion objective (Fig. 16-27).

POTASSIUM HYDROXIDE PREPARATION (KOH)

This has been the traditionally recommended preparation for detecting fungal elements in the skin, hair, nails, and tissue. Addition of a 10% solution of KOH reagent clears the specimen, making the fungi more easily visible. On a glass slide, a drop of the specimen is mixed with a drop of 10% KOH, a coverglass is applied, and the slide is scanned for fungal elements using the low-power objective. Any fungi present will be seen, because the KOH reagent has dissolved the keratin and cellular material in the specimen. If the specimen is extremely viscous, an overnight incubation of the wet-mounted slide in a humidified chamber may be necessary. If the slide appears cloudy, warming may help to clear it for viewing the fungi.

POTASSIUM HYDROXIDE WITH CALCOFLUOR WHITE

Calcofluor white, a fluorescent dye, can be mixed with KOH; a drop is mixed with the specimen on the glass slide, a coverslip applied, and a fluorescence microscope used for observation. Use of this preparation detects the presence of fungi rapidly (in 1 minute) by visualization of a bright apple-green or blue-white fluorescence, depending on the filters used in the microscope. The calcofluor white binds to cell walls of fungi. This method does require a fluorescence microscope, but fungi exhibit an intense, easily recognizable fluorescence with this type of microscopy.

INDIA INK

A drop of India ink may be added to a drop of cerebrospinal fluid sediment from the centrifuged specimen and the specimen examined under high-power magnification. This is a negative staining method, whereby the budding yeast *Cryptococcus neoformans* will be seen surrounded by a large clear area against a black background and is presumptive evidence of an infection with *C. neoformans* (Fig. 16-28). This clear area is due to the capsule that surrounds this yeast and can be referred to as a *halo*. The India ink stain is a rapid test for *C. neoformans*, but the cryptococcal antigen test on cerebrospinal fluid is more sensitive.

ACID-FAST STAIN

The acid-fast stain is used to detect mycobacteria but can also detect *Nocardia* (see also Smear Preparation and Stains Used in Microbiology). In mycology, the acid-fast stain is primarily used to differentiate *Nocardia* spp. from other actinomycetes. *Nocardia* spp. are gram-positive bacilli that appear as branching filamentous forms. They cause mycetomas (infection of subcutaneous tissues) and pulmonary infections. The subcutaneous infections resemble fungal infections of the same type.

Culture of Fungi

Specimens to be cultured for fungi should be inoculated on a general-purpose medium with and without cycloheximide (see next section). Mold cultures should be handled in a class II biological safety cabinet to prevent aerosol dissemination of fungal elements. Yeast cultures can be handled on a regular benchtop with no extra protection other than the usual standard precautions for safety. Numerous species of *Candida* and other yeasts have been identified. Laboratories will differ in their protocols for choosing media for fungal culture. Usually a medium with and without cycloheximide can be used, with the addition of a blood-enriched medium.

CULTURE MEDIA

Sabouraud dextrose agar with antimicrobials (SAB) favors growth of fungi over bacteria and is recommended for primary isolation of fungi. The addition of the antimicrobial agents cycloheximide and chloramphenicol inhibits contaminating fungal and bacterial growth, respectively; Mycosel and mycobiotic agars are two examples of media containing these agents. Media with a combination of SAB and brain-heart infusion (BHI) agar, called *SABHI*, have proved to be useful for isolation of clinically significant fungi. Most specimens for fungal identification are also contaminated with bacteria and other rapidly growing fungi, and it is important that antibacterial and antifungal agents be included in the culture medium. Some fungi require the presence of blood in the medium (sheep blood).

Culture dishes or screw-capped culture tubes are used for satisfactory recovery of fungi.

Examination of the Culture

Fungal cultures are incubated at 30°C for 4 to 6 weeks and examined weekly or twice a week for growth before being reported as negative. One of the first determinations is whether the microorganism is a yeast or a mold. Characteristic gross culture growth and microscopic features are observed to make this determination. Gross features, such as colony color, texture, and growth rate, are necessary initial observations.

MICROSCOPIC EXAMINATION OF ISOLATED MICROORGANISM

Once the organism has been isolated, a direct mount is usually done and examined microscopically. Identification of yeasts requires that certain microscopic features be present, as well as the use of biochemical tests to confirm the species identification. Identification of molds also requires that certain microscopic morphologic features be present (see Characteristics of Fungi).

Yeasts are usually unicellular microorganisms that reproduce asexually by budding; the appearance of the colony is a collection of distinct, individual organisms that resemble the appearance of bacterial colonies on the agar surface. On culture

media, *Candida albicans* colonies appear heaped and dull. Some yeasts may have pseudohyphae, which project from the edges of the colony as filamentous extensions. In contrast, molds are filamentous fungi with tubelike projections or hyphae. Hyphae continue to grow, forming an intertwined mass (mycelia). Different types of hyphae, reproductive structures, and colony morphology can be examined to identify the various types of molds. Identification can be difficult, and laboratories that perform identification of molds have experienced staff to accomplish this task.

GERM-TUBE TEST

Another test done to specifically identify *Candida albicans* is the germ-tube test. This test depends on *C. albicans* being able to produce germ tubes from their yeast cells when placed in 0.5 mL of sheep or rabbit serum and incubated at 35°C for no longer than 3 hours. It is important that the incubation time be limited to 3 hours, because other species will begin to form structures resembling germ tubes with prolonged incubation. Examine under low-power magnification. This allows an early identification of the most common and important yeast pathogen. A **germ tube** is a hyphal-like extension of the yeast cell without having any constrictions at the point where the extension originates[12]; germ tubes are the beginnings of true hyphae (Fig. 16-29).

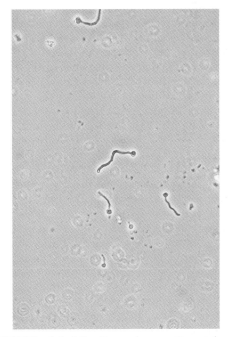

FIGURE 16-29 **Germ-tube test. Germ tubes are true hyphae that are produced by *Candida albicans* in sheep or rabbit serum.** (From Forbes BA, Sahm DF, Weissfeld AS: Bailey and Scott's diagnostic microbiology, ed 12, St Louis, 2007, Mosby.)

Biochemical Screening Methods

Biochemical tests are necessary for yeast identification, but microscopic confirmation is also important. For rapid testing of yeasts, the germ tube (positive test: *C. albicans*) and urea agar (positive test: *C. neoformans*) are typically used (see Common Types of Media). Commercially available yeast identification systems are used by many laboratories, in conjunction with morphology of yeast on cornmeal agar with Tween 80. These methods are usually rapid, and the results are available within 72 hours. These systems use a large database of information based on thousands of yeast biotypes and consider a number of variations and reaction patterns when presenting the result. One method uses a number of biochemical tests, monitoring reactions through various indicator systems after adding a reagent to certain substrates. This system is designed to provide identification within 4 hours. Some systems take longer for the final identification process. In general, these commercial identification systems are easy to use and easy to interpret.

TESTS FOR PARASITES (PARASITOLOGY)

Human parasitic infections occur worldwide, although these problems arise more often in tropical areas. Parasites live in or on their hosts, and by this action they derive a benefit. Some parasites cannot survive without their designated host. Other parasites can exist in a free-living state or as a parasite. Still others live commensally, where the parasite and the host exist together with no harm coming to the host, and the relationship is beneficial to both. Many of the diseases diagnosed in parasitology (study of parasites) are serious infections and have a negative effect on the host.

Parasites as a Source of Infection

Because many persons have lived or traveled in tropical areas, and because of the great influx of refugee populations, many organisms endemic elsewhere are being seen in people now living in the United States. Another consideration is the increasing number of immunocompromised patients, who are at great risk for certain parasitic infections.

Human parasites belong to different divisions. These are the subkingdom Protozoa (amebae, flagellates, ciliates, sporozoans, coccidia, microsporidia), the phylum Nematoda (roundworms), and the phylum Platyhelminthes (flatworms), which can be further separated into the trematodes (flukes) and cestodes (tapeworms). Parasites can also belong to the phylum Arthropoda, which includes insects, spiders, mites, and ticks as members.

Parasitic infections are usually diagnosed by detecting and identifying the **ova** (parasite eggs), **larvae** (immature form), or adults of some types of parasites, usually the helminths, and the cysts (inactive stage) or **trophozoites** (actively feeding and reproducing forms) of others, usually the protozoa. Most protozoa have two developmental stages, the cyst, usually found in formed stool, and the trophozoite, usually found in loose or watery stools. Finding protozoan cysts usually indicates that the infection is in an inactive or carrier state, whereas finding trophozoites usually indicates an active infectious disease.

Identifying the various types of parasitic organisms depends on morphologic criteria; a number of immunologic tests are now available to detect parasitic infections. It is important that the infecting organism be identified specifically, because treatment depends on the type of parasite found and its site of infestation. Any identification process first depends on correct specimen collection and adequate fixation. Specimens for parasitic identification include stool, urine, blood, sputum, and tissue biopsies.

The patient's symptoms and clinical history, including travel, are significant sources of information to be collected and shared with the clinical laboratory. Good lines of communication between the laboratory and the physician will ensure that the appropriate specimen is collected and handled properly. The field of medical parasitology is vast, so medical parasitology textbooks should be consulted for in-depth studies. Excellent resource textbooks and other references contain the specific morphologic criteria needed to identify the more common parasites correctly. The focus of this text will be to introduce information on parasitology such as collection, processing ova and parasite examinations, and common parasite identification.

Collection of Specimens for Parasite Identification

Specimens for parasite identification come primarily from the intestinal tract as fecal specimens, from the urogenital tract as a vaginal or urethral discharge or as a prostatic secretion, from sputum, from cerebrospinal fluid, or from biopsy material from other body tissues. Blood can also be examined for malarial parasites such as *Plasmodium*. Each specimen has unique morphologic criteria for the particular parasites inhabiting the area. Inadequate or improper specimen collection may result in misidentification or failure to identify the infecting organism.

Stool Specimens

Identification of intestinal parasites, particularly protozoa, requires that specific collection protocol be followed; the quality of the specimen being analyzed is directly related to the ability to detect and identify intestinal parasites. Specimen requirements for the identification process should be consulted. A single stool specimen may not be sufficient to isolate an intestinal parasite, for example, because many intestinal parasitic organisms shed eggs or cysts on a variable schedule. The recommended protocol is to collect three stool samples 1 or 2 days apart, but all within a 10-day period, to provide optimal detection of intestinal parasites.

Collection of stool samples for parasites should always be done before radiologic studies involving barium sulfate; the use of barium will affect the sample for at least a week. Certain medications can also affect the detection of parasites in stool samples.

A clean, dry, waterproof container with a tight-fitting lid is an appropriate collection container for a stool sample for parasite studies. Contaminating the specimen with water or urine should be avoided. The sample should be sent to the laboratory as soon as possible; commercial transport systems are available that will preserve the stool sample when the specimen cannot be transported quickly. Any stool sample should be handled carefully because it is a potential source of infection.

Blood Specimens

Thick and thin blood smears are made to allow for better detection of parasites found in blood, such as *Plasmodium* spp. (malaria). The thick smear is used to screen a larger volume of blood; the thin smear is used to identify the parasite because the parasites are not as distorted as with the thick smear. The Giemsa hematologic stain can be used to detect the blood parasites (see Blood and Tissue Microorganisms).

Methods for Detection of Parasites

Methods for parasite detection vary with the specimen and its source. Because many parasitic infections are diagnosed through identification of eggs or larvae in a stool sample, methods of detection in stool are discussed more completely than detection using other specimens. Examination of a direct wet mount of a stool specimen is used to detect the presence of motile protozoan trophozoites and flagellates. A fecal concentration method, either sedimentation or flotation, can be done to enhance the detection of smaller numbers of parasites. Commercial products are available for the

specimen collection and detection of some parasites. Permanent stained smears are made to confirm identification. Quality assurance of detection and identification results begins with the use of properly collected specimens (see Common Parasites Identified).

Wet Mount, Direct Smear

A fresh specimen is necessary for microscopic observation of motile trophozoites and larvae by direct wet mount. A smear is prepared by mixing a small amount of the sample with a drop of physiologic saline on a glass slide with a coverslip. This is repeated using iodine, and both slides are examined for trophozoites, helminth ova (eggs), larvae, and protozoan cysts. Motility is also observed.

Common Parasites Identified

Trichomonas Vaginalis

Trichomonas vaginalis is a parasite that can inhabit the urogenital system of both males and females. It is considered a pathogenic parasite; *T. vaginalis* is the cause of vaginitis, urethritis, and prostatitis. *T. vaginalis* infection is usually considered a sexually transmitted disease. The motile trophozoite is found in freshly voided urine of both sexes, in prostatic secretions, and in vaginal wet preparations (Fig. 16-30). The diagnosis is usually made by observation of the motile trophozoite—a pear-shaped, elongated form—in fresh urine and urogenital specimens. The parasites are observed to move with a jerky and undulating motion; they are approximately the size of a neutrophil.

Motile trophozoites of *T. vaginalis* can be identified microscopically only in very fresh urine specimens and fresh genital secretions. They cannot be identified in old urine specimens or dry vaginal or prostatic secretions, because they are no longer motile or viable, and their morphology generally has changed, becoming "rounded up" and resembling a white blood cell or a transitional epithelial cell. For this reason, proper specimen collection and immediate transportation to the laboratory for analysis are important in the identification process (see Chapter 14). Wet preparations of genital secretions are diluted with a drop of saline and examined under low and high power for motility (appears as jerky motion).

The most sensitive method for identification of *T. vaginalis* is culture, and commercial products are available for this purpose.[7] One product is a self-contained system, the InPouch TV System (BioMed Diagnostics), used for detection of the organism by both culture and direct microscopic examination (Fig. 16-31, *B*). An open plastic viewing frame comes with the system, which allows for correct positioning and viewing of the pouch under the microscope.

A number of commercial products are available for rapid antigen detection of *T. vaginalis*. The OSOM *Trichomonas* Rapid Test (Genzyme Diagnostics, Cambridge, Mass.) is a dipstick method that is both rapid and easy to perform (see Fig. 16-31, A). These antigen-detection methods are more sensitive than the wet preparation for *T. vaginalis* described earlier.

Intestinal Ova and Parasites

Many parasitic infections are diagnosed through identification of their eggs (ova) or larvae in a fecal sample; the parasites are residing in the intestinal tract. Stool specimens for ova and parasite studies must be preserved or fixed immediately. Most commercial collection kits for these

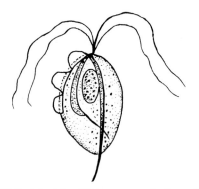

FIGURE 16-30 *Trichomonas vaginalis* trophozoite. (From Forbes BA, Sahm DF, Weissfeld AS: Bailey and Scott's diagnostic microbiology, ed 12, St Louis, 2007, Mosby.)

tests contain the appropriate preservative and pH indicator. The preservative-fixative for specimens to be tested for ova and parasites is formalin or polyvinyl alcohol (PVA). These can be toxic and difficult to dispose of; newer commercial products are available that are considered safer environmental replacements for PVA. These commercial products are EcoFix (Meridian Diagnostics, Cincinnati, Ohio) and Proto-Fix (Alpha-Tec Systems, Vancouver, Wash.). It is important to be aware of possible collection problems, such as with barium (radiologic studies), mineral oil, bismuth, some antidiarrheal preparations, antimalarials, and some antibiotics. Contamination with urine should also be avoided.

MACROSCOPIC EXAMINATION

Macroscopic examination includes observation of the consistency of the specimen. A fecal specimen of normal consistency, in which the moisture content is decreased, will more likely yield cyst stages because the protozoan parasite has encysted to survive. In a soft or liquid sample, the trophozoite stages are more likely to be found. Occasionally, adult helminths can be seen on the surface of the feces. The presence of blood should be noted; dark feces may indicate bleeding high in the gastrointestinal tract, whereas bright red feces indicates bleeding at a lower level.

MICROSCOPIC EXAMINATION

Direct wet mounts of the specimen are observed to detect helminth eggs and motile trophozoite stages of the protozoa. It is not sufficient to identify the protozoa by using only the direct wet mount preparation. Permanent stained smears should also

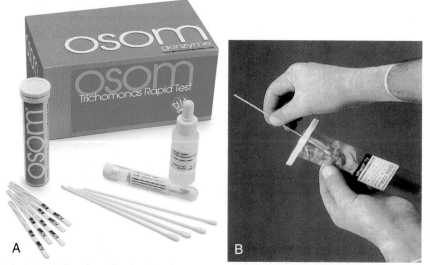

FIGURE 16-31 **A,** Rapid test for the identification of *Trichomonas vaginalis*. **B,** Self-contained system for culturing *T. vaginalis*. (From Forbes BA, Sahm DF, Weissfeld AS: Bailey and Scott's diagnostic microbiology, ed 12, St Louis, 2007, Mosby.)

be examined to confirm the identification of the parasitic organism.

The microscopic identification of intestinal protozoa and helminth ova is based on recognition of specific morphologic characteristics by personnel experienced in parasitology. In these studies, it is imperative that a good microscope with a good light source be used. The microscope should be equipped with a calibrated ocular micrometer to measure the size of the ova and parasites seen.

To observe the sample microscopically, a small amount of the sample is mixed with a drop of physiologic saline on a glass slide, and a coverslip is applied over the mixture. Correct light adjustment, as for unstained urine sediment, is needed to see the motile trophozoite stages of the protozoa because they are very pale and transparent.

After examination of the wet preparation is complete, a drop of weak iodine solution can be placed at the edge of the coverslip. This stained preparation will assist in the identification of protozoan cysts that stain with iodine. These will be seen as cysts with yellow-gold cytoplasm, brown glycogen material, and paler refractile nuclei. Other stains are used to reveal nuclear detail in the trophozoite stages of the protozoa. A permanent stained smear is used to confirm the identification of intestinal protozoa.

CONCENTRATION PROCEDURES

Concentration of fecal material should be included in a complete ova and parasite examination (O&P exam). Concentration procedures allow the visualization of small numbers of parasitic organisms that may be missed if only a direct mount is observed. Various concentration procedures are used, most often sedimentation or flotation techniques.

Sedimentation procedures use gravity or centrifugation and allow recovery of all protozoa, eggs, and larvae present in the specimen.

Flotation procedures allow the separation of protozoan cysts and certain helminth eggs. A reagent with a high specific gravity is used, such as zinc sulfate. The parasitic elements will be in the surface layer of the mixture, and the debris will be in the bottom layer. Some helminth or protozoan eggs do not concentrate well with the flotation method.

PERMANENT STAINED SMEARS

Confirming the identification of intestinal protozoa requires the preparation of a permanent stained smear. Permanent smears also provide a permanent record of the examination. To prepare slides for staining, fixation and preservation are first required. Fresh feces fixed in Schaudinn fixative or a PVA-preserved sample can be stained.

Commercial preparations are available, and stool can be added directly; then the permanent slide can be made from this preparation. Permanent stains used include iron hematoxylin and trichrome. Trichrome stains are most often used.

DIRECT ANTIGEN DETECTION

Many commercial kits are available to detect antigens for both *Giardia lamblia* and *Cryptosporidium* in the same product kit. *G. lamblia* is one of the most common parasites causing infection in the United States, and *Cryptosporidium* is an important parasite in waterborne outbreaks. An O&P examination can be lengthy, and use of these commercial products can save time in identification. The sensitivity of these kits is comparable to microscopy, and many clinical laboratories have adopted their use.

Enterobius vermicularis (Pinworm)

Enterobius vermicularis, the pinworm, is a common parasite in children worldwide. It is a roundworm whose adult female migrates during the night, depositing her eggs in the perianal region. A fecal sample is not the optimal specimen, because the eggs may not be observed in feces. Most laboratories use the clear cellophane tape method to collect and prepare the specimen for examination.

CELLOPHANE TAPE COLLECTION METHOD

The cellophane tape method is often used to collect the pinworm specimen. A piece of clear cellophane tape (not frosted tape), with the sticky side toward the patient, is pressed against the skin across the anal opening to collect any eggs, using even, thorough pressure. The sticky side of the tape is then placed down against the surface of a clean glass slide with a glass coverslip. The slide should be labeled with the patient's name and any other identifying data. Commercial collection kits are available with sticky paddles, simplifying the collection process. These specimens must be collected when the patient awakens in the morning, before bathing, defecating, or urinating. Negative findings must be confirmed with more tests done on subsequent days. The slide is scanned for the characteristically shaped eggs of the organism, using low-power and high-power magnification. *E. vermicularis* eggs are ellipsoid (football shaped) with one slightly flattened side (Fig. 16-32).

Blood and Tissue Microorganisms

Malaria is one of the most common infectious disease worldwide, and its rapid laboratory diagnosis is important. Diagnosis depends on clinical

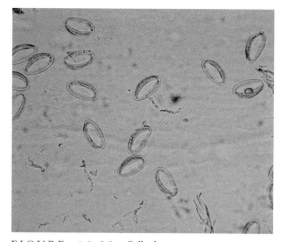

FIGURE 16-32 Cellophane tape preparation of *Enterobius vermicularis* (pinworm) eggs. (From Forbes BA, Sahm DF, Weissfeld AS: Bailey and Scott's diagnostic microbiology, ed 12, St Louis, 2007, Mosby.)

symptoms (headache, fever, chills, sweats, nausea) and identification of the *Plasmodium* malarial parasites in the RBCs. The malarial parasite enters the human through the bite from an infected *Anopheles* mosquito.

Tickborne infectious agents can cause disease; these infections include babesiosis, Lyme disease, and ehrlichiosis. Babesiosis is a disease that clinically resembles malaria. Babesia organisms are tickborne sporozoan parasites. Diagnosis of babesiosis is made through identification of *Babesia* parasites in the RBCs. In Lyme disease, the etiologic agent is the bacterium *Borrelia burgdorferi*. Transmission occurs by inoculation through the bite of a tick of the genus *Ixodes*. Diagnosis of Lyme disease depends on finding antibodies in the serum or spinal fluid. Ehrlichiosis is another infectious process that is tickborne. The organism, *Ehrlichia chaffeensis*, is a gram-negative, obligate intracellular parasite that multiplies in monocytic white cells (human monocytic ehrlichiosis). Diagnosis is made by direct visualization of clusters (morulae) of the organisms in white cells using Giemsa stain, by indirect immunofluorescence for detection of antibodies, and with polymerase chain reaction (PCR) techniques. Human granulocytic ehrlichiosis, now called *human granulocytic anaplasmosis*, is caused by *Anaplasma phagocytophilum*.

Lung tissue or secretions can be infected with *Pneumocystis jiroveci* (formerly *Pneumocystis carinii*), which usually is symptomatic only in immunosuppressed individuals. *P. jiroveci* pneumonia is seen in patients with acquired immunodeficiency syndrome (AIDS) and is a leading cause of death for AIDS patients. More recent DNA technologies have shown that *P. jiroveci* is a fungus. Traditionally, this organism is included in parasitology.

MALARIAL PARASITES

The malarial parasites enter the bloodstream and invade RBCs. Thin and thick smears are prepared, stained with Wright's or Giemsa stain, and examined for the blood parasites. The thick smears are more difficult to interpret but increase the sensitivity. The thin smears are used to better identify the species of the malarial parasite. Correct therapy depends on identification of the specific species of malarial organism present in the blood.

CASE STUDIES

CASE STUDY 16-1

A mother brings her 10-year-old daughter to the clinic; the child is complaining of a sore throat and has a low-grade fever (99.6°F). The mother states that the child has had a runny nose and a cough for the last few days. On examination, the physician notes that the child's pharynx appears red and that her tonsils are slightly swollen; no exudate is noted. Blood is drawn for a complete blood count (CBC), and a rapid strep test is done.

Laboratory Data
Hemoglobin: Normal
White blood count (WBC): High normal
Rapid strep test: Negative
Confirmation culture: Negative for group A β-hemolytic streptococci

1. What is the most likely diagnosis for this patient's condition?
   a. Viral infection, the cause of most cases of pharyngitis
   b. Strep throat infection; treat with antibiotics for 10 days.
2. On what information in the case history and other findings is this diagnosis based? (List findings.)

CASE STUDY 16-2

A 50-year-old man comes to the emergency room (ER) complaining of right-sided chest pain each time he breathes and a cough that has produced a rust-colored sputum. He also states that his symptoms began abruptly with chills the day before this visit to the ER; he had previously been healthy. Examination by the physician shows a fever of 102°F and coarse breathing sounds in the right anterior chest. A chest radiograph shows a right upper lobe infiltrate. Blood is drawn for a CBC, and a sputum sample is collected, Gram stained, and cultured.

Laboratory Data
CBC:
Hemoglobin: 14.5 g/dL (normal)
WBC: Elevated

Differential: 90% neutrophils
Sputum:

Gram stain: Gram-positive lancet-shaped diplo-cocci (cocci in pairs)

Culture report: *Streptococcus pneumoniae*
The diagnosis is pneumonia caused by *S. pneumoniae*.

1. What findings (history, physical exam, laboratory results) support the diagnosis? (List findings.)

2. The observation of which cells on the Gram-stained smear will assure the laboratorian that a sputum specimen has been collected and tested?

   a. Greater than 10 squamous epithelial cells per low-power field (10×)

   b. Fewer than 10 squamous epithelial cells per low-power field (10×)

CASE STUDY 16-3

A 20-year-old female presents to her family practice physician for a routine pelvic examination. It has been several years since her last visit to this clinic, when she was diagnosed and treated for a nongono-coccal sexually transmitted disease (STD). She is now sexually active only with her fiancé but has had sexual encounters with others in the past. She now wants to become pregnant. There are no apparent physical abnormalities, but the physician decides to culture the cervical discharge for gonorrhea and to perform a DNA test (Gen-probe) for chlamydia and gonorrhea. A serum sample is also collected for HIV testing. All laboratory tests are normal, with the exception of the test for chlamydia, which is positive.

Note: Symptoms of chlamydial infections include dysuria and vaginal/urethral discharge, symptoms similar to those of gonorrhea. Many cases of infected patients exhibit no symptoms of a chlamydial infection.

1. What are some of the findings (history, physical exam, laboratory test results) that would lead to the diagnosis of an STD? (List findings.)

2. Which of the following is the test of choice for the laboratory diagnosis of chlamydial infections?

   a. Nucleic acid amplification

   b. Immunofluorescent antibody test

   c. Enzyme immunoassay (EIA)

   d. Culture

CASE STUDY 16-4

A disoriented 58-year-old male patient with a history of poorly controlled diabetes mellitus and chronic obstructive pulmonary disease comes to the ER. The patient has been smoking cigarettes for many years. He has been taking steroid medications for his pulmonary disease. Physical examination shows that he is slightly febrile, lethargic, and in respiratory failure. A diagnosis of meningitis is being considered. A lumbar puncture is done and cerebro-spinal fluid (CSF) collected for a smear and culture.

Laboratory Data
A cytocentrifuged preparation of the CSF is done and stained, using calcofluor reagent specifically for yeast by staining the yeast cell walls. The smear shows encapsulated budding yeasts. A cryptococcal antigen test is done and is positive. The culture of CSF identifies *Cryptococcus neoformans*.

1. What observations (history, physical exam, laboratory findings) support the diagnosis of meningitis caused by this type of infectious organism? (List findings.)

2. Fungi are widespread in the environment but only rarely cause central nervous system (CNS) infection. *C. neoformans* is the most common cause of fungal meningitis. It is especially common among immunocompromised patients. This type of infection is known as which of the following?

   a. Nosocomial infection

   b. Opportunistic infection

   c. Community-associated infection

   d. Health care–associated infection

CASE STUDY 16-5

An 18-year-old female college student complains of fever, chills, headache, and vomiting. She goes to the college health service emergency department, where she is examined. She appears lethargic, and her temperature is 102°F. Blood is drawn for a CBC and culture, urine is collected for analysis, and a serum chemistry profile is ordered. A lumbar puncture is performed, and cloudy CSF is collected.

Laboratory Data
CBC:

WBC: 20.0×10^9 (increased)

Differential: Marked neutrophilia with shift to immature forms (shift to the left)
CSF results:

WBC: 1200 cells/mL with 95% neutrophils (reference value: 0-5 lymphocytes)

Glucose: 25 mg/dL (decreased, compared with blood glucose value)

Protein: 150 mg/dL (increased)

Gram stain: Many neutrophils, gram-negative diplococci in pairs

Urinalysis: Increased protein, few RBC, few granular casts

Serum chemistries: Within reference values
NOTE: *Haemophilus influenzae* (gram-negative coccobacillus) type B was the most common cause of meningitis in children 1 to 6 years of age before the vaccine now available. *Streptococcus pneumoniae* (gram-positive diplococcus) is a causative agent of meningitis in adults. *Neisseria meningitidis* (gram-negative diplococci) is most frequently identified as the causative organism for meningococcal infections in adolescents and young adults and has occurred in epidemics in the United States.

From the history and laboratory results, all but which one of the following findings in the blood and CSF substantiate a bacterial rather than a viral meningeal infection?

a. Decreased CSF glucose

b. Increased WBC in CSF, with neutrophils predominating

c. Gram stain showing gram-negative diplococci

d. Increased protein, few RBCs, few granular casts in urine

REFERENCES

1. Centers for Disease Control and Prevention/Division of Healthcare Quality Promotion/National Center for Preparedness, Detection, and Control of Infectious Diseases, Healthcare-associated infections (HAIs), http://www.cdc.gov/ncidod/dhqp/healthDis.html, date accessed August 8, 2009.

2. Centers for Disease Control and Prevention/Division of Healthcare Quality Promotion/National Center for Preparedness, Detection, and Control of Infectious Diseases, Community-associated MRSA, http://www.cdc.gov/ncidod/dhqp/ar_mrsa_ca.html, date accessed August 8, 2009.

3. Centers for Disease Control and Prevention: Bioterrorism agents/diseases, http://emergency.cdc.gov/agent/agentlist.asp, date accessed August 8, 2009.

4. US Department of Health and Human Services/CDC and National Institutes of Health: In Chosewood LC, Wilson DE, editors: Biosafety in microbiological and biomedical laboratories (BMBL), ed 5, Washington, DC, 2007, US Department of Health and Human Services.

5. Department of Energy: Specification for HEPA filters used by DOE contractors, DOE-STD 3020-97, Washington, DC, 1997, US Department of Energy.

6. Clinical and Laboratory Standards Institute: Procedures for the collection of diagnostic blood specimens by venipuncture; approved standard, ed 6, Wayne, 2007, Pa, CLSI Document H03-A6.

7. Murray PR, Baron EJ, Jorgensen JH, et al: Manual of clinical microbiology, ed 9, Washington, DC, 2007, ASM Press, pp 307, 293, 1025, 2105.

8. Clinical and Laboratory Standards Institute: Quality control for commercially prepared microbiological culture media: approved standard, ed 3, Wayne, 2004, Pa, CLSI Document M22-A3.

9. Difco & BBL manual: Becton Dickinson, New Jersey, 2009, Franklin Lakes.

10. REMEL technical manual, 2007, REMEL, Lenexa, Kansas.

11. Pezzlo MT: Laboratory diagnosis of urinary tract infections: current concepts and controversies, Infect Dis Clin Pract 2:469, 1993.

12. Forbes BA, Sahm DF, Weissfeld AS: Bailey and Scott's diagnostic microbiology, ed 12, St Louis, 2007, Mosby, pp 700, 781, 782, 786.

13. Clinical and Laboratory Standards Institute: Principles and Procedures for Blood Cultures; approved guideline, Wayne, 2007, PA, CLSI Document M47-A.

14. Clinical and Laboratory Standards Institute: Methods for dilution antimicrobial susceptibility tests for bacteria that grow aerobically: approved standard, ed 7, Wayne, 2006, Pa, CLSI Document M7-A7.

15. Clinical and Laboratory Standards Institute: Performance standards for antimicrobial disk susceptibility tests: approved standard, ed 9, Wayne, 2006, Pa, CLSI Document M2-A9.

16. Bondi A, Spaulding EH, Smith ED, et al: A routine method for the rapid determination of susceptibility to penicillin and other antibiotics, Am J Med Sci 214:221, 1947.

17. Bauer AW, Kirby WWM, Sherris JC, et al: Antibiotic susceptibility testing by a standardized single disc method, Am J Clin Pathol 45:493, 1966.

BIBLIOGRAPHY

Clinical and Laboratory Standards Institute: Development of in vitro susceptibility testing criteria and quality control parameter; approved guideline, ed 3, Wayne, 2008, Pa, CLSI Document M23-A3.

Forbes BA, Sahm DF, Weissfeld AS: Bailey and Scott's Diagnostic: Microbiology, ed 12, St. Louis, 2007, Mosby.

Gen-Probe: Package insert, San Diego, 2009, APTIMA Combo 2 assay, Gen-Probe.

Gen-Probe: Package insert, San Diego, 2008, PACE 2 assay, Gen-Probe.

Larone DH: Medically important fungi, ed 4, Washington, DC, 2002, ASM Press.

Murray PR, Baron EJ, Jorgensen JH, et al: Manual of Clinical Microbiology, ed 9, Washington, DC, 2007, ASM Press.

Murray PR, Rosenthal KS, Pfaller MA: Medical Microbiology, ed 5, St Louis, 2005, Elsevier Mosby.

REVIEW QUESTIONS

1. **Microbiology laboratory-acquired infections from an aerosol:**

   a. largely occur in persons who are new to the job.

   b. can occur from an accidental needle puncture wound.

   c. can cause disease with an organism of usually low infectivity.

   d. are associated with improper venting of air in the laboratory setting.

2. **Prevention of aerosolization can best be accomplished by:**

   a. disinfecting the work areas with a bleach solution.

   b. using puncture-proof sharps discard containers.

   c. using a biological safety cabinet when working with specimens or when forming aerosols.

   d. discarding all specimen-contaminated materials in a biohazard bag.

3. **Media that contain dyes, antibiotics, or other chemical compounds that inhibit certain bacteria while allowing others to grow are called:**

   a. enrichment media.

   b. differential media.

   c. supportive media.

   d. selective media.

4. **Media that contain factors (e.g., carbohydrates) that give colonies of particular organisms distinctive characteristics are called:**

   a. enrichment media.

   b. differential media.

   c. supportive media.

   d. selective media.

5. Media that are used to permit the normal rate of growth of most nonfastidious organisms are called:
   a. enrichment media.
   b. differential media.
   c. supportive media.
   d. selective media.

6. Which of the following is not a selective medium?
   a. CNA
   b. Thayer-Martin agar
   c. Sheep blood agar
   d. EMB

7. Which of the following is used to promote the growth of gram-negative organisms while inhibiting the growth of gram-positive organisms?
   a. MacConkey agar
   b. Sheep blood agar
   c. Thayer-Martin agar
   d. Chocolate agar

8. Which of the following is used to promote the growth of *Neisseria gonorrhoeae* and *Neisseria meningitidis*?
   a. MacConkey agar
   b. Sheep blood agar
   c. Thayer-Martin agar
   d. Phenylethyl alcohol agar

9. Automated microbiology systems have generally been designed to replace:
   a. manual antibiotic susceptibility procedures.
   b. manual procedures that are repetitive and that are performed daily on a large number of specimens.
   c. manual procedures that are done infrequently but are labor intensive.
   d. all manual procedures done in the microbiology laboratory.

10. The lowest concentration of antimicrobial agent that will visibly inhibit the growth of the organism being tested is known as the:
    a. minimum inhibitory concentration (MIC).
    b. minimum bactericidal concentration (MBC).
    c. agar disk diffusion test.
    d. dilution test.

11. Use of triple sugar iron agar or Kligler's iron agar can identify all but which one of the following characteristics of members of the Enterobacteriaceae family (common enteric intestinal pathogens)?
    a. Ability to ferment gas from sugars
    b. Ability to produce hydrogen sulfide gas
    c. Ability to produce ammonia
    d. Ability to ferment lactose

12. Pathogenic *Shigella* spp. characteristically are:
    a. non-lactose-fermenters.
    b. lactose-fermenters.
    c. coagulase positive.
    d. oxidase positive.

13. MacConkey agar is quantitatively inoculated with a urine specimen and incubated appropriately. Results are 100,000 CFU/mL urine of gram-negative lactose-fermenting organisms. Which of the following would be statistically the most likely organism to cause this urinary tract infection?
    a. *Escherichia coli*
    b. *Proteus* spp.
    c. *Staphylococcus aureus*
    d. *Klebsiella* spp.

14. What color are gram-negative bacteria after the decolorizing step in the Gram stain method?
    a. Purple
    b. Red
    c. Purple-red
    d. Colorless

15. Which of the following organisms can be recognized by its spreading growth appearance on sheep blood agar?
    a. *Escherichia coli*
    b. *Proteus* spp.
    c. *Staphylococcus aureus*
    d. *Klebsiella* spp.

16. Urogenital swabs to be cultured for gonococci should be plated onto culture media:
    a. immediately; at the bedside preferably.
    b. within 2 hours of collection.
    c. within 4 hours of collection.
    d. within 24 hours of collection.

17. In culturing a throat swab for group A β-hemolytic streptococci testing, which of the following media is preferred?
    a. Sheep blood agar
    b. HE agar
    c. MacConkey agar
    d. Chocolate agar

18. What is the purpose of making cuts in the sheep blood agar when a throat culture is plated?
    a. To count the colonies growing after incubation
    b. To observe the appearance of any hemolysis present
    c. To determine whether the organism is lactose positive or negative
    d. To note the morphologic appearance of the colony growth

19. In some people, untreated pharyngitis infections with group A β-hemolytic streptococci can eventually result in:
    a. chronic pyelonephritis.
    b. acute pyelonephritis.
    c. chronic glomerulonephritis.
    d. scarlet fever.

20. In observing a sheep blood agar plate inoculated with a sputum sample showing the presence of alpha or green hemolysis after incubation, what test can be done to determine whether the organism is viridans streptococci, part of the normal respiratory flora, or *Streptococcus pneumoniae?*
    a. Bile solubility test, in which most S. *pneumoniae* colonies would be dissolved by the reagent used and inhibited by optochin disk
    b. Bile solubility test, in which most viridans streptococci colonies would be dissolved by the reagent used and inhibited by optochin disk
    c. Bacitracin susceptibility test, in which most S. *pneumoniae* colonies would be inhibited by the bacitracin disk
    d. Bacitracin susceptibility test, in which most viridans streptococci colonies would be inhibited by the bacitracin disk

21. In identifying the presence of most group A β-hemolytic streptococci, versus those that are non–group A, which of the following tests can be done?
    a. Bile solubility test, in which most group A β-hemolytic streptococci colonies would be inhibited by an optochin disk
    b. Bile solubility test, in which most non–group A β-hemolytic streptococci colonies would be inhibited by an optochin disk
    c. PYR test, in which most group A β-hemolytic streptococci colonies would produce a bright red color after addition of the PYR reagent to the filter paper
    d. PYR test, in which most non–group A β-hemolytic streptococci colonies would produce a bright red color after addition of the PYR reagent to the filter paper

22. Which of the following antimicrobial agents is used to inhibit nonpathogenic fungi from growing in media that have been designed to promote growth of pathogenic fungi (e.g., Mycosel)?
    a. Penicillin
    b. Streptomycin
    c. Chloramphenicol
    d. Cycloheximide

23. A Gram-stained sputum smear shows 40 to 50 squamous epithelial cells per low-power (10×) field, along with gram-positive cocci, many gram-negative rods, and many gram-positive cocci in pairs using the oil-immersion objective. How should the laboratorian report the result for this smear?
    a. Call physician directly to report life-threatening situation.
    b. Report gram-positive cocci, many gram-negative rods, and many gram-positive cocci in pairs, as well as many squamous epithelial cells.
    c. Subculture must be done to confirm; report pending.
    d. No report; request another specimen because this one is contaminated with mouth flora (probably saliva, not sputum), as evidenced by the large number of squamous epithelial cells.

24. "Clue cells" are best seen in which of the following specimens?
    a. Wet preparation of vaginal discharge
    b. Gram stain of vaginal discharge
    c. KOH–wet preparation of vaginal discharge
    d. KOH–Gram stain of vaginal discharge

25. When antibiotic therapy is needed, specimens for culture and organism identification should be collected:
    a. at any time; administration of antibiotics does not affect the tests.
    b. while the antibiotics are being administered.
    c. before the antibiotics have been administered.
    d. after the antibiotics have been administered.

26. If the antibiotic does not inhibit the growth of an organism, the organism is said to be which of the following?
    a. Susceptible
    b. Sensitive
    c. Resistant
    d. Intermediate

27. The best method for finding pinworm organisms in children is:
    a. ova and parasite (O&P) examination.
    b. rectal swab.
    c. cellophane tape collection.
    d. blood.

28. **What are the requirements for collection of an appropriate specimen for the detection of chlamydia?**
    a. Examine the collected specimen while it is still fresh, when the organisms are still motile.
    b. First use a large swab to remove secretions present, then use a second swab to collect the specimen.
    c. Use the cellophane tape collection procedure on the skin area around the anal opening.
    d. Culture at the bedside is preferred, using chocolate agar and sheep blood agar.

29. **What are the requirements for collection of an appropriate specimen for the optimal detection of *Trichomonas vaginalis*?**
    a. Examine the collected specimen while it is still fresh, when the organisms are still motile.
    b. First use a large swab to remove secretions present, then use a second swab to collect the specimen.
    c. Cleanse the site carefully before any collection is done.
    d. Culture at the bedside is preferred, using chocolate agar and sheep blood agar.

30. **Collection of fecal samples for identification of intestinal parasites should be done:**
    a. after radiologic studies using barium sulfate have been completed.
    b. before radiologic studies using barium sulfate have been done.
    c. in the morning, before the patient has bathed, defecated, or urinated.
    d. before the onset of an acute phase of the intestinal disease.

IMMUNOLOGY AND SEROLOGY

Learning Objectives

At the conclusion of this chapter, the student will be able to:

- Define the term *immunology*.
- Describe the first line of defense against infection.
- Name and explain the components of natural immunity.
- Compare the cellular and humoral components of adaptive immunity.
- Contrast the functions of natural immunity and adaptive immunity.
- Name the three immunologically functional groups of leukocytes.
- Name and describe the five steps and general activities of phagocytosis.

- Name the various types of lymphocytes, and explain the function of each type.
- Define the terms *antigen* and *antibody*.
- Describe the general characteristics of antigens.
- Explain the general characteristics of antibodies.
- Identify and compare the five classes of antibodies.
- Diagram and explain the general configuration of an IgG antibody molecule.
- List and discuss characteristics of the five major classes of immunoglobulins.

Continued

- Illustrate and explain the characteristics of the four phases of an immune response.
- Define the term *immune complex.*
- Compare the terms *monoclonal* and *polyclonal antibodies.*
- Describe the production of monoclonal antibodies.
- Describe the characteristics of agglutination.
- Explain the mechanism of particle agglutination.
- Compare the grading of agglutination reactions.
- Name and compare the principles of latex agglutination, coagglutination, liposome-mediated agglutination, direct bacterial agglutination, and hemagglutination.
- Compare the characteristics of precipitation versus flocculation.
- Explain the action and application of lysis in serologic reactions.
- Name and compare immunofluorescent assays.

- Identify and compare various enzyme immunoassays.
- Briefly describe the applications of polymerase chain reaction (PCR), Southern blot, Northern blot, Western blot, and DNA chip technology.
- Compare the two phases of testing for antibody levels.
- Define the term *antibody titer,* and explain the procedure for the serial dilution of serum.
- Explain the principles of immunologic tests for pregnancy.
- Describe the pathophysiology and immunologic testing in infectious mononucleosis.
- Describe the pathophysiology and screening tests for antinuclear antibody (ANA) in systemic lupus erythematosus (SLE).
- Describe the pathophysiology and laboratory testing for rheumatoid factor (RF) in patients with rheumatoid arthritis (RA).
- Explain the rationale and outcomes of syphilis testing.

OVERVIEW OF IMMUNOLOGY AND SEROLOGY

Immunology is defined as the study of the molecules, cells, organs, and systems responsible for the recognition and disposal of nonself substances; the response and interaction of body components and related interactions; and the way the immune system can be manipulated to protect against or treat diseases. **Serology** is a division of immunology that specializes in laboratory detection and measurement of specific antibodies that develop in the blood during a response to exposure to a disease-producing antigen. **Immunohematology,** or blood banking, uses serologic methods to determine blood groups and unexpected antibodies in the blood of persons donating or receiving blood (see Chapter 18).

The function of the immune system is to recognize "self" from "nonself" and to defend the body against nonself substances. Nonself materials can be as diverse as life-threatening infectious microorganisms or a lifesaving organ transplant. Desirable consequences of immunity include natural resistance to, recovery from, and acquired resistance to infectious disease. A deficiency or dysfunction of the immune system can cause many disorders, such

as acquired immunodeficiency syndrome (AIDS). Undesirable consequences of immunity include allergies, rejection of transplanted tissue or organs, and development of an autoimmune disorder, a condition in which the body attacks itself as a foreign substance (e.g., insulin-dependent diabetes, pernicious anemia).

Many factors, including general health and age of an individual, are important considerations in the defense against disease. The ability to respond immunologically to disease is age related. Although nonspecific and specific body defenses are present in the fetus and newborn, many defenses are incompletely developed at birth, which increases the risk of developing infectious disease. Other factors that can influence body defenses are genetic predisposition to many disorders, nutritional status, and an individual's method of coping with stress.

Body Defenses Against Microbial Disease

Before a pathogen can invade the human body, it must overcome the general resistance provided by the body's immune system, which consists of nonspecific and specific defense mechanisms.

TABLE 17-1

Two Types of Acquired Immunity		
Type	Mode of Acquisition	Antibody Produced by Host
Active	Natural infection	Yes
	Artificial vaccination	Yes
Passive	Natural transfer in vivo or colostrums	No
	Artificial infusion of serum or plasma	No

TABLE 17-2

Acquired Immunity		
	Humoral-Mediated Immunity	Cell-Mediated Immunity
Mechanism	Antibody mediated	Cell mediated
Cell type	B lymphocytes	T lymphocytes
Mode of action	Antibodies in plasma soluble products	Direct cell-to-cell contact or secreted by cells

First Line of Defense

The first line of defense or first barrier to infection is unbroken skin and mucosal membrane surfaces. These surfaces are extremely important because they form a physical barrier to many microorganisms. Normal biota, previously called *normal flora*, consists of bacteria that are usually found in certain parts of the body, such as the throat and intestines. These microorganisms deter penetration or facilitate elimination of foreign microorganisms from the body. Other types of first-line defenses against microbial invasion include secretions such as mucus, earwax (cerumen), lactic acid in sweat, stomach acid, saliva, and tears. The constant motion of the ciliated epithelial cells provides additional protection to the respiratory tract.

Natural Immunity

Natural (innate or inborn) resistance is one of the two ways the body resists infection if microorganisms have penetrated the first line of defense. Natural immunity is characterized as a nonspecific mechanism. This second line of defense consists of particular cells (neutrophils, tissue basophils, macrophages) and soluble substances in the blood (complement, lysozyme, interferon). Neutrophils, monocytes, and macrophages can engulf invading foreign material such as bacteria. Complement proteins, soluble protein components, are the major **humoral** (fluid) component of natural immunity. Lysozymes and interferon are sometimes referred to as *natural antibiotics*. Interferon is a family of proteins produced rapidly by many cells in response to viral infection; it blocks the replication of viruses in cells.

Acquired or Adaptive Immunity

Acquired (adaptive) resistance forms a third line of defense that allows the body to recognize, remember, and respond to a specific stimulus, an antigen. The two types of acquired immunity are active and passive (Table 17-1). **Active immunity** can result from natural exposure in response to an infection

or from an intentional vaccination with an antigen-bearing microorganism. Active immunity should stimulate the production of antibodies in a person with the disease.

Acquired immunity consists of cellular components (T and B lymphocytes, plasma cells) and humoral components (antibodies, cytokines) (Table 17-2). Lymphocytes selectively respond to nonself substances, or antigens, which leads to immune memory and a permanently altered pattern of response or adaptation in immunocompetent individuals. The immunocompetent host is able to recognize a foreign antigen and build specific antigen-directed antibodies, retaining permanent antigenic memory.

The condition of cellular memory, acquired resistance, allows the body to respond more effectively if reinfection with the same microorganisms occurs. The actions of the adaptive response (cell-mediated immunity, humoral-mediated immunity) take place because of the interaction of antibody with complement and phagocytic cells of natural immunity and of T lymphocytes with macrophages.

Humoral-Mediated Immunity

The purpose of humoral-mediated immunity is to act as a primary defense against bacterial infection. If the reaction is natural and active, the person builds antibodies as the result of an infection with a microorganism. If the reaction is natural but artificial, the person builds antibodies after being vaccinated. Vaccines may be composed of living suspensions of weak or attenuated cells or viruses, killed cells or viruses, or extracted bacterial products, such as altered, formerly poisonous toxoids used to immunize against diphtheria and tetanus. Periodic booster vaccinations may be needed to expand the pool of memory cells.

If the reaction is natural and passive, a newborn receives antibodies in vivo or in colostrum produced by the mother. If the reaction is artificial and passive, a person receives antibodies by the infusion of serum or plasma made by another person.

Immediate hypersensitivity reactions are a subset of the body's antibody-mediated mechanisms.

Immediate hypersensitivity involves the reactions of immunoglobulin E (IgE) with tissue basophils (mast cells). Antigen interaction with antigen-specific IgE bound to the surface of the cells release potent chemical mediators from the cells which in turn act on various organs. The most dramatic and devastating systemic manifestation of immediate hypersensitivity is anaphylaxis, a type I hypersensitivity reaction. This type of reaction can be caused by intravenous penicillin injection, bee stings, and food allergies (e.g., peanuts) in allergic individuals.

Cell-Mediated Immunity

Cell-mediated immunity (delayed hypersensitivity, T-lymphocyte–dependent type IV hypersensitivity reaction) is responsible for body defense in the following immunologic events:

- Contact sensitivity (e.g., poison ivy dermatitis)
- Immunity to viral and fungal antigen
- Immunity to intracellular organisms
- Rejection of foreign tissue grafts
- Elimination of tumor cells bearing neoantigens
- Formation of chronic granulomas with nondegradable material sequestered in a focus of concentric macrophages that also contains some lymphocytes and eosinophils

Under some conditions, the activities of cell-mediated immunity may not be beneficial. Immunosuppression, the suppression of the normal adaptive immune response through the use of chemotherapeutic drugs (e.g., steroids) or by other means (e.g., radiation), may be necessary in autoimmune disorders or bone marrow transplantation.

Cell-mediated immunity is moderated by the link between T lymphocytes and phagocytic cells (e.g., monocytes-macrophages). A T lymphocyte does not directly recognize the antigens of microorganisms. Recognition of an antigen takes place when the antigen is present on the surface of an antigen-presenting cell, such as a macrophage. Lymphocytes are immunologically active by various types of direct cell-to-cell contact and by the production of soluble factors (e.g., cytokines).

Cells and Cellular Activities of the Immune System

The entire leukocyte (white blood cell) system is designed to defend the body against disease. Each cell type has a unique function and in many cases acts in cooperation with other cell types. Leukocytes (WBCs) can be functionally divided into the following general categories:

- Granulocytes
- Monocytes-macrophages
- Lymphocytes–plasma cells

Granulocytes and Mononuclear Cells

The primary phagocytic cells are the granulocytic polymorphonuclear neutrophil leukocytes (PMNs) and cells of the mononuclear-macrophage system. Macrophages also participate in antigen presentation and induction of the immune response, as well as secretion of biologically active molecules.

Phagocytosis

The process of phagocytosis (Fig. 17-1) can be divided into the following steps:

1. Chemotaxis
2. Adherence
3. Engulfment
4. Phagosome formation and fusion
5. Digestion and destruction

The physical occurrence of damage to tissues, either by trauma or microbial invasion, releases substances to initiate phagocytosis. Neutrophilic granulocytes continually circulate in the blood and can be found at the site of injury in less than 1 hour. Monocytes move more slowly; macrophages are embedded in the tissues or wandering. Cells are guided to the site of injury by chemoattractants. Adherence brings the phagocyte in contact with the microorganism. On reaching the site of infection, phagocytes engulf the foreign matter and destroy it. Digestion is accomplished because granules of the phagocytes contain degradatory enzymes. Unfortunately, the release of digestive enzymes also kills the phagocyte **(cytolysis).**

If invading bacteria are not phagocytized and destroyed, they may establish themselves in secondary sites in the body, producing a secondary inflammation. If bacteria escape from secondary tissue sites, a bacteremia will develop. If a patient is unresponsive to antibiotic therapy, this situation may be fatal.

Lymphocytes and Plasma Cells

Lymphocytes are derived from a common stem cell in the bone marrow. T and B lymphocytes and plasma cells are the cornerstones of the immune system. Lymphocytes participate in body defenses primarily through the recognition of foreign antigen and production of antibody. About 80% of the lymphocytes circulating in the blood are T lymphocytes; about 20% of the circulating lymphocytes are B lymphocytes. Mature T lymphocytes survive for several months or years, whereas the B lymphocytes survive for only a few days. **Plasma cells,** not normally found in the blood, arise as the end stage of B-cell differentiation into large, activated cells. The function of plasma cells is the synthesis and excretion of immunoglobulins (antibodies).

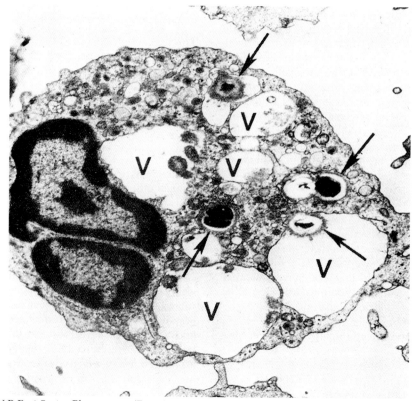

FIGURE 17-1 **Phagocytosis.** (From Bauer JD: Clinical laboratory methods, ed 9, St Louis 1982, Mosby.)

Natural killer (NK) and K-type lymphocytes are a subpopulation of circulating lymphocytes.

Lymphocyte Maturation and Function

T Lymphocytes

T cells arise in the thymus from fetal liver or bone marrow precursors that seed the thymus during embryonic development. These CD34+ progenitor cells develop in the thymic cortex. **T lymphocytes** function in cell-mediated immune responses such as delayed hypersensitivity, graft-versus-host reactions, and allograft rejection. They make up the majority of the lymphocytes circulating in the peripheral blood. In the periphery of the thymus, T cells further differentiate into multiple different T-cell subpopulations with different functions, including cytotoxicity and the secretion of soluble factors, termed *cytokines*. Many different cytokines have been identified, including 25 interleukin molecules and more than 40 chemokines. Their functions include growth promotion, differentiation, chemotaxis, and cell stimulation.

B Lymphocytes

B cells are derived from hematopoietic stem cells by a complex series of differentiation events that occur in the fetal liver and, in adult life, in the bone marrow. **B lymphocytes** most likely mature in the bone marrow and function primarily in antibody production or the formation of immunoglobulins. B cells constitute about 10% to 30% of the blood lymphocytes. B-lymphocyte differentiation is complex and ends in the generation of mature, end-stage, nonmotile cells, the plasma cells. Some activated B cells differentiate into memory B cells, long-lived cells that circulate in the blood. Memory B cells may live for years, but mature B cells that are not activated only live for days.

ANTIGENS AND ANTIBODIES

An **antigen** is a substance that stimulates antibody formation and has the ability to bind to an antibody. Cellular antigens of importance in immunology are major histocompatibility complex (MHC) tissue antigens (or human leukocyte antigens, HLA), autoantigens, and blood group antigens. In most cases, the normal immune system responds to foreign antigens by producing antibodies. **Antibody** produced in response to the foreign antigen is found in the plasma and in other body fluids and reacts with the foreign antigen in some observable way. Antibody is usually specific for the antigen against which it is formed.

The significance of antigens and antibodies is basic to the study of immunity and immunology.

Various microorganisms have antigenic properties and elicit an antibody response when introduced into an immunocompetent host. The antibody formed in response to the foreign antigen (in this case, the microorganism) usually protects the individual from subsequent infections by that specific organism.

Foreign antigenic substances are recognized by lymphoid and plasma cells. Each specific type of antigen stimulates the production of equally specific antibodies by various body tissues. If an antibody has been formed against a foreign antigenic substance, one good way to identify the infecting organism is to identify the antibody produced in response to it. This is the basis for immunologic and serologic determinations. Research has demonstrated that if a known antigen, such as a certain bacterium, is exposed in a test tube to a patient's serum containing antibodies against that antigen, a serologic or immunologic reaction will be observed. If the specific antibody is not present in the patient's serum, no reaction will be observed.

Antibodies that have been produced in response to a specific antigenic stimulus can be identified in the serum. This serologic reaction produces an observable change in the mixture in one of several ways, such as precipitation or agglutination reactions. The reaction takes different forms because of variations in the technique being used and the type of antigen being assayed.

Nature of Antigens

An antigen is generally described as a substance that, when injected into an animal, is recognized as foreign and, provided immunologically active cells are present, provokes an immune reaction or response. As stated previously, this immune response is the production of antibodies, substances that usually protect the body against the foreign antigen. At times, antibodies are not protective (e.g., hay fever, anaphylactic shock). Antigenicity is not confined to proteins. Certain nonantigenic, nonprotein substances known as **haptens** may bind themselves to protein, and the resulting hapten-protein complex is antigenic.

Antigenicity is influenced by molecular size, foreignness, shape of the molecule, and chemical composition. In addition, the antigenicity of a foreign substance is also related to the route of entry. Intravenous and intraperitoneal routes are stronger stimuli than subcutaneous and intramuscular routes.

Characteristics and Production of Antibodies

Antibodies are proteins and are produced in response to foreign antigenic stimuli. Whether a cell-mediated response or an antibody response

TABLE 17-3

Immunoglobulins in Serum or Plasma		
Immunoglobulin Class	Molecular Weight (Daltons)	Proportion of Total Immunoglobulin
IgA	160,000-500,000	13%
IgD	180,000	1%
IgE	196,000	Trace
IgG	150,000	80%
IgM	900,000	6%

takes place depends on the way in which the antigen is presented to the lymphocytes; many immune reactions display both types of response.

Antibodies (immunoglobulins) are found in the gamma globulin fraction of serum or plasma. Some antibodies occur in humans naturally as a result of exposure throughout life to bacteria and plant material through inhalation and ingestion. Antibodies can also be produced in response to natural infections (e.g., typhoid fever organisms), or their production can be artificially stimulated by the injection of antigens in vaccine form. Newborns do not form antibodies but may have received them passively from the mother across the placenta. Infants begin forming antibodies at about 3 months and usually have a normal gamma globulin level by 6 months. This is important when serum from newborns is tested for antibodies, such as testing for ABO blood groups.

When antibodies result from exposure to antigenic material from another species, they are referred to as *heteroantibodies*. When antibodies result from antigenic stimulation within the same species, they are referred to as *alloantibodies* or *isoantibodies*.

Classes of Immunoglobulins (Antibodies)

Five immunoglobulin (Ig) classes of antibodies with different molecular weights and biological activity occur in human blood and body fluids: IgM, IgG, IgA, IgD, and IgE (Table 17-3).

Antibody Structure

All the immunoglobulins have a similar chemical structural configuration, as shown in Fig. 17-2. The common configuration consists of a monomer composed of two identical heavy chains and two identical light chains connected by disulfide bonds or bridges in the hinge region. The chemical structure of the heavy chains is responsible for the differences in the various classes of antibodies. Light chains are of only two types (kappa and lambda) and are common to all classes of immunoglobulins.

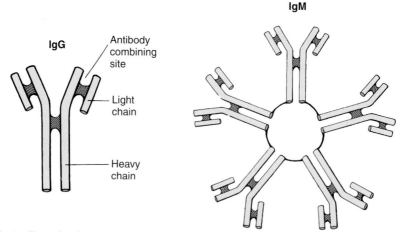

FIGURE 17-2 *Examples of antibody molecular structure. Left,* Immunoglobulin G (IgG) is a simple monomer composed of two heavy chains and two light chains connected by disulfide bonds or bridges. *Right,* Immunoglobulin M (IgM) is in the form of a pentamer. Each monomer has reactive sites capable of combining with corresponding antigens.

Environmentally Stimulated and Immune Antibodies

Environmentally stimulated antibodies (sometimes called *natural antibodies*) appear to exist without intentional antigenic stimulus. In contrast, immune antibodies are the result of stimulation by specific foreign antigens. Examples of environmentally stimulated isoantibodies in blood are the anti-A and anti-B antibodies found in the ABO blood group system (see Chapter 18). Immune antibodies are also referred to as "unexpected antibodies" and are usually the result of specific antigenic stimulation. These antibodies can result from immunization through pregnancy, transfusion, or injection of transfused red blood cells bearing a foreign antigen.

Antibody Response

The response to an antigenic or "foreign" substance is referred to as an **immune response.** An antibody response (Fig. 17-3) has four phases:
1. Lag phase: no detectable antibody
2. Log phase: antibody titer increases logarithmically
3. Plateau phase: antibody titer stabilizes
4. Decline: antibody is broken down (catabolized)

Immunity is not immediate; when first infected, the person is ill or incapacitated by the disease. Antibodies require about 2 weeks to develop sufficiently, after which subsequent exposure to the antigen will elicit an effective secondary anamnestic antigen-antibody response, resulting in protective immunity.

PRIMARY RESPONSE

When a foreign antigen is first introduced, the antibody cannot be detected immediately in the serum or plasma. It is observed about 10 to 14 days after antigenic stimulation, and the antibody titer (the concentration of antibody), is greatest at about 20 days, after which it gradually decreases. This is known as the **primary response.** The subclass of antibody associated with the primary response is IgM.

SECONDARY RESPONSE

A second exposure to the same antigen creates a more rapid response. Detectable amounts of IgM appear first, followed by IgG antibody in the plasma or serum. A memory phenomenon elicited by the lymphocytes results in an immediate antibody response on the second exposure or subsequent exposures. This **secondary anamnestic response** also produces a higher and longer-lasting titer of IgG antibody. An anamnestic response differs from a primary antibody response in the following important aspects:
- Time: a secondary response has a shorter lag phase, a longer plateau phase, and a more gradual decline in antibody titer.
- Type of antibody: IgM-type antibodies are the principal class of antibody formed in a primary response. Although some IgM antibody is formed in a secondary response, the IgG class is the predominant type formed.
- Antibody titer: in a secondary response, antibody concentrations reach a higher titer. The plateau levels in a secondary response are typically tenfold or more than the plateau levels in the primary response.

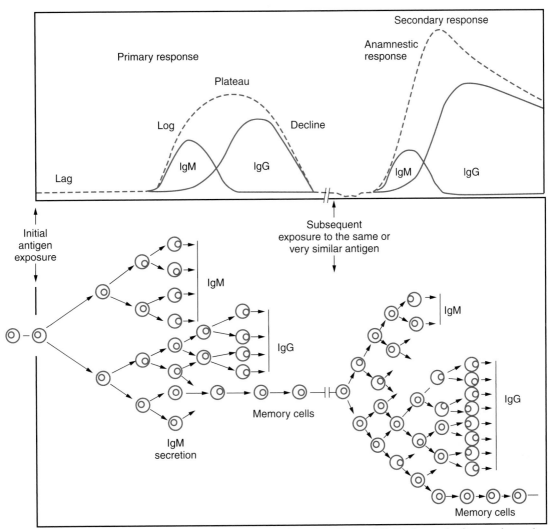

FIGURE 17-3 **Four phases of an immune response.** (Redrawn from Turgeon ML: Fundamentals of immunohematology, ed 2, Baltimore, 1995, Williams & Wilkins.)

Immune Complexes

The noncovalent bonding of an antigen with its respective, specific antibody is called an **immune complex.** An immune complex may be small and soluble or large and precipitating, depending on the nature and proportion of antigen and antibody. Antibody can react with antigen that is fixed or localized in tissues or with antigen that is released or present in the circulation. In the circulation, an immune complex is usually removed by phagocytic cells. Under normal circumstances, this process does not lead to a pathologic consequence. In fact, it can be viewed as a major host defense against the invasion of foreign antigens. In unusual circumstances, an immune complex persists and is deposited in endothelial or vascular structures, where it causes inflammatory damage. This damage can occur in organs (e.g., kidneys) in systemic lupus erythematosus and other immunologic disorders.

Monoclonal and Polyclonal Antibodies

Monoclonal antibodies (mAbs) are purified antibodies cloned from a single cell. These antibodies exhibit exceptional purity and specificity; mAbs are able to recognize and bind to a specific antigen. They are secreted into the serum in large quantities when associated with malignant proliferation of plasma cells or their precursors, as in multiple myeloma. Monoclonal antisera, produced by hybridization, are used as reagents in diagnostic testing because of their greater diagnostic precision. They are also used for cancer therapy.

Polyclonal antibodies are usually produced by immunizing animals with the antigen being studied and then isolating and purifying the antibody from the animal's serum. These antibodies are heterogeneous and lack the specificity of mAbs.

COMPLEMENT

Complement is a heat-labile series of 18 plasma proteins. Proteins of the classic activation pathway and their terminal sequence are called *components.* Normally, complement components are present in the circulation in an inactive form. When an antigen and matching antibody join one another, the classic complement activation pathway is triggered. This cascading pathway results in the ultimate formation of the membrane-attack complex (MAC), which disrupts cellular membranes. The complement system is of importance in transfusion medicine because incompatible ABO blood transfusions can trigger complement and result in a hemolytic transfusion reaction. Complement components, such as C3 and C4, may be assayed as diagnostic testing for disorders (e.g., SLE).

PRINCIPLES OF IMMUNOLOGIC AND SEROLOGIC METHODS

Principles of Agglutination

Agglutination and precipitation are the visible expression of the aggregation of antigens and antibodies through the formation of a framework in which antigen particles or molecules alternate with antibody molecules (Fig. 17-4). **Agglutination** (clumping) is the term used to describe the aggregation of particulate test antigens. **Precipitation** is the term applied to aggregation of soluble test antigens. If a solution is allowed time to settle in a test tube, precipitates (clumps) will fall to the bottom of the tube.

Agglutination occurs only if the antigen is in the form of particles such as bacteria, red blood cells (RBCs), latex particles, white blood cells (WBCs), or any substance that appears cloudy when suspended in saline. Slide agglutination tests are performed less frequently than in the past and have been replaced by the immunoassay technique in most point-of-care tests.

Mechanism of Particle Agglutination

Agglutination is the clumping of particles that have antigens on their surface (e.g., erythrocytes) by antibody molecules that form bridges between the antigenic determinants. This is the endpoint for most tests involving erythrocyte antigens. Agglutination is influenced by a number of factors and is believed to occur in two stages: sensitization and lattice formation.

Sensitization

The first phase of agglutination, **sensitization,** represents the physical attachment of antibody

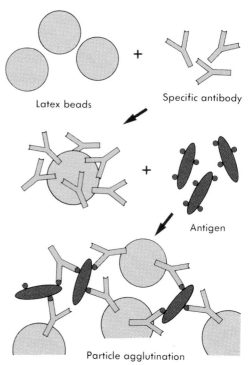

FIGURE 17-4 **Alignment of antibody molecules bound to the surface of a latex particle and latex agglutination reaction.** (From Forbes BA, Sahm DF, Weissfeld AS: Bailey and Scott's diagnostic microbiology, ed 12, St Louis, 2007, Mosby.)

molecules to antigens on the erythrocyte membrane. Physical conditions that affect the amount of antigen-antibody binding include (1) the pH, (2) temperature, (3) length of time of incubation of the coated particles with the patient's serum (or other source of antibody), and (4) the antigen-antibody ratio.

pH (HYDROGEN ION CONCENTRATION)

A pH of 7.0 is used for routine laboratory testing. It is known that some antibodies react best at a lower pH.

TEMPERATURE

The optimum temperature needed to reach equilibrium in an antibody-antigen reaction differs for different antibodies. IgM antibodies are "cold reacting," with a thermal range of 4°C to 22°C, and IgG antibodies are "warm reacting," with an optimum temperature of reaction at 37°C.

LENGTH OF INCUBATION

In laboratory testing, incubation times range from 15 to 60 minutes. The optimum time of incubation varies, depending on the class of immunoglobulin and how tightly an antibody attaches to its specific antigen.

Lattice Formation

Lattice formation, or the establishment of cross-links between sensitized particles (e.g., erythrocytes) and antibodies, resulting in aggregation, is a much slower process than the sensitization phase. The formation of chemical bonds and resultant lattice formation depend on the ability of a cell with attached antibody on its surface to come close enough to another cell to permit the antibody molecules to bridge the gap and combine with the antigen receptor site on the second cell.

Reading Agglutination Reactions

Observation of agglutination occurring in a test tube is initially made by gently shaking the test tube containing the serum and cells and viewing the lower portion, the button, with a magnifying glass as it is dispersed. Because agglutination is a reversible reaction, the test tube must be treated delicately, and hard shaking must be avoided; however, all the cells in the button must be resuspended before an accurate observation can be determined. The observer should also note whether discoloration of the fluid above the cells, the supernatant, is present. If the erythrocytes have been ruptured or hemolyzed, this is as important a finding as agglutination.

The strength of agglutination, called *grading*, uses a scale of 0 or negative (no agglutination) to 4+ (all the erythrocytes are clumped) (Table 17-4). **Pseudoagglutination,** or false appearance of clumping, may rarely occur because of the presence of rouleaux formation. To disperse pseudoagglutination, a few drops of physiologic sodium chloride (saline) can be added to the reaction tube and the solution remixed and reexamined.

Microplate Agglutination Reactions

Serologic testing is now more often being performed with automated instruments as a microtechnique. Micromethods for RBC antigen and antibody testing are either hemagglutination or solid-phase adherence assays. These methods are also considered simpler to perform. Use of microplates allows for the performance of many tests on a single plate, which eliminates time-consuming steps such as labeling test tubes.

Immunofluorescent Assays

Immunofluorescent assays are very popular methods for rapid antigen detection (see Chapter 6). A fluorescent substance, when absorbing light of one wavelength, emits light of another (longer) wavelength.

TABLE 17-4

Grading Agglutination Reactions	
Grade	Description
Negative	No aggregates
Mixed field	Few isolated aggregates; mostly free-floating cells; supernatant appears red
Weak (+/−)	Tiny aggregates that are barely visible macroscopically; many free erythrocytes; turbid and reddish supernatant
1+	A few small aggregates just visible macroscopically; many free erythrocytes; turbid and reddish supernatant
2+	Medium-sized aggregates; some free erythrocytes; clear supernatant
3+	Several large aggregates; some free erythrocytes; clear supernatant
4+	All erythrocytes combined into one solid aggregate; clear supernatant

Fluorescent labeling is a method of demonstrating the reaction of antigens and antibodies. Fluorescent molecules are used as substitutes for radioisotope or enzyme labels. The **fluorescent antibody (FA)** technique consists of labeling antibody with fluorescein isothiocyanate (FITC), a fluorescent compound with an affinity for proteins, to form a conjugate. This conjugate is able to react with antibody-specific antigen. FITC emits a bright apple-green fluorescence when excited.

FA techniques are extremely specific and sensitive. **Immunofluorescence** can also be used to identify specific antigens on live cells in suspension (i.e., flow-cell cytometry). When a live, stained-cell suspension is put through a fluorescent active-cell sorter (FACS) which measures the fluorescent intensity of each cell, the cells are separated according to their particular fluorescent brightness. This technique permits the isolation of different cell populations with different surface antigens (e.g., various types of lymphocytes). Fluorescent conjugates are used in the basic methods of **direct immunofluorescent assay (DFA)** and **indirect immunofluorescent assay (IFA).**

Direct Immunofluorescent Assay

In the direct technique, a conjugated antibody is used to detect antigen-antibody reactions that can be seen with a fluorescent microscope. This technique can be applied to tissue sections or in smears for microorganisms. In DFA, the antigen-specific labeled antibody is applied to the fixed specimen, incubated, and washed. A counterstain may be applied as a last step before viewing the slide with a fluorescence microscope.

Indirect Immunofluorescent Assay

The serologic method most widely used for the detection of diverse antibodies is the IFA. The indirect method is based on the fact that antibodies (immunoglobulins) not only react with homologous antigens but also can act as antigens and react with antiimmunoglobulins.

If the specific antibody in question is present in the serum, the antibody will bind to the specific antigen. To remove any unbound antibody, the slide is washed. In the second part of this process, anti–human globulin that has been conjugated to the fluorescent dye is placed on the slide. The conjugated marker will bind to any antibody already bound to the antigen on the slide. This will serve as a marker for the antibody when the slide is viewed under a fluorescence microscope. The dye marker fluoresces apple green. If antibody is absent, the anti–human globulin dye marker will be removed during the washing procedure, and no fluorescence will be seen. As with DFA, a counterstain may be applied as a last step before viewing the slide with a fluorescence microscope. The fluorescence does not fade appreciably for a few days if the stained slides have coverslips applied with a drop of buffered glycerol and if the slides are kept refrigerated in the dark. It is best to examine the prepared slides immediately after staining.

Other Labeling Techniques

Chemiluminescence is being pursued as the technology of choice by most immunodiagnostics manufacturers. Chemiluminescence has excellent sensitivity and dynamic range. In immunoassays, chemiluminescent labels can be attached to an antigen or an antibody. Chemiluminescent labels are being used to detect proteins, viruses, oligonucleotides, and nucleic acid sequences.

Other emerging labeling technologies include quantum dots (Q dots), squid technology, luminescent oxygen channeling immunoassay (LOCI), fluorescent in situ hybridization (FISH), signal amplification techniques, and magnetic labeling technology.

Enzyme Immunoassays

Enzyme immunoassay (EIA) provides an alternative to immunofluorescent assays. Rather than tagging an antibody with a fluorochrome, EIA uses enzyme molecules that can be conjugated to specific monoclonal or polyclonal antibodies. This type of testing includes the enzyme-linked immunosorbent assay (ELISA). EIA is a popular method for waived over-the-counter testing.

The EIA method uses a nonisotopic label, which offers the advantage of safety and demonstrates specificity, sensitivity, and rapidity. Some EIA procedures provide diagnostic information and measure immune status (e.g., detect either total antibody IgM or IgG). EIAs can detect extremely small quantities of antigen-antibody reactants. The conversion of a colorless substrate to a colored product allows for either visual or colorimetric detection.

Direct and Indirect Sandwich Technique

One type of EIA method involves the use of a direct or indirect sandwich technique. If the target antigen is present in a specimen, it will form a stable complex with the antibody bound to the matrix. Unbound specimen is removed by washing, and a second antibody specific for the antigen is added. In the direct method, the second antibody is conjugated to an enzyme. In the indirect method, a second nonconjugated antibody is added and washed, and a third antibody that is specific for the second antibody is added. The third antibody is conjugated to the enzyme and directed against the Fc portion of the unlabeled second antibody.

Membrane-Bound Technique

Most commercially developed EIA applications require physical separation of the specific antigens from nonspecific complexes found in clinical samples. If the antibody directed toward the agent being assayed is fixed firmly to a solid matrix, either to the inside of the wells of a microdilution tray or to the outside of a spherical plastic or metal bead or some other solid matrix, the system is called a *solid-phase immunosorbent assay* (SPIA).

A modification of SPIA uses a disposable plastic cassette consisting of the antibody-bound membrane and a small chamber to which the specimen can be added. An absorbent material is placed below the membrane to wick the liquid reactants through the membrane. This helps separate nonreacted components from the antigen-antibody complexes being studied. Flow-through EIAs are popular for influenza and group A *Streptococcus* testing because they are easy to use.

Optical Immunoassays

Optical immunoassays (OIA) rely on the alteration of thickness of inert surfaces because of antigen-antibody complexes interaction. The increased thickness causes the surface to appear a different color to the naked eye. This method of testing is used for detection of group A *Streptococcus* and influenza A.

Molecular Techniques

Beginning with **polymerase chain reaction (PCR),** an in vitro method to amplify low levels of specific DNA sequences in a sample to higher quantities suitable for further analysis, molecular techniques continue to find new clinical applications. PCR analysis can lead to the detection of gene mutations that signify the early development of cancer; identification of viral DNA associated with specific cancers, such as human papillomavirus (HPV), a causative agent in cervical cancer; and detection of genetic mutations associated with a wide variety of diseases.

The **Southern blot** and **Northern blot** are used to detect deoxyribonucleic acid (DNA) and ribonucleic acid (RNA), respectively. Single-base mutations that can be determined by Southern blot include sickle cell anemia and hemophilia A. The derivation of this technique from the Southern blot used for DNA detection has led to the common use of the term *Northern blot* for the detection of specific messenger RNA (mRNA). The Northern blot is not routinely used in clinical molecular diagnostic techniques.

Western blot is a technique in which proteins are separated electrophoretically, transferred to membranes, and identified through the use of labeled antibodies specific for the protein of interest. Western blot is used to detect antibodies to specific epitopes. Specific assays using the Western blot technology are used to detect antibodies to human immunodeficiency virus (HIV), the causative agent of AIDS. Before an HIV result using a screening EIA is considered positive, the result should be confirmed by the use of at least one additional test. A current standard test for confirming positive HIV-1 tests uses Western blot technology.

Microarrays (DNA chips) are basically the product of bonding or direct synthesis of numerous specific DNA probes on a stationary, often silicon-based, support. Microarrays are miniature gene fragments attached to glass chips. These chips are used to examine gene activity of thousands or tens of thousands of gene fragments and to identify genetic mutations using a hybridization reaction between the sequences on the microarray and a fluorescent sample. Applications of microarrays in clinical medicine include analysis of gene expression in malignancies (e.g., mutations in BRCA-l, mutations of tumor suppressor gene p53, genetic disease testing, viral resistance mutation detection).

SPECIMENS FOR SEROLOGY AND IMMUNOLOGY

Immunologic testing is done in many areas of the clinical laboratory, including microbiology, chemistry, toxicology, immunology, hematology, surgical pathology, cytopathology, and immuno-hematology (blood banking), and a great variety of specimens are tested. With the advent of procedures devised to give rapid, accurate results—especially those based on the use of mAbs and EIA technology—many clinical constituents can be determined immunologically. Many types of body fluids can be evaluated by using immunologic technology. It is always important to determine the specimen of choice for each procedure being considered. The many commercial kits available for the various assays will state specific specimen requirements and acceptable criteria for collection.

Testing for Antibody Levels

In obtaining specimens for serologic testing, it is important to consider the phase of the disease and the condition of the patient at the time of the specimen collection. This is especially important in assays for diagnosis of infectious diseases. If serum is being tested for antibody levels for a specific infectious organism, generally the blood should be drawn during the **acute phase** of the illness—when the disease is first discovered or suspected—and another sample drawn during the **convalescent phase,** usually about 2 weeks later. Accordingly, these samples are called *acute serum* and *convalescent serum*. A difference in the amount of antibody present, or the antibody titer, may be noted when the two different samples are tested concurrently. An important concept in any serologic testing is the manifestation of a rise in titer.

Antibody Titer

The **antibody titer** is defined as the reciprocal of the highest dilution of the patient's serum in which the antibody is still detectable. That is, the titer is read at the highest dilution of serum that gives a positive reaction with the antigen. If a serum sample has been diluted 1:64 and reacts positively with the antigen suspension used in the testing process, and the next-highest dilution of 1:128 does not give a positive reaction, the titer is read as 64. A high titer indicates that a relatively high concentration of the antibody is present in the serum. For some infections, the titer of antibody rises slowly, even months after the acute infection, as in patients with legionnaires' disease. For most pathogenic infections, an increase in the patient's titer of two doubling dilutions, or from a positive result of 1:8 to a positive result of 1:32 over several weeks, is an indication of a current infection. This is known as a "fourfold" rise in the antibody titer.

TABLE 17-5

Preparation of a Serial Dilution									
	Tube 1	Tube 2	Tube 3	Tube 4	Tube 5	Tube 6	Tube 7	Tube 8	Tube 9	Tube 10
Saline (mL)	—	1	1	1	1	1	1	1	1	1
Serum (mL)*	1	1	1 of 1:2	1 of 1:4	1 of 1:8	1 of 1:16	1 of 1:32	1 of 1:64	1 of 1:128	1:256
Final dilution	—	1:2	1:4	1:8	1:16	1:32	1:64	1:128	1:256	1:512

*Or milliliters of diluted serum.
To prepare a twofold dilution:
1. Label tubes 1-10 and place in a test-tube rack.
2. Add 1 mL of 0.9% saline to tubes 2 through 10.
3. Add 1 mL of patient's serum to tubes 1 and 2.
4. With the same pipet, mix the contents of tube 2 by drawing the contents up into the pipet. The process of drawing up and blowing out is considered one mixing. Repeat this process four times. Note that tube 1 contains **only undiluted serum** and tube 2 contains half **the amount of the serum** because 0.1 mL of undiluted serum was diluted with 0.1 mL saline = diluted 1:2.
5. Continue the serial diluting by transferring 1mL of diluted serum from tube 2 to tube 3 and mixing with 1.0 mL of saline. Mix four times as described above. Continue this dilution process until reaching tube 10. It can be extended to even higher dilutions if needed to achieve a non-reactive tube, e.g., no agglutination or hemolysis after observing visible agglutination or hemolysis.
Follow Up:
6. Specified quantities e.g., 0.1mL of a specific antigen, e.g., red blood cells demonstrating A antigen, would be added to each tube. The serially diluted tubes would be shaken to mix the contents, centrifuged, and finally examined for visible agglutination or hemolysis.

Twofold Dilutions

The standard dilution technique most frequently used in the serology laboratory is a "twofold" dilution. The basis of this type of dilution is that each tube contains half serum and half diluent, e.g., saline. The first tube of the twofold dilution series usually contains a specified quantity of undiluted patient's serum. To dilute a serum specimen serially, progressive regular increments of serum are diluted (Table 17-5). This means each dilution is half as concentrated as the preceding one and the total volume is the same in each tube. Serially, the second tube contains half the amount of serum and therefore half the amount of antibody; the third tube contains a quarter of the amount of antibody, the fourth tube contains an eighth, etc. As previously noted, titers are usually reported as the reciprocal of the last dilution showing the desired reaction, such as agglutination, lysis, or a change in color.

Antigen-Antibody Ratio

The **antigen-antibody ratio** is the number of antibody molecules in relation to the number of antigen sites per cell (Fig. 17-5). Under conditions of decreased antigen-antibody ratio, an antibody excess may exist. The outcome of excessive antibody concentration is known as the **prozone phenomenon,** which can produce a false-negative reaction (Table 17-6). This phenomenon can be overcome by serially diluting the antibody-containing serum until optimum amounts of antigen

and antibody are present in the test system. The **zone of equivalence** is the range of dilutions where the relative concentration of antibody and antigen produce maximal binding of antigen to antibody. In the zone of equivalence, agglutination is observable. After this range of dilutions is exceeded, the post-prozone range of weaker dilutions no longer exhibits visible agglutination. An excess of antigen occurs, resulting in no lattice formation in an agglutination reaction.

Types of Specimens Tested

The majority of immunology tests are done on serum. Blood is collected in a plain tube and allowed to clot completely before being centrifuged. Serum should be removed from the clot as soon as possible after processing. Lipemia, hemolysis, or any bacterial contamination can make the specimen unacceptable. Icteric or turbid serum may give valid results for some tests but may interfere with others. Blood specimens should be collected before a meal to avoid the presence of chyle, an emulsion of fat globules that often appears in serum after eating, during digestion. Contamination with alkali or acid must be avoided; these substances have a denaturing effect on serum proteins and make the specimens useless for serologic testing. Excessive heat and bacterial contamination are also avoided. Heat coagulates the proteins, and bacterial growth alters protein molecules. If the test cannot be performed immediately, the serum should be refrigerated. If the testing cannot be done within 72 hours, the serum specimen must be frozen.

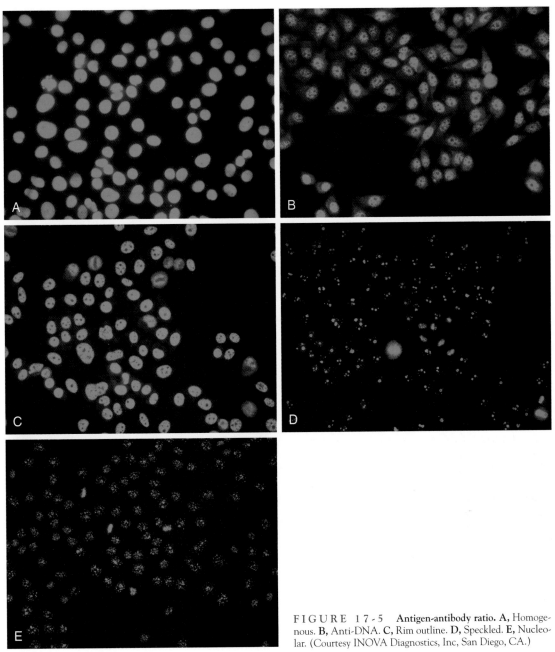

FIGURE 17-5 **Antigen-antibody ratio. A,** Homogeneous. **B,** Anti-DNA. **C,** Rim outline. **D,** Speckled. **E,** Nucleolar. (Courtesy INOVA Diagnostics, Inc, San Diego, CA.)

TABLE 17-6

Prozone and Postzone Phenomenon											
Zones	Prozone		Equivalence								Postzone
Serum dilution	None	1:2	1:4	1:8	1:16	1:32	1:64	1:128	1:256		1:512
Strength of agglutination	Neg	Neg	1+	2+	3+	4+	3+	2+	1+		Neg

TABLE 17-7

			Examples of Non–Instrument-Based Point-of-Care Tests		
Type of Test	Analysis	Type of Specimen	Assay Principle	Format
Qualitative	Occult blood	Feces	Chemical reaction	Impregnated paper
	Pregnancy testing	Urine	Immunochromatography	Single-use, dry-reagent
	Cardiac markers	Blood	Optical immunoassay	cartridge
	Chlamydia	Swab		
	Strep A, strep B, influenza	Swab		Single-use, dry-reagent cartridge
Semiquantitative	Urinalysis (e.g., pH, glucose, protein, blood)	Urine	Chemical/enzymatic reactions	Impregnated strips
	Glucose	Blood		
Quantitative	Therapeutic drugs	Blood	Immunochromatography	Single-use, dry-reagent cartridge

For some testing, the serum complement must first be inactivated. To inactivate complement, the tubes of serum are placed in a heat block at 56°C for 30 minutes. If the protein complement is not inactivated, it will promote lysis of the RBCs and other types of cells and can produce invalid results. Complement is also known to interfere with certain tests for syphilis.

Other specimens include urine for pregnancy tests and tests for urinary tract infections. It is important that the urine specimen be collected after thorough cleaning of the external genitalia to prevent contamination for any microbiological assays. Urine for the human chorionic gonadotropin assay (pregnancy test) must be collected at a suitable time after fertilization to allow the concentration of the hormone to rise to a significant detectable level. Specimens must be collected into a suitable container to prevent in vitro changes that could affect the assay results. Proper handling and storage of the specimen until testing is done are essential. Immunologic assays are also done on cerebrospinal fluid, other body fluids, and swabs of various body exudates and discharges. The established protocol for each specific assay must be followed in terms of specimen collection requirements and conditions for the assay itself.

COMMON IMMUNOLOGIC AND SEROLOGIC TESTS

The advent of monoclonal antibody (mAb) technology has given rise to the development of many new, highly specific and sensitive immunoassays. Classic serologic testing has been an important part of some diagnostic tests in the clinical laboratory for many years; traditional serologic tests have been done for viral and bacterial diseases. Common serologic and immunologic tests important in clinical laboratory diagnoses include tests

for pregnancy, infectious mononucleosis, and syphilis.

Non–Instrument-Based Point-of-Care Testing

Point-of-care testing (POCT) may be done by manual rapid test methods (e.g., pregnancy, occult blood). More rapid tests are being developed for the identification of infectious organisms (e.g., group A *Streptococcus*, HIV) and cardiac markers (e.g., troponin). Instant-ViewTn (Alfa Scientific Designs) is an example of a Food and Drug Administration (FDA)-approved immunoassay for the detection of cardiac markers (free and complex troponins) in emergency rooms, hospital settings, and point-of-care situations.

Most non–instrument-based tests (Table 17-7) apply the principles of competitive and noncompetitive immunoassay, enzymatic assay, or chemical reactions with a visually read endpoint. Tests for pregnancy (see procedure at http://evolve.elsevier.com/Turgeon/clinicallab), drugs of abuse, cardiac markers, and occult fecal blood (see procedure at http://evolve.elsevier.com/Turgeon/clinicallab), as well as those using blood glucose strips, urine dipsticks, and various microbial agents (e.g., Rapid West Nile Virus IgM Assay [Spectral Diagnostics]), are included in this category. Manual entry of data into the medical record is the only mechanism available for non–instrument-based POCT systems.

POCT assays usually assay whole blood, but urine, feces, saliva, or throat swabs can be tested. An example of a recently CLIA-waived assay for HIV that can test oral fluid, as well as plasma and whole blood, is OraQuick (Abbott Diagnostics, http://www.abbottdiagnostics.com/). This rapid antibody test is a single-use, qualitative immunoassay to detect antibodies to HIV types 1 (HIV-1) and 2 (HIV-2).

Pregnancy Tests

Pregnancy tests are designed to detect minute amounts of human chorionic gonadotropin (hCG), a glycoprotein hormone secreted by the trophoblast of the developing embryo that rapidly increases in the urine or serum during early stages of pregnancy. Many pregnancy test kits contain mAb directed against the beta subunit of the glycoprotein (β-hCG) to increase the specificity of the reaction.

Beta–Human Chorionic Gonadotropin

For the first 6 to 8 weeks after conception, β-hCG helps maintain the corpus luteum and stimulate the production of progesterone. In a normal pregnancy, detectable amounts of about 25 mIU/mL β-hCG are secreted 2 to 3 days (48 to 72 hours) after implantation, or approximately 8 to 10 days after conception or fertilization. Peak levels are reached approximately 2 to 3 months after the last menstrual period. Levels rise rapidly after conception. If a test is negative at this stage, the test should be repeated within a week. Most specimens will contain enough β-hCG for detection by the twelfth day after a missed period. Some test methods (e.g., ELISA) use serum and detect increases in β-hCG much earlier, often within days of conception.

Specimen Collection

Most of the kits currently can be used for both serum and urine β-hCG but show better sensitivity with serum, because the concentration of β-hCG in serum is not subject to the wide variation found in urine β-hCG as a result of changes in urine concentration. The first morning urine specimen is required because it contains the highest concentration of hormone. It should have a specific gravity of at least 1.015. The urine specimen is collected in a clean glass or plastic container. It may be refrigerated for up to 2 days or frozen at −20°C for at least 1 year. Thaw frozen samples by placing the frozen specimen in a water bath at 37°C, and then mix thoroughly before use. If turbidity or precipitation is present after thawing, filtering or centrifuge is recommended. Specimens containing blood, large amounts of protein, or excessive bacterial contamination should not be used. Do not refreeze.

Types of Pregnancy Tests

Immunologic pregnancy tests are done in one of several ways. Generally, these tests are easy to perform with blood or urine samples. A variety of commercial kits are available.

Enzyme Immunoassays

Several ELISA tests are available as a result of mAb technology. In these tests, two types of mAb are used.

One is a β-hCG–specific antibody bound to a membrane or other solid support medium. This can be a membrane in a tube or on a disk. The characteristics of nitrocellulose, nylon, or other membrane material can be used to enhance the speed and the sensitivity of ELISA reactions. An absorbent material below the membrane can help pull the liquid reactants through the membrane and help separate components that have not reacted from those that have formed antigen-antibody complexes and have bound to the membrane during the testing process. The washing steps are simplified in this way. When a specimen containing β-hCG is added (urine, plasma, serum, or whole blood can be used), the β-hCG molecules present are bound to the antibodies on the solid support membrane.

The second mAb is a β-hCG antibody that has been linked to a specific enzyme (alkaline phosphatase). This enzyme-linked antibody is added to the testing system and will bind to a different site on the β-hCG molecule, creating a sandwich of bound antibody–β-hCG–enzyme-labeled antibody. After an incubation period, any unbound enzyme-labeled antibody is washed free. A chromogenic substrate reagent is next added, which undergoes a specific color change in the presence of the alkaline phosphatase enzyme, indicating the presence of β-hCG. The color change is often to blue. Variations in these tests include the use of impregnated membranes and strips.

Test results should be reported as "β-hCG positive" or "β-hCG negative," not as "pregnancy positive" or "pregnancy negative," because of the possibility of a false-positive pregnancy test reaction. False-positive results are less common with the ELISA tests. ELISAs are very sensitive, giving positive reactions as early as 10 days after conception.

Infectious Mononucleosis Testing

The Epstein-Barr virus (EBV) was first discovered in 1964 as the cause of infectious mononucleosis (IM). EBV is widely disseminated; it is estimated that 95% of the world's population is exposed to EBV, which makes it the most ubiquitous human virus known. EBV is a DNA herpesvirus.

IM is usually an acute, benign, and self-limiting lymphoproliferative condition that can cause Burkitt's lymphoma (malignant tumor of lymphoid tissue occurring mainly in African children), nasopharyngeal carcinoma, and other neoplasms. Most individuals demonstrate antibodies to EBV without significant clinical signs or symptoms of disease. Immunocompetent persons maintain EBV as a chronic latent infection. Although this viral disorder can affect anyone, IM typically manifests in young adults.

The incubation period of IM is from 10 to 50 days; once fully developed, it lasts for 1 to 4 weeks. Clinical manifestations include extreme fatigue, malaise, sore throat, fever, and cervical lymphadenopathy. Splenomegaly occurs in about 50% of patients. Jaundice is infrequent, although the most common complication is hepatitis.

Heterophil Antibodies

These antibodies represent a broad class of antibody. **Heterophil antibodies** are defined as antibodies that are stimulated by one antigen and react with an entirely unrelated surface antigen present on cells from different mammalian species. Heterophil antibodies may be present in normal individuals in low concentrations (titers), but a titer of 1:56 or greater is clinically significant in suspected cases of IM.

The IgM type of heterophil antibody usually appears during the acute phase of IM, but the antigen that stimulates its production remains unknown. IgM heterophil antibody is characterized by the following features:

1. Reacts with horse, ox, and sheep erythrocytes
2. Absorbed by beef erythrocytes
3. Not absorbed by guinea pig kidney cells
4. Does not react with EBV-specific antigens

Rapid slide tests based on the principle of agglutination of horse erythrocytes are available. The use of horse erythrocytes appears to increase the sensitivity of the test.

Diagnostic Evaluation

In addition to clinical signs and symptoms, laboratory testing is necessary to establish or confirm the diagnosis of IM.

Hematologic studies reveal a leukocyte count ranging from 10 to 20 × 10^9/L in about two-thirds of patients; about 10% of the patients with IM demonstrate leukopenia. A differential leukocyte count may initially disclose a neutrophilia, although mononuclear cells usually predominate as the disorder develops. Typical relative lymphocyte counts range from 60% to 90% with 5% to 30% variant lymphocytes. These variant lymphocytes exhibit diverse morphologic features and persist for 1 to 2 months and as long as 4 to 6 months.

If the classic signs and symptoms of IM are absent, a diagnosis of IM is more difficult to make. A definitive diagnosis of IM can be established by serologic antibody testing. The antibodies present in IM are heterophil and EBV antibodies. A positive slide test in a patient with the appropriate clinical signs and symptoms is strong evidence of acute IM.

Rapid Slide Tests

Rapid slide tests have been developed by several manufacturers (see procedure at http://evolve.elsevier.com/Turgeon/clinicallab). Most screening tests use fine suspensions of guinea pig kidney for the rapid differential absorption and horse red cells (RBCs) for the sensitive detection of IM heterophil antibodies. These rapid screening tests are based on the following general principles:

1. The use of horse RBCs instead of sheep RBCs makes the test more sensitive and thus is especially valuable for low-titer serum found in the early stages of the disease.
2. The unwashed, preserved horse RBC reagent remains in a usable condition for at least 3 months and gives stronger and quicker agglutination with IM serum than horse RBCs preserved with formalin.
3. Some non-IM serum also has a high horse agglutinin titer, and therefore serologic tests cannot depend on titers alone.
4. Fine suspensions of guinea pig kidney give satisfactory instant absorption of antibodies and a clear-cut differentiation between infectious and noninfectious mononucleosis serum. Before any reagents are used for the test, the reagent test cells should be shaken well to provide a homogeneous mixture. The reagents should be used at room temperature.

For many of these rapid tests, serum, plasma, or whole blood (capillary or anticoagulated venous blood) from the patient can be used. As part of the test, it is mixed thoroughly with guinea pig kidney on one section of the slide to absorb or neutralize any Forssman antibodies present, because both IM antibodies and Forssman antibodies will agglutinate the horse RBCs in the test reagent (both are heterophil antibodies). The IM antibodies, if present, will remain reactive and will agglutinate the test horse RBCs when they are added to the absorbed serum mixture. The test reagents are available commercially as part of the specific test kit being used. Directions must always be followed carefully for each specific product. Agglutination is observed at a specific time after the final mixing, generally after 1 minute of mixing. If agglutination is observed, the test is positive. If no agglutination is observed, the test is negative. Specific instructions about interpretation of a test are included with the product information. One commercially available test kit using this principle is MonoSlide.

This product uses specially treated horse RBCs that provide color enhancement to increase the specificity, sensitivity, and readability of the test.

When serum is used for the rapid IM screening tests, the presence of hemolysis in the specimen makes it unsuitable for testing. If testing cannot be done immediately, serum or plasma may be stored at 2°C to 8°C for several days after being collected.

Most of the widely used rapid immunologic assays for IM are highly sensitive. It is still necessary, however, to use adequate and proper control programs as the only dependable method of detecting sources of technical errors. Using both a positive and negative control specimen, control sera should be tested once during each shift of use to ensure proper kit performance. When the results are not clear-cut, it is always important to repeat the test and conduct additional serologic tests if needed.

False-negative slide tests may be obtained in patients with a low heterophil titer. This can occur early, in the first 1 or 2 weeks after onset of symptoms. False-negative tests may also be seen in patients who do not mount a heterophil antibody response to the infection, especially young children. The slide test can be repeated at a later date, or an EBV titer for IgM can be performed to help establish the diagnosis for these patients.

False-positive tests for heterophil antibody have been reported in cases of cytomegalovirus (CMV) infections, rubella infections, leukemia, Hodgkin's disease, Burkitt's lymphoma, rheumatoid arthritis, viral hepatitis, and multiple myeloma.

Systemic Lupus Erythematosus Testing

Systemic lupus erythematosus (SLE) is the classic model of autoimmune disease. Autoimmunity represents a breakdown of the immune system's ability to discriminate between self and nonself. More than 40 autoimmune diseases occur in 5% to 10% of the general population. The term *autoimmune disease* is used when demonstrable immunoglobulins (autoantibodies) or cytotoxic (T) cells display specificity for self-antigens, or autoantigens, and contribute to the pathogenesis of the disease. The Lupus Foundation of America estimates that approximately 1.4 million Americans have a form of lupus. Lupus is most common in females during the reproductive years. No single cause has been identified for SLE, which is a disease of acute and chronic inflammation. Circulating immune complexes are the hallmark of SLE.

Demonstrable antibodies include antibodies to nuclear components; cell surface and cytoplasmic antigens of polymorphonuclear and lymphocytic leukocytes, erythrocytes, platelets, and neuronal cells; and IgG. The antinuclear antibody (ANA)

procedure is an important screening tool for SLE. Detection of autoantibodies by immunofluorescence has become an extremely valuable method. Immunofluorescence is extremely sensitive and may show positive results in cases where ANA procedures (e.g., complement fixation or precipitation) give negative results. At present, the immunofluorescent method is the most widely used technique for ANA screening. Serologic testing frequently reveals high levels of anti-DNA antibodies, reduced complement levels, and the presence of complement breakdown products of C3 (C3d and C3c). In addition, cryoglobulins, which represent immune complexes in some cases, are frequently present in the serum of patients with SLE. The level of cryoglobulins correlates well with the severity of SLE. Assays helpful in assessing renal disease associated with SLE involve antibody to double-stranded DNA, levels of C3 and C4, and cryoglobulins.

Rapid Slide Test for Antinucleoprotein

The SLE Latex Test (Wampole Laboratories) provides a suspension of polystyrene latex particles coated with deoxyribonucleoprotein (DNP). When the latex reagent is mixed with serum containing the ANAs, binding to the DNP-coated latex particles produces macroscopic agglutination. The procedure is positive in SLE and systemic rheumatic diseases such as rheumatoid arthritis, scleroderma, and Sjögren's syndrome.

Antinuclear Antibodies

Antinuclear antibodies (ANAs; Fig. 17-5) are immunoglobulins that react with the whole cell nucleus or with nuclear components (e.g., nuclear proteins, DNA, histones) in the tissue of the host. ANAs are found in other diseases (e.g., rheumatoid arthritis), are associated with the use of certain drugs, and are found in aging persons without disease. Thus the assays for ANAs are not specific for SLE, but ANAs are present in more than 95% of persons with SLE. Because the detection of ANAs is not diagnostic of SLE, their presence cannot confirm the disease, but their absence can be used to help rule out SLE. The significance of the presence of ANAs in a patient's serum must be considered in relation to the patient's age, gender, clinical signs and symptoms, and other laboratory findings. Fluorescent ANA techniques are often used in screening tests for SLE; many are indirect.

Indirect Immunofluorescent Tests

Indirect immunofluorescent tests for ANA are based on the use of fluorescein-conjugated antiglobulin. These methods are extremely sensitive.

TABLE 17-8

Antinuclear Antibody Patterns	
Pattern	Interpretation
Negative reaction: no green or gold fluorescence observed	Normal
Nuclear rim (peripheral)	SLE, SLE activity, and lupus nephritis
Homogeneous (diffuse)	SLE or another connective tissue disorder
Speckled	Many diseases, including SLE
Nucleolar patterns	Progressive systemic sclerosis and Sjögren's syndrome

SLE, Systemic lupus erythematosus.
NOTE: The degree of positive fluorescence may be semiquantitated on a scale of 1+ to 4+.

In one assay the serum specimen is delivered into a well on a microscope slide that contains a mouse liver substrate. Substrates of rat or mouse liver or kidney or cell-cultured fibroblasts can also be used as the antigen and are fixed to the slides. If antibody is present in the patient's serum, the unlabeled antibody will attach to the nuclei of the cells in the substrate. After the substrate is washed in buffer, the slide is incubated with fluorescein-labeled goat antihuman immunoglobulin. If the patient antibodies have attached themselves to the nuclear antigens in the substrate, the fluorescein-tagged goat antihuman immunoglobulin will attach to these antibodies. Fluorescence will be seen microscopically using ultraviolet light. The slides should be examined as soon as possible. If immediate examination is not possible, the slides can be stored in the dark at 4°C for up to 48 hours before being read.

Several different patterns of fluorescence reactivity are seen, depending on whether the ANAs have reacted with the whole nucleus or with nuclear components, such as the nuclear proteins, DNA, or histone (a simple protein). This difference in nuclear fluorescence pattern reflects specificity for various diseases (Table 17-8). After ensuring that the results for positive and negative control specimens are giving the expected reactions, the results for the patient are reported. Results from the screening tests are reported as positive or negative. Patterns are described as being diffuse or homogeneous, peripheral, speckled, or nucleolar fluorescence.

Rheumatoid Arthritis Testing

Rheumatoid arthritis (RA) is a chronic inflammatory disease, primarily affecting the joints and joint tissues. Evidence indicates that immunologic factors are involved in both the articular and the extraarticular manifestations of RA. RA may represent an unusual host response to one or perhaps many etiologic agents. An infectious etiology is possible. It is a highly variable disease that ranges from a mild illness of brief duration to a progressive, destructive polyarthritis associated with a systemic vasculitis. Felty's syndrome is the association of RA with splenomegaly and leukopenia. A high-titer rheumatoid factor assay, a positive ANA assay, and rheumatoid nodules are frequently found in patients with Felty's syndrome. Patients have a propensity for bacterial infections. Juvenile rheumatoid arthritis (JRA) is a condition of chronic synovitis beginning during childhood. The etiologic hypotheses are similar to those proposed for adult RA. Subgroups of JRA include Still's disease, polyarticular onset, pauciarticular onset, and RA.

Two pathogenic mechanisms have been hypothesized in RA. The extravascular immune complex hypothesis proposes an interaction of antigens and antibodies in synovial tissues and fluid. The alternate hypothesis is that RA results from cell-mediated damage because of the accumulation of lymphocytes, primarily T cells, in the rheumatoid synovium, resembling a delayed-type hypersensitivity reaction. The presence of cytokines, involved in both articular inflammation and articular destruction, supports this hypothesis.

Immunofluorescent technique reveals that the rheumatoid synovium contains large amounts of IgG and IgM, alone or together. Immunoglobulins can also be observed in synovial lining cells, blood vessels, and interstitial connective tissues. B cells make immunoglobulin in the synovium of patients with RA. As many as half the plasma cells that can be located in the synovium secrete an IgG rheumatoid factor that combines in the cytoplasm with similar IgG molecules (self-associating IgG). The cause of the various vascular and parenchymal lesions of RA suggests that the lesions result from injury induced by immune complexes, especially those containing antibodies to IgG.

Rheumatoid Factor

The identification of **rheumatoid factor (RF)** in the serum or synovial fluid of patients with clinical features of RA assists in confirming the diagnosis. The serum of most patients with RA has detectable soluble immune complexes. Anti–gamma globulins of the IgG and IgM classes are an integral part of these complexes. RF belongs to a larger family of antiglobulins usually defined as antibodies with specificity for antigen determinants on the Fc fragment of human or certain animal IgG. Rheumatoid factors have been associated with three major immunoglobulin classes: IgM, IgG, and IgA.

RF is present in many but not all persons with RA. RF can be present in other diseases (e.g., tuberculosis, bacterial endocarditis, hepatitis), but the highest titers are found in persons with RA. RF that appears in chronic diseases virtually disappears when the infectious process is treated with the appropriate therapy; RF that is present in RA persists indefinitely. RF is not found in degenerative joint diseases such as osteoarthritis or in gout or infectious joint diseases. The determination of the presence of RF is important in the prognosis and management of RA. High titers of RF are indications of greater amounts of joint destruction, possible increased systemic involvement, and generally more severe disease. RF can also be detected in synovial fluid, but its significance is little more than that of RF in serum.

The tests for RF are based on the reaction between antibodies in the patient's serum (RF) and an antigen derived from gamma globulin. Generally, all tests are designed to detect antibodies to immunoglobulins. A latex-coated suspension with albumin and chemically bonded with denatured human gamma globulin serves as the antigen in one common test for RF. If RF is present in the serum, macroscopic agglutination will be visible when the latex reagent is mixed with serum. Latex agglutination procedures have a 95% correlation with a clinical diagnosis of probable or definite RA. False-positive results may be obtained if the serum is lipemic, hemolyzed, or heavily contaminated with bacteria, or if the test result is read after the specified time (2 minutes). False-positive tests are possible with other rheumatic diseases (e.g., SLE), in chronic infectious diseases (e.g., hepatitis, tuberculosis, syphilis), and in cirrhosis and sarcoidosis. Other RF tests use sensitized sheep cells in hemagglutination procedures. The latex agglutination and sheep cell agglutination tests are the most widely used routine tests for RF.

Rapid Latex Agglutination Test

Serum is usually the specimen used for the rapid latex agglutination test for RA (see procedure at http://evolve.elsevier.com/Turgeon/clinicallab). If the test cannot be performed immediately, the specimen should be refrigerated. If the test cannot be performed within 72 hours, the specimen should be frozen. Frozen serum should be thawed rapidly at 37°C before testing. Before the test is done, the specimen should be at room temperature. All reagents used for the rapid slide RF tests must also be at room temperature. It is always important to follow carefully all instructions provided with the testing product.

Syphilis Testing

Syphilis is caused by a spirochete, *Treponema pallidum*. In 1906, the first diagnostic blood procedure was developed to detect this disease. Syphilis in humans is ordinarily transmitted by sexual contact. In males, the microorganism is transmitted from lesions on the penis or discharged from deeper sites with semen. Lesions in females are usually located in the perineal region or on the labia, vaginal wall, or cervix. In a small percentage of cases, the primary infection is extragenital, usually in or around the mouth.

Untreated syphilis is a chronic disease with subacute, symptomatic periods separated by asymptomatic intervals, during which the diagnosis can be made serologically. The progression of untreated syphilis is generally divided into three main stages from the time of contact and initial infection: primary syphilis, secondary syphilis, and late (tertiary) syphilis. A latent period may develop between the secondary and tertiary stages.

Approximately one-third of untreated individuals with primary syphilis will progress to the second stage (secondary syphilis). This usually occurs at about 2 to 8 weeks after the appearance of the original painless sore (chancre), and in some patients the chancre may still be present.

Secondary syphilis is the most contagious stage of syphilis; the bacteria have spread in the bloodstream and reached their highest numbers. The most common symptom is skin rash, but additional symptoms can be fever, malaise, loss of appetite, and swollen lymph nodes. Although it usually resolves within weeks, in some patients the second stage may last up to a year.

The serum in about a third of patients with syphilis becomes serologically reactive after 1 week and serologically demonstrable in most patients after 3 weeks. The reagin titer increases rapidly during the first 4 weeks and then remains stationary for approximately 6 months. Within 2 to 8 weeks after the appearance of the primary chancre, a patient enters the stage of secondary syphilis. Serologic tests for syphilis are positive. The late (tertiary) stage is usually seen 3 to 10 years after primary infection. In about one-fourth of untreated patients, the tertiary stage is asymptomatic and recognized only by serologic testing.

Classic serologic tests for syphilis measure the presence of two types of antibodies: treponemal and nontreponemal. Treponemal antibodies are produced against the antigens of the organisms themselves. Nontreponemal antibodies, often called **reagin antibodies,** are produced by infected patients against components of their own or other mammalian bodies. Darkfield microscopy is the test of choice for symptomatic patients with primary syphilis. The widely used nontreponemal serologic test is the rapid plasma reagin (RPR) method. The RPR procedure and older Venereal Disease Research Laboratories (VDRL) test produces visible clumps when they are agglutinated by antibody. Specific treponemal serologic tests include the fluorescent treponemal antibody absorption (FTA-ABS) test and the microhemagglutination *Treponema pallidum* (MHA-TP) test. Another procedure, the *Treponema pallidum* immobilization (TPI) test, is obsolete.

Nontreponemal Antibody Tests

Nontreponemal antibodies (reagin antibodies) are produced by infected persons against components of their own or other mammalian bodies. Reagin antibodies are almost always produced by persons with syphilis, but they can also be produced in other infectious diseases, such as leprosy, tuberculosis, malaria, measles, chickenpox, IM, and hepatitis. The reagin antibodies can also be seen in noninfectious disorders such as autoimmune conditions and rheumatoid disease and in nondiseases such as pregnancy and old age. The RPR test is based on an agglutination or flocculation reaction in which soluble antigen particles are coalesced to form larger particles that are visible as clumps when aggregated by the antibody. This nontreponemal screening test can be confirmed by another testing method, usually the FTA-ABS or the MHA-TP test, tests for the presence of specific treponemal antibody.

Treponemal Antibody Tests

Treponemal antibodies are produced against the antigen of the *T. pallidum* organism itself. The FTA-ABS and MHA-TP tests are used to confirm that a positive nontreponemal test result has been caused by syphilis rather than one of the other biological conditions that can also produce a positive nontreponemal test result. In the FTA-ABS test the patient's serum is first absorbed with non–*T. pallidum* treponemal antigens to reduce any nonspecific cross-reactivity. Then a fluorescein-conjugated anti-human antibody reagent is applied as a marker for specific antitreponemal antibodies in the patient's serum. The test slide is examined with a fluorescence microscope and the intensity of fluorescence noted.

Rapid Plasma Reagin Card Test

In the RPR card test, the patient's serum is mixed with an antigen suspension of a carbon-particle cardiolipin antigen on the special disposable card provided with the test kit (see procedure at http://evolve.elsevier.com/Turgeon/clinicallab). If the suspension contains reagin, the antibody-like substance present in the serum of persons with syphilis, flocculation occurs with coagglutination of the carbon particles of antigen. This flocculation appears as black clumps against the white background of the plastic-coated RPR card. This reaction is observed and graded macroscopically. A diagnosis of syphilis cannot be made solely based on a positive RPR card test, without clinical signs and symptoms or supportive history. Positive reactions are occasionally seen with other infectious conditions or inflammatory states, thus necessitating confirmation of all positive results with the qualitative RPR test. Various manufacturers produce RPR kits, and the instructions included with the kits must be followed carefully. Positive and negative control sera should be tested daily to ensure the accuracy of the test antigen reagent.

CASE STUDIES

CASE STUDY 17-1

A 25-year-old woman comes to the clinic for pregnancy testing. She reports that her last menstrual period was 30 days ago. A random urine specimen is collected for testing. The result for this test is reported as negative. The physical examination indicates that the woman is pregnant.

1. What is a possible reason for the false-negative test result?
   a. The specific gravity was greater than 1.015.
   b. The lack of agglutination seen on the test slide was interpreted as a negative test result.
   c. The concentration of hCG present in the specimen is too low to be detected.
   d. The patient had ingested an excessive amount of aspirin.

2. If conception is estimated to have taken place about 2 weeks before her visit to the clinic, and if this is an average pregnancy, what would be the normal average serum hCG concentration at the time of this patient's visit?
   a. 25 mIU/mL
   b. 50 mIU/mL
   c. 500 mIU/mL
   d. 30,000 mIU/mL

3. If this patient was not pregnant, a reason for a false-positive result could be:
   a. a urine specific gravity of less than 1.015.
   b. treatment for infertility with an hCG injection.
   c. conducting the assay at 1 week of gestation.
   d. use of a random urine specimen.

CASE STUDY 17-2

A 45-year-old woman comes to a clinic with complaints of morning stiffness in her ankle joints, worse on rising in the morning and improving during the day. Her discomfort is responsive to aspirin. She has also been fatigued and weak. During the last week, she has noticed that her wrist and ankle joints on both sides of her body are also painful and swollen.

Blood is drawn to test for rheumatoid factor (RF) and antinuclear antibody (ANA). Synovial fluid is aspirated and analyzed. Results from analysis of the synovial fluid rule out crystal deposition diseases, such as gout and pseudogout, and no infectious microorganisms are seen. Results of immunologic blood tests for RF and ANA are:

RF: Positive

ANA: Negative

1. What are possible causes of a positive or false-positive RF assay?
   a. Serum specimen is lipemic, hemolyzed, or heavily contaminated with bacteria.
   b. Reaction time is longer than the specified 2 minutes.
   c. The patient has systemic lupus erythematosus.
   d. All of the above

2. RF is not found in:
   a. Osteoarthritis
   b. Gout
   c. Infectious joint disease
   d. Infectious mononucleosis

3. Based on the findings, the patient is likely to have which of the following?
   a. Degenerative arthritis
   b. Rheumatoid arthritis
   c. Systemic lupus erythematosus with joint involvement
   d. Joint disease from a gonococcal infection

CASE STUDY 17-3

A male college freshman is seen at the college health service complaining of general fatigue, a sore throat, and swollen lymph nodes in his neck. A throat culture is done, and blood is drawn for hematology studies and a rapid MonoSlide test.

Hematology results show a normal hemoglobin value and a slight increase in the white cell count, with many large, reactive lymphocytes seen in the differential. A rapid strep test is negative, but a second swab is cultured on sheep blood and incubated, with the result to be read in 18 hours. The result from the MonoSlide test is positive.

1. From these findings, what is the probable diagnosis for this patient?
   a. Systemic lupus erythematosus
   b. Infectious mononucleosis
   c. Strep throat; infection with group A β-hemolytic streptococci
   d. Viral infection

2. What result would you expect from the 18-hour incubated throat culture?
   a. Normal throat biota (flora); no β-hemolytic streptococci seen on sheep blood

   b. Only group A β-hemolytic *Streptococcus* seen on sheep blood
   c. Heavy growth of pathogenic *Staphylococcus* on sheep blood
   d. Normal throat biota (flora) and β-hemolytic *Streptococcus* seen on sheep blood

3. What can cause agglutination of horse erythrocytes used in the rapid test?
   a. Heterophil antibodies
   b. Forssman antibodies
   c. Particles in the serum being tested
   d. All of the above

BIBLIOGRAPHY

Baines W, Nobele P: Sensitivity limits of latex agglutination tests, Am Clin Lab 12(3):14, 1993.

Craft DW: Direct microbial antigen detection. In Mahon CR, Manuselis G, editors: Textbook of diagnostic microbiology, ed 2, Philadelphia, 2000, Saunders.

Forbes BA, Sahm DF, Weissfeld AS: Bailey and Scott's diagnostic microbiology, ed 12, St Louis, 2007, Mosby.

Turgeon ML: Fundamentals of immunohematology, ed 2, Baltimore, 1995, Williams & Wilkins.

Turgeon ML: Immunology and serology in laboratory medicine, ed 4, St Louis, 2009, Mosby.

REVIEW QUESTIONS

1. **Which immunoglobulin is typically found in external secretions such as saliva and tears?**
   a. IgA
   b. IgE
   c. IgG
   d. IgM

2. **Which of the following substances gain antigenicity only when coupled to a protein carrier?**
   a. Agglutinins
   b. Agglutinogens
   c. Haptens
   d. Opsonins

3. **Which of the following antibodies result from exposure to antigenic material from another species?**
   a. Heteroantibodies
   b. Alloantibodies
   c. Isoantibodies
   d. More than one of the above

4. **Which of the following is the visible result of an antigen-antibody reaction between a soluble antigen and its specific antibody?**
   a. Sensitization
   b. Precipitation
   c. Agglutination
   d. Complement fixation

5. Which of the following is true about immunoglobulins?
   a. Produced by T lymphocytes
   b. Produced by B lymphocytes
   c. Purified (cloned) from a single ancestral cell
   d. Derived from the thymus and influenced by thymic hormones

6. Which of the following is used to confirm a positive screening result in testing a patient for HIV antibody?
   a. ELISA
   b. Immunofluorescent assay
   c. Western blot
   d. Northern blot

7. Which of the following immunoglobulins can cross the placenta and therefore provides passive immunity to the infant for the first few months of life?
   a. IgA
   b. IgD
   c. IgG
   d. IgM

8. Which of the following immunoglobulins is found in the greatest amounts in the serum but is the smallest in size?
   a. IgA
   b. IgD
   c. IgG
   d. IgM

9. When the antigen-antibody complex occurs, agglutination takes place only if the antigen:
   a. is a particle such as a bacterium or blood cell.
   b. is soluble.
   c. both of the above.
   d. neither of the above.

10. The rheumatoid factor in rheumatoid arthritis cannot be associated with which immunoglobulin?
    a. IgA
    b. IgM
    c. IgG
    d. All of the above

11. The most specific assays for human chorionic gonadotropin (hCG) use antibody reagents against which subunit of hCG?
    a. Alpha
    b. Beta
    c. Gamma
    d. Chorionic

12. The concentration of hCG is generally at a particular level in serum about 2 to 3 days after implantation. This is the concentration at which most sensitive laboratory assays can give a positive serum hCG result. What is the lowest level of hormone for which most current serum hCG tests can give a positive result?
    a. 25 mIU/mL
    b. 50 mIU/mL
    c. 100 mIU/mL
    d. 100,000 mIU/mL

13. The heterophil antibody produced in infectious mononucleosis is of which immunoglobulin class?
    a. IgA
    b. IgD
    c. IgG
    d. IgM

14. Which of the following is *not* a characteristic of heterophil antibodies produced in infectious mononucleosis?
    a. Absorbed by guinea pig kidney cells
    b. *Not* absorbed by guinea pig kidney cells
    c. Absorbed by beef red cells
    d. React with horse, ox, and sheep red cells

15. Which of the following does *not* characterize T-lymphocyte function?
    a. Produce and secrete immunoglobulins
    b. Develop killer cells that produce cytokines
    c. Suppresse the immune response
    d. Develop helper cells

16. The primary requirement for a substance to be an antigen in a particular individual is that it must:
    a. have a large molecular weight.
    b. be composed of protein and polysaccharide.
    c. be different from "self."
    d. have several different combining sites.

17. Of the circulating lymphocytes in peripheral blood, which are in the greatest percentages (80%)?
    a. B lymphocytes
    b. T lymphocytes

18. In certain disease states, what is the process in which antibodies are made to self-antigens?
    a. Autoimmune disease
    b. Infection
    c. Inflammatory response
    d. Phagocytosis

CHAPTER 18

IMMUNOHEMATOLOGY AND TRANSFUSION MEDICINE

Learning Objectives

At the conclusion of this chapter, the student will be able to:

- Define the terms *immunohematology*, *blood banking*, and *transfusion medicine*.

- Describe donor selection and blood processing, including assays for bloodborne infectious diseases.

Continued

OVERVIEW OF BLOOD BANKING

The practice of transfusion medicine is regulated by several different agencies in the United States. These include the National Center for Drugs and Biologics of the U.S. Food and Drug Administration (FDA), the Centers for Medicare and Medicaid Services (CMS), the Occupational Safety and Health Administration (OSHA), and the state departments of health, which perform inspections to ensure regulatory compliance. The AABB is a professional association that provides the scientific leadership and mechanisms to deal with progress and change by providing the *AABB Technical Manual*. In addition, the AABB, College of American Pathologists (CAP) and the Joint Commission (TJC) each has written standards and conducts voluntary inspections by peers.

Therapeutic replacement of blood or its components is indicated in many cases when the potential benefit outweighs any potential harm to the patient. Potential harm includes the risk of transfusion-transmitted disease (e.g., viral hepatitis, human immunodeficiency virus [HIV] or acquired immunodeficiency syndrome [AIDS]) and possible a, significantly changing the practice of transfusion medicine. How blood is tested before transfusion, the way donors are selected, and the nature of the blood component or derivative used for transfusion are now vigilantly regulated for safety.

The field of immunohematology has advanced rapidly. In 1951, nine independent blood group systems were known. These historically important systems and the approximate dates of discovery are ABO (1900), MN (1927), P (1927), Rh (1939), Lutheran (1945), Kell (1946), Lewis (1946), Duffy (1950), and Kidd (1951). At present, more than 350 antigens have been identified and organized into 29 different blood group systems, more accurately referred to as *red blood cell* (RBC) *group systems*. The complexity of the RBC membrane and its antigenic polymorphism seems almost endless, and it is expected that as methodology for studying RBC antigen-antibody reactions improves, the boundaries of knowledge will continue to expand. A study of the immunologic reactions of blood (RBCs) is critical when therapeutic replacement of red blood cells is necessary. The many possible antigen-antibody reactions that can occur must be anticipated and tested for using the procedures available in the blood bank laboratory. Therapeutic administration of red blood cells may be indicated in various clinical situations. Acute or chronic loss of blood impairs the ability of the circulatory system to deliver adequate amounts of oxygen to the body cells and critically upsets the delicate homeostatic water and acid-base balance of body fluids. Red blood cell loss may be caused by hemorrhage, excessive destruction of RBCs, or the body's inability to replenish its own red blood cell supply. In specific cases, administration of blood or its components is indicated.

The procedures involved in collecting, storing, and processing blood and the distribution of RBCs and blood components are called **blood banking.** The academic knowledge and procedures involving the study of the immunologic responses to blood components are called **immunohematology.** The medical practice and techniques associated with replacement of RBCs and blood components is known as **transfusion medicine.**

Immunohematology and transfusion medicine are unlike other fields of clinical laboratory investigation. Although accuracy is critically important in the laboratory, it is absolutely essential in transfusion medicine. Even the smallest error can directly result in the death of a patient from a hemolytic transfusion reaction. As R.R. Race said, "RBC group tests are different from most other laboratory tests used in medicine in a vital way—the reported result must be correct, for the wisest physician cannot protect his patient from the consequences of a RBC grouping error."[1]

This chapter is a general introduction to the subject of blood banking and transfusion medicine. The best comprehensive reference is the *AABB Technical Manual.*[2]

BENEFITS AND REASONS FOR TRANSFUSION

There are many indications for the transfusion of RBCs and blood components. In general, these can be divided into four major categories, and the component to be transfused will depend on which category applies:

1. Transfusion may be used to restore or maintain oxygen-carrying capacity or hemoglobin. This is best done by the transfusion of RBCs with plasma removed. The transfusion of whole blood is both unnecessary and contraindicated, because the inclusion of plasma will increase blood volume with possible circulatory overload.
2. Transfusion can be used to restore or maintain blood volume. This is necessary in cases of acute blood loss, as seen with massive bleeding, to prevent shock. In actively bleeding patients who have lost more than 25% to 30% of their blood volume, RBCs and a volume expander (e.g., crystalloid [electrolyte] solutions such as 0.9% sodium chloride [isotonic saline]) or thawed plasma are used. Additional need for hemoglobin can be replaced later with packed RBCs, although in most patients, about 20% of blood volume can be replaced with crystalloid solutions alone.

3. Transfusion can replace coagulation factors to maintain hemostasis. This is done with a variety of blood components, which vary with the particular situation. Components include platelet concentrates and cryoprecipitate.
4. Transfusion may be indicated to restore or maintain leukocyte function. Although rare, this may be necessary for severely granulocytopenic patients with infections that do not respond to antibiotics.

BLOOD DONATION: DONORS, COLLECTION, STORAGE, AND PROCESSING

Donor Selection and Identification

The selection and proper identification of the potential blood donor are essential in ensuring that the blood collected for transfusion is safe and will be of benefit to the recipient. On March 2, 2009, the American Red Cross revised donor criteria. There may have been some changes to these criteria since the last revision date. The most up-to-date eligibility information can be obtained by contacting the American Red Cross or visiting www.arc.com or refer to the latest edition of the AABB Standards for Blood Banks and Transfusion Services (26th edition, 2009) or the latest edition of the Code of Federal Regulations 21CFR 640.3 (Suitability of Donor) (published every year).

The selection of the RBC donor involves a medical history and abbreviated physical examination. Two considerations must be kept in mind when selecting the donor: whether the procedure might be harmful to the donor and whether the donor's blood might be harmful to the recipient. The selection process involves a series of questions to ensure safety to both the donor and recipient. Medical guidelines and requirements for donor selection have been developed by the FDA, the AABB, and the American Red Cross (ARC). It is essential that guidelines and requirements be established for each transfusion service and be codified in its own standard operating procedures manual.

The general guidelines to donate blood for transfusion to another person are that you must:
- Be healthy
- Be at least 17 years old, or 16 years old if allowed by state law
- Weigh at least 110 pounds
- Not have donated whole blood in the last 8 weeks (56 days) or double red cells in the last 16 weeks (112 days)

"Healthy" means that you feel well and can perform normal activities. If you have a chronic

TABLE 18-1

Examples of Donor Acceptability	
Condition	Comments
Acupuncture	Acceptable
Piercing (ears, body), electrolysis	Acceptable so long as the instruments used were sterile or single-use equipment
Tattoo	Wait 12 months after a tattoo if the tattoo was applied in a state that does not regulate tattoo facilities. This requirement is related to concerns about hepatitis.
Allergy	Acceptable so long as donor feels well, has no fever, and has no problems breathing through the mouth
Antibiotics	Acceptable after finishing oral antibiotics for an infection (bacterial or viral). May have taken last pill on the date of donation. Antibiotic by injection for an infection acceptable 10 days after last injection. Acceptable if donor is taking antibiotics to prevent an infection (e.g., prior to dental procedures or for acne). Some conditions which require antibiotics to prevent an infection must still be evaluated at the time of donation by the responsible medical director.
Asthma	Acceptable so long as not having difficulty breathing at the time of donation and feeling well. Medications for asthma do not disqualify.
Birth control	Acceptable
Bleeding condition	Donors with clotting disorder from factor V who are not on anticoagulants are eligible to donate; all others must be evaluated by the health historian at the collection center.
Blood pressure	Acceptable so long as below 180 systolic and below 100 diastolic at the time of donation. Acceptable so long as donor feels well on arrival to donate
Cancer	Depends on type of cancer and treatment history
Chronic illnesses	Acceptable so long as donor feels well
Cold, flu	Not acceptable if donor does not feel well on the day of donation
Dental procedures and oral surgery	Acceptable after dental procedures, so long as there is no infection present. Wait until after finishing antibiotics for a dental infection. Wait for 3 days after having oral surgery.
Diabetes	Acceptable if well controlled on insulin or oral medications. NOTE: Donors with diabetes who since 1980 ever used bovine (beef) insulin made from cattle from the United Kingdom are ineligible to donate. This requirement is related to concerns about bovine spongiform encephalitis.
Hormone replacement therapy (HRT)	Women on hormone replacement therapy for menopausal symptoms and prevention of osteoporosis are eligible to donate.
Immunization, vaccination	Acceptable if vaccinated for influenza, tetanus, or meningitis, provided donor is symptom free and fever free. Includes the Tdap vaccine. Acceptable if donor received an HPV vaccine (example, Gardasil). Wait 4 weeks after immunizations for German measles (rubella), MMR (measles, mumps, and rubella), chicken pox, and shingles. Wait 2 weeks after immunizations for red measles (rubeola), mumps, polio (by mouth), and yellow fever vaccine. Wait 21 days after immunization for hepatitis B, so long as donor is not given the immunization for exposure to hepatitis B. Wait 8 weeks (56 days) from the date of having a smallpox vaccination with no complications.
Malaria	Wait 3 years after completing treatment for malaria. Wait 12 months after returning from a trip to an area where malaria is found. Wait 3 years after living in a country or countries where malaria is found.
Pregnancy, nursing	Persons who are pregnant are not eligible to donate. Wait 6 weeks after giving birth.

Modified from Miller YM: Blood eligibility guidelines, American Red Cross, March 2009. http://www.redcrossblood.org/donating-blood/eligibility-requirements/eligibility-criteria-topic#considerations_health.

condition such as diabetes or high blood pressure, "healthy" also means that you are being treated and the condition is under control. Specific questions are asked to comply with regulations (Table 18-1).

Other aspects of each potential donor's health history are discussed as part of the donation process before any blood is collected. Each donor receives a brief examination during which temperature, pulse, blood pressure, and blood count (hemoglobin or hematocrit) are measured.

Making donations for your own use during surgery (autologous blood donation) is considered a medical procedure that requires a written prescription; the rules for eligibility are less strict than for regular volunteer donations.

Complete, permanent, legible records must be kept of every sequence of the many steps involved in collection and administration of blood components. Manual or computerized record-keeping systems may be employed. Manual results and observations are always entered directly on the permanent record in ink and never recopied, because recopying will invariably result in error at some time. If changes are made to computerized results, they must be appropriately documented in the computer.

Collection of Red Blood Cells

Blood for transfusion must be collected and handled under strictly sterile conditions to prevent contamination. According to the AABB, blood is collected only by trained personnel working under the direction of a qualified licensed physician. The collection must be aseptic, must use a sterile closed collection system, and must use a single venipuncture. If more than one venipuncture is done, a new container and donor set must be used for each skin puncture. The AABB also requires that the phlebotomist sign or initial the donor record, whether or not a full unit is collected. The usual amount of blood drawn for 1 unit of whole blood is 450 mL. This is added to 63 mL of citrate phosphate dextrose (CPD, CP2D) or CPD adenine (CPDA-1) anticoagulant solution, which brings the total volume of a unit of blood to about 500 mL. When the proper amount has been collected, extra tubes and segments must be filled with up to 30 mL of blood for the various testing procedures required before the blood can be used.

Anticoagulants and Preservatives

Infused blood, or blood that is administered by transfusion, must be anticoagulated. Blood must be collected into an FDA-approved container. The RBCs must be pyrogen free, sterile, and contain anticoagulant sufficient for the amount of blood to be collected. The anticoagulant and preservative solution is generally a combination of citrate and dextrose. Citrate is used as an anticoagulant, which binds calcium, thus preventing activation of the coagulation cascade. Dextrose is used to provide an energy source for the RBCs. Inorganic phosphate buffer is added to increase adenosine triphosphate (ATP) production, which increases RBC viability. CPD and CP2D are approved by the FDA for 21-day storage of red cells at 1°C to 6°C. CPDA-1 is approved for storage of RBCs for up to 35 days at 1°C to 6°C. In addition, three saline-adenine-glucose (SAG) solutions are now approved for use with the primary bag anticoagu-

lants: AS-1 (SAG plus mannitol, SAGM) coupled with CPD, AS-3 (SAG plus sodium phosphate, sodium citrate, and citric acid) coupled with CP2D, and AS-5 (ADSOL). These additives increase the 21-day storage of the primary anticoagulant to 42 days.

Labeling

Conversion to the International Society of Blood Transfusion (ISBT) "128" blood labeling has begun in the United States. ISBT 128 is an international information standard for blood, tissue, and cellular therapy products. In the U.S. this working group is the Americas Technical Advisory Group (ATAG) of ICCBBA. The document, The United States Industry Consensus Standard for the Uniform Labeling of Blood and Blood Components[6] using ISBT 128, provides specific instructions for the U.S. where there is flexibility in the ISBT 128 Standard Technical Specification.

Specific information about product coding may be found in a document called Product Code Structure and Labeling–Blood Components. Specific information about the terminology used in product coding is found in a document called Standard Terminology for Blood, Cellular Therapy, and Tissue Product Descriptions. Version 3.0.0 of this document is considerably reorganized and expanded from Version 2.0.0. Many more examples of labels and text are included to help U.S. users standardize labels while meeting the requirements of the FDA, AABB, and the ISBT 128 Standard. Documents important to ISBT 128, will be subject to a continual revision process.

At this time, both ISBT128 and Codabar blood product labeling formats are in use in the United States.

Proper labeling of the collecting container is essential. According to the AABB, each unit of blood or blood component must include at least the following information:

- Name of the product (i.e., whole blood, RBCs)
- Type and amount of anticoagulant
- Volume of the unit
- Required storage temperature
- Name address of the collecting facility including FDA registration or license number
- Expiration date
- Unique donor identification number
- Whether donor a volunteer, autologous, or paid
- Statements: (1) Properly Identify Intended Recipient; (2) Rx Only; (3) See *Circular of Information* for indications, contraindications, cautions, and methods of infusion.

The ABO blood group and Rh type are also shown on the label, once these tests are completed.

The pilot tubes and segments for testing must also be properly labeled. A stoppered or sealed sample of donor RBCs must be retained and properly stored by the transfusion service for at least 7 days after transfusion.

Storage of Blood

Preserved RBCs must be stored in a refrigerator with a constant temperature of 1°C to 6°C. Some type of alarm must be available that will go off whenever the temperature is not within these limits. A thermometer for recording the temperature must be installed. Packed RBCs stored in AS-1, AS-3, or AS-5 can be stored for 42 days. Once the unit has passed this date, the blood is outdated and must be removed from the blood supply.

Stored packed blood is inspected daily for color, turbidity, appearance of clots, and presence of hemolysis. RBC units are removed when they do not meet the appearance criteria established by the transfusion service.

Blood-Processing Tests

The FDA (www.fda.gov) is responsible for ensuring the safety of the nation's blood supply. A blood supply with zero risk of transmitting infectious disease may not be possible, but there are several measures taken by FDA to protect and enhance the safety of blood products. Because of the improvements in donor screening procedures and the use of a variety of new tests in the last few years, the blood supply is safer from infectious diseases than it has been at any other time.

The blood safety system established by FDA is dependent upon:

1. Accurate and complete educational material for donors so they can assess their risk
2. Sensitive communication of the donor-screening questions
3. Donor understanding and honesty
4. Quality-controlled infectious marker testing procedures
5. Appropriate handling and distribution of blood and blood products for patient use

The most important consideration in ensuring that blood is free of transmissible diseases is the careful screening of a blood donor (for the latest regulations see FDA-approved and AABB Donor History Questionnaires at www.fda.gov and aabb.org). The virtual elimination of paid blood donation in the United States has significantly decreased the risk of hepatitis. This, together with procedures to allow for self-deferral

of donors who have risk factors for HIV, the causative agent of AIDS, has done much to ensure the safety of the blood supply. In addition, the following high-risk groups are usually not eligible to donate blood:

- Anyone who has ever used injection drugs not prescribed by a physician
- Men who have had sexual contact with other men since 1977
- Anyone who has ever received clotting factor concentrates such as hemophilia factor
- Anyone with a positive test for HIV/AIDS
- Men and women who have engaged in sex for money or drugs since 1977
- Anyone who has had hepatitis since his or her 11th birthday
- Anyone who has had babesiosis or Chagas disease
- Anyone who has taken etretinate (Tegison) for psoriasis
- Anyone who has risk factors for Creutzfeldt-Jakob disease (CJD) or who has a blood relative with CJD
- Anyone who has risk factors for variant Creutzfeldt-Jakob disease (vCJD)
- Anyone who spent 3 months or more in the United Kingdom from 1980 through 1996
- Anyone who has spent 5 years in Europe from 1980 to the present

Routine Blood Screening Tests

Blood is routinely screened for transmissible disease. The number of routine screening tests has increased dramatically in the past few years (Table 18-2). In addition, donors of viable, leukocyte-rich concentrates must be tested for Cytomegalovirus with an FDA-cleared screening test for anti-CMV (total IgG and IgM).

TESTS FOR SYPHILIS

A serologic test for syphilis continues to be required, although it has been questioned for years. It is now used as a surrogate marker for detecting donors who might be high risk for transmitting transfusion-related disease.

TESTS FOR HEPATITIS

Transmission of hepatitis remains a risk in transfusion. From 80% to 90% of posttransfusion hepatitis is caused by hepatitis C virus (HCV). Hepatitis B virus (HBV) is responsible for about 10%, and a small percentage is caused by cytomegalovirus (CMV), and Epstein-Barr virus (EBV). For this reason, donated blood is screened with several tests for hepatitis virus. At present, these include a test for hepatitis B surface antigen (HBsAg) and

Text continued on p. 554.

TABLE 18-2

Complete List of Donor Screening Assays for Infectious Agents and HIV Diagnostic Assays

Format	Sample	Use	Manufacturer	Approval Date
Antibody to Hepatitis B Surface				
EIA	Serum/plasma/ cadaveric serum	Donor screen & conf kit	Abbott Laboratories Abbott Park, IL U.S. License 0043	4/1/1985
EIA	Serum/plasma/ cadaveric serum	Donor screen & conf kit	Bio-Rad Laboratories Redmond, WA U.S. License 1109	1/23/2003
EIA	Serum/plasma	Donor screen/diagnosis & conf kit	Ortho-Clinical Diagnostics, Inc Raritan, NJ U.S. License 1236	4/23/2003
Chemiluminescent Immunoassay (ChLIA)	Serum/plasma	Donor screening test to detect HBsAg. Also for use in testing blood and plasma to screen organ donors when specimens are obtained while the donor's heart is still beating, and intesting blood specimens to screen cadaveric (non-heart-beating) donors.	Abbott Laboratories Abbott Park, IL U.S. License 0043	7/18/2006
Anti-HIV-1 Oral Specimen Collection Device				
Oral specimen collection device	Oral fluid	For use with HIV diagnostic assays that have been approved for use with this device.	OraSure Technologies Bethlehem, PA	12/23/1994
Anti-HIV-1 Testing Service				
Dried blood spot collection device	Dried blood spot	Diagnostic	Home Access Health Corp Hoffman Estates, IL	7/22/1996
Hepatitis B Surface Antigen (Anti-HBs Assay)				
EIA	Serum/plasma	Anti-HBs	Abbott Laboratories Abbott Park, IL U.S. License 0043	11/18/1982
Hepatitis B Virus Core Antigen (Anti-HBc Assay)				
EIA	Serum/plasma	Donor screen	Abbott Laboratories Abbott Park, IL U.S. License 0043	3/19/1991
EIA	Serum/plasma	Donor screen	Ortho-Clinical Diagnostics, Inc Raritan, NJ U.S. License 1236	4/18/1991
Chemiluminescent Immunoassay (ChLIA)	Serum/plasma	Donor screen	Abbott Laboratories Abbott Park, IL U.S. License 0043	10/13/2005

Continued

TABLE 18-2

Complete List of Donor Screening Assays for Infectious Agents and HIV Diagnostic Assays—cont'd				
Format	Sample	Use	Manufacturer	Approval Date
Hepatitis C Virus Encoded Antigen (Anti-HCV Assay)				
EIA	Serum/plasma/ cadaveric serum	Donor screen	Abbott Laboratories Abbott Park, IL U.S. License 0043	5/6/1992
EIA	Serum/plasma	Donor screen	Ortho-Clinical Diagnostics, Inc Raritan, NJ U.S. License 1236	5/20/1996
SIA	Serum/plasma	Donor supplemental	Chiron Corp Emeryville, CA U.S. License 1106	2/11/1999
Chemiluminescent Immunoassay (ChLIA)	Serum/plasma	Donor screening test for the qualitative detection of antibodies to hepatitis C virus (anti-HCV) in human serum and plasma specimens. Also intended for use in testing blood and plasma to screen organ donors when specimens are obtained while the donor's heart is still beating, and in testing blood specimens to screen cadaveric (non-heart-beating) donors.	Abbott Laboratories Abbott Park, IL U.S. License 0043	7/11/2007
Nucleic Acid Testing				
PCR	Plasma	Prognosis/patient management HIV-1 viral load Assay	Roche Molecular Systems, Inc Pleasanton, CA	3/2/1999
NASBA	Plasma	Prognosis/patient management HIV-1 viral load assay	bioMerieux, Inc Durham, NC	11/19/2001
PCR	Plasma	Donor screen expanded indications for use: source plasma donors, other living donors, and organ donors	Roche Molecular Systems, Inc Pleasanton, CA U.S. License 1636	12/20/2002
HIV-1/HCV nucleic acid test (TMA)	Plasma	Donor screen expanded indications for use: source plasma donors, living organ donors and cadaveric samples	Gen-Probe San Diego, CA U.S. License 1592	6/4/2004
HIV-1 genotyping	Plasma	Patient monitoring	Siemens Medical Solutions Diagnostics Berkeley, CA	4/24/2002
PCR	Plasma	Donor screen	National Genetics Institute Los Angeles, CA 92121	9/18/2001
HIV-1 genotyping	Plasma	Patient monitoring	Celera Diagnostics Alameda, CA	6/11/2003

TABLE 18-2

Complete List of Donor Screening Assays for Infectious Agents and HIV Diagnostic Assays—cont'd				
Format	Sample	Use	Manufacturer	Approval Date
Signal amplification nucleic acid probe	Plasma	Patient monitoring	Siemens Medical Solutions Diagnostics Berkeley, CA	9/11/2002
PCR	Plasma	Donor screen expanded indications for use: source plasma donors, other living donors, and organ donors	Roche Molecular Systems, Inc Pleasanton, CA U.S. License 1636	12/3/2002
PCR	Plasma	Donor screen indications for use: source plasma donors, other living donors, and organ donors	Roche Molecular Systems, Inc Pleasanton, CA U.S. License 1636	4/21/2005
Nucleic acid test (TMA)	Plasma	Qualitative detection of West Nile virus (WNV) RNA from volunteer donors of whole blood and blood components, screen organ donors when obtained while donor's heart is still beating, and test blood specimens to screen cadaveric donors	Gen-Probe San Diego, CA U.S. License 1592	12/1/2005
HIV-1 and HCV/ nucleic acid pooled testing/ synthetic	Plasma	For use as an aid in diagnosis of HIV-1 infection, including acute or primary infection	Gen-Probe, Inc U.S. License 1592	10/4/2006
Nucleic acid test (TMA)	Plasma and serum	Qualitative detection of human immunodeficiency virus type 1 (HIV-1) RNA and hepatitis C virus (HCV) RNA from volunteer donors of whole blood and blood components, screen organ donors when obtained while donor's heart is still beating, and test blood specimens to screen cadaveric donors. 8/12/2008 Additional indication: revision of intended use to include an HBV screening claim for individual samples and pooled samples of up to 16 individual donations. An intended use to include testing of pools of up to 16 donations from donors of Hematopoietic Progenitor Cells (HPCs) or Donor Lymphocytes for Infusion (DLI).	Gen-Probe San Diego, CA U.S. License 1592	10/3/2006
PCR	Plasma	Qualitative detection of HCV ribonucleic acid (RNA) in pools of human source plasma comprised of equal aliquots of not more than 512 individual plasma samples.	BioLife Plasma Services, L.P. Deerfield, IL U.S. License 1640	2/9/2007
PCR	Plasma	Qualitative detection of HIV-1 ribonucleic acid (RNA) in pools of human source plasma comprised of equal aliquots of not more than 512 individual plasma samples.	BioLife Plasma Services, L.P. Deerfield, IL U.S. License 1640	1/31/2007

Continued

TABLE 18-2

		Complete List of Donor Screening Assays for Infectious Agents and HIV Diagnostic Assays—cont'd		
Format	Sample	Use	Manufacturer	Approval Date
PCR	Plasma	Quantitation of human immuno-deficiency virus type 1 (HIV-1) on the automated m2000 System. Not intended to be used as a donor screening test.	ABBOTT Molecular, Inc Des Plaines, IL	5/11/2007
PCR	Plasma	Quantitation of human immunodeficiency virus type 1 (HIV-1) nucleic acid. Not intended to be used as a donor screening test.	Roche Molecular Systems, Inc Pleasanton, CA	5/11/2007
PCR	Plasma	For the qualitative detection of West Nile virus (WNV) RNA in plasma specimens from individual human donors, donors of whole blood and blood components, and other living donors. Also intended for use in testing plasma specimens to screen organ donors when specimens are obtained while the donor's heart is still beating.	Roche Molecular Systems, Inc Pleasanton, CA U.S. License 1636	8/28/2007
Human Immunodeficiency Virus Type 1 (Anti-HIV-1 Assay)				
EIA	Serum/plasma	Donor screen	Bio-Rad Laboratories Redmond, WA U.S. License 1109	6/29/1998
WB	Serum/plasma	Donor supplemental	Calypte Biomedical Corp Berkeley, CA U.S. License 1207	1/3/1991
WB	Serum/plasma	Donor supplemental	Bio-Rad Laboratories Redmond, WA U.S. License 1109	11/13/1998
IFA	Serum/plasma	Donor supplemental	Waldheim Pharmazeutika GmbH Vienna, Austria U.S. License 1150	2/5/1992
EIA	Dried blood spot	Diagnostic	Abbott Laboratories	4/22/1992
EIA	Urine screen	Diagnostic	Calypte Biomedical Corp	8/6/1996
EIA	Dried blood spot	Diagnostic	Bio-Rad Laboratories Redmond, WA	6/29/1998
WB	Urine	Diagnostic supplemental	Maxim Biomedical, Inc	5/28/1998
WB	Dried blood spot	Diagnostic supplemental	Bio-Rad Laboratories Redmond, WA	11/13/1998
WB	Oral fluid	Diagnostic supplemental	OraSure Technologies Bethlehem, PA	6/3/1996

TABLE 18-2

Complete List of Donor Screening Assays for Infectious Agents and HIV Diagnostic Assays—cont'd				
Format	Sample	Use	Manufacturer	Approval Date
IFA	Dried blood spot	Diagnostic supplemental	Waldheim Pharmazeutika GmbH	5/14/1996
Rapid immunoassay	Serum/plasma	Diagnostic	MedMira Laboratories, Inc Halifax, Nova Scotia, Canada B3S 1B3	4/16/2003
Rapid immunoassay	Serum/plasma/ Whole Blood (venipuncture and fingerstick)	Diagnostic	Trinity Biotech, plc Bray Co., Wicklow, Ireland	12/23/2003
Human Immunodeficiency Virus Types 1 & 2 (Anti-HIV-1/2 Assay)				
EIA	Serum/plasma/ cadaveric Serum	Donor screen	Abbott Laboratories Abbott Park, IL U.S. License 0043	2/14/1992
EIA	Serum/plasma/ cadaveric serum	Donor screen	Bio-Rad Laboratories Redmond, WA U.S. License 1109	8/5/2003
Rapid immunoassay	Plasma/serum	Diagnostic	Bio-Rad Laboratories Redmond, WA	11/12/2004
Rapid immunoassay	Whole blood, plasma, oral fluid	Diagnostic	OraSure Technologies Bethlehem, PA	6/22/2004
Chemiluminescent Immunoassay (ChLIA)	Serum/plasma/ cadaveric serum	To be used to screen individual human donors, including volunteer donors of whole blood and blood components and other living donors, for the presence of anti-HIV-1 Groups M and O and/or anti-HIV-2. The assay is also intended for use in testing blood and plasma specimens to screen organ donors when specimens are obtained while the donor's heart is still beating, in testing blood specimens to screen cadaveric (non–heart-beating) donors.	Abbott Laboratories	9/18/2009
Microparticle Chemiluminometric Immunoassay	Plasma/serum	Diagnostic for qualitative determination of antibodies to the human immunodeficiency virus type 1, including Group O, and/or type 2 in serum or plasma	Siemens Medical Solutions Diagnostics Tarrytown, NY	5/18/2006
Rapid immunoassay	Fingerstick & venous whole blood, serum, plasma	Diagnostic	Chembio Diagnostic Systems, Inc Medford, NY	5/25/2006
Human Immunodeficiency Virus Type 2 (Anti-HIV-2 Assay)				
EIA	Serum/plasma	Donor screen	Bio-Rad Laboratories Redmond, WA U.S. License 1109	4/25/1990

Continued

TABLE 18-2

Complete List of Donor Screening Assays for Infectious Agents and HIV Diagnostic Assays—cont'd				
Format	Sample	Use	Manufacturer	Approval Date
Human T-Lymphotropic Virus Types I & II (Anti-HTLV-I/II Assay)				
EIA	Serum/plasma	Donor screen	Abbott Laboratories Abbott Park, IL U.S. License 0043	8/15/1997
Chemiluminescent Immunoassay (ChLIA)	Serum/plasma	To be used as a screening test for individual human donors, including volunteer donors of whole blood and blood components, and other living donors for the presence of anti-HTLV-I/HTLV-II. It is also intended for use in testing blood and plasma to screen organ donors when specimens are obtained while the donor's heart is still beating.	Abbott Laboratories Abbott Park, IL U.S. License 0043	1/16/2008
Trypanosoma cruzi (T. cruzi) (Anti- T. cruzi Assay)				
EIA	Serum/plasma	Donor screening test to detect antibodies to T. cruzi in plasma and serum samples from individual human donors. Also intended for use to screen organ and tissue donors when specimens are obtained while the donor's heart is still beating.	Ortho-Clinical Diagnostics, Inc Raritan, NJ U.S. License 1236	12/13/2006

From www.FDA.gov, updated April 10, 2010.
ChLIA, Chemiluminescent immunoassay; *EIA*, enzyme immunoassay; *PCR*, polymerase chain reaction; *TMA*, transcription-mediated amplification; *WB*, western blot.

antibody tests for HCV and hepatitis B core antibody (HBc).

TESTS FOR HIV/AIDS

Because of the long incubation period of HIV, donor selection methods and self-deferral of donors are essential in the screening of blood for HIV. All donated blood is tested for HIV.

TESTS FOR HTLV

Units of blood must also be tested for human T-cell lymphotropic virus types I and II (HTLV-I/II) antibody. A combination test is used.

WEST NILE VIRUS

Qualitative detection of West Nile Virus (WNV) RNA from volunteer blood donors is required. In addition, living organ donors and cadaveric donors must be screened.

TRYPANOSOMA CRUZI

Donor screening test to detect antibodies to *Trypanosoma cruzi*, T. cruzi, in plasma and serum samples from individual human donors. Also intended for use to screen organ and tissue donors when specimens are obtained while the donor's heart is still beating.

OTHER TYPES OF BLOOD DONATIONS

Autologous Transfusions

The safest blood a recipient can receive is his or her own blood. Not only does this prevent transfusion-transmitted infectious diseases, but it also eliminates the formation of antibodies to antigens in transfused RBCs from others and the possibility of graft-versus-host disease. Blood donation also stimulates erythropoiesis by repeated preoperative phlebotomy.

Patients who meet certain criteria are encouraged to donate blood for themselves before anticipated surgery if they are likely to need a transfusion. There is a significant problem with outdating of blood donated for autologous purposes because it is frequently not used. Intraoperative autologous transfusion or cell salvage techniques are alternatives to autologous donation.

Directed Transfusions

In directed transfusions, the patient directly solicits blood for transfusion from family or friends. Directed transfusion is the public's response to concern about AIDS, but it is based on a false assumption that blood donated by family or friends is safer than that from the regular volunteer donor population. This has not been found to be true, because the directed donor is under significantly more pressure to donate than an anonymous donor. It is also thought that the extra paperwork and other logistics increase the probability of clerical errors.

WHOLE BLOOD, BLOOD COMPONENTS, AND DERIVATIVES FOR TRANSFUSION

Whole Blood

Whole human blood consists of:
- **Formed elements**—red blood cells (RBCs), white blood cells (WBCs), and platelets—which make up about 45% of the total blood volume
- **Plasma,** which makes up about 55% of the total volume

The blood volume of normal adults is approximately 5 to 6 L. In transfusion medicine, reference is often made to a "unit" of blood. For practical purposes, a unit may be considered about 450 to 500 mL of whole blood or a smaller volume of RBCs. Whole blood is rarely transfused and has been replaced with an equivalent dose of RBCs and other volume expander solution if needed.

Whole blood is rarely used when transfusion is indicated. Rather, a variety of preparations including RBCs, plasma, albumin, platelet concentrates, leukocytes, and other preparations and derivatives are used (Table 18-3). Products prepared from whole blood by mechanical methods, especially by centrifugation, are called **components.** Products separated by more complex automated processes are called **blood derivatives** or **fractions.**

In cases of severe hemorrhage, whole blood may be used to replace RBCs and plasma. Whole blood is rarely available or used for transfusion. It is generally separated into various components and derivatives to ensure economic use of a valuable resource and for clinical appropriateness.

Packed Red Blood Cells

Blood component preparation begins with the separation of plasma from whole blood, leaving the RBCs. Red cells for transfusion can be prepared by sedimentation or centrifugation. The technique used must maintain the sterility of both the plasma and the RBCs. If the container is not entered when the red cells are prepared, the expiration date for the cells remains the same as for the original whole blood. If the container is entered, the RBCs are

TABLE 18-3

Blood Components and Derivatives	
Blood Component or Derivative	Use
Red blood cells (RBCs)	To increase RBC mass (e.g., therapy for anemia); use with colloids or crystalloids in active bleeding or massive transfusion
Solution added	Similar to RBCs or whole blood
Leukocytes removed*	To increase RBC mass and avoid febrile and allergic reactions from leukocytes or plasma proteins; to prevent anaphylactic reactions
Deglycerolized	To extend storage of RBCs with rare blood types and autologous transfusion; to prevent HLA sensitization
Platelets†	Functional or quantitative platelet defects
Granulocytes, apheresis	Rare; for septic, severely granulocytopenic patients who do not respond to antibiotic therapy after 48 hours
Fresh frozen plasma	In bleeding patients with multiple coagulation defects; also for treatment of factor V or VI deficiency
Cryoprecipitate	Treatment of von Willebrand disease, factor XIII deficiency, or hypofibrinogenemia
Factor VIII concentrate	For hemophilia A (factor VIII deficiency)
Factor IX concentrate	For hereditary deficiency of factors II, VII, IX (hemophilia B), or X
Albumin/plasma protein fraction (plasma substitutes)	For volume expansion and colloidal replacement without risk of hepatitis or AIDS
Immune serum globulin	For treatment or prophylaxis of hypogammaglobulinemia; to prevent or modify hepatitis A and non-A, non-B hepatitis
Rh immune globulin	To prevent hemolytic disease of the fetus and newborn in Rh-negative women exposed to Rh-positive RBCs

*By centrifugation, washing, or filtration.
†Platelet concentrates, platelet-rich plasma, random or single donor by apheresis.

considered usable for only 24 hours. Packed RBCs are effectively used when oxygen-carrying capacity is diminished or lost, such as in treating certain anemic conditions.

Packed RBCs have essentially replaced whole blood in transfusion except in the case of massive bleeding, when more than 25% to 30% of circulating blood volume is lost. In most cases, even in massive bleeding, RBCs together with isotonic saline or plasma substitutes are preferred.

Red cells may be further treated by removing leukocytes by centrifugation, washing, or filtration. RBCs may also be treated with additive solutions consisting of saline, adenine, glucose, or mannitol. In this case, maximum amounts of plasma are removed shortly after phlebotomy, and additive solutions are used to maintain RBC function. This process extends the shelf life of RBCs to 42 days. Rejuvenation solutions have also been licensed to extend the life of stored RBCs for immediate use, or the blood can be frozen for transfusion later. This is especially useful for rejuvenating outdated units of autologous donor blood.

Plasma

When the RBCs are removed from whole blood, plasma remains. It is the liquid portion of whole blood that has been anticoagulated. Slightly more than half the volume of whole blood is plasma. Plasma should not be used to replace lost blood volume or protein, because much safer products exist, including plasma substitutes (e.g., albumin), synthetic colloids, and balanced salt solutions. These solutions have the advantage of not transmitting disease or causing allergic reactions. Plasma is appropriately used to replace coagulation factors.

FRESH FROZEN PLASMA

When plasma is used, it is often in the form of fresh frozen plasma. Fresh frozen plasma is a good source of labile clotting factors and can be used to replace those coagulation factors. It is especially useful in treating multiple coagulation deficiencies, as seen with liver failure, disseminated intravascular coagulation (DIC), vitamin K deficiency, warfarin toxicity, or massive transfusions.

FACTOR VIII

Plasma is no longer used for the preparation of factor VIII. This blood component is now produced utilizing monoclonal antibody technology. The use of monoclonal antibodies reduces the risk of transmission of infectious diseases.

Plasma Substitutes

Plasma substitutes include albumin and plasma protein fraction which are prepared by the chemical fractionation of pooled plasma. These products are heat treated to eliminate the risk of infectious diseases. They are used to treat patients who need replacement of blood volume. Alternatively, crystalloid (either saline or electrolyte) solutions are used.

Platelets

Many U.S. laboratories use an automated apheresis process to harvest platelets. Platelet concentrates can also be prepared from random-donor whole-blood units by differential centrifugation shortly after donation. These concentrates are used for patients who are bleeding as a result of low platelet counts or, occasionally, abnormally functioning platelets.

Massive transfusions may also result in thrombocytopenia and require platelet concentrates. Occasionally, patients develop human leukocyte antigen (HLA) antibodies that make transfused platelet concentrates ineffective. Crossmatched platelets are a resource for patients who are refractory to platelet transfusions. In such cases, it may be necessary to select HLA-matched donors and prepare platelets by apheresis.

Bacterial contamination is a problem encountered with the platelet blood component.

ANTIGENS AND ANTIBODIES IN IMMUNOHEMATOLOGY

Transfusion medicine is based on a knowledge of antigens and antibodies. An **antigen** is defined as a foreign substance or a nonself antigen. If a foreign antigen is introduced into an immunocompetent individual, a protein called an **antibody** can be produced. The significance of antigens and antibodies is not limited to transfusion medicine (see Chapter 17).

Red Blood Cell Groups

Each species of animal, humans included, has certain antigens unique to that species and usually present on the red cell membranes of members of that species. Some blood group antigens are found not only on RBCs but also in other body fluids (e.g., saliva, plasma).

If the RBCs of sheep, for example, are transfused into a human, an antisheep substance (antibody) will be produced in the plasma (by the B lymphocytes) of the human. The antisheep substance will destroy any sheep red cells that are subsequently introduced. This cellular destruction is what is meant by an "incompatible hemolytic transfusion reaction," and it can result in the death of the recipient.

It is also known that certain antigens are more common. If RBCs containing a foreign antigen are transfused into a recipient whose red cells do not contain that antigen, the recipient can form an antibody. Antibodies from different members of the same species are referred to as **alloantibodies.**

Antigens that exist on a person's red cells within a particular blood group system represent that person's type for that system, such as the ABO system. The number of possible types within one system varies. The more complex Rh-Hr system has more than 100 possible types. Taking all systems and type combinations into account, more than 500 billion different types of RBCs are possible.

Although no two individuals are exactly alike, except identical twins, only certain antigens are likely to create transfusion problems (i.e., incompatible Adverse Effects of Transfusion). There is always the possibility that an unknown or untested-for antigen may create a potential problem. The antigens most likely to cause reactions are in the ABO and Rh-Hr systems and must be tested for whenever blood is administered. In certain circumstances (e.g., presence of alloantibody in a patient, specific antigens screened or in donor RBCs), patients who receive an antigen not present on their red cells may produce an alloantibody in their plasma. These alloantibodies can react with the corresponding foreign antigen in subsequent transfusions. The presence of an alloantibody and its corresponding antigen can be demonstrated by agglutination in vitro or destruction of the red cell containing the foreign antigen in vivo. These two terms—in vivo (in the living body) and in vitro (in a laboratory setting)—are often used in discussing biological reactions.

Inheritance of Red Blood Cell Groups

Genes

The antigens present on a individual's red cell, white blood cell and platelet membranes are inherited. Each antigen is controlled by a gene, which is the unit of inheritance. If the gene for a particular antigen is present, that antigen would be expected to be expressed.

Red blood cell antigens and HLAs conform with Mendelian laws of inheritance and are easily identifiable. Although molecular DNA methods are replacing antigen-antibody testing, knowledge of inheritance related to antigen inheritance is important. Genetic markers such as antigens can be used in paternity testing and exclude a man who is not the father. In direct exclusion, a child who possesses a genetic marker not possessed by either the mother or the alleged father allows for exclusion of the alleged father, as seen in this table:

	Mother	Alleged Father	Child
Phenotype	Group O	Group B	Group A
Genotype	O/O	B/B or B/O	A/O

Conclusion: The alleged father is not the father of this child.

Chromosomes

Each cell, except for mature RBCs, consists of cytoplasm and a nucleus. If the nucleus is observed under the microscope at approximately the time of cell division, several long, threadlike structures will be visible. These structures are referred to as **chromosomes.** Each species has a specific number of chromosomes, and the chromosomes occur in pairs. Humans have 46 chromosomes (23 chromosome pairs). The paired chromosomes are similar in size and shape and have their own distinct functions. A complete set of 23 chromosomes is inherited from each parent. Chromosomes occur in pairs in somatic (body) cells but not in sex cells (sperm and ovum), which contain 23 single chromosomes.

Gene Location (Linkage)

Because the gene is the unit of inheritance, it must also be located within the nucleus. Genes are exceedingly small particles that, when associated in linear form, make up the chromosome. They are too small to see under the normal brightfield microscope but together are visible as the chromosome. Genes are made up of deoxyribonucleic acid (DNA). Each trait that is inherited is controlled by the presence of a specific gene. The genes responsible for a particular trait always occur at exactly the same point or position on a particular chromosome; this position is referred to as the *locus* of the gene.

Research in the field of genetics is continually revealing new information about the location or sequence of genes on the chromosome and about diseases that are genetically inherited or environmentally induced. If genes for different inherited traits are known to be carried on the same chromosome, they are said to be *syntenic*. This term is useful in referring to genes on a single chromosome that are too far apart to display absolute linkage in inheritance. Genes that are located on the same chromosome and are normally inherited together are known as **linked genes.** The closer the loci of the genes, the closer is the **linkage.**

Alleles

Inherited traits are somewhat variable within a species. For example, eye color varies, and it is known to be inherited. Therefore, each possible eye color must be the result of a gene for that color. Variants of a gene for a particular trait are referred to as **alleles** for that trait. Because we have only two genes (one pair) for any given trait, our cells will have only two alleles. However, the number of possible alleles for a trait varies. A person who has identical alleles for a trait is said to be **homozygous** for that trait. For example, a person with blue eyes carries two blue-eye genes and is homozygous for blue eyes.

A person who has two different alleles for a trait is **heterozygous** for that trait—for example, having a blue-eye gene in addition to a brown-eye gene.

Certain alleles may be stronger than or mask the presence of other alleles. In the case of eye color, brown-eye genes mask the presence of blue-eye genes and are said to be dominant over blue-eye genes. Individuals who have one brown-eye gene and one blue-eye gene have eyes that appear brown. Blue-eye genes are then said to be recessive in relation to brown-eye genes. One must have two blue-eye genes to have blue eyes. In transfusion medicine, the various alleles for a particular blood group system are equally dominant, or codominant. If the gene is present (and there is a suitable testing solution available), it will be detected.

Phenotypes and Genotypes

Two other genetic terms often used in transfusion medicine are *phenotype* and *genotype*. The **phenotype** is what is seen by tests made directly on the RBCs, even though other antigens may be present. The **genotype** refers to the actual total genetic makeup of an individual. It is usually impossible to determine the complete genotype in the laboratory; this usually requires additional studies, especially family studies.

Isoantibodies and Immune Antibodies

Antibody classification in immunohematology includes environmentally acquired and immune antibodies. The **isoantibodies** result from internal (e.g., bacterial) or external antigenic stimulus. Substances very similar to RBC group antigens A and B are so widely distributed in nature that the antibody will develop in a person if the antigen is not present. Certain bacteria and foods may have A-like or B-like antigens.

In comparison, **immune antibodies** result from stimulation by specific blood group antigens. Examples of isoantibodies are the anti-A and anti-B antibodies found in the ABO blood group system. In this system, if the red cell lacks the A antigen, anti-A antibody will be found in the serum, and if the red cell lacks the B antigen, anti-B antibody will be found in the serum. Anti-A and anti-B antibodies are routinely used in testing for the ABO blood group. These antibodies are usually immunoglobulin M (IgM) antibodies.

Immune antibodies are also referred to as *unexpected antibodies*. They are usually the result of specific antigenic stimulation from RBCs. These

antibodies are the result of immunization caused by pregnancy or prior blood transfusion. Immune antibodies are of the immunoglobulin G (IgG) type.

Means of Detecting Antigen-Antibody Reactions

A biological reaction that normally occurs in vivo may be demonstrated in vitro.

Antisera

To determine a person's blood type, some type of substance must be available to show what antigens are present on the red cell. The substance used for this purpose is referred to as an **antiserum** (plural antisera) or reagent. An antiserum is a prepared and highly purified solution of antibody and is named based on the antibody it contains. For example, a solution of anti-A antibodies is called *anti-A antiserum*.

PREPARATION OF ANTISERA

Most of the antisera used in transfusion medicine are prepared commercially and purchased by the blood bank. In general, antiserum is prepared as follows:

1. Monoclonal antisera are produced by hybridization, a fusion of a single clone of human neoplastic antibody-producing cells with sensitized splenic lymphocytes obtained from a rodent species.
2. Animals are deliberately inoculated with antigen, and the resulting serum, which contains antibody, is purified and standardized for use as an antiserum.

ANTISERA REQUIREMENTS

Antiserum must meet certain requirements to be acceptable for use. It must be specific for the antigen to be detected, that is, specific under the manufacturer's recommended test conditions. It must have a sufficient concentration, or titer, to detect antigen. Antiserum must have a certain avidity for, or strength of reaction with, corresponding RBCs. It must also be sterile, clear, provided in a good container with a dropper, and stable. Antiserum should be marked with an expiration date and must not be used after this date. In addition, it must be stored at 4°C when not in use.

Exact requirements for antisera are defined by the FDA Center for Biologics Evaluation and Research (CBER). When commercial antisera are used, the manufacturer's directions must be followed carefully and quality assurance procedures established and documented. For antisera that are produced locally and are unlicensed, there must be records of reactivity and specificity, as described in the *AABB Technical Manual*.

REACTION OF ANTISERA WITH RED CELLS

When antiserum is mixed with RBCs, an antigen-antibody reaction may or may not occur. If a reaction does occur, the corresponding antigen must be present on the red cell, and the result is a positive reaction. If a reaction does not occur, the antigen is absent, and the result is negative. For example: a positive reaction with anti-A antiserum demonstrates the presence of the A antigen on the red cell.

In the original definition of antibody, it was stated that antibody resulting from antigenic stimulation would react with the antigen in an observable manner. In transfusion medicine, two types of observable reactions may occur: agglutination and hemolysis.

Agglutination

Agglutination is clumping of RBCs caused by the reaction of a specific antibody and antigen on the cells. A positive antigen-antibody reaction results in an immediate combination of antibody and antigen on the red cell, followed by the visible agglutination, which takes longer to form. The IgG antibody, for example, is thought to be a somewhat Y-shaped structure with a reactive site at the end of each arm of the Y (Fig. 18-1). Each reactive site is capable of combining with corresponding antigen. Agglutination is thought to be the result of bridging of the RBCs by antibody reacting with antigen sites on adjacent RBCs. This bridging causes the RBCs to stick together. Several such bridges result in visible clumping. The degree of agglutination varies. Very strong agglutination forms a large mass of cells that can be easily seen macroscopically. Less strong agglutination results in correspondingly smaller clumps of cells that can also be seen macroscopically, and finally in clumps of cells that can be seen only microscopically. Various strengths of agglutination can be observed.

Hemolysis

Hemolysis is the result of lysis, or destruction, of the red cell by a specific antibody. The antigen-antibody reaction causes the activation of complement, which results in the rupture of the cell membrane and the subsequent release of hemoglobin. The result is a clear, cherry-red solution, with no cloudiness because no cells are present. Hemolysis can be complete, when no intact RBCs remain in the solution, or partial, leaving some RBCs intact. Partial hemolysis is particularly difficult to interpret. It is important that blood bank testing be performed on serum or plasma that is free of hemolysis and that whenever hemolysis occurs, it is interpreted as a positive reaction.

Role of Complement in Hemolysis

For hemolysis to occur, a group of protein components called *complement* must be present in the serum being tested. **Complement** is a complex substance with 18 plasma protein components. It is important in transfusion medicine because some antigen-antibody reactions require the presence of complement to be demonstrated in vitro. Almost all normal sera contain complement when fresh, but it is destroyed by heat. For complement to be active, serum must be either fresh or stored correctly. Complement will remain active if stored for

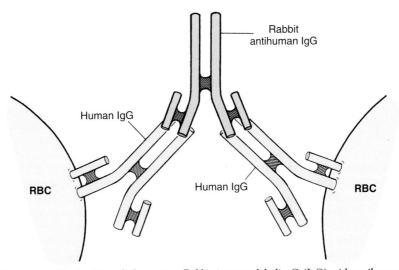

FIGURE 18-1 Antiglobulin (Coombs') reaction. Rabbit immunoglobulin G (IgG) with antihuman IgG specificity is shown combining or reacting with human IgG on human red blood cells (RBCs).

24 to 48 hours at 4°C or for 2 months when stored at −50°C.

If the traditional classic complement pathway is activated by an antigen-antibody reaction, complement components will react sequentially in a cascade that terminates in a membrane attack complex that punctures the cell membrane. If the cell is a red blood cell, hemolysis will result, with hemoglobin spilling out through the punctured membrane.

Note that it is highly questionable that any red cell antibodies will be undetectable even without active complement. That is why it is acceptable to use plasma in antibody screen, ID and crossmatch procedures. Even without complement, it is possible to detect antibodies and incompatibility. Some antibody specificities will also bind complement if it is present and can cause hemolysis in-vivo, these antibodies will still react at RT (ABO antibodies) or at AHG (Kidd antibodies).

Blood-Banking Techniques

The portion of blood used for testing procedures (typing and crossmatching) can be either serum (clotted) or plasma (anticoagulated). The specimen of choice for all blood bank testing has become plasma (AABB Technical Manual 16th ed 2008, Chapter 15 Pretransfusion Testing p441 Specimen Requirements). Plasma may cause some technical problems for tube tests (e.g., small fibrin clots may be present in the plasma and may be incorrectly interpreted as a positive result), but plasma is generally the sample of choice for the newer gel tests. This is more likely to occur in clotted specimens that are incompletely clotted or from patient on some level of anticoagulation therapy.

The detection of antigen on RBCs requires the demonstration of a positive reaction of the cells with a specific solution of antibodies (antiserum). The techniques by which RBCs and antiserum are brought together varies.

Traditionally, RBC group tests are performed in test tubes, although newer techniques, such as dextran-acrylamide gel and solid-phase technology in microplates, have become increasingly popular. When test tubes are used, they are 10 × 75 or 12 × 75 mm. Results are seen as agglutination or hemolysis, as previously described. Other methods of detecting antigen-antibody reactions include inhibition of agglutination, immunofluorescence, enzyme-linked immunosorbent assay (ELISA), and solid-phase RBC adherence tests using indicator RBCs (see Chapter 17).

Many factors affect RBC agglutination, which is thought to occur in two stages: sensitization and agglutination. The first stage involves the physical attachment of antibody to RBCs and is referred to as *sensitization*. Sensitization is affected by temperature, pH, incubation time, ionic strength, and the antigen-antibody ratio. These factors are influenced by the testing medium that is employed: isotonic saline solution, low-ionic-strength saline, or albumin solution.

The second stage of agglutination involves the formation of bridges between sensitized RBCs to form the lattice that is seen as agglutination. Factors that influence this stage include the distance between the cells, the effect of enzymes, and the effect of positively charged molecules such as hexadimethrine (Polybrene).

Factors that affect the reactions used to detect an antigen-antibody reaction include:
- Use of adequate serum and RBCs
- Correct concentration of cell suspensions
- The testing medium
- Proper temperature and duration of incubation
- Proper use of centrifugation
- The condition and correct use of reagents
- Accurate reading and interpretation of agglutination reactions

Correct conditions are essential for reliable tests. Development of correct techniques requires thorough knowledge of these considerations as well as of the RBC groups. The technique will also depend on the brand of antiserum that is used and the manufacturer's directions.

Other Methods of Detecting Antigen-Antibody Reactions

Recent advances in technology have led to other methods beside test tube reactions to detect antigen-antibody reactions. These methods, that may be manual or automated, include gel technology, microplate testing, and solid-phase red blood cell adherence methods.

GEL TECHNOLOGY

In 1985, Yves Lapierre developed gel technology. This led to commercial development by Micro Typing Systems, Inc. (Pompano Beach, Fla.) and FDA approval for use in 1994 followed by ProVue manufactured by Ortho Diagnostics. Essentially, the method uses dextran acrylamide gel particles to trap agglutinated RBCs (Fig. 18-2).

Testing is performed in a prefilled card containing gel mixed with the appropriate reagent. A credit card–sized gel card contains six microtubes. Each microtube contains an upper reaction chamber and a section containing predispensed gel and reagents. Individual gel cards are available for ABO and Rh typing, and AHG cards for indirect testing (e.g., compatibility testing, antibody screening, antibody identification) and direct antiglobulin testing (DAT). A foil strip on the top of the card prevents spillage or drying out of the contents.

Testing involves adding measured volumes of RBCs and plasma/serum to the reaction chamber of the microtube. Incubation allows antigen-antibody reactions to occur. Centrifugation follows to promote maximum contact between antigens and antibodies. A positive reaction demonstrates trapping of RBCs at various levels in the microtube. Larger aggregates of RBCs are trapped at the tip of the gel microtubes and do not travel through the gel when centrifuged. Smaller aggregates travel through the gel microtubes and may be trapped in either the top or bottom half of the tube. A negative reaction is demonstrated by the presence of a button of RBCs on the bottom of the microtube. Nonagglutinated cells travel without difficulty through the length of the tube and form a button at the tip after being centrifuges.

The ID-Micro Typing System (ID-MTS) Gel Test is suitable for a broad range of blood bank applications, including antibody screening and identification, ABO blood grouping and Rh phenotyping, compatibility testing, reverse serum grouping and antigen typing, all using proven serologic methods.

Perceived advantages that this technology offers over tube testing are:

- Improved sensitivity and specificity
- No-wash antiglobulin procedure
- Standardized procedures
- Improved turnaround time
- Enhanced regulatory compliance

MICROPLATE TESTING METHODS

Automated microplate testing has been popular for routine testing in large blood donor centers. The technique can be used for RBC antigen testing and serum antibody detection. After addition of reagents, a microplate is centrifuged and resuspended to read. A positive reaction is demonstrated by a concentrated button of RBCs; a negative reaction is represented by well-dispersed RBCs throughout the well.

SOLID-PHASE RED BLOOD CELL ADHERENCE METHODS

The solid-phase red blood cell adherence serologic method has been available since the late 1980s. A commercially available system, Galileo, is manufactured by Immucor (Norcross, Ga.). Solid-phase technology is presently licensed for compatibility testing, antibody screening, and antibody identification. In this method, RBC screening cells are bound to the surface of a polystyrene microplate. When serum from a patient or donor is added, and low ionic-strength saline is added to the wells, the RBCs capture antibodies during the incubation phase. Subsequently, the plates are washed to remove unbound antibodies, and indicator cells are added to the wells of the microplate. The microplate is centrifuged to bring antigens and potential antibodies together (Fig. 18-3). A positive reaction is demonstrated by observing indicator RBCs being attached to the sides and bottom of the well. A negative reaction is demonstrated by the appearance of a red cell button on the bottom of the wells.

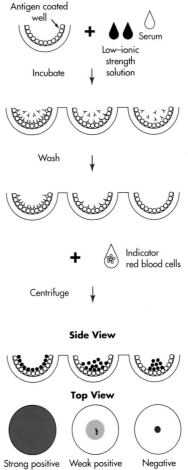

FIGURE 18-3 **Solid-phase red blood cell adherence procedure.** (Courtesy Immucor, Norcross, GA.)

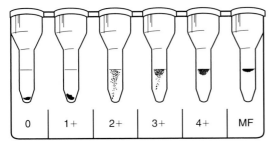

Range of reactions

FIGURE 18-2 **Range of reactions in gel testing.**

ABO RED BLOOD CELL GROUP SYSTEM

The ABO blood group system was first discovered and described in 1900 and 1901 by Karl Landsteiner, who divided RBCs into three groups: A, B, and O. In 1902 the fourth group, AB, was discovered by two of Landsteiner's pupils.

ABO Phenotypes

The ABO system consists of the groups, or phenotypes, A, B, AB, and O. These four groups may be explained by the presence of two antigens on the RBC surface, the A antigen and the B antigen. If a person belongs to group A, the A antigen is present on the red cell. Group B persons have B antigen on their cells. Group AB individuals have both A and B, whereas group O people have neither A nor B.

ABO Genotypes

Genes on the chromosomes determine the antigen present on the red cell. Three allelic genes can be inherited in the ABO system: the A, B, and O genes. Because each person has two genes for any trait (one from each parent), the following combinations of alleles are possible: AA, AO, AB, BB, BO, and OO. These combinations represent the possible genotypes in the ABO system.

If the A gene is present on the chromosome, A antigen will be present on the RBCs. Presence of the B gene results in B antigen on the red cell. If both the A and B genes are present on the chromosome, A and B antigens will be expressed on the RBCs. In addition, A substance will be demonstrated in body fluids. The presence of O gene results in neither antigen on the red cell.

In addition to the A and B genes, expression of the A and/or B antigens as A and/or B substance depends on another gene, H, at a different chromosomal location, to produce H substance, a precursor substrate for the production of the A and B antigens. Most H substance is converted to A and B antigen if the A gene and/or B gene are inherited. Group O individuals have a significant amount of H substance on their RBCs because none of the H substance is converted to A and B antigens because of the lack of A and/or B genes.

ABO Typing Procedures

When the ABO group is to be determined, both the cells and serum should be typed as described. The antigen and antibody typing results should then be compared to be sure mistakes have not occurred and that the results are consistent. This is an excellent way to guard against errors in ABO grouping. ABO typing procedures are divided into front typing and reverse grouping procedures (Table 18-4).

Front Typing

Typing reactions that employ undetermined RBCs and known antibody or antisera are referred to as *antigen, cell, direct,* or *front typing reactions.*

Reverse Grouping

Testing that employ undetermined serum and known RBC antigens is referred to as antibody, serum, indirect, or back typing reactions.

Red Cell Typing for Antigen

In testing RBCs for the ABO group, a suspension of RBCs in saline is prepared. This suspension is tested by mixing one portion with anti-A antiserum (anti-A antibodies), stored at 2°C to 8°C. A second portion is mixed with anti-B antiserum (anti-B antibodies). The mixtures are then observed for a reaction. A positive reaction is the occurrence of agglutination or hemolysis. A negative reaction is

TABLE 18-4

			Antigen, Front, or Direct Typing		Antibody, Back, or Indirect Typing		
Blood Group	Antigens on Red Cells	Antibody in Serum	Reaction of Undetermined Cells With Anti-A Antiserum	Reaction of Undetermined Cells With Anti-B Antiserum	Reaction of Undetermined Serum With A1 Cells	Reaction of Undetermined Serum With B Cells	Possible Genotype
A	A	Anti-B	1	2	2	1	AA, AO
B	B	Anti-A	2	1	1	2	BB, BO
AB	A and B	Neither	1	1	2	2	AB
O	Neither	Anti, A, anti-B	2	2	1	1	OO

the absence of agglutination or hemolysis. Results may be grouped as follows:

- Group A blood (RBCs): positive reaction of cells with anti-A antiserum
- Group B blood (RBCs): positive reaction of cells with anti-B antiserum
- Group O blood (RBCs): negative reaction of cells with both anti-A and anti-B antiserum
- Group AB blood (RBCs): positive reaction of cells with both anti-A and anti-B antiserum

In these typing reactions, the RBCs are merely tested for the presence or absence of A and B antigens. No direct test is made for the presence or absence of the O gene. This is phenotyping, or typing by means of tests made directly on the RBCs. Because blood is tested only for the A and B antigens, genotypes AA and AO will both type as RBC group A. Genotypes BB and BO both contain B antigen and will type as RBC group B. Genotype AB will type as group AB because both antigens are present to react with the appropriate antisera. Genotype OO, will type as blood group O and will not react with either anti-A or anti-B antiserum.

Landsteiner's Rule

Corresponding antigens and antibodies cannot normally coexist in the same person's RBCs. An individual who is group A will not normally form anti-A antibodies and will not have anti-A antibodies in their serum. In the ABO system, unlike other blood group systems, if the A or B antigen is lacking on the red cell, the corresponding antibody will be found in the serum. These are the so-called isoantibodies. Adults lacking group A antigen will be found to have anti-A antibody in their sera. The sera of adults with RBCs lacking B antigen have anti-B antibody. This occurrence of anti-A or anti-B antibody when the corresponding antigen is lacking from the RBC is known as **Landsteiner's rule.** It exists only in the ABO system.

Serum Typing for Antibody

The presence of these environmentally stimulated, anti-A and anti-B antibodies in the serum/plasma of immunocompetent individuals makes the ABO system unique among RBC groups.

The A and B antibodies are very potent, and transfusing RBCs with the antigen to a person with the antibody (ABO incompatible) would result in an immediate and severe hemolytic transfusion reaction that could result in death. It is absolutely essential that the correct ABO blood type be transfused. For these reasons, in addition to testing RBCs with known antibody, the serum is tested

with known group A_1^* and group B reagent RBCs stored at 2°C to 8°C (reverse typing) to determine what antibodies are present in the serum. If there is a positive reaction with known group A_1 cells, the serum contains anti-A antibodies. If there is a positive reaction with known group B cells, the serum contains anti-B antibodies. If the serum reacts with both A_1 and B cells, both anti-A and anti-B antibodies are present. If no reaction occurs with either cell type, both antibodies are lacking. In the ABO system, the serum should contain the corresponding antibody for the A or B antigen lacking from the RBCs of the individual.

The results may be grouped as follows:

- Group A blood (RBCs): positive reaction of serum with group B cells
- Group B blood (RBCs): positive reaction of serum with group A_1 cells
- Group O blood (RBCs): positive reaction of serum with both A_1 and B cells
- Group AB blood (RBCs): no reaction with either A_1 or B cells

Isoantibodies of ABO System

One cause of cell and serum discrepancies in ABO typing procedures in adults involves the expected isoantibodies. These antibodies are not manifested in newborns because infants do not normally begin to produce antibodies until they are 3 to 6 months of age. The titer (concentration) of isoantibodies normally increases gradually through adolescence and then decreases gradually. For this reason, serum grouping results may also show discrepancies in elderly patients, who may have low concentrations of antibodies.

Variation in Titer

The antibody titer varies in the population; in general, the anti-A titer is higher than the anti-B titer. In the laboratory, the antibody titer of serum will only rarely approach the antibody titer of commercially prepared antiserum. For this reason, reactions with cell grouping tests are generally stronger and easier to read than serum grouping reactions.

Subgroups

The occurrence of subgroups of group A or group B antigen might also result in discrepancies between cell and serum grouping reactions. The classification of RBCs in the ABO system into groups A, B, AB, and O is an oversimplification. Both group

---

*A_1 is a subgroup of A antigen. For this discussion, A_1 may be considered synonymous with A antigen.

A and group B may be further classified into subgroups. The most important subdivision is that of group A into A_1 and A_2. Both A_1 and A_2 cells react with anti-A antisera. However, anti-A_1 reagent can be prepared from group B human serum or with the lectin of *Dolichos biflores* seeds. This anti-A_1 antibody will react with A_1 cells only. Practically, the subgroups should be kept in mind when there is difficulty in ABO grouping or compatibility testing.

H Substance

H substance is a precursor of A and B blood group antigens. The ABO system is concerned with substances A, B, and H. Genetically, the ABO system is controlled by at least three sets of genes. We have described one set—the A, A_1, B, and O gene set—which occupies a specific locus or position on corresponding chromosomes.

Another set is described as H and h, which are alleles for another locus or position. The H gene is extremely common; over 99.9% of the population inherits the H gene. Very few people carry an h allele, and the hh genotype, called Bombay or Oh, is extremely rare. It is a cause of unexpected blood-typing reactions because the cells type as group O. However, the serum of these Bombay individuals reacts strongly with group O red cells because of the presence of a potent anti-H antibody. Anti-H antisera are also prepared from the lectin of *Ulex europeaus*. Anti-H antisera will not agglutinate RBCs from Bombay individuals but will give a strong reaction with group O RBCs.

Finally, the Se and se alleles occupy a third locus. The Se and se genes regulate the presence of A, B, and H antigenic material in the body secretions. About 78% of the population has inherited the Se gene (SeSe or Sese). These persons are secretors who have H, A, or B substance produced by their secretory cells. Corresponding H, A, or B substance can be found in the saliva of these persons.

Because of the existence of subgroups, A_1 test cells must be used in ABO serum grouping. Subgrouping tests will involve the use of other reagents.

If a discrepancy is demonstrated between the results of cell and serum grouping, it must be resolved before a blood type can be determined and before type specific blood is transfused.

Immune Antibodies of ABO System

Only environmentally stimulated anti-A and anti-B antibodies have been discussed, but anti-A and anti-B antibodies may also be of the immune type. Serum may contain immune antibodies in addition to the isoantibodies. Isoantibodies are normally found in the serum of adults if the RBC lacks the corresponding antigen. These antibodies arise from the stimulation by ABH substances that are widely distributed in nature. Immune anti-A or anti-B antibodies result from specific antigenic stimulation. This stimulation may occur through incompatible transfusion, pregnancy, or injection of ABH substances or substances having ABH activity.

Physical and Chemical Properties

Immune antibodies and isoantibodies differ in physical and chemical properties and in their serologic behavior. In addition, ABO isoantibodies react best if the RBCs are suspended in saline solution and the test is carried out at room temperature or 4°C. Immune antibodies differ in that they react better if cells are suspended in albumin or serum and incubated at 37°C. Other differences exist in mode of reaction in the laboratory and must be taken into account when the occurrence of an immune-type anti-A or anti-B antibody is suspected or possible—for example, in patients with hemolytic disease of the fetus and newborn (HDFN) who have ABO incompatibility and in screening RBCs for low titers of anti-A and anti-B.

Size and Characteristics of Antibodies

An isoantibody is a large molecule, usually IgM, with a molecular weight of about 900,000 daltons. The immune antibody, generally IgG, has a molecular weight of about 150,000 daltons. IgM antibodies are unable to cross the placental barrier, but IgG antibodies can cross the barrier. This is important in the etiology of HDNF.

Universal Donors and Recipients

One concept that must be discussed in conjunction with the ABO system is that of the "universal donor" and the "universal recipient." These terms are familiar to most people, but the concept is oversimplified and used only in cases of extreme emergency.

When blood products are to be transfused, two questions must be kept in mind:

1. Does the patient's serum contain an antibody against an antigen on the transfused red cell?
2. Does the serum to be transfused contain an antibody against an antigen on the patient's red cells?

The first situation is the more serious one and must be kept in mind whenever RBCs are the transfusion product. It can result in a major reaction and in the death of the patient; the transfused RBCs will be destroyed by antibody in the patient's circulatory system, resulting in accumulation of toxic waste products and probably in severe renal failure and death.

The second situation, in which the donor serum contains antibody against the patient's RBCs, is not as serious. This situation may occur when transfusing plasma products such as fresh frozen plasma or platelet concentrates. A minor reaction might occur, depending on the amount of plasma infused and its ratio to the total blood volume of the recipient.

The terms **universal donor** and **universal recipient** pertain to the transfusion of packed RBC products in emergency situations. The universal donor is the person with group O RBCs. Group O red cells can be safely transfused into a person with any ABO blood type because the donor cells do not contain the A or B antigens and therefore will not react with the patient's A or B antibodies. The universal recipient is the patient with group AB RBCs. Their serum does not contain either anti-A or anti-B, and therefore these patients could receive RBC transfusion of any ABO blood type.

ABO type-specific RBCs should be used whenever possible. The major problem with transfusing non–type-specific RBCs is that the patient's true blood type can be obscured and can produce problems with subsequent transfusions and documentation of the patient's true blood type. Transfusion of non–type-specific RBCs includes situations in which group-specific blood is not available and RBCs must be transfused, or there may not be enough time to type the patient's blood and test for compatibility, or the patient's RBC group cannot be accurately determined.

In patients with ABO HDNF, group O red cells are generally used. This may also be the case in unusual circumstances such as disasters or military situations in which blood cannot be typed for use before it is transfused.

RH RED BLOOD CELL GROUP SYSTEM

Historical Background

The discovery of the Rh system was based on work by Landsteiner and Wiener in 1940 and by Levine and Stetson in 1939. A woman who delivered a stillborn fetus was studied by Levine and Stetson. The woman had never received a blood transfusion; after delivery, however, she was transfused with her husband's RBCs. Both the woman and her husband were group O. After the transfusion, the woman experienced a severe hemolytic reaction.

Similar Adverse Effects of Transfusion had previously been known to follow the first transfusion after childbirth, and they did not seem to be associated with the ABO system. Levine and Stetson developed an explanation of their patient's transfusion reaction that proved to be correct. They explained the reaction by proposing that the woman's RBCs did not contain a "new" antigen. However, the child inherited this new antigen from the father, and the fetal cells containing it found their way into the mother's circulatory system. This resulted in the formation of antibody to the new antigen. When the woman was transfused with her husband's RBCs, her serum contained an antibody to the new antigen present on her husband's red cells. It was also found that the woman's serum agglutinated not only her husband's RBCs but also the red cells of 80 of 104 ABO-compatible RBCs. Levine and Stetson did not name this new antigen.

The naming of this new antigen eventually resulted from studies by Landsteiner and Wiener in 1940. They inoculated rabbits and guinea pigs with the RBCs of rhesus monkeys and found that the resulting rabbit antibody agglutinated the RBCs of rhesus monkeys and, more important, the RBCs of about 85% of samples of the white population of New York City. The 85% of the cells that were agglutinated by the anti-rhesus serum were called "Rh positive," and the remaining 15% not agglutinated were called "Rh negative." Later it was shown that an antibody found in the serum of certain patients who had hemolytic reactions after transfusion of ABO-compatible blood was apparently the same as the antibody in the anti-rhesus serum. It was also found that the antibody contained within the serum of the women studied by Levine and Stetson in 1939 was similar to the antibody in the anti-rhesus serum.

Definition of Rh Antigens and Inheritance

Rh Antigens

The Rh blood group system is the most complex of the red cell antigen systems. There are over 50 antigens defined and more than 150 variations of the two genes that are known to control the system. There are however, five antigens, D, C, c, E, and e, and their corresponding antibodies that are of primary importance in routine blood bank testing and transfusion medicine. Of these five, the D antigen is the most important. The presence or absence of the D antigen identifies a person's cells as being Rh positive or Rh negative.

Because the Rh alleles are inherited in groups of paired antigens, and each person has two chromosomes for the Rh antigens, each person has a total of five Rh antigens. This means that eight possible combinations of antigens can be carried on a particular chromosome. These possible combinations of antigens in CDE notation and the corresponding Rh notation, with their approximate frequency, are given in Table 18-5. These frequencies are for the white population and differ for other races and

TABLE 18-5

Comparative Nomenclature of Rh Antigens				
CDE System (Fisher-Race)	Rh System (Wiener)		Numerical System (Rosenfield et al.)	
D	d	Rh_O	Hr_O	Rh1	
C	c	rh'	hr'	Rh2	Rh4
E	e	rh″	hr″	Rh3	Rh5

TABLE 18-6

Rh Chromosomes and Approximate Frequency		
CDE Notation (Fisher-Race)	Rh-Hr Notation (Wiener)	Approximate Frequency in White Population*
CDe	R^1	Common
cDE	R^2	Common
CDE	R^z	Rare
cDe	R^o	2%
Cde	r'	1%
cdE	r″	1%
CdE	r^y	Extremely rare
cde	r	Common

*Data from Stratton F, Renton PH: Practical blood grouping, Springfield, Ill, 1958, Charles C Thomas, Publisher, p 154.

ethnicities. They are included to give a general idea of the relative frequencies that might be encountered. For more definitive frequencies, consult the *AABB Technical Manual.* One of the eight possible Rh-Hr gene combinations is inherited from each parent, so the total Rh-Hr genotype for a person would be denoted as CDE/ce or CDe/cDe, and so on. In Wiener's Rh-Hr notation corresponding to the CDE system, uppercase *R* refers to the presence of D (Rh_O) antigen, and lowercase *r* refers to the absence of D. The superscript in Wiener's notation refers to the antigens C, c, E, and e.

Nomenclature

In the 1940's and 50's when knowledge of the new system was just beginning to be formed, two different nomenclatures were developed. Each system supported the theory of inheritance put forth by the authors. Although it is now known that both early theories were incorrect, the nomenclatures have remained and are still in wide use today. The CDE system of Fisher-Race is the more preferred and is most frequently used in written text. The Rh-Hr system of Weiner easily conveys the inherited haplotype both verbally and in writing. As the complexity of the system grew and the number of antigens assigned to the system increased, a numerical system was developed by Rosenfeld in the 1960's which assigned each antigen a number based on the order in which the antigen was discovered or assigned to the system. Although not frequently used for the more common antigens, many of the high or low frequency antigens are referred to by their numerical designation only (e.g., Rh23, Rh35, Rh54, etc) (Table 18-6).

Rh System Biochemistry (Tippett)[7,8]

It is now known that there are two genes, *RHD* and *RHCE*, located closely together on chromosome 1 that encode for two amino acid proteins that cross thru the red cell membrane multiple times (trans membrane). The *RHD* gene produces the protein upon which the D antigen resides while the *RHCE* gene produces the protein that contains the CcEe antigens in various combinations. The location of the two genes on Chromosome 1 is close enough

that the genes exhibit linkage and as a result some Rh haplotypes are more common than others. Rh positive individuals possess at least one *RHD* gene and therefore produce the RhD protein and the D antigen on their red cells. Rh negative individuals on the other hand, lack the RhD protein and the D antigen. It appears that the two genes may have developed from a common ancestor gene by duplication and that many of the haplotypes we see today were produced by point mutations, recombination and gene conversions.

A third gene *RHAG*, located on chromosome 6, encodes for another protein RhAG (Rh-associated glycoprotein) and is associated with the production of the Rh_{null} phenotype.

Rh-Positive and Rh-Negative Status

It is now known that the new antigen described by Levine and Stetson is the D (or Rh_O) antigen. Persons whose RBCs contain D antigen either in the homozygous or heterozygous state are now termed **Rh positive;** they represent approximately 85% of the population. In other words, the antibody responsible for several adverse effects of transfusion is the anti-D (anti-Rh_O) antibody. Persons whose RBCs lack the D (Rh_O) antigen are termed **Rh negative;** they represent about 15% of the population. The great majority of Rh-negative persons are cde/cde. This genotype is what is meant by a truly Rh-negative person. Other very rare genotypes that lack the D antigen must also be considered Rh-negative as blood recipients.

Characteristics of Rh Antigens

C, D, E, c, and e are antigenic. This means they are capable of stimulating the production of antibodies if introduced into the body of a person whose RBCs completely lack them. The Rh antigens are permanent inherited characteristics that remain constant throughout life. However, not all the Rh antigens are equally antigenic. The D (Rh$_O$) antigen is the strongest and will generally result in immunization if introduced into a foreign host. For this reason, the term *Rh positive* merely refers to the presence of D antigen without respect to the other Rh antigens. The antigenic strength of D also makes it imperative that RBCs be tested for Rh type before transfusion. Rh-negative persons should not be transfused with Rh-positive (D-positive) RBCs, because they will certainly develop anti-D antibodies more than 80% of the time, according to the *AABB Technical Manual*. This would not be harmful at the first transfusion, but subsequent transfusions with D-positive RBCs would result in a transfusion reaction. In the woman cited earlier who was sensitized by an Rh-positive fetus, transfusion with D-positive RBCs resulted in a hemolytic reaction with the first transfusion.

Although D is the most antigenic of the Rh antigens, the other antigens are also antigenic. If strength is considered in terms of antibody frequency, anti-c is the next most common, followed by anti-E, anti-C, and finally anti-e. Combinations of antibodies in the same RBCs are also seen.

Weak Expression of D Antigen

Not all RBCs that contain D antigen react equally well with anti-D blood grouping reagent. Some of these cells may even appear to be D negative, depending on methodology. This weak reactivity with anti-D sera is referred to as *weak D*.

Characteristics of Rh Antibodies

The Rh antibodies are made from the gamma globulin portion of the blood plasma and are predominantly IgG in structure. They are specific for the antigen against which they were formed. Unlike the ABO antibodies, the Rh antibodies are immune or unexpected antibodies. No environmentally stimulated antibodies occur as Rh antibodies. They result from specific antigenic stimulation, whether by transfusion, pregnancy, or injection of antigen. The typing methods in this system depend on antigen-typing or cell-typing procedures involving unknown antigen and known antiserum.

Types of Rh Typing Reagents (Antisera)

Many types of commercially available reagent antisera can be used for routine Rh testing. The reagents can be high-protein, low-protein,

chemically modified, saline-reactive, monoclonal, or monoclonal blends. The most common reagents currently used are the monoclonal-polyclonal blends and monoclonal blends.

High-Protein Antisera

Commercial antisera of the high-protein variety contain IgG-type antibodies. In general, the albumin-active antisera are more avid preparations, so many of them may be used with a slide method or the rapid tube technique. In addition, the reaction takes place in less time than with saline-active antibody, and the incubation time is shortened. The high-protein reagents in rapid tube tests will generally give strong reactive results with D-positive cells at the immediate-spin, room-temperature phase. In general, most Rh antibodies are IgG in form and will not react unless the test is warmed or incubated at 37°C. High-protein reagents are labeled "for slide or rapid tube test (or modified tube test)," and it is essential to follow the manufacturer's directions.

There are several causes of false-positive results when high-protein antisera are used. A high-protein control must always be included. There may be spontaneous agglutination of IgG-coated RBCs, or factors in the patient's own serum may affect the test, which often uses unwashed RBCs suspended in the patient's own serum or plasma. Other causes of false-positive results include:

- Strong autoagglutinins
- Abnormal serum protein that causes rouleaux formation
- Antibodies against an additive in the reagent itself

The best control consists of an immunologically inert control reagent, generally the diluent used for manufacturing the particular antiserum. It is important to use the high-protein control provided by the same manufacturer as the maker of the antiserum.

Low-Protein Antisera

Antibody of the saline type is labeled "for saline tube tests." When this preparation is used, reactions must be carried out on saline suspensions of RBCs, and the test must be performed in a test tube. Slide tests cannot be performed.

The first Rh antibodies discovered were active in saline solution. These reagents use IgM forms of anti-D. Anti-C and anti-E antisera (in addition to anti-D) are normally available in a saline-active form. Antisera of this type will be labeled "for saline tube tests," and the tests must be performed in test tubes. Weak-D testing cannot be performed using this reagent.

Chemically Modified Antisera

These reagents use the IgG form of the antibody but are chemically modified by breaking some of the disulfide bonds at the hinge region so the antibody molecule can stretch longer distances and cause RBC agglutination (positive reaction) in a low-protein medium. This antiserum has the advantage of a low-protein reagent with less false-positive reactions and no need for a specific Rh control reagent. In addition, these chemically modified reagents will react with the D antigen at the immediate-spin, room-temperature phase of testing and can be used for slide and tube testing.

Monoclonal Antisera

Monoclonal antisera have become the reagents of choice. They can be used in slide, tube, microplate, and automated testing methods. They have the same advantages of the chemically modified reagents, and because they are prepared from hybridoma cell cultures rather than human sources, monoclonal reagents carry no risk of disease transmission. Because of the complexity of the D antigen and the narrow specificity of the monoclonal antibodies, most commercial anti-D reagents are prepared by blending antibody from several clones.

Nature of Rh Antibody Molecule

The differences in reactivity among antibodies depend on the length of the antibody molecule. The molecules that are reactive in saline suspensions of cells are of the larger IgM type. Their length is sufficient to cause bridging of adjacent cells in suspension (agglutination). However, RBCs in suspension are known to carry an electrical charge, the zeta potential, which causes them to repel each other. The IgM-type antibody molecules are so long that they extend beyond the range of the zeta potential and can react with antigenic sites on adjacent cells. Molecules of the smaller IgG type are so short that they do not extend beyond the zeta potential and cannot react with adjacent cells. To demonstrate the existence of IgG molecules by means of agglutination, the repulsion caused by the zeta potential must be overcome or reduced. It can be reduced by suspending the cells in a sufficiently high protein medium (either their own serum or a commercial protein preparation, or both). Other techniques for the demonstration of IgG include high-speed centrifugation and enzyme methods.

Typing Blood for Transfusion

When RBCs are to be transfused, the patient must be tested for the presence or absence of the D (Rh$_O$) antigen. This is because the D antigen is so antigenic that most persons who are D negative (Rh$_O$ negative) may produce an anti-D antibody if transfused with D-positive RBCs. Individuals who are D negative (d/d) must be transfused with Rh-negative RBCs, but Rh-positive persons can be transfused with Rh-negative RBCs without adverse consequences.

Because the D (Rh$_O$) antigen is the most antigenic of the Rh antigens, laboratories test only for the presence or absence of this antigen and transfuse Rh-positive or Rh-negative RBCs accordingly. In most cases, this is sufficient because other Rh antibodies are comparatively rare and are tested for indirectly by compatibility testing or antibody screening techniques. RBCs that are negative at the immediate-spin phase should be further tested for the presence of weak D by means of incubation at 37°C and the antihuman globulin (Coombs') test. The use of appropriate positive and negative controls is mandatory.

By performing additional Rh tests, the complete Rh phenotype may be determined, or the most probable genotype may be determined by consulting the frequency charts available from these typing reactions. This may be useful in determining the probability of HDNF in mothers negative for an antigen that the father possess. In such cases, both the mother and the father are typed, and the most probable genotypes are determined.

OTHER BLOOD GROUP SYSTEMS

Human blood groups were discovered in 1900. In addition to the antigens of the ABO and Rh systems, the ISBT has defined 30 blood group systems (Table 18-7), with numerous associated antigens in these systems (Table 18-8). Some of these antigens are common (high frequency); others are uncommon or rare (low frequency). All antigens receiving ISBT numbers must have been shown to be inherited.

ANTIHUMAN GLOBULIN REACTION (COOMBS' TEST)

Antibodies detectable by the antihuman globulin (AHG) test react with red cells, but the reaction is not observable by direct agglutination. The antibodies coat the RBCs by reacting with antigenic sites on the RBC surface, but the other arm of the antibody molecule is unable to react with antigen on an adjacent red cell to demonstrate agglutination. To demonstrate the coating of RBCs by antibody, some sort of reagent must be available to demonstrate that the cells have reacted with antibody, as seen in Fig. 18-1. These antibodies are capable of reacting in the body and, if present, may result in a severe transfusion reaction.

TABLE 18-7

No.	System Name	System Symbol	Gene Name(s)*	Chromosomal Location	CDNumbers
001	ABO	ABO	ABO	9q34.2	
002	MNS	MNS	GYPA, GYPB, GYPE	4q31.21	CD235
003	P	P1		22q11.2–qter	
004	Rh	RH	RHD, RHCE	1p36.11	CD240
005	Lutheran	LU	LU	19q13.32	CD239
006	Kell	KEL	KEL	7q34	CD238
007	Lewis	LE	FUT3	19p13.3	
008	Duffy	FY	DARC	1q23.2	CD234
009	Kidd	JK	SLC14A1	18q12.3	
010	Diego	DI	SLC4A1	17q21.31	CD233
011	Yt	YT	ACHE	7q22.1	
012	Xg	XG	XG, MIC2	Xp22.33	CD99†
013	Scianna	SC	ERMAP	1p34.2	
014	Dombrock	DO	ART4	12p12.3	CD297
015	Colton	CO	AQP1	7p14.3	
016	Landsteiner-Wiener	LW	ICAM4	19p13.2	CD242
017	Chido/Rodgers	CH/RG	C4A, C4B	6p21.3	
018	H	H	FUT1	19q13.33	CD173
019	Kx	XK	XK	Xp21.1	
020	Gerbich	GE	GYPC	2q14.3	CD236
021	Cromer	CROM	CD55	1q32.2	CD55
022	Knops	KN	CR1	1q32.2	CD35
023	Indian	IN	CD44	11p13	CD44
024	Ok	OK	BSG	19p13.3	CD147
025	Raph	RAPH	CD151	11p15.5	CD151
026	John Milton Hagen	JMH	SEMA7A	15q24.1	CD108
027	I	I	GCNT2	6p24.2	
028	Globoside	GLOB	B3GALT3	3q26.1	
029	Gill	GIL	AQP3	9p13.3	
30	Rh-associated glycoprotein	RHAG	RHAG	6p21-qter	CD241

*As recognized by the HUGO Gene Nomenclature Committee: http://www.genenames.org/.
†MIC2 product.

Developing a reagent to demonstrate the coating of antibody on RBCs is based on antibodies being some form of human globulin. The reagent need only be an antibody to human globulin. This is the basis of the antiglobulin, or Coombs', sera. The reagent is an antibody to human globulin, or antihuman globulin antibody. This antiglobulin antibody will react with any antibody coating a red cell. Because it is sufficiently long (it is actually an IgM-type antibody), it will react with antibody coating adjacent RBCs, resulting in bridging or agglutination of the RBCs.

Preparation and Nature of Antihuman Globulin Reagent

Antihuman globulin reagent is produced commercially by the companies that produce blood group antisera. The AHG reagent may be prepared by inoculating laboratory animals (usually rabbits) with human serum or a purified globulin fraction of human serum. The laboratory animals produce an antibody to the human globulin, or AHG antibody. The animal is bled and the serum collected. This

TABLE 18-8

System		Antigen Number											
		001	002	003	004	005	006	007	008	009	010	011	012
001	ABO	A	B	A,B	A1	—							
002	MNS	M	N	S	s	U	He	Mi^a	M^c	Vw	Mur	M^g	Vr
003	P	P1	—	—									
004	RH	D	C	E	c	e	f	Ce	C^w	C^x	V	E^w	G
005	LU	Lu^a	Lu^b	Lu3	Lu4	Lu5	Lu6	Lu7	Lu8	Lu9	—	Lu11	

Table of Blood Group Antigens Within Systems

From http://ibgrl.blood.co.uk. Partial listing, accessed August 5, 2009.

serum is purified by various techniques until it is specific for human globulin. The antihuman serum is often prepared in such a way that it reacts with both gamma globulin and complement. The antiglobulin portion of the serum is anti-IgG globulin. Some antibodies must be detected by the AHG. It has been found that some of these other antibodies use complement in their reaction or fix complement.

Monospecific and polyspecific reagents are available. Examples of monospecific reagents include anti-IgG with no anticomplement activity and anti-C3d and other complement components with no antiimmunoglobulin activity. These monospecific reagents may be produced through the injection of purified fractions of human serum into rabbits or by the production of murine (mouse) monoclonal antibodies. Monospecific antibodies may be pooled to form polyspecific reagents.

Antihuman globulin reagent that contains both anti-IgG and anticomplement antibodies is called *polyspecific AHG reagent*. Currently, polyspecific AHG reagents require antibody to human IgG and the C3d component of human complement. Current polyspecific reagents are a blend of polyclonal IgG antibodies against human subclasses of IgG and monoclonal antibodies against C3b and C3d complement components.

Antihuman Globulin Test Procedures

The antiglobulin test is performed in two ways: the direct AHG and the indirect AHG methods. Neither the indirect nor the direct antihuman globulin test is specific for a particular antibody.

Direct Antihuman Globulin Test

The direct AHG test, or direct antiglobulin test (DAT), is performed on RBCs suspected of being coated with antibody. The DAT is used to demonstrate antibody that has coated or reacted with the RBCs in the patient's body (in vivo). RBCs coated with antibody in vivo are removed from the

circulation by the mononuclear phagocytic system. The net effect is a shortened life span for the RBCs. The DAT is used to investigate Adverse Effects of Transfusion and to diagnose autoimmune hemolytic anemia, HDNF, and drug-induced hemolytic anemia.

Indirect Antihuman Globulin Test

The indirect AHG test, or indirect antiglobulin test (IAT), is used to detect antigen-antibody reaction that occurs in the test tube (in vitro). It tests for antibodies that are freely circulating in the plasma or antisera and reacts with specific antigens on RBCs in vitro. It is used for detecting antibody in the patient/donor serum (antibody screen), identifying the presence of antibody in the patient's serum against the donor unit cells (crossmatching), and identifying antigens present on the patient's RBCs, such as weak D and Kell (phenotyping).

COMPATIBILITY TESTING AND CROSSMATCHING

Compatibility Testing: Definition and General Considerations

Whenever red blood cells are to be transfused, two considerations must be kept in mind:
1. RBCs must be selected that will not be harmful to the patient or result in a transfusion reaction.
2. RBCs must be selected that will be of maximum benefit to the patient.

Whenever blood is to be transfused, it must be tested for compatibility between the donor and the recipient (patient). Compatibility testing is much more than crossmatching, which is just one part of the testing procedures. Compatibility testing involves a series of tests that must include:
1. Correct identification of donor and recipient
2. A review of the patient's past history and blood bank records for type and the presence of unexpected antibodies

3. ABO and Rh typing of both donor and recipient
4. Testing of serum (or plasma) of the donor and recipient for the presence of unexpected antibodies (antibody screen)
5. Identification of unexpected antibodies and management of previous antibodies identified
6. Crossmatching of the donor's RBCs with the patient's serum

In general, compatibility testing is used to help detect:

- Unexpected antibodies in the patient's serum
- Some ABO incompatibilities
- Some errors in labeling, recording, or identifying patients or donors

Unfortunately, crossmatching and compatibility testing will not prevent all transfusion problems. The most frequent causes of incompatible blood transfusions are preanalytical errors of an organizational or clerical nature. Although these errors may be detected by means of compatibility testing and the crossmatch, this is not always the case. The laboratory must always work with great care to avoid mistakes. It requires diligent effort and attention to established policies and procedures to ensure the best possible transfusion outcome for each patient.

Incompatibility in the crossmatching procedure will be discovered only if the patient's serum contains an unexpected antibody to the donor's RBCs. Compatibility testing will not prevent immunization if the patient is transfused with foreign antigen. For example, an Rh-negative person who has never been exposed to Rh-positive antigenic material will not show incompatibility if crossmatched with Rh-positive RBCs, but the person may develop an anti-D antibody. Errors of Rh typing will be detected only if the recipient's serum contains an Rh antibody.

No single crossmatching procedure or antibody screening procedure will detect all unexpected antibodies that may be present in the patient's serum. Even if the blood is found to be compatible, testing procedures will not ensure the normal survival of donor RBCs. The blood must be processed and stored correctly.

ABO and Rh Typing of Donor and Recipient

When blood is selected for transfusion, the patient and donor are tested for ABO type and the presence or absence of the D (Rh_O) antigen. The ABO group is matched and the Rh type selected with respect to the D antigen. Patients whose cells contain the D antigen are given red cells positive for the D antigen (Rh-positive RBCs), and patients who are negative for the D antigen are always given red cells negative for the D antigen (Rh-negative RBCs). The other antigens that collectively make up a person's complete blood type are not matched when RBCs are to be transfused.

Unexpected Antibody Screening and Identification

Antibody Screening

Antibodies known by various names—atypical, unexpected, or irregular antibodies—may be produced by an individual who has been exposed to foreign RBC antigens as the result of prior RBC transfusion or pregnancy. A screening procedure for such antibodies is routinely done for patients requiring transfusion, pregnant women, blood donors, and patients with a suspected transfusion reaction.

Antibody screening with known reagent RBCs allows for testing of the patient's serum in advance of the actual transfusion, allowing for selection of antigen negative donor RBCs when necessary (Figs. 18-4 and 18-5).

The group O RBCs for antibody screening are available as commercially prepared products. Each vial is from an individual donor. They are supplied in sets of two or three vials, suspended in a preservative solution, and must be stored at 2°C to 8°C when not in use. Commercial manufacturers will type for other additional antigens.

To see the screening procedure, go to http://evolve.elsevier.com/Turgeon/clinicallab.

The antibody screen test is an indirect antiglobulin/Coombs test. It consists of testing two drops of patient serum and one drop from each vial of reagent

Cell	Rh							MNSs				P_1	Lewis		Lutheran		Kell		Duffy		Kidd				
	D	C	E	c	e	f	C^w	M	N	S	s	P_1	Le^a	Le^b	Lu^a	Lu^b	K	k	Fy^a	Fy^b	Jk^a	Jk^b			
I R1R1 (56)	+	+	0	0	+	0	0	+	+	0	+	0	+	0	0	+	+	+	+	0	+	+			
II R2R2 (89)	+	0	+	+	0	0	0	0	+	+	0	+	0	+	0	+	0	+	0	+	+	0			

FIGURE 18-4 Screening cell antigram. Diagrams the antigens present on the red cells in each bottle, for the lot number indicated. +, Antigen present; 0, antigen absent. (From Blaney KD, Howard PR: Basic & applied concepts of immunohematology, ed 2, St Louis, 2009, Mosby.)

	Result					Tentative interpretation

Antibody screen

1.

Cell	IS	37º C	AHG	CC
I	0	0	0	✓
II	0	0	2+	NT

1. Alloantibody
2. IgG
3. Single specificity

Direct antiglobulin test

Poly		IgG	C3
0	✓	NT	NT

Antibody screen

2.

Cell	IS	37º C	AHG	CC
I	0	0	3+	NT
II	0	2+	3+	NT

1. Alloantibody
2. IgG
3. Multiple specificities

Direct antiglobulin test

Poly		IgG	C3
0	✓	NT	NT

Antibody screen

3.

Cell	IS	37º C	AHG	CC
I	1+	0	0	✓
II	2+	0	0	✓

1. Alloantibody
2. IgM specificity
3. Single specificity showing dosage

Direct antiglobulin test

Poly		IgG	C3
0	✓	NT	NT

Antibody screen

4.

Cell	IS	37º C	AHG	CC
I	1+	0	0	✓
II	1+	0	0	✓

1. Autoantibody
2. IgM specificity
3. Cold autoantibody

Direct antiglobulin test

Poly		IgG	C3
2+	0	✓	1+

Antibody screen

5.

Cell	IS	37º C	AHG	CC
I	0	0	2+	NT
II	0	0	2+	NT

1. Autoantibody/transfusion reaction
2. IgG
3. Warm autoantibody with possible underlying alloantibodies

Direct antiglobulin test

Poly	IgG	C3
2+	2+	0

FIGURE 18-5 Screen interpretations. Tentative interpretations that can be made following testing of the antibody screen and direct antiglobulin test. *IS,* Immediate spin; 37ºC, 37°C incubation; *AHG,* antiglobulin test; *CC,* check cells; 0, no agglutination or hemolysis; ✓, check cells agglutinate; *NT,* not tested; *Poly,* polyspecific antiglobulin reagent; *C3,* anti-complement reagent. (From Blaney KD, Howard PR: Basic & applied concepts of immunohematology, ed 2, St Louis, 2009, Mosby.)

RBCs. The mixture is centrifuged and observed for agglutination or hemolysis at room temperature. This is the immediate spin, room temperature phase followed by the addition of an enhancement media (e.g., LISS) and incubation of the tubes at 37°C. After incubation, AHG antisera is added, and the tubes are centrifuged and read. Agglutination or hemolysis indicates that an antigen and its corresponding antibody are present. To determine a preliminary identity, the antigram (a listing of the identified antigens present on the RBCs in each vial representing one donor) is consulted for the RBC antigens and the expected phases of reactivity (Table 18- 9). Once the preliminary screening cell study has been completed and the probable antibody or antibodies have been identified, a large panel of RBCs (ten or more) representing multiple donors can be tested with the patient or donor's serum for antibody identification. In some cases, the patient or donor RBCs are tested to confirm the absence of the antigen on the patient's or donor's

RBCs. The absence of antigen makes it feasible to build the corresponding antibody if there is a history of prior foreign RBC exposure due to RBC transfusion or pregnancy (Table 18-10).

Crossmatching

A well-defined compatibility testing regimen is required whenever blood is to be transfused. If compatibility testing has been performed with strict adherence to the procedures established by the particular transfusion service, transfusion of RBCs can be a relatively safe procedure with tremendous benefit to the patient.

The major crossmatch involves testing the donor's RBCs with the patient's serum to detect any antibody in the patient's serum that will react with the donor's RBCs. The presence of such antibody in the patient's serum would certainly result in a major transfusion reaction, because the infused donor

TABLE 18-9

Antibody Screening Antigram			
Blood Group	Antigen	I R1R1	II R2R2
Rh	D	+	+
	C	Neg	+
	E	Neg	+
	c	+	Neg
	e	+	Neg
	f	Neg	Neg
	C^W	Neg	Neg
MNSs	M	+	Neg
	N	+	+
	S	Neg	+
	S	+	Neg
P1	P1	Neg	+
Lewis	Le^a	+	Neg
	Le^b	Neg	+
Lutheran	Lu^a	Neg	+
	Lu^b	Neg	+
Kell	K	+	Neg
	k	+	+
Duffy	Fy^a	+	Neg
	Fy^b	+	Neg
Kidd	Jk^a	+	+
	Jk^b	+	Neg

NOTE: Positive (+) antigen is present on the commercial RBCs, Neg(−) negative-the antigen is absent on the commercial RBCs. Each vial contains the RBCs of one donor.

TABLE 18-10

Screening Cells				
Blood Group	Antigen	I R1R1	II R2R2	Patient Results
Rh	D	+	+	Neg
	C	Neg	+	Neg
	E	Neg	+	Neg
	c	+	Neg	+
	E	+	Neg	Neg
	F	Neg	Neg	Neg
	C^W	Neg	Neg	Neg
MNSs	M	+	Neg	Neg
	N	+	+	Neg
	S	Neg	+	Neg
	S	+	Neg	Neg
P1	P1	Neg	+	Neg
Lewis	Le^a	+	Neg	Neg
	Le^b	Neg	+	Neg
Lutheran	Lu^a	Neg	+	Neg
	Lu^b	Neg	+	Neg
Kell	K	+	Neg	Neg
	K	+	+	Neg
Duffy	Fy^a	+	Neg	Neg
	Fy^b	+	Neg	Neg
Kidd	Jk^a	+	+	Neg
	Jk^b	+	Neg	Neg

NOTE: Positive (+) antigen is present on the commercial RBCs, Neg (−) negative-the antigen is absent on the commercial RBCs. Each vial contains the RBCs of one donor. Probable unexpected antibody is anti-c.

cells would be destroyed by the patient's antibodies. Even if the patient's serum did contain an unexpected antibody, it would be detected only if the donor's cells contained the corresponding antigen. For this reason, an antibody screening is performed.

Crossmatch Procedure

The traditional crossmatch involves mixing serum and a 2% to 4% suspension of cells in saline solution in a test tube. An immediate centrifugation is performed, and the test tubes are observed for the presence of agglutination or hemolysis. At this stage, ABO incompatibility will be observable, as will incompatibility caused by antibodies of the P, MNSs, Lewis, Lutheran, or Wright systems.

If the test is negative at this point, the test tube is incubated at 37°C for a sufficient time and observed again. Saline solution–reacting antibodies of the Rh-Hr and Lewis systems will be detected, and antibodies of the P, MNSs, and Kell systems may sometimes react at this stage. If the crossmatch is still negative, it may be further tested using the AHG crossmatch.

Antihuman Globulin Crossmatch

The AHG crossmatch is an extension of the traditional crossmatch procedure. After incubation at 37°C, the cells are thoroughly washed with saline solution. The AHG serum is added and the test carried out as recommended by the manufacturer. This is an indirect test between the patient and the prospective donor. The crossmatch will detect most Rh antibodies. In addition, it may be the only means of detecting some antibodies, especially in the Duffy, Kidd, and Kell blood group systems. The AHG crossmatch is no longer necessary when the patient's serum has been previously screened for unexpected antibodies with reagent cells and has no previous history of clinically significant antibodies.

Abbreviated Crossmatch

For an abbreviated (immediate spin) crossmatch, only a crossmatch procedure designed to detect ABO incompatibility is required. This consists of testing the donor cells and patient serum (major crossmatch) at room temperature by immediate spin or by centrifugation after incubation for 5 minutes.

Other Crossmatching Techniques

As in typing procedures, several other techniques may be applied to crossmatching and antibody screening. Gel technique can be used. Low-ionic-strength (LIS) salt solution may be used to ensure the formation of antigen-antibody complexes. Hexadimethrine has been used as a rapid and sensitive crossmatch method. It is useful in detecting ABO incompatibility when the patient has demonstrated a negative antibody screen. Microplate methods for antibody detection using LIS salt solution are also used to screen large numbers of sera for unexpected antibodies. A technique that uses polyethylene glycol (PEG) is also used for antibody detection and identification. This may be used as a supplement to more conventional methods when weak reactions are encountered.

Electronic Crossmatching

Computer crossmatching may be used in transfusion services when it is permissible to omit the AHG phase of the crossmatch and perform only a procedure to detect ABO compatibility. The computerized selection of RBCs may be used if regulatory requirements met.

Fully automated systems (e.g., Ortho Provue) are based on column agglutination gel testing. Systems such as this use bar-coding technology for total automation of blood typing, antibody screening, and crossmatching. The crossmatch is referred to as an *electronic crossmatch*.

Adverse Effects of Transfusion

Clinically, the result of RBC destruction is a transfusion reaction. The signs and symptoms of a transfusion reaction vary from patient to patient. Generally, chills, high temperature, pain in the lower back, nausea, vomiting, and shock, as indicated by decreased blood pressure and rapid pulse, characterize an immediate reaction. These first effects of the reaction are rarely fatal, but the byproducts of RBC destruction pose many problems, primarily severe renal involvement. A patient may eventually die from kidney failure.

Although the most life-threatening transfusion reaction is the hemolytic reaction that occurs with the destruction of incompatible RBCs by antibodies in the patient's serum (usually ABO incompatibility), several other forms of transfusion reaction exist, with varying severity to the patient. Adverse effects of transfusion (Table 18-11) can generally be characterized as **immune** or **nonimmune**. Both immunologic and nonimmunologic types can occur as **immediate adverse effects of transfusion.**

Immediate Immunologic Adverse Reactions

More than 850 patients receive transfusions intended for someone else each year in the United States, and at least 20 of these patients die from complications.[4] Most of these errors result from

TABLE 18-11

Immunologic Adverse Effects of Transfusion		
Type of Reaction	Examples	Characteristic of Reaction
Immediate immune	Hemolytic, febrile, allergic, anaphylactic, and TRALI	Manifested as abrupt lysing of blood cells due to antigen-antibody reaction
Immediate nonimmune	Bacterial contamination, nonimmune hemolysis, circulatory overload	
Delayed immune	Alloimmunization, delayed hemolytic GVHD	Manifested as decrease in normal RBC survival due to coating of RBCs by antibodies and removal of these cells by mononuclear phagocytic system
Delayed nonimmune	Iron overload, disease transmission	

clerical rather than technical errors. A new monitoring technology called *radiofrequency identification* (RFID) is being introduced in transfusion medicine. RFID allows patients to wear wristbands that transmit their blood type by tiny radio signals. Microchips are embedded into both the wristband and the unit of blood. If sensors detect a difference between the signals coming from the wristband and from the microchip in the blood bag, a computer will flash a message. Another safety system is the bar coding of patient wristbands and blood bags (see Chapter 3).

Other immediate immunologic Adverse Effects of Transfusion include febrile nonhemolytic reactions, usually a reaction to the donor's granulocytes. Anaphylaxis from antibody to IgA, urticaria (hives) from antibody to plasma proteins, and noncardiac pulmonary edema from antibody to leukocytes or complement activation are other immediate immunologic causes of Adverse Effects of Transfusion.

Transfusion-related acute lung injury (TRALI) has been identified as a life-threatening complication of transfusion, with significant morbidity and mortality. It is reported to be the third most common cause of fatal effects of transfusion.[5] TRALI is thought to result from the interaction of specific leukocyte antibodies with leukocytes.

Immediate Nonimmunologic Adverse Reactions

Immediate nonimmunologic transfusion reactions include marked fever with shock from bacterial contamination, congestive heart failure from increased blood volume, and hemolysis of infused RBCs from the physical destruction of cells, such as from freezing or overheating or mixing nonisotonic solutions with RBCs.

Delayed Adverse Reactions

Delayed hemolysis may occur from prior sensitization to RBC antigens by antibodies that are not present or detectable in the RBCs immediately before transfusion. Graft-versus-host disease may result from engraftment of transfused functional lymphocytes. Purpura (presence of purple patches on skin and mucous membranes) from bleeding may be caused by the development of antiplatelet antibodies. Also, the patient may be sensitized and may form antibodies to donor antigens on red cells, white cells, platelets, or plasma protein. Other delayed nonimmunologic adverse effects include iron overload from multiple (>100) transfusions and disease transmission as a result of transfusion (e.g., hepatitis, HIV, protozoan infections).

HEMOLYTIC DISEASE OF THE FETUS AND NEWBORN (HDFN)

Pathophysiology

Hemolytic disease of the fetus and newborn (HDFN) occurs when a baby inherits an antigen for which the mother is negative. The disease most often involves antigens of the Rh and ABO blood group systems, although it may result from incompatibilities in virtually any RBC group system. For HDNF to occur, the fetus must be positive for an antigen and the mother must be negative.

This condition develops while the fetus is in the uterus. The mechanism involves sensitization or immunization of the mother to foreign antigen present on her child's RBCs. Although the circulatory systems of a mother and her child are separate, and only small molecules such as nutrients can cross the placenta, some seepage of fetal RBCs can occur into the mother's circulatory system, most likely very late in pregnancy or at birth. If any incompatible fetal RBCs enter the mother's circulatory system, she can develop an antibody to the antigen on them. If immunization occurs, it is permanent. The antibody formed by the mother is of the IgG type, and it can cross the placenta into the circulatory system of the fetus, where it reacts with corresponding antigen on the RBCs of the fetus, with resultant destruction of the cells. HDNF is the condition that exists when maternal antibody crosses the placenta and reacts with antigen on fetal RBCs. This was the cause of stillbirth of the child delivered by a woman studied by Levine and Stetson in 1939, which led to the discovery of the Rh blood group system.

ABO Antigens

HDFN most often occurs as a result of antigens in the ABO system. In this case the mother is usually group O and the child inherits the A or B antigen from the father. Group O individuals have a relatively high concentration of IgG anti-A and anti-B in addition to IgM anti-A and anti-B antibody. This immune IgG antibody can cross the placenta and react with the corresponding antigen on the RBCs of the fetus. Although ABO sensitization may occur often, hemolytic disease caused by ABO incompatibility is less severe. The child may be only mildly affected and may require little or no treatment.

Rh Antigens

Severe HDNF most often involves the Rh blood group system (e.g., D antigen) followed by anti-c and anti-Kell. In the case of Rh incompatibility, the mother is negative for D (d/d), and the father is positive for D. The child inherits this antigen from the father and is D positive (D/d). If any of the D-positive RBCs of the fetus cross into the mother's circulatory system, she may develop an immune anti-D antibody. This IgG crosses the placenta and reacts with the RBCs of the fetus.

Sensitization usually occurs only very late in pregnancy or at delivery, so the first child is rarely affected by HDNF. Subsequent pregnancies with children who are D negative theoretically are not affected by anti-D antibody in the mother's circulatory system. For this reason, determining the most probable genotype of the parents in possible cases of HDNF may be useful in predicting the chance of occurrence of the disease. For example, if the father is heterozygous for the D antigen (D/d) and the mother is D negative (d/d), chances are that only half the children will inherit the D antigen (Fig. 18-6). On the other hand, if the father is homozygous for D (D/D), the children will inherit the D antigen, and there is a 100% chance of HDNF. About 1 in 10 pregnancies involve an Rh-negative mother and an Rh-positive father.

The first child is rarely affected by HDNF. Fewer than 20% of Rh-negative women actually become immunized during pregnancy. Although a woman can have one or two children who are both Rh positive and encounter no difficulties, her immunization is permanent. Once the disease develops in one child, subsequent children positive for the

FIGURE 18-6 Chance for development of hemolytic disease of the fetus and newborn (HDFN). Chance is based on genotypes for the D antigen.

antigen are likely to be affected at least as severely. If a woman has been sensitized before pregnancy as a result of transfusion of incompatible RBCs or injection of antigenic material, even the first child can be severely affected. Anti-D antibody is the most common cause of HDNF. Other antibodies causing the disease include anti-c, anti-K (Kell), anti-E, and even incompatibilities in the ABO system.

Laboratory Tests

Many laboratory tests are performed in cases of HDNF, on the parents' (primarily the mother's) RBCs before birth and on the child's RBCs after birth. The first step is to type the mother for ABO and Rh early in pregnancy. The mother's serum is usually screened by means of the indirect AHG test to see if an antibody exists. If an antibody is found, it is identified and the titer determined. This titer is rechecked throughout pregnancy as a monitor of the possible severity of the disease. An increasing titer indicates an active immune response.

After birth, several tests can be performed on the child's red cells, in addition to further tests on the maternal serum. Initially, a sample of umbilical cord RBCs is tested for ABO group and Rh type, and a direct AHG test is performed. Other laboratory tests that may be performed on the child's RBCs include hemoglobin determinations, blood smear examination and differential, reticulocyte count, and serum bilirubin determination.

The decision to perform exchange transfusion will depend on a combination of laboratory results and the clinical condition of the child. Preparation can and should be made before birth so the exchange can be done as soon as possible if necessary.

Detection of Fetal Hemoglobin

Fetal hemoglobin, or hemoglobin F (Hb F), can be measured by various techniques; most measure the amount of Hb F. Techniques used include:

- Acid elution technique (modified Kleihauer-Betke test)
- Chromatography

- Ion-exchange high-performance liquid chromatography (HPLC) for hemoglobins
- Reverse-phase HPLC for globin chains
- Flow cytometry based on antibodies against Hb F

ACID ELUTION STAIN (MODIFIED KLEIHAUER-BETKE METHOD)

This stain is based on the fact that fetal hemoglobin is resistant to acid elution (separation of a substance by extraction), whereas adult hemoglobin is not. That is, when a thin blood smear is exposed to an acid buffer, the adult RBC loses its hemoglobin into the buffer, leaving only the RBC stroma, but the fetal RBC is unaffected and retains its hemoglobin. The smears are examined under the microscope after staining, and the percentage of fetal cells in the maternal RBCs is used to calculate the approximate volume of fetal hemorrhage into the maternal circulation.

FLOW CYTOMETRY

Flow cytometric analysis permits the distinction of true fetal cells, which contain Hb F as the major form of hemoglobin, from maternal circulating F cells, which have lower cellular Hb F content.[3]

Treatment

When HDNF does occur, it varies considerably in severity. In its most severe form (anti-D) the infant may be stillborn or severely affected at birth. In other cases (e.g., ABO incompatibility) a baby is usually mildly affected. Severely affected infants are exposed to the products of RBC destruction and develop anemia. The cell destruction results in a hemolytic anemia accompanied by abnormal levels of serum bilirubin, with the clinical appearance of jaundice. The accumulation of bilirubin can result in irreversible brain damage (kernicterus) if present in extremely elevated concentration. If the child survives and is not treated adequately, the brain damage will result in severe mental retardation.

Treatment for infants with severe HDNF includes RBC exchange transfusion. In an exchange transfusion, a significant proportion of the child's RBCs is replaced with transfused red cells. The exchange transfusion corrects the anemia and removes the abnormal levels of serum bilirubin, at least temporarily, and can prevent brain damage. The procedure may need to be repeated several times, depending on the level of bilirubin accumulation.

The type of RBCs used for transfusion depends on the antibody responsible for the disease. Use of O-negative red cells is the most common

selection. The RBCs must be negative for the antigen against which the antibody has been formed. The child is given blood that is compatible with the mother. In HDNF caused by the formation of anti-D antibody in the mother's serum, the child is transfused with RBCs that are specific for the child's own ABO type but negative for the D antigen. This is because not all the child's blood is replaced at the time of exchange, and some maternal antibody is left. RBCs are given that will not react with the remaining antibody and will not harm the child. In cases of ABO incompatibility that require exchange, the mother is usually group O and the child group A or B. In such cases, the child is transfused with group O RBCs of the child's Rh type.

In cases of severe HDNF, it is sometimes necessary to attempt to treat the fetus before birth. This intrauterine transfusion may be necessary to correct severe anemia and prevent death in utero (stillbirth) when the risk of early delivery is too great. In such cases, based on maternal antibody titer, obstetric history, and ultrasound, an amniocentesis is performed. The amniotic fluid is tested for bilirubin level and fetal maturity. If the fetus appears to be severely affected, an intrauterine transfusion may be indicated. In an intrauterine transfusion, packed RBCs are infused through the fetal abdominal wall into the peritoneum. Direct transfusion into the umbilical vein may also be attempted.

Prevention of Rh Immunization (Use of Rh Immune Globulin)

In the 1960s a dramatic decrease in the incidence of HDNF was seen in the United States and other developed countries following the introduction of **Rh immune globulin (RhIG),** which could prevent immunization to the D antigen during and immediately after pregnancy. This was an extremely important advance, and the incidence of immunization by pregnancy to the Rh antigen D is very different now. It was found that if RhIG is injected within 72 hours of delivery into Rh-negative women who deliver Rh-positive babies, they are well protected against Rh problems in subsequent pregnancies.

The use of RhIG is based on interference with recognition of the Rh antigen on the fetal cells by the mother's immune system. This blocking interference prevents immunization (sensitization) by the fetus Rh-positive RBCs. The mother is passively immunized by the administration of RhIG when recognition of foreign antigen on the maternal RBCs (sensitization) by fetal RBCs is most likely. Most exposure to fetal blood occurs at delivery.

RhIG is injected intramuscularly within 72 hours of delivery in mothers (1) who are D negative, (2) who have no detectable anti-D antibody, and (3) whose newborns are D positive.

Antepartum treatment at 28 weeks' gestation has also been advocated by the American College of Obstetricians and Gynecologists. If done, a sample of RBCs obtained immediately before treatment should be tested for ABO group, Rh type, antibody screen, and identification of antibody, if present.

RhIG is supplied as a sterile, clear, approximately 1-mL solution to be injected intramuscularly. It is a concentrated solution (300 µg/mL) of IgG anti-D that may be derived from human plasma. It does not transmit hepatitis, HIV, or other detectable infectious diseases.

The anti-D antibody can be detected 12 to 60 hours after the administration of RhIG and is sometimes found for as long as 5 months thereafter. If it is detected 6 months after delivery, active immunization and failure of the RhIG can be assumed. Such failures are infrequent, but they can occur if RhIG is given too late or in too small a dose, or if Rh immunization has already occurred during the pregnancy. Most of the D-positive fetal cells enter the maternal circulation at delivery. The amount of fetal RBCs present in the maternal circulation is important for the RhIG dosage.

If the amount of Rh-positive fetal RBCs entering the mother's circulation is greater than 30 mL of whole blood, the standard dose of RhIG is not enough to prevent anti-D antibody formation. Thus, it is important to determine the presence and amount of fetomaternal hemorrhage. This may be done by acid elution or enzyme-linked antiglobulin testing.

CASE STUDIES

CASE STUDY 18-1

A well-hydrated male infant was 1 day old when the neonatologist observed he was beginning to appear jaundiced. This baby was the first child of a 30-year-old computer analyst who had no previous obstetric history or history of prior blood transfusion. The pregnancy had been normal.

Total bilirubin, hemoglobin/hematocrit, blood type/Rh, and direct antiglobulin tests were ordered for the baby. A cord blood sample had not been collected at delivery. Blood grouping and Rh testing and a screening test for unexpected antibodies were requested for the mother.

Laboratory Data
Neonatal results:
   Total bilirubin: 10.8 mg/dL
   Hemoglobin: 16.9 g/dL
   Hematocrit: 52%
   Blood group and Rh: A, Rh positive
   Direct antiglobulin test: Negative
Maternal results:
   Blood group and Rh: O, Rh negative
   Unexpected antibody screen: Negative

Treatment
The baby was immediately started on phototherapy. Subsequent total bilirubin tests were no higher than the 24-hour value and continued to decrease over the next 48 hours. At discharge, the total bilirubin was 6.9 mg/dL.

1. The most probable cause of the infant's jaundice is:
   a. prematurity.
   b. dehydration.
   c. milk allergy.
   d. blood group incompatibility between mother and baby.

2. The treatment of choice is:
   a. phototherapy.
   b. exchange transfusion.
   c. rehydration with electrolytes.
   d. all of the above.

3. What is the most likely diagnosis?
   a. ABO incompatibility between mother and baby
   b. Rh incompatibility between mother and baby
   c. Hemolytic disease of the fetus and newborn (HDFN)
   d. Both a and c

CASE STUDY 18-2

This 18-year-old man was admitted with multiple injuries after he and a passenger were in a motorcycle accident. After receiving 50 mL of the first unit of RBCs, he developed shaking chills and became hypotensive with a falling blood pressure. The unit of cells was immediately discontinued, and the transfusion service was notified of the situation.

A recheck of testing was requested immediately.

Laboratory Testing
Clerical check: No evidence of clerical errors
Hemoglobinemia: Slight hemolysis observed
Direct Antiglobulin Test
   Patient pretransfusion: Negative
   Patient posttransfusion: Weakly positive
Recheck of Blood Grouping
   Patient pretransfusion: A positive
   Patient posttransfusion: O positive
   Donor: A positive
Repeat Crossmatches
   Patient pretransfusion + Donor red blood cells = Compatible
   Patient posttransfusion + Donor red blood cells = Incompatible

1. What is the most probable cause of the incompatible crossmatch?
   a. A mix-up in the patient specimens
   b. A mix-up in the transfused units
   c. Rh incompatibility
   d. None of the above

2. What type of transfusion reaction did the patient experience?
   a. Immediate hemolytic
   b. Delayed hemolytic
   c. Immediate nonhemolytic
   d. Delayed nonhemolytic

3. Could this type of transfusion reaction be fatal?
   a. Yes
   b. No

REFERENCES

1. Dunsford I, Bowley CC, editors: Techniques in blood grouping, Edinburgh, 1955, Oliver & Boyd, Preface.
2. Brecher ME, editor: AABB technical manual, ed 14, Bethesda, Md, 2002, American Association of Blood Banks.
3. Fibach E: Flow cytometric analysis of fetal hemoglobin in RBC and their precursors, www.enco.co.il (retrieved December 2005).
4. Allen S: System targets blood-type mix-ups, www.boston.com (retrieved July 2005).
5. MacLennan S: Transfusion related acute lung injury (TRALI), April 2003, National Blood Service Transfusion Medicine Clinical Policies Group, Washington, DC.
6. ISBT 128 The Global Standard www.iccbba.org/
7. Petrides M, et al: Practical guide to transfusion medicine, ed 2, Bethesda, MD, 2007, AABB Press.
8. AABB technical manual, ed 16, Bethesda Md, 2008, American Association of Blood Banks.

BIBLIOGRAPHY

American Association of Blood Banks (AABB): Technical Manual, ed 15, Bethesda, MD, 2005, AABB.
Blaney KD, Howard PR: Basic and applied concepts of immunohematology, ed 2, St. Louis, 2009, Mosby.
Henry JB: Clinical diagnosis and management by laboratory methods, ed 21, Philadelphia, 2007, Saunders.
Malloy D, editor: Immunohematology methods, Rockville, MD, 1993, American National Red Cross.
Rudmann SV: Textbook of blood banking and transfusion medicine, ed 2, Philadelphia, 2005, Saunders.

REVIEW QUESTIONS

Questions 1-8: Match each of the following terms with its definition (a to h).

1. ___ Allele

2. ___ Transfusion medicine

3. ___ Red blood cell (RBC) and fresh frozen plasma

4. ___ Genotype

5. ___ Immune antibody

6. ___ Immunohematology

7. ___ Isoantibody

8. ___ Phenotype
   a. Actual genetic makeup; may not be evident by direct tests.
   b. Antibodies that appear to exist without antigenic stimulus, such as anti-A and anti-B antibodies in ABO system.
   c. RBC (blood) type, as determined direct tests.
   d. The procedures involved in collecting, storing, processing, and distributing blood and its components.
   e. The technique of replacing whole blood and its components.
   f. The techniques and procedures involving the study of the immunologic responses of blood (RBCs).
   g. Unexpected antibodies that result from specific antigenic stimulation.
   h. Variants of a gene for a particular trait.

Questions 9-13: Indicate whether the following statements are A = True or B = False.

9. ___ A positive reaction in transfusion medicine procedures is seen as hemolysis or agglutination.

10. ___ Agglutination is clumping caused by the presence of any antigen present on red cells.

11. ___ An antiserum is a solution of antigens.

12. ___ Blood (RBC) group tests in general may be performed either on a microscope slide or in a test tube.

13. ___ For hemolysis to be seen as a positive reaction in transfusion medicine procedures, complement must be present in the serum.

Questions 14-17: Match the genotypes in the ABO blood group system with the corresponding phenotypes (a to c). (An answer may be used more than once.)

14. ___ AO

15. ___ BO

16. ___ BB

17. ___ AB
   a. AB
   b. A
   c. B

18. When blood is to be transfused, the most important consideration is:
   a. Does the donor's serum contain an antibody against the patient's RBCs?
   b. Do the patient's RBCs contain an antigen against the donor's serum?
   c. Does the donor's serum contain an antibody against the patient's RBCs?
   d. Does the patient's serum contain an antibody against the donor's RBCs?

19. Patients are generally described as Rh positive or Rh negative based on the presence of which of the following antigens on the RBCs?
   a. C
   b. c
   c. D
   d. E
   e. e

Questions 20 and 21: *Match the type of antiglobulin test with the statement concerning antihuman globulin testing (a and b).*

20. ___ Direct antiglobulin test (DAT)

21. ___ Indirect antiglobulin test
   a. Test performed on RBCs suspected of being coated with antibody.
   b. Test performed on serum suspected of containing antibodies.

22. The most important reason for the decrease in the number of cases of hemolytic disease of the fetus and newborn (HDFN) is the:
   a. acid elution stain.
   b. more correct Rh typing.
   c. use of improved typing procedures.
   d. use of Rh immune globulin.

Questions 23-27: *A = True; B = False.*
   Which of the following is part of usual compatibility testing?

23. ___ ABO and Rh typing of donor and recipient.

24. ___ Correct identification of donor and recipient.

25. ___ Crossmatching of the donor's RBCs with the patient serum.

26. ___ Crossmatching of the patient's RBCs with the donor serum.

27. ___ Testing of the patient's serum with a panel of group O cells for unexpected antibodies.

28. Compatibility testing is used to help detect:
   a. some ABO incompatibilities.
   b. some errors in labeling, recording, or identification.
   c. unexpected antibodies in the patient's serum.
   d. all of the above.

29. Which of the following are generally characterized as a transfusion reaction?
   a. Hemolytic
   b. Febrile
   c. Allergic
   d. All of the above

30. Which of the following tests is required in the screening of potential blood donors for transfusion-transmitted disease?
   a. Hepatitis B surface antigen (HBsAg)
   b. Hepatitis C antibody (HCV)
   c. Hepatitis B core antibody (HBc)
   d. All of the above

Questions 31-36: *Match each of the following components or blood derivatives with the use or statement (a to f).*

31. __ Factor VIII

32. __ Crystalloid solutions or plasma substitutes

33. __ Fresh frozen plasma

34. __ Packed red blood cells

35. __ Platelet concentrates

36. __ Whole blood
   a. Bleeding caused by low or dysfunctional platelets.
   b. Rarely, if ever, used in transfusion.
   c. Restore or maintain blood volume.
   d. Restore or maintain oxygen-carrying capacity.
   e. Source of labile clotting factors.
   f. Treatment of severe von Willebrand's disease.

APPENDIX A

NAACLS CLINICAL ASSISTANT COMPETENCIES

With permission NAACLS

CORE MODULE

These competencies describe duties at a level below that of the established Clinical Laboratory Technician/ Medical Laboratory Technician. As a member of the health care delivery team, the clinical assistant works under the supervision of an appropriate qualified person. Note: The instructional content appropriate to the achievement of these Competencies should be consistent with the entry level job responsibilities.

1.0 Define the role of the clinical assistant in the healthcare delivery system as it relates to the point of care or clinical laboratory environment.

2.0 Use common medical terminology.

3.0 Demonstrate knowledge of infection control and safety practices.

    3.1 Demonstrate accepted practices for infection control, isolation techniques, aseptic techniques and methods for disease prevention.

    3.2 Comply with federal, state and locally mandated regulations regarding safety practices.

        3.21 Use the OSHA Universal Precaution Standards.

        3.22 Use prescribed procedures to handle electrical, radiation, biological and fire hazards.

        3.23 Use appropriate practices, as outlined in the OSHA Hazard Communication Standard, including the correct use of the Material Safety Data Sheet as directed.

4.0 Follow standard operating procedures to collect specimens.

4.1 Demonstrate basic knowledge of the circulatory, urinary, and other body systems necessary to perform assigned specimen collection tasks.

4.2 Describe the difference between whole blood, serum, and plasma.

4.3 Identify and use blood collection equipment.

    4.31 Identify the additive by the evacuated tube color.

    4.32 Identify and properly use equipment needed to collect blood by venipuncture and capillary (skin) puncture.

4.4 Collect blood specimens by venipuncture.

4.5 Collect blood specimens by capillary (skin) puncture.

4.6 Identify special precautions necessary during blood collections by venipuncture and capillary (skin) puncture.

4.7 List and apply the criteria that would lead to rejection or recollection of a patient sample.

4.8 Instruct patients in the proper collection and preservation for various samples, including:

- blood.
- sputum.
- stools.

5.0 Prepare blood and body fluid specimens for analysis according to standard operating procedures.

5.1 Follow standard operating procedures for labeling, transport, and processing of specimens, including transport to reference laboratories.

5.2 Describe and follow the criteria for specimens and test results that will be used as legal evidence.

6.0 Prepare/reconstitute reagents, standards and controls according to standard operating procedure.

6.1 Follow laboratory protocol for storage and suitability of reagents standards and controls.

6.2 Recognize and report contamination and/or deterioration in reagents, standards, and controls.

7.0 Perform appropriate tests at the clinical assistant level, according to standard operating procedures.

7.1 Compare test results to reference intervals.

7.2 Record results by manual method or computer according to laboratory protocol.

7.3 Report STAT results of completed tests according to laboratory protocol.

7.4 Recognize critical values and follow established protocol regarding reporting.

7.5 Clean glass and plastic labware.

7.6 Use pipetting equipment.

7.7 Use measurement equipment such as beakers and flasks.

8.0 Perform and record vital sign measurements.

8.1 Perform and record blood pressure measurement.

8.2 Perform and record pulse rate.

8.3 Perform and record body temperature.

8.4 Recognize and report abnormal values for vital sign measurement, using predetermined criteria.

9.0 Follow established quality control protocols to include maintenance and calibration of equipment.

9.1 Perform quality control procedures.

9.2 Record quality control results.

9.3 Identify and report control results that do not meet predetermined criteria.

10.0 Communicate (verbally and nonverbally) effectively and appropriately in the workplace.

10.1 Maintain confidentiality of privileged information about individuals.

10.2 Value diversity in the workplace.

10.3 Interact appropriately and professionally with other individuals.

10.4 Discuss the major points of the American Hospital Association's Patient's Bill of Rights or the Patient's Bill of Rights from the institution.

10.5 Model professional appearance and appropriate behavior.

10.6 Follow written and verbal instructions in carrying out testing procedures.

11.0 Use information systems necessary to accomplish job functions.

12.0 Identify and report potential preanalytical errors that may occur during specimen collection, labeling, transporting, and processing.

CHEMISTRY MODULE

These competencies describe duties at a level below that of the established Clinical Laboratory Technician/Medical Laboratory Technician. As a member of the health care delivery team, the clinical assistant works under the supervision of an appropriate qualified person. Note: The instructional content appropriate to the achievement of these Competencies should be consistent with the entry level job responsibilities. In developing this module, please refer to the competencies in the Core Module.

1.0 Use common clinical chemistry terminology as it relates to the point-of-care or clinical laboratory environment.

2.0 Prepare, store, and dispose of specimens for chemistry analysis according to standard operating procedures.

3.0 Determine suitability of specimens for chemistry procedures according to:
- the test requested.
- appropriate patient preparation/method of collection.
- time of collection/processing.
- storage.
- hemolysis/lipemia and interfering substances.

4.0 Assemble/prepare reagents, standards and controls for chemistry tests.

5.0 Perform appropriate tests at the clinical assistant level.

6.0 Recognize technical testing errors for each test performed.

7.0 Report results of procedures using predetermined criteria.

8.0 Follow established quality control procedures specific to chemistry tests, including maintenance and instrument calibration.

9.0 Maintain inventory control and supplies for chemistry tests.

DONOR ROOM COLLECTION/ SCREENING AND COMPONENT PROCESSING MODULE

These competencies describe duties at a level below that of the established Clinical Laboratory

Technician/Medical Laboratory Technician. As a member of the health care delivery team, the clinical assistant works under the supervision of an appropriate qualified person. Note: The instructional content appropriate to the achievement of these Competencies should be consistent with the entry level job responsibilities.

1.0 Use common donor room, collection processing, and component preparation terminology as it relates to the point-of-care or clinical laboratory environment.

2.0 According to standard operating procedures, perform donor screening.
   2.1 Complete donor medical/social history.
   2.2 Complete measurement of donor temperature.
   2.3 Complete donor hemoglobin measurement.
   2.4 Complete blood pressure measurement.
   2.5 Perform donor pulse rate.

3.0 Perform unit collection procedures as defined by established regulations.
   3.1 Follow the procedure for donor identification.
   3.2 Follow the proper skin preparation procedure, and describe its importance.
   3.3 Perform donor collection, donor assessment during and after collection, and troubleshooting actions for inadequate blood flow and donor reaction.
   3.4 Strip unit tubing, mix and package for transport.

4.0 Follow procedures for the component preparation system.
   4.1 Prepare components according to established regulations.
   4.2 Follow the procedure for packing and shipping of collected blood bags and testing tubes.
   4.3 Receive and distribute collected blood components.
   4.4 Prepare packed red blood cells, plasma, platelets, and cryoprecipitates.
   4.5 Follow storage requirements for blood and blood components.

5.0 Follow established quality control procedures specific to donor room collection/component screening, including maintenance and instrument calibration.
   5.1 Comply with current Good Manufacturing Practices (GMP).
   5.2 Determine suitability of specimens according to predetermined criteria.

6.0 Follow predetermined criteria for unit suitability and lot release.

7.0 Maintain inventory control and supplies for donor screening, collection processing, and component preparation.

HEMATOLOGY MODULE

These competencies describe duties at a level below that of the established Clinical Laboratory Technician/Medical Laboratory Technician. As a member of the health care delivery team, the clinical assistant works under the supervision of an appropriate qualified person. Note: The instructional content appropriate to the achievement of these Competencies should be consistent with the entry level job responsibilities. In developing this module, please refer to the competencies in the Core Module.

1.0 Use common hematology terminology as it relates to the point-of-care or clinical laboratory environment.

2.0 Prepare, store, and dispose of specimens for hematology analysis according to standard operating procedures.

3.0 Determine suitability of specimens for hematology procedures related to:
   • the test requested.
   • appropriate patient preparation/method of collection.
   • time of collection/processing.
   • storage.
   • interfering substances.

4.0 Assemble/prepare reagents, standards, and controls for hematology tests.

5.0 Prepare and stain slides for further analysis.

6.0 Perform hematology procedures at the clinical assistant level.

7.0 Recognize technical testing errors for each test performed.

8.0 Follow established quality control procedures specific to hematology tests, including maintenance and instrument calibration.

9.0 Maintain inventory control and supplies for hematology tests.

IMMUNOLOGY MODULE

These competencies describe duties at a level below that of the established Clinical Laboratory Technician/Medical Laboratory Technician. As a member of the health care delivery team, the clinical assistant works under the supervision of an appropriate qualified person. Note: The instructional content appropriate to the achievement of these Competencies should be consistent with the entry level job responsibilities. In developing this module, please refer to the competencies in the Core Module.

1.0 Use common immunology terminology as it relates to the point-of-care or clinical laboratory environment.

2.0 Prepare, store, and dispose of specimens for immunology testing according to standard operating procedures.

3.0 Determine suitability of specimens for immunology procedures related to:
- the test requested.
- appropriate patient preparation/ method of collection.
- time of collection/processing.
- storage.
- interfering substances.

4.0 Assemble/prepare reagents, standards, and controls for immunology tests.

5.0 Perform immunology tests at the clinical assistant level.

6.0 Recognize technical testing errors for each test performed.

7.0 Report results of tests using predetermined criteria.

8.0 Follow established quality control procedures specific to immunology tests, including maintenance and instrument calibration.

9.0 Maintain inventory control and supplies for immunology tests.

MICROBIOLOGY MODULE

These competencies describe duties at a level below that of the established Clinical Laboratory Technician/ Medical Laboratory Technician. As a member of the health care delivery team, the clinical assistant works under the supervision of an appropriate qualified person. Note: The instructional content appropriate to the achievement of these Competencies should be consistent with the entry level job responsibilities. In developing this module, please refer to the competencies in the Core Module.

1.0 Use common microbiology terminology as it relates to the point-of-care or clinical laboratory environment.

2.0 Follow special safety procedures and aseptic technique required for processing microbiology specimens.

3.0 Prepare, store, dispose of, and properly transport specimens for microbiology testing according to standard operating procedure.

4.0 Determine suitability of specimens for microbiology procedures related to:
- the test requested.
- appropriate patient preparation/ method of collection.
- time of collection/processing.
- storage.
- interfering substances.

5.0 Assemble/prepare reagents, standards, and controls for microbiology procedures.

6.0 Prepare and stain slides for further analysis.

7.0 Perform microbiology testing at the clinical assistant level.

8.0 Recognize technical errors for each test performed.

9.0 Report results of procedures using predetermined criteria.

10.0 Perform predetermined quality control procedures specific to microbiology testing, including maintenance and instrument calibration.

11.0 Maintain inventory control and supplies for microbiology procedures.

URINALYSIS MODULE

These competencies describe duties at a level below that of the established Clinical Laboratory Technician/ Medical Laboratory Technician. As a member of the health care delivery team, the clinical assistant works under the supervision of an appropriate qualified person. Note: The instructional content appropriate to the achievement of these Competencies should be consistent with the entry level job responsibilities. In developing this module, please refer to the competencies in the Core Module.

1.0 Use common urinalysis terminology as it relates to the point-of-care or clinical laboratory environment.

2.0 Prepare, store, dispose of, and properly transport specimens for urinalysis testing according to standard operating procedure.

3.0 Instruct patients in the proper collection and preservation for various urine samples, including:
- mid-stream.
- random.
- clean catch.
- timed collections.
- collections for drug screening.
- urine pregnancy tests.

4.0 Determine suitability of specimens for urinalysis procedures related to:
- the test requested.
- appropriate patient preparation/ method of collection.
- time of collection/processing.
- storage.
- interfering substances.

5.0 Assemble/prepare reagents, standards, and controls for urinalysis testing.

6.0 Prepare slides for microscopic examination.

7.0 Perform urinalysis tests at the clinical assistant level.

8.0 Recognize technical errors for each test performed.

9.0 Report results of tests using predetermined criteria.

10.0 Perform predetermined quality control procedures for urinalysis tests, including maintenance and instrument calibration.

11.0 Maintain inventory control and supplies for urinalysis testing.

APPENDIX B

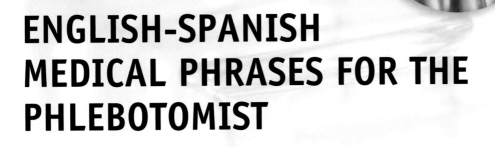

ENGLISH-SPANISH MEDICAL PHRASES FOR THE PHLEBOTOMIST

Medical Phrases	Frases Médica
Common Terms and Phrases	
Hello	¡Hola!
Good morning	Buenos días
Good afternoon	Buenas tardes
Good evening	Buenas noches
Please, come in	Por favor., pase usted
My name is	Me llamo es _____.
Who is the patient?	¿Quién es el (la) paciente?
What is your name?	¿Cómo se llama usted?
It is nice to meet you.	Mucho gusto en conocerle.
How are you?	¿Cómo está usted?
I need for you to sign this form.	Necesito que usted firme este formulario.
Please	Por favor
Thank you	Gracias
Yes	Sí
No	No
Did you come alone?	¿Vivo usted solo(a)?
Who brought you?	¿Quién le trajo?
Where were you born?	¿Dónde nació usted?
Where do you live?	¿Dónde vive usted?
What is your address?	¿Cuál es su dirección?

Medical Phrases	Frases Médica
Specimen Collection	
I'm going to take a blood sample.	La presión sanguinea.
I need to prick your finger to obtain a specimen.	Necesito pincharle el dedo para obtener una muestra.
Are you comfortable?	¿Está usted confortable?
I need to apply a tourniquet around your arm.	Tengo que ponerle un torniquete alrededor del brazo.
You're going to feel a needlestick.	Usted va a sentir un piquete de aguja.
This glucometer is used to measure your blood sugar.	Este glucómetro se usa para medir el azúcar en la sangre.
You need to provide a urine specimen.	Tiene usted que darnos un espécimen de orina.
Phlebotomy Complications	
Please, bend over forward.	Por favor, inclínese usted hacia atrás.
Please, lean forward.	Por favor, inclínese usted hacia atrás.
Please, lie down.	Por favor, acuéstese usted.
Please, lie on your back.	Por favor, acuéstese usted boca arriba.
Do you need a blanket?	¿Necesita usted una manta (cobija)?
You can use the emesis basin if you need to vomit.	Usted puede usar esta cubeta si tiene que vomitar.

Adapted from McElroy OH, Grabb LL: Spanish-English, English-Spanish medical dictionary, ed 3, Baltimore, 2005, Lippincott Williams & Wilkins, and English & Spanish medical words & phrases, ed 3, Springhouse, Pa, 2004, Lippincott Williams & Wilkins.

APPENDIX C

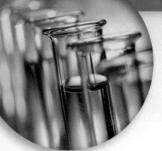

PREFIXES, SUFFIXES, AND STEM WORDS

Every specialty has a vocabulary of its own. The clinical laboratory is no different. Progress in learning the vocabulary of the laboratory and of medicine in general will come with experience, but some introductory information is important for anyone coming into the laboratory for the first time.

Most modern medical words are made up of parts derived from Greek or Latin, some with changes that have gradually been made over the years as the ancient words were adopted into English. All but the simplest medical terms are made up of two or three parts. For example, *pathology* is the study of disease. The root word is *pathos-*, from the Greek, meaning "disease." The suffix *-logy* is from the Greek word *-logia*, from *logos*, meaning "the study of." By examining the root or stem word along with the prefix or suffix, the meaning of most medical words can be understood.

Many of the common prefixes, suffixes, and stem words are listed below.

Prefix/Stem Word	Meaning
a-, an-	lack, not
ab-, a-	away from, outside of
ad-	to, toward
ambi-, ambo-	both
amyl-, amylo-	starch
angi-, angio-	vessel, vascular
ante-	before, preceding, in front of
arteri-, arterio-	artery, arterial
arthr-, arthro-	joint
aur-, auri-, auro-	ear
bi-	two, twice, double
bi-, bio-	life
brachi-, brachio-	arm, brachial
brady-	slow
bronch-, broncho-	bronchus, bronchial

Prefix/Stem Word	Meaning
cardi-, cardia-, cardio-	heart, cardiac
cephal-, cephalo-	head
cerebr-, cerebri, cerebro-	cerebrum, cerebral, brain
cervic-, cervico-	neck, cervix, cervical
chol-, chole-, cholo-	bile, gall
circum-	around, about
co-, com-, con-, cor-	with, together
col-, coli-, colo-	colon
contra-, counter-	against, opposite
crani-, cranio-	cranium, cranial
cyan-, cyano-	dark blue, presence of the cyanogen group
cyst-, cysti-, cysto-	gallbladder, urinary bladder, pouch, cyst
de-	undoing, reversal
dec-, deca-	ten, multiplied by ten
deci-	tenth, one tenth of
derm-, derma-, dermo-	dermis, dermal, skin
dextr-, dextro-	toward, of, or pertaining to the right
di-, dis-	two, twice, double
dipl-, diplo-	twofold, double, twin
dis-, di-	separation, reversal, apart from
dys-	abnormal, diseased, difficult, painful, unlike
en-, em-	in, inside, into
end-, endo-	within, inner, internal
enter-, entero-	intestine, intestinal
ep-, epi-	upon, beside, among, above
erythr-, erythro-	red
eu-	good, well, normal, true
ex-, e-, ef-	out, away, without
extra-	outside of, beyond the scope of

Prefix/Stem Word	Meaning
ferri-	ferric, containing iron III
ferro-	ferrous, containing iron II
fibr-, fibro-	fiber, fibrous
gastr-, gastro-	stomach, gastric
gluc-, gluco-	glucose
glyc-, glyco-	sweet, sugar, glucose, glycine
gyne-	female, woman
hem-, hema-, hemo-	blood
hemi-	half, partial
hepat-, hepato-	liver, hepatic
heter-, hetero-	other, another, different
hex-, hexa-	six
hom-, homo-	common, like, same
hydr-, hydro-	water, hydrogen
hyp-, hypo-	deficiency, lack, below
hyper-	excessive, above normal
hyster-, hystero-	uterus, uterine, hysteria
icter-, ictero-	icterus, jaundice
immuno-	immune, immunity
in-, im-	not, in, into
inter-	between, among
intra-	within, inside
is, iso-	equality, similarity, uniformity
juxta-	near, next to
kerat-, kerato-	horn, horny, cornea
ket-, keto-	presence of the ketone group
kilo-	thousand
lact-, lacti-, lacto-	milk, lactic
lapar-, laparo-	flank, abdomen
laryng-, laryngo-	larynx, laryngeal
latero-	lateral, to the side
leuk-, leuc-, leuko-, leuco-	white, colorless, leukocyte
levo-	left, on the left
lith-, litho-	stone
lymph-, lympho-	lymph, lymphatic
macr-, macro-	large, great, long
mal-	wrong, abnormal, bad
mamm-, mammo-	breast
medi-, medio-	middle, medial, median
meg-, mega-, megal-	large, extended, enlarged, one million times as large as
micr-, micro-	small, minute, one millionth
mon-, mono-	single, one, alone
morph-, morpho-	form, structure
multi-	many, much, affecting many parts
my-, myo-	muscle
myel-, myelo-	marrow
nas-, naso-	nose, nasal
ne-, neo-	new, recent

Prefix/Stem Word	Meaning
necr-, necro-	death
nephr-, nephro-	kidney
neur-, neuro-	neural, nervous, nerve
nitr-, nitro-	nitrogen
non-	not, ninth, nine
normo-	normal
nucle-, nucleo-	nucleus, nuclear
oo-	egg, ovum
orth-, ortho-	straight, direct, normal
ost-, oste-, osteo-	bone
ot-, oto-	ear
oxy-	oxygen
par-, para-	near, beside, adjacent to
path-, patho-	pathologic
peri-	about, beyond, around
phag-, phago-	eating, feeding
pharyng-, pharyngo-	pharynx, pharyngeal
phleb-, phlebo-	vein, venous
phon-, phono-	sound, speech, voice
phot-, photo-	light
physi-, physio-	natural, physical, physiologic
phyt-, phyto-	plant, vegetable
plasm-, plasmo-	plasma, protoplasm, cytoplasm
pneum-, pneumo-	air, gas, lung, respiratory
poly-	multiple, compound, complex
post-	after, behind
pre-	before
pro-	front, forward, before
proct-, procto-	rectum, anus
prot-, proto-	first, primitive, early
pseud-, pseudo-	false, deceptively resembling
psych-, psycho-	psyche, psychic, psychology
pulmo-	lung, pulmonary
py-, pyo-	pus
pyel-, pyelo-	renal, pelvic
pykn-, pykno-, pycn-, pycno-	compact, dense
pyr-, pyro-	fire, heat
radio-	radiation, radioactivity
re-	again, back
ren-, reni-, reno-	kidney, renal
retro-	back, backward, behind
rhin-, rhino-	nose, nasal
rubr-, rubri-, rubro-	red
sarc-, sarco-	flesh, fleshlike, muscle
semi-	half
ser-, seri,- sero-	serum, serous
sub-	under, less than
super-	above, upon, extreme
supra-	upon, above, beyond, exceeding

Prefix/Stem Word	Meaning
syn-, sym-	together, with
tachy-	rapid, quick, accelerated
thorac-, thoraci-, thoracio-, thoraco-	thorax, thoracic
thromb-, thrombo-	clotting, coagulation, blood platelets
thyr-, thyreo-, thyro-	thyroid
tox-, toxi-, toxo-	toxic, poisonous
trache-, tracheo-	trachea, tracheal
trans-	through, across
trich-, tricho-	hair, filament
un-	not, without
uni-	one
ur-, uro-	urine, urinary
uter-, utero-	uterus, uterine
vas-, vasi-, vaso-	vessel, vascular
ven-, vene-, veni-, veno-	vein, venous

Suffix/Stem Word	Meaning
-algia	a painful condition
-ase	enzyme
-ation	action, process
-blast	sprout, shoot, germ, formative cell
-cele	tumor, hernia, pathologic swelling
-cyte	cell
-desis	binding, fusing

Suffix/Stem Word	Meaning
-ectomy	surgical removal
-emia	blood
-ethesia	feeling, sensation
-gram	drawing, record
-graph	something written, recorded
-itis-	inflammation
-logy	field of study
-lysis	dissolving, loosening, dissolution
-megaly	abnormal enlargement
-oma	tumor, neoplasm
-opia, -opy	defect of the eye
-osis	process, state, diseased condition
-pathy	disease, therapy
-penia	deficiency
-phil, -phile	having an affinity for
-plasty	plastic surgery
-rrhage, -rrhagia	abnormal or excessive discharge
-scope	viewing instrument
-scopy	inspection, examination
-stoma	mouth, opening
-stomy	operation establishing an opening into a part
-tomy	cutting, incision, section
-uria	of or in the urine

APPENDIX D

ABBREVIATIONS

ADH	antidiuretic hormone
AGN	acute glomerulonephritis
AGT	antiglobulin test or reaction
AHG	antihuman globulin
AIDS	acquired immunodeficiency syndrome
AIN	acute interstitial nephritis
ANA	antinuclear antibody
APTT	activated partial thromboplastin time
ASCLS	American Society for Clinical Laboratory Science
ASCP	American Society of Clinical Pathologists
ASO	antistreptolysin O
BAP	blood agar (plate)
BT	bleeding time
CAP	College of American Pathologists
CBC	complete blood count
CDC	Centers for Disease Control and Prevention
CFU	colony-forming unit
CFU-C	colony-forming unit, culture
CFU-L	colony-forming unit, lymphoid
CFU-S	colony-forming unit, spleen
CLA	clinical laboratory assistant
CLIA '88	Clinical Laboratory Improvement Amendments of 1988
CLSI	Clinical and Laboratory Standards Institute (formerly NCCLS)
CLT	clinical laboratory technician
COLA	Commission on Office Laboratory Accreditation
CPD	citrate phosphate dextrose
CPDA-1	citrate phosphate dextrose with adenine
CPU	central processing unit
CQI	continuous quality improvement
CRT	cathode ray tube

CSF	colony-stimulating factor; cerebrospinal fluid
DAT	direct antiglobulin test
DIC	disseminated intravascular coagulation
DNA	deoxyribonucleic acid
EA	early antigen
EBV	Epstein-Barr virus
EDTA	ethylenediaminetetraacetic acid
EIA	enzyme immunoassay
ELISA	enzyme-linked immunosorbent assay; enzyme-labeled immunosorbent assay
EMB	eosin–methylene blue agar
ESR	erythrocyte sedimentation rate
FIA	fluorescence (fluorescent) immunoassay
Hb, Hgb	hemoglobin
HBV	hepatitis B virus
HCFA	Health Care Financing Administration
Hct, Ht	hematocrit
HCV	hepatitis C virus; formerly non-A, non-B hepatitis virus
HDN	hemolytic disease of newborn
HHS	Department of Health and Human Services
HIS	hospital information system
HIV	human immunodeficiency virus
HLA	human leukocyte antigen
HMWK	high-molecular-weight kininogen
IAT	indirect antiglobulin test
IDDM	insulin-dependent (type 1) diabetes mellitus
IF	intrinsic factor
Ig	immunoglobulin
IL	interleukin
IM	infectious mononucleosis
IU	international unit
IV	intravenous
L	liter

LAP	leukocyte alkaline phosphatase	PKK	plasma prekallikrein
LIS	laboratory information system	PMN	polymorphonuclear neutrophil (leukocyte)
LISS	low-ionic-strength saline solution		
		PPM	provider-performed microscopy
m	meter	PRP	platelet-rich plasma
Mac	MacConkey (agar)	PT	prothrombin time
MBC	minimal bactericidal concentration	PTT	partial thromboplastin time
		PV	predictive value
MCH	mean cell hemoglobin	QA	quality assurance
MCHC	mean cell hemoglobin concentration	QC	quality control
		RAM	random-access memory
MCV	mean cell volume	RBC	red blood cell
MIC	minimal inhibitory concentration	RCF	relative centrifugal force
		RDW	red cell distribution width
MKC	megakaryocyte	RES	reticuloendothelial system
MLA	medical laboratory assistant	RF	rheumatoid factor
MLT	medical laboratory technician	RhIG	Rh immune globulin
mol	mole	RIA	radioimmunoassay
MPV	mean platelet volume	RTF	renal tubular fat
MSDS	material safety data sheets	SB	sheep blood (agar)
MT	medical technologist	SEM	scanning electron microscope, microscopy
NA	numerical aperture		
NAD$^+$	nicotinamide adenine dinucleotide, oxidized form	SI	International System of Units (le Système International d'Unités)
NADH	nicotinamide adenine dinucleotide, reduced form		
		SLE	systemic lupus erythematosus
NBS	National Bureau of Standards	SPIA	solid-phase immunosorbent assay
NCA	National Certification Agency for Medical Laboratory Personnel		
		TEM	transmission electron microscope, microscopy
NCEP	National Cholesterol Education Program	TJC	The Joint Commission
		TLC	thin-layer chromatography
NIDDM	non–insulin-dependent (type 2) diabetes mellitus	TQI	total quality improvement
		TT	thrombin time
OFB	oval fat body	VAD	vascular access device
OGTT	oral glucose tolerance test	VDRL	Venereal Disease Research Laboratories (test for syphilis)
OSHA	Occupational Safety and Health Administration		
		vWD	von Willebrand disease
PCT	postcoital test	vWF	von Willebrand factor
PCV	packed cell volume	WBC	white blood cell
PEP	postexposure prophylaxis		

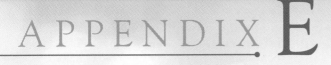
APPENDIX E

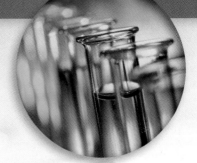

QUICK REFERENCE VALUES

Selected reference values for common clinical laboratory tests follow. Values will differ slightly with individual laboratories and methodology. Reference values must be established for each laboratory.

HEMATOLOGY[1]

Values are for adults, unless indicated otherwise (M, male; F, female).

Hemoglobin	M	13.5-17.5 g/dL
	F	12.0-16.0 g/dL
Hematocrit[2]	M	41.5%-50.4%
	F	36%-45%
RBC count	M	$4.5\text{-}5.9 \times 10^{12}/L$
	F	$4.5\text{-}5.1 \times 10^{12}/L$
MCV	M/F	80-96.1 fL
MCH	M/F	27.5-33.2 pg
MCHC	M/F	33.4-35.5 g/dL
RDW	M/F	11.5%-14.5%
WBC count	M/F	$4.5\text{-}11.0 \times 10^9/L$ (>21 years)
Platelets	M/F	$150\text{-}450 \times 10^9/L$
Reticulocyte count[3]		
Adult		0.5%-2.5%
Newborn		2.5%-6.0%

Leukocyte differential cell count (M/F, ≥21 years)

		Mean absolute count $\times 10^9/L$
Neutrophils	40-74	1.4-6.5
Band	0-3.0	0-0.17
Lymphocytes	22-40	1.2-3.4
Monocytes	2-6	
Eosinophils	1-4	
Basophils	0.5-1	

Erythrocyte sedimentation rate (ESR)[4]

	<50 years	>50 years
Male	0-10 mm/hr	0-15
Female	0-13 mm/hr	0-20

URINALYSIS[5]

Specific Gravity

Random urine	1.001-1.035
Normal diet and fluid	1.016-1.022

Chemical Screen

pH	5-7
Protein	Negative
Blood	Negative
Glucose	Negative
Ketones	Negative
Nitrite	Negative
Leukocyte esterase	Negative
Urobilinogens	To 1 EU/dL
Bilirubin (conjugated)	Negative

Sediment Examination

(12:1 concentration; *hpf*, high-power field; *lpf*, low-power field.)

RBC	0-2/hpf
WBC	0-5/hpf (female > male)
Casts	0-2 hyaline/lpf
Squamous epithelial cells	Few/lpf
Transitional epithelial cells	Few/hpf
Renal tubular epithelial cells	Few/hpf
Bacteria	Negative
Yeast	Negative
Abnormal crystals	Negative

CHEMISTRIES, SERUM (ADULT)[6]

Alanine aminotransferase (ALT)	10-35 U/L
Alkaline phosphatase	
Male	30-90 U/L
Female	20-80 U/L
Aspartate aminotransferase (AST)	10-40 U/L
Bicarbonate	22-29 mmol/L
Bilirubin	
Total	0.3-1.2 mg/dL
Direct, conjugated	0.0-0.2 mg/dL
Calcium, total	8.5-10.2 mg/dL
Chloride	98-107 mmol/L
Cholesterol	
Desirable	<200 mg/dL
Borderline/moderate risk	200-239 mg/dL
High risk	>240 mg/dL
Creatinine	
Male	0.7-1.3 mg/dL
Female	0.6-1.1 mg/dL
Creatinine clearance	
Male (<40 years)	90-139 mL/min/1.73 m^2
Female (<40 years)	80-125 mL/min/1.73 m^2
Creatine kinase (CK)	
Male	15-105 U/L
Female	10-80 U/L
Glucose (fasting)	70-105 mg/dL
Iron	
Male	65-170 µg/dL
Female	50-170 µg/dL
Total iron-binding capacity	250-450 µg/dL

% saturation of iron	
Male	20%-55%
Female	15%-50%
pH (arterial blood)	7.35-7.45
Potassium	3.8-5.0 mmol/L
Protein, total	6.4-8.3 g/dL
Protein, albumin	3.9-5.1 g/dL
Sodium	136-145 mmol/L
Triglyceride (10- to 12-hour fast required)	
Male	40-160 mg/dL
Female	35-135 mg/dL
Urea	5-39 mg/dL
Urea nitrogen	7-18 mg/dL
Uric acid	
Male	0.5-7.2 mg/dL
Female	2.6-6.0 mg/dL

REFERENCES

1. Greer JP: Wintrobe's clinical hematology, ed 11, Philadelphia, 2004, Lippincott Williams & Wilkins, pp 2697–2719.
2. Clinical and Laboratory Standards Institute (CLSI, NCCLS): Procedure for determining packed cell volume by the microhematocrit method: approved standard, ed 2, Villanova, Pa, 1993, NCCLS Document H7–A2.
3. Williams WJ, et al: Hematology, ed 4, New York, 1990, McGraw-Hill.
4. McPherson RA, Pincus MR: Henry's clinical diagnosis and management by laboratory methods, ed 21, Philadelphia, 2006, Saunders.
5. Reference values established for Fairview University Medical Center, University Campus, Minneapolis, Minn.
6. Burtis CA, Ashwood ER, Bruns DE, editors: Tietz fundamentals of clinical chemistry, ed 6, St Louis, 2008, Saunders.

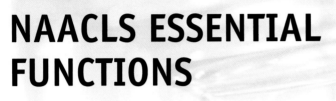

APPENDIX F

NAACLS ESSENTIAL FUNCTIONS

With permission NAACLS

In order to participate in a clinical laboratory science educational program, students must be able to comply with program-designated essential functions or request reasonable accommodations to execute these essential functions. Requirements include a sound intellect; good motor skills such as eye-hand coordination and dexterity; effective communication skills; visual acuity to perform macroscopic and microscopic analyses or read procedures, graphs, and the like; professional skills such as the ability to work independently, manage time efficiently, and comprehend, analyze, and synthesize various materials; and sound psychological health and stability.

ASCLS MISSION/VISION STATEMENT

ASCLS serves as the voice of all clinical laboratory professionals, creating a vision for the advancement of the clinical laboratory practice field and advocating the value and role of the profession in ensuring safe, effective, efficient, equitable, and patient-centered health care.

Core Values

- Promoting the value of the profession to healthcare and the public;
- Uniting the profession to speak with one voice;
- Advocating on behalf of the profession;
- Promoting professional independence;
- Enhancing quality standards and patient safety;
- Ensuring workplace safety;
- Providing professional development opportunities;
- Promoting expanded roles and contributions of clinical laboratory professionals to the healthcare team;
- Increasing the diversity in the profession and expanding the voice and role of underrepresented individuals and groups.

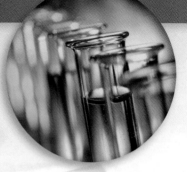

Answers to Review Questions

CHAPTER 1

1. c
2. b
3. e
4. c
5. a
6. d
7. d
8. c
9. a
10. b
11. d
12. b
13. d
14. b
15. d
16. a
17. a
18. b
19. c

CHAPTER 2

1. a
2. c
3. d
4. b
5. b
6. b
7. d
8. d
9. c
10. d
11. a
12. b
13. c
14. d
15. d

16. a
17. c
18. b
19. a
20. b
21. a
22. a
23. a
24. b
25. a
26. d
27. c
28. d
29. a
30. c
31. b
32. a
33. b

CHAPTER 3

1. d
2. a
3. c
4. b
5. b
6. b
7. d
8. b
9. d
10. c
11. a
12. e
13. b
14. a
15. d
16. c
17. a
18. c

19. b
20. d
21. d
22. d
23. d
24. d
25. a
26. b
27. a
28. c
29. a
30. a
31. a
32. a

CHAPTER 4

1. c
2. a
3. b
4. c
5. c
6. b
7. c
8. a
9. b
10. a
11. a
12. a
13. d
14. a
15. b
16. d
17. a
18. a
19. b
20. a
21. a
22. a
23. b
24. b
25. c

CHAPTER 5

1. a-stand, b-neck/arm, c-stage, d-clips/mechanical
2. b
3. a
4. c
5. c
6. b
7. a
8. c
9. b
10. a

11. d
12. b
13. a
14. b
15. d
16. c
17. d
18. d
19. b
20. a
21. a
22. a
23. a
24. a
25. a

CHAPTER 6

1. c
2. b
3. d
4. a
5. b
6. b
7. a
8. c
9. a
10. b
11. c
12. b
13. a
14. c
15. b
16. a
17. b
18. b
19. a
20. b
21. b
22. c
23. a
24. c
25. b
26. a
27. a
28. b
29. c
30. d
31. d
32. a
33. d
34. c
35. a
36. a

37. b
38. c
39. a
40. b
41. a
42. a
43. b
44. c
45. b
46. a
47. c
48. d
49. b
50. d
51. d
52. d
53. d
54. a

CHAPTER 7

1. d
2. a
3. c
4. b
5. a. 6.3   b. 15.6   c. 10.0   d. 26   e. 24
6. b
7. b
8. b
9. b
10. c
11. b
12. c
13. a
14. d
15. a
16. b
17. c
18. c
19. c
20. a
21. d
22. b
23. b
24. c
25. b

CHAPTER 8

1. a
2. d
3. b
4. c
5. b
6. a

7. c
8. a
9. a
10. b
11. b
12. d
13. c
14. a
15. e
16. a
17. b
18. a
19. c
20. b
21. b
22. a
23. a
24. a

CHAPTER 9

1. a
2. a
3. a
4. a
5. a
6. a
7. b
8. b
9. a
10. a
11. a
12. a
13. a
14. a
15. a

CHAPTER 10

1. d
2. a
3. a
4. a
5. a
6. b
7. a
8. e
9. d
10. c
11. d
12. c
13. d
14. d
15. b
16. a

17. c
18. b
19. d

CHAPTER 11

Answers to Case Studies

Case 11-1: a

The normal (reference range for creatinine clearance for this patient is male (<40 years of age) 90-139 mL/min/1.73 mm^2

Case 11-2: b

Case 11-3: b

Case 11-4: a

Case 11-5: d

Case 11-6: 1. a   2. d

1. a
2. d
3. b
4. b
5. d
6. a
7. d
8. b
9. c
10. b
11. b
12. a
13. d
14. b
15. a
16. a
17. b
18. c
19. d
20. d
21. d
22. d
23. d
24. a
25. a
26. d
27. b
28. d
29. d
30. c
31. d
32. b
33. b
34. c
35. a
36. d
37. c
38. d
39. a
40. c
41. c
42. b
43. a
44. c
45. b
46. a
47. c
48. b
49. a
50. a
51. b

CHAPTER 12

Answers to Case Studies

Case 12-1:   1. a   2. a   3. c   4. a   5. a

Case 12-2:   1. c   2. b   3. a   4. d   5. b

Case 12-3:   1. b   2. b   3. b   4. d   5. b

Case 12-4:   1. a   2. c   3. c   4. d   5. a

Case 12-5:   1. b   2. c   3. c   4. a   5. d   6. c

1. a
2. c
3. d
4. b
5. c
6. c
7. b
8. a
9. a
10. a
11. b
12. b or c
13. b
14. d
15. a
16. c
17. b
18. f
19. a
20. c
21. e
22. d
23. d
24. e
25. c
26. d
27. a
28. b
29. a
30. c

31. a
32. b
33. c
34. b
35. a
36. a
37. a
38. b
39. b
40. a
41. d
42. c
43. b
44. a
45. b
46. c
47. a
48. b
49. a
50. b
51. g
52. g
53. e
54. f
55. d
56. d
57. a
58. a
59. c
60. d
61. c
62. b
63. d
64. a
65. d
66. c
67. c
68. c
69. a
70. a
71. b
72. a
73. a
74. a
75. d
76. c
77. b
78. d
79. b
80. a
81. d
82. b
83. d

CHAPTER 13

Answers to Case Studies

Case 13-1: a
Case 13-2: d
Case 13-3: b

1. c
2. b
3. b
4. a
5. a
6. b
7. a
8. a
9. a
10. a
11. b
12. b
13. b
14. a
15. a
16. b
17. a
18. a
19. c
20. a
21. a
22. a
23. b
24. a
25. b
26. b
27. a
28. a
29. c
30. a
31. a
32. a
33. b
34. b
35. b

CHAPTER 14

Answers to Case Studies

Case 14-1: 1. a 2. b 3. b 4. c
Case 14-2: 1. a 2. d 3. a 4. b 5. a
Case 14-3: 1. d 2. b 3. c 4. a 5. c 6. d
Case 14-4: 1. d 2. d 3. d 4. e
Case 14-5: 1. b 2. a 3. c 4. c
Case 14-6: 1. a 2. d 3. d 4. d

1. d
2. a

3. d
4. b
5. a
6. e
7. d
8. c
9. b
10. e
11. g
12. a
13. d
14. i
15. h
16. f
17. j
18. c
19. b
20. a
21. a
22. b
23. a
24. b
25. a
26. b
27. a
28. a
29. d
30. d
31. c
32. b
33. a
34. a
35. b
36. a
37. b
38. a
39. b
40. a
41. a
42. d
43. b
44. c
45. b
46. a
47. a
48. b
49. f
50. d
51. i
52. b
53. b
54. c
55. h

56. a
57. g
58. b
59. a
60. c
61. d
62. g
63. c
64. h
65. e
66. a
67. f
68. b
69. c
70. f
71. e
72. g
73. a
74. c
75. b
76. b
77. a
78. a
79. b
80. a
81. a
82. b
83. b
84. a
85. a
86. a
87. b
88. b
89. b
90. b
91. d
92. a
93. b
94. c
95. a
96. c
97. d

CHAPTER 15

Answers to Case Studies

Case 15-1: 1. a 2. b   3. b   4. a
Case 15-2: 1. a 2. c

1. a
2. a
3. f
4. a
5. b

6. c
7. d
8. e
9. a
10. a
11. e
12. c
13. b
14. f
15. d
16. h
17. i
18. g
19. a
20. b
21. e
22. b
23. c
24. a
25. b
26. d
27. d
28. e
29. a
30. c
31. a
32. d
33. a
34. c
35. b
36. a
37. b
38. a
39. b
40. a
41. b
42. b
43. a
44. b

CHAPTER 16

Answers to Case Studies

Case 16-1:

1. a
2. Findings that support diagnosis include normal CBC results, negative rapid strep test, absence of exudates in throat, presence of low-grade fever, cough, and runny nose.

Case 16-2:

1. Findings that support diagnosis of a bacterial pneumonia include productive cough (sputum produced), blood-tinged sputum, chest pain, x-ray, laboratory findings: elevated WBC with increased percentage of neutrophils, Gram stain, and culture.
2. b

Case 16-3:

1. Findings that support diagnosis of a sexually transmitted disease include sexual history (classic patient profile includes history of multiple sex partners and having had other sexually transmitted diseases), positive chlamydial antigen test.
2. a

Case 16-4:

1. Findings that support diagnosis of cryptococcal meningitis include positive cryptococcal antigen test (Cryptococcus neoformans is a common cause of fungal meningitis, especially among immunocompromised patients), poorly controlled diabetes (metabolic disturbances also predispose to fungal meningitis), chronic pulmonary condition, a smoker of long duration, on steroid medications—all factors that influence the status of the immune system; patient is immunocompromised; patient's physical findings, including lethargy and disorientation, suggest a CNS effect.
2. b

Case 16-5: d

1. d
2. c
3. d
4. b
5. c
6. c
7. a
8. c
9. b
10. a
11. c
12. a
13. a
14. d
15. b
16. a
17. a
18. b
19. d
20. a
21. c
22. d
23. d
24. a
25. c

26. c
27. c
28. b
29. a
30. b

CHAPTER 17

Answers to Case Studies

Case 17-1:   1. c   2. a   3. b
Case 17-2:   1. d   2. d   3. b
Case 17-3:   1. b   2. a   3. a

1. a
2. c
3. a
4. b
5. b
6. c
7. c
8. c
9. a
10. d
11. b
12. a
13. d
14. a
15. a
16. c
17. b
18. a

CHAPTER 18

Answers to Case Studies

Case 18-1:   1. d   2. a   3. a
Case 18-2:   1. a   2. a   3. a

1. h
2. d
3. e
4. a
5. g
6. f
7. b
8. c
9. a
10. b
11. b
12. a
13. a
14. b
15. c
16. c
17. a
18. d
19. c
20. a
21. b
22. d
23. a
24. a
25. a
26. b
27. a
28. d
29. d
30. d
31. f
32. c
33. e
34. d
35. a
36. b

Glossary

A

absolute cell count (absolute numbers): Concentration of a cell type expressed as a number per volume of whole blood, usually per liter; obtained by multiplying the relative percentage value by the total leukocyte count per liter.

absorbance: Amount of light that is absorbed or retained and therefore not able to pass through or be transmitted through a solution.

absorbance spectrophotometry: Methodology that utilizes Beer's law, whereby the amount of light absorbed by a solution is directly proportional to the concentration of the solution; this measurement can be made only by mathematical calculation from the transmission data obtained by use of a quantitative analytical method, such as spectrophotometry.

absorbance units: Units of measure for light that is absorbed by a colored solution.

absorbed light: Light that is not transmitted.

acceptable control range: Statistically determined range of values within which a test result must fall to be considered acceptable; it is a means of quality control or assurance.

accuracy: Correctness of a result, freedom from error, or how close the answer is to the "true" value.

accurate and precise technology (APT): "Easy" or automated quantitative tests or easy qualitative tests for which the manufacturer of the automated instrument has been granted special standing under CLIA '88 definitions of laboratory tests.

acholic stool: Absence of bile; results in formation of colorless, chalky-appearing fecal specimens.

acid crystals: Crystals seen in urine of an acidic pH, less than pH 7.0.

acid-base balance: Maintenance of a constant balance between acids and bases; maintenance of constant pH.

acid-fast bacteria (AFB): Bacteria that retain staining dye and make the decolorization step difficult.

acid-fast stain: Used to detect organisms that are difficult to decolorize, even with acid-alcohol solutions; typical organisms are those that cause tuberculosis or leprosy.

acidophilic: Acid loving; on blood films, the cell components that stain with the acidic portion of Wright or Wright-Giemsa stain, such as hemoglobin and eosinophilic granules, which stain orange to pink.

acidosis: Decrease in blood pH.

activated partial thromboplastin time (APTT): A test sensitive to heparin; useful in detecting deficiencies in intrinsic and common pathway factors.

active reabsorption: A form of reabsorption that requires the expenditure of energy. This is usually against a concentration gradient, from a region of lower to one of higher concentration.

acute glomerulonephritis (AGN): Also postinfectious glomerulonephritis. A disease of the kidney glomerulus that is an immunologic sequela of a bacterial infection. Characteristics include, oliguria, edema, proteinuria, with red blood cell or granular casts, and hematuria.

acute interstitial nephritis (AIN): An inflammation of the interstitial tissue of the kidney that is an immunologic, adverse reaction to certain drugs, such as sulfonamide or methicillin. The condition is characterized by fever, rash, proteinuria, and the presence of eosinophils in urine.

acute phase: Early in the course of a disease, when the disease is first suspected; blood is drawn (acute phase serum) when little or no antibody has had time to develop and is compared with antibody level in convalescent serum.

acute-phase reactants: Group of glycoproteins associated with nonspecific inflammatory conditions.

acute pyelonephritis: An infection of the pelvis and parenchyma of the kidney; usually the result of an ascending infection from the lower urinary tract.

additives, anticoagulants: Additives usually are anticoagulants that prevent coagulation of the blood specimen. Several different anticoagulants are available for different testing purposes. Some laboratory tests require the use of plasma or whole blood for the assay, and these must be anticoagulated during the collection process.

aerobes: Microbes that require oxygen for growth.

aerosols: Infectious particles that are airborne; fine mist in which particles are dispersed.

agar: A seaweed extract that is liquid when heated and solid when cooled; used as base medium for preparation of culture plates, slant tubes, and stab tubes.

agar disk diffusion tests: Tests that employ antibiotic-impregnated disks placed on an agar culture plate inoculated with the organism to be tested.

agar slant: Tubes of agar media that are solidified on a slant (the surface of the medium is on an incline); useful for particular cultures.

agglutination: Visible clumping or aggregation of red cells or any particles; used as an indication of a specific antigen-antibody reaction.

agglutinins: Antibodies that form visible clumps, or agglutinate, with their specific antigens.

agglutinogens: Antigens that form visible clumps, or agglutinate, with their specific antibodies.

aggregometer: Instrument that measures platelet aggregation in platelet dysfunction studies.

albuminemia: Decreased blood albumin.

albuminuria: Presence of albumin in urine.

aldosterone: Hormone that controls the sodium-potassium pump, the primary mechanism for sodium reabsorption in the kidney; regulator of blood sodium and potassium levels.

alignment: Microscope adjustment that ensures that the light path from the light source throughout the microscope and ocular is physically correct.

aliquot: One of a number of equal parts.

alkaline crystals: Crystals seen in urine of an alkaline pH; generally pH 7.0 and above.

alkalosis: Increase in blood pH.

alleles: Variants of a gene for a particular trait.

alloantibodies: Antibodies resulting from antigenic stimulation within the same species.

alpha hemolysis: Incomplete or partial hemolysis (appears green).

ambulatory patient: A patient not confined to bed; example, an outpatient or clinic patient.

American Standard Code for Information Interchange (ASCII): Standardized codes allowing the keyboard of the computer to be used to enter alphanumeric as well as numerical data into the computer.

Americans with Disabilities Act (ADA): Mandates that specific plans be developed for any person with a disability employed by a clinical laboratory, to ensure that the person is working in a safe atmosphere.

amorphous material: Crystalline material seen in the urine sediment as granules without shape or form.

anaerobes: Microbes that cannot grow in an atmosphere of oxygen; special steps must be taken to provide an oxygen-free atmosphere for incubation and growth of these organisms.

analog computation: Measurement derived directly from an instrument signal.

analytical balance: Instrument used to weigh substances to a high degree of accuracy (e.g., chemicals used in the preparation of standard solutions).

analytical functions: Process whereby analytical analyses are carried out; includes generating work lists, doing the analyses, entering the results, quality control measures, and results verification.

analyzer: In polarizing microscopy, a polarizing filter located above the specimen, between the objective and the eyepiece.

anemia: A condition in which there is a decrease in hemoglobin in the blood and therefore in the amount of oxygen reaching the tissues and organs. May be the result of a decrease in the number of erythrocytes (decreased red cell mass), decreased hemoglobin concentration, or abnormal hemoglobin.

anion gap: Concentration of unmeasured anions; calculated as the difference between measured cations and measured anions.

anisocytosis: A general term indicating increased variation in the size of red cells in the blood film.

antibiotic resistance: Exists if the growth of a microorganism is not inhibited by the presence of an antibiotic; the organism is resistant to the antibiotic.

antibiotic sensitivity or susceptibility: Ability of the antibiotic to inhibit growth of a microorganism.

antibody: Protein substance, found in the plasma or other body fluids, that is formed as the result of antigenic stimulation and is specific for the antigen against which it is formed. In blood banking, antibodies are present in commercially prepared serum called *antiserum*.

antibody titer: Amount of antibody present or required to produce a reaction with a particular amount of another substance; concentration of antibody.

anticoagulant: Prevents coagulation of blood.

antidiuretic hormone (ADH): A hormone that regulates urine volume by increasing the amount of water reabsorbed by the kidney.

antigen: Foreign (different from "self") substance that, when introduced into the body of a person lacking the antigen, results in an immune response and formation of a corresponding antibody. In blood banking, antigens are generally but not always found on the red cell membrane.

antigen-antibody ratio: Number of antibody molecules in relation to the number of antigen sites per cell.

antihuman globulin (AHG) test (AGT) or reaction: Method of detecting the presence of all human isoantibodies by using a specially prepared antiserum to human immunoglobulin and/or complement. May be a direct (DAT) or indirect (IAT) test. Also known as the *Coombs' reaction* or *Coombs' test*.

antinuclear antibodies (ANA): Circulating immunoglobulins that react with the whole nucleus or nuclear components; frequently assayed by using indirect fluorescent antibody (IFA) techniques.

antiserum: Serum containing antibodies. In blood banking, a special highly purified preparation of antibodies used as a reagent to show the presence of antigen on red blood cells.

anuria: The complete absence of urine formation.

aperture iris diaphragm: The part of the microscope located at the bottom of the Abbé condenser, under the lens but within the condenser body; controls the amount of light passing through the material under observation; can be opened or closed to adjust contrast by means of a lever.

aplastic: Condition when the bone marrow is suppressed or unable to function normally in cell production.

Apt test: Test for maternal hemoglobin ingestion in newborn infants.

arithmetic logic unit: A component of the central processing unit (CPU) of a computer.

arthrocentesis: Collection of synovial fluid from a joint by needle aspiration.

ASCII: See American Standard Code for Information Exchange.

ascorbic acid (vitamin C): A strong reducing substance that may interfere with several of the reagent strip tests used in urinalysis, especially tests for blood and glucose.

atherosclerosis: Condition of "hardening of the arteries," in which plaques of cholesterol, lipids, and cellular debris collect in the inner layers of the walls of large- and medium-sized arteries.

autoantibodies: Antibodies directed against self-antigens.

autoclave: Apparatus for effecting sterilization by using steam under pressure; when it is used with an automatic regulating pressure gauge, the degree of heat to which the contents are subjected is automatically regulated also.

automated cell counters: Instruments designed to repeatedly and automatically count the numbers of formed cellular elements present in a blood specimen, usually the erythrocytes, leukocytes, and platelets.

automated differential counters: Instruments designed to repeatedly and automatically determine the types and percentages of leukocytes present in a blood specimen.

automated hematocrit: The hematocrit result obtained when a multiparameter instrument is used for hematology determinations. The result is computed from measured red cell volume.

automatic pipettes: Devices used to repeatedly and accurately measure volumes of standard solutions, reagents, specimens, or other liquid substances.

automatic pipetting devices: See automatic pipettes.

azotemia: Significantly increased concentrations of urea and creatinine in the blood.

B

B lymphocyte: Blood cell that matures in the bone marrow; undergoes transformation to plasma cell that produces antibodies or immunoglobulins.

bacilli: Rod-shaped bacteria.

bacteremia: Presence of bacteria in blood; bacteria can be cultured from the blood.

bacteriology: The study of bacteria.

bacteriuria: Presence of bacteria in the urine.

balance the centrifuge: To make certain that weight is distributed evenly on opposite sides of the centrifuge to prevent breakage of contents being centrifuged.

bar-code readers: Optical reading devices that convert a series of black lines into a sequence of numbers or letters for entry into a computer (e.g., names of patients, identification numbers, tests requested).

bar coding: A sample recognition system whereby the bar codes—a series of black lines or bars on a label, for example—can be electronically read. Bar codes contain information such as name, hospital number, date, and other patient demographic data; see bar-code readers.

barrier precautions: Personal protective devices (e.g., gloves, gowns) placed between blood or other body fluid specimen and the person handling it, to prevent transmission of infectious agents borne by specimens. See also personal protective equipment.

basic first aid: Immediate care given after an injury, before treatment is started by trained medical personnel.

basophilia: An increase in the number of basophils.

basophilic: Base loving. The acidic cell components, such as nuclei and cytoplasmic RNA, that stain blue-violet by methylene azure in polychrome stains.

basophilic stippling: The presence of dark blue granules evenly distributed throughout the red cell in Wright-stained blood films.

batch or run: A collection of any number of specimens to be analyzed at any one time, plus control specimens, standard solutions, and so forth.

batch analyzers: Analyzer that can test a batch of samples simultaneously for one particular analyte at a time; are designed to analyze a number of different analytes, but only one at a time.

bedside testing: Capillary blood samples can be used to perform rapid testing procedures (many are utilizing commercial products) at the bedside; a common test is the glucose blood test, done for management of diabetes mellitus patients; see also point-of-care testing (POCT).

Beer's law, Beer-Lambert law: In a solution, color intensity at a constant depth is directly proportional to concentration.

Benedict's qualitative test: A copper reduction test for reducing sugars (substances) in urine; the basis of the Clinitest Tablet Test.

beta hemolysis: Clear or complete hemolysis.

bilirubin: Vivid yellow pigment; major byproduct of normal red blood cell destruction.

bilirubin glucuronide, direct bilirubin, conjugated bilirubin: Water-soluble form of bilirubin; formed by conjugation with glucuronic acid in the liver.

biochemical properties and reactions: Properties are characteristics (e.g., molecular weight, melting point) present in various types of chemicals; reactions involve the conversion of one chemical species, the reactant, to another chemical species, the product.

biohazard symbol: Symbol or term denoting any infectious material or agent that presents a possible health risk.

biohazard containers: All infectious materials are handled as potential biohazards. These special containers should be used for all blood, other body fluids, and tissues, and disposable materials contaminated with them; they should be tagged "Biohazard" or bear the standard biohazard symbol.

biohazard waste: See infectious waste.

biometrics: The science of statistics applied to biological observations.

biosafety cabinet: Protective workplace device used to control the presence of infectious agents in the air.

birefringence: Ability of an object or crystal to rotate or polarize light.

blank solution: Solution containing all the components, including solvents and solutes, except the compound to be measured.

bleeding time (BT): The time required for cessation of bleeding after a standardized capillary puncture to a capillary bed; dependent on capillary integrity, numbers of platelets, and platelet function.

blood banking: The procedures involved in collecting, storing, processing, and distributing blood.

blood spot collection: Collection of capillary blood onto a filter paper; example, spot collections for neonatal screening programs.

blood transfusion: Technique of replacing whole blood and/or its components.

bloodborne pathogens: Infectious agents or pathogens carried by blood and blood products.

Board of Registry of the American Society of Clinical Pathologists (ASCP): Offers an examination and certification for medical laboratory personnel.

body cavity fluids: Fluids normally found in small amounts in various cavities or body spaces (e.g., cerebrospinal, pleural, abdominal, pericardial, peritoneal, and synovial fluid). In certain conditions, such fluid is aspirated and assayed.

body tube: The part of the microscope through which the light passes to the ocular.

brightfield microscope: Illumination system used in the common clinical microscope.

broth media: Culture media that are in a broth or liquid form in a tube.

buffy coat: One of the three layers of normal anticoagulated blood. A thin grayish-white layer on top of the packed red blood cells, consisting of leukocytes and platelets, which normally makes up 1% of the total blood volume.

buret: Long, cylindrical graduated tube with a stopcock delivery closing on one end, used to control the delivery of the flow of liquid from the device; used to deliver measured quantities of fluid or solutions.

C

calibrated cuvettes: Tubes or cuvettes that have been optically matched so that the same solution in each will give the same reading on the photometer.

calibration: Means by which glassware or other laboratory apparatus is checked to determine the exact units it will measure or deliver by relating them to a known concentration of an analyte.

calibration mark: Mark on volumetric glassware that indicates the point from which the volume is measured.

calculi: Kidney or renal stones.

CAP quality assurance program: Provided by CAP to assist a laboratory in organizing and managing its quality assurance program under CAP.

capillary blood (peripheral blood) collection: Blood drawn from the capillary bed by means of puncturing the skin; example, a finger or heel puncture.

capillary pipette: Small glass or plastic tube used to collect small amounts of capillary blood, usually directly from a capillary puncture.

capillary tube density gradient: Method of cell enumeration whereby cells, upon centrifugation, settle in different layers because of their different densities; they are further expanded, stained, and magnified to derive the results of the counts.

carcinogens: Substance that can cause the development of cancerous growths in living tissues.

casts: Structures that result from solidification of Tamm-Horsfall mucoprotein in the lumen of the kidney tubules; they form a mold, or cast, of the tubule and trap other material that may be present when they are formed. Several types exist. They represent a biopsy of the kidney and are clinically significant.

catabolism: The phase of metabolism in which fats are broken down for energy.

cathode ray tube (CRT), terminal, video display unit: Television-like screen device used to monitor input, output, and general status of a computer system.

cell-mediated (cellular) response: Involves actions of T lymphocytes and their subsets, together with plasma cells and macrophages.

Celsius scale: Scale used to measure temperature in the metric system; outdated term for this scale is *centigrade*.

Centers for Disease Control and Prevention (CDC): Carries out mandated public health laws and reporting requirements.

central memory: A component of the central processing unit (CPU) of a computer; provides storage and rapid access for information (data).

central processing unit (CPU): The part of the computer that controls and performs the execution of programs or instructions.

centralized laboratory: A central location in a health care facility where all laboratory testing is done.

centrifugation: Separation of a solid material from a liquid by application of increased gravitational force by rapid rotating or spinning.

cerebrospinal fluid (CSF): Extravascular fluid that surrounds the brain and spinal cord. Formed by the choroid plexus in the ventricles of the brain and found within the subarachnoid space, the central canal of the spinal cord, and the four ventricles of the brain.

cervical mucus test: See Fern test.

chain of custody: When results of laboratory testing are to be used in a court of law, a specific chain of documentation is required, whereby all steps of the testing are recorded, from specimen collection to the issuing of the results report.

chemical hygiene plan: Outlines the specific work practices and procedures necessary to protect workers from any health hazards associated with use of hazardous chemicals.

chloride shift: When carbon dioxide leaves the plasma and chloride diffuses or shifts out of the red cells to replace it; can take place when plasma and red cells are not separated in a timely manner.

chromasia: Term used to describe the staining reaction of red cells in the Wright-stained blood film.

chromatography: Method of analysis in which the solutes, dissolved in a common solvent, are separated from one another by differential distribution of the solutes between two phases (a mobile phase and a stationary phase).

chromosome: Threadlike structure within the nucleus of each cell, made up of genes. Chromosomes exist in pairs in all cells except sex cells. Each species has a specific number of paired chromosomes.

chylomicrons: Small droplets of lipoproteins that give blood specimens a characteristic milky appearance when present.

CLIA '88: See Clinical Laboratory Improvement Amendments of 1988 (CLIA '88).

clinical assistant (CLA): See Appendix A.

clinical immunology: Study of antigen-antibody reactions in vitro.

Clinical Laboratory Improvement Amendments of 1988 (CLIA '88): Standards set for all laboratories to ensure quality patient care; provisions include requirements for quality control and assurance, for the use of proficiency tests, and for certain levels of personnel to perform and supervise work done in the clinical laboratory.

clinical laboratory scientist: See MLS.

clinical laboratory technician: See MLT.

clinical pathology: Medical discipline by which clinical laboratory science and technology are applied to the care of patients.

clone: Cell originating from a single ancestral parent cell.

clot: Formation of a fibrin network; a thrombus.

clot retraction: Clot becomes smaller.

clue cells: Vaginal squamous epithelial cells that are covered or encrusted with *Gardnerella vaginalis*.

coagglutination: To enhance visibility of agglutination, antibodies are bound to a particle.

coagulation: Mechanism whereby after injury to a blood vessel, plasma coagulation factors, tissue factors, and calcium work together on the surface of platelets to form a fibrin clot.

coagulation cascade: Process of coagulation in which a series of biochemical reactions occur, converting inactive substances to active forms that in turn activate other substances; carefully controlled process responding to injury while maintaining normal blood circulation.

coagulation factors: Proteins engaged in formation of a fibrin clot from fibrinogen.

coagulation system: See coagulation cascade.

cocci: Bacteria that are round.

coefficient of variation (CV): Used to compare the standard deviations of two samples; in percent, the CV is equal to the standard deviation divided by the mean.

cofactors: Proteins that accelerate the reactions of the enzymes involved in the coagulation process.

College of American Pathologists (CAP): Professional organization of pathologists; one responsibility is to certify clinical laboratories.

colony forming unit, culture (CFU-C): Multipotential hematopoietic (myeloid) stem cell.

colony forming unit, lymphoid (CFU-L): Committed lymphoid stem cell.

colony forming unit, spleen (CFU-S): Uncommitted pluripotential stem cell; also colony forming unit, lymphoid-myeloid (CFU-LM).

colony forming units (CFU): In microbiology, colony count; in hematology, a pluripotential, undifferentiated stem cell that is stimulated to proliferate and differentiate into colonies of a specific cell type.

colony stimulating factor (CSF): Factor required for hematopoietic stem cells to multiply and differentiate.

colorimetry: Technique used to determine the concentration of a substance by the variation in intensity of its color.

commensal state: Situation in which parasite and host exist together with no harm coming to the host.

Commission on Office Laboratory Accreditation (COLA): Provides accreditation for physician office laboratories; has been deemed HCFA approved.

common pathway: Final stages of the coagulation cascade, beginning with the convergence of the extrinsic and intrinsic pathways (factor X) and ending with formation of the fibrin clot.

community-acquired infection: Infection from organisms residing or incubating in the patient before admission to a health care facility.

compatibility testing: All of the tests performed before a transfusion to ensure that the transfused blood or component will benefit and not harm the recipient. These include tests on both recipient and donor blood, including a crossmatch between patient serum and donor red blood cells.

compensated polarized light: Modification of the polarizing microscope in which a compensator (first-order red plate or filter) is inserted between the two crossed polarizing filters and positioned at 45 degrees to the crossed polarizer and analyzer to determine the type of birefringence. In the clinical laboratory, especially useful in examination of synovial fluid.

complement: Group of serum proteins that can produce inflammatory effects and lysis of cells when activated.

complement fixation: When complement is tied up or bound (fixed) to an antigen-antibody complex, it is no longer available to be activated.

complete blood count (CBC): Hematologic tests basic to the initial evaluation and follow-up of the patient. Generally includes measurement of hemoglobin, hematocrit, red blood cell count with morphology, white blood cell count with differential, and platelet estimate; specific tests vary with the facility.

components: Portions of whole blood prepared for transfusion by physical means, especially centrifugation.

concentration of solution: The amount of solute in a given volume of solution. May be expressed in different ways; example, moles of solute per volume of solution, with use of liter as the reference value.

condenser: The part of the microscope that directs and focuses the beam of light from the light source onto the material under examination; positioned just under the stage and can be raised or lowered by means of an adjustment knob.

confidence limits (confidence interval): A value used to express or estimate a statistical parameter; an example is when the reference range is set using values 2 SD on either side of the mean, with 95% of the values falling above and below the mean; see also 95% confidence interval.

conjugated bilirubin, direct bilirubin, bilirubin glucuronide: Bilirubin that has been conjugated with glucuronate in the liver; exists in plasma unbound to any protein, as contrasted to unconjugated bilirubin; is water soluble, and high blood levels are excreted in the urine.

Continuous Quality Improvement (CQI): See Total Quality Improvement (TQI).

continuous-flow analyzer: Instrument that constantly pumps reagent and sample through tubing and coil, forming a continuous stream.

control specimen: Material or solution with a known concentration of the analytes being measured; used for quality control when the test result for the control specimen must be within certain limits in order for the unknown values run in the same "batch" to be considered reportable.

convalescent phase: About 2 weeks after the acute phase of illness, convalescent serum is tested and the antibody titer compared with that of the acute phase serum; an important phase of serology testing is the manifestation of a rise in antibody titer during the course of a disease.

Coombs' test: See antihuman globulin test.

cortex (kidney): Outer anatomical portion of the kidney; consists of the glomerular portions of the nephron and the proximal convoluted tubules.

coulometry: Technique in which the charge required to completely electrolyze a sample is measured.

Coulter principle: Means of counting particles and measuring their size or volume by impedance change caused by the particle in a current-conducting fluid (electrolyte); this principle is applied in many of the blood cell counters used in hematology laboratories (Coulter counter).

creatinine clearance: Estimate of the function of the glomerular filtration rate; obtained by measuring the amount of creatinine in plasma and its rate of excretion in the urine.

crenated: Appearance of red blood cells when present in a hypertonic solution (i.e., in urine of a high specific gravity). The cells appear shrunken, with little spicules or projections.

critical or panic values: See panic or critical values.

crossmatch: A procedure used to determine the compatibility of a donor's blood with that of a recipient after the specimens have been matched for major blood type. One part of compatibility testing.

crystalluria: The presence of crystals in the urine sediment.

crystals, abnormal: Urinary crystals of metabolic or iatrogenic origin that are generally of pathologic significance and require chemical confirmation.

crystals, normal: Urinary crystals that may be found in normal urine specimens of an acid or alkaline pH; generally are not pathologic and can be reported on the basis of morphologic appearance.

culture: Growing of microorganisms or living tissue cells in special, artificial medium.

culture medium: Mixture of nutrients on which a microorganism is grown; see culture.

culture plate: Petri dish or plate in which the medium is placed; where a culture of an organism grows.

cuvette: Tube or receptacle used in a photometer for holding the sample to be measured.

cyanide-nitroprusside reaction: Qualitative test used to confirm the presence of cystine crystals in urine.

cyanosis: Bluish discoloration of the skin and mucous membranes.

cylindroids: A type of hyaline cast with one end that tapers off to a tail or point.

cysts: Inactive form of a microorganism, as a parasite cyst.

cytocentrifugation: Special slow centrifugation method used to prepare permanent microscope slides of fluids (e.g., urine, other body fluids), resulting in better morphologic preservation than by other centrifugation or preparation methods.

cytocentrifuge: Uses a slow centrifuging speed, a low inertia, which rapidly spreads monolayers of cells across a special slide; used for critical morphologic studies.

D

data: Information or results.

database: Systematic store of information (data) that can be accessed by the operator or user of a computer system.

decontamination: Process of eliminating something that has become contaminated or mixed with something that makes it impure; as cleaning a work surface after blood or other potentially infectious material has been spilled on it.

deionization: Process of removing ionized substances from water.

deionized water: See deionization.

density: Amount of matter per unit volume of a substance.

Department of Health and Human Services (HHS): Department of the U.S. government under which the Health Care Financing Administration (HCFA) is managed. Responsible for implementation of laws and writing of regulations that provide details of how various laws are to be carried out; publishes details of proposed regulations in the *Federal Register*, an official government document.

derivatives: Blood products prepared from whole blood by more complex methods than components are. Also referred to as *fractions*.

dextrose: Glucose; a simple sugar.

diabetes mellitus: Chronic metabolic syndrome of impaired carbohydrate, fat, and protein metabolism that is secondary to insufficiency of insulin secretion or to the inhibition of the activity of insulin; characterized by increased concentration of glucose in the blood and urine.

diabetic coma: State of unconsciousness due to a high glucose concentration.

diazo reaction: Coupling of a diazonium salt with another aromatic ring to give an azo dye.

difference check: Computer comparison of current patient result with a previous result for that same patient.

differential media: Media containing dyes, indicators, or other constituents that give colonies of particular organisms distinctive and easily recognizable characteristics.

differential stain: Stain used to differentiate specific cellular details in a microorganism; more than one stain is used to produce the end result. Gram stain is an example of a differential stain.

digital computation: Calculations that involve data available in the form of discrete units or numbers.

dilution factor: Reciprocal of the dilution made; multiply the result by the reciprocal of the dilution to correct for the dilution used.

dilutions: Weaker solutions made from a stronger solution. The term describes the relative concentrations of the components of a mixture; the preferred method is to refer to the number of parts of the material being diluted in the total number of parts of the final product.

diopter: A metric unit of measure for the refractive power of a lens. The focus of a microscope is adjusted for the microscopist by means of the diopter adjustment in the ocular.

direct agglutination: Showing visible agglutination when the constituent (antibody) being measured is present to react with the antigen, as with antigen-coated latex particles in latex agglutination assays.

discrete sample analyzer: Instrument that compartmentalizes each sample reaction.

disinfectant: Cleaning solution that removes pathogenic organisms but not necessarily bacterial or other spores; example, household bleach.

distilled water: As water is boiled, the steam is cooled, condensed, and collected as distilled water; this process removes minerals such as iron, magnesium, and calcium.

diuresis: Any increase in urine volume, even if temporary.

documentation: An important aspect of quality assurance; CLIA '88 regulations mandate that any problem or situation that might affect the outcome of a test result must be recorded and reported, with follow-up monitored.

dry film reagent technology: Instruments or tests that use a dry film layered device that supplies the necessary reagents for the reaction to take place when the serum sample is added to it; the specimen (serum) provides the solvent (water) necessary to rehydrate the dry reagents on the film.

duplicate determinations: Specimens are measured in duplicate to check technique used; a measure of precision or repeatability of the method.

dysmorphic: Distorted or misshapen. Red cells in urine that are dysmorphic may indicate glomerular disease.

E

edema: The abnormal accumulation of fluid in the interstitial spaces of tissues, resulting in generalized swelling.

effusion: Abnormal accumulation of any of the extracellular fluids. Fluid escapes from the blood or lymphatic vessels into the tissues or body cavities (e.g., serous cavities: pericardium, peritoneum, or pleura) or the joints.

Ehrlich's aldehyde reaction: Reaction of urobilinogen, porphobilinogen, and other Ehrlich-reactive compounds with *p*-dimethylaminobenzaldehyde in concentrated hydrochloric acid to form a colored aldehyde.

electrical resistance cell counter: Cell counter that uses electrical resistance. Blood cells passing through an aperture through which an electric current is being passed cause a change in the electrical resistance; this change is counted as voltage pulses.

electrolyte battery or profile: Collection of tests for common electrolytes: chloride, bicarbonate, sodium, and potassium. These four electrolytes often are measured at the same time because changes in the concentration of one almost always is accompanied by changes in one or more of the others.

electronic cell-counting device: Automatic instrument that counts cellular elements in the blood (usually erythrocytes, leukocytes, and platelets) repeatedly and accurately.

electrophoresis: Movement of charged particles in an electrical field; technique used to separate mixtures of ionic solutes by the differences in their rates of migration in an electrical field.

employee "right to know" rule: Designed to ensure that laboratory workers are fully aware of the hazardous chemicals being used in the workplace.

enrichment media: Media that permit one organism to grow rapidly while inhibiting the growth of other organisms.

enumeration of formed elements: Counting of cellular elements of the blood (usually erythrocytes, leukocytes, and platelets).

enzyme immunoassay (EIA): Uses enzymes as immunochemical labels in detection of antigen-antibody reactions.

enzyme-linked (or labeled) immunosorbent assay (ELISA): Immunoassay or test that uses an enzyme conjugated to antibodies or antigens to produce a visible end point; diagnostic test used to detect antigens or antibodies in a patient's specimen.

enzymology: The study of the various biological materials (proteins) that have catalytic activity; the study of enzymes present in the blood.

eosinopenia: A decrease in the absolute number of eosinophils below normal limits.

eosinophilia: An increase in the absolute number of eosinophils above normal limits.

epithelial cells: Cells that make up the covering of the various internal and external organs of the body, including the lining of the blood vessels.

equivalent (equiv) weight (or mass): Mass in grams that will liberate, combine with, or replace 1 gram of hydrogen ion; generally is the molecular weight divided by the valence.

erythrocyte: Red blood cell, one of the formed elements of the peripheral blood; chief role is to transport oxygen to the tissues.

erythrocyte sedimentation rate (ESR): Rate in millimeters at which the red blood cells fall, or sediment, in a given unit of time (usually 1 hour).

ethics: The discipline dealing with good and bad or a set of moral principles.

etiologic agent: Agent causing a disease.

eukaryote: Fungi, algae, protozoa; more complex than prokaryotes; contain membrane-enclosed organelles such as mitochondria, lysosomes, and a true membrane-enclosed nucleus.

exfoliated: Sloughed off tissue or cells.

exponents: Superscript numbers used to indicate how many times a number must be multiplied by itself.

exposures to hazardous chemicals: OSHA standards seek to minimize occupational exposures of this type.

extravascular component: Tissue surrounding the blood vessels.

extravascular fluid: Body cavity fluid other than blood or urine.

extrinsic system of coagulation: Coagulation pathway that is activated by tissue thromboplastin; necessary components are factor VII and calcium.

exudate: Effusion that results from inflammatory conditions, such as infections and malignancies, that directly affect the membranes lining a cavity.

eyepiece (ocular): Microscope lens that magnifies the image formed by the objective.

F

facultative microorganism: Organism that can grow under either aerobic or anaerobic conditions.

facultative parasite: Parasite that can exist in a free-living state, as a commensal, or as a parasite; see commensal parasite.

false negatives: Those subjects who have a negative test yet do have the disease.

false positives: Those subjects who have a positive test but do not have the disease.

fastidious: Said of a microorganism that is sensitive to changes; usually requires protected culture conditions.

fasting blood glucose: Blood glucose test performed on a fasting specimen; see fasting state.

fasting state: Eight to twelve hours of refraining from consumption of food and liquids other than water. Example is when blood is collected after a 12-hour fast for some tests. Additional patient restrictions are sometimes also necessary, such as no smoking or administration of certain drugs during the fasting period.

federal regulations: Standards existing to meet objectives, such as safety regulations. For the clinical laboratory, see Clinical Laboratory Improvement Amendments of 1988 (CLIA '88).

Fern test (cervical mucus test): Test used to determine ovulation in fertility studies and for contraception and rupture of membranes in pregnancy by observing the appearance of dried cervical mucus on a glass microscope slide.

fibrin: End product of coagulation. Forms a visible clot, a fibrin mesh, to entrap the blood cells. Is derived from fibrinogen, a plasma protein, by the action of thrombin.

fibrin clot: See fibrin.

fibrinogen, coagulation factor I: Plasma protein that is the substrate for thrombin action in the formation of fibrin. Manufactured by the liver; is not vitamin K dependent; is the soluble precursor of the clot-forming protein, fibrin.

fibrinolysis: Destruction of the fibrin clot by plasmin activity to keep the vascular system free from clots; under normal conditions, coagulation and fibrinolysis are kept in balance.

fibrinolytic system: Functions to keep the vascular system free of fibrin clots or deposited fibrin; see fibrinolysis.

fibronectin: Assists in bonding platelets to substrate; is secreted by endothelial cells.

field diaphragm: The part of the microscope through which light passes up to the condenser. Located in the light port in the base of the microscope, it controls the area of the circle of light in the field of view when the specimen and condenser have been properly focused.

first morning urine specimen: First urine voided in the morning. It is generally the most concentrated specimen of the day, because less fluid or water is excreted during the night, yet the kidney has maintained excretion of a constant concentration of solid or dissolved substances.

fistula: An abnormal connection, such as between the colon and the urinary tract.

fixed angle–head centrifuge: A centrifuge in which the cups are held in a rigid position and at a fixed angle.

flame emission photometry: Atoms of certain elements, when sprayed into a hot flame, become excited and emit energy at wavelengths characteristic for those elements (commonly lithium, sodium, and potassium). Utilizes a device (flame photometer) to measure the intensity of the colored flame. Solution containing metal ions is sprayed into a flame, and the intensity and color of the flame are proportional to the amount of substance present in the solution.

flame photometer: Instrument used to measure the energy emitted by certain elements when they are sprayed into a flame in the photometer; see flame emission photometry.

flocculation: Clumping of fine particles to form visible masses.

floppy disks or diskettes: Diskettes that can store information not needed on a hard drive.

flow cytometers: Used to identify and enumerate the blood cells in a given patient sample; see flow cytometry.

flow cytometry: Enumeration and differentiation of blood cells by passing them through a focused beam of a laser.

fluorescent antibody (FA): Assay that uses antibodies labeled with fluorescein compounds, which cause microscopic fluorescence as an indication of an antigen-antibody complex being formed.

fluorescent antinuclear antibody (FANA): Screening assay for SLE; see fluorescent antibody.

focal length: Slightly less than the distance from an objective being examined microscopically to the center of the objective lens; practically, equal to the working distance.

Food and Drug Administration (FDA): Issues certification and licensure requirements, which are an external control for clinical laboratory standards.

Forssman antibody: A heterophil antibody.

free bilirubin, unconjugated bilirubin, indirect bilirubin: Water-insoluble form of bilirubin that is carried through the blood bound to albumin.

fungemia: Presence of fungi in the blood.

G

galactosuria: The presence of galactose in urine.

galvanometer: Measures and records the amount of current (in the form of electrons) reaching it.

Gaussian curve or distribution: Particular symmetric statistical distribution, also known as a "normal" distribution; a statistical tool used to set reference ranges.

genitourinary tract specimens: Specimens collected from the genital or urinary tract (e.g., vaginal cervix and perineal area in women, anterior urethra in men).

genotype: Actual total genetic makeup. Often impossible to determine by laboratory testing but requires additional family studies.

genus: Members of the same genus share common biological characteristics; the next larger classification after species.

germ tube: An appendage on yeast cells, the beginning of true hyphae.

gestational diabetes: Glucose intolerance that occurs during some pregnancies.

glitter cells: Large, swollen neutrophilic leukocytes that appear in hypotonic urine with a specific gravity of about 1.010 or less. The cells show Brownian motion of granules in the cytoplasm, giving a glittering appearance.

glomerular filtrate: Ultrafiltrate of blood formed as blood is filtered through the glomerular capillaries of the glomerulus into Bowman's capsule. First step in urine formation; basically blood plasma without protein or fat.

glomerulus: Part of the nephron; made up of a tuft of blood vessels.

gluconeogenesis: Glucose from fat and protein that is provided to the blood.

glucose oxidase: Enzyme that allows for the oxidation of glucose to gluconic acid; the basis of the reagent strip tests for glucose in urine.

glucose tolerance test: Measures the response of the body to a challenge load of glucose; used to aid in the diagnosis of diabetes mellitus.

glucosuria, glycosuria: Abnormally high concentration of glucose in urine.

glycated hemoglobin: Hemoglobin derivative, also known as *hemoglobin* A_{1c}; formed when glucose and hemoglobin combine; tests used to monitor long-term blood glucose concentration in blood of diabetics measures diabetes control.

glycogenesis: Formation of glycogen from glucose.

glycolysis: Breakdown or oxidation of glucose.

glycosuria: Presence of glucose in the urine.

grades of chemicals: Varying qualities of production criteria that are placed on the manufacture of chemicals for laboratory use, depending on the use to which the chemical is put; the grade indicates the level of quality.

graduated pipette, measuring pipette: Cylindrical tube used to deliver a measured volume of liquid between two calibration (or graduation) marks on the tube; has several graduation or calibration marks on the tube, allowing a variety of measurements with the same device.

gram-molecular weight: One gram-molecular weight equals the sum of all atomic weights in a molecule of compound, expressed in grams.

gram negative: See Gram staining reaction.

gram positive: See Gram staining reaction.

Gram staining reaction (Gram stain): With the Gram staining method, microorganisms retaining the violet (purple) color of the primary stain (crystal violet-iodine complex) are considered gram "positive"; microorganisms having the red-pink color of the counterstain (safranin) are considered gram "negative." Use of these properties serves to classify or differentiate organisms in microbiology; Gram stain is a differential stain.

gram-stained smear: Used routinely to determine Gram staining characteristics; see Gram staining reaction.

granulocyte: Leukocyte that contains prominent cytoplasmic granules; neutrophils, eosinophils, and basophils.

gravimetric analysis: Analysis by measurement of mass.

Griess test: A test for nitrite that involves a diazo reaction; basis of the reagent strip tests for nitrite in urine.

group A β-hemolytic streptococci: Microorganisms that account for most infectious "strep throat." Organisms are isolated from throat swabs by one of several methods (e.g., culture plates, rapid slide agglutination procedures).

gum guaiac: Phenolic compound that turns blue when oxidized. Commonly used as the chromogen in tests for the detection of occult blood in feces.

H

hand washing: The most important means of interrupting the transmission of infectious pathogens.

Hansel's stain: Stain containing eosin and methylene blue; used to stain for the presence of eosinophils.

hapten: Nonantigenic, nonprotein substance that binds to protein, making a hapten-protein complex that is antigenic.

haptoglobin: Protein-bound form of hemoglobin by which hemoglobin is carried through the bloodstream.

hard copy: Computer-generated data printed on paper.

hard disks or hard drive: Revolving disks in a computer with a magnetic surface that can be easily accessed; data are stored in tracks, a series of concentric circles on the disks.

hardware: Physical elements of a computer system (e.g., central processing unit, printer, terminal).

hazard identification system: Provides in words, symbols, and pictures information on presence of potential laboratory materials considered hazardous (e.g., flammable, health risk, chemical reactivity).

Health Care Financing Administration (HCFA): Agency of the U.S. Department of Health and Human Services; regulates and administers funding under the Health Insurance for the Aged Act of 1965 (Medicare); regulates reimbursement for Medicare-related activities. Medicare and Medicaid amendments to the Social Security Act authorize the regulation of specific laboratory services if the government is authorized to pay for these services to the aging and needy population of the United States. HCFA coordinates its regulatory functions with the Centers for Disease Control and Prevention (CDC).

hemagglutination (HA): Agglutination of red cells as indicator of antibody-antigen complex formation.

hematocrit: Ratio of packed red blood cell volume to whole blood volume, expressed as a percent or ratio unit.

hematoma: Collection of blood under the skin.

hematopoiesis: Blood cell production.

hematuria: Presence of red blood cells in urine.

heme: An iron complex containing one iron atom. The iron-containing portion of the hemoglobin molecule.

hemocytometer: Counting chamber used to perform manual cell counts.

hemoglobin: Iron-containing protein portion of the red blood cells that carries oxygen to the tissues; four globin chains, each containing a heme moiety.

hemoglobin variants: Different structural forms of hemoglobin, which vary in the content and sequence of amino acids in the globulin chains.

hemoglobinopathies: Disorders in which the presence of structurally abnormal hemoglobins is considered to play an important role pathologically.

hemoglobinuria: The presence of free hemoglobin in urine.

hemolysis: Rupture of the red cell membrane and release of hemoglobin into the suspending medium or plasma; the plasma or serum appears reddish. In blood banking and other immunologic reactions, hemolysis is used as an indicator of an antigen-antibody reaction.

hemolysis, alpha: In microbiology, partial destruction (lysis) of red blood cells in a blood agar plate; greenish color appears around the bacterial colony producing the alpha hemolysin.

hemolysis, beta: In microbiology, complete destruction (lysis) of red blood cells around a colony on a blood agar plate; leads to a completely clear zone surrounding the colony producing the beta hemolysin.

hemolytic jaundice: Type of jaundice that results from increased destruction of red cells.

hemolyzed serum: Serum with lysed red blood cells in it; appears pink or red.

hemophilia: Hereditary deficiency of plasma coagulation proteins; results in varying degrees of bleeding disorders, mild to severe, depending on the specific deficiency.

hemophilia A: Classic bleeder's disease; sex-linked deficiency of the coagulant component of factor VIII (antihemophilic factor); see Hemophilia.

hemophilia B: Christmas disease; sex-linked deficiency of factor IX; see Hemophilia.

hemosiderin: Iron-containing granules that may occur in urine after a hemolytic episode. Stain blue with Prussian blue stain for iron.

hemostasis/hemostatic mechanism: Cessation of blood flow from an injured blood vessel, with final intent to stop the bleeding. The state of equilibrium in which the supply is equal to the demand between all the fluid and cellular elements that make up the blood.

hemostatic plug: Result of activation of the hemostatic system; formation of platelet plug.

hepatic jaundice (hepatocellular jaundice): Jaundice that results from conditions that involve the liver cells directly and prevent normal excretion of bilirubin, including failure in conjugation and failure in transport (regurgitation).

hepatitis B virus (HBV): Virus that can be directly transmitted by the blood, causing hepatitis, an acute viral illness. Hepatitis is an inflammation of the liver that is endemic worldwide. Complete recovery is usual; some patients, however, remain carriers or can develop chronic hepatitis.

hepatitis C virus (HCV): Previously known as *non-A, non-B hepatitis virus*. Can be transmitted directly by the blood, causing acute viral hepatitis. This infection does not show the serologic markers of hepatitis A or hepatitis B.

heteroantibodies: Antibodies resulting from exposure to antigenic material from another species.

heterophil antibodies: Antibodies stimulated by one antigen that react with entirely unrelated antigens on the red cells from different mammalian species; examples are Forssman, infectious mononucleosis, and serum sickness antibodies.

heterozygous: Having different alleles for a given trait.

high-complexity tests: CLIA '88 regulations define a certain group of tests in this category; they require technical personnel of the highest degree of experience and training to be responsible for the testing.

high-power objective: Usually a 40× magnification objective, used for more detailed examination of wet preparations.

histiocyte: A cell of the reticuloendothelial system; called a *macrophage* when it has begun to phagocytose.

Hoesch test: Inverse aldehyde reaction used for the detection of porphobilinogen in urine.

homozygous: Having identical alleles for a given trait.

horizontal-head centrifuge: A centrifuge in which cups holding tubes of material to be centrifuged occupy a vertical position when the centrifuge is at rest but assume a horizontal position when the centrifuge revolves.

hospital information system (HIS): Main hospital database; contains the base of information about the patient, established when the patient was first admitted or registered by the hospital or clinic. This database can be accessed by the laboratory information system (LIS) as necessary.

household bleach: See disinfectant.

human chorionic gonadotropin (hCG): Hormone produced by the placenta during pregnancy; constituent measured in most rapid pregnancy tests.

human immunodeficiency virus (HIV): Virus that can be transmitted by the blood and some body fluids; can cause HIV infection or acquired immunodeficiency syndrome (AIDS).

humoral response: Involves antibodies produced by the B lymphocytes along with complement.

hyaluronate (hyaluronic acid): High-molecular-weight mucopolysaccharide found in synovial fluid, responsible for its normal viscosity. Secreted by the synovial fluid cells that line the joint cavity.

hyperglycemia: Increase in concentration of blood glucose.

hyperkalemia: High concentration of potassium in the serum or blood.

hypernatremia: High concentration of sodium in the serum or blood.

hypertonic: Solution or diluent that is more concentrated than that inside of the red cell.

hyphae: Tube-like projections, a part of the basic structure of molds; also called *mycelia*.

hypochromic: Said of red cells with decreased hemoglobin content, which appear very pale and show an increased area of central pallor on the peripheral blood film.

hypoglycemia: Low concentration of glucose in blood.

hypokalemia: Low concentration of potassium in the serum or blood.

hyponatremia: Low concentration of sodium in the serum or blood.

hypotonic: Solution or diluent that is less concentrated than that inside of the red cell.

hypoxia: Lack of oxygen.

I

iatrogenic: The result of medication or treatment; inadvertently caused by the physician.

icterus: See jaundice.

immune antibodies: Result from stimulation by a specific foreign antigen.

immune response: Any reaction demonstrating specific antibody response to antigenic stimulus.

immunoassays: Assays utilizing antigen-antibody reactions to detect the presence of a specific constituent.

immunofluorescence: Technique used for rapid identification of an antigen by treating it with a known antibody tagged with a fluorescent dye and observing the resulting characteristic antigen-antibody reaction; will appear luminous in ultraviolet light projected using a fluorescent microscope.

immunoglobulins (Ig): Antibodies; proteins of the gamma globulin type; produced by B lymphocytes (plasma cells).

immunohematology: The study of antigen-antibody reactions and their effects on blood. Includes blood transfusion medicine and blood banking.

immunoprophylaxis: Recommended after exposure to blood that is known to contain or might contain hepatitis B antigen; immune globulin is given in a single dose as soon as possible after the exposure, within 24 hours if practical.

impaired glucose tolerance: When there is an abnormal glucose tolerance test but no measured hyperglycemia; a midway position between normal and a state of diagnosed diabetes mellitus.

input devices: Allow communication between the user and the CPU.

in situ monitoring: Monitoring in place or on site.

in vitro antigen-antibody reactions: Reactions between antigens and antibodies in a test tube or on a slide (outside the living body; *in vitro* is a Latin term meaning "in glass").

incidence: The number of subjects found to have a disease within a defined period of time, such as within a particular year.

indirect agglutination: Assays that show agglutination when no positive constituent is present.

indwelling lines: Devices used to administer therapeutic products (e.g., fluids, medications, blood products) to patients over long periods. With careful training, it is also possible to collect blood samples from these lines. Also called *vascular access devices* (VAD).

infection control: Set policy or program within a health care institution to prevent exposure to biological hazards.

infection control program: Program whereby laboratory sets up specific steps to prevent contamination from biohazardous specimens in the collection steps, transportation to the laboratory, and processing and testing steps.

infectious waste: Waste that contains biohazardous specimens, such as blood and blood products, contaminated materials, or other potentially infectious products.

informed consent: Legal consent granted by the patient whereby he or she is made aware of, understands, and agrees to the nature of the testing or services to be done.

infusion set: Allows collection of blood from patients with small, fragile, or rolling veins.

inoculate: To place the specimen on the medium in the plate or tube.

inoculating loop or needle: Metal loop or needle attached to a long handle, used to inoculate culture media with specimens or to transfer colonies for subculture. Metal loops must be flamed between uses. Disposable varieties of these loops are available.

inoculum: What is being inoculated onto the medium—plate or tube; usually the specimen is the inoculum; in antimicrobial susceptibility tests, the isolated organism to be tested is prepared in a specific way, depending on the methodology being used.

input device: Any device allowing data or instructions to be placed into a computer system.

insulin shock: State of unconsciousness due to a low blood glucose concentration.

interfacing data: Communications link that allows the transfer of data between the user and the computer system or between another processor and the computer system.

interleukins (IL): Hematopoietic growth factors that contribute to the control of hematopoiesis.

internal standard: Chemical compound of known amount added to a specimen and carried through all steps of an analytical procedure to provide a basis for accurate quantitation, despite variations in the procedural steps; is similar chemically and structurally to the substance being assayed; frequently used in gas chromatography and high-pressure liquid chromatography assays.

International Bureau of Weights and Measures: Responsible for maintaining the standards on which the SI system of measurement is based; see also International System of Units.

International Committee on Nomenclature of Blood Clotting Factors: Establishes and maintains standardized terminology for the various coagulation factors.

international normalized ratio (INR): The PT ratio that would have been obtained if the WHO international reference standard preparation was used as the source of thromboplastin in the PT assay; compares the patient's PT to a mean, normal PT; ensures that results for PT tests done in any laboratory can be compared.

international sensitivity index (ISI): Mathematical indicator of the responsiveness of the PT testing systems to deficiencies of vitamin K coagulation factors; WHO reference standard is assigned an ISI of 1.0.

International System of Units: (SI units, from Système International d'Unités); standard international language of measurement.

interpretive report: Reporting of laboratory results in a usable format, including information about reference ranges or flagging of abnormal values, so the physician can find the results for the requested analyses in an efficient, concise manner.

interpupillary distance: The distance between the two oculars of a binocular microscope; must be adjusted for the microscopist.

intravascular component: Platelets and coagulation proteins that circulate in the blood vessels.

intravascular devices: Devices used to obtain specimens of blood from blood vessels.

intravascular hemolysis: Hemolysis or abnormal destruction of red blood cells in the bloodstream.

intrinsic system of coagulation: Utilization of plasma contact factors to initiate coagulation, beginning with the activation of factor XII; all necessary factors required are contained in the circulating blood.

ionic concentration: In urinalysis, a measure that is related to specific gravity. The principle of the reagent strip test for specific gravity; substances must ionize in order to be measurable with this method.

ionized calcium: Calcium that participates in the coagulation process; necessary to activate thromboplastin and to convert prothrombin to thrombin.

ion-selective electrodes: Indicator electrodes used in potentiometry devices to respond to specific ions in the solution.

iris diaphragm: The part of the microscope located at the bottom of the Abbé condenser, under the lens but within the condenser body; controls the amount of light passing through the material under observation; can be opened or closed to adjust contrast by means of a lever.

isoantibodies: Antibodies resulting from antigenic stimulation within the same species.

isolated colonies: When streak plates are properly made, isolated, or individual, colonies may be seen in specific sections of the plate; enables pure cultures to be made.

iso-osmolar: Two solutions having the same solute concentration, such as the glomerular filtrate and plasma, are normally iso-osmolar with each other.

isotonic: Situation when the concentration of fluid or diluent outside the red cell is the same as it is inside the red cell.

J

jaundice: Accumulation of bilirubin pigment in the tissues and blood; skin and sclera of eyes become jaundiced, or yellow.

jaundiced serum: Increased concentration of bilirubin in the blood (serum) and accumulation of bilirubin pigment in the tissues; serum appears brownish yellow.

The Joint Commission (TJC): Voluntary organization, not governmental, made up of representatives from various health care associations (e.g., hospital, physician, dentist). Mission of JCAHO is to enhance the quality of health care provided to the public, and the organization is dedicated to improving the process to carry out this mission. One important function of JCAHO is accreditation of U.S. hospitals. Standards and guidelines are set for hospitals, and accreditation is carried out and monitored through a continual process of site visits, surveys, and reports. The organization also monitors other health care facilities (e.g., mental health facilities, nursing homes, home health agencies, hospices, managed care and ambulatory care organizations).

K

kernicterus: Results when unconjugated bilirubin passes into the brain and nerve cells and is deposited in the nuclei of these cells; can result in cell damage and death.

ketoacidosis: Acidosis resulting from the presence of increased ketone bodies.

ketogenic diet: A diet containing more than 1.5 g of fat per 1.0 g of carbohydrate; this will result in ketone accumulation, with ketosis and ketonuria.

ketonemia: Increased concentration of ketones in the blood.

ketonuria: Increased concentration of ketones in the urine.

ketosis: Increased concentration of ketones in blood and urine.

kilogram (kg): Standard unit for measurement of mass (and weight).

L

labile factor: Factor V; essential for prompt conversion of prothrombin to thrombin in clotting mechanism; is involved in common pathway of both intrinsic and extrinsic clotting pathways.

laboratory information system (LIS): Computer system designed for use by the clinical laboratory; includes collection of patient information, generation of test results, assembly of data output, production of ancillary reports, and storage of data.

laboratory medicine: Medical discipline by which clinical laboratory science and technology are applied to the care of patients.

laboratory procedure manual: Collection of information about the specific procedures for all analytical assays performed by the laboratory; includes information about specimen requirements and special collection or processing details, test request information, procedural information (how to perform the test, reagents used for the assay, control specimens used), calibration of instruments, quality control data, details about reference values and reporting of results, and any information about bibliographical resources.

laboratory report: Information about results of various assays performed by the laboratory; should be presented in a usable format; see interpretive report.

Landsteiner's rule: In the ABO blood group system, if the A or B antigen is lacking on the red cell, the corresponding antibody will be found in the serum.

larvae: Immature form, as in parasite larvae.

latex agglutination: Particles of latex are used to visualize an antigen-antibody agglutination reaction; test latex particles are coated with a specific antibody and clump together (agglutinate) when the specific antigen is present in the specimen being assayed.

latex-microparticle enzyme immunoassay (MEIA): An immunoassay technology.

lattice formation: In process of agglutination, results in the visible aggregation or clumping reaction.

LE (lupus erythematosus) factor: Present in blood of persons with SLE; has ability to depolymerize the nuclear chromatin of PMNs, making them capable of being ingested by an intact PMN (thus creating the LE cell).

leukemia: Progressive malignant disease of the blood-forming organs, characterized by abnormal proliferation of leukocytes and their precursors in body tissues. Peripheral blood cells and bone marrow cells are changed quantitatively and qualitatively.

leukoblastic reaction: The presence of white blood cell forms more immature than bands in the peripheral blood.

leukocyte: White blood cell; one of formed elements found in peripheral blood.

leukocyte differential: Classification and recorded percentages of various types of leukocytes as seen on a stained blood film or as obtained from an electronic counting device.

leukocyte esterase: Enzyme present in the azurophilic or primary granules of the granulocytic leukocytes; presence of this enzyme in urine indicates urinary tract infection.

leukocytosis: An increase in the white cell count above the normal upper limit.

leukoerythroblastotic reaction: The presence of younger forms of leukocytes and red cells than are normally found in peripheral blood.

leukopenia: A decrease in the white cell count below the normal lower limit.

Levey-Jennings control chart: See quality control chart.

light absorbed: Light that is absorbed by a colored solution; measured as absorbance units or optical density (OD).

light transmitted: Light that passes through a colored solution; measured as percent transmittance units (%T).

light-emitting diode (LED): Readout device found in digital computerized equipment; a semiconductor device visualized as a glowing readout.

linear graph paper: Graph paper with a linear scale on both axes.

linkage (linked genes): Genes for different traits located on the same chromosome, positioned so closely that they are inherited as a unit.

lipemic serum: Serum with presence of fats or lipids; appears white or milky.

liter (L): Standard unit of volume.

lithiasis: Kidney stone formation.

low-power objective: Usually a 10× magnification objective; used for the initial scanning and observation in most routine microscopic work.

lymphocytosis: An increase in the absolute number of lymphocytes above normal limits.

lysin: Antibody that causes lysis.

lysis: Hemolysis of the red cells, rupture of the red cell membrane, and release of hemoglobin; an indicator of an antigen-antibody reaction.

M

macrophage: Any phagocytic cell of the reticuloendothelial system. Thought to be derived from both monocytes and histiocytic cells.

malabsorption: Inadequate, incomplete, or impaired absorption from the gastrointestinal tract; may be associated with presence of increased fat in the feces.

mass per unit mass: See weight per unit weight.

material safety data sheets (MSDS): Information about the hazards of each chemical are provided by the supplier or manufacturer of the chemical; any hazardous chemicals used in a laboratory should be accompanied by this information.

mean (X-bar): Statistically calculated mathematical average value for a valid series of numbers, as for a series of test results, for example; the series of values is totaled and divided by the number in the series; also called the *X-bar*.

measurement of mass or weight: Gravimetric analysis; commonly, measurement of weight by using various types of balances for preparation of laboratory reagents and standard solutions.

meconium: Viscid, elastic, greenish black material composed of amniotic fluid, biliary and intestinal secretions, and epithelial cells; passed from the intestine by newborn infants within the first 24 hours after delivery.

median: The middle value of a body of data; the point that falls halfway between the highest and lowest in position.

median cubital vein: Vein in the antecubital area, most commonly used as site for venipuncture collection of venous blood.

medical laboratory scientist (MLS): Formerly known as medical technologist (MT) or clinical laboratory scientist (CLS), usually a bachelor of science degree holder.

medical laboratory technician (MLT): Formerly clinical laboratory technician (CLT), usually an associate degree program.

medical technologist (MT): See clinical laboratory scientist (CLS).

medulla (kidney): Central anatomic portion of the kidney; consists of the loop of Henle, the distal convoluted tubules, and the collecting tubules.

melena: Black or tarry fecal specimens; dark color is due to the presence of blood, which is changed to a black substance as it passes through the gastrointestinal tract.

meniscus: Curvature in the top surface of a liquid.

menu: Programs or functions (options) offered by a system.

meter (m): Standard unit for measurement of length or distance.

metric system: System of weights and measures based on a decimal system, or divisions and multiples of tens; based on a standard unit of length, the meter.

microalbuminuria: The presence of very small amounts of albumin in the urine.

microorganisms: Microscopic organisms; organisms seen only with the use of a microscope (e.g., bacteria, viruses, fungi, protozoa).

micropipette, micropipettor: Device used to measure very precise, very small volumes; micropipettes are usually calibrated to contain a specific volume, and the entire contents is part of the measurement.

microsampling: Obtaining very small amounts of blood or other body specimens (e.g., capillary blood, cerebrospinal fluid); usually requires micromethods for assay.

milliequivalent: Relates to the equivalent; see milliequivalent weight.

milliequivalent weight: The equivalent weight in milligrams equals 1 milliequivalent (mEq).

milligram-molecular weight: Molecular weight expressed in milligrams.

millimole (mmole): One milligram-molecular weight is equal to a millimole (mmole).

minimum bactericidal concentration (MBC): Minimum concentration of antimicrobial agent needed to kill an organism.

minimum inhibitory concentration (MIC): Minimum concentration of antimicrobial agent needed to prevent visually discernible growth of a bacterial or fungal suspension.

mode: The value that occurs most commonly in a mass of data.

moderate-complexity tests: CLIA '88 regulations place most laboratory tests in this category. Complexity is based on the analyte tested and the method or instrumentation used to perform the test.

molarity: Gram-molecular mass or weight of a compound per liter of solution.

molecular diagnostics: The use of principles of basic molecular biology in the practice of laboratory medicine.

monoclonal antibody: Highly specified antibody derived entirely from a single ancestral antibody-forming parent cell. Produced by hybridization; used in diagnostic testing.

multiple-reagent strips: Plastic strips that contain one or more chemically impregnated test sites on an absorbent pad. When a chemical reaction occurs, it is indicated by a color change. The basis for chemical screening in urinalysis, for example. Also referred to as *dipsticks*.

mycelium: See hyphae.

mycology: The study or science of fungi.

myeloid: Of or pertaining to the bone marrow. The granulocytic leukocytes come from the myeloid series of development and include neutrophils, eosinophils, basophils, and monocytes.

myoglobinuria: The presence of myoglobin in the urine.

N

National Bureau of Standards (NBS): Agency of the U.S. government. Maintains and supplies standard reference materials needed for the preparation of primary standard solutions; develops reference methods and reference materials.

National Cholesterol Education Program (NCEP): Program established to set standards for the detection and classification of individuals at high risk for coronary heart disease (CHD).

National Committee for Clinical Laboratory Standards (NCCLS): Nonprofit educational organization that sets voluntary consensus standards for all areas of clinical laboratories.

natural antibodies: Exist without antigenic stimulus; examples are anti-A and anti-B in ABO groups.

negative birefringence: Pattern of birefringence seen when a crystal appears yellow when the long axis of the crystal is parallel to the slow wave of vibration of a full-wave compensator and blue when the long axis is perpendicular to the slow wave.

negative exponent: Indicates the number of times the reciprocal of the base is to be multiplied by itself; indicates a fraction.

negative predictive value (PV): Indicates the number of patients with a normal test result who do not have a disease compared with all patients with a normal (negative) result.

neonatal physiologic jaundice: Type of jaundice that results from an enzyme deficiency in the immature liver of the newborn.

neonatal screening programs: Approved testing laboratories test for specific diseases or pathologies in newborns; capillary blood is usually collected onto filter paper and sent to the reference laboratory for testing; see also blood spot collections.

nephelometry: Measurement of light that has been scattered when it strikes a particle in a liquid; the nephelometer measures the amount of light scattered.

nephron: Working unit of the kidney, where urine is formed; includes glomerulus, Bowman's capsule, proximal and distal convoluted tubules, and loop of Henle.

nephrotic syndrome: An abnormal kidney condition characterized by heavy or massive proteinuria (albuminuria), decreased blood albumin (hypoalbuminemia), and edema.

neutropenia: A reduction of the absolute neutrophil count below normal limits.

neutrophilia: An increase in the absolute number of neutrophils present in blood above normal limits.

95% confidence interval: Numerical limits within which a sample must fall to be part of the normal distribution of values; determined statistically, and is the basis for quality control "rules" for the acceptance or rejection of certain results; based on a gaussian curve, whereby 95% of the population have observations within 2 standard deviations.

nocturia: The excretion of over 400 mL of urine at night.

nomenclature of blood clotting factors: International Committee on Nomenclature of Blood Clotting Factors ascertains consistency in terminology used; standardizes the complex nomenclature for the various clotting factors.

nonglucose reducing substances (NGRS): Substances other than glucose (including several sugars) that may be present in the urine and that have the ability to reduce heavy metal from a higher to a lower oxidation state. NGRS are not detected by the reagent strip tests specific for glucose.

normal flora: Organisms that inhabit the human body normally and do not cause disease.

"normal" range or value: See reference range or value.

normality: Number of equivalent weights per liter of solution.

normochromic: Said of red cells with normal hemoglobin content.

nosepiece: The part of the microscope on which the objectives are mounted. Usually on a pivot to allow for a quick change of objectives.

nosocomial infection: Infection acquired in a hospital or health care facility.

numerical aperture (NA): Index or measurement of the resolving power of a microscope. Also an index of the light-gathering power of a lens that describes the amount of light entering the objective. As the numerical aperture increases, resolution decreases.

O

objective: The major part of the magnification system of the microscope. Most commonly used microscopes have three objectives: low power, high power, and oil immersion. Usually mounted in a rotating nosepiece that enables a quick change of objectives.

obligate parasite: A parasite that cannot survive without its designated host.

obstructive jaundice, posthepatic jaundice, regurgitative jaundice: Type of jaundice that results from obstruction of the common bile duct by stones, tumors, spasms, or stricture.

occult blood: Blood not observable by the naked eye; requires use of a chemical test to be detected.

Occupational Health and Safety Act of 1970: Created the Occupational Health and Safety Administration within the U.S. Department of Labor to set levels of safety and health for all workers in the United States. A federal agency.

Occupational Health and Safety Administration (OSHA): See Occupational Health and Safety Act of 1970.

ocular (eyepiece): The part of the microscope that magnifies the image formed by the objective.

oil-immersion objective: Generally a 100× magnification lens with a relatively short working distance of 1.8 mm. Requires the addition of a special immersion oil placed between the objective and the slide or coverglass. Cannot be used with wet preparations.

oliguria: Abnormally small excretion of urine; less than 500 mL/24 hours.

opportunistic pathogen: Organism that does not usually cause disease in persons with an intact immune system but does cause disease in immunocompromised persons.

optical density (OD): Term used to express the amount of light being absorbed when being passed through a solution; see absorbed light.

optical methods, cell counters: Automated cell counters with focused laser beams whereby cells cause a change in the deflection of a beam of light, which is converted to measurable pulses by a photomultiplier tube.

oral glucose tolerance test (OGTT): Oral glucose is consumed and blood tested for glucose concentration; test measures the ability of a person to respond appropriately to a heavy load of glucose.

order entry: The first step in the laboratory information system is the test ordering or order entry.

organized sediment: The biological part of the urine sediment; includes cells, fat of biological origin, casts, organisms, and microorganisms.

orthostatic proteinuria: Proteinuria that is present when persons are engaged in normal activity but disappears when they lie down or recline.

OSHA standards: See Occupational Health and Safety Act of 1970.

osmolarity: Number of osmoles of solute per liter of solution.

osmosis: The passage of a solvent through a membrane from a dilute solution into a more concentrated one.

osmotic fragility: Test to determine the ability of the red blood cells to withstand hypotonic or hypoosmotic solutions. Measure of the resistance of the red cell membrane to rupture; cells with membrane defects (hereditary spherocytosis) have increased fragility.

output/output device: Any device that allows information generated by a computer system to be used (e.g., results of calculations for a laboratory assay). Information output can be printed, displayed, or transferred to another processor.

ova: Eggs, as in parasite eggs.

oval fat body (OFB), renal tubular fat (RTF) body: Renal epithelial cell (and possibly macrophage) filled with fat droplets.

P

packed cell volume (PCV): The hematocrit. A macroscopic measurement of the percentage volume of packed red cells.

panic or critical values: Possibly life-threatening laboratory values that must be noted and communicated to the physician as quickly as possible; automated instruments flag or highlight these results for the laboratory personnel.

parasitism: Result of parasite injuring its host by its actions.

parasitology: The study or science of parasites.

pathogens: Microorganisms that cause disease.

pathologist: A licensed physician with special training in clinical and/or anatomic pathology.

patient demographics: Information about the patient such as name, gender, age or birth date, referring or attending physician.

Patient's Bill of Rights: Document drawn up by a health care institution that declares certain rights for all patients being cared for in that facility. Being considerate of these rights constitutes good patient care. In the laboratory context, the Patient's Bill of Rights must be considered in collecting the various patient specimens needed for testing.

percent: Parts per hundred parts.

percent solution: Somewhat outdated expression of concentration based on parts per hundred parts (e.g., 10% sodium chloride, which is 10 g NaCl diluted to 100 mL with deionized water; currently expressed as 10 g/dL).

percent transmittance: Amount of light that passes through a colored solution compared with the amount of light that passes through a blank solution.

percent transmittance units: Units used to measure the amount of light transmitted through a solution.

pericardial fluid: Extravascular fluid that surrounds the heart.

peripheral blood film: Blood smear prepared on a glass microscope slide using circulating peripheral blood. Blood is usually obtained by venipuncture or finger puncture.

peritoneal fluid: Extravascular fluid that surrounds the abdominal and pelvic cavities.

peroxidase: Enzyme that catalyzes release of free oxygen from hydrogen peroxide. Peroxidase activity of the heme portion of the hemoglobin molecule is the basis of the reagent strip tests for blood.

personal protective equipment: OSHA requires facilities to provide their personnel with protective equipment, such as protective clothing, gloves, eyewear, protective shields and barriers, and respiratory devices, for their safety in the workplace.

Petri dish or plate: Shallow, flat glass or plastic plate with a loose-fitting deep cover, used to hold culture media.

pH: Unit that describes the acidity or alkalinity of a solution.

phagocytosis: A process in which a cell engulfs and disposes of foreign material.

phase contrast: Microscope illumination system that uses a special condenser with an annular diaphragm with a matched absorption ring in the corresponding objective. Used to give additional contrast in wet preparations; especially useful for counting platelets and observing urinary sediment.

phenotype: Observable genetic makeup that can be determined by direct testing (i.e., blood type).

phlebotomist: Person trained in drawing blood. Primarily trained to draw blood by venipuncture but also trained to perform capillary collections and to do skin punctures of various types. Drawing blood specimens from indwelling lines is an additional technique performed by a trained phlebotomist.

photoelectric cell, photodetector: Electronic device that measures the intensity of light being transmitted by a solution; produces electrons in proportion to the amount of light reaching it.

photometry: Technique used to determine the quantitative concentration of a substance by measuring the variation in its color intensity by use of a photometer.

physical properties: In urinalysis, color, transparency, odor, foam, and specific gravity of a urine specimen.

physician office laboratory (POL): A laboratory in a physician's office or clinic where tests are done only on the patients coming to the practice or group.

physiologic jaundice: Can result from a deficiency of an enzyme that transfers glucuronate groups onto bilirubin or from liver immaturity; can result in jaundice that occurs in some infants during the first few days of life; also called *neonatal jaundice*; see jaundice.

plan for evacuation: Routes for exiting the laboratory site in an emergency must be readily available to all persons working in the laboratory area.

plasma: Liquid portion of blood after it has been anticoagulated and centrifuged or otherwise allowed to settle.

plasma cell, plasmacyte: Derivative of the B lymphocyte. Large, with a round or oval eccentric nucleus. Specialized for production of antibodies; rarely is seen in the peripheral blood.

plasmin: Proteolytic enzyme that breaks down fibrin; is generated by the activation of a plasma precursor, plasminogen.

platelet adhesion, platelet adherence: Test that measures the ability of platelets to adhere to glass surfaces; essential requirement for primary hemostasis.

platelet aggregation: Massing or clumping of platelets with one another; test for platelet function.

platelet plug: Formation of an aggregate or mass of platelets that physically plug or slow down the flow of blood at the site of an injury to a blood vessel; result of activation of the hemostatic system.

pleural fluid: Extravascular fluid that surrounds the lungs.

pluripotential stem cell (PSC): Stem cell that is uncommitted to any specific cell line; stimulation results in differentiation and maturation.

point-of-care testing (POCT): Tests performed at the bedside of the patient or near the site where the patient is; a decentralized form of laboratory testing—the laboratory testing comes to the patient.

polarize: To bend or rotate light.

polarized light: Light that is propagated so that radiation waves occur in only one direction rather than at random.

polarizer: A filter that allows the passage of light waves in only one orientation.

polarizing microscope: Microscope illumination system that employs two crossed polarizing lenses, extinguishing the passage of light through the microscope. Used to detect objects or crystals that bend or polarize light, making them visible when viewed with crossed polarizing filters.

polychromasia: Many colors. A property of red cells that show a faint blue or blue-orange color when stained with Wright stain, because of the presence of both blue RNA and red hemoglobin in young red cells.

polyclonal antibodies: Antibodies derived from multiple ancestral clones of antibody-producing cells; characteristically produced in infectious diseases.

polydipsia: Excessive thirst.

polyphagia: Excessive, constant hunger.

polyuria: Excessive urination.

porphobilinogen: An unstable intermediary product in the synthesis of heme; a significant increase in the urine can be seen in acute intermittent hepatic porphyria.

porphyrias: A group of inherited disorders that are characterized by an increased production of porphyrins; some forms result in the presence of porphobilinogen in urine.

positive birefringence: Pattern of birefringence seen when a crystal appears blue when the long axis of the crystal is parallel to the slow wave of vibration of a full-wave compensator and yellow when the long axis is perpendicular to the slow wave.

positive exponent: Indicates the number of times the base is to be multiplied by itself.

positive predictive value (PV): Indicates the number of patients with an abnormal test result who have a disease compared with all patients with an abnormal result.

postanalytical function: Includes functions that occur after the analysis itself, such as generating chart reports, printing result reports as needed, archiving results, and billing.

postcoital test (PCT): Test that evaluates cervical mucus; scored on a scale of 1 to 15 by assessment of spinnbarkeit, ferning, consistency, and pH.

postexposure prophylaxis (PEP): For HIV exposure, the degree of risk for infection must be assessed and the worker followed by the health care facility's infection control department and offered postexposure prophylaxis immediately.

posthepatic jaundice: See obstructive jaundice.

postprandial: Directly after a meal; a postprandial blood specimen is one collected directly after a meal.

postprandial specimen, 2-hour: Blood that is drawn 2 hours after a meal.

postrenal azotemia: Azotemia resulting from obstruction whereby urea is reabsorbed into the circulation; see azotemia.

potentiometry: Technique in which the potential difference between two electrodes is measured under equilibrium.

pour plates: A specimen is inoculated in a liquid medium, which is then mixed and poured into a culture plate, where it solidifies.

preanalytical functions: Functions in testing protocol that occur before the actual analyses—test ordering, specimen collection, and so forth.

precipitation (precipitate): Visible result of an antigen-antibody reaction between a soluble antigen and its specific antibody.

precipitin: An antibody that reacts with a soluble antigen to form a precipitate.

precision, reproducibility: Measure of the closeness of the results obtained when analysis on the same sample is repeated; agreement between replicate measurements.

predictive value (PV): Means or ability to predict the results of an analysis of the same data by using another test instrument or measurement; contributes to the validity of a test.

prerenal azotemia: Azotemia resulting from poor perfusion of the kidneys; see azotemia.

prevalence: The proportion of a population that has a disease.

primary culture: The initial or first culture done with a specimen.

primary hemostasis: Involves platelets and the vascular response.

primary response: First antibody response to foreign antigen.

proenzymes: Enzyme precursors or zymogens.

proficiency testing (PT) or survey: Program under which samples are sent to a group of laboratories for analysis; results are compared with those of other laboratories participating in the program. Included as a component of quality assurance programs.

proficiency testing programs: See proficiency testing (PT) or survey.

program: Set of commands or steps that instruct the computer to perform a certain task.

program for infection control: See infection control.

prokaryote: Small bacterium containing DNA in a single, circular chromosome.

prophylaxis: To prevent exposure.

proportion: Two or more ratios having the same relative meaning but with different numbers.

proportioning: A combination of predetermined amounts of reagent and sample in an automated laboratory instrument.

protective immunity: Provided by antibodies that after formation will protect from subsequent exposure to the antigen.

protective isolation: Measures used to protect a patient from infectious agents.

protein error of pH indicators: Color change of a pH indicator due to the presence of protein rather than hydrogen ion concentration.

protein-free filtrate: After preparation of a specimen to remove the protein, the filtrate, free from protein, remains.

proteinuria: Presence of protein, usually albumin, in urine.

prothrombin, coagulation factor II, prethrombin: Produced by the liver; is vitamin K dependent.

prothrombin time (PT): Time it takes for the plasma to clot after an excess of thromboplastin and an optimal concentration of calcium have been added; measures functional activity of the extrinsic and common pathways of coagulation.

protoplasts: Unusually long, rod-shaped forms of bacteria with central swelling; the result of damage to the cell wall by antibiotics.

provider-performed microscopies (PPM): Specific microscopies (mostly wet mounts) usually performed by the physician or provider for his or her own patients; these tests are a special subcategory of the moderately complex CLIA '88 tests.

prozone phenomenon: An excess of antibody; can result in a false-negative reaction.

pseudocasts: False casts. Structures in the urine sediment that appear like, and might be mistaken for, casts.

pseudohyphae: False hyphae. Elongated yeast cells that may be branched and have terminal buds and resemble the mycelia of true fungi.

Public Health Service Act: Act under which Medicare and Medicaid are licensed.

puncture-resistant sharps containers: Used for disposal of sharps such as needles, lancets, and broken glass.

pure culture: Culture in which each colony is from a single isolated originating bacterial cell.

pyuria: Presence of pus (leukocytes) in the urine; indicates a possible urinary tract infection.

Q

quality assurance (QA): Comprehensive set of policies, procedures, and practices necessary to make sure that a laboratory's results are reliable. QA includes record keeping, calibration and maintenance of equipment, quality control, proficiency testing, and training.

quality assurance indicators: Indicators that monitor the performance of a laboratory and are evaluated as part of CQI; see continuous quality improvement.

quality assurance program: Plan to carry out policies and practices necessary to comply with quality assurance standards set by accreditation agencies to make certain that a laboratory's results are reliable and that these results are used in the best interest of the patient. See also total quality improvement (TQI).

quality control (QC): Set of laboratory procedures designed to ensure that a test method is working properly and that the results meet the diagnostic needs of the physician. QC includes testing control samples, charting the results, and analyzing them statistically.

quality control chart: Visual documentation of information derived from using control specimens; values for control specimen assays used for a particular substance are plotted on the chart on a regular basis and are statistically analyzed for trends of change.

quality control program: Plan to carry out procedures established to make certain that laboratory assay methods are working properly and that assay results meet the diagnostic needs of the physician; makes use of control specimens and standard solutions.

quality control specimen: See control specimen.

quantitative analysis: A very precise means of measurement of the quantity of a substance.

quantitative transfer: Process of transferring the entire amount of a weighed or measured substance from one vessel to another; usually used in the process of reagent preparation, in which the weighed substance (chemical) must be transferred in its entirety to a volumetric flask for dilution with deionized water.

quantitative urine culture methods: Traditional method of detecting urinary tract infection, in which urine is cultured on an appropriate medium and identified.

R

random access analyzer: Instrument that does all the selected determinations on one sample before going on to the next sample.

random access memory (RAM): Central memory in the central processing unit (CPU) of a computer; commonly used as a means of storage of information that is frequently altered, changed, or updated.

rapid streptococcal antigen detection: Basis for rapid tests for detection of "strep throat" caused by group A β-hemolytic streptococci.

ratio: Amount of something in proportion to an amount of something else; always describes a relative amount.

reactive lymphocytes: Altered lymphocytes associated with viral infections, especially infectious mononucleosis; also referred to as *atypical* or *variant lymphocytes.*

reagent: Any substance employed to produce a chemical reaction.

reagin antibodies: Antibody-like proteins that react in some serologic tests for syphilis.

recovery solution: A measured amount of a substance being quantitated is added to a specimen; theoretically, the amount of substance added should be recovered at the end of the determination if the method is an accurate one.

red blood cell indices: In hematology, the calculated values for red cell measurements such as mean cell volume (MCV), mean cell hemoglobin (MCH), and mean cell hemoglobin concentration (MCHC).

reducing sugars: Sugars (including glucose) that have the ability to reduce copper ions from Cu^{2+} to Cu^+ in the presence of alkali and heat.

reference laboratory: Laboratory setting where specimens are sent that require more complex testing methodologies and for tests that are infrequently ordered.

reference range, normal range, normal values, reference values: Range of values that includes 95% of the test results for a healthy reference population; see gaussian curve.

reflectance photometry or spectrophotometry: Photometric technique whereby light reflected from the surface of a colorimetric reaction is used to measure the amount of unknown colored product generated in the reaction;

a beam of light is directed at a flat surface, and the amount of light reflected is measured.

refractive index: A measure of solute concentration. The ratio of the velocity of light in air to the velocity of light in solution.

refractometer: Temperature-compensated instrument used to measure refractive index.

relative centrifugal force (RCF): Expression of the number of revolutions per minute and the centrifugal force generated; method of comparing the forces generated by various centrifuges, taking into account the speed of rotation and the radius from the center of rotation.

relative numbers (cell count): The concentration of a cell type expressed as a percentage.

reliability: Ability of a laboratory assay to produce consistent results when testing is repeated successively.

renal azotemia: Azotemia resulting primarily from diminished glomerular filtration; see azotemia.

renal threshold: Level above which a substance cannot be reabsorbed by the renal tubules and is thus excreted into the urine.

renal tubular fat (RTF): See oval fat bodies.

reproducibility: See precision, reproducibility.

resolution: Limit of usable magnification; tells how small and how close individual objects can be and still be recognized.

reticulocyte: Young red blood cell that has just extruded its nucleus. Characterized by the presence of RNA; becomes a normal, mature red cell when all the RNA is lost; stains with a supravital stain.

reticuloendothelial system (RES): A functional system of the body involved primarily in defense against infection and in disposal of the products of the breakdown of cells by phagocytosis.

Rh immune globulin (RhIG): Concentrated and purified form of anti-D antibody, used to immunosuppress Rh-negative women who deliver Rh-positive babies, to prevent sensitization of the mother by her child's red blood cells.

Rh negative: Red blood cells lacking the D antigen (d/d).

Rh positive: Red blood cells containing the D antigen (D/D or D/d).

rhabdomyolysis: Acute destruction of muscle fibers.

rheostat: Control used to adjust the amount of light entering a microscope.

rheumatoid factor (RF): Autoantibodies present in the serum of patients with clinical features of rheumatoid arthritis; circulating complexes of immunoglobulins, known collectively as *rheumatoid factor*.

rhinitis: Inflammation of the mucous membranes of the nose, usually accompanied by swelling of the mucosa and nasal discharge.

rickettsiology: The study or observation of rickettsia.

rounding off a number: To bring a digit (number) to the chosen number of significant figures.

Rous test: A wet Prussian blue stain for iron; used to confirm the presence of hemosiderin in the urine sediment.

S

safety manual: Current compilation of all safety practices and procedures, kept in a readily available format for use by all persons in a specific laboratory setting; anything that could pose a potential safety hazard for persons in the laboratory must be described in this manual.

safety program: Required by OSHA for every clinical laboratory.

sampling procedure: Only a very small amount of sample is usually used in laboratory measurements; sampling difficulties can lead to fluctuations and variations in results reporting; affects reliability of the procedure.

scanning electron microscope (SEM): A type of electron microscope that looks at the surface of a specimen and produces a three-dimensional image by striking the sample with a focused beam of electrons.

secondary hemostasis: Response by coagulation proteins.

secondary response: Response to second exposure to the same antigen; rapid amounts of detectable antibody in the serum or plasma.

sediment: Solid material that has settled out of suspension (e.g., urinary sediment).

selective media: Substances present in these media selectively inhibit growth of certain microorganisms and permit growth of others.

semilogarithmic graph paper: Graph paper with a logarithmic scale on one axis and a linear scale on the other; allows the plotting of a straight line when percent transmittance readings are plotted against concentration.

sensitivity: The proportion of cases having a specific disease or condition that give a positive test result.

sensitivity to antimicrobial agents: The situation that exists when an organism's growth is inhibited in the presence of certain antibiotics (antimicrobial agents).

sensitization: Process in which an individual is made sensitive to a foreign antigen through exposure. Once sensitization has occurred, the individual responds to a repeated exposure with an accentuated immune response.

septicemia, sepsis: Bacteria in the blood or toxin produced by the bacteria is causing harm to the patient.

serial dilutions: Progressive dilutions of a substance in a series of tubes in predetermined ratios to give concentrations of a specific amount.

serologic pipette: Much like a graduated pipette but is graduated to the end of the delivery tip; allows for a faster delivery and is less precise for this reason.

serologic reaction: The observed reaction when an antigen-antibody reaction has taken place.

serology: The division of immunology specializing in detection and measurement of specific antibodies that develop in blood (serum) during a response to exposure to a disease-producing antigen.

serotonin: Vasoconstricting substance.

serous fluids: The fluid within the closed cavities of the body (e.g., pleural, pericardial, peritoneal).

serum: The fluid portion of blood that remains after coagulation. Preferable to plasma when typing or otherwise testing blood for compatibility.

serum separator collection tubes: See serum separator gel.

serum separator gel: Additive used to assist in obtaining serum after centrifuging a whole blood specimen. A special silicon gel layer is added to the collection tubes that moves to form a barrier between the cells and serum during centrifugation; the gel hardens to form an inert barrier, allowing easy serum separation or removal after the centrifugation process.

sharps containers: Used disposable needles and other sharp objects must be safely discarded in these containers, which are made of rigid plastic, metal, or stiff paperboard. The containers must be conveniently located, easily recognizable, and marked as a biohazard. All skin lancets, needles, scalpel blades, and bleeding time devices must be discarded properly in a sharps container, with extreme caution.

shift cells: Nucleated red cells or polychromatic macrocytes (reticulocytes) in the peripheral blood.

shift to the left: The release into the peripheral blood of immature cell forms that are normally present only in the bone marrow.

significant figures: Digits of whole numbers or in decimal form, beginning with the leftmost nonzero digit and extending to the right; numbers should contain only digits necessary for the precision of the determination or measurement; the digits of a number that are known to be reliable.

simple stain: One stain that colors everything in the cell the same color.

single dilution: When one unit of original specimen is diluted to a final volume of 2, 5, or 10, and so on; when a concentrated specimen or solution needs a single dilution, usually expressed as a ratio; examples are 1:2, 1:5, and 1:10.

skin puncture: Capillary puncture for blood microsampling, such as finger puncture or heel puncture.

slant culture, tube: The surface of the medium is inclined at an angle.

slide agglutination: Used in assay to determine antigen-antibody reaction; usually employs latex agglutination.

software: Series of instructions or commands that direct the operation of a computer system.

solute: Substance dissolved in a solution; usually the substances being measured in clinical laboratory analyses are the solutes, these being dissolved in blood.

solvent: Substance in which a solute is dissolved; usually deionized water in laboratory reagents.

species: Basic unit of the biological world; used in nomenclature.

specific gravity: Ratio of the density of a solution to the density of an equal volume of water at a constant temperature; depends on the weight and number of particles in a solution.

specificity: The proportion of cases with absence of a specific disease or condition that gives a negative test result.

spectrophotometer: Device that quantitatively provides the relationship between the intensity of the color of an unknown solution and that of a standard solution; see photometry.

spectrophotometry: Quantitative measuring technique in which the color of a solution of an unknown concentration is compared with the color of a similar solution of known concentration.

spermatozoa: Mature male germ cells.

spores: An inert stage of a microorganism that the organism can revert to in a hostile environment.

spring-activated skin puncturing device: Device used to collect capillary blood; makes a clean, rapid incision of a consistent depth.

spun microhematocrit method: Hematocrit measurement method that utilizes a high-speed centrifuge in a relatively short centrifugation time.

stab tube: A tube of medium that is inoculated by stabbing or passing through the medium with an inoculating needle, leaving the specimen behind in the medium.

stable factor: Factor VII; presence monitored by thrombin time.

standard calibration curve: Plotting of percent transmission or absorbance readings on graph paper for several known standard solutions of varying concentrations will enable construction of a "standard curve" for a particular assay.

standard deviation (SD): Statistical measurement of the degree of variation from the mean of a series of measurements; measure of precision or reproducibility.

standard precautions: Recommended safety policies used for handling all biological (patient) specimens. Potential infectivity of any patient's blood or body fluids is unknown; therefore all blood and body substances (fluids) are considered equally infectious; also called *universal precautions*.

standard solution: Reference material of the substance being assayed that is of fixed and known chemical composition and can be prepared in a pure form for use in the laboratory; certified reference material that is generally accepted or officially recognized as the unique standard for the assay, regardless of the purity of the analyte content.

steatorrhea: Presence or increased quantities of fat in the feces.

stem cell: The common progenitor or uncommitted pluripotential stem cell from which all types of blood cells are derived.

stercobilin: Pigment derived from bilirubin; responsible for normal color of the feces.

stercobilinogen: Colorless degradation product of urobilinogen; is formed in the intestine and oxidized to the colored pigment stercobilin.

Sternheimer-Malbin Stain: A crystal violet and safranin stain commonly used in the microscopic analysis of the urine sediment.

sterile: Free from living microorganisms.

sterilization: Killing or destroying all microorganisms.

streak plate: Culture plate prepared by inoculating so as to spread out colonies as much as possible so that single, isolated colonies may be observed after incubation.

subculture: A colony from the primary culture plate that is picked up with an inoculating loop or needle and transferred to a second medium for further culturing.

supportive media: Media that contain nutrients that allow most nonfastidious organisms to grow at their normal rates.

synovial fluid: Extravascular fluid that surrounds the joints of the body.

syringe and needle collection system: Separate syringes and needles of appropriate size and gauge are used to collect some blood specimens. Blood in the syringe is carefully added to the appropriate collection tube containing the necessary additive.

T

T lymphocyte: Blood cell that is derived from the thymus; functions in cell-mediated responses; makes up the majority of the lymphocytes in the peripheral blood.

Tamm-Horsfall protein: Mucoprotein secreted by the renal tubular cells and not derived from the blood plasma. This protein forms the matrix of urinary casts.

taxonomy: Biological classification system of microorganisms on the basis of their natural relationships and, from this, giving them suitable names.

telescoped sediment: Urine sediment that contains all, or most, types of casts (hyaline, cellular, granular, and waxy) in one sediment.

test tube culture: Culture medium dispersed in test tubes, such as slants or liquid broth.

therapeutic drug monitoring: Testing of blood level of a drug to monitor or keep track of its medical effectiveness in treatment of a disease.

thin-layer chromatography: Method of chromatography often used to do therapeutic drug monitoring tests; the stationary phase is a thin layer of an adsorbent coated on a glass plate or sheet of plastic; the mobile phase is a solvent or a solvent mixture.

throat swab: Sterile fibrous material (commonly Dacron or rayon) fixed to a stick; used to collect material from the back of the throat for culture or rapid detection tests for diagnosis of "strep throat."

thrombin: Activated form of factor II that acts as a serine proteolytic enzyme to cleave fibrinogen and form fibrin; is a reagent to test platelet aggregation.

thrombin time (TT): Measurement of the time required for change of fibrinogen to fibrin.

thrombocyte, platelet: One of the formed elements in the peripheral blood; chief function is its role in coagulation of blood.

thromboplastin: Substance with ability to convert prothrombin to thrombin.

thrombosis: Formation of a thrombus or fibrin clot.

thrombus: Result of activation of the hemostatic system; formation of platelet plug.

timed urine collection: Urine collected over time (e.g., 2, 12, or 24 hours). Collection commonly is preserved by refrigeration between voidings, and is used when a quantitative assay is needed. It is important to adhere to specific time requirements and be certain that the collection time is noted on the container. Entire timed collection must be sent to the laboratory in the container.

titration: Quantitative volumetric technique of measuring the concentration of an unknown solution by comparing it with a measured volume of a solution of known concentration.

to-contain pipettes: Pipettes calibrated to contain a specific amount of liquid; to ensure that all the liquid is emptied from the pipette, it must be rinsed well with a diluting solution.

to-deliver pipettes: Pipettes calibrated to deliver a specified volume when filled properly and the liquid is allowed to drain completely into a receiving vessel.

tolerance: Form of resistance to an antimicrobial agent. In volumetric glassware, the degree of acceptable variability of volume delivery from that stated on the glassware; the tolerance increases with the capacity of the pipette.

torsion balance: Laboratory balance commonly used to weigh chemicals; is assembled as a single flexible structure by means of highly tensed torsion bands of watch-spring alloy; has no knife edges to dull, or other loose parts.

Total Quality Improvement (TQI): Internal monitoring programs to improve the quality of services performed by the clinical laboratory.

Total Quality Management (TQM): See total quality improvement (TQI).

tourniquet: Elastic strip or cuff that can be tightened when applied around the arm, usually just above the elbow; allows the vein to become more prominent so that venipuncture can be more easily done.

toxicology: Study of the origin, nature, and effects of poison. Toxicologic analyses are used to detect the amounts of substances that could be poisonous or toxic at certain concentrations.

transfer needle: See inoculating loop or needle.

transfusion reaction: Any adverse effect of transfusion; generally characterized as hemolytic, febrile, allergic, or circulatory overload.

transmission-based precautions: Precautions coming from the CDC that apply to patients (1) with known specific infection or suspected to be infected with specific microorganisms spread by airborne, droplet, or contact routes or (2) during the incubation period of certain easily transmitted diseases.

transmission electron microscope (TEM): A type of microscope that illuminates the specimen with a beam of electrons produced by an electron gun; the electrons are accelerated by a high voltage potential and passed through a condenser lens system (usually two magnetic lenses). The electron microscope allows for significantly greater magnification (up to 50,000 times magnification) than the brightfield microscope.

transmitted light: Light that is not absorbed.

transudate: An effusion formed as the result of filtration through a membrane.

traumatic tap: The presence of blood in a body fluid specimen, such as cerebrospinal fluid, as a result of bleeding at the site of entry as the fluid is collected. First tube appears bloody while subsequent tubes show lesser concentrations of blood.

triple-beam balance, "trip" balance: Three-beamed balance. Each beam provides a different weighing scale; scales are provided with movable weights. Used commonly in preparation of laboratory reagents.

trophozoite: Motile form of a parasite.

true negatives: Those subjects who have a negative test and who do not have the disease.

true positives: Those subjects who have a positive test and who have the disease.

tuberculosis control: OSHA requires use of special masks and/or respirators for persons who are exposed to patients with known or suspected pulmonary tuberculosis.

turbidimetry: Measurement of the loss in light intensity transmitted through a solution because of the light being scattered as a result of the turbidity of the solution.

type 1, or insulin-dependent, diabetes mellitus (IDDM): Insulin injection is required because insufficient amounts of insulin are secreted by the pancreas.

type 2, or non-insulin-dependent, diabetes mellitus (NIDDM): The activity of the insulin present is not sufficient; patients are usually not dependent on insulin injections.

typing: Testing of suspensions of red cells with known antibody solutions (antisera) to determine the identity of antigens, known as the *blood type.*

U

ultracentrifuge: High-speed centrifuge; generally used for research.

ultrafiltrate of plasma: Filtrate of plasma over a membrane, whereby extremely small particles such as proteins are restricted, or not filtered.

unconjugated bilirubin, indirect bilirubin, free bilirubin: Water-insoluble form of bilirubin that is formed as a breakdown product from heme by the reticuloendothelial system and carried in the bloodstream bound to albumin. Because of its insolubility, this form cannot be excreted by the kidney or found in the urine.

unexpected antibody: Antibody that results from specific antigenic stimulus. In blood banking, the result of stimulation from pregnancy, transfusion, or injection of red cells. Also referred to as an *immune antibody.*

universal blood and body substance technique (UBBST): See standard precautions.

universal precautions: See standard precautions.

Unopette system: Commercially available disposable self-filling pipette and diluent-reservoir system used to measure and dilute blood for testing purposes.

unorganized sediment: The chemical part of the urine sediment, includes crystals of chemicals and amorphous material.

urea nitrogen/creatinine ratio: Useful relationship in diagnosis of renal function disorders. Normal ratio for a person on a normal diet is between 12 and 20.

uremia: Abnormally high concentration of urea nitrogen in the blood.

urinalysis: The physical, chemical, and microscopic analysis of urine.

urinary system: Consists of two kidneys and two ureters plus the bladder and the urethra.

urine: Fluid composed of the waste materials of blood; formed in the kidney and excreted from the body by way of the urinary system.

urobilin: An orange-yellow pigment found in normal urine. Urobilin is an oxidation product of the colorless urobilinogen.

urobilinogen: Group of colorless chromogens that are formed in the intestine from the reduction of bilirubin by the action of bacteria present in the normal bacterial flora; normal product of bilirubin metabolism.

urochrome: A yellow pigment found in normal urine.

uroerythrin: A red pigment found in normal urine.

V

vaccination: The process of introducing a foreign antigen, e.g., attenuated live or killed organism into a person to stimulate immune antibodies (immunize).

vacuum tube and needle collection system: Blood collection system consisting of evacuated collection tubes with appropriate additives, double-ended needles, and needle holders; allows blood collection directly from the vein into the tube.

valence: Expression of the total combining power of an element whereby it can combine chemically with atoms of hydrogen or their equivalent.

variance (or error): Fluctuation in the measurement of a substance; factors causing variance can be limitations of the procedure itself or can be related to the sampling mechanism.

vascular access device (VAD): Device or indwelling line used to administer therapeutic products over a long period; see indwelling line.

vascular component: Activity of the blood vessels themselves.

vasoconstriction: Constriction of blood vessels; most immediate response of the body to bleeding.

venipuncture: Process of collecting blood from a vein.

venous blood: Blood collected from a vein by venipuncture.

verified: Results must be verified, or approved or reviewed, before the data are released to the patient report.

virology: The study or science of viruses.

visible spectrum: The range of light that is visible to the human eye, generally from wavelengths of 380 to 750 nm.

visual colorimetry: Determination or comparison of color intensity of a solution by use of the human eye; has all but been replaced by photoelectric colorimetry and spectrophotometry instrumentation.

voided midstream urine specimen: Noncatheterized urine specimen collected after the first few milliliters have been deposited in the urinal or toilet; the urine is free flowing, and the mid-portion of the collection is saved in a specimen container.

volume per unit volume: Measured volume of a liquid added to a specific volume of another liquid (v/v); usually expressed as milliliters per milliliter (mL/mL) or milliliters per liter (mL/L).

volumetric glassware: Glassware that has been manufactured of good-quality glass and calibrated under strict conditions to hold, contain, or deliver a specific volume of liquid (e.g., volumetric pipette, flask, buret).

volumetric (or transfer) pipette: Extremely accurate, single-line pipette used to measure specimens, controls, and standard solutions, or anything requiring precise measurement.

von Willebrand disease (vWD): Deficiency of vWF; prolonged bleeding time results; see vWF.

von Willebrand factor (vWF): Subendothelial factor (factor VIII:vWF); acts as the glue necessary for optimal platelet-collagen binding to occur; factor is required for normal platelet adhesion to endothelium.

W

waived laboratory tests: CLIA regulations specify that the FDA has cleared these tests; that is, the tests are so simple that the likelihood of erroneous results is negligible, or no risk is posed to the patient if the tests are performed incorrectly.

waste disposal program: OSHA standards mandate implementation of a specific plan for disposal of medical wastes to prevent transmission of infectious agents and accidental exposure to possibly hazardous material.

Watson-Schwartz test: Test for urobilinogen and porphobilinogen, based on the Ehrlich aldehyde reaction; basis of the Multistix reagent strip test for Ehrlich reacting substances.

wavelength of light: Linear distance traveled by one complete wave cycle of a particular beam of radiant energy.

weight (mass) per unit volume (w/v): Measured weight of a substance added to a specific volume of a diluent, usually deionized or distilled water. The usual way is as grams per liter (g/L) or milligrams per milliliter (mg/mL).

weight per unit weight (w/w): Mass per unit mass; used when the desired chemical to be weighed is a solid and is mixed with or diluted with another solid.

Western blot technology: Antigenic proteins or nucleic acids are separated by gel electrophoresis and transferred or blotted onto membrane filter paper antiserum from the patient is allowed to react with the filter paper, and by use of labeled anti-antibody detectors, the specific antibody bound to its homologous antigen is detected.

wet reagent chemistry: Assay utilizing wet reagents. Traditional manual chemistry assays use wet reagent chemistry. Compare with dry reagent technology.

white blood cell differential: Determination of the percentage of each white blood cell type present in a peripheral blood film.

Wintrobe hematocrit method: A macromethod for hematocrit determination; has been generally replaced by the microhematocrit or calculated hematocrit.

work list: Defines the workload for a laboratory for a defined time period—for the day, for example.

working distance: In microscopy, the distance from the bottom of the objective to the material being studied.

Wright stain: A mixture of eosin and methylene blue used to observe cellular morphology of blood cells in examination of blood films; a polychromatic Romanovsky-type stain.

Wright-Giemsa stain: Variation of Wright stain. See Wright stain.

X

xanthochromia: Yellowish discoloration; used to describe the supernatant spinal or other serous fluid, indicating the presence of previous hemorrhage. Strictly speaking, xanthochromia represents a yellow color; however, the term is applied to pale pink to orange or yellow in describing fluids.

xenoantibodies: Antibodies resulting from exposure to antigenic material from another species.

Z

Zymogens: Enzyme precursors or proenzymes.

Index

Note: Page numbers followed by "f" refer to illustrations; Page numbers followed by "t" refer to tables; Page numbers followed by "b" refer to boxes.